Tecklin's

Pediatric Physical Therapy

SIXTH EDITION

Tecklin's

Pediatric Physical Therapy

SIXTH EDITION

Elena McKeogh Spearing, PT, DPT

Board-Certified Pediatric Clinical Specialist
Owner
Dynamic Physical Therapy Solutions, LLC
Hartsville, Pennsylvania
Adjunct Faculty
Arcadia University
Physical Therapy Program
Former Manager of Physical Therapy
The Children's Hospital of Philadelphia
Philadelphia, Pennsylvania

Eric S. Pelletier, PT, DPT

Board-Certified Pediatric Clinical Specialist
Department of Physical Therapy
Assistant Professor of Physical Therapy
University of the Sciences
Philadelphia, Pennsylvania

Mark Drnach, PT, DPT, MBA

Board-Certified Pediatric Clinical Specialist
Department of Physical Therapy
Clinical Professor of Physical Therapy
Wheeling University
Wheeling, West Virginia

Wolters Kluwer

Philadelphia · Baltimore · New York · London
Buenos Aires · Hong Kong · Sydney · Tokyo

Acquisitions Editor: Matt Hauber
Senior Development Editor: Amy Millholen
Editorial Coordinator: Nancy Antony
Production Project Manager: Catherine Ott
Marketing Manager: Phyllis Hitner
Manufacturing Manager: Margie Orzech
Designer: Stephen Druding
Prepress Vendor: S4Carlisle Publishing Services

Sixth Edition

9 8 7 6 5 4 3 2 1

Printed in China

Library of Congress Cataloging-in-Publication Data

Names: Spearing, Elena McKeogh, editor. | Pelletier, Eric S., editor. |
   Drnach, Mark, editor.
Title: Tecklin's pediatric physical therapy / [edited by] Elena McKeogh
   Spearing, Eric Pelletier, Mark Drnach.
Other titles: Pediatric physical therapy (Tecklin) | Pediatric physical
   therapy
Description: Sixth edition. | Philadelphia: Wolters Kluwer Health, [2022]
   | Preceded by Pediatric physical therapy / [edited by] Jan S. Tecklin.
   Fifth edition. [2015] | Includes bibliographical references and index.
Identifiers: LCCN 2021005646 | ISBN 9781975141578 (paperback)
Subjects: MESH: Physical Therapy Modalities | Child | Infant
Classification: LCC RJ53.P5 | NLM WB 460 | DDC 615.8/2—dc23
LC record available at https://lccn.loc.gov/2021005646

shop.lww.com

CCS0421

We dedicate this sixth edition to Jan Stephen Tecklin.

We thank Jan for entrusting us with his passion.

The faith and confidence he had in us gave us a tremendous sense of

responsibility to continue this work.

We have taken his faith in us very seriously.

Jan, we hope this effort has made you proud.

We also dedicate this edition to the many children

and families we have worked with in our

collective 90 years of practice.

You have taught us so much more than we have taught you.

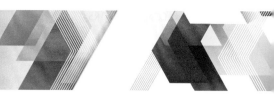

Joseph Ableman, PT, DPT
Physical Therapist
Acute Care Therapy Services
Legacy Emanuel Medical Center—Oregon Burn Center
Portland, Oregon

Karl Barner, CPO/L
Certified Prosthetist Orthotist
Department of Orthotics and Prosthetics
Children's Healthcare of Atlanta
Atlanta, Georgia

Jason Beaman, PT
Cerebral Palsy Team Lead Therapist
Therapeutic and Rehabilitation Services
Nemours/Alfred I. duPont Hospital for Children
Wilmington, Delaware

Anjana Bhat, PT, PhD
Assistant Professor in Kinesiology
Physical Therapy Program
University of Connecticut
Storrs, Connecticut

Jamie Bradford, PT, DPT
Physical Therapist III
Department of Physical Therapy
The Children's Hospital of Philadelphia
Philadelphia, Pennsylvania

Heather Lever Brossman, PT, DHSc(c), DPT, MS
Board-Certified Cardiovascular and Pulmonary Clinical Specialist
Board-Certified Pediatric Clinical Specialist
Physical Therapist
GRIT Physical Therapy, LLC
Richboro, Pennsylvania
Bucks County Intermediate Unit #22
Doylestown, Pennsylvania

Deborah Bubela, PT, PhD
Board-Certified Clinical Specialist in Pediatric Physical Therapy
Associate Professor in Residence
Doctor of Physical Therapy Program
Kinesiology Department
University of Connecticut
Storrs, Connecticut

Jill Cannoy, PT, DPT
Board-Certified Pediatric Clinical Specialist
Children's Healthcare of Atlanta
Atlanta, Georgia

Stacey DiBiaso Caviston, PT, DPT
Board-Certified Pediatric Clinical Specialist
Education and Development Coordinator
The Children's Hospital of Philadelphia
Philadelphia, Pennsylvania

Kathleen Coultes, PT, MSPT
Board-Certified Pediatric Clinical Specialist
Trinity Health Mid-Atlantic MCMC
Mercy Fitzgerald Campus
Darby, Pennsylvania

Mark Drnach, PT, DPT, MBA
Board-Certified Pediatric Clinical Specialist
Department of Physical Therapy
Clinical Professor of Physical Therapy
Wheeling University
Wheeling, West Virginia

Brian P. Emling, MSPO, CPO, LPO
Certified Prosthetist Orthotist
Orthotics and Prosthetics Department
Children's Healthcare of Atlanta
Atlanta, Georgia

Jean M. Flickinger, PT, MPT
Board-Certified Pediatric Clinical Specialist
Physical Therapist III
Department of Physical Therapy
The Children's Hospital of Philadelphia
Philadelphia, Pennsylvania

Rita Geddes, PT, MEd, DPT
Physical Therapist
Department of Early Childhood Education
Bucks County Intermediate Unit
Doylestown, Pennsylvania
Bensalem Township School District
Bensalem, Pennsylvania

Courtney L. Ginter, PT, DPT
Physical Therapist
Department of Physical Therapy
Seattle Children's Hospital
Seattle, Washington

Allan M. Glanzman, PT, DPT
Board-Certified Pediatric Clinical Specialist
Co-Chair, Research and Scientific Review Committees
Department of Physical Therapy
The Children's Hospital of Philadelphia
Philadelphia, Pennsylvania

Elliot M. Greenberg, PT, PhD, DPT
Board-Certified Orthopedic Clinical Specialist
Physical Therapist/Clinical Research Scientist
The Children's Hospital of Philadelphia Sports Medicine and
    Performance Center
Philadelphia, Pennsylvania

Eric T. Greenberg, PT, DPT
Board-Certified Sports Clinical Specialist
Assistant Professor
Department of Physical Therapy
New York Institute of Technology
Old Westbury, New York

Alison Hayward, PT, DPT
Lead Acute Physical Therapist
Acute Care Therapy Services
Legacy Emanuel Medical Center
Oregon Burn Center
Portland, Oregon

Rebecca Hernandez, CPO, LPO
Certified/Licensed Prosthetist/Orthotist
Clinical Supervisor
Orthotics and Prosthetics Department
Children's Healthcare of Atlanta
Atlanta, Georgia

Jennifer Jones, PT, DPT
Board Certified Clinical Specialist
Department of Physical Therapy
Children's Hospital of Philadelphia
Philadelphia, Pennsylvania

Karen A. Josefyk, PT, MSR
Board-Certified Pediatric Clinical Specialist
Staff Physical Therapist
Outpatient Therapy Services
Nemours/Alfred I. duPont Hospital for Children
Wilmington, Delaware

Faithe R. Kalisperis, PT, MPT, DPT, C/NDT
Pediatric Physical Therapist
Gait Lab Clinical Specialist
Nemours/Alfred I. duPont Hospital for Children
Wilmington, Delaware

Lori Kile, PTA
Physical Therapist Assistant III
Department of Physical Therapy
The Children's Hospital of Philadelphia
Philadelphia, Pennsylvania

Alison Kreger, PT, EdD, DPT
Board-Certified Pediatric Clinical Specialist
Associate Clinical Professor
Department of Physical Therapy
Wheeling University
Wheeling, West Virginia

Rebecca Landa, PhD, CCC-SLP
Founder and Executive Director, Center for Autism and Related
    Disorders
Vice President
Kennedy Krieger Institute
Professor
Department of Psychiatry and Behavioral Science
John's Hopkins School of Medicine
Baltimore, Maryland

Jessica Laniak, PT, DPT
Board-Certified Orthopedic Clinical Specialist
Site Manager
Good Shepherd Penn Partners
Penn Therapy & Fitness
Philadelphia, Pennsylvania

Kirsten H. Malerba, PT, DPT
Board-Certified Pediatric Clinical Specialist
Department of Rehabilitation
Center for Advanced Pediatrics
Children's Healthcare of Atlanta
Atlanta, Georgia

Kathleen Miller-Skomorucha, OTR/L, C/NDT
Occupational Therapist
Department of Therapeutic and Rehabilitative Services
Nemours/Alfred I. duPont Hospital for Children
Wilmington, Delaware

Christine G. Paris, PT, MS
Board-Certified Pediatric Clinical Specialist
Outpatient Therapy and Medical Clinics Manager
Easterseals Eastern Pennsylvania
Reading, Pennsylvania

Eric S. Pelletier, PT, DPT
Board-Certified Pediatric Clinical Specialist
Department of Physical Therapy
Assistant Professor of Physical Therapy
University of the Sciences
Philadelphia, Pennsylvania

Megan Ryninger, PT, DPT
Board Certified Pediatric Clinical Specialist
Physical Therapist
Department of Physical Therapy
Children's Hospital of Philadelphia
Philadelphia, Pennsylvania

Elena McKeogh Spearing, PT, DPT
Board-Certified Pediatric Clinical Specialist
Owner
Dynamic Physical Therapy Solutions, LLC
Hartsville, Pennsylvania
Adjunct Faculty
Arcadia University
Physical Therapy Program
Former Manager of Physical Therapy
The Children's Hospital of Philadelphia
Philadelphia, Pennsylvania

Meg Stanger, MS, PT
Board-Certified Pediatric Clinical Specialist
Manager of Physical Therapy and Occupational Therapy
UPMC Children's Hospital of Pittsburgh
Pittsburgh, Pennsylvania

Gerald Stark, PhD, MSEM, CPO/L, FAAOP(D)
Senior Clinical Specialist
Adjunct Instructor
Ottobock Healthcare
Northwestern University
University of Tennessee at Chattanooga
Signal Mountain, Tennessee

Elena Tappit-Emas, PT, MHS
Private Practice, Early Intervention
Philadelphia, Pennsylvania
Former Senior Staff
Myelomeningocele Clinic
Lurie Children's Hospital
Chicago, Illinois

Diane Versaw-Barnes, PT, MS, DPT
Board-Certified Pediatric Clinical Specialist
Physical Therapy Supervisor, Newborn/Infant Intensive Care Unit
Director, Physical Therapy Neonatology Fellowship Program
The Children's Hospital of Philadelphia
Philadelphia, Pennsylvania

Leslie F. Vogel, PT, MSPT
Clinical Therapist/Researcher at Seattle Children's Hospital
Clinical Faculty Appointment
Rehabilitation Medicine Department at the University of
    Washington
Seattle, Washington

Lauren B. Ward, PT, MSPT
Board-Certified Pediatric Clinical Specialist
Certified Lymphedema Therapist
Physical Therapist III
The Children's Hospital of Philadelphia
Philadelphia, Pennsylvania

Richard Welling, Jr., MSPO, CPO
Lead Prosthetist
Limb Deficiency Team
Orthotics & Prosthetics Department
Children's Healthcare of Atlanta
Atlanta, Georgia

Terri Wonsettler, OTR/L
Assistive Technology Professional
Senior Occupational Therapist
UPMC Children's Hospital of Pittsburgh
Pittsburgh, Pennsylvania

Audrey Wood, PT, MS, DPT
Board-Certified Pediatric Clinical Specialist
Physical Therapist III
Newborn/Infant Intensive Care Unit
The Children's Hospital of Philadelphia
Philadelphia, Pennsylvania

ACKNOWLEDGMENTS

In 1987, Jan Stephen Tecklin set out to put together a comprehensive pediatric textbook for entry-level and new practitioners. Now, 34 years later, we are humbled and honored to bring to you the sixth edition of *Tecklin's Pediatric Physical Therapy*. Developing this book has been an enlightening and rewarding adventure. We have enjoyed working together and are excited to bring you this excellent resource.

We would like to acknowledge the skill, creativity, knowledge, determination, and *generosity* of the authors who contributed chapters to this sixth edition. We appreciate the support and patience that our contributors afforded us as we found our way. We thank Kirsten H. Malerba, Diane Versaw-Barnes, Audrey Wood, Rita Geddes, Jason Beaman, Faithe R. Kalisperis, Kathleen Miller-Skomorucha, Elena Tappit-Emas, Allan M. Glanzman, Jean M. Flickinger, Jennifer Jones, Elliot M. Greenberg, Eric T. Greenberg, Kathleen Coultes, Heather Lever Brossman, Anjana Bhat, Deborah Bubela, Rebecca Landa, Meg Stanger, and Christine G. Paris, who worked on previous editions and continued to provide us with their expertise for this edition. We welcome and are so grateful to the new contributors including Terri Wonsettler, Jill Cannoy, Brian P. Emling, Gerald Stark, Karl Barner, Rebecca Hernandez, Richard Welling, Jr., Alison Kreger, Lori Kile, Jamie Bradford, Jessica Laniak, Karen A. Josefyk, Courtney L. Ginter, Leslie F. Vogel, Megan Ryninger, Stacey DiBiaso Caviston, Lauren B. Ward, Alison Hayward, and Joseph Ableman. You have added a new level of energy and fresh information to the content. We truly feel this book includes the most outstanding clinicians, mentors, scholars, and caregivers to children.

We are deeply indebted to the authors for all the hard work that we know has been put into making this the best edition yet. Thank you for your patience in navigating and responding to last-minute e-mail and deadline requests. We know how busy everyone is, but you always gave us exactly what we needed. Thank you from the bottom of our hearts.

We acknowledge the support of the staff at Wolters Kluwer. First and foremost, Mr. Matt Hauber, our acquisitions editor, who was the driving force behind getting this edition off the ground. Your guidance and encouragement helped us turn our thoughts and ideas into reality. Thank you to Ashley Pfeiffer and Nancy Antony, our editorial coordinators, who worked diligently and patiently to put this book into production. Finally, to Amy Millholen, our senior development editor, who not only worked tirelessly to keep it all running smoothly but was always available to answer questions or give advice, no matter what time of day it was. To each and every one who had anything to do with the production of this book, we offer our heartfelt appreciation and thanks.

Finally, we want to thank our families. The Spearing, Pelletier, and Drnach family members have been a constant source of support and strength throughout this whole process. We couldn't have done this without them.

Elena McKeogh Spearing
Eric S. Pelletier
Mark Drnach

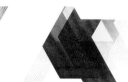

The sixth edition of *Tecklin's Pediatric Physical Therapy* brings the same level of high-quality, cutting-edge information that has made previous editions of *Pediatric Physical Therapy* so popular with entry-level physical therapy programs in the United States and abroad.

The mission of this book is to provide a current description of the major areas of practice in pediatric physical therapy for entry-level students and novice practitioners. This edition, as in each previous edition, strives to prepare entry-level students and new practitioners to practice in pediatric physical therapy care with content that is evidence based, provides knowledge and insight within specific diagnostic categories, and offers tools by which to initiate care and make sound clinical decisions for children and adolescents.

≫ Organization

The book is organized into several sections based on the practice of pediatric physical therapy and the more common groups of disorders seen in infants and children.

Part I, Foundations of Pediatric Physical Therapy, describes the overarching themes of working with children with any diagnosis. Chapter 1, revised by Eric S. Pelletier, focuses on the basics of chronologic motor development with a strong emphasis on the biomechanical aspects of gross motor development. Chapter 2, written by Kirsten H. Malerba, updates the description of the most utilized tests and measures of development in the pediatric population. Chapter 3, updated by Elena McKeogh Spearing, reviews principles of family-centered care that are so important in the provision of pediatric physical therapy.

Part II, Examination and Intervention along the Pediatric Continuum of Care, outlines the provision of pediatric physical therapy from the Neonatal Infant Care Unit to the Pediatric Acute Care and Rehabilitation units to the Outpatient and School Age practice settings. This section provides a comprehensive description of the settings in which physical therapists provide care. Chapter 4 brings the expertise of Diane Versaw-Barnes and Audrey Wood again to the book. Meg Stanger adds Chapter 5 with an important update to the book with Physical Therapy in the Medical Setting (Acute Care, Inpatient and Outpatient Rehabilitation). Chapter 6, Physical Therapy in the Educational Setting: From Early Intervention to School Age, discusses these areas of pediatric practice and was written once again by Rita Geddes. Terri Wonsettler has revised Chapter 7, entitled Adaptive Equipment. In addition, new to this book is a chapter dedicated to pediatric orthotics and prosthetics written by a team of professionals including

Jill Cannoy, Karl Barner, Brian P. Emling, Rebecca Hernandez, Gerald Stark, and Richard Welling, Jr.

Part III, Pediatric Neuromuscular Disorders, is a compilation of chapters including Chapter 9, Cerebral Palsy, by Jason Beaman, Faithe R. Kalisperis, and Kathleen Miller-Skomorucha. Chapter 10, Spina Bifida, is authored by Elena Tappit-Emas, who has contributed to this book since its first edition. Alison Kreger updated Chapter 11, Traumatic Brain Injury, as well as Chapter 12, Spinal Cord Injury. Allan M. Glanzman, Jennifer Jones and Jean M. Flickinger, once again, bring a comprehensive description of Muscular Dystrophy to the book in Chapter 13. Chapter 14 provides an exciting and new chapter, Pain and Regional Pain Disorders, written by Lori Kile and Jamie Bradford.

Part IV, Pediatric Musculoskeletal Disorders, offers current information in this area. Karen A. Josefyk and Jessica Laniak revised Chapter 15, Orthopedic Conditions. Elliot M. Greenberg and Eric T. Greenberg have authored Chapter 16, Sports Injuries. Chapter 17, Juvenile Idiopathic Arthritis and Other Rheumatic Disorders, was updated and expanded by Courtney L. Ginter and Leslie F. Vogel.

Part V, Pediatric Cardiovascular and Pulmonary Disorders, has important updates. Heather Lever Brossman updated Chapter 18, Cardiac Conditions, and Chapter 19, Pulmonary and Respiratory Conditions. Chapter 20, Fitness and Prevention, was also revised, once again, by Kathleen Coultes.

Part VI, Other Medical/Surgical Disorders include chapters on several important and diverse groups of disorders. Stacey DiBiaso Caviston, Megan Ryninger, and Lauren B. Ward updated Chapter 21, Oncologic Disorders. Chapter 22, Burn Injuries, was revised by Alison Hayward and Joseph Ableman. Anjana Bhat, Deborah Bubela, and Rebecca Landa have updated information and discussion in Chapter 23, Autism Spectrum Disorders. Chapter 24 highlights information on Down Syndrome and Intellectual Disorders by Christine G. Paris.

Part VII, Considerations in the Provision of Pediatric Physical Therapy Services, with Chapter 25, by Mark Drnach, concludes the book with a discussion of transition to adulthood. This is an exciting addition to this book and provides information important to all physical therapists regarding recommendations for our clients as they become adults.

≫ Features

Extensive **Chapter Outlines** are provided to guide students and instructors to focus on specific information in the chapter. **Displays** have been included in an effort to provide greater depth of knowledge, allowing information to be more inclusive without necessarily lengthening the text of the chapters. **Chapter Summaries** encapsulate and recapitulate the major points of information presented in each chapter. **Case Studies** help students hone their clinical decision-making skills with real-world situations.

» Ancillaries

An interactive website is also included with this edition of *Tecklin's Pediatric Physical Therapy.* Instructors will have access to an Image Bank and PowerPoint lecture outlines. All of these resources are available at thePoint.lww.com/ Spearing6e.

The sixth edition of *Tecklin's Pediatric Physical Therapy* is much more than a timely update. It includes four entirely new chapters and major updates for virtually all other chapters. In addition to the updates, all authors in this edition have extensive experience in clinical care and regularly teach at the full-time faculty level or as an associated faculty member, and most have participated in clinical research. The authors in this edition represent the best in pediatric physical therapy practice.

CONTENTS

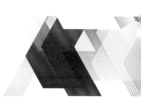

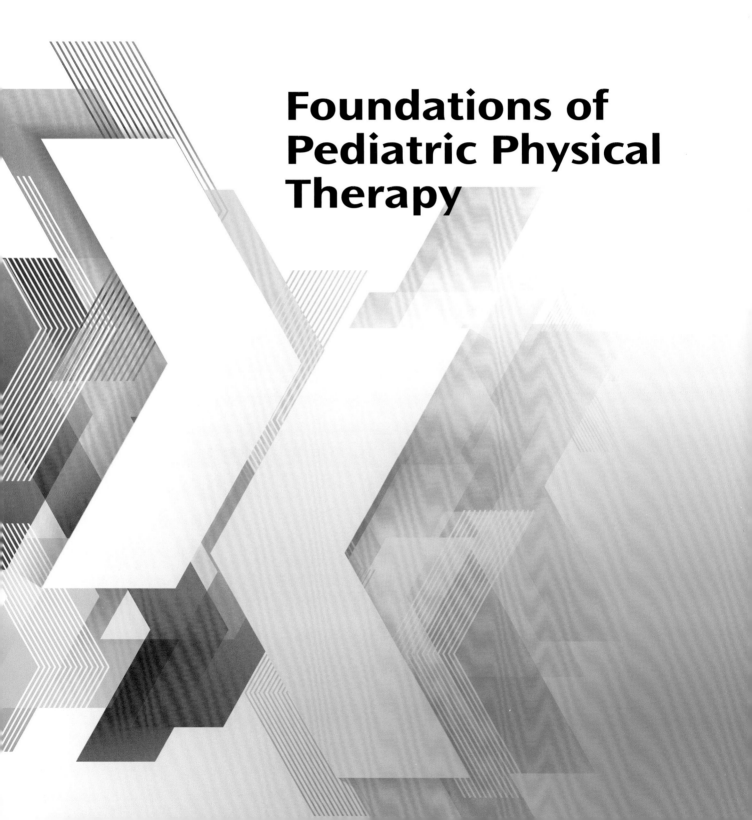

Foundations of Pediatric Physical Therapy

Typical Development

Eric S. Pelletier

>> Introduction

Typical development of abilities and skills in humans begins at the moment of conception. In normal conception and pregnancy, the embryo (third through the eighth week of gestation) and the fetus (the ninth week of gestation until birth) develop according to a sequence and timing common to all humans.[1] Birth typically occurs at 40 weeks of gestation or 10 lunar months after conception, plus or minus 2 weeks.[2,3] Infants considered to be term or full term have a gestational age of 38 to 42 weeks.[2,3] Postpartum development of human behaviors is the continuation of that which began at conception. A person's development occurs over their life span as the body undergoes change. Human development is an ongoing process that continues throughout the lifespan.

After a child is born, change occurs at a relatively rapid rate compared to the many changes that occur in adulthood. Particularly notable during the first 24 months of life is the acquisition of and changes in gross and fine motor skills.

Although novel gross and fine motor skills are learned and refined after the age of 2, many of these new and refined motor behaviors occur as the child or adult learns new skills required for play, sports, and/or work. Also, new motor skills are acquired and refined as needed when the individual has particular age-appropriate functional requirements. Milani-Comparetti has referred to these as *appointments with function.*[4] Some of these appointments with function occur

at relatively typical times in life, such as learning to independently don and doff one's jacket in time to begin kindergarten, learning to drive at 16 years of age, or learning to tie one's own necktie when moving away from home to attend college. The chronologic ages of achievement of motor behaviors and skills are influenced by these appointments with function and numerous intrinsic and extrinsic factors, which occur both prenatally and postnatally.[5]

Gestational and postgestational motor development usually occurs according to a typical sequence, pattern, and timing. Extrinsic factors such as the opportunity to learn and practice a skill, exposure to environmental pollutants, inadequate nurture and bonding, and parental and cultural child-rearing practices may modify the age of skill acquisition and possibly the sequence and pattern of the motor behaviors. As the child ages, more latitude must be allowed for the expression of differences in development as a result of the many and varied extrinsic factors (Table 1.1).

Behaviors that develop in the human include gross motor, fine motor, cognitive, language, and personal–social behaviors. Although the emphasis of this chapter is on chronologic motor development, a thorough appreciation for and understanding of a child's development stems from knowledge regarding all developmental domains, as well as growth parameters such as strength and range of motion. In addition, the development of and changes in the various systems of the body have an influence on the timing of skill acquisition.

TABLE 1.1.	Examples of Extrinsic Factors That Affect Motor Development
Factor	**Example**
Opportunity	Stair climbing develops earlier in a child who must contend with stairs in the home, compared with children who are not permitted on stairs.
Environmental pollutants	Children raised in an environment of smoke from cigarette smoking may be delayed in developing motor skills and may have stunted growth.
Inadequate nurture and bonding	Infants who are not held to be fed may experience motor delay as well as failure to thrive.
Parental and cultural child-rearing practices	Children placed supine to sleep may be slower to develop head control in prone and upright, prone-on-elbows position, and rolling prone to supine.

All of these areas interact together as the child matures, grows, and develops.

The focus of this chapter is on typical gross and fine motor development in the infant, toddler, and young child. The motor developmental sequence offers physical therapists a foundation for studying and understanding not only typical development but also aberrant or atypical development of the child. This developmental sequence may be used as a basis for examining, evaluating, assessing, and treating motor delays and deficiencies in both children and adults. The sequence, in particular, can play an important role in evaluating and treating people of all ages because identifiable components of motor behavior begin to evolve in specific aspects of the sequence. For example, in the prone-on-elbows or -forearms position, typical of a 4-month-old infant, once the child is able to assume the position, the child begins to shift weight while maintaining this position. Weight shifting in prone contributes to the emergence of movement components such as elongation of the trunk on the side bearing more weight (i.e., to the side the weight is shifted), unilateral weight bearing in the upper extremities to allow for visually directed reaching, and early accidental rolling from prone to supine. If the prone-on-elbows position is not achieved or is delayed, the evolution of some movement components may be delayed, or the components may not develop at all.

Each stage of the motor developmental sequence has a purpose and contributes to the overall development of the child. Therefore, various aspects of the sequence can be used in therapy, for adults and children, to facilitate the evolution of different movement components. In the evaluation and assessment of children, the typical timing of the acquisition of specific motor skills is linked to the determination of a *motor age*. Ideally, as an infant or toddler develops, the assessed motor age will be congruent with the child's chronologic age. A gap between the child's chronologic age and motor age, assessed according to established standards for age of skill or milestone development, is undesirable.[6-9] The greater the gap between chronologic age and motor age, the more likely that the child is exhibiting a possible developmental problem.

In the *habilitation* of a developing child, established norms for the sequence, timing, and patterns of motor behaviors can be used not only to evaluate and assess the child but also to set treatment goals and develop a treatment plan. This is not to suggest that the typical sequence must be followed in some strict manner when habilitating or rehabilitating a child or an adult. Rather, the sequence can be used as a guide, and it informs the therapist's understanding of the need for particular movement components to develop and refine specific functional motor skills.

Care must be taken when using the terms *normal* and *typical* when speaking about the motor development of a child, especially regarding age of milestone acquisition. Normal is defined as conformity with the established standards for humans.[10] Typical is defined as having the qualities of a particular group, in this case, human infants and children, so completely as to be representative of that group.[10] The reader should keep in mind that what is normal or typical motor behavior of humans at various ages is generally described in ranges. Such ranges exist because both motor development and individual motor skills are affected by numerous factors, in addition to the intrinsic biologic nature of the human. Even the intrinsic anatomy and physiology of a human are, in many ways, uniquely his or her own. For the purposes of this chapter, the terms normal and typical are used synonymously.

Normative values for age of skill acquisition, based on a defined subject pool, are set forth in numerous norm-referenced developmental instruments.[6-9,11-14] Because the norms are based on a limited, albeit large, group of subjects and therefore established with certain cultural bias, extrinsic factors such as cultural customs, parental practices, and opportunity to learn skills may detract from or improve a child's score.[15-24] Therefore, this text emphasizes a rather broad range of achievement ages, based on several norm-referenced evaluation and assessment tools. Also, it is important to note that typical ages of achievement are usually based on full-term gestation in humans, which is 40 weeks.[2,3] Table 1.2 shows approximate expected ages of acquiring specific motor milestones for full-term infants.

» The variability of human growth and development

Although human birth, growth, and development have long histories, our understanding of these processes has increased and been refined over time. In the study of human development, one characteristic clearly stands the test of time. Human development is characterized by variability. In fact, lack of variability, either within one individual or when comparing an individual with textbook standards, is often a red flag. The less variable and more stereotypical a child's movements

TABLE 1.2. Ages of Motor Milestone Acquisition in Typical Full-term Infants		
Milestone	Typical Age	Age Range
Physiologic flexion	Birth	N/A
Turns head to side in prone	Birth	N/A
Attempts to lift head in midline	1 mo	1–2 mo
Automatic stepping	Birth	N/A
Fencer's position	2 mo	1–4 mo
Astasia	2 mo	N/A
Abasia	2 mo	N/A
Rolling supine to side-lying nonsegmentally	3 mo	2–4 mo
Beginning midline head control	3 mo	2–3 mo
Prone-on-elbows, head to 90 degrees, chin tuck	4 mo	3–5 mo
Hands to midline	4 mo	3–5 mo
Unilateral reaching prone-on-elbows	5 mo	4–6 mo
Prone-on-extended-arms	5 mo	4–6 mo
Pivot prone position	5 mo	4–6 mo
Beginning intra-axial rotation	5 mo	4–5 mo
Rolling prone to supine, segmentally	5 mo	4–6 mo
Head lifting in supine	5 mo	4–6 mo
Supine, hands to knees and feet	5 mo	4–6 mo
Supine, hands to feet	5 mo	4–6 mo
Supine, feet to mouth	5 mo	4–6 mo
Propped sitting	5 mo	5–6 mo
Supine bridging	5 mo	5–7 mo
Rolling supine to prone, segmentally	6 mo	5–7 mo
Ring sitting, unsupported with full trunk extension and high guard	6 mo	5–7 mo
Transferring objects hand to hand	6 mo	5–7 mo
Independent sitting with secondary curves	8 mo	7–9 mo
Beginning quadruped	8 mo	7–9 mo
Beginning pull-to-standing	8 mo	7–9 mo
Creeping	10 mo	9–11 mo
Plantigrade position	10 mo	10–12 mo
Plantigrade creeping	10 mo	10–12 mo
Pulls to standing and lowers self	10 mo	9–12 mo
Cruising	10 mo	9–11 mo
Pulls to standing through half-kneeling	12 mo	10–13 mo
Walking independently	12 mo	10–15 mo
Creeps up stairs*	15 mo	14–18 mo
Walks up stairs with help or handrail*	18 mo	16–20 mo

*Age of achievement of ascending and descending stairs depends greatly on motivation, opportunity, and experience.

are, the more likely that his or her development and movement are atypical.[25-27]

Motor development and motor behaviors vary because of the influence of numerous intrinsic (endogenous) and extrinsic (exogenous) factors, many of which can be difficult or impossible to influence or control. However, many intrinsic and extrinsic factors can be controlled and manipulated to optimize fetal and infant development. For example, it is now known that fetal exposure to alcohol of unknown quantities can result in a child who has fetal alcohol syndrome (FAS), alcohol-related neurodevelopmental disorder (ARND), or alcohol-related birth defects (ARBDs).[28-33] Children who have been exposed to alcohol or illicit drugs in utero have been found to exhibit delayed mental, motor, and/or behavioral development when compared with standardized norms at 1, 4, 12, and 18 months and 2, 3, and 5 years of age.[34-41] Furthermore, prenatal alcohol effects on fetal, infant, and child development are not totally known, and the effects can be compounded by other pre-, peri-, and postnatal risk factors.[35,40,42-45] Fetal alcohol exposure can be controlled (i.e., eliminated) during pregnancy, thereby effectively eliminating the potential adverse effects of alcohol on growth and development. To the contrary, if a woman unexpectedly develops a disease process during pregnancy, the disease may impact the fetus and child negatively. However, this insult to the developing embryo or fetus may not have been preventable.

The variability of human motor development has been the subject of much study. Scientists and therapists have attempted to explain the differences in motor development between one person and another, and have tried to discover ways to optimize those factors that produce healthy motor behaviors and minimize those that have a negative impact.

A number of theories about how humans develop motor and other behaviors have been proposed. Brief descriptions of some of these theories follow. The reader should keep in mind that just as no two humans develop exactly alike, it is most likely that no single theory can explain how development occurs.

» Developmental theories

Developmental theories have been applied to all aspects of infant and child development, including physical, psychosocial, and cognitive. To effectively work with children, physical therapists need to have a broad understanding of all areas of infant and child development. However, physical therapists most definitely need a broad and deep understanding of the physical aspects of growth and development. Therefore, those developmental theories that adequately address a child's physical development are easiest to apply in physical therapy. Those theories will be emphasized in this brief discussion.

Maturational Theories

Maturational theories, also referred to as hierarchical theories, have been developed and advanced by researchers such as Piaget, Gesell, Bayley, and McGraw, beginning in the early 1900s. The works of these developmental theorists continue to contribute heavily to the understanding of child development today.[6,29,46-50] Their legacies are seen in the clinics worldwide. For example, Nancy Bayley's early work from the 1930s produced standardized scales for mental and motor development.[51-53] Her work continues to be a powerful clinical tool for assessing a child's mental and/or motor development, with several editions of the *Bayley Scales of Infant Development* having been published.[6]

Maturational theories of development emphasize a *normal developmental sequence* that is common to all fetal, infant, and child mental and motor development. According to *maturationists*, the normal sequence of development evolves as the central nervous system (CNS) matures, and is the major driving force of development.[50,53-56] Hierarchical theory has been interpreted by some to suggest a strict, invariant sequence of development in all *normal* children.[50,51] However, others have interpreted hierarchical development in a less stringent manner, including many physical therapists who have practiced since the 1970s and understand the hierarchy of motor skills to be merely, but consistently, a roadmap. Nonetheless, many of these same therapists believe in the primacy of the CNS in dictating developmental sequence and timing.

Behavioral Theories

A behavioral theory of development is rooted in the works of Pavlov, Skinner, and Bandura, with emphasis on conditioning behavior through the use of a stimulus–response approach.[51,54] Behavior theory advocates modifying behavior through manipulating stimuli in the environment to create a response that positively or negatively reinforces a particular behavior.[51,57,58] This type of theory is used by physical therapists when they control the environment to elicit a predictable behavior. For example, a therapist may move a very distractible child from the physical therapy gym to a quiet room, to control or improve the child's ability to stay on task. Therapists also use a stimulus–response approach when they manipulate parameters such as intensity, rate, and frequency of application of a given treatment modality.[59] Regarding motor development, some of a child's motor behaviors (responses) are conditioned by positive or negative feedback to particular behaviors.[60,61] For example, a child may demonstrate to a therapist a preference to use an atypical pattern of creeping on his or her hands and feet versus the typical pattern of creeping on hands and knees. The conditioning aspect of the preference for the atypical pattern was determined by environmental factors presented to the child while learning the skill. Those factors included learning the skill of creeping on an outdoor rough concrete patio surface while wearing shorts. The discomfort of the surface on the skin of the child's shins caused the child to move to a hands and feet position, thus learning the skill in an atypical manner, while remaining able to move about and explore the environment.

Dynamic Systems Theories

The dynamic systems theory is based on the original work of Bernstein in 1967 and has been modified by numerous others more recently, including Thelen et al., Horak, Heriza, and Shumway-Cook and Woollacott.[5,50,51,53,54,62] Unlike the longitudinal and hierarchical maturation theories, which consider the CNS to be the predominate factor and manager, organizer, and regulator of development, dynamic systems theories see infant and child development as nonlinear and the result of many factors, both intrinsic and extrinsic, that impact the developing fetus and child. According to the dynamic systems theory, no one system (such as the CNS in the maturational theories) is the preeminent director of development. Instead, each fetus and child develops certain characteristics and skills based on the confluence of many factors.[5,50,51,53-55,62-64] Although motor behaviors do seem to develop in the fetus, infant, and toddler according to a basic scheme, the sequence, timing, and quality of developmental milestones may be modified by numerous factors in any one fetus or child.

Factors that influence motor development in the human include genetic inheritance, errors and mutations in genetic transmission, maternal/fetal and child nutrition, fetal and infant exposure to toxins and other chemical substances, race, ethnicity, presence or absence of quality prenatal care, child-rearing practices, socioeconomic level (which may have immense bearing on several of the other factors mentioned here), disease processes, and trauma. In addition, opportunity, cognitive abilities, level of stimulation, and motivation affect the learning of new motor skills in children and adults, as do the motor task at hand, the functional outcome desired, and the context for using a particular motor skill.[5,15,19-21,28,29,34,42,46,49-51,65-77]

In a dynamic systems view of growth and development, the CNS is merely one, albeit very important, influential system. Unlike a purely hierarchical or maturational viewpoint, a dynamic systems approach to development considers the profound influences of other body systems on the anatomic, physiologic, and behavioral qualities of the fetus and child (the organism). These other systems include the peripheral nervous, musculoskeletal, cardiopulmonary, and integumentary systems.

Central Pattern Generators

"Today the existence of networks of nerve cells producing specific, rhythmic movements, without conscious effort and without the aid of peripheral afferent feedback, is indisputable for a large number of vertebrates. These specialized neural circuits are referred to as 'neural oscillators' or 'central pattern generators' (CPGs)."[78] It is known that the brain stem has CPGs for rhythmic functions such as chewing, breathing, and swallowing.[50,78-80] The spinal cord has CPGs for functional locomotion.[78,81]

In the absence of afferent input, the CPGs can still produce stereotypic, rhythmic movements such as locomotion. This is not to say that sensory feedback is not an important factor in normal locomotion.[78] However, the idea that motor output can occur without first having sensory input is contrary to early thinking in this field of study.[59]

Which Developmental Theory Is Correct?

Motor development in humans and motor behaviors have been shown to be under the influence of supraspinal structures, spinal structures, peripheral sensory input, CPGs, dynamic environmental features, and neuromodulatory influences. Supraspinal centers that control human locomotion include the sensorimotor cortex, cerebellum, and basal ganglia.[78] Sensory afferents, from the periphery, are important regulators of movement, helping modify the patterns generated centrally so that movements can be constantly adapted to the environment, task, and task context.[78] Neuromodulators such as serotonin and dopamine are also thought to influence centrally generated locomotion in some vertebrates, but their role is not yet completely understood.[78]

Among the many theories of development, including those affecting motor development, probably no single theory can ever be considered the one and only correct theory. Rather, many different theories can be called upon to explain and predict fetal and child motor development. Principles from different theories can be combined to analyze, interpret, and even predict motor development. Many aspects of the dynamic systems approach probably come closest to being the dominant theory of motor development used by physical therapists in the 21st century, because this approach, in itself, considers the impact of many variables on the creation, growth, and development of a human biologic system. However, given the multitude of environments in which children have grown and developed over time, the similarities in the *normal developmental sequence* and motor milestone acquisition among infants and toddlers are simply too great to be ignored.

» Preterm infants

Because of the prematurity, a *preterm* or *premature* infant, defined as one with a gestational age of less than 38 weeks, may not exhibit motor skills consistent with his or her chronologic age.[3] The child born too early may demonstrate motor delays equivalent to the number of weeks premature.[82,83] To distinguish between delays that are the natural result of not having enough in utero time and delays caused by abnormal pathophysiology, the premature infant is evaluated and assessed according to an *adjusted age*. Adjusted age is determined by subtracting the *gestational age* of the child, the number of weeks and days in utero, from 40 weeks. This remainder is then subtracted from the child's actual *chronologic age*, which is calculated from the date of the child's birth.[82,83] A sample adjusted age calculation is shown in Display 1.1.

» Developmental direction

Studying the typical sequence of motor development reveals a developmental direction that applies to most of development, although there are exceptions. Pertinent exceptions

are noted in the following discussion. Ten sequences of developmental direction are listed in Table 1.3, with examples of how these sequences are revealed in normal development. A few of these principles deserve additional attention to develop an understanding of the typical emergence of motor skills in humans.

Motor behavior in humans is at first reflexive in nature. As the organism matures, motor behaviors become more complex and eventually come under *cortical* or *volitional* control. This is an example of *reflex to cortical* developmental direction. In addition, primitive reflex responses tend to be more generalized rather than are localized responses. This *generalized or total movement before the development of localized movement* in a given area of the body is another example of developmental direction. A good example of a generalized response is the response seen in the *flexor withdrawal reflex*. This reflex is a *primitive reflex* that is present at birth and produces a total flexion response in the limb, either upper or lower, when the hand or foot, respectively, is exposed to a *noxious* or *nociceptive* stimulus (Fig. 1.1). The response to the stimulus in this reflex, because it is primitive and generalized, does not permit selective or isolated movements at the various joints of the limb when elicited. The flexor withdrawal reflex is present at birth and becomes partially integrated by 2 months of age.[46] However, vestiges of this reflex remain throughout life as a protective mechanism for the hands and feet. The flexor withdrawal reflex is controlled at the level of the spinal cord in the CNS.[46] Most early or primitive reflexes are spinal cord reflexes, whereas the mature postural and balance responses are mediated in the midbrain and the

TABLE 1.3.   Examples Reflecting Principles of Developmental Direction

Principle	Earliest Control/Response	Control/Response with Maturation
Reflex control before cortical control	Asymmetrical tonic neck reflex causes limbs to move in response to the head position.	Child volitionally moves limbs independent of head position.
Total response before localized response	Neonate moves upper extremities in wide sweeps and at random.	Child gains control of individual joints to stabilize the shoulder for precise, visually directed reach and grasp.
Proximal control before distal control	Child develops shoulder and hip stability.	Elbow, then wrist, and knee, then ankle, stability develop.
Cephalic control before caudal control	Shoulders develop control and stability.	Hips develop control and stability.
Medial control before lateral control	Three ulnar fingers dominate first grasp.	Thumb and index finger dominate pincer grasp. Forefinger dominance develops.
Cervical control before rostral control	Child has motor control of mouth at birth.	Child develops ability to fix eyes and focus.
Gross motor control before fine motor control	Child stabilizes the shoulders and holds a baby bottle with both hands.	Child picks up tiny pellets and puts them in a small bottle.
Flexor muscle tone develops before extensor muscle tone	Neonate is dominated by physiologic flexion.	Flexor tone loses dominance, and extensor tone is more manifest to balance tone.
Extensor antigravity control develops before flexor antigravity control	Child lifts head in prone at 4 months of age.	Child lifts head in supine at 5 months of age.
Weight bearing occurs on flexed extremities before on extended extremities	Child bears weight on upper extremities flexed at elbows in prone-on-elbows.	Child bears weight on extended elbows in prone-on-extended-arms and quadruped.

cortex of the brain. The stimulus for a spinal cord reflex is an *exteroceptive* stimulus.[5] The receptors for exteroceptive stimuli are "peripheral end organs of the afferent nerves in the skin or mucous membrane, which respond to stimulation by external agents."[1,5,84,85] Another example of a *total response* developing before *localized response* is neonatal kicking. When the infant is born, the infant first moves in

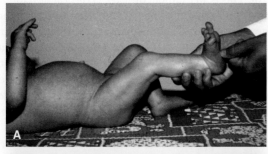
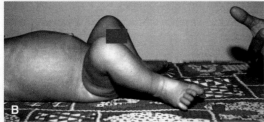

FIGURE 1.1. Flexor withdrawal reflex. **A:** Nociceptive stimulus to the sole of the foot. **B:** Flexor withdrawal response, total lower extremity flexion.

random total patterns. In fact, full-term neonates, when compared with preterm neonates, exhibit a variety of neonatal kicking patterns, with differences in frequency, reciprocal movements, and intralimb *coupling*.[86-88] Coupling is defined by Heathcock et al. as similar timing of movement between joints within the same limb.[86] Heathcock et al. also found that full-term neonates were able to exhibit task-specific and purposeful lower extremity control compared with their preterm cohorts.[86] When some *neonates* kick, both lower limbs often move together, the infant being unable to consistently *dissociate* one lower extremity from the other. Also, when kicking, the pelvis frequently moves with the lower extremities, another example of lacking dissociation. In this case, the lack of dissociation is between the hips and pelvis. As the infant matures, he or she is consistently able to move the lower extremities while keeping the pelvis stable, and the right and left limbs can move independently of each other as well as reciprocally, all examples of dissociation. The ability to move the limbs independent of each other allows for *reciprocal kicking*, alternating kicks of the lower extremities. At this point, the infant is also able to move one lower extremity without moving the other and to move a joint within an extremity independent of the other joints in that extremity.

A third principle of developmental direction is *cephalocaudal* development. Generally, this principle is demonstrated in the development of motor control in that the head, upper trunk, and upper extremities develop motor control before the lower trunk and lower extremities. An example of

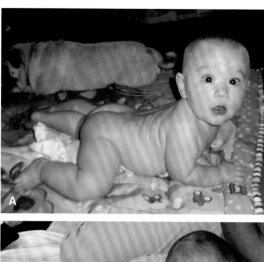

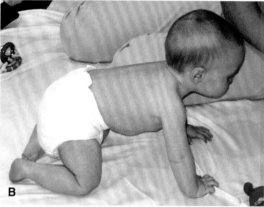

FIGURE 1.2. Cephalocaudal development in prone. **A:** Prone-on-elbows position with prestance positioning of lower extremities; the more cephalic shoulder girdle exhibits stability. **B:** Quadruped position; the more caudal hip exhibits stability as well.

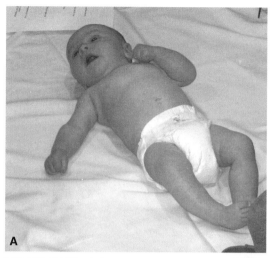

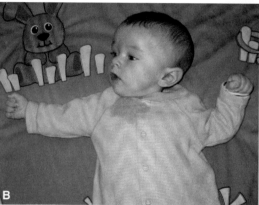

FIGURE 1.3. Asymmetric tonic neck reflex (fencer's position) with head turned to right; note the extension of the face-side limbs and flexion of the skull or occiput-side limbs. **A:** Fencer's position seen here in an infant 2 months of age. **B:** Fencer's position waning.

cephalocaudal development of motor control is the development of stability of the scapulae and shoulders to maintain the prone-on-elbows position, before the development of stability of the pelvis and hips as needed for the quadruped position (Fig. 1.2). An exception to cephalocaudal development is the development of muscle tone in the fetus. Studies of premature infants have shown that muscle tone develops in the lower extremities and lower body before tone in the upper extremities and upper body develops.[89]

Motor control also develops from *medial to lateral*; that is, control develops close to the median or midline of the body before developing more laterally. Midline stability of the neck and trunk develop before the more lateral shoulder and hip stability. During the first few weeks of life, the infant is relatively symmetric, with the exception of the head, which is turned to one side or the other in prone and supine. The second through fourth months of life are characterized in the typical term infant by asymmetry, as a result of the influence of reflex activity, most notably the *asymmetric tonic neck reflex (ATNR)*[90] (Fig. 1.3). The ATNR influence diminishes over those first months, thereby reducing reflex dominance and allowing the development of volitional control. Volitional control and developing stability begin medially in

what is termed *midline activity*. As the ATNR wanes, the child is able to bring his or her head into midline and maintain it there, instead of being in the asymmetric cervical extension pattern of the ATNR, by 4 months of age. In addition, the child begins bringing his or her hands to midline, relying on the newly developed shoulder stability to use the hands together in midline (Fig. 1.4). Thus, by 6 months of age, the child demonstrates good symmetry.

Another example of this medial-to-lateral development is the development of grasp. Consider and visualize the body in the standard anatomic position. The ability to grasp and manipulate objects with the hands begins with predominant use of the ulnar fingers, which are more medial, before using the more lateral index finger (radial finger) and thumb.[91]

Control of the flexors and extensors also develops in a particular developmental direction and occurs in a general sequence. Development of flexors and extensors differs depending on whether the infant is developing muscle tone, antigravity control, or weight-bearing function. Dominant **muscle tone** throughout the body develops in flexor muscles

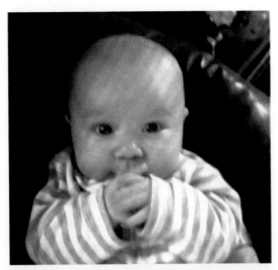

FIGURE 1.4. Notable symmetry of the infant; head and hands are stable in midline.

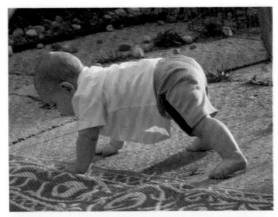

FIGURE 1.5. Plantigrade position with weight bearing on palms of hands and soles of feet; this is a transition position between being on the floor and erect standing and may also be used as a locomotive form called plantigrade creeping.

before that in the extensor muscles, as readily seen in the full-term neonate who is born with *physiologic flexion*.[47,48,92] This physiologic flexion is a dominant flexor tone in all positions when at rest and with passive or active movement. Even in the absence of physiologic flexion, as seen in infants born preterm, extensor tone is relatively low.

In each position, the development of antigravity movements and control occurs first in extensor muscles at a particular joint, before the development of the antagonist flexor muscles at that joint. For example, the infant learns to use the cervical extensors in the controlled antigravity movement of lifting the head in prone before being able to lift the head against gravity in supine, which requires antigravity flexor control. However, to develop full and balanced control at a joint, both antigravity extensors and antigravity flexors are needed. Cephalocaudally developing trunk extensors for antigravity work develop before the flexors of the trunk. Therefore, the child is able to get into a prone-on-elbows position by 4 months of age, using midline antigravity extensors, before being able to bring his or her feet to the mouth in supine at 5 months of age. The foot-to-mouth activity requires antigravity flexor control of the trunk.

The weight-bearing function of the extremities occurs on flexed limbs before weight bearing occurs on extended limbs. In prone-on-elbows, the infant bears weight on the flexed upper extremities, with relatively passive lower extremities. Prone-on-elbows occurs before quadruped, wherein weight bearing is on extended upper extremities (the elbows) and on flexed lower extremities (knees and hips) (see Fig. 1.2). The plantigrade creeping position calls for weight bearing on the open hands and soles of the feet (Fig. 1.5). This position is an example of weight bearing on extended upper extremities (elbows) and extended lower extremities (knees). In addition to exemplifying the rule of weight bearing, this progression from prone-on-elbows to the plantigrade creeping position is also an example of cephalocaudal development.

Gross motor skills develop before fine motor skills, the infant being able to stabilize the shoulder with the large muscles of the shoulder before gaining control of the small muscles of the fingers and hand for fine motor skills. This exemplifies not only the *gross-to-fine* principle of developmental direction, but also the *proximal-to-distal* principle. Proximal refers to the part of an extremity, upper or lower, that is closest to the midline of the body. Distal refers to the part of the extremity farthest from the midline.

The neck and trunk muscles and all major joints of the extremities (i.e., shoulders, elbows, wrists, hips, knees, and ankles) develop according to certain stages of motor control. They develop mobility, stability, controlled mobility, and skill, as described by Sullivan et al.[85] This sequence was first described with different terminology, in the early 1960s by Margaret Rood.[59] In the upper extremity, the sequence unfolds in the following manner. The shoulder first develops mobility, the ability to move the upper extremity in space with the distal end, the hand, free. This is referred to as an *open-chain* movement.[93] The early movement of the infant is random and poorly controlled initially, but evolves over the first few weeks of life. Success with this ability to move the upper extremity at the shoulder in an open-chain activity paves the way for the shoulder to stabilize in the *closed-chain* activity of prone on elbows and prone on forearms.[93] The distal segments of the extremity (i.e., the forearm, hand, and fingers) are not free in space. Rather, the extremity is performing a weight-bearing function, described by Rood as the stability aspect of motor behavior. Next, the infant demonstrates the ability to move the proximal joint, the shoulder in this example, over the distal extremity while the extremity is in a closed chain. This movement is seen as the development of weight shifting in the various weight-bearing positions of the upper extremities. Rood and others have described this phase as controlled mobility.[59,85] Eventually, the child is able to shift the weight entirely onto one or the other upper

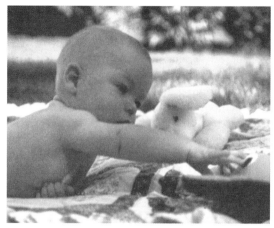

FIGURE 1.6. Unilateral weight bearing in prone-on-elbows position with weight shift to the skull side and one upper extremity freed for reaching.

extremities for unilateral weight bearing. Then the infant begins to stabilize the non–weight-bearing shoulder with the hand free (open-chain activity), as the fingers move to grasp and manipulate an object, as seen in Figure 1.6. This represents the skill level denoted by Rood.[59,85]

The lower extremities follow the same sequence for developing mobility, stability, controlled mobility, and functional distal control. This sequence plays out again and again, for both the upper and lower extremities, in each of the developmental positions of prone-on-elbows, prone-on-extended-arms, sitting, quadruped, and erect standing. In sitting

without support and erect standing, the upper extremities play a vital role in providing stability of the upper body, even though they are not performing a weight-bearing function.

» The neonate

The neonatal period in the infant is the first 28 days of postpartum life.[3] Full-term infants are born with *physiologic flexion*, as described earlier, a prime example of muscle tone developing in flexor muscles before extensor muscles. This results in generalized moderate flexion in all positions of the neonate, prone, supine, held in sitting, vertical or horizontal suspension, and held in standing.[47,48,91,92] This flexor tone gradually diminishes over the first month of life in these full-term infants.

Infants who are preterm exhibit less physiologic flexion or the flexion is absent, depending on the infant's gestational age.[94,95] The more weeks the infant is preterm, the less likely he or she is to have the physiologic flexion. Instead, preterm infants are born with limbs and trunk relatively extended. This extension is not a dominance of extensor tone, but rather a lack of or diminished flexor tone. The reasons for this lack of flexor tone in the preterm infant are unknown. Several theories have been suggested, including intrauterine positioning and maternal hormonal influences.

In addition to lack of physiologic flexion in preterm infants, other differences between full and preterm infants are noted at birth. These differences have been well described by Dubowitz and others, and a few of the major differences are shown in Table 1.4.[2]

TABLE 1.4.	Differences between Full-term and Preterm Neonates	
Tone and Movement Patterns	**Preterm Neonate (<32 wk)**	**Full-term Neonate (>36 wk)**
Position	Full extension	Physiologic flexion (full flexion)
Scarf sign: arm passively moved across chest of child in supine with head midline	No resistance to passive movement	Resistance to passive movement before reaching midline
Popliteal angle: passively move knee to chest; extend knee	Angle of extension between lower leg and thigh is 135–180 degrees.	Angle of extension between lower leg and thigh is 60–90 degrees.
Ankle dorsiflexion: infant supine, passively flex foot against shin	Angle between lower leg and foot is 60–90 degrees.	Angle between lower leg and foot <30 degrees
Slip through: infant in vertical suspension, holding under axillae	Completely slips through hands, does not set shoulders	Sets shoulders and does not slip through
Pull to sit: child supine, pull to sitting by pulling gently on both upper extremities	Complete head lag	Head held in alignment with body
Rooting reflex: child supine in midline, stroke corner of mouth	Absent	Head turns toward stimulus and mouth opens.
Sucking reflex: put nipple or clean finger in child's mouth	Weak or absent sucking response	Strong rhythmic sucking
Grasp reflex: place finger horizontally in child's palm	Absent	Sustained flexion and traction
ATNR: child supine with head in midline, passively turn head to one side	Absent	Upper and lower extremities on face side extend; extremities on skull-side flex.

» Motor development goals

One goal of typical motor development is control of the body against gravity.[4] These antigravity movements generally develop first in the head, followed by development in the trunk (cervical to thoracic to lumbosacral), then in the lower extremities. Antigravity control in the lower extremities includes control at the three major joints of the hip, knee, and ankle. Although the overall development of antigravity control is cephalocaudal, as revealed by the development of head control, then midline trunk control, and then lower extremity control, control at the various joints of the lower extremities may be occurring simultaneously, very close together in timing, or with the ankle being the lead joint.

Antigravity movements must develop in both extension and flexion movements. However, in mature, erect standing, the major body extensor groups are the antigravity muscles, as compared with their flexor antagonists. That is, the midline neck and trunk extensors, hip extensors, and knee extensors are the primary muscle groups that keep humans from surrendering to the force of gravity when upright.

A second goal of development is the ability to maintain the body's center of mass within the base of support.[4] The center of mass when standing is gradually and progressively rising as humans grow in height. Learning to maintain the body's center of mass within the base of support is accomplished as the infant and toddler develop righting, equilibrium, and tilting reactions. Although these reactions develop and continue to be activated automatically, the typically developing child can eventually control these automatic responses volitionally, as long as there are no intrinsic or extrinsic barriers to such control.

A third goal of motor development is the performance of intrasegmental and intersegmental isolated movements.[4] For example, even though various joints of the upper extremity move in a coordinated manner to produce an upper extremity functional skill, the individual joints, such as the elbow joint, must learn to move independently while the other upper extremity joints do not move. This is intrasegmental dissociation. Intersegmental dissociation, such as moving the head without moving the extremities or moving one lower extremity into flexion while moving the contralateral lower extremity into extension, must develop as well.

» The developmental progressions

Rather than discussing motor development as a timeline of chronologically occurring events, this text presents the sequence of occurrences that leads to the development of various components of movement. This sequence includes various motor milestones and positions and movement within these positions. Because these events in the typical infant and toddler develop in an orderly sequence in each position, these sequences are referred to as *progressions*. One of the earliest developmentalists, Myrtle McGraw, defined

these progressions.[47] Prone, supine, rolling, sitting, and erect standing progressions are presented, as well as various forms of locomotion in each progression.

Stabilizing in various positions is termed *static position* and is in contrast to dynamic position, the translation of those static positions into movement for locomotion, transitions between positions, and prehension.[48] These static and dynamic positions are often referred to as *motor milestones*. Particularly significant ages of performing certain milestones are discussed. More detail of the age ranges for the achievement of these motor milestones can be found in Table 1.2. An important point to note is that the ages of acquisition of certain skills fall within ranges rather than at exact points in the developing child. Each developing child is unique, both in the intrinsic factors, biologic structure and function, and in the extrinsic factors that affect his or her development. This uniqueness must be remembered and considered, even though basic commonalities of anatomy, physiology, sequential development, and pathology exist.

Prone Progression

Prone Lying

At birth, the healthy, full-term neonate has physiologic flexion, which dominates the prone position.[96] In prone, the head is turned to one side (Fig. 1.7). This turning of the head to one side is the result of two primary influences. The first influence is a survival instinct, which allows the infant to turn the head to the side to clear the mouth and nose to breathe in prone, and the second is the influence of the ATNR.[46,97] Although the normal infant can be moved out of this pattern easily, the ATNR continues to influence head position in all positions, including prone, until the influence has completely subsided by approximately 4 months of age. Encountering considerable resistance to moving the child out of this ATNR-dominated fencer's position may be an indication of atypical neuromotor development.[98,99]

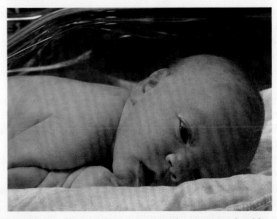

FIGURE 1.7. Neonate in prone; note the extreme shoulder adduction of the upper extremity with the elbow caudal to the shoulder in this infant only 2 hours after birth.

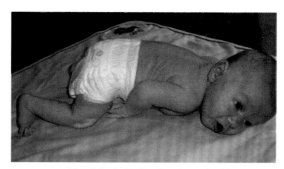

FIGURE 1.8. Physiologic flexion in a 3-week-old neonate; note that the shoulder adduction has decreased, and the hips and knees are still flexed with the buttocks up in the air.

The hip flexion aspect of physiologic flexion is particularly strong in prone lying and is accompanied by a relative anterior tilt of the pelvis. The infant's knees are drawn underneath the body with the buttocks up in the air, and the exaggerated hip flexion and anterior tilt are preventing the pelvis from lying flat on the surface (Fig. 1.8). The infant's weight is shifted forward onto the upper chest and face. When the head is turned to one side, the weight shifted onto the head is borne by the infant's cheek on that side. The upper extremities are adducted into the side of the body with the elbows caudal to the shoulders. Hands are generally fisted, owing to the strong influence of the hand grasp reflex. However, the hands frequently and spontaneously will open and can be opened passively in the typically developing infant. Persistently fisted hands that never open may indicate atypical sensorimotor development.[98] Persistently fisted hands with the thumb flexed into the palm and held by the fingers is often a sign of pathology.[100-102]

As physiologic flexion diminishes over the first month, the infant begins falling more and more into gravity in both prone and supine. In prone, hip flexion decreases, allowing the buttocks to come down and the anterior pelvis to lie flat against the surface. Weight shifts away from the face, caudally toward the trunk and lower extremities. However, a relative anterior pelvic tilt is still present, albeit decreased (Fig. 1.9A to C). The diminished nature of the anterior pelvic tilt is not due to an active posterior tilt at this point, but results simply from the loss of the physiologic flexion that kept the hips and knees flexed underneath the infant's body.

As physiologic flexion disappears completely, the infant lies flat on the surface in prone (Fig. 1.10). The hips are now passively extended and prepared for the beginning of active posterior pelvic tilt, which is an indication of the activation and development of the abdominal muscles (the trunk flexors) and the hip extensors. Without the buttocks in the air, the infant's weight is no longer shifted forward onto the chest and cheek, but instead is borne over all the body segments that are in contact with the surface. The infant at this point has no active antigravity control, with the exception of cervical extension, which is beginning to emerge.

In the ensuing prone position, the lower extremities are positioned in hip abduction, partial extension, and external

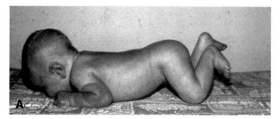

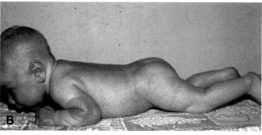

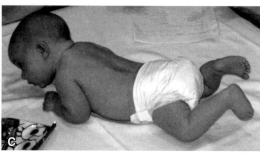

FIGURE 1.9. Neonate in prone. **A:** Note the anterior pelvic tilt and hip flexion, with buttocks up in the air; position prevents infant from lifting his head from the surface. **B:** As physiologic flexion diminishes, the pelvis comes down toward the mat with decreasing hip flexion and anterior pelvic tilt; the pelvis is flatter on the surface as caudal weight shifting evolves, making it easier for the child to begin to lift the head in prone. **C:** As anterior tilt continues to decrease, weight continues to shift caudally from head and upper chest to pelvis and lower extremities, improving attempts to lift head and attain prone-on-elbows, but pelvis is still in a relative anterior tilt, and upper extremities are held close to the sides with the elbows too caudal for weight bearing.

rotation (Fig. 1.11). Knees are semiflexed and feet are dorsiflexed. This position of the lower extremities is the precursor to the position of the lower extremities in initial standing. Beginning at approximately 5 months of age, the typically developing infant can stand, with hands held or holding onto something such as the crib rails, with this same wide base

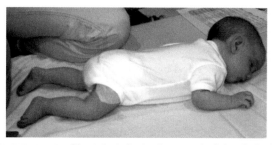

FIGURE 1.10. Physiologic flexion is gone; the infant is flat in prone with elongated hip flexors and a relatively neutral pelvis.

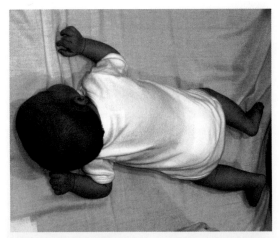

FIGURE 1.11. Once physiologic flexion has disappeared, lower extremities exhibit a prestance position in prone, which includes hip external rotation with slight flexion and abduction, slight flexion of the knee, and dorsiflexion of the ankle.

of support, hips, knees, and feet mimicking the early lower extremity position seen in prone.

Prone-on-Elbows

To achieve the *prone-on-elbows* or prone-on-forearms position, the next step in the prone progression, three abilities must be present: (1) stabilization of the pelvis, (2) head lifting with cephalocaudally progressing antigravity extensor control, and (3) movement of the upper extremities out of the neonatal position.

Head control in prone is the earliest antigravity control to develop. For the infant to begin experimenting with head control, the infant must move the head away from the support of the surface. To lift the head, the infant must actively contract the cervical extensors. At birth, the typically developing infant was able to lift his or her head only briefly in prone to turn the head to the side for breathing. The first truly active attempts at lifting the head in prone are tenuous, at best (see Fig. 1.9). Body proportions of infants are different from those in older children and adults. In the infant, the head makes up approximately one-quarter of the body in length, causing the head to be proportionally large and heavy.[103] This compares with the body proportions of an adult, in whom the head is only one-eighth of height.[103] Maturation and practice of the skill of head lifting strengthen the cervical extensor muscles so that the infant can eventually lift the heavy head (Fig. 1.12). This ability depends on the cervical flexors, the anterior muscles, to lengthen through reciprocal inhibition.

Even with cervical extensors increasing in strength, the child is not able to lift the head without stabilizing in another part of the body. When the buttocks were elevated and the head was down, weight was shifted toward the head. If the head is to be lifted antigravity, the buttocks must be down, the weight must be shifted caudally, and the pelvis must stabilize for head and midline upper trunk lifting. If one thinks

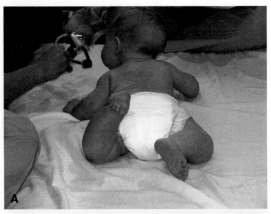

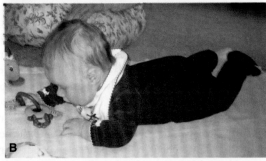

FIGURE 1.12. Infant has a relative posterior pelvic tilt, which promotes the use of the antigravity cervical extensors for head lifting in prone. **A:** Note the more abducted and forward position of the upper extremities and the prestance position of the lower extremities. **B:** Improved head lifting so that the face is at a 45-degree angle.

of the infant's head and upper trunk as being a lever arm, the fulcrum around which the lever arm turns for this movement is the pelvis, so the pelvis must be stabilized. This stabilization of the pelvis is achieved by recruiting abdominal muscles to tilt the pelvis posteriorly and hold it stable in a posterior tilt. With the help of the abdominal muscles to stabilize the pelvis in a relative posterior tilt, the infant begins actively lifting the head at approximately 2 months of age. By 3 months, cervical extension is adequate to lift the head such that the infant's face is at a 45-degree or greater angle with the surface, and head control is mostly due to antigravity extensor muscles (Figs. 1.12B and 1.13). As development of the spinal extensors progresses cephalocaudally, the upper thoracic extensors begin to strengthen and gain antigravity control. By 4 months, the infant is able to lift the head to 90 degrees. However, the chin of the infant who is able to lift his or her head to 90 degrees tends to jut forward slightly, with the neck hyperextended, during early successes in the prone-on-elbows and prone-on-extended-arms positions (Fig. 1.14). Although the infant has control of the cervical and upper thoracic antigravity extensors to lift the head to this face vertical position, one element of head control remains absent. Control at any joint in the body depends on a balance of synergistic muscles surrounding that joint. Therefore, head control is not complete until the antigravity cervical flexors have been

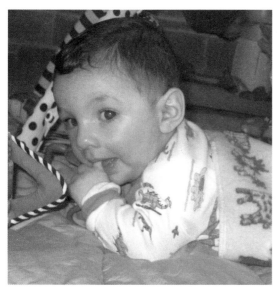

FIGURE 1.13. At 3 months of age, the child attains prone-on-elbows with the face at an angle greater than 45 degrees, not yet 90 degrees; note the forward position of elbows.

activated and strengthened to balance the antigravity cervical extensors.

The infant's ability to use midline cervical extensors to lift his or her head is a sign of the diminishing ATNR and the development of active cervical flexors. Although the strength of the ATNR diminishes during the first 4 months, the waning influence continues to provide slight cervical asymmetric extension. Once the infant begins to develop active cervical flexors to balance the extensors, the head is more easily brought to midline for lifting against gravity in prone. Continued strengthening of the cervical flexors, along with the activation of the serratus anterior muscles in the prone-on-elbows position, contributes to what Bly refers to as a *chin tuck* when the head is lifted to 90 degrees so that the face is vertical (Fig. 1.2A).[104]

The infant who is 4 months of age and has stable control of the head at 90 degrees, with the chin tucked, displays

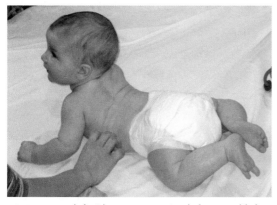

FIGURE 1.14. Infant in prone-on-extended-arms with face vertical (at 90 degrees), but with mild cervical hyperextension and without chin tuck.

balanced cervical extensors and flexors. By comparison, head control of the 3-month-old child during head lifting is dominated by extensors that are not balanced by antigravity flexors, helping produce a chin that is not tucked.

Chin tuck appears, therefore, as a result of three developmental occurrences: (1) activation and strengthening of the cervical flexors, (2) reduction of the ATNR, and (3) activation and strengthening of the serratus anterior muscles. The infant uses the serratus anterior muscles to protract the shoulder girdle and push the elbows into the surface. Without the protraction provided by these muscles, the child may exhibit what Bly and others have termed *TV shoulders*.[104] In TV shoulders, the child's upper extremities are not worked into the surface. Rather, the shoulders elevate and the neck hyperextends, with the infant's occiput resting on his posterior cervical soft tissue, chin jutting forward. The face, in this position, is not at 90 degrees or vertical, and the child does not have active head control. With the shoulders elevated at the sides of the head, close to the ears, the head is passively supported. Consequently, persistence of the TV shoulders interferes with the development of active, antigravity head control and lateral head righting. TV shoulders also make it difficult to swallow, talk, and breathe, because of the cervical hyperextension.

If at 4 months of age the child exhibits cervical hyperextension with the occiput of the skull resting on the upper back, the cervical flexors and/or serratus anterior muscles are not activated, nor do they have insufficient strength. This is an example of how the developmental sequence and the movement components might be used to determine a plan of treatment. If a child exhibits TV shoulders while prone-on-elbows, the strength of the serratus anterior muscles and that of the cervical flexor and extensor muscles should be examined. Weakness of any of these muscles may account for the cervical hyperextension, at least in part. If the cervical extensors are weak, it is likely that they are too weak to maintain the head upright, and once the head is lifted, the infant compensates for the inability to actively stabilize the neck. The head falls backward into hyperextension as a response to gravity. This is a pattern frequently seen in children who have delayed or abnormal sensorimotor development, such as children with cerebral palsy or other brain disorders. In such a case, one component of the physical therapy treatment plan would include strengthening the muscles that are weak and practicing control over those muscles.

The third element necessary for the child to achieve the prone-on-elbows milestone is a forward position of the elbows. The upper extremities, in the full-term neonate, are adducted closely into the body, or even slightly under the body, and extended at the shoulders, causing them to have a mechanical disadvantage in trying to lift the upper trunk and head (see Fig. 1.8). During the second month, at the time when the infant is first attempting to lift his or her head, upper extremity control at the shoulder begins to develop. The infant gradually abducts and flexes the shoulders, bringing the elbows from underneath the body forward, more to a position underneath or just anterior to the shoulders. This enables the infant to bear weight on the elbows and forearms when the head is lifted. Figures 1.7 through 1.9, and 1.12 and 1.13, show this progression. One important component of movement that begins to develop in this process is *scapulohumeral* elongation. Scapulohumeral elongation refers to the elongation of the axillary region because the humerus is flexed and/or abducted away from the body and therefore away from the scapulae. Without the ability to elongate this region, the infant will not be able to get the elbows into position underneath the shoulders for the prone-on-elbows position. Failure to elongate the axillary region will also interfere with reaching out in space, such as when an older child reaches out to grasp an object while sitting at their desk.

Although the upper extremities are typically envisioned as limbs with important mobility functions, such as reach and grasp, and the lower extremities are visualized in terms of their weight-bearing functions, such as standing, all four extremities have both weight-bearing and mobility functions to perform. Before assuming the prone-on-elbows position, the upper extremities have exhibited only mobility functions. The prone-on-elbows position is the first call for the upper extremities to be weight bearing. This ability to weight-bear through the forearms, elbows, and shoulders foreshadows the weight bearing that will follow in the quadruped position.

Once the infant has achieved a stable prone-on-elbows position, to be functional he or she must be able to translate the position into movement while maintaining stability at the proximal joint, the shoulder. The infant begins to shift weight from side to side, increasing the amount of weight bearing on each upper extremity as the weight is shifted to that side. Shifting weight side to side soon becomes shifting of weight in all directions, including forward, backward, and diagonally. This weight shifting is a feature of all the milestone positions once the stability of each position has been established. It is critical for the development of equilibrium and tilting responses for maintaining balance, as well as for functional use of the upper extremity. In the prone-on-elbows position, if the infant does not learn to shift his or her weight, the upper extremities will not be able to develop controlled mobility functions. Essentially, the infant will be stuck. Without the appropriate development of weight shifting, the controlled mobility functions of reaching (open chain) and the closed-chain propulsion function of the upper extremities, needed for crawling and creeping, will not develop.

Weight shift is necessary for reasons other than developing controlled mobility and unweighting a limb for movement. Weight shift encourages elongation of muscles on one side of a joint or joints while the antagonist muscles shorten. In typical sensorimotor development, this elongation during weight shift occurs in the lateral trunk muscles on the side that is weight bearing or bearing most of the weight. For example, when the infant shifts his or her weight while in quadruped resulting in unilateral weight bearing on an upper extremity, the lateral trunk on the side bearing the weight is elongated (relaxed and stretched), whereas the lateral trunk

on the side of the free upper extremity shortens (contracts), with lateral bending or flexion to that side (Fig. 1.15). Figures 1.16 through 1.21 show this elongation on the weight-bearing side in different positions and at different ages.

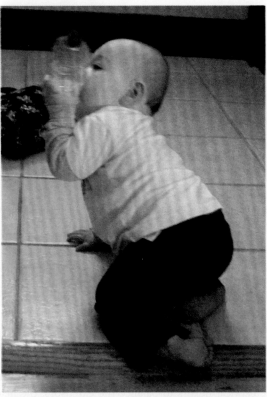

FIGURE 1.15. Unilateral weight bearing in the upper extremities from quadruped with elongation of the child's trunk on the side bearing the most weight, in this case the right side.

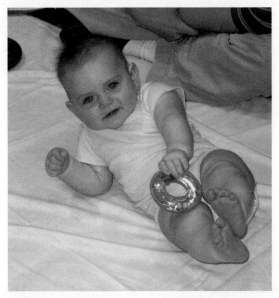

FIGURE 1.16. Weight shift to side-lying with elongation on the right (weight-bearing side).

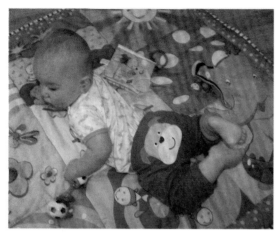

FIGURE 1.17. Prone-on-elbows with weight shift to skull side for unilateral weight bearing with elongation on the weight-bearing side.

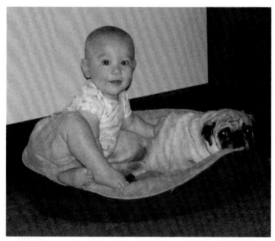

FIGURE 1.18. Sitting with weight shifted to the child's left side with elongation of the weight-bearing side; note the crossing of midline with the lower extremity.

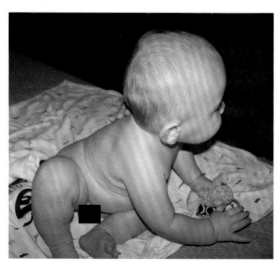

FIGURE 1.19. Sitting, shortening of the right side with weight shift to the left side; note the high degree of intra-axial rotation.

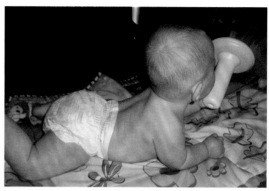

FIGURE 1.20. Prone-on-elbows, elongation on the child's right side with reaching with the left hand.

Weight shift also introduces the infant to vestibular stimulation, which is under his or her control, as opposed to the vestibular stimulation of being moved by another person or an object (rocking chair) or watching another person or object move (the crib mobile). Finally, when in full unilateral weight bearing, weight shift increases the amount of weight borne, and therefore joint compression, on a particular side or limb, up to twice the normal customary weight and compression. This increased weight on one limb or on one side of the trunk facilitates the recruitment of motor units in the working muscles.[59,105]

Weight shifting in prone-on-elbows has another subtle, yet significant, effect on the infant's development. Infants are born with their forearms in relative pronation and are unable to supinate the forearms actively, even though the forearms can be moved passively into supination. As the infant shifts from side to side in prone-on-elbows, the weight shifting causes the forearm on the side to which the infant shifts weight to supinate, whereas the forearm on the side away from which the weight shifts pronates. The proprioceptive feedback from this reciprocal pronation and supination lays the foundation for emerging, active forearm supination.

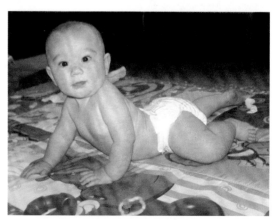

FIGURE 1.21. Prone-on-extended-arms with muscles of the weight-bearing anterior trunk, pelvis, and lower extremities elongated; also note the slight weight shift to the child's right side with shortening of left lateral trunk musculature.

Without the ability to supinate the forearms, the infant would not develop the ability to reach for, grasp, and visually engage an object. With the forearm in pronation, the first two steps can be accomplished, but the dorsum of the hand blocks the infant's view of the object grasped (Fig. 1.22). Lack of supination of the forearm is also responsible for spillage when children first attempt to feed themselves with a spoon. The child holds the spoon and captures the food with the forearm in pronation. As the child brings the spoon toward the mouth, the child needs to supinate to keep the bowl of the spoon level. Until the child develops full active supination, spillage will continue to occur (Fig. 1.23). Many other functional activities across the life span depend on the ability to supinate the forearms, such as donning a shirt, buttoning and unbuttoning a shirt, turning a door knob, turning a steering wheel, and tying a bow.

As the infant practices weight shift in prone-on-elbows, he or she begins to take an interest in reaching for toys from this

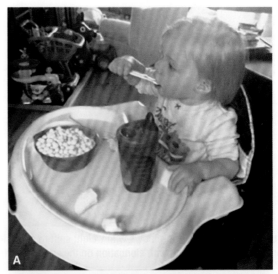

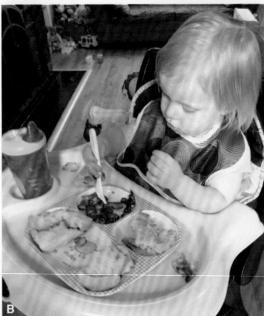

FIGURE 1.23. A: Lack of forearm supination when bringing the spoon to the mouth causes spillage. **B:** With the development of forearm supination, a child is able to use a spoon with very little spillage.

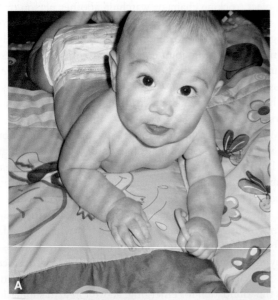

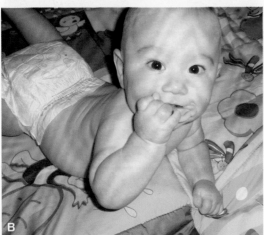

FIGURE 1.22. A: With forearm in pronation, visual examination of toy grasped in hand is blocked by the dorsum of the hand. **B:** The development of forearm supination allows visual examination of an object and putting the object in the mouth with ease.

position. First attempts at reaching while prone-on-elbows often fail because the child shifts weight onto the side to which he or she is looking (Fig. 1.24). Eventually, the child learns to shift weight away from the limb needed for reaching for the toy they see. With practice of weight shifting in this position and through trial and error, the infant is eventually able to shift weight to one elbow and forearm while looking in the opposite direction, thereby establishing visually directed reaching (Fig. 1.25).

Prone-on-Extended-Arms

Having secured the prone-on-elbows position and having learned to shift their weight in different directions, infants

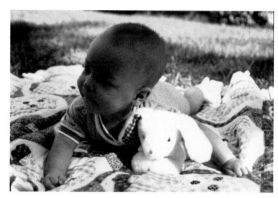

FIGURE 1.24. First attempts at visually directed reaching in prone-on-elbows or extended-arms are often unsuccessful because the child shifts weight in the direction that he or she is looking, and the arm nearest the object is not freed.

begin to lift themselves farther from the surface. They push themselves up into prone-on-extended-arms, working their open hands into the surface, using the triceps to extend the elbows, and actively using the serratus anterior muscles to protract and stabilize the shoulder girdle (Fig. 1.26A). The trunk extensors, continuing to activate and strengthen in a cephalocaudal direction, assist in this antigravity movement. The anterior thoracic muscles must elongate. The elbows, in the prone-on-extended-arms position, illustrate the principle of weight bearing on extended limbs after first weight bearing on flexed limbs. In addition to the extended elbows, this position is noted for increased antigravity extension using midline thoracic extensors, increased scapulohumeral elongation, a pelvis still in a relative posterior tilt to stabilize the lifted head and upper trunk, and comparatively passive lower extremities.

Although the lower extremities are decidedly passive in prone-on-elbows and prone-on-extended-arms, the position assumed by the lower extremities in these positions is predictive of later development and active use of the lower

extremities. It is the same lower extremity position seen in the infant after the loss of physiologic flexion (see Figs. 1.2A and 1.26A).

Once the infant has begun to push into prone-on-arms with extended elbows, he or she begins to weight-shift in that position, as done in the prone-on-elbows position. Weight shifting produces increased stability at the shoulder joints because more weight is accepted onto one or the other shoulder during weight shifting. Weight shifting to the side eventually produces unilateral weight bearing with the ability to reach and grasp, with the accompanying elongation of the trunk on the weight-bearing side. Posterior weight shift may actually cause the infant to move backward in this position, increasing scapulohumeral elongation. While pushing backward, the infant may lift the buttocks from the surface, continuing to push weight backward over the knees and into the quadruped position, with weight on the open hands. If the infant pushes with enough force, the weight may shift backward onto the toes, rather than on the flexed knees, in a "push-up" position (Fig. 1.26B). Eventually, the infant

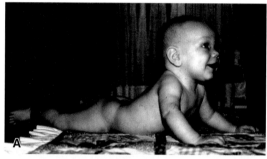

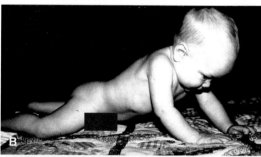

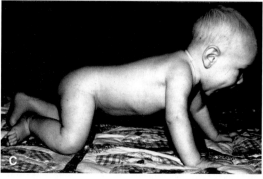

FIGURE 1.26. Transition from prone-on-extended-arms to quadruped. **A:** Prone-on-extended-arms. **B:** Push-up transition position. **C:** Quadruped.

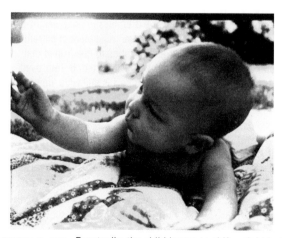

FIGURE 1.25. Eventually, the child learns to shift weight to the skull-side limb, freeing the appropriate arm for reaching the object as he or she looks at it.

succeeds in getting the weight shifted posteriorly onto the knees for hands-and-knees weight bearing (quadruped or four-point). The infant is definitely pleased with this accomplishment (Fig. 1.26C).

Pivot Prone

At approximately 5 months of age, the infant develops an interesting skill that contributes to pelvic and scapular mobility. The pivot prone position or pattern, as seen in Figure 1.27, uses cephalocaudally progressing extension to extend the neck, midline trunk, and lower extremities. The pelvis is in an anterior tilt, with hips hyperextended. The upper extremities assume the *high guard* position with the scapulae adducted by the rhomboid muscles. The upper limbs are horizontally abducted at the shoulders and flexed at the elbows. This *retraction* of the shoulder girdle with the posturing of the upper extremities enhances the trunk extension. To assume the pivot prone pattern, the anterior musculature must elongate.

Once the infant develops stability in the pivot prone position, he or she will playfully move alternately between pivot prone and prone-on-elbows. In this manner, the infant practices scapular and pelvic mobility. The shoulder girdle alternates between *protraction* in prone-on-elbows and retraction in pivot prone. The pelvic girdle moves between the posterior tilt of prone-on-elbows and the anterior tilt of pivot prone. Often, out of exuberance, the infant actually pivots the body in a circle and kicks the legs, or quickly alternating between these two positions.

Quadruped

As in other positions, early attempts at the hands-and-knees position are generally not refined, often because the lower extremities are not positioned optimally to accept weight (Fig. 1.28). But with practice, the infant soon masters another new skill. Refer again to Figure 1.2B. Note that the infant's open hands are aligned under flexed shoulders, and the knees are aligned under flexed hips. The active participation of the lower extremities in *quadruped*, also called *four-point*, requires stability around the hip joints caused by co-contraction of the hip musculature. The principles of developmental direction are illustrated well in quadruped.

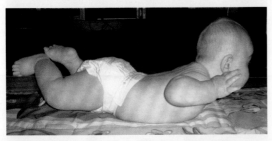

FIGURE 1.27. Pivot prone position with elongation of anterior trunk and lower extremity musculature and retraction of shoulder girdle; only mid and lower trunk are in contact with the supporting surface.

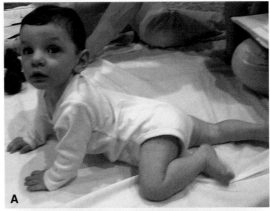

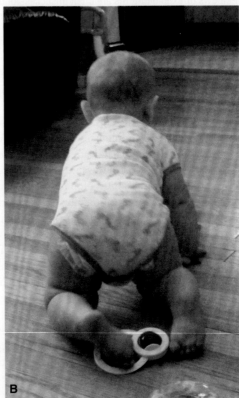

FIGURE 1.28. Immature quadruped position with hip abduction and external rotation, lower extremities in poor weight-bearing alignment; reciprocal and contralateral movement of extremities. **A:** Note the lumbar lordosis, an indication in quadruped that the abdominals are weak or not being activated. **B:** Improved quadruped position, but base of support is still wide, interfering with lateral weight shift for creeping.

Weight bearing on flexed elbows has given way to weight bearing on extended elbows. True to cephalocaudal development, the lower extremities now participate actively, unlike when in the prone-on-elbows position. Stability in quadruped increases, as it does in prone-on-elbows and prone-on-extended-arms, as the child moves into the weight-shifting phase of the quadruped position. When weight is shifted posteriorly, with the upper extremities fixed in a closed chain, scapulohumeral elongation is facilitated. The base of support in quadruped may be wide in initial attempts, particularly because of excessive abduction of the lower extremities (Fig. 1.28B). This wider base of support helps the infant to be more stable. However, it interferes with adequate lateral weight shift, which is needed to achieve unilateral weight bearing. Unilateral weight bearing is necessary in both the upper and lower body to free one upper and one lower limb for the forward movement of creeping.

A stable quadruped position requires not only stable hips and shoulders but also a stable trunk. Trunk flexors and extensors must balance each other to produce a flat back in the four-point position. When the child first achieves the quadruped position, he or she generally displays the lumbar lordosis of the young infant whose abdominal musculature is not yet developed and strong. This is due to underdeveloped abdominal muscles and strong contraction of the hip flexors to stabilize. Overly active hip flexion is progravity fixing to increase muscle tone around the hip joints, and therefore stability. Increased hip flexion posturing leads to increased lumbar lordosis or anterior pelvic tilt. Development of the abdominals begins when the infant first acquires the posterior tilt, which was essential for lifting of the head in prone. Concurrent with the achievement of a stable prone-on-elbows position, with its posterior pelvic tilt resulting from activation of abdominal muscles, changes are taking place in the supine position to further recruit and strengthen abdominal muscles. Abdominal musculature continues to develop to balance the extensors of the trunk. With the balance of lumbar flexors and extensors, the quadruped position with a flat back is achieved (see Fig. 1.2B).

Locomotion in Prone

Locomotion is defined as movement from one place to another.[1] Six modes of locomotion develop in the prone position typically. In the order of development, they are scooting, crawling, pivoting in prone, rolling, creeping, and plantigrade creeping. Some locomotive forms may develop and be used nearly simultaneously, such as crawling and pivoting in prone, at approximately 5 months of age. Also, it is not unusual for one or more modes of locomotion not to develop in a given child. No long-term negative effects result from this lack of development. However, it is important for the child to develop, in other ways, any components of movement that typically develop or improve in the different forms of prone locomotion.

As early as a few days of age, the infant is able to move in the crib by wiggling and scooting. This is the first form of locomotion. Inevitably, an infant placed in the middle of a crib for a nap will find the way to a corner of the crib. It is thought that the closeness and security offered by a corner is comforting to the child, especially after 40 weeks in the close spaces of the womb. Because infants are able to wiggle and scoot, not even the youngest of infants should be left unattended on a raised surface such as a sofa, an adult bed, a changing table, or a mat table.

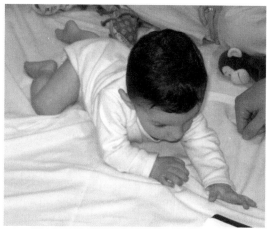

FIGURE 1.29. Crawling with reciprocal use of upper extremities.

During the first 2 months, when an infant is in prone or supine, he or she will wiggle and scoot as the chief form of locomotion. Once the infant attains and is stable in the prone-on-elbows position, he or she may locomote by crawling, moving the body forward by digging elbows and forearms into the surface and extending the shoulders. *Crawling* is a locomotive form that infants may use from 3 months to 8 or 9 months of age. Crawling is defined as moving "slowly by dragging the body along the ground."[10,47,48,106] First attempts at crawling often produce a backward motion as the infant flexes the shoulders, instead of extending them. Once the infant achieves a forward progression, the infant may crawl by moving both forearms forward at the same time, or may crawl using reciprocal motions of the upper extremities (Fig. 1.29). This reciprocal motion is a precursor to reciprocal creeping, plantigrade creeping, and walking with reciprocal arm swing.

The defining component of crawling is that the infant's abdomen is in contact with the floor. This compares with *creeping*, which means to move across the floor on hands and knees without the trunk being in direct contact with the surface.[10,46-49,106] Although this distinguishing component may seem inconsequential, especially when the lay public often uses the terms synonymously, differentiating between crawling and creeping is important in the health care professions so that terminology is used consistently, leaving no room for misunderstanding.

In crawling, the lower extremities are basically passive while the upper extremities move either together or reciprocally. Crawling with nonreciprocal use of the upper extremities requires no trunk rotation, whereas reciprocal crawling does require rotation within the body axis. In **rotation** of the trunk, either the upper or the lower trunk moves while the rest of the trunk remains stable. Rotation of the upper trunk means the upper trunk moves on a stable, nonmoving lower trunk. The converse is true as well. Reciprocal, contralateral creeping requires counterrotation, a progressively more complex movement. This contralateral movement requires counterrotation within the trunk. *Counterrotation* is defined as rotating the upper trunk to one side, while rotating the lower trunk in the opposite direction. Counterrotation of the trunk is a different movement from simple rotation of the trunk.

Pivoting in prone, as described previously, is a form of locomotion that some infants use in conjunction with crawling or rolling to move intentionally in a particular direction. For example, if the infant wants to reach a toy that is out of his or her immediate space, the infant will often use a combination of these movements appropriately to reach the toy.

Rolling from prone to supine and supine to prone, another means of locomotion, develops in the infant by 5 to 6 months of age. Still lacking an efficient locomotive form, once the infant achieves rolling from prone to supine and supine to prone, the infant may use a combination of rolling and crawling to move in a specific direction across the floor.

At 6 to 7 months of age, while prone-on-extended-arms, the infant begins pushing the body backward, raising the buttocks into the air in an attempt to get into quadruped (hands-and-knees position). This position, also called four-point, is the position from which the next locomotive form, **creeping**, will develop. Both the upper and lower extremities participate equally in creeping (Fig. 1.30).

Once the infant is stable on hands and knees, the usual process of weight shifting in various directions occurs. With controlled weight shift, the infant is able to lift one limb at a time, eventually lifting one upper extremity and the opposite lower extremity at once. This movement leads to creeping on hands and knees at approximately 9 to 11 months of age. Typical and refined creeping is both reciprocal and contralateral. In other words, the child advances one arm and the opposite leg at the same time (contralateral), reciprocating with the other arm and leg, which also move together. This contralateral movement requires not only rotation of the trunk, but also counterrotation. The reciprocal activity of creeping helps to refine intra-axial rotation and reciprocal use of the limbs, strengthening counterrotation for use in the higher levels of locomotion.

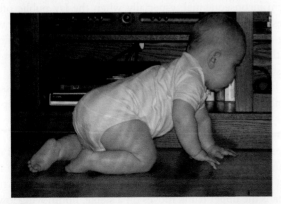

FIGURE 1.30. Creeping with reciprocal use of upper and lower extremities; note the loss of lumbar lordosis, an indication that lumbar flexors and extensors are co-contracting (compare with Fig. 1.28).

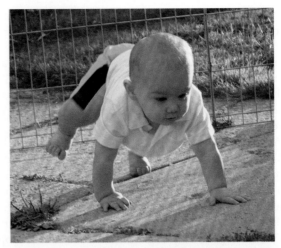

FIGURE 1.31. Plantigrade creeping, also called bear walking.

Plantigrade creeping, sometimes referred to as bear walking, is more of a transitional position than a form of locomotion. However, some children do use the plantigrade position, open hands and plantar surfaces of the feet in closed-chain contact with the ground, to locomote. In many cases, this type of creeping may be the result of an environmental factor. For example, the child may choose plantigrade creeping over creeping in quadruped if the knees are bare and the child is creeping on a concrete or other rough surface (see Fig. 1.31). This illustrates the dynamic nature of development. Many factors, in addition to maturation, influence the development of motor skills.

As a transitional position, the plantigrade position is used by the child as one means of getting to standing from the prone position. In early attempts, the child may rely on being near furniture or a wall for assistance as they rise to standing, moving through the plantigrade position to the upright standing position.

Supine Progression

Supine Lying and Pull to Sitting

Like the prone progression, development in the supine position proceeds in a known sequence. The full-term neonate in supine is dominated by physiologic flexion, expressed in slight cervical flexion, with the head held toward midline, elbow flexion, posterior pelvic tilt, hip adduction, and hip and knee flexion. The feet are typically in the air and not touching the surface. Hands are held loosely fisted, but do open frequently, both at rest and with the infant's random movements (Fig. 1.32). When the infant is *pulled to sitting*, the examiner gently pulls the infant's upper extremities at the wrists, the head is held in plane with the body and the infant exhibits no *head lag*, mimicking active head control. Over the first month, as the physiologic flexion gradually disappears, the head falls away from midline to the side, elbows relax, and the hip and knee flexion dissipate, bringing the infant's feet down to the surface (Fig. 1.33). As the feet come down

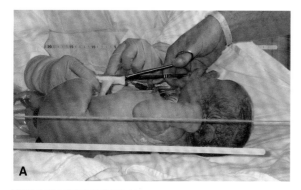

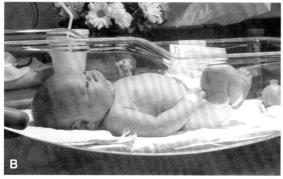

FIGURE 1.32. Physiologic flexion in supine in the full-term neonate; note that the feet are held above the supporting surface, and the hands and fingers are inconsistently in a fist. **A:** Physiologic flexion seen in an infant only minutes old. **B:** Physiologic flexion in supine in an infant 24 hours after birth. Note the inconsistently fisted hands of the neonate in both **A** and **B**.

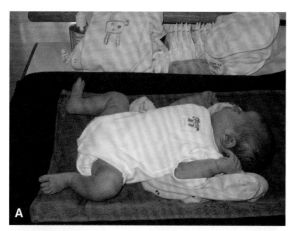

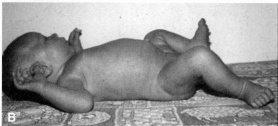

FIGURE 1.33. As physiologic flexion diminishes, the hip and knee flexion gradually decrease **(A)**, allowing the feet to rest on the supporting surface **(B)**.

to the surface, the pelvis is pulled into a relative anterior tilt by gravity, now unopposed by physiologic flexion. Increasing hip abduction and external rotation begin to evolve. When pulled to sitting, head lag is present. This means that the infant's head, no longer being supported by the physiologic flexion, lags behind the rest of the body as the child is pulled toward the sitting position. Antigravity flexors have yet to develop. Without active head control, the child's head falls backward into gravity when he or she is pulled toward the sitting position. Over time, as the antigravity cervical flexors become stronger and active head control develops, the infant exhibits less and less head lag when pulled to sitting. After the initial period of head lag, which follows the loss of physiologic flexion, the infant will begin to hold the head in alignment with the body. Then the infant learns to lead with the head as soon as the stimulus of being pulled to sitting occurs. Next in the sequence, the lower extremities begin to flex actively at the hips during the pull-to-sitting maneuver. Finally, the pull-to-sitting stimulus recruits cervical flexors, trunk flexors, and hip flexors. Figure 1.34 shows the pull-to-sitting sequence.

In supine, after the first month, the infant usually has the head turned to one side or the other, influenced by the ATNR. The ATNR is manifested in infants during wakefulness and sleep and diminishes over time, as seen in Figure 1.3. This reflex begins prenatally and is manifested by asymmetric extension of the neck, with accompanying predictable limb movements. Under the influence of the ATNR, when the head is turned to one side in slight hyperextension, cervical proprioceptors are stimulated. This causes the *face limbs*, the ipsilateral upper and lower extremities on the side to which the head is turned, to extend. The contralateral limbs, the *skull limbs* or *occiput limbs*, flex. The upper extremity manifestations of the ATNR are usually stronger than are the lower extremity manifestations. The ATNR is seen in normal infants during the first 4 months of life, more as an attitude or assumed position than as a strong obligatory position. This position is frequently termed the *fencer's position* (see Fig. 1.3). Although this fencer's position is evident in nearly all infants during this period and is seen repeatedly in supine and supported sitting, the ATNR is not so strong in typical infants that it limits voluntary or passive movement of the extremities or head. If the ATNR presents stereotypically, is obligatory during those first months, or produces strong flexor or extensor tone in the extremities, this may be an indication of atypical neuromotor development. In the typical infant, the strength of the ATNR reflex is noted to diminish over time such that by 4 months it is evident inconsistently and finally integrates.[96,98,99,107]

The ATNR is evidence of the infant's lack of dissociation. *Dissociation* is the ability of the human to move limbs independently from the head, move limbs independently from each other, move joints within the same limb independently, and move the body independently from the head. Head and limbs lack dissociation in an infant manifesting an ATNR. The proprioceptors of the neck influence the position of the

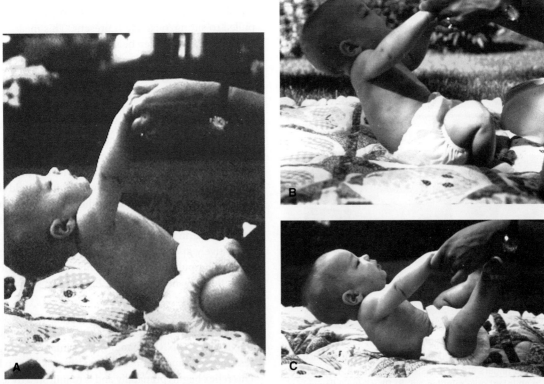

FIGURE 1.34. Pull-to-sitting sequence. **A:** Head lag when pulled to sitting, denoting lack of antigravity control of cervical flexor muscles. **B:** No head lag when pulled to sitting; as the child matures and control of antigravity cervical flexors develops, the child holds the head in the same plane as the body. **C:** Cervical, trunk, and hip flexors exhibit active antigravity control when the child is pulled to sitting.

limbs, resulting in the position as described. As the infant matures and the ATNR loses its influence, the limbs no longer assume specific positions based on the position of the head, thereby demonstrating dissociation.

Another reflex that affects the supine and prone positions is the tonic labyrinthine reflex. The role of the tonic labyrinthine reflex in typical neuromotor development is not well understood, although it appears to provide an underlying predisposition for flexion tone in prone and extension tone in supine.[96,98,99,107] The receptors for this reflex are in the labyrinths of the ears and are responsive to the continuous forces of gravity. The basic functional skills of lifting the head in prone and supine and performing total body antigravity extension in prone (the pivot prone pattern) and antigravity flexion in supine (the feet-to-mouth pattern) are accommodated in the typical infant because resting tone and tone with initiation of movement are not excessive. However, the infant with atypical development may be influenced negatively by the tonic labyrinthine reflex, exhibiting extensor or flexor hypertonus that may prevent the development of antigravity contraction of the antagonist muscles in either or both positions. If tone is excessive in extensors in supine, for example, the flexor antagonists are not able to contract because the extensor muscles are not able to relax. This loss of *reciprocal inhibition*, the ability of antagonist muscles to relax or

lengthen while agonist muscles contract or shorten, may be strong enough to cause sensorimotor impairment.

As the ATNR diminishes, the infant begins to appear more symmetric in supine (Fig. 1.35). The ability to bring the head to midline and hold it there is a significant milestone. Two processes interact to allow head-to-midline movement.

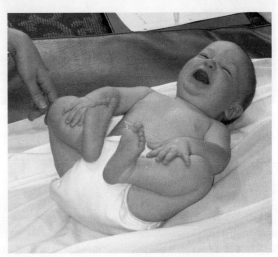

FIGURE 1.35. Postural symmetry exhibited by 6 to 7 months of age.

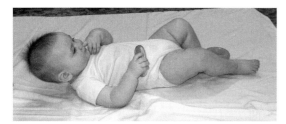

FIGURE 1.36. Lifting head in supine, an indication of well-developed antigravity cervical flexion.

Because the ATNR is an asymmetric influence on the position of the head, as the ATNR diminishes the cervical extensors no longer contract as a reflex response. Rather, they relax, no longer keeping the head to one side. At the same time, this passive factor occurs in supine, the cervical flexors begin to work as antigravity muscles, helping to actively bring the head to midline. Eventually, the cervical flexors are strong enough to bring the head to midline and to lift the infant's head from the surface in supine (Fig. 1.36). These developmental achievements in supine are occurring during the second to fourth months, at the same time that the cervical extensors are emerging as antigravity muscles in prone. Complete development of lifting of the head in prone (4 months) develops shortly before full lifting of the head in supine (5 months). When the cervical flexors contract to lift the head into flexion while in supine, the cervical extensors must elongate. This is another example of reciprocal inhibition. Children with neuromotor pathologies may lack the ability to lengthen or relax the cervical extensors.

As cephalocaudal development continues in supine, controlled movement of the upper extremities begins with volitional movement and subsequent stabilization of the shoulder joints. The achievement of prone-on-elbows aids in developing the stability of the shoulder girdle in a weight-bearing function (closed chain), whereas the supine position permits the development of shoulder stability for non–weight-bearing function (open chain).

During the first 3 months of life, the infant has little control over the placement and holding of the upper extremities in space. Attempts at grasping an object are made with the hands close to the body, because the child lacks the shoulder girdle stability and the strength to use the hands in space away from the body (see Fig. 1.4). With shoulder adduction, the upper extremities are held against the sides of the infant's body, providing stability in the only way the infant knows at this point. This process is referred to as *fixing*. Fixing is a normal process of development that occurs with first attempts to stabilize the body, relative to gravity, in all positions. These first attempts are not true antigravity stability. Instead, they are a temporary means of stabilizing by fixing into gravity (*progravity*), until the appropriate muscles in a particular position learn to stabilize or fix against gravity (*antigravity*).

Without the eventual emergence of muscle groups strong enough to work as antigravity muscles, development will be delayed. Fundamentally, antigravity muscle work is what keeps a person upright against gravity, whether in sitting, kneeling (tall kneeling or knee standing), quadruped, or standing erect. In normal mature bipedal movement, extensor muscles are the main antigravity muscles that keep humans upright. These include the erector spinae, gluteus maximus, proximal hamstrings, and quadriceps muscles. In the supine position, however, the flexors act as antigravity muscles. Specific flexor muscles include the cervical flexors, abdominal muscles, and hip flexors.

Once the infant develops shoulder stability using co-contraction of all of the muscles around the shoulder joint, the infant is able to reach out to grasp toys (Fig. 1.37A), and thus begin the skills of grasp and manipulation. This process of fine motor development will take approximately 18 months to refine and will not be complete until approximately 30 months of age. Development of grasp and prehension is discussed elsewhere in this chapter.

Hands to Knees and Feet, Feet to Mouth

Another developmental landmark occurs when the infant reaches upward against gravity while in supine. As the pectoral muscles are being activated, so are the abdominals. The pectoral muscles are partially responsible for reaching the upper extremity toward the ceiling in supine (Fig. 1.37B).

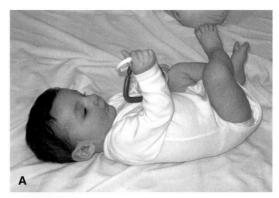

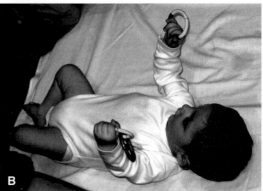

FIGURE 1.37. Reaching with upper extremities. **A:** Once stability is achieved in the shoulder girdle, the child can reach into space to grasp a toy; note the midline orientation of the head and hands. **B:** Reaching well into space using antigravity control of the serratus anterior muscles; note the supine symmetry and concurrent but separate use of hands.

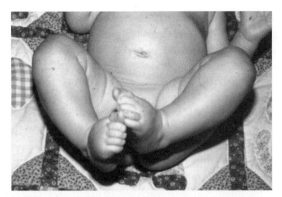

FIGURE 1.38. Supine at 5 months, foot-to-foot contact.

For this movement to occur, the serratus anterior muscles act in synergy, and the rhomboid muscles must elongate. These muscles, acting in concert, cause the shoulder girdle to protract. It is now that one sees the infant's ability to reach for the caregiver's face while being diapered or dressed. Active use of the pectorals with reciprocal inhibition of the rhomboids, along with the recent inhibition of the ATNR, allows the infant to reach upward and also to bring his or her hands to midline.

In supine at 5 months of age, as infants continue to gain ever-increasing control of their antigravity flexors, with reciprocal lengthening of antagonist extensor muscles, they begin to actively lift their lower extremities from the surface. Some foot-to-foot contact usually occurs (Fig. 1.38). Next, infants begin to reach for their knees and then their feet. At first, they reach their hand to the ipsilateral knee and foot, as seen in Figure 1.35. Eventually, they are able to cross midline with their upper extremities, placing a hand on the contralateral knee and/or foot (Fig. 1.39). This contact of the infant with his or her own body is important to the process of developing *body image* or *body scheme*.[97]

As the infant flexes the hips to bring his or her feet toward the hands and head, the abdominals and hip flexors are gaining strength. Active contraction of the abdominal muscles causes the pelvis to tip posteriorly and the gluteus maximus and proximal hamstrings to elongate. The hips are in moderate flexion, abduction, and external rotation. The knees are flexed, and the feet are dorsiflexed and supinated (Fig. 1.40A).

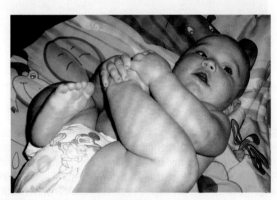

FIGURE 1.39. Supine, hand to contralateral foot.

The natural progression of hands to knees and hands to feet leads to the infant bringing the feet to his or her mouth. At 5 months of age, an infant is very interested in oral stimulation. No longer under the influence of the rooting and sucking reflexes, the infant begins to use the mouth for more than eating. As he or she brings a foot toward the mouth, the infant exhibits feed-forward anticipation of putting the toes into the mouth (Fig. 1.40B). Putting the foot in the mouth, seen in Figure 1.40C, further develops body image. This activity also facilitates cognitive development. Infants learn about objects through touch, including the touch that accompanies placing objects in the mouth, a process referred to as *mouthing* (Fig. 1.41).

Pelvic stability, in a posterior pelvic tilt, is needed in prone for the infant to begin lifting the head in prone. In supine, at 5 months of age, the infant puts his or her feet in the mouth, further enhancing the active posterior pelvic tilt. Once the posterior pelvic tilt is achieved and

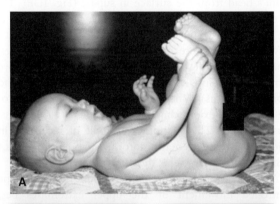

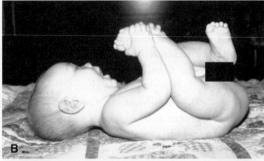

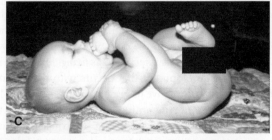

FIGURE 1.40. Foot-to-mouth sequence at 5 months of age. **A:** Note the elongation of posterior musculature and visually directed reaching to foot. **B:** Movement of foot toward mouth, child opening the mouth with feed-forward anticipation. **C:** Child puts foot into the mouth, one way of learning about the body.

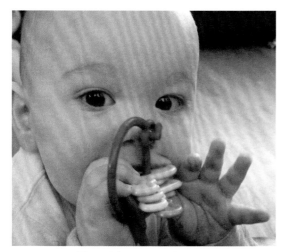

FIGURE 1.41. The activity of mouthing helps the infant develop form and shape perception as well as body image.

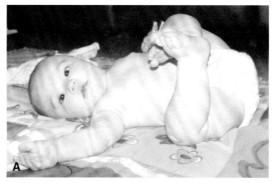

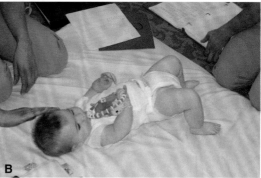

FIGURE 1.42. Development of pelvic mobility in supine. **A:** Feet toward head with posterior pelvic tilt. **B:** Bridging with anterior pelvic tilt.

strengthened, the infant begins to develop pelvic mobility. That is, the infant moves back and forth in supine between a posterior pelvic tilt and an anterior pelvic tilt. This is often observed during spontaneous play in supine, as children bring their feet to their mouth with a posterior pelvic tilt. Then they lower their feet to the surface, with a relative anterior tilt. Sometimes when they lower their feet to the surface, they continue with active lumbar extension into the *bridging* position, which requires more of the relative anterior tilt. In doing this, children work their feet into the surface (Fig. 1.42A and B). Developing pelvic mobility in supine allows the infant to move back and forth between these two positions, in tandem with activities occurring in prone. At about the same time in development, approximately 5 months of age, the infant practices pelvic mobility in prone. This requires alternating between the posterior tilt of prone on forearms and the anterior tilt of the pivot prone position, as discussed previously.

Rolling Progression

Nonsegmental Rolling

Rolling develops in a two-stage progression. From birth to 6 months of age, the infant performs *nonsegmental rolling.* *Segmental rolling* develops at approximately 6 months of age. Nonsegmental rolling, also referred to as *log rolling,* allows the infant to roll from supine to side-lying. This movement is based on one of the infant reflexes, the *neck-righting reaction.* In the neck-righting reaction, the stimulation of proprioceptors in the neck as the infant's head is turned actively or passively to one side causes the body to follow in one complete unit, without rotation within the vertebral column.[46,107] The neck-righting reaction gradually diminishes over time as another reaction, the *body-righting reaction acting on the body,* evolves.[46,107]

Segmental Rolling

The body-righting reaction acting on the body is a predominant factor in movement by 6 months of age. When the head is rotated to one side, the body reacts to the proprioceptive stimulus to the neck by following in the direction of the head turning, thus rolling toward that side. Now the movement within the vertebral column is segmental. That is, the different segments, the trunk, shoulder girdle, and pelvic girdle, as well as the upper and lower extremity on one side, are seen to respond sequentially, rather than moving as one unit (Fig. 1.43A). The sequence of movement of the various body segments is not identical in all infants, nor is it always the same sequence in an individual infant. The infant may lead with the head, a lower extremity, an upper extremity, the pelvic girdle, or the shoulder girdle, and the other segments follow the lead segment (Fig. 1.43B to D). Segmental rolling requires rotation within the body axis, the vertebral column. This rotation is referred to as *intra-axial rotation* and is facilitated by the body-righting reaction acting on the body, permitting the infant to roll from prone to supine and supine to prone.

Rolling Prone to Supine and Supine to Prone

Before the infant attempts to roll volitionally, rolling from prone to supine and supine to prone often occurs accidentally. Early on, the infant may roll accidentally from prone to supine because he or she pulls the knees underneath and the buttocks are elevated. If the center of mass gets high

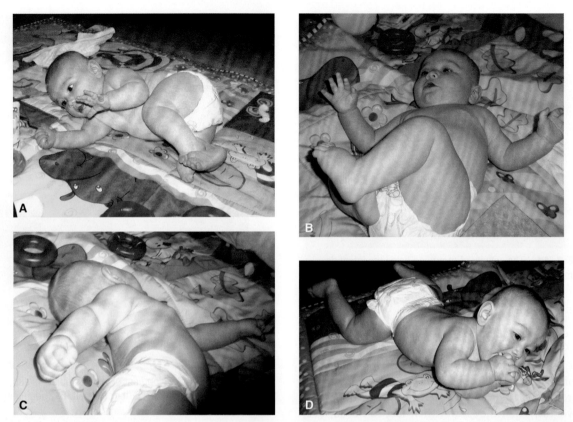

FIGURE 1.43. A: Intra-axial rotation develops, in part, as the result of the body righting acting on the body response. **B:** Segmental rolling, supine to prone, leading with the lower extremity; **C:** prone to supine, leading with the upper extremity; **D:** prone to supine, leading with the head.

enough, as a result of the elevated buttocks, the infant may roll accidentally (Fig. 1.44). Accidental rolling, from prone to supine, may also occur as spinal extension progresses caudally, and the infant achieves prone-on-elbows and prone-on-extended-arms. In this case, the center of mass becomes higher through the lifting of the head and upper trunk. Experimenting with the prone-on-elbows and prone-on-extended-arms positions, the infant becomes rather top-heavy and therefore may roll to supine accidentally. When this happens, the infant may attempt to replicate the movement. Once able to replicate the movement, the infant will practice this movement. Through trial and error and the increasingly strong body-righting reaction acting on the body, the infant learns to roll segmentally from prone to supine, usually by 5 months of age (Fig. 1.45).

Rolling supine to prone also may occur as an involuntary movement initially. When the infant is in supine around the age of 4 or 5 months, he or she may lift the pelvis from the surface by plantar flexing the feet, working the feet into the surface. This bridging type of maneuver raises the center of mass, through the lower trunk, and may cause the infant to roll to one side or the other as he or she pushes a little harder into the surface with one foot, the foot

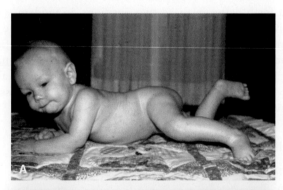

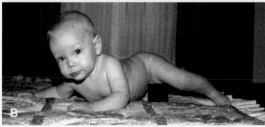

FIGURE 1.44. Accidental rolling prone to supine. **A:** In prone, the child lifts buttocks from the surface. **B:** As he or she lifts buttocks higher off the surface and pushes into the supporting surface with the foot, the child may accidentally roll prone to supine.

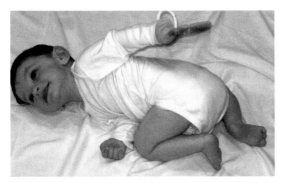

FIGURE 1.45. Segmental rolling prone to supine, leading with upper extremity.

contralateral to the direction to which he or she accidentally rolls. Trial-and-error practice, along with the strong body-righting reaction acting on the body, combines with other factors such as motivation, allowing the infant to volitionally roll supine to prone by 6 months of age, using intra-axial rotation (Fig. 1.46). Although the age of acquisition of rolling skills may vary slightly, volitional rolling usually occurs from prone to supine before supine to prone, at 5 and 6 months, respectively.

Once an infant is able to roll volitionally, it is important that he or she learns to roll toward both left and right sides when in prone or supine. This will occur naturally in most cases, unless the infant encounters an obstacle to rolling to either left or right. Furniture, the side of the crib, or other

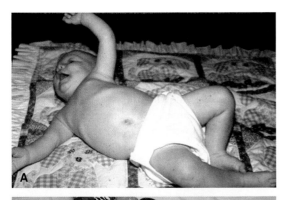

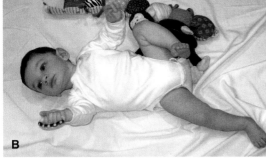

FIGURE 1.46. Segmental rolling supine to prone using intra-axial rotation. **A:** Rolling leading with upper extremity; note the scapulohumeral elongation. **B:** Segmental rolling leading with lower extremity; note the crossing of midline.

environmental barriers may cause the infant to always roll toward the same side. However, if such is the case, attentive parents and other caregivers can make sure the infant is placed away from environmental obstacles and encouraged to roll toward both left and right sides during play. An infant unable to roll toward one or the other side in the absence of environmental barriers or lack of opportunity may be exhibiting signs of neuromotor or musculoskeletal pathology. In such cases, the inability to roll in both directions should be viewed as a red flag, but is not in itself diagnostic.

The functional activity of rolling helps develop and secure several components of movement, as well as being a functional motor milestone in its own right. As the infant learns to roll segmentally from prone to supine, the asymmetric cervical extension that he or she uses to initiate rolling during early attempts gives way to extension of the neck with lateral flexion and rotation. As the infant gets to supine, he or she completes the roll using slight cervical flexion.

If the infant leads with the upper extremity when rolling supine to prone, he or she typically will bring one upper extremity across the chest, reaching toward the side to which he or she is rolling. This movement requires and encourages scapulohumeral elongation at the shoulder of the leading extremity (Fig. 1.46A). Rolling supine to prone using intra-axial rotation also requires the lead upper or lower extremity, along with the other ipsilateral extremity, to cross midline (Fig. 1.46A and B). The ability to roll demonstrates dissociation of the right and left extremities as well as dissociation of the extremities and the head. If the upper or lower extremities are dependent on movements of the head to function, segmental rolling likely will not occur. In such a case, the ATNR may be influencing the limb movements. That is, turning the head to one side to roll supine to prone causes the face-side extremities, upper more than lower, to extend in a pathologic pattern that blocks the ability to roll toward that side. Persistence of a primitive or obligatory ATNR may contribute to an infant's inability to roll supine to prone. However, such reflex activity may actually be used by the infant to roll prone to supine, using the abnormal asymmetric extensor tone of the ATNR and an elevated center of mass. This is also an atypical and pathologic pattern and is another red flag, particularly if the infant does not have dissociation of the head and extremities and/or intra-axial rotation.

Sitting Progression

Supported Sitting

Preparation for sitting begins in the prone and supine positions as the infant develops early components such as cephalocaudally progressing antigravity extension of the spine, pelvic mobility, intra-axial rotation, scapular mobility, and weight bearing on the upper extremities. During the neonatal period when the infant is held in sitting, the position is remarkable for extreme flexion of the spine, caused by the lack of antigravity extensor muscle control. In this position, seen in Figure 1.47A, the infant's trunk exhibits what is termed a *complete C-curve*. The head is forward, with chin resting on the chest. Even though the infant is at the mercy of gravity at this time and must be supported in sitting, the pelvis of the typical infant is perpendicular to the surface on which he or she sits (Fig. 1.47A). That is, the infant should be bearing weight on the ischial tuberosities. If the pelvis is perpendicular to the surface, the very top portion of the gluteal cleft is

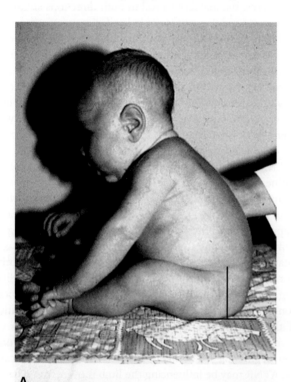

A

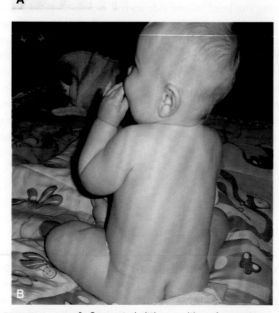

B

FIGURE 1.47. A: Supported sitting position of neonate; note the lack of antigravity spinal extension and that the pelvis is perpendicular to the supporting surface. **B:** Sitting with full back extension, visible gluteal cleft indicates pelvis is perpendicular to surface.

visible (Fig. 1.47B). If the infant is bearing weight, instead, on the sacrum, the pelvis is not perpendicular and the gluteal cleft is hidden from view. This weight bearing on the sacrum, referred to as *sacral sitting*, is a red flag and may be indicative of pathology. Regardless of an infant's age and stage of development, it is atypical to sit with the extreme posterior pelvic tilt exhibited in sacral sitting, even when the spine is in the immature C-curve characteristic of the neonate. Note the position of the pelvis in all of the figures of children sitting in this chapter.

As the infant develops, antigravity extension of the neck and trunk in sitting begins to appear. First, the cervical spine develops antigravity control, counteracting the infant's forward head position and lifting the head so that the face is vertical and the mouth is horizontal. As head control develops in supported sitting over the first 3 to 4 months, the infant is also gaining increased antigravity extension in the prone position. At the same time, in the supine position, the infant is developing antigravity flexion control. Thus, head control, as provided by a balance of cervical flexors and extensors, evolves to keep the head upright against gravity when sitting. In addition, the development of the chin tuck in the prone and supine positions secures the stable head in sitting by 4 months of age, even though the infant still depends on external support to remain in a sitting position (Fig. 1.48).

Propped Sitting

At approximately 5 months of age, the infant begins to exhibit the first abilities for sitting without the external support of either being held or sitting with a backrest. When placed in the sitting position, the infant attempts to prop with the upper extremities. With the weight shifted forward, the infant's hands are able to make contact with the surface. The *hand grasp reflex* has diminished and generally disappeared by 4 months of age, allowing the infant's open hands to be placed on the floor, anteriorly. Thus, the infant begins the adventure of sitting, with the lower extremities out in front

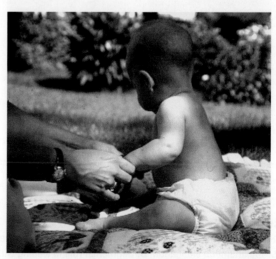

FIGURE 1.48. Supported sitting with full spinal extension; note the position of pelvis and stable head and neck.

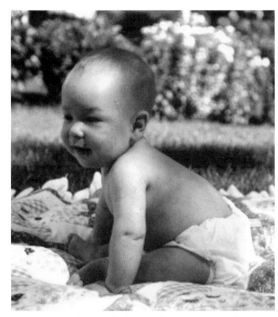

FIGURE 1.49. Propped sitting using the upper extremities to create a large base of support; note that pelvis is perpendicular to the supporting surface.

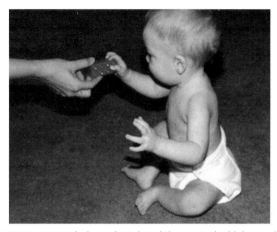

FIGURE 1.50. Independent ring sitting; note the high guard position of the upper extremities, used by the child to enhance trunk stability.

and the upper extremities once again performing in a major weight-bearing role. The two hands and the buttocks create a tripod base, which gives the infant a larger and more stable base of support than if the infant were to attempt to sit without the propping support of the upper extremities. This *propped sitting* position is typical of an infant who is 5 months of age. As the infant feels increasingly secure in this position, he or she will begin to rotate the neck to look around at the surroundings (Fig. 1.49). During propped sitting, the infant fixes progravity, strongly contracting the hip flexors to increase stability. The infant has not learned yet that the antigravity extensors will serve him or her better for remaining upright.

Mature stability against the forces of gravity in upright positions such as sitting and erect standing is attained through activation and strengthening of extensor muscles primarily. This antigravity extension of the trunk, hips, and knees develops over time in various positions. However, initial attempts at stability in upright positions are through the use of progravity contractions of trunk, hip, and knee flexors. Using progravity-stabilizing motor behaviors is referred to as *fixing into gravity* rather than *fixing against gravity*.

Ring Sitting

One major disadvantage of propping with the upper extremities while sitting is that the infant cannot use the upper extremities for reaching and grasping objects. As the trunk extensors become stronger, the infant is eventually able to rely less on the upper extremity support and the wide base, until finally is able to lift the hands from the surface on which he or she sits. This new sitting position is termed *ring sitting* because of the position of the lower extremities (Fig. 1.50).

Now the infant is sitting more erect, the pelvis still perpendicular to the surface, utilizing the ever-increasing trunk extensors to remain upright against gravity. Although by this time, approximately 6 months of age, the infant has adequate spinal extension to resist the pull of gravity while in sitting, he or she probably feels less stable in that position. To secure trunk extension even more when sitting without propping or other external support, the infant holds the upper extremities in the *high guard* position (see Fig. 1.50). The retraction of the shoulders in this position is analogous to the positioning of the upper extremities in the pivot prone position and serves as an adjunct to the spinal extension. Contraction of the rhomboids increases the overall muscular activity in the infant's posterior trunk, better securing him or her against gravity. This high guard position, using the rhomboid muscles to increase midline trunk stability against the pull of gravity, is seen again in the initial performance of tall kneeling and erect standing, as the child's center of mass moves higher in space relative to the supporting surface. However, the upper extremities, in the high guard position, are rendered virtually useless in terms of reaching for, grasping, and manipulating objects.

The lower extremities in ring sitting are flexed and externally rotated at the hips and flexed at the knees. The plantar surfaces of the feet are nearly touching or touching each other. The ankles may be pushed into moderate passive supination by contact with the surface. Ring sitting provides a relatively wide base of support because the externally rotated hips allow the lower extremities to rest on the floor. With the wider base of support and the high guard position, the infant is able to sit independent of external support at this point, but lacks the ability to independently achieve the sitting position from the prone or supine positions. Rather, when placed in sitting, the infant is able to remain stable without falling as long as he or she does not attempt much movement while in this position, which will disturb the balance.

Other Independent Sitting Positions

As the child experiences increasing stability in independent sitting, he or she begins to move the lower extremities out of the ring position, into either a *half–ring* position or *long sitting* (Figs. 1.51 and 1.52). The ability to have one lower extremity placed in front with relatively neutral hip rotation and an extended knee, while the other hip is still in flexion and external rotation with a flexed knee, is a sign of developing dissociation between the two lower limbs. The child moves in and out of this position, varying which leg is extended, and is often seen to be in simple long sitting. In mature long sitting, the base of support is narrowed mediolaterally, allowing lateral weight shifting with ease.

The child develops a series of increasingly advanced sitting positions that do not require external support, including ring sitting, half–ring sitting, long sitting, and side sitting. The child also develops short sitting (sitting with knees and hips flexed to ~90 degrees) on a child-sized chair, climbing onto higher surfaces such as a child's high chair to sit, and getting into and sitting on an adult-sized chair (Fig. 1.53). Depending on the environment and the individual child's motivation and opportunity, once the child achieves propped sitting followed by ring sitting, these various, more mature sitting positions may develop at different times for each child, sometimes nearly concurrently. In each new sitting position, the child repeats a series of motor behaviors that take them from a stable position when placed, through being able to move in and out of the position (the **transition**), to using the hands for prehension and object manipulation in each

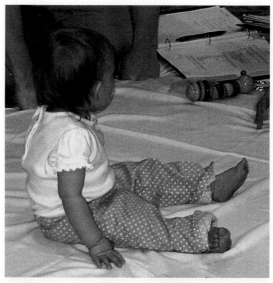

FIGURE 1.52. Long sitting with narrowed mediolateral base of support.

position. These motor behaviors include antigravity performance, antigravity stabilization, weight shifting, intra-axial rotation, and transition between positions. Weight shifting in each position is accompanied by elongation on the weight-bearing side.

As the child becomes more secure in ring sitting, he or she gradually relaxes the rhomboid muscles and lowers the upper extremities. No longer dependent on the upper extremities for stability in sitting, the child is able to volitionally protract and retract the shoulder girdle to reach for and grasp objects (Fig. 1.54). At about the same time, the child feels confident enough in sitting that he or she is able to rotate the head and neck to look around and begin performing visually directed reaching. The stability that results from the wide base of support in ring sitting, however, is gained at the expense of lateral weight shifting. The wider the base of support in any position, the more difficult it is to shift weight. Consequently, the child must move beyond ring-sitting to sitting positions with narrower bases of support.

At 6 months of age, the child's forearms are pronated such that, as the child looks toward and reaches for an object, he or she will grasp the object with the forearm pronated. Being unable to supinate volitionally, the child is unable to inspect the object visually once it is in the hand (Fig. 1.50). It is also difficult or impossible to inspect the object with the mouth. By 8 months of age, the child develops volitional supination and reciprocal pronation and supination of the forearms and is able to look at the object that he or she has secured and put it in the mouth. The ability to reach, grasp, and supinate with either upper extremity makes it possible for the child to take an object presented to him or her, inspect it, manipulate it by transferring the object from one hand to the other, and put it in the mouth. This bilateral hand activity also requires working in midline and crossing the midline of the body

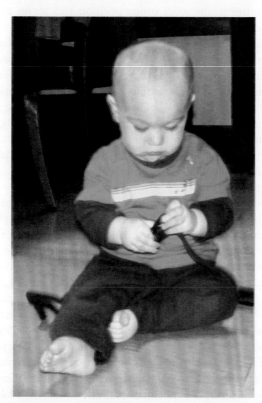

FIGURE 1.51. Half–ring sitting.

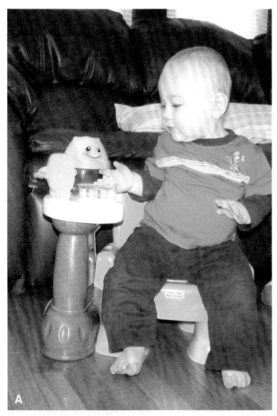

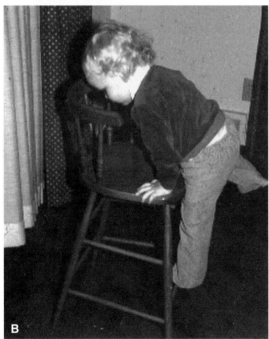

FIGURE 1.53. Sitting on surfaces of various heights. **A:** Short sitting on child-sized chair. **B:** Climbing onto a high chair.

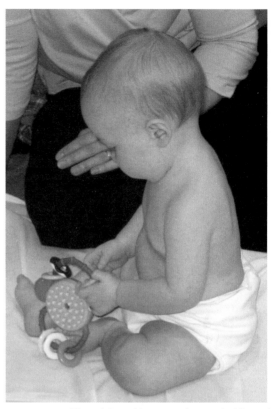

FIGURE 1.54. Ring sitting with no guard; note the bilateral use of the hands in midline.

with the upper extremities, head, and eyes. By the time the typical child has achieved the ring-sitting position, the child is no longer influenced by the ATNR, so keeping the head in midline, using two hands in midline, and crossing midline with the head, eyes, and hands are easily achieved.

In propped sitting and ring sitting, the feet and ankles are notable for their passive positioning in supination (see Figs. 1.49 and 1.50). Therefore, at 5 and 6 months of age, these sitting positions reflect the supinated feet, hip flexion and external rotation, and knee flexion seen in the supine position when the child is bringing the feet to the mouth at 5 months of age. Also notable in the propped and ring-sitting positions is the child's tendency for progravity stabilization, using the hip flexors and abdominal muscles.

Once the child is stable in ring sitting and is able to move the head and limbs, he or she begins to use intra-axial rotation in sitting. This intra-axial rotation develops and strengthens by 5 to 7 months of age in prone and supine, allowing for segmental rolling. The intra-axial rotation also allows the child to make transitions between positions, thus broadening the repertoire of sitting positions and increasing independence as the child learns to move from supine and prone to sitting and vice versa, using intra-axial rotation. See Figure 1.55 for one example of this transition from sitting to prone. Intra-axial rotation also serves to increase the accessibility of the space around the child, making more of the environment available for interaction as the child uses rotation to transition to quadruped and perhaps to creep (Fig. 1.56).

By 8 months of age, the child is able to sit independently. The child has developed not only full antigravity extension of the back but, by the eighth month, the sitting position is characterized by the completion of the secondary curves of

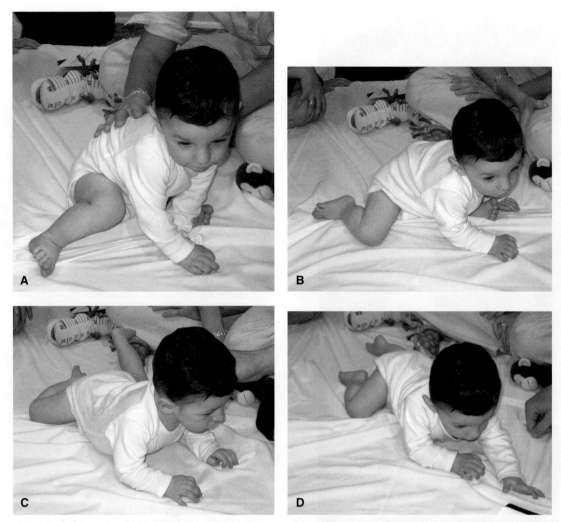

FIGURE 1.55. A–C: Sequence of transition from sitting to prone-on-elbows using intra-axial rotation. **D:** Reciprocal and contralateral crawling.

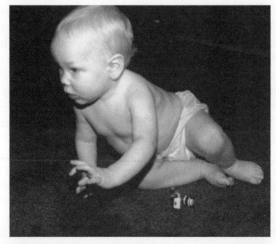

FIGURE 1.56. Intra-axial rotation is also used to increase the accessibility of the child's environment and for the transition between sitting and quadruped.

the spine (Fig. 1.57). These anterior–posterior curves, developing cephalocaudally, are the *cervical lordosis* and the *lumbar lordosis*. Now the child is able to move from prone or supine to sitting and return to prone or supine. The child is also able to move in and out of the various sitting positions using the intra-axial rotation and can pull up into standing.

Side sitting is a mature sitting position that requires a number of motor components and abilities, including intra-axial rotation, dissociation, weight shifting, and elongation of the trunk on the weight-bearing side (Fig. 1.58). In side sitting, dissociation of the lower extremities is present, as evidenced by the hip external rotation and abduction of one lower extremity with internal rotation and adduction of the other hip. Sitting on a child-sized chair requires the child to use another component of movement, eccentric contractions. Eccentric or lengthening contractions of the quadriceps, proximal hamstrings, and gluteus maximus muscles allow the child to transition from stance to sit, lowering slowly into

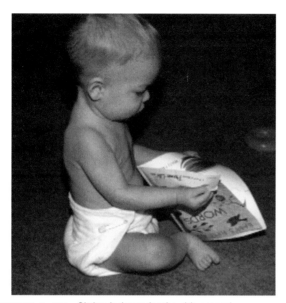

FIGURE 1.57. Sitting independently with secondary curves, the cervical and lumbar lordoses.

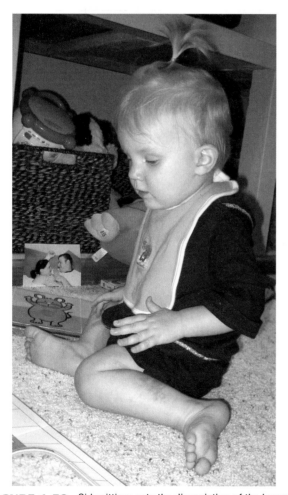

FIGURE 1.58. Side sitting; note the dissociation of the lower extremities.

a seated position in a chair. As the child moves to sit, he or she shifts the weight posteriorly from the forefoot to the heel of the foot. Rising to standing from a small chair requires an anterior weight shift and concentric contractions of these same muscles.

Sitting on an adult-sized chair, such as a sofa, is accomplished through a combination of several movements. This activity is often the first function that reveals a child's developing climbing skills. When a child begins to climb onto an adult-sized chair, he or she usually uses considerable lateral trunk flexion to one side while the child abducts and flexes the opposite hip. After months of practice, the child begins to use more weight shifting to one side with accompanying elongation of the lateral trunk on that weight-bearing side, intra-axial counterrotation, and hip flexion of the opposite lower extremity. Figure 1.59 shows a series of movements used by a child to get into an adult-sized chair.

Locomotion in Sitting

Once children exhibit dissociation of the two lower extremities and are stable in half–ring sitting, some children actually develop a locomotive form in this position called **hitching**. Hitching is when a child, while sitting on the floor, uses either foot to dig into the surface to scoot forward on the buttocks. Many children use hitching as a means of moving around in their environments before they learn to creep efficiently and can become quite adept at this form of locomotion.

Erect Standing Progression

Supported Standing

When held in standing during the neonatal period, the infant bears partial weight on the lower extremities, which appear stiff because of muscle co-contraction, and the base of support is very narrow, with the feet supinated. Head control is absent, and the neck is flexed with the chin resting on the chest (Fig. 1.60). While in supported standing, tilting the infant forward slightly will produce reflex stepping (automatic stepping) (Fig. 1.61).

By the end of 2 months of age, most infants lose the reflex stepping ability. Early developmentalists believed that the cessation of automatic stepping was simply a function of maturation of the infant's CNS.[107] However, the groundbreaking studies of Esther Thelen in the early 1980s found that reflex stepping in infants whose lower extremities were weighted artificially was diminished. Infants who were held in standing in water increased their stepping rather than ceasing to step, presumably due to the effect of buoyancy on the lower extremities, and the stepping persisted beyond the usual age of dissolution of the stepping reflex. The conclusion drawn from these studies was that reflex stepping typically ceased at approximately 2 months of age, not because of programming and maturation of the CNS, but because the mass of the infant's lower extremities became such that it was too difficult for the infant to lift the heavy lower extremities.[108]

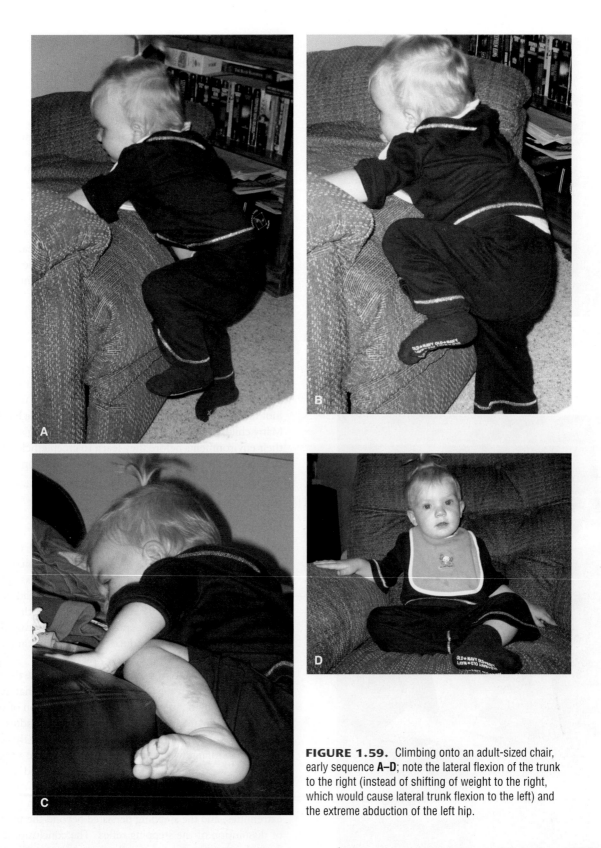

FIGURE 1.59. Climbing onto an adult-sized chair, early sequence **A–D**; note the lateral flexion of the trunk to the right (instead of shifting of weight to the right, which would cause lateral trunk flexion to the left) and the extreme abduction of the left hip.

Regardless of the theory that one accepts for the cessation of automatic stepping, by the end of 2 months the typical infant no longer produces this reflex stepping and will often cease to take weight on the lower extremities when held in standing. This absence of automatic stepping is referred to as *abasia*, derived from the Greek words that mean *without*

step.[1] The next stepping abilities will be volitional. The lack of weight bearing through the lower extremities, which occurs typically during the third and fourth months, is the stage of *astasia*, literally meaning *without standing*.[1] This stage is temporary during normal development and may not be seen in all children.

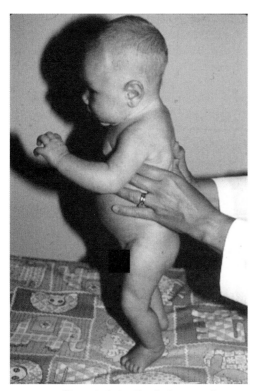

FIGURE 1.60. Supported standing in the neonate.

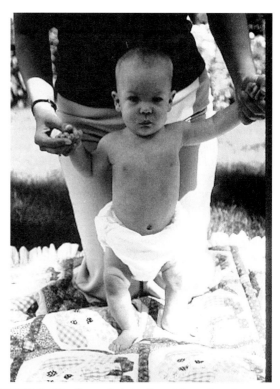

FIGURE 1.62. Supported standing at 5 months of age; note the flexed hips and knees.

During the first 4 months, head control has been developing in all positions, as control and balance of the antigravity cervical extensors and flexors progressed. By 5 months of age, the head is secure in space, and the infant volitionally begins to accept partial weight on the lower extremities during supported standing (Fig. 1.62). This milestone is

characterized by moderate abduction, flexion, and external rotation of the hips, with knee flexion and pronation of the feet. This 5-month position becomes even more exaggerated by 7 months of age, at which time the child is volitionally bearing full weight on the lower extremities (Fig. 1.63).

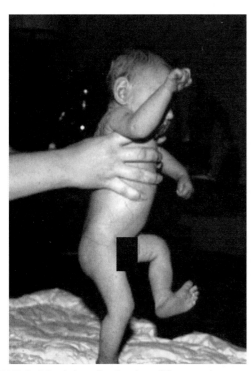

FIGURE 1.61. Automatic stepping of the neonate.

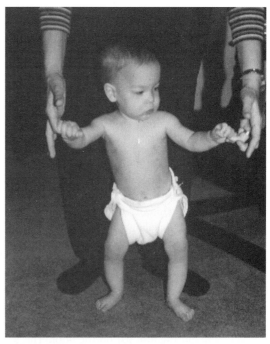

FIGURE 1.63. Supported standing at 7 months of age; note the wide base of support, hip and knee flexion, and pronation of feet.

At 7 months, the child's poor anterior–posterior weight-bearing alignment and underdeveloped balance responses prevents him or her from standing alone without external support. The child can stand and walk with the hands held (Fig. 1.63). Gait is characterized by hip external rotation and moderate abduction, giving the child a wide base of support, and extremely pronated feet. The greater the abduction and external rotation of the hips, the more the feet pronate. Typically, a fat pad masks the longitudinal arch of each foot, in infants and toddlers, increasing the pronated appearance of the feet. Hips and knees are flexed, creating continued poor anterior–posterior alignment for standing without support. In correct mature weight-bearing alignment for standing, an imaginary straight line can be drawn in a parasagittal plane through the ear, shoulder, hip, knee, and lateral malleolus (Fig. 1.64A). In the immature standing position, the imaginary line falls through the ear and shoulder but anterior to the hip joint and often slightly posterior to the knee joint, due to the flexion of the hips and knees (Fig. 1.64B and C).

The child begins pulling to stance in the crib at about this time (7 to 8 months). At first, this is accomplished using the newly developed strength of the upper extremities, while the lower extremities remain essentially passive. Once standing, the child will frequently hold onto the crib rails for support while he or she bounces and experiments with this newly discovered standing ability. During the earliest attempts at supported standing in the crib, the child finds that returning to a seated position is challenging. Lowering slowly to the mattress requires strong eccentric control of the hips and knees, something that the child has not fully developed. Frustrated and tired of standing, the child may simply let go of the crib rails and drop to sitting, owing to gravity, or may begin to cry, signaling to the caregivers the need for help. The caregiver will come and either take the child from the crib or place him or her in prone or supine. Once this has happened, the child may realize that these actions resulted in attention by the caregiver, so the child will pull to stance once again, and the sequence of events repeats. This is great fun for the child to repeat these behaviors, as he or she discovers that the action causes effects, oftentimes predictable effects.

Independent Standing

By 10 months of age, the child pulls to stance at furniture, such as a sofa or low table. As seen in the sequence in Figure 1.65, the child achieves standing by moving through the knee-standing (tall-kneeling) and half-kneeling positions and are adept at lowering back down with control. In the tall-kneeling position, the base of support is kept relatively wide as the child's center of mass moves farther away from the floor. To achieve the half-kneeling position, the child must shift the weight to one side, elongating the trunk on that side, so that the child is able to bring the unweighted limb forward and put the foot flat on the floor. This action, the transition between the tall-kneeling and standing positions, requires intra-axial rotation, just as all transitional

positions do. Once in half-kneeling, the child uses the lower extremity muscles, particularly the hip extensors and knee extensors, to raise up against gravity. The child relies very little on the strength of the upper extremities as in past pull-to-standing attempts. Instead, the lower extremities do most of the work and the upper extremities help with balance. The same half-kneeling and tall-kneeling positions are used to get down to the floor from standing. With practice, these movements become very controlled and fast. Occasionally, the child may simply let go of the support and drop quickly to the floor.

Cruising

Once standing at furniture, the child will play for long periods, going back and forth between the floor and the furniture, squatting and rising to stand repeatedly. The child moves in and out of the various positions. Soon the child begins stepping sideways while holding onto the furniture. This supported walking, seen at 10 months of age, is called **cruising** (Fig. 1.65C). The child is able to work his or her way back and forth along the sofa or table and eventually begins to reach to other pieces of furniture to move around the room. Meanwhile, the child's anterior–posterior alignment is improving, with decreasing hip and knee flexion.[97] While standing at furniture, the child can be seen to lift one or the other hand from the support, sometimes rotating the trunk to one side or the other while still maintaining balance. Often, as the child cruises around the furniture and reaches for the next piece of furniture, he or she will briefly stand and maybe even take one or two steps without support from either upper extremity. At times the child stands briefly without touching the supporting surfaces. However, when walking forward without furniture for support, the child still needs someone to hold onto his or her hand(s), but they are fast approaching the day when the child will walk forward without holding the furniture or someone's hand. During the cruising phase of development, in addition to practicing walking, the child's cruising movements contribute to the development and strengthening of hip abduction/adduction and eversion/inversion of the ankles as they side-step (Fig. 1.66). Even though the child walks, supported by holding onto furniture or someone's hand, the *plantar grasp reflex* may still be positive at 10 months of age, although considerably diminished and present inconsistently. The plantar grasp reflex is manifested by curling of the toes when the examiner places a finger horizontally at the base of the toes (Fig. 1.67). A positive plantar grasp causes the toes to flex or curl.[16,107] This reflex can also be observed spontaneously as curling of the toes when the child is in supported standing. Usually the complete dissolution of this reflex must occur before independent walking without support will develop. Gradually, over the next several weeks, the child will let go of the adult's hand or the furniture, often standing independently for brief periods. When this happens, the child's upper extremities usually assume the high guard position for increased trunk stability.

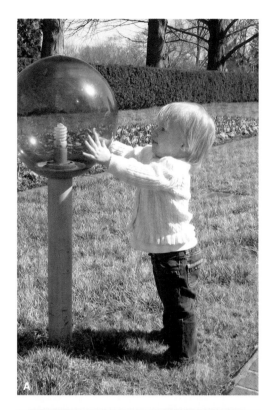

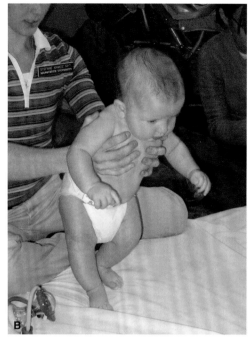

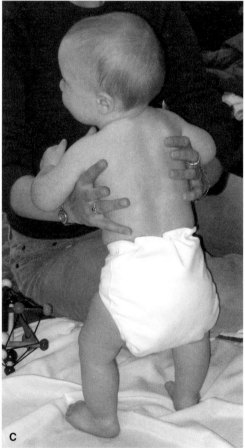

FIGURE 1.64. Ear-to-heel postural alignment for standing. **A:** Mature alignment; **B:** inadequate and immature weight-bearing alignment for independent standing; note that the ear-to-heel weight line falls anterior to the hips and posterior to the knees, and also note the narrow base of support with supination of the feet. **C:** Improved postural alignment, but alignment is still inadequate for standing independently.

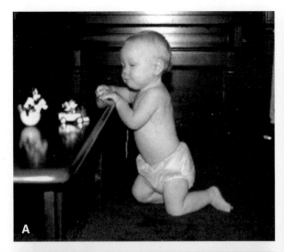

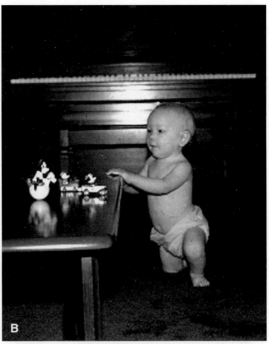

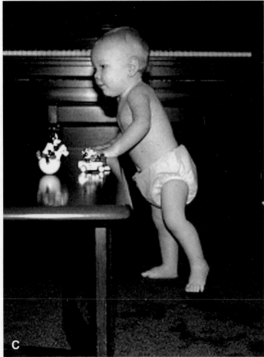

FIGURE 1.65. Pull-to-standing at furniture sequence. **A:** Tall kneeling. **B:** Half-kneeling; note the intra-axial rotation and the dissociation of the lower extremities. **C:** Erect standing at low table with cruising.

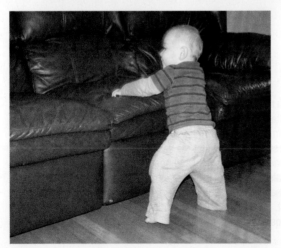

FIGURE 1.66. Cruising helps develop hip abduction for both mobility and stability (weight-bearing) functions.

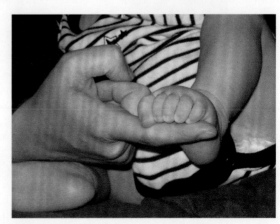

FIGURE 1.67. Plantar grasp, positive response.

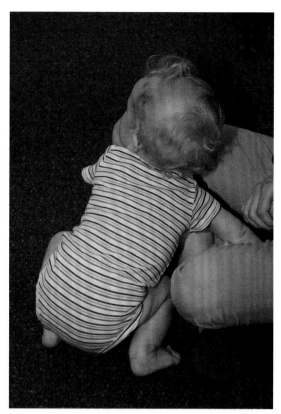

FIGURE 1.68. Squatting. The child frequently performs active squat to stand and back to squat and uses squat position as a play position.

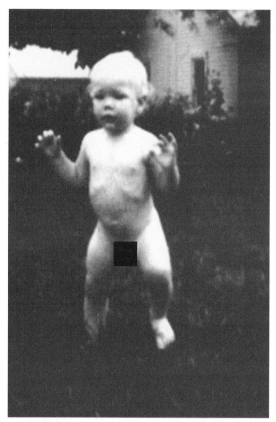

FIGURE 1.69. First independent walking with high guard positioning of upper extremities.

During the development of standing, cruising, and walking, the child develops the ability to squat to play as well as squatting to pick up an object (Fig. 1.68). Often, while standing at furniture, such as a sofa, the child can be seen to squat to pick up a toy, stand and place the toy on the sofa, and repeat this process many times. Also, the child is able to spend great lengths of time in the squat position while playing. Squatting, therefore, is both a movement used to transition between positions and a position in itself. Some have theorized that the active squat-to-stance-to-squat sequence facilitates co-contraction, and therefore stability, of the muscles surrounding the ankle joint. The theory is that the prolonged and maximal stretch to the muscle spindles of the ankle musculature activates both primary and secondary afferent endings.[59]

Independent Bipedal Locomotion

Independent forward walking generally occurs between 10 and 15 months of age, with the typical child walking at 12 months of age, plus or minus a month. At first, the child holds the upper extremities in the high guard position, the same position the arms were held during the child's first independent sitting, in an attempt to increase stability against gravity by adducting the scapulae (Fig. 1.69). Position is characterized by improving but continuing poor, vertical alignment, with hips and knees flexed. Abduction and external

rotation of the hips continue to provide a wide base of support. The child does not have heel strike initially, and the feet are still in considerable pronation.

As forward independent gait progresses over the next months, the shoulders lose much of the flexion of the high guard position, assuming a low guard position with elbows still flexed and hands just above the waist; fingers may be pointed upward or the shoulders are adducted, and the hands are stabilized against the body, as shown in Figure 1.70. Then the upper extremities relax into full shoulder extension and hang at the child's sides. Over the next few weeks, reciprocal arm swing during gait is attained (Fig. 1.71).

With practice, the anterior–posterior postural alignment continues to improve with increasing hip and knee extension, decreasing hip abduction with narrowing of the base of support, and lessening of external rotation of the hips. Eventually, the child walks with good postural alignment, a narrow base of support, neutral pronation/supination of the feet, heel strike, push off, and reciprocal arm swing. The plantar fat pad does not completely disappear until approximately 2 years of age, at which time the longitudinal arches become visible.

Bipedal locomotion will continue to improve and progress over the next 2 to 4 years. Gait parameters for the 3-year-old child differ from early gait parameters at age 1 year.[109] These parameters include alignment of the lower extremities as

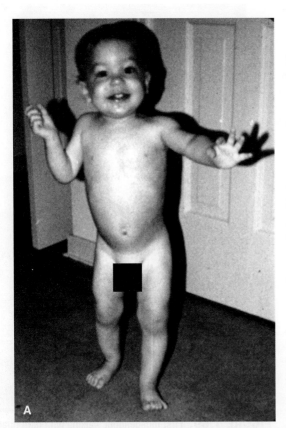 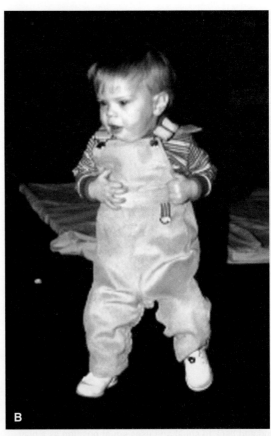

FIGURE 1.70. Independent walking. **A:** Note that the high guard position is decreasing, with the right upper extremity still in high guard, the left upper extremity being lowered with shoulder girdle protraction. **B:** Walking independently with a low guard to enhance upright trunk stability.

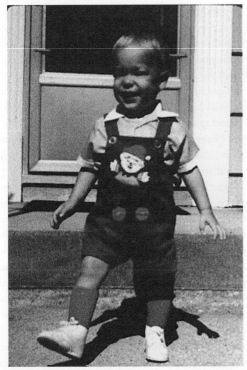

FIGURE 1.71. Mature independent walking with heel strike and reciprocal arm swing.

well as various aspects of the gait cycle. As the child's gait matures, mediolateral alignment at the hip progresses from hip abduction to adduction, until the feet are approximately shoulders' width apart. At the knees, mediolateral alignment moves from genu varus at birth to approximately 12 degrees of genu valgus at 3 years of age. Then between 4 and 7 years of age, the valgus resolves to only 7 to 10 degrees. This change in alignment of the knees affects the mediolateral alignment of the hips, ankles, and feet as well.[109] Other gait parameters that change with growth and maturation are cadence, step and stride length, and velocity.[109] *Cadence*, the number of steps per minute, starts out very high in first independent walking. The 1-year-old child spends a decreased amount of time in single limb stance, compared with the 3-year-old and the adult. This is because the 1-year-old child has less strength and stability in the hip muscles. Consequently, the child takes more steps per minute, resulting in less time in single limb support.[109]

Gait *velocity*, the distance one covers in a specified amount of time, starts low and increases as the child ages.[109] Velocity is related to the length of one's step or stride. A *step* is measured from heel strike of one lower extremity to heel strike of the opposite lower extremity. *Stride length*, measured from heel strike of one foot to heel strike of the same foot, is approximately twice the step length.[109] However, in a

TABLE 1.5. Gait Parameters in 1- and 3-Year-Old Children			
Gait Parameter	1 Year of Age	3 Years of Age	Direction of Change
Base of support (pelvic span to ankle spread)	<1	≥1	↓
Step length	20 cm	33 cm	↑
Stride length (double the step length)	40 cm	66 cm	↑
Single limb stance	32% of gait cycle	35% of gait cycle	↑
Cadence (step frequency)	180 steps per minute	154 steps per minute	↓
Velocity (speed)	60 cm/sec	105 cm/sec	↑

From Long TM, Toscano K. *Handbook of Pediatric Physical Therapy.* Lippincott Williams & Wilkins; 2001.

case where the step length of the two extremities differs considerably because of pathology affecting only one limb, to be accurate, both step and stride length must be measured, instead of calculating stride length by multiplying the step length by two.

From 1 to 3 years of age, a child's step length and stride length increase, as do velocity and single limb stance time.[109] Single limb stance increases with increasing strength and balance abilities. Length of step and/or stride, and therefore gait velocity, increases as the child's lower extremities continue to grow in length, even well after age 3. Otherwise, gait at age 3 is considered to have parameters similar to those of an adult.[109] Various gait parameters at ages 1 year and 3 years are shown in Table 1.5.

Even though a toddler is able to walk fast, and the parents often insist that the toddler is running, true running does not develop until 3 to 4 years of age. A **true run** is characterized by having both feet off the ground at the same time, unlike walking, where one foot does not leave the ground until the other foot makes initial contact.

Stair Climbing

Stairs present a considerable challenge to toddlers. The typical **rise** of a step in a flight of stairs is 7 to 8 inches. For a 15-month-old toddler to negotiate stairs in erect standing would be the equivalent of an adult attempting to climb stairs with a knee-high rise (Fig. 1.72).

The ability to ascend and descend stairs is affected by a number of factors, most particularly, opportunity. Therefore, the age of achieving this milestone has considerable variability, although the sequence of achievement is much the same from one child to the next. A child who lives in a home without stairs, or at least without stairs that the child is permitted to climb, often develops stair-climbing skills at a later age than does the child who has frequent daily encounters with stairs to get to and from the bedroom and/or toys.

The first ability to ascend and descend stairs is usually in the quadruped position (Fig. 1.73). The child learns to go up the stairs on hands and knees, followed soon by coming down the stairs backward on hands and knees. Sometimes

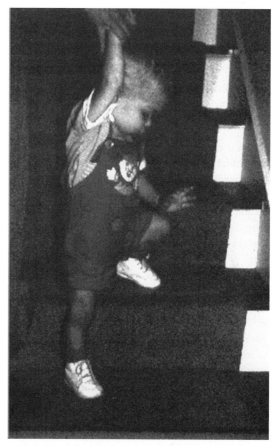

FIGURE 1.72. Descending stairs with hand held; note the rise of the step in relationship to the length of the child's lower extremity.

children, in their first attempts at descending stairs, will try to do so in quadruped, but head first, with disastrous results if a caregiver is not nearby. With a bit of coaching, the child quickly learns through trial and error to descend the stairs backward on hands and knees.

Ascending stairs generally develops to a more skillful level before descending stairs develops to the same level of skill. This sequence generally repeats itself in bipedal locomotion after the child has developed the ability to go up and

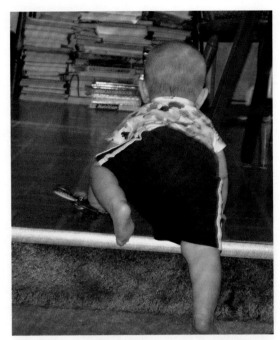

FIGURE 1.73. Ascending a step in quadruped.

down stairs using quadrupedal locomotion. Another feature of stair climbing that develops in a rather typical pattern is apparent once the child is climbing stairs while standing. Initially, bipedal stair climbing is performed by placing both feet on each step, in a manner that is called *marking time*.[48] Generally, the child will not begin to ascend steps, one step over the other (i.e., only one foot to each step) until they are close to 3 years of age, depending on how much trial and error and practice on negotiating stairs. This pattern of the feet is also dependent on the type of upper extremity support that is available. Stair climbing progresses as the upper extremity support decreases from using one handrail and/or an adult hand for support, to needing a handrail but no adult, and finally to needing no upper extremity support (Fig. 1.74). The speed with which the child develops increasingly more skillful stair-climbing abilities varies greatly, and like other skills, the ability to locomote on stairs may temporarily digress as unique and/or challenging circumstances, such as unusually steep stairs or the absence of a handrail, present themselves.

» Balance

Maintaining balance, that is, keeping the center of mass within the base of support and effectively compensating when balance is disturbed, is a challenge to the developing child as he or she attempts and learns new motor skills. Following the achievement of a particular milestone or developmental position, a child must develop the ability to maintain balance in that position. Usually, as the child is bravely moving toward the next developmental position in the hierarchy, the child continues to practice the newest learned position, thereby developing new balancing skills in each successive

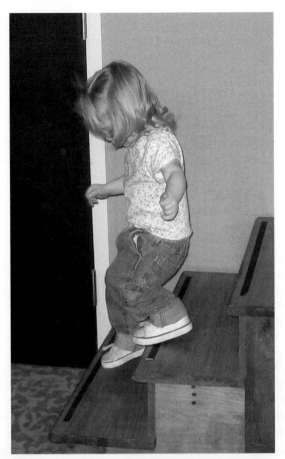

FIGURE 1.74. Descending stairs without upper extremity support.

position. Balance skills make up the normal postural reflex mechanism. These balance skills are divided into four subgroups: righting reactions, tilting reactions, equilibrium reactions, and protective reactions. Each subgroup has a defined aspect of balance for which it is responsible. These subgroups operate on a continuum such that when the body's balance is challenged, the reactions occur in a predictable order (see Display 1.2).

Righting reactions are responsible for securing the head in space and must develop in all planes.[46,107] When there is a disturbance in the child's center of mass in any position, *head-righting reactions*, also termed *labyrinthine righting reactions*,

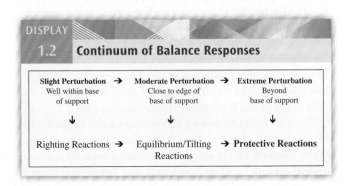

DISPLAY 1.2   Continuum of Balance Responses

Slight Perturbation →	Moderate Perturbation →	Extreme Perturbation
Well within base of support	Close to edge of base of support	Beyond base of support
↓	↓	↓
Righting Reactions →	Equilibrium/Tilting Reactions	→ **Protective Reactions**

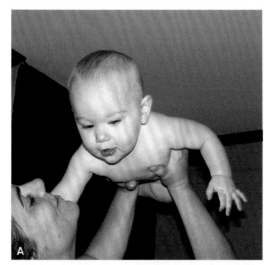

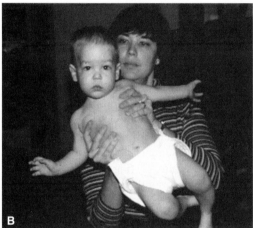

FIGURE 1.75. Positive labyrinthine righting reflex (head righting); face is maintained vertical with mouth horizontal in response to **A:** ventral suspension and **B:** a lateral tilt to the child's right.

come into play first. If the disturbance is only slight and does not come close to moving the child's center of mass outside the base of support, the head-righting reactions suffice in bringing the body back into balance. When the child's body is tilted in any direction, the head automatically rights itself; that is, no matter what the position of the body, the head moves to an upright position wherein the mouth is horizontal and the face is vertical, referenced to the floor or ground[46,107] (Fig. 1.75). If the disturbance is large enough to move the center of mass very near the edge of the child's base of support, then head righting occurs automatically, but it is not enough to maintain balance. Help is needed from the tilting or equilibrium reactions.

Tilting and equilibrium reactions, responsible for securing the position of the body in space when balance is challenged, are identical responses, but are elicited by slightly different stimuli. A *tilting reaction* is the correct term to use when the surface on which the child is seated, standing, or otherwise positioned is moved, thus causing the child's center of mass to shift. When this happens, head righting occurs immediately. If the body senses that head righting is insufficient, the tilting reactions are elicited. The response looks like this. When on a balance board, ball, or other moveable surface, if the child is tilted to the left far enough to elicit the tilting reactions, lateral bending toward the right side occurs. If viewing the spine from a posterior vantage point, the vertebral column curves to the right, away from the direction toward which the child was tilted (Fig. 1.76). This returns the body's mass toward the center of the base of support. If the stimulus and the response are strong enough, the limbs enter into the response. In this case, the right shoulder and hip abduct, in an effort to help bring the body mass into the center of the base of support once again. An **equilibrium reaction** is identical to the tilting reaction, but the stimulus differs in

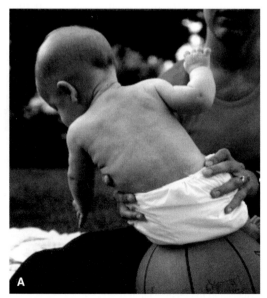

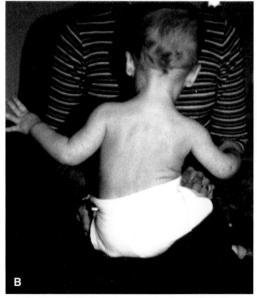

FIGURE 1.76. Test for tilting reaction in sitting. **A:** Response to a tilt to the left is negative but age appropriate because the child does not right the trunk. **B:** Response to the same tilt is positive in an older child, who laterally flexes the trunk away from the direction of the tilt.

that the child is on a stationary surface instead of on a mobile surface, and the force of the perturbation is directed at the child's body rather than at the surface.[46,107] Tilting and equilibrium reactions develop in each successive position shortly after the child develops stability in that position and while he or she is beginning to experiment with and work on the next higher position.

The final type of balance response is the protective response. In typical development, the protective response is responsible for regaining balance when the center of mass has been pushed beyond the borders of the base of support. When this happens, head-righting and tilting/equilibrium responses are elicited, but are insufficient to regain control. Automatically, the child protects himself or herself from the inevitable fall by moving the upper or lower extremity, extending the distal joints, toward the direction of the movement (Fig. 1.77). This motion effectively moves the borders of the base of support outward, enlarging the base. In this manner, the body's mass is once again within the base of support, not because the body returned to being inside the base of support, as in the tilting/equilibrium reactions, but because the base of support has enlarged to once again capture the center of mass within its borders. The following example shows how protective responses are used in one of two ways to maintain balance and sometimes prevent injury. When a person is standing in the aisle on a moving bus, and the driver suddenly applies the brakes, if head-righting and tilting responses, both of which are elicited first, do not suffice in regaining balance, a person probably will do one of two things. Either the person will take a step with one foot to increase the size of his or her base of support enough to regain balance within the base of support or the person

will fall forward. If the person falls, as he or she nears the floor of the bus, one or both arms will reach out to help break the fall, creating a new and larger base of support and hopefully protecting the head and face from the potential impact. This second response is the reason people often fracture the distal end of the radius in a fall, referred to as a Colles fracture.[1]

» Fine motor development

Grasp

A discussion about motor development cannot be complete without attention to the development of grasp. Earlier in this chapter, the importance of proximal stability to the development of grasp and prehension was discussed. As with gross motor development, fine motor development occurs, in most typical cases, in a predictable order.

At birth, the full-term neonate has a hand grasp reflex. This reflex, which began in utero, is a reflex closing of the hand when stimulated by touch to the palmar surface with stretch of the intrinsic muscles of the hand. The response to this two-part stimulus is reflex grasping of the stimulating object. As long as the stimulus is in contact with the neonate's hand, the fist remains closed. The grasp reflex is usually tested by the examiner placing his or her index finger into the neonate's palm[46,107] (Fig. 1.78).

During the early months of life, the grasp reflex is intact, although it gradually weakens until disappearing at approximately 4 months of age. This means that until the reflex becomes naturally inhibited with time, anything that stimulates the palm of the infant's hand will elicit a reflex behavior. Such reflex grasp preempts voluntary grasping of objects. Therefore, attempts by the infant at voluntary grasp will not be successful until the hand grasp reflex has diminished and then disappeared. Even though this may

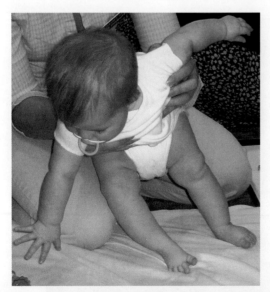

FIGURE 1.77. Protective extension of the upper extremity to the side.

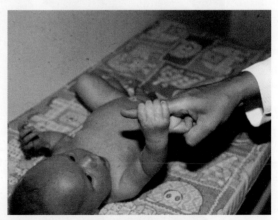

FIGURE 1.78. Hand grasp reflex is positive in response to tactile and proprioceptive stimuli from the examiner's finger being placed in the infant's palm.

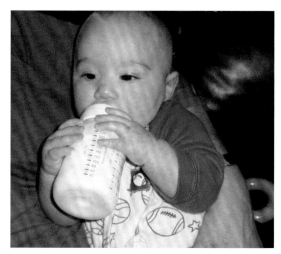

FIGURE 1.79. Volitional grasp to hold a bottle.

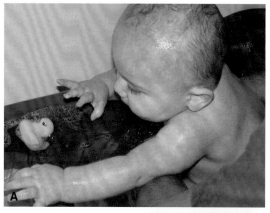

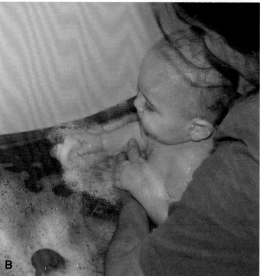

FIGURE 1.80. Sufficient shoulder stability to **A:** reach away from the body to grasp the object; **B:** note the pronated forearm with immature grasp.

mean that the infant's early attempts at voluntary grasp are essentially thwarted, little is lost during those 4 months of active reflex behavior. This is because until approximately 3 to 4 months of age, the infant still lacks the stability in the shoulder joint needed for skillful reaching for and grasping of objects at will.

During the first 4 months, while the infant's grasp reflex diminishes, the infant is gradually developing the ability to volitionally grasp an object, as seen in Figure 1.79 with the infant beginning to hold a bottle. The infant also develops the ability to stabilize the shoulders to reach for objects with some degree of accuracy and hold the upper extremity stable while grasping an object (Fig. 1.80A and B). The development of this shoulder stability is followed by the development of the infant's ability to control the extremity enough to bring the object toward himself or herself for a closer look, to put it in the mouth, or to examine it with two hands (Fig. 1.81). Shoulder stability and the ability to perform a controlled reach arise from the infant's increasingly skillful weight bearing and weight shifting in the prone-on-elbows position. It is complemented by such activities in supine as bringing the hands to midline (inhibition of the ATNR), reaching hands to knees and eventually hands to feet, and reaching up to touch the caregiver's face during dressing and feeding activities. Accomplishing these motor behaviors in prone and supine requires activation of the pectoralis major and serratus anterior muscles, with concurrent lengthening of the rhomboid muscles, allowing protraction of the shoulders. Before the development of these particular components of motor behavior, the infant is unable to reach into space and stabilize the shoulder for grasp and prehension. Consequently, at 3 months of age, the infant will take a toy such as a rattle only if it is presented close to the body, within 2 or 3 inches. This is because the infant cannot stabilize the shoulders when reaching into space, but

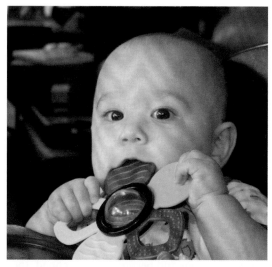

FIGURE 1.81. Bilateral use of hands in midline with mouthing; note beginning supination of forearms.

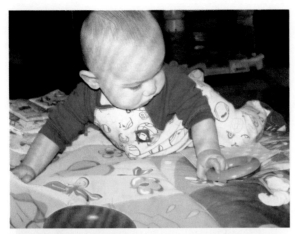

FIGURE 1.82. Reach and grasp with pronation of the forearm.

can stabilize them by adducting and fixing the upper arms into the body.

At 4 to 5 months of age, the infant actively and successfully reaches for objects in space and can grasp them, at will, using the whole hand in a palmar grasp. The thumb is inactive initially. Once the infant grasps the object, he or she can bring it close to the face, but is not able to put it into the mouth or visually inspect it with one hand. This is because the infant has not developed the ability to actively supinate the forearm (Fig. 1.82). Consequently, the dorsum of the hand is between the mouth and/or eyes and the object, and the object is essentially hidden from view. At 4 months of age, with a stable prone-on-elbows position, the infant is beginning to shift weight. As mentioned earlier in this chapter, weight shifting in prone-on-elbows is the beginning of supination, and the ability to pronate and supinate the forearm reciprocally. As active, controlled supination develops and improves, the infant begins to engage an object with the eyes, reach for the object, and grasp it. The infant then supinates the forearm as he or she brings the object close to the face. Now the infant can put the object into the mouth, visually inspect it, touch it with both hands at once, and/or transfer the object from one hand to the other. (Fig. 1.83)

Although voluntary grasp at first is crude and palmar, the development of refined grasp progresses rather quickly. Sitting in a high chair with an object on the chair tray, a child at first will pick up the object by crudely raking it into the palm of the hand, using just the fingers, with the ulnar two fingers predominating.[48,110] This ulnar activity occurs long before the active participation of the thumb (radial activity), and it is a good example of the medial-to-lateral principle of developmental direction. In the anatomic position, the ulnar fingers are medial and the thumb is lateral.

As grasp develops and becomes more refined, the child continues to use the fingers to palm the object, ulnar fingers still predominating, but radial fingers also participating. The thumb is still inactive. This type of grasp progresses to

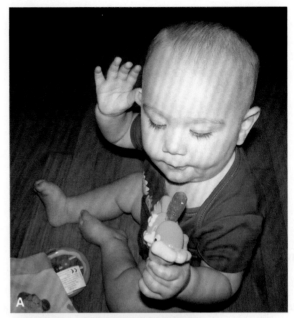

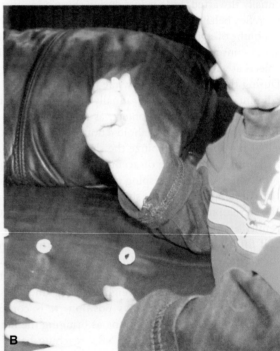

FIGURE 1.83. Forearm supination had developed, allowing **A:** visual inspection of object and **B:** putting objects in the mouth with ease.

increasing dominance by the first two fingers. By 10 months of age, the child begins using a very active forefinger (index finger or first finger), and will explore objects with that index finger.[17,51] This is the time when a child will poke a finger in the nose, eyes, and ears. This poking with the forefinger continues to dominate fine motor activities for many months, as seen in the 15-month-old child in Figure 1.84. This obsession with the forefinger occurs at about the same time the thumb is becoming very active. At 10 months of

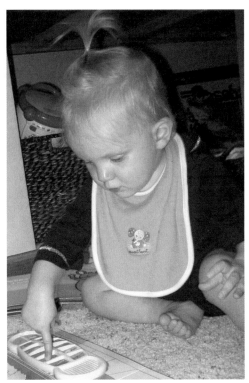

FIGURE 1.84. Forefinger (index finger) dominance, poking and prodding.

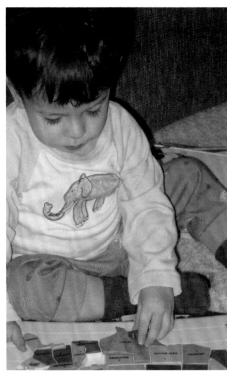

FIGURE 1.86. Three-jaw chuck grasp, using thumb, index finger, and second finger in a triangular pattern.

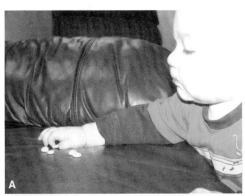

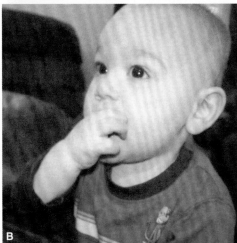

FIGURE 1.85. Pincer grasp to **A:** pick up dry cereal and **B:** put it in the mouth.

age the child has a *pincer grasp*, using the thumb and first finger pad to pad.[48,110] Finger foods are very important to the child at this time as he or she develops the ability to pick up dry cereal pieces and put them in the mouth with considerable accuracy (Fig. 1.85). Also around 10 months of age, the child begins to use a *three-jaw chuck* type of grasp for larger objects, using the thumb, index, and second fingers[48,110] (Fig. 1.86).

Release

The development of release lags somewhat behind the development of grasp. Volitional release begins at approximately 11 months of age. Until that time, a child lets go of an object simply by relaxing the finger flexion. Not until 11 months of age does the child begin to intentionally release by actively extending the fingers.[48] The inability to actively and accurately release an object during those first 10 to 12 months of life is the root cause of the tendency to knock down the tower when trying to stack blocks. Until the child begins to gain some control over the release, he or she is able to place one block on top of another, but causes the tower to fall when the child tries to withdraw the hand.[48]

By 18 months of age, a child can grasp a pencil in the center using the pads of the fingers, put tiny pellets in a small bottle, stack a tower of three blocks, and mark with a crayon while holding the paper with the other hand[6,48,110] (Fig. 1.87). See Table 1.6 for approximate times of development of various fine motor skills.

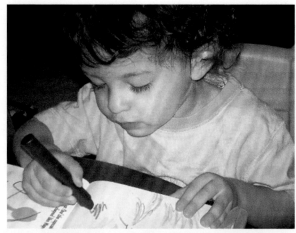

FIGURE 1.87. Using a crayon with the opposite hand holding the paper.

TABLE 1.6. Development of Fine Motor Skills	
Skill	**Age of Achievement**
Hand grasp reflex	Birth to 4–5 mo
Visual regard	Birth to 2 mo
Swipes with whole hand	2–3 mo
Visually directed reaching	3–5 mo
Midline clasping of hands	3–5 mo
Reaches out to grasp object	4–5 mo
Plays with feet; bangs objects together	5 mo
Crude palming, ulnar fingers predominating	5–7 mo
Transfers object from one hand to the other	6 mo
Lateral scissors grasp	8–9 mo
Pincer grasp, forefinger and thumb in opposition	10–11 mo
Forefinger dominance: poking and prodding with index finger	10–11 mo
Holds crayon	11 mo
Beginning voluntary release	11 mo
Uses graded pressure; varies pressure depending on object; uses fingertip with thumb opposition in fine pincer grasp	12 mo
Precision grasp with fine pincer and controlled release	15 mo
Scribbles on paper	15–18 mo
Holds paper with other hand when scribbling	18 mo
Puts object in container and dumps contents	18 mo
Builds tower of three cubes	18 mo
Turns pages of book, perhaps two or three at a time	21 mo
Turns pages of a book one at a time	24 mo
Unscrew jar lid	24 mo
Builds tower with eight cubes	30 mo

TABLE 1.7. Advanced Motor Skills and Approximate Ages of Acquisition	
Motor Skill	**Age of Acquisition**
Stands on low balance beam	2 yr
Walks straight line	3 yr
Walks circular line	4 yr
Balances on one foot for 3–5 sec	5 yr
Walks backward	18 mo
Jumps from bottom step	2 yr
Jumps off floor with both feet	28 mo
Hops 3 times	3 yr
Hops 8–10 times on same foot	5 yr
Hops distance of 50 feet	5 yr
Gallops	4 yr
Skips	6 yr
Catches ball using body and hands	3 yr
Catches ball using hands only	5 yr
Attempts to kick ball	18 mo
Kicks ball	2–3 yr
Hurls ball 3 feet	18 mo
Throws ball	2–3 yr
Fast walk	18 mo
True run with nonsupport phase	2–3 yr

» The 2-to-7-year-old child

During the first 2 years of life, the typical child develops the motor skills required for ordinary mobility and prehension. Further gross and fine motor development occurs after the first 2 years, but these later-attained skills are more specific to a child's play and work. These more advanced motor skills are developed and perfected more intentionally by each individual. Table 1.7 lists some of these more advanced skills and the approximate ages of acquisition.

Summary

Typical motor development in humans usually occurs according to a particular sequence and timing. The sequence and timing are important to the clinician and can be used as guides in the physical therapy evaluation and treatment of children and adults. A thorough understanding of typical motor development is particularly germane to the study of atypical neuromotor development in children. Although all humans share a common anatomy, physiology, and developmental sequence, many intrinsic and extrinsic factors, including pathology and culture, affect the sequence and timing of motor development in an individual.

REFERENCES

1. Dirckx JH. *Stedman's Concise Medical Dictionary for the Health Professions: Illustrated.* 4th ed. Lippincott Williams & Wilkins; 2001.

2. Cowlin AF. *Women's Fitness Program Development.* Human Kinetics; 2002.

3. Bale JR, Stoll BJ, Lucas AO, eds. *Improving Birth Outcomes: Meeting the Challenge in the Developing World.* The National Academies Press; 2003. Accessed January 20, 2021. http://www.nap.edu/catalog/10841.html

4. VanSant AF. Should the normal motor developmental sequence be used as a theoretical model to progress adult patients? In: *Contemporary Management of Motor Control Problems: Proceedings of the II STEP Conference.* Bookcrafters, Inc; 1991:95-97.

5. Shumway-Cook A, Woollacott MH. *Motor Control: Translating Research into Clinical Practice.* 5th ed. Wolters Kluwer; 2016.

6. Bayley N. *Bayley Scales of Infant and Toddler Development, Fourth Edition (Bayley-4).* Pearson; 2019.

7. Stuberg WA, Dehne P, Miedaner J, et al. *The Milani-Comparetti Motor Development Screening Test.* 3rd ed rev. University of Nebraska Medical Center; 1992.

8. Piper MC, Darrah J. *Alberta Infant Motor Scale.* WB Saunders; 1994.

9. Folio MR, Fewell RR. *Peabody Developmental Motor Scales, Second Edition (PDMS-2).* Pearson; 2000.

10. Friend JH, Guralnik DB, eds. *Webster's New World Dictionary of the American Language. (College ed).* The World Publishing Company; 1960.

11. Provost B, Heimerl S, McClain C, et al. Concurrent validity of the Bayley Scales of Infant Development II Motor Scale and the Peabody Developmental Motor Scales-2 in children with developmental delays. *Pediatr Phys Ther.* 2004;16(3):149-156.

12. Connolly BH, McClune NO, Gatlin R. Concurrent validity of the Bayley-III and the Peabody Developmental Motor Scale-2. *Pediatr Phys Ther.* 2012;24(4):345-352.

13. Campbell SK, Kolobe THA, Wright BD, et al. Validity of the Test of Infant Motor Performance for prediction of 6-, 9- and 12-month scores on the Alberta Infant Motor Scale. *Dev Med Child Neurol.* 2002;44(4):263-271.

14. Spittle AJ, Doyle LW, Boyd RN. A systematic review of the clinimetric properties of neuromotor assessments for preterm infants during the first year of life. *Dev Med Child Neurol.* 2008;50(4):254-266.

15. McClain C, Provost B, Crowe TK. Motor development of two-year-old typically developing Native American children on the Bayley scales of infant development II motor scale. *Pediatr Phys Ther.* 2000;12(3):108-113.

16. Valentini NC, Saccani R. Brazilian validation of the Alberta Infant Motor Scale. *Phys Ther.* 2012;92(3):440-447.

17. Jeng S, Yau K, Chen L, et al. Alberta infant motor scale: reliability and validity when used on preterm infants in Taiwan. *Phys Ther.* 2000;80(2):168-178.

18. Sanhueza AD. Psychomotor development, environmental stimulation, and socioeconomic level of preschoolers in Temuco, Chile. *Pediatr Phys Ther.* 2006;18:141-147.

19. Mayson TA, Harris SR, Bachman CL. Gross motor development of Asian and European children on four motor assessments: a literature review. *Pediatr Phys Ther.* 2007;19:148-153.

20. Tripathi R, Joshua AM, Kotian MS, et al. Normal motor development of Indian children on Peabody Developmental Motor Scales-2 (PDMS-2). *Pediatr Phys Ther.* 2008;20:167-172.

21. Santos DCC, Gabbard C, Goncalves VMG. Motor development during the first year: a comparative study. *J Genet Psychol.* 2001;162(2):143-153.

22. Kelly Y, Sacker A, Schoon I, et al. Ethnic differences in achievement of developmental milestones by 9 months of age: the millennium cohort study. *Dev Med Child Neurol.* 2006;48(10):825-830.

23. Keller H, Yovsi RD, Voelker S. The role of motor stimulation in parental ethnotheories: the case of Cameroonian Nso and German women. *J Cross Cult Psychol.* 2002;3:398-414.

24. Kolobe THA. Childrearing practices and developmental expectations for Mexican-American mothers and the developmental status of their infants. *Phys Ther.* 2004;84(5):439-453.

25. Dusing SC, Harbourne RT. Variability in postural control during infancy: implications for development, assessment, and intervention. *Phys Ther.* 2010;90:1838-1849.

26. Vereijken B. The complexity of childhood development: variability in perspective. *Phys Ther.* 2010;90:1850-1859.

27. Hadders-Algra M. Variation and variability: key words in human motor development. *Phys Ther.* 2010;90(12):1823-1837.

28. Streissguth AP. *Fetal Alcohol Syndrome: A Guide for Families and Communities.* Paul H. Brookes; 1997.

29. Edelman C, Mandle CL. *Health Promotion Throughout the Lifespan.* 5th ed. Mosby, Inc; 2002.

30. Landgren M, Svensson L, Strömland K, et al. Prenatal alcohol exposure and neurodevelopmental disorders in children adopted from Eastern Europe. *Pediatrics.* 2010;125(5):e1178-e1185. doi:10.1542/peds.2009-0712

31. Committee on Substance Abuse and Committee on Children with Disabilities. Fetal alcohol syndrome and alcohol-related neurodevelopmental disorders. *Pediatrics.* 2000;106(2):358-361.

32. Stratton K, Howe C, Battaglia F, eds. *Fetal Alcohol Syndrome: Diagnosis, Epidemiology, Prevention and Treatment.* National Academy Press; 1996:4-21.

33. Astley SJ. Comparison of the 4-digit diagnostic code and the Hoyme diagnostic guidelines for fetal alcohol spectrum disorders. *Pediatrics.* 2006;118(4):1532-1545.

34. Kartin D, Grant TM, Streissguth AP, et al. Three-year developmental outcomes in children with prenatal alcohol and drug exposure. *Pediatr Phys Ther.* 2002;14:145-153.

35. U.S. Department of Health and Human Services. *Healthy People 2010.* U.S. Department of Health and Human Services/Office of Public Health and Science; 1998.

36. Singer LT, Moore DG, Min MO, et al. One-year outcomes of prenatal exposure to MDMA and other recreational drugs. *Pediatrics.* 2012;130:407-413.

37. Lester BM, Tronick EZ, La Gasse L, et al. The maternal lifestyle study: effects of substance exposure during pregnancy on neurodevelopmental outcome in 1-month-old infants. *Pediatrics.* 2002;110(6):1182-1192.

38. Fetters L, Tronick EZ. Neuromotor development of cocaine-exposed and control infants from birth through 15 months: poor and poorer performance. *Pediatrics.* 1996;98(5):938-943.

39. LaGasse LL, Derauf C, Smith LM, et al. Prenatal methamphetamine exposure and childhood behavior problems at 3 and 5 years of age. *Pediatrics.* 2012;129(4):681-688.

40. Koseck K, Harris SR. Changes in performance over time on the Bayley Scales of Infant Development II when administered to infants at high risk of developmental disabilities. *Pediatr Phys Ther.* 2004;16(4):199-205.

41. Simmons RW, Thomas JD, Levy SS, et al. Motor response programming and movement time in children with heavy prenatal alcohol exposure. *Alcohol.* 2010;44(4):371-378.

42. LaGasse LL, Seifer R, Lester BM. Interpreting research on prenatal substance exposure in the context of multiple confounding factors. *Clin Perinatol.* 1999;26:39-54.

43. Messinger DS, Bauer CR, Das A, et al. The maternal lifestyle study: cognitive, motor, and behavioral outcomes of cocaine-exposed and opiate-exposed infants through three years of age. *Pediatrics.* 2004;113(6):1677-1685.

44. Arendt R, Angelopoulos J, Salvator A, et al. Motor development of cocaine-exposed children at age two years. *Pediatrics.* 1999;103(1):86-92.

45. Frank DA, Jacobs RR, Beeghly M, et al. Level of prenatal cocaine exposure and scores on the Bayley scales of infant development: modifying effects of caregiver, early intervention, and birth weight. *Pediatrics.* 2002;110(6):1143-1152.

46. Illingworth RS. *The Development of the Infant and Young Child: Normal and Abnormal.* Churchill Livingstone; 1980.

47. McGraw MB. *The Neuromuscular Maturation of the Human Infant.* Hafner Publishing; 1945.

48. Gesell A, Ilg FL. *Infant and Child in the Culture of Today.* Harper and Brothers Publishers; 1943.

49. Cech DJ, Martin ST. *Functional Movement Development Across the Life Span.* 2nd ed. W.B. Saunders; 2002.

50. Keshner EA. How theoretical framework biases evaluation and treatment. In: Lister MJ, ed. *Contemporary Management of Motor Control Problems: Proceedings of the II STEP Conference.* Bookcrafters, Inc; 1991:37-47.

51. Effgen SK. *Meeting the Physical Therapy Needs of Children.* 2nd ed. F.A. Davis; 2013.

52. Bayley N. *The California Infant Scale of Motor Development.* University of California; 1936.

53. Tecklin JS, ed. *Pediatric Physical Therapy.* 3rd ed. Lippincott Williams & Wilkins; 1998.

54. Horak FB. Assumptions underlying motor control for neurologic rehabilitation. In: Lister MJ, ed. *Contemporary Management of Motor Control Problems: Proceedings of the II STEP Conference.* Bookcrafters, Inc; 1991:11-27.

55. Sugden D. Current approaches to intervention in children with developmental coordination disorder. *Dev Med Child Neurol.* 2007;49(6):467-471.

56. Salihagic-Kadic A, Medic M, Kurjak A. Neurophysiology of fetal behavior. *Ultrasound Rev Obstet Gynecol.* 2004;4(1):2-11.

57. Nader K, Bechara A, van der Kooy D. Neurobiological constraints on behavioral models of motivation. *Annu Rev Psychol.* 1997;48: 85-114.

58. Holland PC. Cognitive versus stimulus–response theories of learning. *Learn Behav.* 2008;36(3):227-241.

59. Stockmeyer SA. An interpretation of the approach of Rood to the treatment of neuromuscular dysfunction. *Am J Phys Med.* 1967;46:900-956.

60. Horne PJ, Erjavec M. Do infants show generalized imitation of gestures? *J Exp Anal Behav.* 2007;87(1):63-87.

61. Hauf P, Aschersleben G. Action-effect anticipation in infant action control. *Psychol Res.* 2008;72(2):203-210.

62. Spence JP, Clearfield M, Corbetta D, et al. Moving toward a grand theory of development: in memory of Esther Thelen. *Child Dev.* 2006;77(6):1521-1538.

63. Pin T, Eldridge B, Galea MP. A review of the effects of sleep position, play position, and equipment use on motor development in infants. *Dev Med Child Neurol.* 2007;49(11):858-867.

64. Bartlett DJ, Fanning JK, Miller L, et al. Development of the daily activities of infants scale: a measure supporting early motor development. *Dev Med Child Neurol.* 2008;50(8):613-617.

65. Rose-Jacobs R, Cabral H, Beeghly M, et al. The movement assessment of infants (MAI) as a predictor of two-year neurodevelopmental outcome for infants born at term who are at social risk. *Pediatr Phys Ther.* 2004;16:212-221.

66. Monson RM, Deitz J, Kartin D. The relationship between awake positioning and motor performance among infants who slept supine. *Pediatr Phys Ther.* 2003;15:196-203.

67. Dudek-Shriber L, Zelazny S. The effects of prone positioning on the quality and acquisition of developmental milestones in four-month-old infants. *Pediatr Phys Ther.* 2007;19:48-55.

68. Ravenscroft EF, Harris SR. Is maternal education related to infant motor development? *Pediatr Phys Ther.* 2007;19:56-61.

69. Abbott AL, Bartlett DJ, Fanning JE, et al. Infant motor development and aspects of the home environment. *Pediatr Phys Ther.* 2000;12(2):62-67.

70. Nervik D, Martin K, Rundquist P, et al. The relationship between body mass index and gross motor development in children aged 3 to 5 years. *Pediatr Phys Ther.* 2011;23(2):144-148.

71. Hanson H, Jawad AF, Ryan T, et al. Factors influencing gross motor development in young children in an urban welfare system. *Pediatr Phys Ther.* 2011;23(4):335-346.

72. Oriel KN, Frazier K, Lebron M, et al. The impact of the back to sleep campaign on gross motor development. *Pediatr Phys Ther.* 2006;18(1):102.

73. Smith MR, Danoff JV, Parks RA. Motor skill development of children with HIV infection measured with the Peabody developmental motor scales. *Pediatr Phys Ther.* 2002;14(2):74-84.

74. Majnemer A, Barr RG. Influence of supine sleep positioning on early motor milestone acquisition. *Dev Med Child Neurol.* 2005;47(6):370-376.

75. Marshall J. Infant neurosensory development: considerations for infant child care. *Early Child Educ J.* 2011;39(3):175-181.

76. Rodrigues LP, Saraiva L, Gabbard C. Development and construct validation of an inventory for assessing the home environment for motor development. *Res Q Exerc Sport.* 2005;76(2):140-148.

77. Bartlett DJ, Palisano RJ. Physical therapists' perceptions of factors influencing the acquisition of motor abilities of children with cerebral palsy: implications for clinical reasoning. *Phys Ther.* 2002;82(3):237-248.

78. MacKay-Lyons M. Central pattern generation of locomotion: a review of the evidence. *Phys Ther.* 2002;82:69-83.

79. Marder E, Calabrese RL. Principles of rhythmic motor pattern generation. *Physiol Rev.* 1996;76:687-717.

80. Jordan M, Brownstone RM, Noga BR. Control of functional systems in the brainstem and spinal cord. *Curr Opin Neurobiol.* 1992;2:794-801.

81. Grillner S. Locomotion in vertebrates: central mechanisms and reflex integration. *Physiol Rev.* 1975;55:247-304.

82. D'Agostino J. An evidentiary review regarding the use of chronological and adjusted age in the assessment of preterm infants. *J Spec Pediatr Nurs.* 2010;15(1):26-32.

83. Palisano RJ. Use of chronological and adjusted ages to compare motor development of healthy preterm and full-term infants. *Dev Med Child Neurol.* 1986;28(2):180-187.

84. Edwards S, ed. *Neurological Physiotherapy.* 2nd ed. Churchill Livingstone; 2002.

85. Sullivan PE, Markos PD, Minor MAD. *An Integrated Approach to Therapeutic Exercise: Theory & Clinical Application.* Reston Publishing Company; 1982.

86. Heathcock JC, Bhat AN, Lobo MA, et al. The relative kicking frequency of infants born full-term and preterm during learning and short-term and long-term memory periods of the mobile paradigm. *Phys Ther.* 2005;85(1):8-18.

87. Piek JP, Carman R. Developmental profiles of spontaneous movements in infants. *Early Hum Dev.* 1994;39:109-126.

88. Thelen E, Ridley-Johnson R, Fisher D. Shifting patterns of bilateral coordination and lateral dominance in the leg movements of young infants. *Dev Psychobiol.* 1983;16:29-46.

89. Morgan A. *Neuro-developmental Approach to the High-risk Neonate.* (Notes from a seminar presented in Williamsburg, VA: November 3-4; 1984.) Cited in: Tecklin JS. *Pediatr Phys Ther.* Lippincott Williams & Wilkins; 1999.

90. Clopton NA, Duvall T, Ellis B, et al. Investigation of trunk and extremity movement associated with passive head turning in newborns. *Phys Ther.* 2000;80(2):152-159.

91. Suzanne SD. *Neurological Development in the Full Term and Premature Neonate.* Elsevier; 1977. Cited in: Bly L. *Motor Skills Acquisition in the First Year: An Illustrated Guide to Normal Development.* Therapy Skill Builders; 1994.

92. Guzzetta A, Haataja L, Cowan F, et al. Neurological examination in healthy term infants aged 3-10 weeks. *Biol Neonate.* 2005;87:187-196.

93. Oatis CA. *Kinesiology: The Mechanics and Pathomechanics of Human Movement.* Lippincott Williams & Wilkins; 2004:106.

94. Piek JP. *Infant Motor Development.* Human Kinetics; 2006.

95. Dubowitz LMS, Dubowitz V, Mercuri E. *The Neurological Assessment of the Preterm and Full-Term Newborn Infant.* 2nd ed. Mac Keith Press; 1999.

96. Capute AJ. Early neuromotor reflexes in infancy. *Pediatr Ann.* 1986;15(3):217-222.

97. Bly L. *Motor Skills Acquisition in the First Year: An Illustrated Guide to Normal Development.* Therapy Skill Builders; 1994.

98. Morgan AM, Aldag JC. Early identification of cerebral palsy using a profile of abnormal motor patterns. *Pediatrics.* 1996;98(4):692-697.

99. Kornhaber L, Ridgway E, Kathirithamby R. Occupational and physical therapy approaches to sensory and motor issues. *Pediatr Ann.* 2007;36(8):484-493.

100. Koman LA, Smith BP, Shilt JS. Cerebral palsy. *Lancet.* 2004;363:1619-1631.

101. Pooh RK, Ogura T. Normal and abnormal fetal hand positioning and movement in early pregnancy detected by three-and four-dimensional ultrasound. *Ultrasound Rev Obstet Gynecol.* 2004;4(1):46-51.

102. Jaffe M, Tal Y, Dabbah H, et al. Infants with a thumb-in-fist posture. *Pediatrics.* 2000;105:e41. Accessed September 20, 2012. http://www.pediatrics.org/cgi/content/full/105/3/e41

103. Haywood KM, Getchell N. *Life Span Motor Development.* 3rd ed. Human Kinetics; 2001.

104. Bly L. Normal and Abnormal Components of Movement. Course notes presented in September 1984, Milwaukee, WI.

105. Umphred DA. *Neurological Rehabilitation.* 4th ed. Mosby, Inc; 2001.

106. Norton ES. Developmental muscular torticollis and brachial plexus injury. In: Campbell SK, Vander Linden DW, Palisano RJ, eds. *Physical Therapy for Children.* 2nd ed. Saunders; 2000:291.

107. Fiorentino M. *Reflex Testing Methods for Evaluating CNS Development.* Charles C. Thomas; 1972.

108. Thelen E, Fisher DM. Newborn stepping: an explanation for a "disappearing" reflex. *Dev Psychol.* 1982;18:760-775.

109. Long TM, Toscano K. *Handbook of Pediatric Physical Therapy.* Lippincott Williams & Wilkins; 2001.

110. Erhardt RP. *Erhardt Developmental Prehension Assessment.* Ramsco Publishing; 1984. Cited in: Bly L. *Motor Skills Acquisition in the First Year: An Illustrated Guide to Normal Development.* Therapy Skill Builders; 1994.

2

Pediatric Assessment Tools

Kirsten H. Malerba

Pediatric physical therapists promote active participation when working with children and their families by assisting each child in reaching their maximal potential for functional independence at home, school, or in community environments.[1] Physical therapists have expertise in movement, motor development, and body function (e.g., strength and endurance). As primary health care providers, physical therapists also promote health and wellness in collaboration with families, communities, and other medical, educational, developmental, and rehabilitation specialists. Therapists use clinical reasoning during examination, evaluation, diagnosis, and intervention for children, youth, and young adults.[1] In doing so, knowledge of motor development is central to the practice of pediatric physical therapy. Understanding the normal, orderly sequence of developmental achievement and patterns of integration is the basis upon which significant deviation in maturation is gauged.[2] From the knowledge of typical development, therapists can determine if a child is functioning at the expected norm for a given age through clinical observations and objective measurements, including developmental testing.

>> Purposes of developmental testing

The purposes of developmental testing include identifying the risk of developmental delay, determining eligibility for services, intervention planning, documenting change over time, determining efficacy of treatment over time, or research purposes.

Developmental tests can be used as screening tools promoting early intervention for children at risk for delays in motor development.[3] The Committee on Children with Disabilities of the American Academy of Pediatrics recommends developmental surveillance be incorporated at every well-child visit and any concerns raised during surveillance should be promptly addressed.[4] Early identification of developmental disorders is critical for the well-being of children and their families. Developmental tests that are discriminative measures are used for determining eligibility for therapy services in early intervention or in school settings. Developmental tests also include evaluative measures, which are designed to measure change over time or response to an intervention.[3] Developmental tests can be used to plan interventions and measure progress over time as with curriculum-based assessments such as the Battelle Developmental Inventory 2 (BDI-2).[5] Finally, developmental tests are used as a clinical research tool when assessing reliability and validity of other developmental tests or for program evaluation.

>> Basic methods of examination

The *Guide to Physical Therapist Practice*[6] offers a model of patient/client management that is designed to maximize patient outcomes through a systematic, comprehensive approach to clinical decision-making. The elements of Examination, Evaluation, Diagnosis, Prognosis, Intervention, and Outcomes serve as a guide for therapists working with children who have been referred for physical therapy examination.

Physical therapy examination is the first element in patient/client management, which consists of obtaining patient/client history, performing a systems review, and selecting and administering tests and measures. The interview process for obtaining pertinent history includes identifying the family's concerns and needs related to the child's development, understanding the family's perception of the problem, and inquiring whether the developmental concerns impact daily family routines. The family's expectations, goals, and desired outcomes for physical therapy are important factors to identify during the interview process.

The review of the child's developmental and medical history provides valuable information and can be obtained through a questionnaire such as a case history form or through parent/client interview. The possible lack of reliability and bias of the parent should be considered in assessing the information gained in the history. When available, the medical records of a child may provide objective information regarding precautions, patient health status, previous medical history, suspected diagnosis, prognosis, medications, and other factors impacting the child's health. Other pertinent history, including information about the family and its genetic history, the pregnancy, labor, and delivery of the child, and the perinatal and neonatal events, should be obtained.

Therapists can gather a plethora of information about the child through clinical observations, often during the interview process. Is the child motivated to explore and move about in the environment, or is he or she more of an observer and active listener preferring to remain close to his or her family? If the child is mobile, what is the quality and symmetry of movement? How does the child's body respond to the effects of gravity? How does the child communicate with the parents and the therapist?

Developing a rapport with the family and child, assuring comfort in the environment, and being flexible and accommodating to the child's temperament, behavior, or special needs are necessary skills for the pediatric physical therapist.

Selection of appropriate tests and measures for the examination depends on the purpose of the examination. Kirshner and Guyatt describe three purposes of examination: (1) Evaluative measures are used to determine change over time or change as the result of intervention; (2) Predictive measures are used to help identify children who will have delays in the future or to predict the outcome of the delay; and (3) Discriminative measures are used to distinguish between children who have a delay, impairment, functional limitation, or atypical development and those who do not.[7,8] Determining the most appropriate developmental test for the physical therapy examination is a key component of a valid developmental assessment.

» Tools for assessment

Guidelines for Selection of Tests

Careful and knowledgeable selection of tests is an important component of the physical therapy examination. If evaluators are unaware of the strengths, weaknesses, limitations, and restrictions of the tests being used, there is a high probability that an inappropriate test could be used, thus resulting in inaccurate or misinterpreted information.[9] Most published tests have some limitations or restrictions to their use, particularly regarding the ages and populations for whom they were developed and on whom they were standardized. These varied restrictions and limitations must be carefully examined and considered by the physical therapist in order to avoid choosing an inappropriate test, which could result in unintended misinterpretation of testing results.

In order to choose an appropriate test, some guidelines by which to evaluate a test are needed. Stangler and associates have proposed six criteria for evaluating a screening test that can be applied to any assessment test: (1) acceptability, (2) simplicity, (3) cost, (4) appropriateness, (5) reliability, and (6) validity. Every test may not fulfill each criterion; however, the test may be used knowledgeably if a therapist is aware of the limitations.[10]

Acceptability is defined as acceptance to all who will be affected by the test, including the children and families screened, the professionals who receive resulting referrals, and the community. *Simplicity* is the ease by which a test can be taught, learned, and administered. *Appropriateness* of screening tests is based on the prevalence of the problem to be screened and on the applicability of the test to the particular population. *Cost* includes the actual cost of equipment, preparation and payment of personnel, the cost of inaccurate results, personal costs to the person being screened, and the total cost of the test in relation to the benefits of early detection. In addition, tests must show both *reliability* and consistency between measurements, as well as *validity*, or the extent to which a test measures what it purports to measure.[10]

Using Questions as Guidelines

The choice of which developmental assessment is most appropriate for the examination depends on the response to the following questions[11]:

1. *For what purpose will the test be used?*
   - For identifying developmental delay
   - For determining eligibility for services
   - For research
   - For measuring the effect of therapy intervention
2. *What are the characteristics of the child?*
   - Age
   - Functional capability
   - Cognitive and language ability
3. *What content areas need to be assessed?*
   - Gross motor
   - Fine motor
   - Speech
   - Comprehensive examination of functional capabilities

4. *What setting will the examination take place in?*
   • The child's natural environment (home, daycare, school)
   • Outpatient rehabilitation setting
   • In-patient hospital setting
   • Follow-up or specialty clinic
5. *What are the external constraints for the examiner?*
   • Time
   • Examiner experience and training
   • Space and equipment
   • Purchasing costs
   • Payor requirements or limitations

>> Definitions

Terms for Understanding Standardized Assessments

An *age-equivalent score* is the mean chronologic age (CA) represented by a certain test score. For example, a raw score of 165 on the Locomotion subtest of the Peabody Developmental Motor Scale 2 (PDMS-2) represents an age equivalent to 53 months. Age-equivalent scores may be especially useful with developmentally delayed children for whom it may be impossible to derive a meaningful developmental index. Age-equivalent scores are easy for parents to understand, but they must be interpreted carefully because they can be misleading.

The *criterion-referenced test* is one in which scores are interpreted on the basis of absolute criteria (e.g., the number of items answered correctly) rather than on relative criteria, such as how the rest of the normal group performed. Such tests are usually developed by the teacher or researcher and can be used for research involving a comparison of groups, just as norm-referenced tests are used. Criterion-referenced tests are used to measure a person's mastery of a set of behavioral objectives. The tests represent an attempt to maximize the validity or appropriateness of the content based on that set of objectives. The *developmental quotient* is the ratio between the child's actual score (developmental age) on a test and the child's CA. An example is motor age / CA equal to the motor quotient (MQ).

Norm-referenced or *standardized tests* use normative values as standards for interpreting individual test scores. The purpose of standardized tests is to make a comparison between a particular child and the "norm" or "average" of a group of children. Norms describe a person's test score relative to a large body of scores that have already been collected on a defined population. Examples of norm-referenced tests include the Bayley Scales of Infant and Toddler Development 4 (Bayley-4), PDMS-2, and the Bruininks–Oseretsky Test of Motor Proficiency, 2nd edition (BOT-2).

The *percentile score* indicates the number of children of the same age or grade level (or whatever is used for a source of comparison) who would be expected to score lower than the child tested. For example, a child who scores in the 75th percentile on a norm-referenced test has done better than 75% of the children in the norm group.

A *raw score* is the total of individual items that are passed or correct on a particular test. On many tests, this will require establishing a basal and ceiling level of performance. The number of items required to achieve a basal or ceiling level varies from one test to another.

Reliability refers to consistency or repeatability between measurements in a series. Types of reliability include interobserver and test–retest. Interobserver reliability describes the relationship between items passed and failed, or the percentage of agreement, between two independent observers. Simply stated, interobserver reliability is an index of whether two different testers obtain the same score on a test. Test–retest reliability is the relationship of a person's score on the first administration of the test to the score on the second administration. Simply stated, this type of reliability determines whether the same or similar scores are achieved when the test is repeated under identical conditions.

Standard error of measurement (SEM) is a measure of reliability that indicates the precision of an individual test score. The SEM gives an estimate of the margin of error associated with a particular test score and is related to the probability of observing a score at a given interval. The SEM can be used to develop confidence intervals for interpreting the accuracy of a test score.

Standard scores are expressed as deviations or variations from the mean score for a group. Standard scores are expressed in units of standard deviation (SD). When using standard scores, information is needed concerning the mean and SD of the standard score.

Validity is an indication of the extent to which a test measures what it purports to measure. *Construct validity* is an examination of the theory or hypothetical constructs underlying the test. *Content validity* assesses the appropriateness of the test or how well the content of the test samples the subject matter or behaviors about which conclusions must be drawn. The sample situations measured in the test must be representative of the set from which the sample is drawn. There are two types of *criterion-related validity*. *Concurrent validity* relates the performance on the test to performance on another well-known and accepted test that measures the same knowledge or behavior. *Predictive validity* means that the child's performance on the test predicts some actual behavior.

Sensitivity can be defined as the ability of a test to identify correctly those who actually have a disorder. High sensitivity results in few false-negative scores.

Specificity refers to the ability of the test to identify correctly those who do not have the disorder. High specificity results in few false-positive scores.

The *positive predictive value* of a test is defined as the proportion of true positives among all those who have positive results. The *negative predictive value* is the proportion of true negatives among all those who have negative screening results.

» Overview of tests

Developmental assessments may be considered in several broad categories. Screening tests are used to identify deficits in a child's performance that indicate the need for further services. Assessments of component functions address specific areas of functioning (e.g., gross motor ability or reflex status). Comprehensive developmental scales evaluate all areas of development. Functional assessments evaluate the essential skills that are required in the child's natural environments of home and school. Outcome and health-related quality-of-life (HRQOL) measures are used to assess patient functioning in multiple life domains.

The rest of the chapter reviews selected tests that are available for physical therapy evaluation. Some of the more widely known standardized evaluative procedures are presented, as are some tests that are not standardized but that have proven useful in clinical practice. The categories just mentioned are used for organization.

Screening Tests

Developmental screening is the process of proactively testing whole populations of children to identify those who are at high risk for clinically significant deviations or delays in development.[12] Screening tests are designed to be a brief assessment to identify children who would benefit from more intensive diagnosis or examination. Screening tests may be parent-completed tools such as the Ages and Stages Questionnaire (ASQ) or the Parents' Evaluation of Developmental Status (PEDS) or directly administered tools by health care practitioners.[13]

Harris Infant Neuromotor Test

The Harris Infant Neuromotor Test (HINT) was developed to be used in clinical and research settings as an early screening for potential developmental disorders in both high- and low-risk infants.[14,15] Infants shown to be at a higher risk for developmental delay based on screening using the HINT would then be referred for more extensive examination of motor delay.[14]

TEST MEASURES AND TARGET POPULATION The HINT measures infant motor behavior, behavioral state, head circumference, and parent/caregiver's concerns about the infant's development. The target population for the HINT is infants from 2.5 to 12.5 months of age and is intended for use by a wide variety of health care professionals, such as community health nurses, physical therapists, occupational therapists, physicians, and early childhood special educators.[16]

TEST CONSTRUCTION AND STANDARDIZATION The HINT was developed based on published research on early identification of neurodevelopmental difficulties, research involving the Movement Assessment of Infants (MAI), and the lead author's clinical experiences over 15 years.[17] The items assessing locomotion, posture, movement, stereotypical behaviors,

behavioral state, and head circumference measurements were selected from previously published predictive validity studies. The parent/caregiver questionnaire was included in the HINT to ensure that parents' concerns are addressed. Normative data have been collected on 412 Canadian infants from five provinces and stratified by gender, maternal education, and ethnicity.[14]

TEST FORMAT Type The test is a norm-referenced neuromotor, cognitive, behavioral screening tool.

Content The test comprises four sections: Section 1—infant's background information; Section 2—five questions assessing caregiver's perception of the infant's movement and play; Section 3—twenty-one items assessing the infant's motor skills in five positions (supine, prone, supine-to-prone transition, sitting, and standing), muscle tone, movement against gravity, cooperation, stereotypical behaviors, and head circumference; and Section 4—the tester's clinical impression of the infant's development[14] shows the HINT test items (Table 2.1).

Administration The test can be administered in approximately 15 to 30 minutes, depending on the infant's behavior and the skill of the administrator. Infant handling is minimal, and the test is meant to be primarily observational.

Scoring Throughout the testing session, the motor behaviors and movements observed are checked off in boxes on the score sheet to the right for each item. The corresponding score is to the right of the description of the behavior. Total scores are derived from a sum of all scores for each of the 21 motor behavior items.

Interpretation Lower HINT total scores indicate a more mature or more optimal infant development. For the HINT assessment, a total score falling within 1 SD of the mean for a particular age group is considered within normal limits. A score that is greater than 1 SD but less than 2 SD above the mean is considered suspect. Scores that are greater than 2 SD above the mean are considered atypical or abnormal.[14]

RELIABILITY AND VALIDITY Reliability and validity of the HINT were reported in a study of two high-risk infant follow-up programs in Vancouver, British Columbia.[16] The interrater, test–retest, and intrarater reliabilities of the total HINT score were all greater than or equal to 0.98, well above the "benchmark" of 0.80. Concurrent validity with the Bayley Scales of Infant Development II (BSID-II) was assessed by comparing HINT total scores to raw scores for BSID-II Mental and Motor Scales. Moderately strong and significant relationships between scores on the HINT and BSID-II Mental Scales were identified, suggesting that HINT may be tapping early cognitive behaviors assessed in the first year of life. Using the Pearson product–moment correlation, the HINT and BSID-II Motor Scales correlated strongly at $r = -0.89$, $p < 0.01$.[16]

Concurrent validity between the HINT and the Alberta Infant Motor Scale (AIMS) was reported in a longitudinal

TABLE 2.1. Harris Infant Neuromotor Test (HINT) Items		
Test Method	**Cognitive or Behavioral Development Items**	**Motor Development Items**
Observation (infant is observed in supine, prone, sitting, and standing positions)	• Behavior and cooperation • Presence of stereotypical behaviors	• Mobility, supine • Neck retraction, supine • Eye muscle control • Head position, prone • Upper extremity position, prone • Head position, sitting • Trunk position, sitting • Locomotion and transition skills • Posture of hands • Posture of feet • Frequency and variety of movements
Testing (infant is provided stimulation or is handled by the examiner to determine scores)	• Head circumference	• Visual following • Asymmetric tonic neck reflex • Reaching from supine position • Passive range of motion in supine position • Head righting in transition from supine to prone to supine positions • Trunk mobility in transitions from supine to prone to supine positions • Passive range of motion in prone position

Items to be tested in Harris Infant Neuromotor Test. With permission from American Physical Therapy Association.

study of 121 typical and at-risk infants.[18] Both the AIMS and the HINT were administered concurrently at two time points, 4 to 6.5 months and 10 to 12.5 months. The HINT total scores were strongly related to the AIMS total scores in at-risk infants at both time periods during the first year of life and in typical infants at ages 4 to 6.5 months. Correlation coefficients for the entire sample exceeded 0.80 at both assessment time points.

Concurrent validity was also studied between HINT and ASQ. Pearson product–moment correlations between the two test scores for 52 infants tested ranged from $r = -0.82$ to -0.84 ($p < 0.05$).[19]

ADVANTAGES/DISADVANTAGES The HINT was designed as a screening test that may appeal to community providers who are frequently involved in screening healthy infants.[18] The inclusion of caregiver comments regarding their level of concern for the infant's movement and play is a strength as it makes the HINT more family centered. The HINT differentiates itself from the AIMS or the Test of Infant Motor Performance (TIMP) screening items as it is aimed at not only identifying motor deficits but also identifying early cognitive delays or behavioral difficulties.

The HINT normative sample is small (412 Canadian infants) relative to other infant motor assessments and covers a narrow age range (2.5 to 12.5 months), which may limit its utility in pediatric settings with a broad age span of children.

Bayley Infant Neurodevelopmental Screener

The Bayley Infant Neurodevelopmental Screener (BINS) is a screening tool designed to identify infants and young children who are at risk for developmental and neurodevelopmental delays.[20] It is mainly used in settings where high-risk infants are followed up, such as developmental follow-up clinics or large-volume clinical and research programs.

TEST MEASURES AND TARGET POPULATION The BINS assesses four conceptual areas of ability: basic neurologic function/intactness (posture, muscle tone, movement symmetry), expressive functions (gross, fine, and oral motor/verbal), receptive functions (visual, auditory, verbal), and cognitive processes (object permanence, goal-directedness, problem solving).[20] This screening test is appropriate for infants and young children from 3 to 24 months.

TEST CONSTRUCTION AND STANDARDIZATION The BINS was constructed from a subset of items from the BSID-II as well as items measuring neurologic status. The BINS was standardized on more than 600 infants, stratified according to age, sex, ethnicity, region, and parent education.

TEST FORMAT

Type The test is a norm-referenced, standardized screening tool.

Content The BINS consists of six item sets assessing basic neurologic functions, receptive, expressive, and cognitive functions. Each set contains 11 to 13 items, depending on the child's age.

Administration/Scoring Each item in the BINS is scored "optimal" (1) or "nonoptimal" (0), and the total number of "optimal" items in each set is added, yielding a summary score. The BINS can be administered in 15 to 20 minutes.

Interpretation For each of the item sets, three established summary cut scores identify an infant's level of risk for developmental delay, yielding three risk groupings: low risk, moderate risk, or high risk. The three-tiered framework is used to determine which infants need to be monitored (infants in the moderate-risk status) and which infants should be enrolled in intervention programs (high risk).

RELIABILITY AND VALIDITY Depending on the age of the child, test–retest reliability for the BINS ranges from 0.71 to 0.84. Interrater reliability was established and ranges from 0.79 to 0.96, with moderate to strong internal consistency.[20] During test standardization, the BINS demonstrated acceptable concurrent validity with the BSID-II.[20]

ADVANTAGES/DISADVANTAGES The BINS is one of the few psychometrically sound screening tests for infants and young children at risk for developmental delay. It is brief and easily administered by a number of health care providers with a variety of backgrounds. The BINS has a high degree of sensitivity and specificity (75% to 86%), which is an important aspect of any screening test.[21] The BINS given to 45 preterm infants between the ages of 3 and 24 months predicted neurodevelopmental status of 7- to 10-year-olds for verbal and performance scores on the Wechsler Intelligence Scale-Revised for children as early as 7 to 10 months of age.[22]

Limitations include difficulty clarifying the need for comprehensive developmental assessment for children whose BINS scores fall in the middle of the three-tiered classification system (those at moderate-risk group) and a need for clarification of criteria for many test items, including muscle tone.

Tests of Motor Function

Physical therapists use motor development assessment tools as part of the physical therapy examination to measure motor development and function. A large number of assessment tools that examine gross and fine motor function are available. TIMP, the AIMS, Gross Motor Function Measure (GMFM), and Gross Motor Function Classification System (GMFCS), PDMS-2, and BOT-2 are described.

Test of Infant Motor Performance

Campbell and colleagues developed the TIMP for physical and occupational therapists to assess posture and movement of infants from 34 weeks postmenstrual age through 4 months corrected age.[23,24]

TEST MEASURES AND TARGET POPULATION The TIMP quantitatively assesses motor development and is used to identify infants who might benefit from early intervention services. It assesses the postural control and alignment needed for age-appropriate functional activities involving movement in early infancy, including changing positions and moving against the force of gravity, adjusting to handling, self-comforting, and orienting the head and body for looking, listening, and interacting with caregivers. The TIMP is intended for use with infants in intensive care nurseries, developmental follow-up clinics, and early intervention programs.[25] The items in the test were designed to reflect the full range of motor maturity from 34 weeks' postconceptual age to 4 months postterm.

TEST CONSTRUCTION AND STANDARDIZATION Version 1 of the TIMP was initially developed by Girolami for use in assessing the efficacy of neurodevelopmental treatment on posture and movement in prematurely born high-risk infants from 34 to 35 weeks' postconceptual age.[26] Several revisions to the original TIMP have occurred, including revision/elimination of test items and reduction in length of the assessment through Rasch analysis, resulting in the 42-item TIMP.[27] Age standards developed from 990 U.S. infants reflecting distribution of race/ethnicity in the U.S. population are available.

TEST FORMAT Type The test is norm-referenced with elicited and observed item components.

Content Version 5.1 of the TIMP contains an observed scale of 13 dichotomously scored items used to examine an infant's spontaneous movements such as head in midline and individual finger and ankle movements. An elicited scale of 29 items tests the infant's movement responses to various positions, sights, and sounds.

According to the test authors, the processes tested by the items include the following:

1. The ability to orient and stabilize the head in space and in response to auditory and visual stimulation in supine, prone, side-lying, and upright positions and during transitions from one position to another
2. Body alignment when the head is manipulated
3. Distal selective control of the fingers, wrists, hands, and ankles
4. Antigravity control of arm and leg movements

Administration/Scoring The test can be administered in 25 to 40 minutes, depending on the child's abilities, behavioral state, physiologic stability, and level of cooperation. Observations of spontaneous emitted behaviors/movements are rated present (1) or absent (0) throughout the course of the examination. Elicited items are administered according to standardized instructions and involve direct handling of the infant. Responses to these items are scored on a 3-, 4-, 5-, or 6-point rating scale that describes specific behaviors to be noted, ranging from less mature or minimal response to mature or full response, as defined individually for each test item. Total raw scores range from 0 to 142.

Interpretation Raw scores are transformed into standard scores and interpreted relative to the mean for the corresponding age group. Score sheets for plotting the infants' scores against percentile ranks provide age-equivalent scores. On the basis of previous research on predictive validity of the TIMP, the authors suggest a −0.5 SD below the mean for identifying infants who may require close monitoring and/or referral for intervention.[25]

RELIABILITY AND VALIDITY Test–retest reliability over a 3-day period is reported at $r = 0.89$ for infants from 34 weeks post conceptual age (PCA) to 4 months of age.[28] Intrarater reliability (intraclass correlation [ICC] = 0.98 to 0.99) and interrater reliability (ICC = 0.95) are excellent.[29] Construct validity was assessed by determining the test's sensitivity for assessing age-related changes in motor skills and correlation with risk for developmental abnormality. The correlation between postconceptual age and TIMP performance measures was 0.83. Risk and age together explained 72% of the variance in TIMP performance ($r = 0.85$; $p < 0.00001$).[30] The relationship between cerebral magnetic resonance imaging (MRI) at term age, and the TIMP and General Movements Assessment at 10 to 15 weeks postterm age was studied in 53 preterm infants (median gestational age 28 weeks). Infants with abnormal white matter were significantly more likely to have both abnormal general movements ($p = 0.01$) and abnormal TIMP scores ($p = 0.001$). Infants with abnormal general movements were significantly more likely to have lower TIMP scores ($p = 0.01$).[31]

ADVANTAGES/DISADVANTAGES The TIMP has excellent test–retest and rater reliabilities and is designed specifically to assess infants born preterm and those at risk for poor motor outcome based on perinatal medical conditions. The predictive validity of TIMP scores at 3- to 12-month AIMS percentiles demonstrates a high sensitivity of 0.92 and a specificity of 0.76.[32] The TIMP scores at 3 months also demonstrate predictive validity for preschool motor performance using the PDMS, with a sensitivity of 0.72 and specificity of 0.91.[33] Because of the age specifications of this test, its clinical utility is limited to settings such as special care nurseries, developmental follow-up clinics, or early intervention services.

Alberta Infant Motor Scale

The AIMS is an observational assessment scale constructed by Piper and Darrah to measure gross motor maturation in infants from birth through independent walking.[34] It was developed to incorporate components of motor development, which are deemed essential to the evaluation and treatment of at-risk infants. The AIMS is designed to (1) identify infants whose motor performance is delayed or aberrant relative to a normative group; (2) provide information to the clinician and parent(s) about the motor activities

the infant has mastered, those currently developing, and those not in the infant's repertoire; (3) measure motor performance over time or before and after intervention; (4) measure changes in motor performance that are quite small and thus not likely to be detected using more traditional motor measures; and (5) act as an appropriate research tool to assess the efficacy of rehabilitation programs for infants with motor disorders.

TEST MEASURES AND TARGET POPULATION The test is an assessment of gross motor performance designed for the identification and evaluation of motor development of infants from term (40 weeks after conception) through the age of independent walking (0 to 18 months of age). The AIMS not only focuses on achievement of motor milestones but also assesses the motor aspects and mechanisms necessary to attain such milestones (e.g., weight-bearing, posture, and antigravity movement).[35] Sequential development of postural control relative to four postural positions—supine, prone, sitting, and standing—is assessed through observation.

TEST CONSTRUCTION AND STANDARDIZATION The AIMS was constructed to fulfill three clinical purposes: the identification of different levels of motor performance, the evaluation of change in motor performance over time (through maturation or intervention), and the provision of useful information for the planning of motor intervention strategies.[34] Test items were obtained through an exhaustive review of existing instruments and descriptive narratives of early motor development. Content validation of the instrument was accomplished through meetings with and a mail survey of Canadian pediatric physical therapists and consultation with an international panel of experts. A total of 58 items were included in the provisional test for reliability and validity testing. The establishment of norms for the AIMS involved data collection on 2,200 Albertan infants stratified by age and sex.[36] Darrah et al. published a reevaluation of infant norms for motor development comparing normative data of the original 2,220 infants to a cross-sectional cohort study of 650 Canadian infants in 2014. The correlation coefficient between the age locations of items on the original and contemporary data sets was 0.99. The mean age difference between item locations was 0.7 weeks. Age values from the original data set when converted to the contemporary scale differed by less than 1 week. **Conclusion:** The sequence and age at emergence of AIMS items has remained similar over 20 years and current normative values remain valid.[37]

TEST FORMAT Type The test is norm-referenced, providing percentile ranks to determine an individual's motor performance relative to the reference group.

Content The test includes 58 items organized into four positions: prone, supine, sitting, and standing. The distribution of these items is as follows: 21 prone, 9 supine, 12 sitting, and 16 standing. For each item, certain key descriptors are identified that must be observed for the infant to pass the items. Each item describes three aspects of motor performance—weight-bearing, posture, and antigravity movements (Fig. 2.1).

Administration/Scoring The administration of the test involves observational assessment, with minimal handling required. The surface of the body bearing weight, posture, and movement are assessed for each item. The scoring is recorded as "observed"/"not observed." For each of the four positions, the least mature and most mature item observed in the assessment is recorded as "observed" and serves as the "window" of the infants' possible motor repertoire. Scores in each area (prone, supine, sitting, standing) are summed to yield a total score of items passed.

Interpretation The infant's total AIMS score is plotted on a graph to determine the percentile ranking of the infant's motor performance compared with the normative age-matched sample. The higher the percentile ranking, the less likely the infant is demonstrating a delay in motor development. As the AIMS is not a diagnostic test, implications of lower percentile rankings (10%) are not definitive, and the examiner's clinical judgment is required for decisions related to ongoing monitoring, referral for further diagnostic workup, and/or recommendations for intervention for motor delay.

RELIABILITY AND VALIDITY The original sample consisted of 506 (285 male, 221 female) normal infants, age stratified from birth through 18 months. One hundred twenty infants were scored on the AIMS, PDMS-2, and Bayley Scales for an assessment of concurrent validity, and 253 infants were each scored two or three times on the AIMS to assess the interrater and test–retest reliability of the AIMS.[36] The authors found an interrater reliability of 0.99 and a test–retest reliability of 0.99. Correlation coefficients reflecting concurrent validity with the Bayley and Peabody Scales were determined to be $r = 0.98$ and $r = 0.97$, respectively.[36] Pin et al. studied

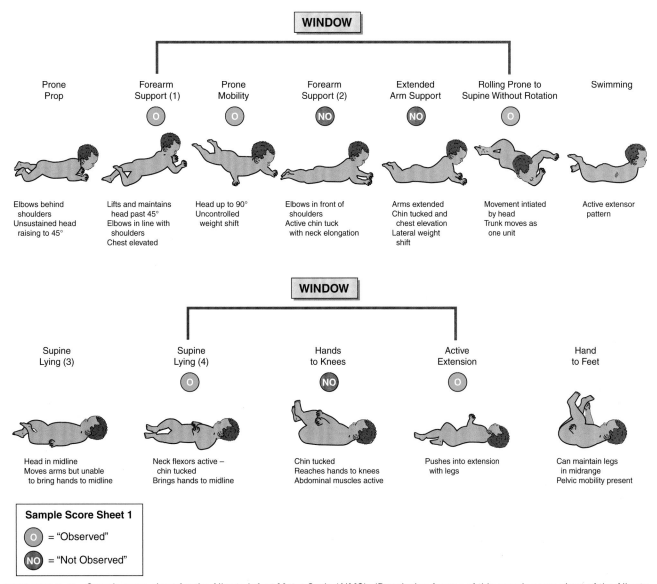

FIGURE 2.1. Sample score sheet for the Alberta Infant Motor Scale (AIMS). (Permission for use of this sample score sheet of the Alberta Infant Motor Scales figure 4-1 in AIMS Manual from Elsevier Publishers.)

the intra- and interrater reliability in infants born at or before 29 weeks gestational age from 4 to 18 months CA.[38] All of the ICC values were greater than 0.75 and the SEM was less than 1.2. Although the AIMS is a reliable measurement tool to be used in this infant population, the ICC values of subscores were low at 4 and 18 months CA because of the limited number of test items at these two extreme ages. The authors caution about using the AIMS for infants younger than 4 months or after the infant has achieved independent walking, because of the limited test items at these time points. The ability of AIMS and the HINT to predict scores on the BSID at age 2 and 3 years was studied to compare predictive validity between the two tests given during the infant's first year of life.[39] Infants with typical and at-risk development were assessed with the HINT and AIMS at 4 to 6.5 months and 10 to 12.5 months and with the BSID at 2 and 3 years. The early (4 to 6.5 months) HINT had higher predictive correlations than the AIMS for 2-year BSID-II motor outcomes and 3-year BSID-III gross motor outcomes. Correlations were identical for the 10- to 12.5-month HINT and AIMS scores and 3-year BSID-III gross motor ($r = 0.58$ and 0.58) and fine motor ($r = 0.35$ and 0.35) subscales.

ADVANTAGES AND DISADVANTAGES The AIMS provides the ability to detect, as early as possible, any deviations from the norm, thereby permitting early intervention to remediate or minimize the effects of dysfunction. Use of percentile ranking should be done with caution because a small change in raw score can result in a large change in percentile ranking.[40]

Gross Motor Function Measure

The GMFM is a clinical measure designed to evaluate change in gross motor function in children with cerebral palsy.[41]

TEST MEASURES AND TARGET POPULATION The test is designed to assess motor function or how much of an activity a child can accomplish. It is an evaluative index of gross motor function and changes in function over time, or after therapy, specifically for children with cerebral palsy. The original validation sample included children 5 months to 16 years old. The GMFM is appropriate for children whose motor skills are at or below those of a 5-year-old child without any motor disability. The Gross Motor Performance Measure (GMPM), an observational instrument assessing quality of gross motor movement, can be used in conjunction with the GMFM to evaluate change over time in specific qualitative features of motor behavior.[42]

TEST CONSTRUCTION AND STANDARDIZATION The GMFM was developed and tested according to contemporary principles of measurement design through a process of item selection, reliability testing, and validation procedures. The selection of items was based on a literature review and the judgment of pediatric clinicians. Items judged to be clinically important and measurable with the potential of showing change in the function of children were included. The original GMFM contains 88 items (GMFM-88). In an effort to improve the interpretability and clinical usefulness of the GMFM, Rasch analysis was applied to the GMFM-88, resulting in the GMFM-66.[43] The authors report that the GMFM-66 provides hierarchical structure and interval scoring that provides a better understanding of motor development in children with cerebral palsy than the older GMFM-88.[44]

TEST FORMAT

Type The GMFM is a criterion-based observational measure.

Content The test includes 88 items that assess motor function in five dimensions: (1) lying and rolling; (2) sitting; (3) crawling and kneeling; (4) standing; and (5) walking, running, and jumping. With emphasis on maximizing a child's potential for independent function, the test measures whether a child can complete the task independently (with or without the use of aids), without any active assistance from another person.

Administration/Scoring For ease of administration, the items are grouped on the rating form by test position and arranged in a developmental sequence. For scoring purposes, items are aggregated to represent five separate areas of motor function. Each GMFM item is scored on a 4-point ordinal scale. Values of 0, 1, 2, and 3 are assigned to each of the four categories; 0 = does not initiate; 1 = initiates (<10% of the task); 2 = partially completes (10% to <100% of the task); and 3 = task completion. A one-page score sheet is used to record results. Specific descriptions for how to score each item are found in the administration and scoring guidelines contained within the test manual. The 66 items that form the GMFM-66 are indicated on the scoresheet by shading and an asterisk. The time required to complete the GMFM-88 is approximately 45 to 60 minutes. As the GMFM-66 has 22 fewer items to be administered, it should require less time to administer the test.

Interpretation Each of the five dimensions contributes equal weight to the total score; therefore, a percent score is calculated for each dimension (child's score/maximum score × 100%). A total score is obtained by adding the percent scores for each dimension and dividing by five. A "goal total score" can also be calculated in order to increase the responsiveness of the measure by narrowing the focus to include selected GMFM dimensions most relevant to the child's goals. In order to interpret scores for the GMFM-66, a computer program, the Gross Motor Ability Estimator (GMAE), is required. The GMFM-66 score differs from the GMFM-88 score in that it has interval (as opposed to ordinal) properties.

RELIABILITY AND VALIDITY The test authors found intrarater reliability for each dimension and the total score to range from 0.92 to 0.99 and interrater reliability to range from 0.87 to 0.99 (ICC).[3] The GMFM-66 is also highly reliable (ICCs = 0.97 to 0.99) and sensitive to change.[44,45]

Construct validity of the GMFM-88 was demonstrated with significant linear relationships between gait speed and dimensions D (standing) (r = 0.91) and E (walking, running, and jumping) (r = 0.93).[46] More recently, the longitudinal construct validity of three scoring options (GMFM-88, GMFM-88 goal total, and GMFM-66) was evaluated in a 5-year follow-up study.[47] Forty-one children with cerebral palsy who were undergoing selective dorsal rhizotomy were monitored with the GMFM for 5 years. All three scoring options showed large longitudinal construct validity in the 5-year study. The GMFM-88 total and goal total scores revealed large changes in gross motor function earlier postoperatively than the GMFM-66 scores. Validity and reliability of two abbreviated versions of the GMFM-66 have also been reported.[48] Both the GMFM-66-IS (item set) and the GMFM-66-B&C (basal and ceiling approach) demonstrate high levels of validity (ICCs of 0.99) and reliability (ICCs >0.98) and can be used in clinical practice or for research purposes.

During the course of validation of the original version of the GMFM, it became evident that a meaningful, valid, and reliable classification of children's functional mobility was needed to enhance communication among families and professionals and to provide a sound basis for stratification of children for research.[49] The GMFCS for Cerebral Palsy, developed by Palisano and colleagues in 1997, was created to classify motor function in children with cerebral palsy into one of five clinically meaningful levels (Table 2.2).[50]

From Level I (most able) to Level V (most limited), the GMFCS describes motor function within four age bands, from before a child's second birthday to between the 6th and 12th birthday. Motor function is described in "word pictures," focusing on function under ordinary circumstances, rather than on capacity as observed with formal tools such as the GMFM or Pediatric Evaluation of Disability Inventory (PEDI). The GMFCS-E&R is the expanded and revised version of the GMFCS, with a revised 6- to 12-year age band, addition of a 12- to 18-year age band, with an expanded conceptual framework to coincide with the International Classification of Functioning, Disability, and Health (ICF).[50] Although utilized in published research on populations other than cerebral palsy, the GMFCS Levels classification was developed and validated for children with cerebral palsy only. In addition, the GMFCS Levels should not be used in children under 1 year of age as it was not validated for this age range.[51]

ADVANTAGES/DISADVANTAGES Debuse and Brace completed a systematic review of outcome measures of activity for children with cerebral palsy.[52] The GMFM-88, GMFM-66, and PEDI were the three outcome measures selected as most appropriate for testing function in children with cerebral palsy. Both the GMFM-88 and the PEDI exhibit high completion rates, confirming the relevance of these outcome measures to the functional ability of children with cerebral palsy. Long completion time and relative unidimensionality (testing only gross motor capacity in a controlled testing environment) were reported as weaknesses or disadvantages of the test. Although the GMFM-66 has 22 fewer items to test, allowing a faster completion time, it has floor effects in children with low motor ability and ceiling effects in children older than 5 years.[44] Careful consideration is required when determining whether to use the GMFM-88 or the GMFM-66 based on the child's motor abilities, ability to complete all test items

TABLE 2.2.	General Headings for Each Level of Gross Motor Function Classification System—Expanded and Revised (GMFCS-E&R)

General Heading for Each Level

LEVEL I—Walks without Limitations
LEVEL II—Walks with Limitations
LEVEL III—Walks Using a Handheld Mobility Device
LEVEL IV—Self-Mobility with Limitations; May Use Powered Mobility
LEVEL V—Transported in a Manual Wheelchair

Distinctions between Levels I and II—Compared with children and youth in Level I, children and youth in Level II have limitations walking long distances and balancing; may need a handheld mobility device when first learning to walk; may use wheeled mobility when traveling long distances outdoors and in the community; require the use of a railing to walk up and down stairs; and are not as capable of running and jumping.

Distinctions between Levels II and III—Children and youth in Level II are capable of walking without a handheld mobility device after age 4 (although they may choose to use one at times). Children and youth in Level III need a handheld mobility device to walk indoors and use wheeled mobility outdoors and in the community.

Distinctions between Levels III and IV—Children and youth in Level III sit on their own or require at most limited external support to sit, are more independent in standing transfers, and walk with a handheld mobility device. Children and youth in Level IV function in sitting (usually supported), but self-mobility is limited. Children and youth in Level IV are more likely to be transported in a manual wheelchair or use powered mobility.

Distinctions between Levels IV and V—Children and youth in Level V have severe limitations in head and trunk control and require extensive assisted technology and physical assistance. Self-mobility is achieved only if the child/youth can learn how to operate a powered wheelchair.

Permission from CanChild Website. https://canchild.ca/en/resources/42-gross-motor-function-classification-system-expanded-revised-gmfcs-e-r

required, and/or the clinician's knowledge and ability to use the GMAE appropriately.

Peabody Developmental Motor Scales— Second Edition

The PDMS-2 is the culmination of over a decade of research by the authors in response to reviewers' suggestions and feedback from examiners for improving the original PDMS.[53]

TEST MEASURES AND TARGET POPULATION The PDMS-2 comprises six subtests that measure the interrelated gross and fine motor abilities that develop early in life. The PDMS-2 can be used by physical and occupational therapists, early intervention specialists, adapted physical education teachers, psychologists, diagnosticians, and others interested in examining the motor abilities of young children. It was designed to assess motor skills in children from birth through 6 years of age.

TEST CONSTRUCTION AND STANDARDIZATION The original PDMS was developed to improve on the existing instruments used for motor evaluation. Test items were obtained from validated motor scales, and new items were created based on studies of children's growth and development. Characteristics of the PDMS-2 include a larger normative sample of 2,003 children stratified by age residing in 46 states and one Canadian province, the addition of studies showing the absence of gender and racial bias, reliability coefficients for subgroups of the normative sample (e.g., individuals with motor disabilities, African Americans, Hispanic Americans, females, and males) as well as for the entire normative sample, and validity studies with special attention devoted to showing that the test is valid for a wide variety of subgroups as well as for the general population.[53]

TEST FORMAT
Type The PDMS-2 is a discriminative measure and is norm-referenced.

Content The PDMS-2 is divided into two components: the Gross Motor Scale and Fine Motor Scale. The Gross Motor Scale contains 151 items divided into four subtests: Reflexes (birth to 11 months), Stationary (all ages), Locomotion (all ages), and Object Manipulation (12 months and older).

The Fine Motor Scale contains 98 items divided into two subtests: Grasping (all ages) and Visual Motor Integration (all ages). Norms are provided for each skill category at each age level, as well as for total scores.

The results of the subtests may be used to generate three global indexes of motor performance called composites—the Gross Motor Quotient (GMQ), the Fine Motor Quotient (FMQ), and the Total Motor Quotient (TMQ).

Administration Both scales can be given to a child in approximately 45 to 60 minutes. To shorten testing time, entry points

and basal and ceiling levels are used on all but one of the subtests (Reflexes). Examiners who give and interpret the PDMS-2 should have a thorough understanding of test statistics; general procedures governing scoring and interpretation; specific information about gross and fine motor ability testing; and development in children who are not progressing typically.[53] In order to achieve valid interpretation of a child's PDMS-2 performance, the scales must be administered exactly as specified in the Guide to Item Administration.

When the purpose of the test is eligibility or placement, instructional, or treatment programming for a child with disabilities, the examiner should administer an item as directed or adapt to fit the child's individual needs while retaining the intent of the item.

Scoring Each item on the PDMS-2 is scored as 0, 1, or 2. Specific criteria are given for each item, as are the general criteria for the numeric scores. Scores are assigned as follows:

0—The child cannot or will not attempt the item, or the attempt does not show that the skill is emerging.

1—The child's performance shows a clear resemblance to the item mastery criteria but does not fully meet the criteria. (This value allows for emerging skills.)

2—The child performs the item according to the criteria specified for mastery.

Scoring may be completed on a written summary sheet or by using the PDMS-2 Online Scoring and Report System.

Interpretation The PDMS-2 yields five types of scores: raw scores, age equivalents, percentiles, standard scores for the subtests, and quotients for the composites. From the raw scores calculated from each subtest, the age-equivalent and standard scores are obtained from the norms tables provided in the manual. The quotients for the fine motor, gross motor, and total motor composites are derived from summing the subtest standard scores and converting them to a quotient. After the standard scores and quotients have been determined, they may be plotted on the Motor Development Profile. This profile provides a means of visually comparing performance on the Gross Motor Scale and Fine Motor Scale and on the skill categories in each scale. Figure 2.2 presents an example of scoring the PDMS-2.

RELIABILITY AND VALIDITY The overall reliability of the PDMS-2 was studied by the test developers for three types of error variance—internal consistency, test–retest reliability, and interscorer reliability. The reliability coefficients for three composites and six subtests (Cronbach's $\alpha = 0.89$ to 0.97, test–retest $r = 0.82$ to 0.93, and interscorer $r = 0.96$ to 0.99) suggest a high degree of reliability. The magnitude of these coefficients strongly suggests that the PDMS-2 possesses little test error and that users can have confidence in its results.[53] A study published in 2019 assessed whether modifying instructions on the PDMS-2 affected scores in children with typical development. Effects for instruction type ($p = 0.03$) and an interaction between instruction type and

Item #	Ages in Months	Item name, Position, and Description	Score Criteria	Score
16	7	ROLLING *(Lying on back)* Shake Rattle at midline 12 in. above child. Lower rattle to surface on child's left, out of child's reach. Repeat procedure on opposite side.	2 Rolls from back to stomach (both sides) 1 Rolls from back to stomach (on side only) 0 Remains on back	2
17	7	ROLLING *(Lying on back)* Attract child's attention to toy by shaking it to side of child. Repeat procedure on opposite side.	2 Rolls from back to stomach, leading with hips and thighs, folllowed by stomach and then shoulders (both sides) 1 Rolls from back to stomach (one side) 0 Remains on back	2
18	8	MOVING FORWARD *(Lying on stomach)* Place toy 5 ft. in front of child. Say, "Get the toy."	2 Moves forward using arms 1 Moves forward at least 2 ft. but less than 3 ft. using arms 0 Moves less than 2 ft.	1
19	9	RAISING SHOULDERS & BUTTOCKS *(Lying on stomach)* Sit 3 ft. in front of child. Hold your hands out to child and say, "Come here."	2 Raises and bears weight on hands and knees for 5 seconds and rocks back and forth for 2 cycles 1 Raises and bears weight on hands and knees for 1–5 seconds 0 Remains on stomach	1
20	9	CREEPING *(Hand and knees)* Place toy on floor 6 ft. in front of child. Say, "Get the toy." Move toy back as child approaches.	2 Creeps forward on hands and knees, using a cross-lateral pattern for 5 ft. 1 Creeps forward on hands and knees using cross-lateral pattern for 4 ft. or creeps without using cross-lateral pattern for 5 ft. 0 Remains stationary or moves on stomach	0
21	9	CREEPING *(Sitting)* Sit beside child on floor. Say, "Watch me." Demonstrate scooting by using your hands to propel your body forward on your buttocks to retrieve toy. Place toy 5 ft. in front of child. Say, "Scoot like I did and get the toy."	2 Maintains sitting posture and uses hands and legs to scoot forward 3 ft. 1 Maintains sitting posture and scoots forward 1–2 ft. 0 Moves less than 1 ft. forward	0

FIGURE 2.2. Peabody Developmental Motor Scale 2 (PDMS-2) item administration sample.

order ($p = 0.02$) were reported. These finding suggest that instruction modification can affect scores, and that if modified instructions are performed, the normative values should not be reported.[54]

According to the authors, the content validity of PDMS-2 is based on established research on normal children's motor development and on other validated tests assessing motor development. The construct validity of the PDMS-2 was established by confirmatory factor analyses, with results demonstrating that the fine motor and the gross motor composites are two separate constructs within general movement. Concurrent validity between the BSID-III and the PDMS-2 was studied in 184 eighteen-month-old children. High correlations were found between total motor ($r = 0.88$), gross motor ($r = 0.88$), and fine motor scores ($r = 0.79$). Both assessments had 93% agreement on classification for motor impairment; 23 children were identified by both assessments as having motor impairments, but 12 children were identified differently on each assessment (7 as impaired on PDMS-2 but average on Bayley-III; 5 as impaired on Bayley-III but average on PDMS-2). Both the Bayley-III and PDMS-2 identify motor delays in children; however, clinicians should be aware of the concurrent validity as each assessment may lead to differing results.[55]

ADVANTAGES/DISADVANTAGES The PDMS-2 is a standardized, reliable, and valid assessment tool with a broad age range for assessing infants and young children. Subtest composites can be scored separately, easing administration, and the 3-point scoring system enables examiners to identify emerging skills and to measure progress in children who are slow in acquiring new skills. Disadvantages of the PDMS-2 include absence of normative data on European children, long administration time for younger children, and the absence of a short form.[56]

Bruininks–Oseretsky Test of Motor Proficiency— Second Edition

The BOT-2 is the second revision of the Bruininks–Oseretsky Test of Motor Proficiency (BOTMP) developed by Dr. Robert H. Bruininks.[57] The BOT-2 provides a comprehensive assessment of motor skills, including differentiated measures of fine and gross motor proficiency.

TEST MEASURES AND TARGET POPULATION The BOT-2 is designed to assess gross and fine motor functioning in children and is used to support diagnosis of motor impairments, screen for motor deficits, assist in educational placement decisions, and can be used as a means for planning and evaluating various motor development curricula. The test is appropriate for children aged 4 through 21.[57]

TEST CONSTRUCTION AND STANDARDIZATION The revision of the BOTMP began in 2002 with a development team consisting of the authors, test directors, and researchers. The revision provided contemporary norms, improved test organization and content, and addressed current user needs. The BOT-2 has been standardized on a sample of 1,520 children from 38 states. Over 11% of the normative sample included children with disabilities. The sample selection was random and stratified across sex, race/ethnicity, socioeconomic status, and disability status within each of the 12 age groups.

TEST FORMAT Type The BOT-2 is norm-referenced, and it involves individually administered tasks with direct observation and assessment of a child in a structured environment.

Content The BOT-2 assesses proficiency in four motor-area composites: Fine Manual Control, Manual Coordination, Body Coordination, and Strength and Agility. These four motor-area composites each comprise two of the eight BOT-2 subtests. The fifth composite, the Total Motor Composite, is devised from all eight subtests.

The relationship of the eight subtests to the composites is shown in Figure 2.3.

Administration The Complete Form can be administered in 40 to 60 minutes, with an extra 10 minutes needed to prepare the testing area. The Short Form (used for screening purposes) can be administered in 15 to 20 minutes, with an additional 5 minutes needed for area setup. The Short Form consists of 14 BOT-2 items carefully selected from all eight subtests and yields a single score of overall motor proficiency. Two short testing sessions are recommended for young children. Procedures for administration and scoring of the test are well written and are shown in the manual. Materials needed to administer the BOT-2 are provided in the standardized test kit with the exception of stopwatch and tape measure.

Scoring Scoring may be completed using the BOT-2 ASSIST™ software or through hand scoring. The child's raw scores are recorded during the administration of the test and are converted first to point scores, then to standard scores, approximate age equivalents, and percentile rank (see Fig. 2.4 for a sample record form for BOT-2). Five descriptive categories are also included on the scoring sheet to assist in communicating test results to examinees, parents, and teachers.

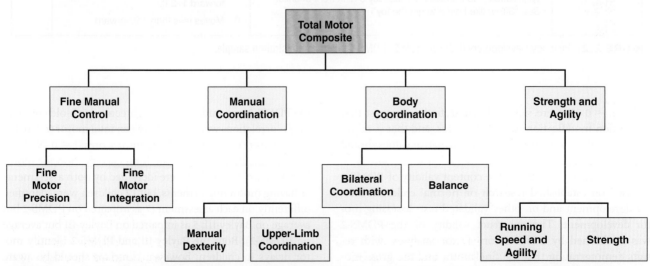

FIGURE 2.3. Relationship of the eight subtests of the Bruininks–Oseretsky Test of Motor Proficiency (BOT) to the BOT-2 composites. (Adapted figures from the Bruininks-Oseretsky Test of Motor Proficiency, Second Edition [BOT-2]. Copyright 2005 NCS Pearson, Inc. Reproduced with permission. All rights reserved. "BOT" is a trademark, in the U.S. and/or other countries, of Pearson Education Inc. or its affiliates.)

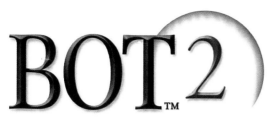

Bruininks-Oseretsky Test
of Motor Proficiency, *Second Edition*
Robert H. Bruininks, PhD, & Brett D. Bruininks

Gross Motor Record Form

	Year	Month	Day
Test Date	___	___	___
Birth Date	___	___	___
Chronological Age	___	___	___

Preferred Foot/Leg:	Right	Left

Norms Used:	■ Female	■ Male	■ Combined

Examinee Name _____   Sex _____   Grade _____

Examiner Name _____   School/Clinic _____

	Total Point Score	Scale Score Mean = 15, *SD* = 5 (Tables B.1–B.3)	Standard Score Mean = 50, *SD* = 10 (Tables B.4–B.6, S.5)	Confidence Interval: 90% *or* 95% (Tables C.1, C.2, S.6)		%ile Rank (Tables B.4–B.6, S.5)	Age Equiv. (Tables B.14–B.16)	Descriptive Category (Table C.13)
				Band	Interval			
4 Bilateral Coordination	___	☐		+ ___ – ___	– ___	___	___	___
5 Balance	___	☐		+ ___ – ___	– ___	___	___	___
Body Coordination	Sum	☐	☐	+ ___ – ___	– ___	___	___	___
6 Running Speed and Agility	___	☐		+ ___ – ___	– ___	___	___	___
8 Strength Push-up: Knee Full	___	☐		+ ___ – ___	– ___	___	___	___
Strength and Agility	Sum	☐	☐	+ ___ – ___	– ___	___	___	___
Gross Motor Composite	Sum		☐	+ ___ – ___	– ___	___	___	___

DIRECTIONS

During the testing session, record the examinee's performance on each item.

After the testing session, convert each item raw score to a point score using the conversion table provided. For items needing two trials, convert the better of the two raw scores. Then, record the point score in the appropriate oval in the Point Score column.

For each subtest, add the item point scores, and record the total in the oval labeled Total Point Score and on the appropriate line on the cover page.

PEARSON

PsychCorp is an imprint of Pearson Clinical Assessment.
Pearson Executive Office 5601 Green Valley Drive Bloomington, MN 55437
800.627.7271 www.PearsonClinical.com
Copyright © 2011 NCS Pearson, Inc. All rights reserved.
Warning: No part of this publication may be reproduced or transmitted in any form or by any means, electronic or mechanical, including photocopy, recording, or any information storage and retrieval system, without permission in writing from the copyright owner.
Pearson, the **PSI logo, PsychCorp,** and **BOT** are trademarks in the U.S. and/or other countries of Pearson Education, Inc., or its affiliate(s).
Portions of this work were previously published.
Printed in the United States of America.
  3 4 5 6 7 8 9 10 11 12 A B C D E

⊕ PsychCorp

Product Number 58043

FIGURE 2.4. Recording form for the eight subtests of the Bruininks–Oseretsky Test of Motor Proficiency. (Adapted figures from the Bruininks-Oseretsky Test of Motor Proficiency, Second Edition [BOT-2]. Copyright 2005 NCS Pearson, Inc. Reproduced with permission. All rights reserved. "BOT" is a trademark, in the U.S. and/or other countries, of Pearson Education Inc. or its affiliates.)

The Total Motor Composite is derived from the sum of the four motor-area composite standard scores and is the most reliable and preferred measure of overall motor proficiency.

Interpretation Tables of norms are provided, and by comparing derived scores with the scores of subjects tested in the standardization program, users can interpret a child's performance in relation to a national reference group.

RELIABILITY AND VALIDITY Test–retest reliability coefficients for the subtests are in the upper 0.70s for examinees aged 4 through 7 and 8 through 12, and 0.69 for examinees aged 13 through 21. The mean of the composite correlation coefficients is in the low 0.80s for examinees aged 4 through 12, and is 0.77 for examinees aged 13 through 21.[57] Internal consistency reliability is high, with the mean subtest reliability in three age groups ranging from the high 0.70s to the low 0.80s.

Interrater reliability coefficients are extremely high at 0.98 and 0.99 for Manual Coordination, Body Coordination, and Strength and Agility composites. The Fine Motor Control composite coefficient is also high at 0.92.

Evidence supporting the use of the BOT-2 to assess gross and fine motor proficiency of individuals aged 4 through 21 is provided through test content, internal structure, clinical group differences, and relationships with other tests of motor skills. Content and construct validity studies comparing BOT-2 scores with scores on the BOTMP, PDMS-2, and the Test of Visual Motor Skills, Revised (TVMS-R) are reported in the manual.

ADVANTAGES AND DISADVANTAGES A review of the BOT-2 by Deitz et al. summarizes the following strengths and limitations of the test. The strengths include the following: (1) the Administration Easel, which provides photos for test items, allowing efficient and standard test administration; (2) test items reflecting typical childhood activities (face validity); (3) the construct validation of the test; (4) current norms reflecting the demographics of the United States; and (5) moderate to strong interrater and test–retest reliabilities of the Complete Form Total Motor Composite and Short Form. The reported limitations include (1) weak test–retest reliability coefficients for some subtests and motor-area composites for some age groups; (2) the scoring process can be time intensive and tedious; and (3) the difficulty of the items for 4-year-old children who are developing typically or 5-year-old children with delays.[58]

RECENT RESEARCH The compatibility and usefulness of the complete (BOT-2 CF) and short form (BOT-2 SF) of the BOT-2 were evaluated on 153 neurotypical middle-school-aged children. Previous studies indicated the BOT-2 SF provides significantly higher results than the BOT-2 CF. In this study, the BOT-2 SF provided a statistically significantly lower standard score, $x = 45.87$ (± 5.41), compared to the BOT-2 CF, $x = 47.57$ (± 8.29), $p < 0.05$, with middle effect size value, Hays' $\omega^2 = 0.09$. The BOT-2 SF does not provide practically significant different results compared to the BOT-2 CF when using a proper scale for comparing both versions. The study authors suggest the BOT-2 SF and BOT-2 CF may not measure the same behavioral domain.[59]

Comprehensive Developmental Scales

Comprehensive developmental scales assess all areas of infant and child development and are well suited for multidisciplinary and area assessment teams. Developmental areas assessed include physical, cognitive, communication, social–emotional, and adaptive language, complying with Part C of Individuals with Disabilities Education Act (IDEA) regulations for service eligibility for early intervention and special education services.[60]

Bayley Scales of Infant and Toddler Development—4th Edition

The Bayley-4[61] is a revision of the Bayley-III[62]. Applications of Bayley-4 include identifying infants and toddlers with developmental delay, assisting practitioners with intervention planning, monitoring a child's progress after intervention, and conducting research. Changes from BSID-III occurred in several areas: Administration and Scoring, Content updates, Norms and clinical studies, Administration time, and Digital delivery.[61]

TEST MEASURES AND TARGET POPULATION The Bayley-4 assesses infant and toddler development across five domains: Cognitive, Language, Motor, Social–Emotional, and Adaptive. The Cognitive, Language, and Motor domains are assessed directly through item administration to the child, whereas the Social–Emotional and Adaptive domains are assessed through caregiver questionnaire. The Bayley-4 is individually administered to infants and children between 16 days and 42 months of age.

TEST CONSTRUCTION AND STANDARDIZATION The original BSID was derived from several infant and child developmental scales and a broad cross-section of infant and child research.[63] The creation of items for the Bayley-4 was based on developmental research and theory that identifies behaviors typical for normal development in young children. Item administration for all four of the Bayley Scales (BSID, BSID-II, Bayley-III, Bayley-4) occurs in a modified power sequence; that is, items are typically ordered according to their degree of difficulty.

The normative information in the Bayley-4 is based on a national standardization sample representative of the U.S. population for infants 16 days through 42 months of age. Normative data were collected from 2017 to 2019. The sample included 1,700 demographically representative children divided into 17 age groups composed of 100 participants for the Cognitive, Motor, and Language Standardization Scale, and 320 children divided into 8 age groups for the Social–Emotional Scale. Seven hundred and fifty children were included in the normative sample for the Social–Emotional

Standardization Scale collected during the Vineland-3 standardization.[61]

TEST FORMAT

Type The test is norm-referenced. Information is obtained by direct observation and interaction with the child.

Content The Bayley-4 contains the following scales: (1) Cognitive-items assess sensorimotor development, exploration and manipulation, object relatedness, concept formation, memory, and other aspects of cognitive functioning; (2) Language-items assess receptive and expressive communication; (3) Motor-items assess fine motor and gross motor skills; (4) Social–Emotional-items assess social and emotional milestones in children based on the Greenspan Social–Emotional Growth Chart: A Screening Questionnaire for Infants and Young Children; and (5) Adaptive Behavior-items assess adaptive skill functioning in Communication, Daily Living Skills, and Socialization based on Vineland Adaptive Behavior Scales—Third Edition (Vineland-3)[64,65] (Display 2.1).

Administration The time required for administration of the Bayley-4 varies with test familiarity, specific strengths and limitations of the child, and test session behavior. The reported completion time ranges from 30 to 70 minutes. Administration is through paper-and-pencil form or digitally through Q-global. Forms include Cognitive, Language, and Motor record Forms, Motor response booklets, and Social–Emotional and Adaptive Behavior questionnaires.

Based on an age-specific start point, the child must receive a score of 2 on the first three consecutive items to move forward (basal level). If the child scores a 0 on the first age-specific item, the examiner goes to previous age-specific item and applies the same rule. The test is discontinued for the particular scale when the child receives scores of 0 for five consecutive items (ceiling level).

Scoring and Interpretation The Bayley-4 uses Polytomous Scoring for the Cognitive, Language, and Motor Scales. For a given test item, the child scores (0) if the response or behavior indicates the skill or behavior is Not Present, (1) if the response or behavior indicates the skill is Emerging, and (2) if the response or behavior indicates Mastery. Certain structured test items are now associated with caregiver questions independent of performance and given the same score values. The raw scores for each subtest are converted to Scaled Scores, Composite Scores, Age Equivalents, Percentile Rank, and Confidence Intervals using tables provided in the manual or through the software on Q-global. Criterion for interpretation can vary by states, but several different criteria are used to diagnose developmental delay including percent delay, SD criterion below the mean, and performance a certain level below CA.

RELIABILITY AND VALIDITY All measures reflect a high degree of reliability in the items, and the Bayley-4 scales are

---

DISPLAY 2.1 Bayley Scales of Infant and Toddler Development 4 (Bayley-4) Items to Be Tested

Adaptive Behavior
- Communication
- Community use
- Functional preacademics
- Home living
- Health and safety
- Leisure
- Self-care
- Self-direction
- Social
- Motor

Cognitive
- Sensorimotor development
- Exploration and manipulation
- Object relatedness
- Concept formation
- Memory
- Habituation
- Visual acuity
- Visual preference
- Object permanence
- Plus other aspects of cognitive processing

Items that measure age-appropriate skills include the following:
- Counting (with one-to-one correspondence and cardinality)
- Visual and tactile exploration
- Object assembly
- Puzzle board completion
- Matching colors
- Comparing masses
- Representational and pretend play
- Discriminating patterns

Language

Expressive communication

Assesses preverbal communications such as:
- Babbling
- Gesturing
- Joint referencing
- Turn taking
- Vocabulary development such as naming objects, pictures, and actions
- Morpho-syntactic development such as use of two-word utterances and use of plurals and verb tense

Receptive communication

Assesses preverbal behaviors and vocabulary development such as:
- The ability to identify objects and pictures that are referenced
- Vocabulary related to morphologic development such as pronouns and prepositions
- Understanding of morphologic markers such as plurals and tense markings

(continued)

2.1 Bayley Scales of Infant and Toddler Development 4 (Bayley-4) Items to Be Tested (*continued*)

Motor

Fine motor

Fine motor skills associated with:
- Prehension
- Perceptual–motor integration
- Motor planning
- Motor speed

Items measure age-appropriate skills including:
- Visual tracking
- Reaching
- Object manipulation
- Grasping
- Children's quality of movement
- Functional hand skills
- Responses to tactile information (sensory integration)

Gross motor

Items assess:
- Static positioning (e.g., head control, sitting, standing)
- Dynamic movement including locomotion (crawling, walking, running, jumping, walking up and down stairs)
- Quality of movement (coordination when standing up, walking, kicking)
- Balance
- Motor planning
- Perceptual–motor integration (e.g., imitating postures)

Social–Emotional
- Determines the mastery of early capacities of social–emotional growth
- Monitors healthy social and emotional functioning
- Monitors progress in early intervention programs
- Detects deficits or problems with developmental social–emotional capacities

List of assessment area domains and subdomains from Bayley N. *Bayley Scales of Infant and Toddler Development (Bayley-4)*. 4th ed. San Antonio, TX: The Psychological Corporation; 2019. Copyright © 2019 NCS Pearson, Inc. Reproduced with permission. All rights reserved. "*Bayley Scales of Infant and Toddler Development*" is a trademark, in the United States and/or other countries, of Pearson Education, Inc. or its affiliates(s).

equally reliable for assessing individuals with different levels of development or individuals with different clinical diagnoses: Internal Consistency for Cognitive, Language and Motor Scale, Subtest Level: range from 0.93 to 0.95; Composite Level: range from 0.95 to 0.96.

Four hundred and twelve children were included to provide evidence of internal consistency for special groups (autism spectrum disorder, developmental delay, Down syndrome, language delay, moderate/late premature, motor impairment, prenatal drug/alcohol exposure, specific language impairment, and very/extreme premature): The reliability coefficients ranged from 0.97 to 0.99; Social–Emotional

Scale, range from 0.85 to 0.91, and Adaptive Behavior Scale, range from 0.91 to 0.98.[61]

Classification accuracy was used in comparing appropriate groups with typically developing peers as measured by the area under the receiver operating characteristic (ROC) curve. ROC area estimates range from 0.50 (chance accuracy) to 1.00 (perfect accuracy). Traditional benchmarks suggest that values greater than or equal to 0.90 are excellent, 0.80 to 0.89 are good, 0.70 to 0.79 are fair, and less than 0.70 are poor. Cognitive and Language scales range between 0.80 and 0.89 (good) and Motor Scales range is 0.90 (excellent).[61]

ADVANTAGES The Bayley-4 is the product of decades of research in infant and child development. The five distinct scales are designed to meet federal and state guidelines for early childhood assessment. The psychometric qualities and clinical utility have improved with the newest revision, while maintaining the basic qualities of the earlier Bayley Scales. The Bayley-4 has fewer items to administer relative to the Bayley-III, reducing administration time, and incorporates parent questions into the scoring items.

DISADVANTAGES Although reduced in total number of items, the time to administer the assessment is lengthy and can be difficult to complete in many health care settings. Future research is needed to assess Bayley-4's ability to estimate developmental status.

Battelle Developmental Inventory—Second Edition Normative Update

The Battelle Developmental Inventory—Second Edition Normative Update (BDI-2NU) is a comprehensive developmental assessment for children used to measure development in children with and without disabilities, to screen for children at risk for developmental delay, and to assist in development of individualized family service plans and individualized education plans.[66] It may be administered by a team of health care professionals or by an individual provider.

TEST MEASURES AND TARGET POPULATION The BDI-2NU measures development in five domains: Adaptive, Personal-Social, Communication, Motor, and Cognitive. Each domain contains subdomains whose entry points in the test are determined by age or estimated ability of the child. The BDI-2NU is appropriate for children from birth to 7 years, 11 months. The BDI-2 Screening Test is also available, consisting of a subset of items from the BDI-2 item pool.

TEST CONSTRUCTION AND STANDARDIZATION The original BDI, developed in 1984,[67] has been used for determining children's eligibility for services as well as measuring change longitudinally in program-based studies, particularly for its assessment in the five domains of development listed in Part C of IDEA. The BDI-2 was the result of a 5-year development process including updating of test items, refining the scoring criteria, revising the domain/subdomain structure, and new normative sampling. The second edition features colorful items and child-friendly manipulatives for all ages, new comprehensive norms, clear and scripted interview items with follow-up probes, computed or hand-scored processing, flexible administration, and an expanded range of items for all ages. The skills comprising the 450 test items were chosen based on their relationship to functional life skills and ability to be impacted by educational intervention. The BDI-2NU has the same test content, items and structure, but new norms based on 2015 U.S. census. Normative data were collected on 2,500 children from birth to 7 years, 11 months, reflecting the changing demographics in the United States in 2015.

TEST FORMAT

Type The BDI-2NU is a norm-referenced and criterion-referenced comprehensive developmental assessment.

Content The five domains with subdomains include (1) Adaptive: Personal Responsibility and Self-Care; (2) Personal-Social: Adult Interaction, Self-Concept and Social Growth, and Peer Interaction; (3) Motor: Fine Motor, Gross Motor, and Perceptual Motor; (4) Communication: Expressive and Receptive; and (5) Cognitive: Perceptual Discrimination/Conceptual Development, Reasoning and Academic Skills, and Attention and Memory.

Administration The BDI-2NU includes modifications that allow it to be used with infants or children with special needs or disabilities, as well as different language versions. There are multiple administration options including structured, play-based activities, observation, and scripted interviews for parents or caregivers. A single provider or a team consisting of multiple disciplines can administer the test. A Spanish User's Guide is available in the Appendix. The complete BDI-2NU can be administered in 60 to 90 minutes, and 10 to 30 minutes for the Screening Test.

Scoring/Interpretation The BDI-2NU can be hand-scored or scored with optional scoring software, BDI-2 Data Manager™. The child's performance is scored based on standardized criteria using a simple 3-point scoring system (2 = mastered milestone, 1 = emerging milestone, 0 = future learning objective). At the subdomain level, norm-referenced scores are provided (scaled scores with a mean of 10; SD = 3; score range, 1 to 19). The subdomain scores combine to form the five BDI-2NU domain scores and the overall BDI-2NU Developmental Quotient (standard scores with a mean of 100, SD = 15, score range from 40 to 160). Percentiles and Confidence Intervals are provided for the domain scores and Developmental Quotient. Additionally, age-equivalent tables are provided. The BDI-2 Data Manager software provides consistency in determining raw score totals and norm-referenced scores. Narrative reports can be generated for parents and professionals, as well as score reports and aggregate reports for program evaluation purposes.

RELIABILITY AND VALIDITY Overall test score reliability is reported in the manual at 0.99.[66] Internal consistency using the split-half method is reported as reliabilities across ages. Reliabilities on domains averaged 0.90 to 0.96, and 0.85 to 0.95 on subdomains. Concurrent and criterion validity was obtained with the original BDI, BSID-II, Woodcock Johnson III (WJ III), Denver II, preschool language scale-4 (PLS-4), Vineland Social-Emotional Early Childhood Scales (Vineland SEEC), and The Wechsler Preschool and Primary Scale of Intelligence (WPPSI-III). The BDI-2 exceeds the recommended level of accuracy for testing (0.75) with a sensitivity of 0.83 and a specificity of 0.85. Spies et al. assessed the use of the BDI-2 as an early screener for autism spectrum disorders and reported high sensitivity (0.94) with a determined cutoff score of 96 (1.5 SD from the mean of the autism spectrum disorders group).[68]

ADVANTAGES/DISADVANTAGES The BDI-2NU has a flexible framework for gathering information and can be used by multiple providers. Specific guidelines for providers working with children with developmental disabilities assist in assessment administration, and the inclusion of a screening test is beneficial in settings with time constraints. The 3-point scoring system of 0, 1, and 2 accounts for emerging and developing skills. The time required to administer the complete battery of items is a limitation, and providers may have difficulty scoring the test when there is disagreement between observation and interview data.

Examination of Functional Capabilities

Functional assessments examine what the child does in the context of daily life across multiple domains. What a child actually does in the community may be entirely different from their physical capability to perform the activity. It is important, therefore, to assess functional performance as well as functional capacity. Functional assessments are often grounded in a similar conceptual framework as the World Health Organization's ICF.[69] The approach is to assess the child's participation in daily routines, the activities performed, and the environmental and personal factors that contribute to the child's daily function.

According to Haley, the concept of disability and functional assessment incorporates the following key concepts:

1. A child may have serious motor impairments that are not always reflected by the level of functional limitation or disability.
2. Functional deficits may or may not lead to a restriction in social activities and important childhood roles.
3. Environmental factors, family expectations, and contextual elements of functional task requirements play an important role in the eventual level of disability and handicap of the child.[70]

Comprehensive functional assessment instruments contain mobility, transfer, self-care, and social function items;

they include measurement dimensions of assistance and adaptive equipment; and they incorporate developmental stages of functional skill attainment.[71] Functional assessments give pediatric physical therapists information on how a child's disability or movement disorder impacts task requirements of daily life routines.

Pediatric Evaluation of Disability Inventory—Computer Adaptive Test

The Pediatric Evaluation of Disability Inventory—Computer Adaptive Test (PEDI-CAT) is a full revision of the PEDI based on years of experience, feedback, and formal research with the original PEDI.[72,73] The PEDI-CAT is intended to be used as an instrument to detect functional deficits or delays, as an evaluative instrument to monitor progress in pediatric rehabilitation programs, and/or as an outcome measure for program evaluation, either in pediatric rehabilitation setting or in an educational setting.

TEST MEASURES AND TARGET POPULATION The PEDI-CAT utilizes preinstalled software to estimate a child's abilities from an item bank of 254 activities, measuring function in four domains: (1) Daily Activities, (2) Mobility, (3) Social/Cognitive, and (4) Responsibility. The revisions to the original PEDI include (1) items extending the functional content assessed in self-care, mobility, and social functioning domains; (2) a 4-point difficulty scale replacing the dichotomous capable/unable scale; (3) addition of illustrations for self-care and mobility items; (4) replacement of Caregiver Assistance section with a "Responsibility" section; and (5) creation of a CAT platform for content administration in each domain.[73] The PEDI-CAT is designed for use with children and youth (birth through 20 years of age) with a variety of physical and/or behavioral conditions (Display 2.2).

TEST CONSTRUCTION AND STANDARDIZATION Content validity of the PEDI-CAT was established through a review of existing adult and pediatric functional assessments and input

from practicing clinicians, parents of children with and without disabilities, and experts in the field of rehabilitation.[74]

The PEDI-CAT's normative standardization sample was recruited through an online panel and resulted in a nationally representative sample of 2,205 parents of children less than 21 years of age in the contiguous United States.

The clinical validation sample of 703 children with disabilities (behavioral, intellectual, and physical) was also recruited through the online panel as well as through two clinical sites in the Northwest Central and Northeastern United States.[73]

TEST FORMAT

Type The PEDI-CAT can be used to identify functional delay (with normative scores), to examine improvement after intervention (scaled scores), or to evaluate and monitor progress in research groups.

Content The PEDI-CAT measures abilities in three functional domains: Daily Activities (68 items), Mobility (75 items), and Social/Cognitive (60 items). The PEDI-CAT's Responsibility domain (51 items) measures the extent to which the caregiver or child takes responsibility for managing complex, multistep life tasks.

Administration The CAT platform allows items to be administered based on previous responses, thus avoiding irrelevant items or items too easy or difficult for the child. Item administration begins in the middle range of difficulty or responsibility, and the response to that item dictates which item will appear next (easier or harder item). With the administration of subsequent items, the score is reestimated and either the assessment ends if a "stopping" rule has been satisfied or continues on with new items until the "stopping" rule has been met. The PEDI-CAT software then calculates and displays results, including an item map, age percentiles, and standard scores.[73] As with the original paper-and-pencil PEDI, the PEDI-CAT can be administered by professional judgment of clinicians or educators who are familiar with the child or by parent report. Two versions of the PEDI-CAT exist: the "Speedy-CAT," which requires only 15 or fewer items per domain to be administered,

---

DISPLAY 2.2 PEDI-CAT Domains

Daily Activities 68 Items	Social/Cognitive 60 Items	Mobility 75 Items	Responsibility 51 Items
• Getting dressed	• Interaction	• Basic movement and transfers	• Organization and planning
• Keeping clean	• Communication	• Standing and walking	• Taking care of daily needs
• Home tasks	• Everyday cognition	• Steps and inclines	• Health management
• Eating and mealtime	• Self-management	• Running and playing	• Staying safe
		• Mobility device specific items	

Three domains aligned with ICF activity dimension: Daily Activities, Social/Cognitive, and Mobility. One domain aligned with ICF participation dimension: Responsibility.
Table created from Fragala-Pinkham M, Shore B, Kramer J. Introduction to the Pediatric Disability Inventory Computerized Adaptive Test (PEDI-CAT) for children with cerebral palsy: a new option for measuring function in Daily Activities, Mobility, Social/Cognitive and Responsibility. From AACPDM 69th Annual Meeting, October 21–24, 2015.

and the "Content-Balanced CAT," which includes approximately 30 items per domain with a balance of item content within each domain.[73]

Scoring Each of the PEDI-CAT domains is self-contained and can be administered individually or in a combination appropriate for assessment of the child. The level of difficulty for each domain is measured using a 4-point response scale: easy, a little hard, hard, and unable.

The Responsibility domain has its own 5-point Responsibility Scale with responses ranging from "Adult/caregiver has full responsibility; the child does not take any responsibility" to "Child takes full responsibility without any direction, supervision, or guidance from an adult/caregiver."

The PEDI-CAT software utilizes item response theory (IRT) statistical models to estimate a child's abilities from a minimal number of the most relevant items or from a set number of items within each domain. All respondents begin with the same item in each domain in the middle of the range of difficulty or responsibility and the response to that item then dictates which item will appear next (a harder or easier item), thus tailoring the items to the child and avoiding irrelevant items. The CAT program then displays the results instantly.

Normative standard scores (provided as age percentiles and T scores) and Scaled Scores are available for 21 age groups (intervals of 1 year).

Interpretation Normative scores provided as age percentiles and T scores are based on a child's CA and intended for use by clinicians so that they may interpret a particular child's functioning relative to others of the same age. Scaled scores provide a way to look at a child's current functional skills and progress in these skills over time. Scaled scores are especially helpful in documenting improvements in functional skills for children not expected to exhibit or regain normative levels of functioning. Scores are displayed instantly at the completion of an assessment. A Detailed Score Report and a Summary Score Report are available. Item Maps represent a reasonable, sequential pattern of functional skills consistent with children's development and recovery of function and transfer of responsibility from adult to child throughout childhood and young adulthood.

RELIABILITY AND VALIDITY Concurrent validity and reliability of the PEDI-CAT mobility domain with the original PEDI Functional Skills Mobility Scale were investigated by Dumas and Fragala-Pinkman.[75] Strong correlations between scaled scores ($r = 0.82$; $p < 0.001$) indicated strong agreement between the PEDI-CAT and the original PEDI, supporting concurrent validity. ICC coefficients ranged from 0.3390 to 1.000, and agreement results ranged from 60% to 100% for eight items measured. Both assessment tools identified children with limitations with functional mobility, with the PEDI-CAT identifying a larger percentage of older children with functional limitations (Display 2.3).

ADVANTAGES AND DISADVANTAGES An advantage of the PEDI-CAT is that it can be used for infants, children, and youth up to 21 years of age, which allows for tracking of function for children with disabilities over a longer period of time. A benefit of a computer adaptive test is that it is not a fixed paper-and-pencil format, and revisions can be made more easily by updating the software. In addition, the PEDI-CAT was developed on a 20 to 80 metric to allow items to be easily added at either end of the scale.[73] Disadvantages include skills tested are at a low end of the continuum, items are focused primarily on home-based activities, making testing difficult without parent input, and license renewal is required annually.

Functional Independence Measure for Children

The Functional Independence Measure for Children (WeeFIM) is the pediatric adaptation of the Functional Independence Measure (FIM) for adults of the Uniform Data System for Medical Rehabilitation (UDS).[76] The WeeFIM measures function in a developmental context and is intended to help monitor children with disabilities as they grow into adults who function at a maximum level of independence. The WeeFIM-II system includes the WeeFIM instrument, the WeeFIM instrument 0–3 Module, and an Internet-based software application with a report generator and quarterly aggregate reports.[77]

TEST MEASURES AND TARGET POPULATION The WeeFIM consists of 18 items within three domains—Self-care, Mobility, and Cognition—and is designed for use with children between the ages of 6 months and 7 years, but may be used with older children with developmental disabilities and mental ages less than 7 years.[76] The WeeFIM is a measure of disability, not impairment, and is intended to measure what a child with a disability actually does, not what they ought to be able to do or might be able to do if circumstances were different. The WeeFIM contains a minimum number of items and is designed to be useful across disciplines by trained clinicians.

TEST CONSTRUCTION AND STANDARDIZATION
The WeeFIM was built on the organizational format of the FIM for adults and is developed as a collaboration among an interdisciplinary team who reviewed gross motor, fine motor, receptive and expressive language, adaptive, cognitive, and educational instruments.[76] A normative sample of 417 children, aged 6 months to 8 years, without developmental delays was studied by Msall et al.[78] A significant correlation was found between the age of the child in months and the total WeeFIM scores for children aged 2 to 5 years ($n = 222$, $r = 0.80$, $p < 0.01$). Normative values for the WeeFIM are presented in the manual in 3-month intervals, with the first grouping from 5 to 7 months and the last grouping for children 83 months and older. Because the WeeFIM total ratings tend to flatten beyond 83 months at a total rating of 120, there is no additional breakdown provided beyond this age range.

TEST FORMAT

Type The test is criterion based and is a descriptive measure of the caregiver and special resources that are required because of functional limitations.

Content The test consists of three domains: Self-care (eight items), Mobility (five items), and Cognition (five items) (Display 2.4).

DISPLAY 2.4 Functional Independence Measure for Children (WeeFIM) Domains

Self-care
1. Eating
2. Grooming
3. Bathing
4. Dressing—upper body
5. Dressing—lower body
6. Toileting
7. Bladder management
8. Bowel management

Mobility
1. Transfer chair, wheelchair
2. Transfer toilet
3. Transfer tub/shower
4. Crawl/walk/wheelchair
5. Stairs

Cognition
1. Comprehension
2. Expression
3. Social interaction
4. Problem solving
5. Memory

Administration/Scoring Assessment using the WeeFIM should be based on direct observation of the child. If direct observation is not possible, assessments may be completed by interviewing parents or caregivers who are familiar with the child's everyday activities. Each of the 18 items to assess the child's function is rated on a 7-level ordinal scale, from (1) total dependence to (7) complete independence (Display 2.5).

The manual describes each of these levels as a general overview of the ratings and also provides specific guidelines for applying the levels scale for each of the 18 items.

Interpretation The WeeFIM measures functional abilities and the "need for assistance" associated with varying levels of disability in children. The scores obtained are utilized as baseline descriptive clinical assessments of severity, assist in selection of treatment goals and evaluation of treatment, and aid in identifying the child and family's need for support. It is designed to track functional status and outcomes over time both in preschool years and in the early elementary school years.

RELIABILITY AND VALIDITY
Test–retest and interrater reliability for the total WeeFIM are 0.99 and 0.95, respectively.[79] Data related to construct and discriminative validity indicate that the WeeFIM is a valid measure of disability related to functional independence.[80] Concurrent validity between WeeFIM and PEDI was reported by Ziviani et al., with Spearman correlation coefficients greater than 0.88 for self-care, transportation/locomotion, and communication/social function, indicating that the two tests measure similar constructs.[81]

ADVANTAGES AND DISADVANTAGES
The WeeFIM has a short administration time from 10 to 15 minutes and is useful for communicating a child's ability to cope with daily living tasks in a common language among health care providers. Use of the WeeFIM does require a subscription fee, and if

---

DISPLAY 2.5 Levels of Function for the Functional Independence Measure for Children (WeeFIM)

No Helper
7 = Complete independence (timely, safely)
6 = Modified independence (device needed)

Helper

Modified Dependence
5 = Supervision
4 = Minimal assist (child = 75%–99%)
3 = Moderate assist (child = 50%–74%)

Complete Dependence
2 = Maximal assistance (child = 25%–49%)
1 = Total assistance (child = 0%–24%)

institutions subscribe to a test database, accreditation of users is required. Information necessary for guiding clinical decision-making may be difficult to extract from documentation of caregiver assistance alone.

School Function Assessment

The School Function Assessment (SFA) was developed by Coster, Deeney, Haltiwanger, and Haley in response to the need for an effective functional performance measure for children attending elementary school.[82] A reliable and valid assessment tool specific to the student's needs and abilities and performance within the school environment is necessary for effective evaluation and service planning.

TEST MEASURES AND TARGET POPULATION The SFA measures a student's performance of functional tasks that support participation in academic and social school-related activities for students in kindergarten through grade 6. The SFA permits students with disabilities to use alternative methods to accomplish functional tasks, recognizing that function is defined primarily by what an individual is able to do.

TEST CONSTRUCTION AND STANDARDIZATION In 2002, Burtner et al. reported that the most frequently used assessment tools used in southwest states' school systems were assessments designed to measure only fine and gross motor skills.[83] In fact, many of the assessment tools utilized provide little information about the school-related abilities of the children being evaluated. Thus, the SFA was developed to fulfill the need for an effective functional assessment of students' performance in the context of the school environment. The SFA was standardized on a sample of 678 students comprising two groups: 363 students with special needs and 315 students in regular education programs at 112 sites in 40 states and Puerto Rico.[84]

TEST FORMAT
Type The SFA is a standardized, criterion-referenced assessment tool.

Content The SFA consists of three sections: Participation, Task Supports, and Activity Performance.[82] Participation is measured in six school activity settings: general or special education classrooms, playground, transportation to/from school, bathroom, transitions to/from class, and mealtimes. The Task Support section measures adaptations made and assistance given to the individual during school-related functions. The four scales in this section include Physical Task Support—Assistance, Physical Task Support—Adaptations, Cognitive/Behavioral Task Support—Assistance, and Cognitive/Behavioral Task Support—Adaptations. The Activity Performance Section contains two major categories: Physical Tasks and Cognitive/Behavioral Tasks, measuring performance in school-related functional activities such as following school rules, using school materials, and communicating needs.

Administration/Scoring In the Participation section, a 6-point rating system (1 = participation is extremely limited to 6 = full participation) is used for each of the six school activity settings to indicate whether the student's participation is similar to that of an age-related/grade peer. In the Task Supports section, a 4-point rating system (1 = extensive assistance/adaptation to 4 = no assistance/adaptation) is used to examine the extent of assistance and adaptations provided to the student. In the Activity Performance Section, the activities are rated on a 4-point scale (1 = does not perform to 4 = consistent performance) with specific criteria defining performance. The raw scores for each section are converted to criterion scores on a 1 to 100 continuum using scoring tables provided in the SFA manual.[82] Criterion scores are then compared with criterion cutoff scores. Detailed guidelines for completion of the assessment are provided in the SFA *Rating Scale Guide* and the *Record Form* (Fig. 2.5).

Interpretation Criterion scores are interpreted as a measure of the student's current functional performance relative to the overall participation, need for services, or functional performance represented in each particular scale. A score of 100 represents a criterion of full grade-appropriate functioning in a particular area. To identify when a student's performance is below what is expected of his or her same-grade peers, the criterion scores are compared with the criterion cutoff scores. The criterion cutoff scores were derived from the sample of students in regular education programs. Five percent or fewer from this population would be expected to have scores below these cutoff points.[84]

RELIABILITY AND VALIDITY Test–retest reliability estimates reported in the SFA manual ranges from $r = 0.90$ to $r = 0.98$ and internal consistency measure estimates (Cronbach's α) range from $\alpha = 0.95$ to 0.98.[82] Validity studies evaluating content were conducted during the development of the SFA. The SFA was determined to contain items that were both relevant and distinct among different levels of function and is both a comprehensive and relevant examination for students with disabilities in elementary school.[84] Hwang et al. examined the known-group validity of the SFA comparing scores of three different groups of children (general education students without disabilities, students with learning disabilities, and students with cerebral palsy).[85] Significant differences were found across all parts of the SFA among the three groups of students supporting validity of the SFA. Interrater reliability between occupational therapists and teachers administering the SFA was assessed on 16 students' ratings. ICCs demonstrated moderate relationships (ICCs from 0.68 to 0.73) between teachers and occupational therapist ratings.[86]

ADVANTAGES/DISADVANTAGES The SFA is based on current models of function and special education legislation, with content reflecting the functional requirements of elementary school environments utilizing transdisciplinary focus and language. The criterion-referenced scales measure meaningful

PART II Task Supports

Directions: Read the description of each task provided below. Then refer to the rating criteria for Part II provided in the *Rating Scale Guide* to determine the rating that best describes the student's needs for additional help or for modifications to perform school-related functional tasks. Circle the appropriate rating next to each task. Sum the ratings within each scale to obtain the total raw score. Record the total raw score for each scale in the appropriate box.

Physical Tasks	ASSISTANCE	ADAPTATIONS
Travel: moving on all different types of indoor and outdoor surfaces; moving around obstacles, through congested or narrow spaces, or in a line; moving all distances required in school, including to and from transportation or playground; keeping pace with peers in all school situations, including evacuating the building as necessary.	1 ② 3 4	① 2 3 4
Maintaining and Changing Positions: moving self to and from positions (including chair or wheelchair, standing, floor, and toilet); maintaining stable seated position on floor or toilet; maintaining functional position in seat for 1/2 hour of class instruction or seat work; boarding and disembarking from all vehicles.	1 ②3 4	① 2 3 4
Recreational Movement: playing games involving physical activity, including throwing and catching during ball games; playing kickball; running, jumping, and climbing; and playing on both low and high playground equipment.	1 2 ③4	① 2 3 4
Manipulation With Movement: transporting materials or belongings within and to and from classroom and in mealtime setting; carrying fragile objects or containers with spillable contents; picking up and setting down large and small objects; retrieving objects from table, storage space, or floor; opening and closing all types of doors.	①2 3 4	1 ②3 4
Using Materials: using all classroom tools effectively, including pencils, erasers, markers, scissors, stapler, tape, and glue; opening, closing, and turning pages in books; folding and securing papers; using art materials; and manipulating small game pieces.	① 2 3 4	①2 3 4
Setup and Cleanup: retrieving, gathering, and putting away materials in classroom and lunchroom; opening food or classroom containers; setting up equipment or materials; disposing of waste; wiping up or tidying table top or desk.	①2 3 4	①2 3 4
Eating and Drinking: using all needed utensils; eating and drinking a typical meal, including drinking from a cup without spilling; using a napkin to wipe face and hands; completing mealtime/snack time tasks in the time allowed; drinking from student-accessible water fountain.	① 2 3 4	1 ②3 4
Hygiene: toileting control; completing toileting tasks including wiping, flushing, or managing equipment; washing and drying hands; completing tasks within typical time limits; managing nose care; covering mouth when coughing or sneezing.	①2 3 4	①2 3 4
Clothing Management: putting on and taking off clothing as required for indoor and outdoor use, including fasteners (e.g., small buttons and zippers) and shoes; managing clothing for toileting purposes.	①2 3 4	①2 3 4
DW Respondent's Initials **Physical Tasks**	*13*	*11*
	Assistance Raw Score	Adaptations Raw Score

Complete any of the following three tasks that are applicable to this student in this school. Record raw scores in the optional tasks section of the Summary Score Form. Do not add these scores to the total raw scores on this page.

	ASSISTANCE	ADAPTATIONS
Up/Down Stairs: moving up and down a full flight of stairs (at least 12 steps); carrying objects up and down stairs; maintaining regular speed on stairs.	①2 3 4	①2 3 4
Written Work: producing written work (letters, words, and numbers) of acceptable quality; organizing items on lines, in columns, or on a page; copying from a textbook or blackboard; sustaining physical effort on written tasks; maintaining speed to keep up with peers.	1 2 3 4	1 2 3 4
Computer and Equipment Use: operating switches; using keyboard or mouse to carry out basic functions; inserting or removing tapes or diskettes; completing work on computer in a timely fashion.	1 2 ③4	①2 3 4

Reminder: Refer to the *Rating Scale Guide* for rating definitions and examples.

4

FIGURE 2.5. Case study form from the School Function Assessment (SFA). (Copyright 1998 NCS Pearson, Inc. Reproduced with permission. All rights reserved.)

functional change, and the separate scales delineate the students' function in specific performance areas. The SFA is useful for prioritizing needs in program planning, IEP development, and documenting progress and effects of intervention. To complete the entire SFA requires a lengthy time commitment up to 1.5 hours, although individual scales are reported to be completed in 5 to 10 minutes. Outcomes for students receiving school-based physical therapy for 6 months, as measured by the SFA, were reported by Effgen et al. in 2016.[87] Criterion scores for many students remained stable (46% to 59%) or improved (37% to 51%), with most students improving in Participation and Maintaining/Changing Positions. Students aged 5 to 7 years showed greater change than 8- to 12-year-olds on five scales. Students with higher gross motor function (GMFCS levels I vs. IV/V and II/III vs. IV/V) showed greater change on nine scales.

Outcome Measures

Pediatric outcome measures and HRQOL measures are used in clinical practice to improve patient–provider communication, improve patient/parent satisfaction, identify hidden morbidities, and assist in clinical decision-making.[88] The development and utilization of HRQOL measures have increased over the last decade in an effort to improve patient health and determine the value of health care services.[89] The incorporation of HRQOL measures in clinical practice serves as a comprehensive evaluation of patient functioning across multiple life domains and can assist in targeting interventions based on patient-perceived needs.

Pediatric Quality-of-Life Inventory

The Pediatric Quality-of-Life Inventory™ (Peds-QL) is a modular instrument designed to measure HRQOL in healthy children and adolescents and those with acute and chronic illnesses.[90] The 23-item Peds-Q Generic Core Scales measure core dimensions of health as delineated by the World Health Organization, as well as school functioning. Peds-Q Condition-Specific and Disease-Specific Modules for asthma, arthritis, cancer, cardiac disease, cerebral palsy, rheumatology, and diabetes are also available for designated clinical populations. The comprehensive list of disease-specific modules continues to be published through MAPI Research Trust with noted additions to include multidimensional fatigue, sickle cell, neuromuscular, and stem cell transplant modules.[91]

TEST MEASURES AND TARGET POPULATION The Peds-QL Generic Core Scales is a multidimensional questionnaire, measuring HRQOL pertaining to physical, emotional, social, and school functioning. Developmentally appropriate forms are available for children 2 to 4, 5 to 7, 8 to 12, and 13 to 18 years of age. The Peds-QL contains a pediatric self-report for children 5 to 18 years and a parent proxy report for children 2 to 18 years.

TEST CONSTRUCTION AND STANDARDIZATION The original Peds-QL 1.0 was designed from a pediatric cancer database as a generic quality-of-life inventory to be used across multiple pediatric populations. Further advancements in the measurement model, including additional constructs and items and a broader age range for child and parent proxy reports, led to additional revisions, with the most recent being Peds-QL 4.0. The initial field trial for the Peds-QL Generic Core Scales was administered to 1,677 families (963 child self-report; 1,629 parent proxy report) recruited from pediatric health care settings.[92,93]

TEST FORMAT

Type The Peds-QL is a norm-referenced HRQOL outcome-measures questionnaire.

Content The Peds-QL contains four multidimensional scales—(1) Physical Functioning (8 items), (2) Emotional Functioning (5 items), (3) Social Functioning (5 items), and (4) School Functioning (5 items)—and provides three summary scores: (1) Total Scale Score (23 items), (2) Physical Health Summary Score (8 items), and (3) Psychosocial Health Summary Score (15 items) (Fig. 2.6).

Administration The Peds-QL Generic Core Scale is presented to the patient (self-report) or the caregiver (parent proxy) to complete, with approximate completion time of 5 minutes or less. The instructions for the Standard Version ask how much of a problem each item has been in the past 1 month. An Acute Version is available for the time interval of the past 7 days.

Scoring Response choices for the questions in each scale include (0) never a problem, (1) almost never a problem, (2) sometimes a problem, (3) often a problem, and (4) always a problem. Items are reverse scored and transformed to a 0- to 100-point scale (0 = 100, 1 = 75, 2 = 50, 3 = 75, 4 = 0), indicating a better HRQOL with higher scale scores. To create Scale Scores, the mean is computed as the sum of the items over the number of items answered. The Psychosocial Health Summary Score is the mean computed as the sum of the items over the number of items answered in the Emotional, Social, and School Scales. The Physical Health Summary Score is the same as the Physical Functioning Scale Score. The Total Scale Score is the mean of the sum of all items over the number of items answered in all scales.

Interpretation In general, the higher the scores, the better the HRQOL. In published studies by the Peds-QL author, children in good health have scores around 83, whereas children in poor health have scores in the mid-60s to low 70s.[94]

RELIABILITY AND VALIDITY Internal consistency reliability for the Total Scale Score ($\alpha = 0.88$ child, 0.90 parent report), Physical Health Summary ($\alpha = 0.80$ child, 0.88 parent report), and the Psychosocial Health Summary Score

The **Child and Parent Reports** of the PedsQL™ 4.0 Generic Core Scales for:

- Young Children (ages 5–7)
- Children (ages 8–12)
- And Teens (ages 13–18)

are composed of 23 items comprising 4 dimensions.

DESCRIPTION OF THE QUESTIONNAIRE:

Dimensions	Number of Items	Cluster of Items	Reversed scoring	Direction of Dimensions
Physical Functioning	8	1–8	1–8	
Emotional Functioning	5	1–5	1–5	Higher scores indicate better HRQOL.
Social Functioning	5	1–5	1–5	
School Functioning	5	1–5	1–5	

SCORING OF DIMENSIONS:

Item Scaling	5-point Likert scale from 0 (Never) to 4 (Almost always) 3-point scale: 0 (Not at all), 2 (Sometimes) and 4 (A lot) for the Young Child (ages 5–7) child report
Weighting of Items	No
Extension of the Scoring Scale	Scores are transformed on a scale from 0 to 100.
Scoring Procedure	**Step 1: Transform Score** Items are reversed scored and linearly transformed to a 0–100 scale as follows: 0=100, 1=75, 2=50, 3=25, 4=0 **Step 2: Calculate Scores** Score by Dimensions: • If more than 50% of the items in the scale are missing, the scale scores should not be computed, • Mean score = Sum of the items over the number of items answered. Psychosocial Health Summary Score = Sum of the items over the number of items answered in the Emotional, Social, and School Functioning Scales. Physical Health Summary Score = Physical Functioning Scale Score **Total Score:** Sum of the items over the numbers of items answered on all the Scales.
Interpretation and Analysis of Missing Data	If more than 50% of the items in the scale are missing, the Scales Scores should not be computed. if 50% or more items are completed: Impute the mean of the completed items in a scale.

FIGURE 2.6. Pediatric Quality-of-Life Inventory (Peds-QL) Version 4.0 example of Child Report (ages 8–12). (http://PedsQLTM.pedsql.org/about_pedsql.html from PedsQL™, Copyright © 1998 JW Varni, Ph.D. All rights reserved.)

($\alpha = 0.83$ child, 0.86 parent report) was reported as acceptable for group comparisons.[94] Construct validity was demonstrated using the known-group methods, between the Peds-QL 4.0 Generic Core Scales and the Peds-QL 3.0 Cancer Module.[93] The Peds-QL 4.0 Generic Core Scales are able to distinguish between healthy children and those with acute or chronic conditions and are related to indicators of morbidity and illness burden. Reliability, validity, and responsiveness to clinical change were also reported for the Peds-QL 4.0 Generic Scales and the Peds-QL Asthma Module Asthma Symptom Scale.[95]

ADVANTAGES/DISADVANTAGES The Peds-QL is a brief, easy-to-administer outcome measures tool that is used internationally across multiple health-related fields. It assessed multiple dimensions of health from both the parent's and the child's perspective and is applicable to several age groups. The Peds-QL measurement instruments (generic and disease-specific) may be utilized as an outcome measure in clinical trials, research, and clinical practice as a measure of HRQOL. Disadvantages for generic quality-of-life measures such as Peds-QL include inability to assess relevant domains of functioning specific to disease processes and decreased sensitivity to measure small but meaningful changes that occur as a result of clinical intervention.[96]

Pediatric Outcomes Data-Collection Instrument

The Pediatric Outcomes Data-Collection Instrument (PODCI), also known as the Pediatric Orthopedic Society of North America (POSNA) instrument, was created by the American Academy of Orthopedic Surgeons (AAOS) and the POSNA in 1997 as a comprehensive measure of musculoskeletal outcomes associated with pediatric orthopedic problems.[97] It was created to measure outcomes that orthopedic treatment could affect: upper and lower extremity motor skills, relief of pain, and restoration of activity.

TEST MEASURES AND TARGET POPULATION The PODCI consists of an Adolescent Self-Report Outcomes Questionnaire, an Adolescent Parent-Report Outcomes Questionnaire, and a Pediatric Outcomes Questionnaire, which measure overall health, pain, and ability to participate in normal daily activities as well as vigorous physical activities. The Pediatric Outcomes Questionnaire is intended to be used for children 2 to 10 years through parent report; the Adolescent Parent-Report Questionnaire is intended for use in children between 11 and 18 years; and the Adolescent Self-Report Questionnaire is intended for youth and children 11 to 18 years who can complete the form independently. For the purposes of this chapter, the Pediatric Outcomes Questionnaire will be reviewed.

TEST CONSTRUCTION AND STANDARDIZATION The original POSNA instrument was constructed by the Pediatric Outcomes Instrument Development Group in 1994 as an outcomes questionnaire based on existing instruments, input from expert panelists, and pilot testing with patients/parents.[97] The instrument was revised after additional pilot testing determined important concepts and domains pertinent to pediatric functional health for the child and parent study group. The Child Health Questionnaire (CHQ), a validated and reliable scale with national norms, was used as a benchmark for validity tests and comparisons for sensitivity to change. In 2002, the AAOS completed a normative data study for all of the outcome instruments to provide general, healthy population scale scores for comparison to patient scores.[98] A total of 20,631 valid responses were included in the study, providing an overall confidence interval of $\pm3\%$ at a 95% confidence level.

TEST FORMAT

Type The PODCI is a norm-referenced functional HRQOL outcome-measures questionnaire.

Content The Pediatric Outcomes Questionnaire consists of eight scales: (1) Upper Extremity and Physical Function Scale, (2) Transfer and Basic Mobility Scale, (3) Sports/Physical Functioning Scale, (4) Pain/Comfort Scale, (5) Treatment Expectations Scale, (6) Happiness Scale, (7) Satisfaction with Symptoms Scale, and (8) Global Functioning Scale. The questionnaire contains 86 questions.

Administration The Pediatric Outcomes Questionnaire is completed by a parent/guardian who has knowledge of the child's condition with approximate completion time of 10 to 20 minutes. Responses to questions are rated on various scales (ranging from 1 to 4, 5, or 6).

Scoring Standardized and normative scores can be calculated for each patient. The standard score is based on the mean of items in each scale. Although scales may have differing item values, for scoring purposes, all items are rescaled to range from 0 to 5 (i.e., 0 = lowest score possible and 5 = maximum score possible). Items comprising a given scale are then averaged over the total number of items answered and multiplied by 20 to have a range from 0 to 100. The final number is then subtracted from 100 to yield the patient's standardized score. Computation through Excel worksheets includes formulae for item recoding, computation of missing items, and known general population means and SDs. Using the actual mean and SD of the 0-to-100 scale from the general, healthy population, a formula is applied to derive the normative score.

Interpretation Standardized scores range from 0 to 100, with 0 representing the *most* disability and 100 representing the *least* disability. The normative score as a measure based on the healthy populations mean provides a numeric measure of disability relative to this population.

RELIABILITY AND VALIDITY Internal reliability ranges from 0.82 to 0.95 in the adult scales and 0.75 to 0.92 in the adolescent scales, and test–retest reliability is 0.71 to 0.97.[97] The scales were correlated with physicians' assessments and the CHQ by patterns of results indicating construct validity. Construct validity between the Activity Scales for Kids (ASK) and the PODCI shows high correlation at $r \geq 0.78$.[99] Concurrent validity is reported between the CHQ (0.60 to 0.81), the GMFM (0.56 to 0.94), and the PEDI (0.50 to 0.81).[80]

ADVANTAGES/DISADVANTAGES As an outcome measure, the PODCI is highly correlated with parents and clinician's global physical function ratings and is able to distinguish between different diseases or different levels of disease severity. It addresses critical components of outcomes in disabled children: pain, physical function, and impact on the child's psyche. The PODCI is used extensively in orthopedic outcomes research in multiple diagnostic categories. Because of its length and complex scoring algorithms, it may not be feasible in some clinical settings. However, correlations between the Peds-QL Global Score and the PODCI Total Score have been reported as Strong in orthopedic patients, suggesting the Peds-QL may be a suitable substitute in high-volume clinics.[100]

» Integration of information

The administration of developmental assessments is just one component of a physical therapy examination, as described by *The Guide to Physical Therapist Practice*[6] model for patient/client management. *Examination* includes history, systems review, and selection of tests and measures. *Evaluation* is the dynamic process of the physical therapists' clinical judgment through analysis and synthesis of information obtained through the examination to develop a plan of care. *Diagnosis*, or physical therapy diagnosis, highlights the activity limitations and participation restrictions. When sharing diagnostic information with the individual and family, therapists are supportive and use strength-based and family-friendly language. Formulating a physical therapy diagnosis helps determine the most appropriate intervention strategies. *Prognosis* pertains to the predicted optimal level of functional improvement and includes the frequency and duration of intervention, plan of care, and discharge criteria. Pediatric physical therapists consider the facilitators and barriers across all domains of the ICF when predicting optimal level of improvement and the time needed to reach that level. Long-term and short-term goals are the objective measurements with time frames for achievement, whereas the expected outcomes included in prognosis are the changes anticipated as the result of implementing the physical therapy plan of care. *Intervention*, the purposeful and skilled interaction of the physical therapist with the patient/client, occurs in several settings: hospital, clinical, and natural settings. Therapists recognize the importance of self-determination for the individual and self-efficacy for the family in determining intervention strategies including procedural interventions (therapeutic exercise, functional training, etc.). Intervention also includes providing information to assist families in negotiating the medical, educational, and community systems and planning for the future. Home or school activity programs are developed collaboratively within the context of daily routines and activities. *Outcomes* described by *Guide to Physical Therapist Practice* may include goal mastery and self-report measures

---

DISPLAY 2.6

Suggested Outline for a Narrative Report on the Results of Development Testing

1. Identification information: child's name, date of birth, current age, date of evaluation
2. Reason for evaluation and source of referral
3. History
   a. Perinatal history
   b. Significant medical history
   c. Developmental history as presented by parents or other historian
4. Clinical observations
   a. Neurologic development: reflex development, muscle tone, equilibrium, and protective responses
   b. Musculoskeletal status: range of motion, manual muscle test, anthropometric measurements
   c. Sensory status: results of sensory testing, pain assessment, visual ability, and auditory ability
   d. Functional abilities: daily activities (e.g., feeding, toileting, dressing), assistive devices
5. Results of developmental assessments: include developmental age
6. Summary of findings
7. Recommendations

---

to ensure that outcomes of physical therapy service reflect a meaningful impact to the individual and family.[6] Reexamination, the process of using tests and measures to evaluate progress and to modify intervention, may be performed periodically to review the appropriateness of the treatment program and to monitor the progress of the child. Reports of physical therapy examination are usually presented in narrative form. The purposes of a report are to clarify what has been heard and observed, to give the data on which recommendations for treatment are based, and to transmit this information in a clear and understandable way to others. Certain information is included for all children, but each child's report should provide a specific description of the distinctive abilities and disabilities of that child.[101] An outline of a narrative report is given in Display 2.6.

Summary

Several clinically useful and commonly used tools for assessment have been described, among which are screening tests, tests of motor function, comprehensive developmental assessments, functional assessments, and HRQOL outcome measures. The information gained from these assessments is combined with history and systems review for the examination of each child as described in the patient/client management model. The guidelines presented for the selection of specific tests will aid the therapist in choosing the test most appropriate for the population to be assessed. Pediatric physical therapists can use the guide's information on tests and measures to select the most appropriate tools categorized by the ICF model to gather information on the child's participation in the home, school, and community; ability to do activities; and the implications of health conditions, personal/environmental factors, and body structures/functions on performance.[6]

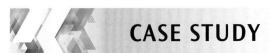

CASE STUDY

ASSESSMENT TOOLS USED IN DEVELOPMENTAL PROGRESS CLINIC

Birth and Medical History:

Taylor was born prematurely at 26 weeks gestation via c-section weighing 690 g. The pregnancy was significant for pregnancy-induced hypertension, eclampsia, and gestational diabetes. APGAR scores were 5, 5, and 8 at 1, 5, and 10 minutes, respectively. Her neonatal course was complicated with respiratory distress, reflux, and feeding difficulties. Cranial ultrasound confirmed ventriculomegaly but no intraventricular hemorrhage. Taylor was discharged home after 254 days in the neonatal intensive care unit (NICU). She had a g-tube and required supplemental oxygen secondary to bronchopulmonary dysplasia. She was referred for physical, occupational, and speech therapy services upon discharge and received outpatient hospital-based services, followed by early intervention services prior to her assessment at a developmental clinic for at-risk infants.

Developmental Progress Clinic and Developmental Testing:

Taylor was referred to the Developmental Progress Clinic, a specialty clinic for babies born prematurely and at risk for developmental delays. At 8 months corrected age, she continued to require oxygen via nasal cannula with noted costal retractions at rest. She had increased tactile hypersensitivity on her hands and feet. Her muscle tone was low normal with muscle weakness globally. Clonus was present bilaterally, left greater than right. The quality of her movement was asymmetric, with increased use of the right hand over the left. Functionally, Taylor could attain and maintain prone on elbows position but could not pivot or commando crawl. In supine, Taylor could grasp toys in midline and transfer objects hand to hand, but was not able to bring feet to hands. She had good chin tuck with pull to sit transfers, but lacked postural control for independent sitting. In supported standing, her hips were posterior to her feet, initially up on toes but she could easily attain foot flat position with support at her hips. Taylor was administered the **Alberta Infant Motor Scale (AIMS)** for her corrected age of 8 months, 17 days. Her total score was 25, with a 5th percentile rank. Concerns included asymmetric movement and generalized weakness, low tolerance, and delay of prone progression skills. Taylor continued

early intervention services where she received weekly services for physical and speech/feeding therapy services.

Taylor presented to the Developmental Progress Clinic for follow-up and additional testing at the age of 20 months corrected. She was progressing well with feeding and PO intake, utilizing the g-tube for thin liquids only. She remained on ¼ L oxygen at night. She had easy work of breathing and normal breath sounds. She presented with increased muscle tone in her ankles with deep tendon reflexes +3 bilaterally. She walked with a wide-based gait and newly acquired preference for toe-walking.

Taylor was administered the **Bayley Scales of Infant and Toddler Development; 3rd edition (Bayley-III)**. Estimates of developmental level were gathered based on parent interview, clinical observation, and test performance. Taylor's results were as follows:

- Social Domain: social and emotional functioning for her age
- Self-Help Domain: 15- to 18-month range
- Gross Motor Test performance was at the 16-month level.
- Fine Motor Test performance was in the 12- to 15-month range.
- Expressive Language Test performance was in the 12- to 15-month range. Parent report and clinical observation suggest this may overrepresent her current abilities, especially with regard to nonverbal communication.
- Receptive Language Test performance at the 14-month level
- Cognitive Test performance at the 15-month level

Following her assessment, she was referred to a neurologist because of continued global delays, asymmetric movement, brisk tendon reflexes, and abnormality of gait (toe-walking). At 22 months corrected age, Taylor was evaluated by a neurologist to review MRI results consistent with mild ventriculomegaly with enlarged extra-axial spaces as indicated on previous cranial ultrasound. Taylor was diagnosed with cerebral palsy, GMFCS Level 1, but did not require tone management at that time. Her plan of care was to continue physical therapy and speech and feeding therapy through early intervention, and transition to special needs preschool upon turning 3 years.

REFERENCES

1. Academy of Pediatric Physical Therapy, American Physical Therapy Association. The ABC's of Pediatric Physical Therapy Fact Sheet. 2019. Accessed January 12, 2021. https://pediatricapta.org/includes/fact-sheets/pdfs/09%20ABCs%20of%20Ped%20PT.pdf?v=1.1
2. Scherzer AL, Tscharnuter I. *Early Diagnosis and Therapy in Cerebral Palsy*. New York, NY: Marcel Dekker; 1982.
3. Russell DJ, Rosenbaum PL, Avery LM, et al. *Gross Motor Function Measure (GMFM-66 and GMFM-88) User's Manual*. London, UK: Mac Keith Press; 2002.
4. The Committee on Children with Disabilities of the American Academy of Pediatrics. Identifying infants and young children with developmental disorders in the medical home: an algorithm for developmental surveillance and screening. *Pediatrics*. 2006;118:405-420.
5. Newborg J. *Battelle Developmental Inventory*. 2nd ed. Itasca, IL: Riverside; 2005.
6. American Physical Therapy Association. *Guide to Physical Therapist Practice*. 3rd ed. Alexandria, VA: APTA. Accessed January 12, 2021. http://www.guidetoptpractice.apta.org

7. Kirshner B, Guyatt G. A methodologic framework for assessing health indices. *J Chronic Dis.* 1985;38:27-36.

8. Long T, Toscano K. *Handbook of Pediatric Physical Therapy.* 2nd ed. Philadelphia, PA: Lippincott Williams & Wilkins; 2002.

9. Lewko JH. Current practices in evaluating motor behavior of disabled children. *Am J Occup Ther.* 1976;30:413-419.

10. Stangler SR, Huber CJ, Routh DK. *Screening Growth and Development of Preschool Children: A Guide for Test Selection.* New York, NY: McGraw-Hill; 1980.

11. Tieman BL, Palisano R, Sutlive AC. Assessment of motor development and function in preschool children. *Ment Retard Dev Disabil Res Rev.* 2005;11:189-196.

12. Rydz D, Shevell MI, Majnemer A, et al. Developmental screening. *J Child Neurol.* 2005;20(1):4-21.

13. Mackrides PS, Ryherd SJ. Screening for developmental delay. *Am Fam Physician.* 2011;84(5):544-549.

14. Harris SR, Megens AM, Daniels LE. *Harris Infant Neuromotor Test (HINT) Test User's Manual Version 1.0 Clinical Edition (2009).* Chicago, IL: Infant Motor Performance Scales LLC; 2010.

15. Harris SR, Daniels LE. Content validity of the Harris Infant Neuromotor Test. *Phys Ther.* 1996;76:727-737.

16. Harris SR, Daniels LE. Reliability and validity of the Harris Infant Neuromotor Test. *J Pediatr.* 2001;139:249-253.

17. Harris SR, Megens AM, Backman CL, et al. Development and standardization of the Harris Infant Neuromotor Test. *Infants Young Child.* 2003;16(2):143-151.

18. Tse L, Mayson TA, Leo S, et al. Concurrent validity of the Harris Infant Neuromotor Test and the Alberta Infant Motor Scale. *J Pediatr Nurs.* 2008;23:28-36.

19. McCoy SW, Bowman A, Smith-Blockley J, et al. Harris Infant Neuromotor Test: comparison of US and Canadian normative data and examination of concurrent validity with the ages and stages questionnaire. *Phys Ther.* 2009;89(2):173-180.

20. Aylward GP. *The Bayley Infant Neurodevelopmental Screener.* San Antonio, TX: The Psychological Corporation; 1995.

21. Aylward GP, Verhulst SJ. Predictive utility of the Bayley Infant Neurodevelopmental Screener (BINS) risk status classifications: clinical interpretation and application. *Dev Med Child Neurol.* 2000;42:25-31.

22. Soysal AS, Gucuyener K, Ergenekon E, et al. The prediction of later neurodevelopmental status of preterm infants at ages 7 to 10 years using the Bayley Infant Neurodevelopmental Screener. *J Child Neurol.* 2014;29(10):1349-1355.

23. Campbell SK, Osten ET, Kolobe THA, et al. Development of the test of infant motor performance. *Phys Med Rehabil Clin N Am.* 1993;4(3):541-550.

24. Campbell SK. *The Test of Infant Motor Performance: Test User's Manual.* Version 2.0. Chicago, IL: Infant Motor Performance Scales, LLC; 2005.

25. Campbell SK, Levy P, Zawacki L, et al. Population-based age standards for interpreting results on the test of infant motor performance. *Pediatr Phys Ther.* 2006;18:119-125.

26. Girolami GL, Campbell SK. Efficacy of a neuro-developmental treatment program to improve motor control in infants born prematurely. *Pediatr Phys Ther.* 1994;6(4):175-184.

27. Campbell SK, Wright BD, Linacre JM. Development of a functional movement scale for infants. *J Appl Meas.* 2002;3(2):190-204.

28. Campbell SK. Test-retest reliability of the Test of Infant Motor Performance. *Pediatr Phys Ther.* 1999;11:60-66.

29. Lekskulchai R, Cole J. Effect of a developmental program on motor performance in infants born preterm. *Aust J Physiother.* 2001;47:169-176.

30. Campbell SK, Kolobe TH, Osten ET, et al. Construct validity of infant motor performance. *Phys Ther.* 1995;75(7):585-596.

31. Peyton C, Yang E, Kocherginsky M, et al. Relationship between white matter pathology and performance on General Movement Assessment and the Test of Infant Motor Performance in very preterm infants. *Early Hum Dev.* 2016;95:23-27.

32. Campbell SK, Kolobe THA, Wright B, et al. Validity of the Test of Infant Motor Performance for prediction of 6-, 9-, and 12-month scores on the Alberta Infant Motor Scale. *Dev Med Child Neurol.* 2002;44:263-272.

33. Kolobe THA, Bulanda M, Susman L. Predicting motor outcomes at preschool age for infants tested at 7, 30, 60, and 90 days after term age using the Test of Infant Motor Performance. *Phys Ther.* 2004;84:1144-1156.

34. Piper MC, Darrah J. *Motor Assessment of the Developing Infant.* Philadelphia, PA: WB Saunders; 1995.

35. Lee LLS, Harris SR. Psychometric properties and standardization of four screening tests for infants and young children: a review. *Pediatr Phys Ther.* 2005;17:140-147.

36. Piper MC, Pinnell LE, Darrah J, et al. Construction and validation of the Alberta Infant Motor Scale (AIMS). *Can J Public Health.* 1992;83(suppl 2):S46-S50.

37. Darrah J, Bartlett D, Maquire TO, et al. Have infant gross motor abilities changed in 20 years? A re-evaluation of the Alberta Infant Motor Scales normative values. *Dev Med Child Neurol.* 2014;56(9):877-881.

38. Pin TW, de Valle K, Eldridge B, et al. Clinimetric properties of the Alberta Infant Motor Scale in infants born preterm. *Pediatr Phys Ther.* 2010;22:278-286.

39. Harris SR, Backman CL, Mayson TA. Comparative predictive validity of the Harris Infant Neuromotor Test and the Alberta Infant Motor Scale. *Dev Med Child Neurol.* 2010;52:462-467.

40. Fetters L, Tronick EZ. Neuromotor development of cocaine-exposed and control infants from birth through 15 months: poor and poorer performance. *Pediatrics.* 1996;98(5):938-943.

41. Russell DJ, Rosenbaum PL, Cadman DT, et al. The Gross Motor Function Measure: a means to evaluate the effects of physical therapy. *Dev Med Child Neurol.* 1989;31:341-352.

42. Can Child—Center for Childhood Disability Research. CanChild Website. Accessed November 15, 2019. http://www.canchild.ca/en/measures/gmpmqualityfm.asp

43. Avery LM, Russell DJ, Raina PS, et al. Rasch analysis of the Gross Motor Function Measure: validating the assumptions of the Rasch model to create an interval-level measure. *Arch Phys Med Rehabil.* 2003;84(5):697-705.

44. Russell DJ, Avery LM, Rosenbaum PL, et al. Improved scaling of the gross motor function measure for children with cerebral palsy: evidence of reliability and validity. *Phys Ther.* 2000;80(9):873-885.

45. Shi W, Wang SJ, Liao YG, et al. Reliability and validity of the GMFM-66 in 0 to 3-year old children with cerebral palsy. *Am J Phys Med Rehabil.* 2006;85(2):141-147.

46. Drouin LM, Malouin F, Richards CL, et al. Correlation between the Gross Motor Function Measure scores and gait spatiotemporal measures in children with neurological impairments. *Dev Med Child Neurol.* 1996;38:1007-1019.

47. Josenby AL, Jarnlo G, Gummesson C, et al. Longitudinal construct validity of the GMFM-88 total score and goal total score and the GMFM-66 score in a 5-year follow up study. *Phys Ther.* 2009;89:342-350.

48. Brunton LK, Bartlett DJ. Validity and reliability of two abbreviated versions of the gross motor function measure. *Phys Ther.* 2011;91:577-588.

49. Rosenbaum PL, Palisano RJ, Bartlett DJ, et al. Development of the Gross Motor Function Classification System for cerebral palsy. *Dev Med Child Neurol.* 2008;50:249-253.

50. Palisano R, Rosenbaum P, Walter S, et al. Gross motor function classification system for cerebral palsy. *Dev Med Child Neurol.* 1997;39:214-223.

51. Towns M, Rosenbaum P, Palisano R, et al. Should the Gross Motor Functional Classification Levels system be used in children without cerebral palsy? *Dev Med Child Neurol.* 2018;60(2):147-154.

52. Debuse D, Brace H. Outcome measures of activity for children with cerebral palsy: a systematic review. *Pediatr Phys Ther.* 2011;23:221-231.

53. Folio MR, Fewell RR. *Peabody Developmental Motor Scales*. 2nd ed. Austin, TX: Pro-Ed; 2000.

54. Fay D, Wilkinson T, Anderson AD, et al. Effects of Modified Instructions on Peabody Developmental Motor Scales, Second Edition, Gross motor scores in children with typical development. *Phys Occup Ther Pediatr*. 2019;39(4):433-445.

55. Gill K, Osiovich A, Synnes A, et al. Concurrent validity of the Bayley-III and Peabody Developmental Motor Scales-2 at 18 months. *Phys Occup Ther Pediatr*. 2019;39(5):514-524.

56. Cools W, De Martelaer K, Samaey C, et al. Movement skill assessment of typically developing preschool children: a review of seven movement skill assessment tools. *J Sports Sci Med*. 2009;8:154-168.

57. Bruininks R, Bruininks B. *Bruininks-Oseretsky Test of Motor Proficiency (BOT-2)*. 2nd ed. Minneapolis, MN: NCS Pearson; 2005.

58. Deitz JC, Kartin D, Kopp K. Review of the Bruininks-Oseretsky Test of Motor Proficiency, second edition (BOT-2). *Phys Occup Ther Pediatr*. 2007;27(4):87-102.

59. Jirovec J, Musalek M, Mess F. Test of Motor Proficiency-Second Edition (BOT-2): compatibility of the complete and short form and its usefulness for middle school aged children. *Front Pediatr*. 2019;7:153.

60. Individuals with Disabilities Education Act Amendments of 1997, Pub L No 105-117, 20 USC, 1400 *et seq*.

61. Bayley N. *Bayley Scales of Infant and Toddler Development (Bayley-4)*. 4th ed. San Antonio, TX: The Psychological Corporation; 2019.

62. Bayley N. *The Bayley Scales of Infant Development-III*. San Antonio, TX: The Psychological Corporation; 2005.

63. Bayley N. *The Bayley Scales of Infant Development*. San Antonio, TX: The Psychological Corporation; 1969.

64. Greenspan S. *Greeenspan Social-Emotional Growth Chart*. San Antonio, TX: The Psychological Corporation; 2004.

65. Sparrow S, Cicchetti D, Saulnier C. *Vineland Adaptive Behavior Scales*. 3rd ed. Bloomington, MN: Pearson; 2016.

66. Newborg J. *Battelle Developmental Inventory, 2nd Edition Normative Update*. Itasca, IL: Houghton Mifflin Harcourt Publishing Company; 2016.

67. Newborg J, Stock JR, Wnek L, et al. *Battelle Developmental Inventory*. Allen, TX: DLM; 1984.

68. Spies M, Matson JL, Turygin N. The use of the Battelle Developmental Inventory–Second Edition (BDI-2) as an early screener for autism spectrum disorders. *Dev Neurorehabil*. 2011;14(5):310-314.

69. World Health Organization. *International Classification of Functioning, Disability, and Health*. Geneva, Switzerland: WHO; 2001.

70. Hayley SM, Coster W, Kao Y. Lessons from use of the Pediatric Evaluation of Disability Inventory: where do we go from here? *Pediatr Phys Ther*. 2010;22:69-75.

71. Haley SM. Motor assessment tools for infants and young children: a focus on disability assessment. In: Forssberg H, Hirschfeld H, eds. *Movement Disorders in Children*. Basel, Switzerland: S. Karger AG; 1992:278-283.

72. Haley SM, Costern J, Ludlons LH, et al. *Pediatric Evaluation of Disability Inventory (PEDI): Development, Standardization and Administration Manual*. Boston, MA: New England Medical Center Hospitals and PEDI Research Group; 1992.

73. Haley SM, Coster WJ, Dumas HM, et al. *PEDI-CAT: Pediatric Evaluation of Disability Inventory-Computer Adaptive Test: Development, Standardization, and Administration Manual*. Boston, MA: CREcare, LLC; 2012. http://pedicat.com.

74. Dumas HM, Fragala-Pinkman MA, Haley SM, et al. Item bank development for a revised Pediatric Evaluation of Disability Inventory (PEDI). *Phys Occup Ther Pediatr*. 2010;30:168-184.

75. Dumas HM, Fragala-Pinkman M. Concurrent validity and reliability of the pediatric evaluation of disability inventory-computer adaptive test mobility domain. *Pediatr Phys Ther*. 2012;24:171-176.

76. Data Management Service of the Uniform Data System for Medical Rehabilitation and the Center for Functional Assessment Research. *Guide for Use of the Uniform Data System for Medical Rehabilitation, Including the Functional Independence Measure for Children (WeeFIM)*. Version 1.5. Buffalo, NY: State University of New York at Buffalo; 1991.

77. *The WeeFIM II Clinical Guide*. Version 6.0. Buffalo, NY: Uniform Data System for Medical Rehabilitation; 2006.

78. Msall ME, DiGaudio K, Duffy LC, et al. WeeFIM normative sample of an instrument for tracking functional independence in children. *Clin Pediatr (Phila)*. 1994;33:431-438.

79. Ottenbacher KJ, Msall ME, Lyon NR, et al. Interrater agreement and stability of the Functional Independence Measure for Children (WeeFIM): use in children with developmental disabilities. *Arch Phys Med Rehabil*. 1997;78:1309-1315.

80. McCarthy ML, Silberstein CE, Atkins EA, et al. Comparing reliability and validity of pediatric instruments for measuring health and wellbeing of children with spastic cerebral palsy. *Dev Med Child Neurol*. 2002;44:468-476.

81. Ziviani J, Ottenbacher K, Shephard K, et al. Concurrent validity of the Functional Independence Measure for Children (WeeFIM) and the Pediatric Evaluation of Disability Inventory (PEDI) in children with developmental disabilities and acquired brain injuries. *Phys Occup Ther Pediatr*. 2002;21:91-101.

82. Coster W, Deeney TA, Haltiwanger JT, et al. *School Function Assessment*. Boston, MA: Boston University; 1998.

83. Burtner PA, McMain MP, Crowe TK. Survey of occupational therapy practitioners in southwestern schools: assessments used and preparation of students for school-based practice. *Phys Occup Ther Pediatr*. 2002;22(1):25-39.

84. *School Function Assessment Technical Report*. Accessed January 12, 2021. https://images.pearsonassessments.com/images/tmrs/tmrs_rg/SFA_TR_Web.pdf?WT.mc_id=TMRS_School_Function_Assessment

85. Hwang J, Davies PL, Taylor MP, et al. Validation of school function assessment with elementary school children. *OTJR*. 2002;22(2):1-11.

86. Davies PL, Soon PL, Young M, et al. Validity and reliability of the school function assessment in elementary school students with disabilities. *Phys Occup Ther Pediatr*. 2004;24(3):23-43.

87. Effgen SK, McCoy SW, Chiarello LA, et al. Outcomes for students receiving school-based physical therapy as measured by the school functional assessment. *Pediatr Phys Ther*. 2016;28(4):371-378.

88. Fayers PM, Machin D. *Quality of Life: Assessment, Analysis and Interpretation*. New York, NY: Wiley; 2000.

89. Varni JW, Burwinkle TM, Lane MM. Health-related quality of life measurement in pediatric clinical practice: an appraisal and precept for future research and application. *Health Qual Life Outcomes*. 2005;3. Accessed January 12, 2021. https://hqlo.biomedcentral.com/articles/10.1186/1477-7525-3-34

90. Varni JW, Seid M, Rode CA. The PedsQL™: measurement model for the Pediatric Quality of Life Inventory. *Medical Care*. 1999;37(2):126-139.

91. MAPI Research Trust. PedsQL (Pediatric Quality of Life Inventory). Accessed January 12, 2021. http://www.pedsql.org/about_pedsql.html.

92. Varni JW, Seid M, Rode CA. The PedsQL™: measurement model for the Pediatric Quality of Life Inventory. *Med Care*. 1999;37:126-139.

93. Varni JW, Burwinkle TM, Katz ER, et al. The PedsQL™ in pediatric cancer: reliability and validity of the pediatric quality of life inventory generic core scales, multidimensional fatigue scale, and cancer module. *Cancer*. 2002;94:2090-2106.

94. Varni JW, Seid M, Kurtin PS. PedsQL™ 4.0: reliability and validity of the pediatric quality of life inventory version 4.0 generic core scales in healthy and patient populations. *Med Care*. 2001;39:800-812.

95. Seid M, Limbers CA, Drscoll KA, et al. Reliability, validity, and responsiveness of the Pediatric Quality of Life Inventory™ (PedsQL™) Generic Core Scales and Asthma Symptoms Scales in vulnerable children with asthma. *J Asthma*. 2010;47:170-177.

96. Lim CMS. *Pain, Quality of Life, and Coping in Pediatric Sickle Cell Disease* [dissertation]. Psychology Dissertations Paper 54. Atlanta, GA: Georgia State University; 2009.

97. Daltroy LH, Liang MH, Fossel AH, et al. The POSNA Pediatric Musculoskeletal Functional Health Questionnaire: report of reliability, validity, and sensitivity to change. *J Pediatr Orthop*. 1998;18:561-571.

98. Hunsaker FG, Cioffi DA, Amadio PC, et al. The American Academy of Orthopaedic Surgeons Outcomes Instruments. *The Journal of Bone & Joint Surgery*. 2002; 84(2): 208-215.

99. Pencharz J, Young NL, Owen JL, et al. Comparison of three outcomes instruments in children. *J Pediatr Orthop*. 2001;21:425-432.

100. Mahan ST, Kalish LA, Connell PL, et al. PedsQL correlates to PODCI in pediatric orthopedic outpatient clinic. *J Pediatr Orthop*. 2014;34(6):e22-e26.

101. Knobloch H, Pasamanick B, eds. *Gesell and Amatruda's Developmental Diagnosis: The Evaluation and Management of Normal and Abnormal Neuropsychologic Development in Infancy and Early Childhood*. Hagerstown, MD: Harper & Row; 1974.

Family-Centered Care

Elena McKeogh Spearing

>> Introduction

The definition of family, in today's society, respects the notion that each family has unique characteristics and variables. Today, the family unit consists of "those significant others who profoundly influence the personal life and health of the individual over an extended period of time."[1] Families today come in all configurations and sizes and are not all traditional, married, two-biologic parent families. The 2010 U.S. Census reports that the number of husband–wife–biologic children family households has decreased over the past 20 years despite increases in the total number of family households. The number of single-parent families, dual-income families, adoptive families, same-sex-parent families, and intergenerational families has steadily increased.[2] This increase is likely to be seen in the 2020 U.S. Census reports as well.

Additionally, there is a "melting pot" of various cultural identities represented in the United States. The U.S. Census Bureau reported that the minority population continued to grow to an all-time high in 2012, with 21.5% of Americans speaking languages other than English outside the home.[3] A total of 13.5% of the population is foreign born, and this is projected to rise in the coming decades.[3] The three fastest growing racial categories continue to be Asian and Pacific Islander, Hispanic, and "other."[3] This cultural factor presents additional challenges to health care providers who care for people with varying cultural and ethnic backgrounds. This is very important to remember when providing physical therapy services to a child.[4,5]

In pediatric physical therapy, there has historically been a change in the developmental theory behind how therapists provide care (Display 3.1). This change has resulted in a shift from a reflex hierarchy model, where a child develops on the basis of a set of primitive reflexes, to one where a child develops as a result of the dynamic interaction of different systems that affect one another in the development of the child. In this dynamic system's model, all systems' components interact to produce meaningful, functional behavior.[6] The child's family is one of those systems. Similarly, pediatric physical therapy care has shifted from being child focused, as in the 1980s, to currently being family focused.[7,8] Today, many center-based physical therapy service delivery models have been replaced by physical therapy service in the natural environment of the home and school. These initiatives help to promote family-centered care practice by the physical therapist. Because a child is dependent on a caretaker, the therapist must address both the child and the caretaker when interacting with a child receiving physical therapy.

DISPLAY 3.1	**The Change in Structure of Pediatric Service Delivery Motor Learning and Function**	
Reflex Hierarchy Model	→	Systems Model
Child-Centered Services	→	Family-Centered Service
Center-Based Delivery	→	Natural Environment

Family-centered care is the foundation of pediatric physical therapy.

The notion of family-centered care extended into the health care policy arena in the 1980s, beginning in pediatric health care facilities, whereas until then, families in the hospital setting functioned more or less as visitors or attendants. Additionally, families of children with intellectual disabilities were encouraged to institutionalize them. Slowly, hospitals began recognizing the importance of open visiting hours, sibling visits, rooming in, and parent advocacy. This philosophy of care then spread to adult hospital units for cancer, mental health issues, maternity wards, and various health care practices, where it is referred to as patient-centered care. Family-centered care is a philosophy that recognizes that the family plays a vital role in ensuring the health and well-being of its members. Family-centered care also empowers the family to participate fully in the planning, delivery, and evaluation of health care services. It supports families in this role by building on the family members' individual strengths.[1,8,9]

Physical therapists who practice in the early intervention setting are mandated by law to provide care that respects a family's individualism. Those therapists have been charged with providing family-centered care since the initiation of Public Law 99-142, in 1975; Public Law 99-457, in 1986; and Public Law 102-119, in 1991.[8] Public Law 107-110, of 2001—No Child Left Behind (NCLB), and PL 108-446, of 2004, The Individuals with Disabilities Improvement Act—have similar mandates.[7,10] These laws placed the focus on revising and enhancing parents' involvement in the habilitation and education of the child.[8,11] Early studies showed that it was difficult to achieve this role on the basis of white middle-class families, and little attention was paid to social or ethnic differences. Additionally, enhancing parents' involvement is based on the assumption that the parents can participate in formal processes and, when necessary, draw on the availability of due process of law. Family-centered care processes are also central to the development of the individualized family service plan (IFSP) and the individualized education program (IEP), the required documentation for early intervention and educational services.

Physical therapists who practice in other pediatric settings, including the medically based inpatient and outpatient arenas, may be bound by health care accreditation standards, which recognize the importance of family-centered care. The Joint Commission on the Accreditation of Healthcare Organizations has standards of care initiatives in place to address the needs of the family.[12] The Joint Commission has also developed publications to assist hospitals with meeting these standards.[13,14]

Collectively, the vision for family-centered care has included increasing support for the emotional and developmental needs of the child. Strategies for this include prehospitalization visits, presurgical education and preparation, 24-hour parental visitation and sibling visitation guidelines, and home care services. These initiatives have shifted from placing the family central not only to the child, but also to the child's plan of care.[15,16] Ultimately, this type of care results in a respect and a value for the parents as the ultimate experts in caring for their child.

Family-centered care involves the following themes[17-19]:

1. Respecting each child and his or her family.
2. Honoring racial, ethnic, cultural, and socioeconomic diversity and its effect on the family's experience and perception of care.
3. Recognizing and facilitating the choices for the child and family even in difficult and challenging situations.
4. Facilitating and supporting the choices of the child and family about approaches to their care.
5. Ensuring flexibility in organizational policies, procedures, and provider practices so services can be tailored to the needs, beliefs, and cultural values of each child and family.
6. Sharing honest and unbiased information with families on an ongoing basis and in ways they find useful and affirming.
7. Providing and ensuring formal and informal support for the child and parent and/or guardian during pregnancy, childbirth, infancy, childhood, adolescence, and young adulthood.
8. Collaborating with families in the care of their individual child at all levels of health care, including professional education, policy making, and program development.
9. Empowering each child and family to discover their own strengths, build confidence, and make choices and decisions about their health care.

The purpose of this chapter is to provide a framework for understanding the principles of family-centered care in order to enable the physical therapist to incorporate principles of family-centered care into their examination, evaluation, and intervention techniques regardless of the pediatric practice setting. Themes of family-centered care cross not only practice settings, but also age and diagnosis. Because these themes are threads across the pediatric spectrum of care, they are also threaded throughout the chapters of this textbook.

» Understanding culture and its influences

Understanding cultural influences on a child and his or her family is central to providing family-centered care. Culture also affects how others view disability, how people with disabilities view themselves, and how people with disabilities are treated. The cultural context within which a disability is perceived is important to understanding the meaning of disability for a person or his or her family. It is also important to know the kinds of services to be provided to families and people with disabilities.

Culture can be defined in many ways. O'Connor defines culture as "the acquired knowledge people use to interpret experience and generate social behavior."[20] Other definitions include "the ever changing values, traditions, social and political relationships and a world view shared by a group of people bound together by a number of factors that can include a common history, geographic location, language, social class and/or religion."[21] An analysis of the various studies of culture yields the emergence of various similar themes[20]:

1. Culture is not innate or biologically inherited but, in fact, learned patterns of behavior.
2. Culture is transmitted from the older people to the young, from generation to generation.
3. Culture serves as a group identity and is shared by other members of the group.
4. Culture provides the individual or the members of a group with an effective mechanism for interacting with each other and their environment.

Cultural Diversity versus Cultural Sensitivity

Many terms are used today to refer to the impact of culture on health care. It is necessary to describe the two most common terms and their fundamental differences. *Cultural diversity* refers to having a range of cultures represented in an organization. This leads to a workforce that is more representative of the general population. In health care, diversity in the workplace leads to the increased potential of having similar cultures represented. By comparison, *cultural sensitivity* and effectiveness is a process of becoming "culturally competent" and striving toward the ability and availability to work effectively within the cultural context of a client, individual, family, or community regardless of the cultural background.[21]

Cultural sensitivity refers to the understanding that cultural differences exist. These differences are not necessarily better or worse, right or wrong, or more or less intelligent, but rather simply differences.[22] It is necessary to examine, in detail, attitude, behavior, and communication, which directly affect health care. It is important to realize that each person within a culture is an individual and should not be characterized or stereotyped on the basis of his or her cultural association. It is only through generalizations that one can gain a frame of reference and become more culturally aware.

Influences on Cultural Identity

There are various things that influence how a person views him or herself with respect to illness and disability. These include nationality, race, and ethnicity. Similarly, socioeconomic status and education also play a role. Society's view of illness and disability also influences the perception of the same. Other things like age, religion, and past experience shape beliefs.

In addition to these, health care providers who were brought up in the U.S. culture are finding that their medical views are in conflict with the views of their patients from differing cultural backgrounds. Care provided in the past was monocultural and suited for the Euro-American culture. Traditionally, in medicine medical professionals have functioned under a "medical culture," one that values a "cure" and the expertise of those in the medical profession.[11]

This traditional model, however, is not as appropriate or relevant for those who are not of that "medical" cultural identity.[11] When this cultural disconnect occurs, the consequence is often disparities in the quality of care received by racial and ethnic minority populations.[11] Fortunately, these disparities are evolving with time, but they still exist. Guerrero et al. found that black children have similar experiences as white children on overall family-centered care in models that adjust for socioeconomic factors. In contrast, differences were still found on dimensions of overall family-centered care between white children and Latino children, irrespective of interview language and even with multivariate adjustment.[23]

Cultural and Parental Expectations

Many studies reveal that culture and acculturation are strong predictors of parental expectations of cognitive and social development.[11] Most studies point to ethnic origin as the differentiating factor. More contemporary literature has determined that Western education and socioeconomic status were more predictive of differential beliefs than ethnic origin. This demonstrates that acculturation has a powerful effect on parenting styles and on parental beliefs about child development. What is even more profound is the difference between the description of the terms "cognitively delayed," "behaviorally disordered," and "learning disabled" between the parents and the professionals. Even negative terms like "retarded" and "low IQ" may still be referred to in some instances. Ethnographic studies have shown that there are sometimes differences related to culture, which emphasized that for some parents a child's cognitive and social functioning has to be more limited for the concept of handicap or disabled to be applied. These statements are then interpreted by the professional as families being in "denial."[22] The following themes occur in a review of the literature on culturally appropriate services in the special education[11]:

1. There are cultural differences in definitions and interpretations of disability.
2. There are cultural differences in family coping styles and responses to disability-related stress.
3. There are cultural differences in parental interaction styles, as well as expectations of participation and advocacy.
4. There are differences in cultural groups' access to information and services.
5. There are negative professional attitudes to, and perceptions of, families' roles in the special education processes.
6. There is dissonance in the cultural fit of educational programs.

» The family dynamics of having a child with an illness or disability

Families' Response to Medical Illness and Disability

When parents are faced with the fact that their child has an illness or disability, their lives must change immediately. Some changes include readjusting the family's expectations and dealing with financial difficulties and health care systems and professionals. The most common initial responses include shock, disbelief, guilt, a sense of loss, and denial. After the period of denial, some parents may experience anger because of the stress of the medical issues as well as spousal disagreement or individual feelings of fault and guilt.[24]

As a result of these responses and concerns, there are many stresses for families with a child with a disability. Families raising a child with a disability will have different responses and means of adaptation. Factors that affect how a family responds include past life experiences, familial reactions to the child and the disability, and knowledge about health care and support systems. Supports can also vary. Sometimes, there is a lack of understanding of the medical implications from those outside the family. There can also be feelings of embarrassment for the family. Professionals can use a cognitive approach to problem solving to help families examine their feelings and develop solutions for their own needs.

The effects of having a child with a disease or disability can not only affect the parents' relationship but can also have varied effects on siblings who also have individualized needs based on gender, birth order, and temperament. Siblings can also have mixed feelings toward their disabled sibling.[25] Some siblings may feel or be expected to have increased responsibility for the care of their siblings. Some siblings may have feelings of jealousy toward the sibling who has special needs.

A child with a disability may experience different effects as a result of his or her disability. By school age, most children are aware of their disability and may need help dealing with their feelings as they transition to school. The transition to school can be eased with education to the classmates prior to the child with a disability entering school. Parents and professionals can assist with this planning. During adolescence, there may be particular new issues that emerge for children with a disability. Feelings of comparing themselves and being part of a peer group are important for all adolescents and can present new challenges for those with chronic or new disabilities. Adolescents should also be acknowledged as having sexual interests. They should be educated on these feelings as well as trained in social skills. They should also be exposed to age-appropriate recreational skills, such as dancing, listening to music, and sports activities. Programs of inclusion help children to develop socialization skills and a good self-image.

Children with a disability or illness may also have varying levels of understanding about their disease process or disability.[16] More recent data in the medical literature demonstrate that children with sickle cell disease provide their parents with information about their pain and assist with decision making. This should be kept in mind with children even as young as 5 years old.

The transition to adulthood is both important and difficult for patients and parents. Those individuals who remain dependent through adolescence tend to remain dependent through adulthood.[26] Adolescents who have the potential for independence but are having difficulties with separation may need assistance. Likewise, the family members may need assistance in supporting their child during this difficult time. Professionals should be partners with the family members and empower them to make decisions.

Disability, as defined by the Americans with Disabilities Act, is "physical or mental impairment that substantially limits one or more of the life activities of an individual, a record of such an impairment, or being regarded as having such an impairment."[27] Advances in medical technology, diagnosis, and treatment have resulted in decreased mortality rates for children with life-threatening conditions to survive well into adulthood.[26] The diagnosis of chronic illness or disability clearly impacts a family. How families respond to the diagnosis is a function of their adaptive capabilities.[24] What makes some families reorganize and become stronger, whereas others decline in function, become symptomatic, and sometimes disintegrate, depends on family resilience according to Ferguson.[24] He describes eight aspects of resilient family processes. These are as follows:

1. Balancing the illness with other family needs
2. Developing communication competence
3. Attributing positive meaning to the situations
4. Maintaining clear family boundaries
5. Maintaining family flexibility
6. Engaging in active coping efforts
7. Maintaining social integration
8. Developing collaborative relationships with professionals

A family's ability to be resilient or the extent of its resiliency is defined largely by society, time, place, and culture.[24]

Additionally, in studies dealing with disability, when looking at reaction to disability, there are three issues that are considered to be universal. They are as follows[28]:

1. The culturally perceived cause of a chronic illness or disability will play a significant role in determining family and community attitudes toward the individual.
2. The expectations for physical survival for the infant or the child with a chronic disability will affect both the immediate care the child receives and the amount of effort expended in planning for future care and education.
3. The social role(s) deemed appropriate for children and adults with an illness or disability will help determine the amount of resources a family and community invests in an individual. This includes issues of education and training, participation in family and social life, and the long-range planning done by, or undertaken for, the

individual over the course of a lifetime. In the history of literature on family reactions to having a child with a disability, there has been a shift in thinking. In the 19th century, with the flourish of specialization, the moral blame for disabilities was often placed on the parents. This set of beliefs most often placed the blame on poor mothers who made bad judgments. Reform schools, asylums, and residential schools all became apparent in the 19th century. This movement also led to special education schools after the turn of the century. The only way to deal with children that weren't "normal" was to turn the parenting over to professionals within the walls of these facilities.[24,28]

There was a major shift in thinking throughout the 20th century that included a reversal of the foregoing assumptions. Professionals shifted to focusing on the damage that children with disabilities caused their families. The medical model began to analyze the family unit with terms such as *guilt, denial,* and *grief* and *role disruption, marital cohesiveness,* and *social withdrawal.*

Over the past few decades, a new approach has developed in regard to the impact of a child's disability on the family. The recent approach includes models of stress and coping (adaptation) and models of Family Life Course Development. The adaptive family describes X—the potential family crisis—as an interaction of three factors: (1) an initial stressful event, combined with (2) a family's resource for dealing with the crisis and (3) the family's definition of the stressor.[24] This approach has allowed researchers to focus on the resiliency of the family and its ability to cope with a potentially stressful situation. There is a level of consensus today that identifies the varying ways that families with children with disabilities deal with stressful situations. There is great similarity to the way that families with children without disabilities deal with similar issues. There are also varying responses to how some deal with stressors. Sometimes, others can view stressors as benefits. Also, the response to stressors is cyclic and cumulative. Each stressor response affects others' responses.[24]

The evolving family concept also accepts that families evolve over time and tries to identify where they are in their developmental process. Similarly, families need to be considered across the continuum of care. This is especially true as their younger children age and approach adulthood. This line of thinking has allowed researchers to look at how and why some families are more resilient than others and also how extended coping with chronic disabilities affects families over time.

The supported family members look at internal and external resources that are available to them. How family members respond to difficulties depends on their supports. This also has roots in societal and cultural assumptions. Recent research on family adaptation shows the following key themes[24]:

- There is a dominant body of literature that shows patterns of adjustment and well-being to be similar across groups of families of children with and without disabilities. This does show, however, that there are some developmental differences over the family life course.
- Additionally, there is an increasing recognition and growing research that a significant number of parents actually report numerous benefits and positive outcomes for their family associated with raising a child with a disability. These include coping skills (adaptability), family harmony (cohesiveness), spiritual growth or shared values, shared parenting roles, and communication.
- There are, obviously, stressors associated with having a child with a disability. Research continues to refine the understanding of why some families are more resilient than others in adapting to stress. Some research has suggested that the level of disability or family structure may not be as crucial as other factors (income, self-injurious behaviors, and so on). There are also differing patterns of adaptation along ethnic and cultural lines.[24]

The Cultural Response to Illness

How one views and responds to health, illness, and death is largely defined by his or her cultural values. Before detailing this, a distinction between disease and illness must be made.

Physicians diagnose and treat diseases, which can be defined as abnormalities in the structure and function of body organs and systems. Illnesses, on the other hand, are experiences of disvalued changes in states of being and cultural reactions to disease or discomfort.[29]

How a person understands and responds to illness is determined by what Kleinman calls "explanatory models." These are defined as "notions about an episode of sickness and its treatment that are employed by all those engaged in the clinical process."[29] Explanatory models address five major issues:

1. Etiology of the problem
2. Time and mode of onset
3. Pathophysiology of illness
4. Course of illness and degree and severity
5. Type of treatment that should be sought[29]

"Illness is culturally shaped in how we perceive, experience, and cope with disease based on our explanations of sickness, explanations specific to the social positions we occupy and systems of meanings we employ."[29] The role of traditional medicine and folk healing is based on cultural values. An estimated 70% to 90% of self-recognized episodes of sickness are managed outside of the formal health care system.[29] As Kleinman states, "[F]olk healers deal with the human experience of illness." They seek to provide meaningful explanations for illness and respond to personal, family, and community issues surrounding it.[29] Illness referred to as "folk illness" (i.e., illnesses that are recognized within a cultural group) may sometimes conflict with the biomedical paradigm.[29]

It is important to understand folk illness because people who experience "folk illness" may present to a medical practitioner and a "folk healer." Additionally, some "folk treatments" are potentially hazardous. Finally, folk illness may be cultural interpretations of states of pathophysiology that may require medical attention. For many chronic problems, patients have reported greater improvement with marginal folk healers than with medical physicians. Kleinman attributes this improvement to folk healers' increased emphasis on "explanation" and a greater concordance of explanatory systems between healer and patient.[29]

For more serious illness, values and beliefs become even more crucial to understanding. Although the biologic manifestations of diseases are the same among cultural groups, individuals differ in the way they experience, interpret, and respond to illness. Explanatory models as well as coping styles have been shown to influence perceptions of illness.[29] Some have suggested that meanings are assigned using characteristic themes resulting from individual coping styles, knowledge, beliefs, and cultural background.[29] Viewing illness as a challenge regards the illness as something to be approached internally and mastered. The proper authorities are consulted, advice is followed, and life goes on. Illness as "God's will" is often perceived as beyond human control and may result in passive acceptance and resignation of what cannot be changed. This set of beliefs may result in less interest in aggressive procedures and may produce depression. Illness as a "strategy" describes using illness to secure attention or nurturing from parents, family, or health care professionals. Illness as a "value" may be the "highest form" of coping, where illness is viewed as an opportunity that can result in important insight into the meaning of life. Although meanings may be influenced by culture, they are not culture specific.[29]

The expectations and perceptions of symptoms, as well as the labels attached to sickness behaviors, are influenced by environment, family, and explanatory models. In addition, the way in which problems are communicated, how symptoms are presented, when and who is visited for care, how long one remains in care, and how care is evaluated are all affected by cultural beliefs.[30,31] Likewise, culture dramatically influences the reaction to and expression of pain, which has been learned throughout childhood.[32]

The Cultural Response to Disability

Research gives strong support to the argument that definitions of disability are socially constructed.[11,22] When disability is severe, studies show that although all groups recognize gross developmental, behavioral, or sensory impairments, their attributions differ widely, as does the extent of stigma or value associated with that condition.[11,33] Responses to impairments vary through time, place, and culture. Over the course of history, societies have defined what did and did not constitute a disability or handicap. The past decade has seen changes in the conceptualization of the meaning of disability and the interplay between the possibility that an impairment becomes a physical handicap. Even more than physical limitations placed on the individual with a disability, attitudinal

concepts and images affect treatment of an individual with a disability. The sources of concepts and images they produce are found in literature and art, television and movies, religious texts, and school books. Because these sources are all artifacts of culture, it is impossible to separate culture from attitudes toward disability.[11]

For children with disabilities, the culturally perceived cause of a chronic illness or disability affects aspects of a family and community's attitudes toward that child.[28] In some cultures, disability is viewed as a form of punishment. Depending on the belief system, the individual with a disability, the family, or an ancestor has been targeted by God, or a god, for having sinned or violated a taboo.[32]

Similarly, inherited disorders can oftentimes be attributed to "running in the blood" or caused by a curse.[30,31] In societies where there is a belief in reincarnation, disability may be seen as the result of a transgression in a previous life by parents of a child with a disability or the child. Some belief systems may emphasize the imbalance of humoral elements in the body as the cause of disability.[28]

All of these perceived causes identify the individual with the disability as responsible for that disability and suggest likely consequences for the person's place in the family. Additionally, where disability is seen as a punishment, the presence of a child with a disability may be a source of embarrassment to the family. Various types of neglect may be apparent, including isolation. In many cultures, the idea of early intervention is not in the mindset for medical and educational professionals.[28] There may also be strong social pressures placed on the family in these instances. Families may be reluctant to participate in therapeutic programs, fearing that these will call attention to their family member's physical and intellectual limitations.[28]

An understanding of traditional expectations for survival is also important. For some cultures, the belief that severely disabled children will simply not survive makes the allocation of medical and parental attention to healthy children more practical. Either neglecting a child with a disability or overprotecting him or her because he or she is alive for only a short period of time can have serious implications for both health care services and psychological development. Moreover, how one is believed to be restored to health can have implications for long-term planning or arranging for special care, with members of some cultures feeling that "maybe God will make your baby all better on its own."[28]

Societies that limit occupational roles and social roles for individuals with disabilities can affect the time, energy, and expense invested in educating a child with a disability. Additionally, a gender bias, common in some cultures, may affect the degree to which a family is willing to spend money in order to obtain medical care. In these cultures, it may be perceived as less justifiable to expend vast amounts of family resources on female children with a disability than male children with a disability.[28]

Failure to fully understand cultural beliefs and values toward disability may influence a family's care toward its disabled child. Consider the family members whose cultural beliefs lead them to feel that it is their responsibility to provide complete and total care for their child with a disability. They may prefer to keep their child at home, unseen by even neighbors. They may hesitate to come forward for aid or advice, for various reasons, which may include poverty, fear, language barriers, or faith in traditional medical practices. When not viewed in a cultural context, this may be construed as neglect—the failure of parents to nurture and provide adequate ongoing education and emotional support.[22]

The Cultural Response to Death and Dying

The number of children with severe and complex neurodevelopmental disabilities and complex medical conditions who are surviving is increasing owing to advances in medical care and technology.[34] There can be conflict between palliative care at the end of life and cure-oriented treatment. Death and the customs surrounding it need to be addressed because they are highly influenced by cultural values. Expressions of grief and coping mechanisms vary from person to person but are related to cultural background.[35] The meaning of death, family patterns, including family roles during periods of grief, and the family's expectations for professional health care need to be understood. Professional attitudes regarding quality of life and appropriateness of care, the uncertainty of prognosis and the unique role of the child with a chronic disability, and the codependence between caregiver and child may all contribute to barriers to end-of-life care in this patient population.

The loss of a child with a chronic disability signifies loss not only of the child but also of a lifestyle. Respecting the family's expertise when it comes to their child will assist with effective advanced care planning and implementation.[34]

» Providing family-centered intervention

The nursing literature has explored the process of cultural competence in the delivery of health care service, including a model for providing culturally competent interventions. This model of cultural competence includes cultural desire, cultural awareness, cultural knowledge, and cultural skill.[36,37]

Cultural Desire

The first requirement for cultural competence is "cultural desire." This is the motivation to "want to" engage in the process of becoming culturally aware, becoming culturally knowledgeable, becoming culturally skillful, and seeking cultural encounters.[37] Rather than doing it because it is required, cultural desire involves doing it because it is personally desired. It includes a genuine passion to be open and flexible with others, to accept differences and build on similarities, and to be willing to learn from others as cultural informants.

Cultural Awareness

Cultural awareness is the next step in achieving cultural competence and has been described as the self-examination and in-depth exploration of one's own cultural background.[36] This awareness involves recognizing one's biases, prejudices, and assumptions about individuals who are different. Without this self-awareness, there is a risk of imposing one's own beliefs, values, and patterns of behavior on one from another culture.

Cultural Knowledge

Cultural knowledge is the process of seeking and obtaining a sound educational foundation about diverse cultural and ethnic groups.[37] Obtaining this information does not refer to learning generalizations but to learning individual differences. Learning generalizations about specific cultural subgroups leads to the development of stereotypes. Understanding that there is as much intracultural difference and intercultural difference because of life experiences, acculturation to other cultures, and diversity within cultures will prevent the imposition of stereotypical patterns on patients and families.

Cultural Skill

Cultural skill is the ability to collect cultural data regarding the patient's problem as well as performing a culturally based physical assessment.[37] There are many tools available to help collect this information via questions. One must also remember that it is a developmental skill to ask questions in a way that does not offend the patient or family. Listening and remaining nonjudgmental are effective and sensitive ways to obtain information. Additionally, having multiple cultural encounters is the way to refine or modify one's own belief about a cultural group and prevent stereotyping. Linguistic assessment is necessary to facilitate accurate communication. The use of specifically medically trained interpreters is important to the assessment process. Untrained interpreters, family members, and, specifically, children and siblings, may pose a problem owing to lack of medical knowledge.

Care must be provided that is not only culturally competent, but that also provides for low literacy skills. It is documented that people who have limited English proficiency experience obstacles when accessing health care.[37] They may experience delays in making appointments and are also more likely to have misunderstandings regarding time, place, date, and location of appointment. People with low literacy skills may have difficulty communicating with the health care professional and employees in the health care institution. These issues are more likely to exacerbate medical problems that require timely treatment or follow-up.[37]

In 1999, the U.S. Department of Health and Human Services (HHS) office of Minority Health developed standards of care within these areas. These standards were revised in 2007 (Display 3.2). In addition, the Office of Civil Rights and

The CLAS standards are primarily directed at health care organizations[40]; however, individual providers are also encouraged to use the standards to make their practices more culturally and linguistically accessible. The principles and activities of CLAS should be integrated throughout an organization and undertaken in partnership with the communities being served.

Standard 1
Health care organizations should ensure that patients/consumers receive from all staff members, effective, understandable, and respectful care that is provided in a manner compatible with their cultural health beliefs and practices and in preferred language.

Standard 2
Health care organizations should implement strategies to recruit, retain, and promote at all levels of the organization a diverse staff and leadership that are representative of the demographic characteristics of the service area.

Standard 3
Health care organizations should ensure that staff at all levels and across all disciplines receive ongoing education and training in CLAS delivery.

Standard 4
Health care organizations must offer and provide language assistance services, including bilingual staff and interpreter services, at no cost to each patient/consumer with limited English proficiency at all points of contact, in a timely manner during all hours of operation.

Standard 5
Health care organizations must provide to patients/consumers in their preferred language both verbal offers and written notices informing them of their right to receive language assistance services.

Standard 6
Health care organizations must assure the competence of language assistance provided to limited-English-proficient patients/consumers by interpreters and bilingual staff. Family and friends should not be used to provide interpretation services (except on request by the patient/consumer).

Standard 7
Health care organizations must make available easily understood patient-related materials and post signage in the languages of the commonly encountered groups and/or groups represented in the service area.

Standard 8
Health care organizations should develop, implement, and promote a written strategic plan that outlines clear goals, policies, operational plans, and management accountability/oversight mechanisms to provide CLAS.

Standard 9
Health care organizations should conduct initial and ongoing organizational self-assessments of CLAS-related activities and are encouraged to integrate cultural and linguistic competence-related measures into their internal audits, performance improvement programs, patient satisfaction assessments, and outcomes-based evaluations.

Standard 10
Health care organizations should ensure that data on the individual patient's/consumer's race, ethnicity, and spoken and written language are collected in health records, integrated into the organization's management information systems, and periodically updated.

Standard 11
Health care organizations should maintain a current demographic, cultural, and epidemiologic profile of the community as well as a needs assessment to accurately plan for and implement services that respond to the cultural and linguistic characteristics of the service area.

Standard 12
Health care organizations should develop participatory, collaborative partnerships with communities and utilize a variety of formal and informal mechanisms to facilitate community and patient/consumer involvement in designing and implementing CLAS-related activities.

Standard 13
Health care organizations should ensure that conflict- and grievance-resolution processes are culturally and linguistically sensitive and capable of identifying, preventing, and resolving cross-cultural conflicts or complaints by patients/consumers.

Standard 14
Health care organizations are encouraged to regularly make available to the public information about their progress and successful innovations in implementing the CLAS standards and to provide public notice in their communities about the availability of this information.

HHS enforce federal laws that prohibit discrimination by health care providers who receive funding from the HHS. Antidiscrimination laws are established by Section 504 of the Rehabilitation Act of 1973, Title VI of the Civil Rights Act of 1964, Title II of the Americans with Disabilities Act of 1990, Community Service Assurance provisions of the Hill–Burton Act, and the Age Discrimination Act of 1975.[38] The laws mandate that providers who accept federal money must "ensure meaningful access to and benefits from health services for individuals who have limited English proficiency."[39] Using an interpreter and translating materials into languages and levels that can be read by those who have literacy deficiencies are important mandated tools.

Adults who have literacy deficiencies face many problems in understanding written and verbal materials that are provided to them. It is important to remember that although some readily admit their limitations in regard to understanding verbal and written information, others may feel ashamed and use strategies to hide their limitations. In these situations, it is appropriate to use oral explanation and demonstration. Pictures, photographs, and visual cues also help to reinforce the information. Some people will also use family members to assist them with reading, a resource that may be important in the education process.

It is possible to identify people with low literacy skills by looking for clues. An example is someone who gives excuses for not being able to read something or who cannot read back information that is provided. Some other strategies to providing information to those with low literacy skills include[39]:

- Remaining nonjudgmental
- Involving the patient/family
- Asking the patient simple questions
- Simplifying instructions
- Repeating the information many times
- Finding various ways to give the same message
- Organizing information so that the most important information is provided first
- Using audiovisual information
- Involving family and friends in the learning and reinforcing of information
- Asking the patient to recall the message in his or her own words or demonstrate the skill that is being taught
- Empowering individuals and families and fostering independence in their programs

Health care professionals and physical therapists should promote the sharing of information and collaboration among patients, families, and health care staff. Offering places such as a family resource center will give families opportunities to educate themselves about their child's needs. Also, developing programs that provide support to families in the community is an important related activity.

Some institutions have instituted family faculty or ambassadors.[40] These families have often been in similar situations and can act to encourage and facilitate parent-to-parent support. They also provide a network for families. Additionally, it is important for health care providers to support family caregiving and decision making and help give families the tools to do so, even if it is not in agreement with one's own preferences. Institutions must involve patients and families in the planning, delivery, and evaluation of health care services. They should take feedback from families and incorporate that into program planning. They should also consider the family needs as well as the child's needs. In summary, one provides culturally competent intervention by asking the right questions.[21]

» Benefits to providing family-centered care

Health care practitioners who practice family-centered care are aware that it can enhance parents' confidence in their roles and, over time, increase the competence of children and young adults to take responsibility for their own health care, particularly in anticipation of the transition to adult services.[41] Family-centered care can improve patient and family outcomes, increase patient and family satisfaction, build on the child and family strengths, increase professional satisfaction, decrease health care costs, and lead to more effective use of health care resources, as shown in the following examples from the literature[42,43]:

- Family presence during health care procedures decreases anxiety for the child and the parents. Research indicates that when parents are prepared, they do not prolong the procedure or make the provider more anxious.
- Children whose mothers were involved in their posttonsillectomy care recovered faster and were discharged earlier than were children whose mothers did not participate in their care.
- A series of quality improvement studies found that children who had undergone surgery cried less, were less restless, and required less medication when their parents were present and assisted in pain assessment and management.
- Children and parents who received care from child life specialists did significantly better than did control children and parents on measures of emotional distress, coping during the procedure and adjustment during the hospitalization, the posthospital period, and recovery, including recovery from surgery.
- A multisite evaluation of the efficacy of parent-to-parent support found that one-on-one support increased parents' confidence and problem-solving abilities.
- Family-to-family support can have beneficial effects on the mental health status of mothers of children with chronic illness.
- Family-centered care has been a strategic priority at children's hospitals all over the country. Families participated in design planning for the new hospital, and they have been involved in program planning, staff education, and other key hospital committees and task forces.

Staff satisfaction also improves with family-centered care initiatives. The following points have been found[44]:

- Staff report valuable learning experiences.
- A Vermont program has shown that a family faculty program, combined with home visits, produces positive changes in medical student perceptions of children and adolescents with cognitive disabilities.
- When family-centered care is the cornerstone of culture in a pediatric emergency department, staff members have more positive feelings about their work than do staff members in an emergency department that does not emphasize family-centered care.
- Coordination for prenatal care in a manner consistent with family-centered principles for pregnant women at risk for poor birth outcomes at a medical center in Wisconsin resulted in more prenatal visits, decreased rate of tobacco and alcohol use during pregnancy, higher infant birth rates and gestational ages, and fewer neonatal intensive care unit days. All these factors decrease health care costs and the need for additional services.
- After redesigning their transitional care center in a way that is supportive of families, creating 24-hour open visiting for families, and making a commitment to information sharing, a children's hospital in Ohio experienced a 30% to 50% decrease in their infants' length of stay.
- In Connecticut, a family support service for children with HIV hired family support workers whose backgrounds and life experiences were similar to those of the families served by the program. This approach resulted in decreases in HIV-related hospital stays, missed clinic appointments, and foster care placement.
- King County, Washington, has a children's managed care program based on a family participation service model. Families decide for themselves how dollars are spent for their children with special mental health needs as long as the services are developed by a collaborative team created by the family. In the 5 years since the program's inception, the proportion of children living in community homes instead of institutions has increased from 24% to 91%. The number of children attending community schools has grown from 48% to 95%, and the average cost of care per child or family per month has decreased from approximately $6,000 to $4,100.

Benefits to the health care professional include[45]:

- A stronger alliance with the family in promoting each child's health and development
- Improved clinical decision making on the basis of better information and collaborative processes
- Improved follow-through when the plan of care is developed by a collaborative process
- Greater understanding of the family's strengths and caregiving capacities

- More efficient and effective use of professional time and health care resources
- Improved communication among members of the health care team
- A more competitive position in the health care marketplace
- An enhanced learning environment for future pediatricians and other professionals in training
- A practice environment that enhances professional satisfaction
- Greater child and family satisfaction with their health care
- Involving patients and families in change efforts in health care institutions helps deliver improvements in care processes, gains in health literacy, and more effective priority setting as well as more cost-effective use of health care and better outcomes.[43,44]

» Barriers to providing family-centered care

Role conflict between families and health care professionals can impede the implementation of family-centered care. Often, this is very evident in the acute care setting. In the past, parents were expected to hand over the care of their child to the professionals and remain separate from the child. Today, parents are expected to stay with their child and participate in their care. This example can also be seen in the home care environment where parents may not be afforded the respite care that they were once able to access.

Role conflict contributes to role stress. Role stress is defined as "a subjective experience that is associated with lack of role clarity, role overload, role conflict, or temporary role pressures."[15] This stress can affect the communication process between health care provider and parent by causing one or the other to focus on the source of the stress as opposed to the underlying issues. Parents can be subjected to role stress owing to their child being ill, with exacerbation of that stress being associated with the child being hospitalized (Display 3.3).[15]

DISPLAY 3.3   Stress-Limiting Strategies

Newton defines strategies that health care providers can use to limit stress for a family by using the acronym LEARN[15]:

Listen sympathetically and with understanding to the family's perception of the situation.
Explain your perception of the situation.
Acknowledge and discuss the similarities and differences between the two perceptions.
Recommend interventions.
Negotiate an agreement on the interventions.

The hospitalization of a child can be extremely stressful for even the most well-organized family. Many studies show that a professional can ease this stress by helping the parents understand the illness, help provide familiarity and comfort with the hospital setting, and encourage negotiating care of the child with health professionals.[15] Building a relationship with families and adapting styles to the individual learning styles, emotional stresses, and culture can lead to more effective intervention.[6] This has also been reported to improve developmental outcome and lead to enhanced cognitive and socioeconomic development in premature babies in the neonatal intensive care unit.[6,46]

Summary

It is important for the health care provider to examine his or her own belief systems to provide family-centered culturally competent care. First, it is necessary to recognize the vital role families play in ensuring the health and well-being of its family members. It has been proposed that family members are equal members of the team. Next, there is a need to acknowledge that emotional, social, and developmental supports are integral components of health care. Third, there is a need to respect the patient's and the family's choices and their values, beliefs, and cultural backgrounds. This can be accomplished by asking questions. Finally, there is a need to acknowledge that families, even those living in difficult circumstances, bring important and unique strengths to their health care experiences. "Family-centered care is a service delivery model that includes the manner in which the services match the needs identified by the family."[8] Although many people practice family-centered care, it is not widespread. Health care professionals must adopt new practices and policies, and families and patients must learn new skills.

Today, there are many government agencies that have been instituted around family-centered care initiatives. The Agency for Healthcare Research and Quality (AHRQ) (www.hhs.gov) and the Institute for Patient and Family Centered Care (www.ipfcc.org) are two examples. These organizations provide recommendations for training programs to educate professionals both pre- and postprofessionally about their role in fostering family-centered care. Historically, these agencies began in an attempt to educate professionals around principles of family-centered care. In 1998, then Vice President Al Gore held a conference in Nashville on families and health. This conference set the stage for initiatives nationwide to recognize the value of family-centered care in the nation's health system. A Family Bill of Rights was originally developed by President Clinton. This Bill of Rights is posted in public areas in health care practices in multiple languages and made available to families as necessary.[17] At the family reunion conference, Vice President Gore also outlined a five-step action plan for bringing the powers of families into our health care system. This action plan can be used as a summary for this chapter. The plan is SMART. Its principles are as follows[17]:

Support families with information, education, understanding, and resources. Some examples of this are family resource centers, family advocacy groups, and family faculty.

Measure the effectiveness of programs. This can be done with outcome measures, qualitatively and quantitatively.

Ask the right questions. Determine the individual needs of the patient and family. This will decrease the tendency to make generalizations based on culture.

Respect that individual differences do occur and that they may be different from that of the professional.

Train early on in the health care profession. Recognize that training is lifelong and ongoing.

Training programs should be in place to educate health care workers both pre- and postprofessionally about their role in fostering family-centered care. There is an urgent need for preservice training in multicultural practices.[17] Coursework for special educators and health professionals should be part of the preprofessional curriculum. Much has been published about specific cultural groups. This type of approach is promising for professionals who are being trained to work with specific groups of people. There is danger, however, in this method of training. It risks the development of stereotypes and assumptions that are not true. No individual training program can possibly address all the differences that are possible within groups. More effective methods of teaching cultural effectiveness include processes for a much broader conceptual approach. Many programs have developed their own methods. All have common themes: self-assessment, culturally effective knowledge of language, and the ability to apply the knowledge at both interpersonal and systems levels. Harry recommends an approach that is a habit of reflective practice that will lead to effective parent–professional collaboration without having a great deal of culturally specific information.[11] The approach includes developing culturally appropriate observation and interviewing skills, including asking questions that are open-ended. The federal government will continue to look at funding systems for programs and enact legislation to ensure that principles are being respected. If these principles are in place with our delivery of physical therapy examination, evaluation, and intervention, it will serve to improve all aspects of the patient experience.[45]

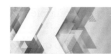

CASE STUDIES

ROSELYN

Roselyn is an 8-year-old girl with cerebral palsy. She lives with her mother, father, two brothers, one sister, grandmother, aunt, and four cousins in a small home in an urban environment. Roselyn's parents moved to the United States when they were teenagers. They have learned to speak English, but it is not their primary language spoken at home. Roselyn is unable to walk and does not attend school. Her family takes care of her every need. She rarely leaves the house except to go to church, where she is carried and doesn't have many friends her own age. She has a close family and enjoys many visits from friends and neighbors. Her family takes her regularly to the major medical center for all her medical care.

The professionals have recommended a special educational setting for Roselyn, where she would receive all her educational needs and therapies. The family has declined such a placement and prefers to homeschool her. She is not receiving any therapy at this time.

Many professionals who have seen Roselyn have tried to get the family to agree to engage outside help for her. They have stressed the importance of teaching her how to function independently. The family members insist that she does not need to do anything, because they will take care of her. They do not even want to get any type of special equipment to help them to take care of her. Roselyn has not had any acute medical issues; however, the team feels that Roselyn could do more for herself.

After many years of team recommendations not being followed by Roselyn's family, a new physical therapist offered to make a visit to the family's home to assess the situation. When she arrived, she found a very crowded living arrangement within a very small home. As she stayed to "visit," she observed a typical day in the life of Roselyn. She was amazed to see the whole family involved. One family member bathed and dressed her. Another family member fed her along with the rest of the family. When the other children went off to school, Roselyn's mother spent a few hours teaching her math and reading and doing "exercises" to make her strong. After lunch, Roselyn was carried outside and taken for a walk around the neighborhood and accompanied her father to the store for some groceries in a homemade wagon. After the children returned from school, Roselyn sat outside on the porch and watched the children as they played. They all included her in their games.

The physical therapist realized that Roselyn's family and neighbors had embraced her care as a team. They had developed strategies to care for her and included her in the family's activities. When speaking to Roselyn's mother, she sensed that she had an enormous sense of responsibility for Roselyn's disability, even referring to "punishment for sins that had been committed by her parents." It was obvious that Roselyn's family took great pride in her caretaking.

When the physical therapist returned from her visit, she shared the information that she had received with the team. She took photos and a video of the house and the equipment that the family used. All agreed that Roselyn was being cared for but that perhaps they were going about helping her in the wrong way. They decided to have a social worker, who was of the same ethnic group, to work with the family on changing its understanding of the disability. Instead of focusing on changing what the family was doing, the team worked to support the family members in what they were doing. Very soon, the family accepted some help from the team. The team was able to give the family members suggestions to make it easier for them to care for Roselyn and also for how she could play a more active role in the family and the community.

Clinic visits were not frustrating anymore as the team took a new approach to making recommendations to the family.

Discussion Points

Was the team being family centered when they first worked with Roselyn and her family?

How did the therapist's visit change the perception of the team?

Why was the family so resistant to the recommendations that they made as a team?

How should the team proceed with their recommendations as Roselyn gets older?

DANIEL

Daniel is a 4-year-old boy who was admitted to the hospital for "a bad cough." His parents were not born in this country and spoke little English. There was no other family member with Daniel who spoke English, so the nurses and doctors attempted to get information to complete their assessment using gestures, pictures, and simple English. It appeared from the examination that Daniel had been ill for quite some time, without medical care. He appeared malnourished and had a severe productive cough with bloody sputum. He also had marks on his chest that appeared to be caused by a small object being rubbed on it. The professionals who examined Daniel felt that there may have been neglect and discussed the appropriate course of action because they are mandated reporters. The attending physicians decided to admit Daniel to the hospital for a workup. He called Social Services because of his concerns about the family and refused to allow the parents to accompany Daniel to his room. The family was left in the emergency room while Daniel was wheeled away, and security was called to restrain them there until Social Services arrived.

The social worker arrived at the situation and first went to speak to the physician. The physician said that he felt the parents neglected Daniel's needs and that he was very concerned for Daniel's welfare. He added that Daniel had signs of abuse on his chest and was malnourished. It was his duty to call child protective services. In the meantime, Daniel was undergoing tests to determine what was wrong with him. The physician left to attend to Daniel as the social worker returned to the emergency room to speak with the parents.

The social worker met the parents and found out by simple cards with different languages what language they spoke. She was then able to get an interpreter through a language service. She collected basic facts about the boy and his current medical situation. She was also able to get a phone number to a neighbor of the family who was bilingual. She was able to convey to the parents that their son was going to have some medical tests to determine why he was sick and how to make him better.

The family's neighbor was able to come to the hospital to help to communicate with the family. It turned out that the boy had been sick for a few weeks and that the family members were using traditional means to care for their son. "Coining," where a coin is rubbed on the ailing part of the body, was performed by the mother to "drive out the cough." The family also believed that a special diet of herbs and natural foods would cleanse his body and bring him back to health. It was very apparent to the social worker that they loved their son very much and were doing everything in their means to make him well.

The social worker determined that the family was not neglectful but did not understand Western medicine and the importance that Americans place on their medical system. She spoke with the doctor and relayed, through the family interpreter, that the boy needed special treatment with medication. The family was scared because they did not trust the medical system. With the help of the interpreter, the nurses spent some time teaching the family some techniques, using pictures. The parents were allowed to be with their son. The nurses allowed the family to set up the child's room to allow "spiritual healing" to occur. They also took the time to explain everything that they were doing to the family.

A member of the family's church came to visit the boy and spoke with the nurses and doctor about some of the family's traditions, and they all decided on a few modifications to these traditions that the family would be able to carry out in the hospital room. For example, instead of prayer with the use of candles, the nurses obtained a battery-operated candle that used a light bulb for the flames. The family was also shown manual airway clearance techniques to perform in place of coining to assist Daniel with coughing.

The team held family meetings with Daniel's family frequently during his admission, with the use of medical interpreters. A mutual trust developed between the team and the family. Daniel began to get well and was discharged home with his family. He was followed as an outpatient and continued to enjoy a healthy and happy life.

Discussion Points

How could the emergency room situation have been handled differently?

How did the social worker's behavior change the situation?

Do you think that Daniel's family was negligent? Why or why not?

Did the physician provide family-centered care? Why or why not?

What would you do if you were responsible for the care of this child?

REFERENCES

1. McGrath JM. Family: essential partner in care. In: Kenner C, Lott JW, eds. *Comprehensive Neonatal Care: An Interdisciplinary Approach*. 4th ed. Saunders Elsevier; 2007:491-509.

2. *Census 2010 Profile*. U.S. Department of Commerce, Economics, and Statistics Administration, U.S. Census Bureau; 2012.

3. Vespa J, Medina L, Armstrong D. Demographic turning points for the United States: population projections for 2020 to 2060. Current Population Reports, P25-1144, U.S. Census Bureau, Washington, DC, 2020.

4. Reynolds D. Improving care and interactions with racially and ethnically diverse populations in healthcare organizations. *J Healthc Manag*. 2004;49(4):237-249.

5. U.S. Department of Health and Human Services. *Health Communication in Healthy People 2010: Understanding and Improving Health*. 2nd ed. U.S. Government Printing Office; 2010. Accessed September 1, 2020. https://www.cdc.gov/nchs/data/hpdata2010/hp2010_final_review.pdf

6. Sweeny J, Heriza CB, Blanchard Y, et al. Neonatal physical therapy. Part II: practice frameworks and evidence-based practice guidelines. *Pediatr Phys Ther*. 2010;22(1):2-16.

7. Iverson M, Shimmel J, Ciacera S, et al. Creating a family-centered approach in early intervention services—perceptions of parents and professionals. *Pediatr Phys Ther*. 2003;15:23-31.

8. O'Neil ME, Palisano R. Attitudes toward family centered care and clinical decision making in early intervention among physical therapists. *Pediatr Phys Ther*. 2000;12:173-182.

9. Kau DZ, Houtrow AJ, Arango P, et al. Family centered care: current applications and future directions in pediatric health care. *Maternal Child Health*. 2012;16:297-305.

10. ED.gov. U.S Department of Education. Accessed September 1, 2020. www.idea.ed.gov

11. Harry B. Trends and issues in serving culturally diverse families of children with disabilities. *J Special Educ*. 2002;36:131-138. Accessed January 26, 2021. https://clintonwhitehouse4.archives.gov/textonly/WH/New/html/19980622-11246.html.

12. *The Joint Commission on the Accreditation of Healthcare Organizations. Comprehensive Accreditation Manual for Hospitals*. Joint Commission Resources, Inc; 2006.

13. Wilson-Stronks A, Lee KK, Cordero CL, et al. *One Size Does Not Fit All: Meeting the Health Care Needs of Diverse Populations*. The Joint Commission; 2008. http://www.ipfcc.org/about/index.htm

14. The Joint Commission on the Accreditation of Healthcare Organization. Facts about advancing effective communication, cultural competence, and patient and family-centered care. 2010. Accessed September 2, 2020. https://www.jointcommission.org/-/media/tjc/documents/resources/patient-safety-topics/health-equity/aroadmapforhospitalsfinalversion727pdf.pdf?db=web&hash=AC3AC4BED1D973713C2CA6B2E5ACD01B.

15. Newton M. Family-centered care: current realities in parent participation. *Pediatr Nurs*. 2000;26:164-169.

16. Mitchell MJ, Lemanmek K, Palermo TM, et al. Parent perspectives on pain management, coping and family functioning in pediatric sickle cell disease. *Clin Pediatr (Phila)*. 2007;46(4):311-319.

17. Harvey J. *Proceedings from the Family Re-Union 7 Conference*. Vanderbilt University; 1998. Accessed October 10, 2020. https://govinfo.library.unt.edu/npr/library/speeches/062498.html.

18. The Institute for Family Centered Care. Patient and family-centered care. Accessed September 1, 2020. https://www.ipfcc.org/.

19. Clay A, Parsh B. Patient and family-centered care: it's not just for pediatrics anymore. *AMA J Ethics*. 2016;18(1):40-44.

20. McMillan A. Relevance of culture on pediatric physical therapy: a Saudi Arabian experience. *Pediatr Phys Ther*. 1995;7(3):138-139.

21. Camphina-Bacote J. Many faces: addressing diversity in health care. *Online J Issues Nurs*. 2003;8(1):3.

22. Anderson PP, Fenichel ES. *Serving Culturally Diverse Families of Infants and Toddlers with Disabilities.* National Center for Clinical Infant Programs; 1989.

23. Guerrero AD, Chen J, Inkelas M, et al. Racial and ethnic disparities in pediatric experiences of family-centered care. *Med Care.* 2012;48(4):388-393.

24. Ferguson P. A place in the family: an historical interpretation of research on parental reactions to having a child with a disability. *J Special Educ.* 2002;36:124-130.

25. Suris JC, Michaud PA, Viner R. The adolescent with a chronic condition. Part I: developmental issues. *Arch Dis Child.* 2004;89:938-942.

26. Blum R. A consensus statement on health care transitions for young adults with special health care needs. *Pediatrics.* 2002;110:1304-1307.

27. Americans with Disabilities Act of 1990, Pub L 101-336.

28. Groce E, Irving Z. Multiculturalism, chronic illness and disability. *Pediatrics.* 1993;91(5):1048-1055.

29. Kleinman A. *Patients and Healers in the Context of Culture: An Exploration of the Borderline Between Anthropology, Medicine, and Psychiatry.* University of California Press; 1980.

30. Parry K. Patient-therapist relations: culture and personal meanings. *Phys Ther.* 1994;2(10):88-345.

31. Pachtner LM. Culture and clinical care: folk illness beliefs and their implications for health care delivery. *JAMA.* 1994;271:690-694.

32. Munet-Vilaro F, Vessey JA. Children's explanation of leukemia: a Hispanic perspective. *Adv Nurs Sci.* 1990;15(2):76-79.

33. Spearing E, Devine J. A qualitative analysis of attitudes towards disability between Hispanic and Anglo-American families of children with chronic disabilities. *Pediatr Phys Ther.* 2004;16(1):65.

34. Graham RJ, Robinson WM. Integrating palliative care into chronic care for children with severe neurodevelopmental disabilities. *J Dev Behav Pediatr.* 2005;26(5):361-365.

35. Lawson LV. Culturally sensitive support for grieving parents. *MCN Am J Matern Child Nurs.* 1990;15(2):76-79.

36. Gartner A, Lipisky D, Turnball A. *Supporting Families with a Child with a Disability.* Paul H. Brooks Publishing Co; 1991.

37. Camphina-Bacote J. A model and instrument for addressing cultural competence in health care. *J Nurs Educ.* 1999;38:203-207.

38. Byrd W, Clayton LA. *An American Health Dilemma: A Medical History of African Americans and the Problem of Race.* Routledge; 2000.

39. *National Standards for Culturally Linguistically Appropriate Services in Health Care.* U.S. Department of Health and Human Services; 2007.

40. The Office of Minority Health. U.S. Department of Health and Human Services. National Standards on culturally and linguistically appropriate services (CLAS). Accessed October 20, 2020. https://minorityhealth.hhs.gov/omh/browse.aspx?lvl=2&lvlid=53.

41. McDowell BC, Duffy C, Parkes J. Service use and family centered care in young people with severe cerebral palsy: a population based, cross sectional clinical survey. *Disabil Rehabil.* 2015;37(25):2324-2349.

42. Best A, Greenhalgh T, Lewis S, et al. Large-system transformation in health care: a realistic review. *Milibank Q.* 2012;90(3):421-456.

43. Everhart J, Haskell H, Khan A. Patient and family centered care: leveraging best practices to improve the care of hospitalized children. *Pediatr Clin N Am.* 2019;66:775-789.

44. Matthew WR, Theodore CS. Pediatric hospital medicine: where we are, where we are headed: state of specialty, looking forward. *Pediatr Clin North Am.* 2019;66(4):891-895.

45. Frank LS, O'Brien K. The evolution of family centered care: from supporting parent-delivered interventions to a model of family integrated care. *Birth Defects Res.* 2019;111(15):1044-1059.

46. Klawetter NM, Klawetter S, Greenfield JC, et al. Mothers' experiences in the NICU before family-centered care and in NICUS: where it is the standard of care. *Adv Neonatal Care.* 2020;20(1):68-79.

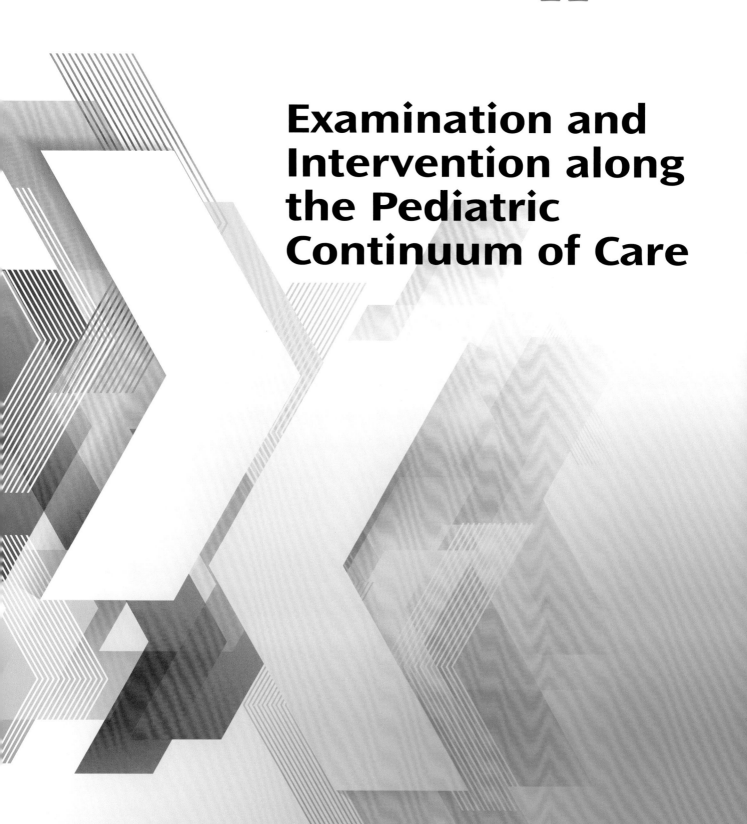

Examination and Intervention along the Pediatric Continuum of Care

II

Physical Therapy in the Neonatal Intensive Care Unit

Diane Versaw-Barnes and Audrey Wood

≫ Introduction

Today newborn infant intensive care is the standard of care in the United States for preterm babies and other newborns with life-threatening diseases. This was not the case at the beginning of the 20th century, when infant mortality was not even monitored.[1] The transformation of health care for infants in the 20th century was a result of several mutually occurring phenomena including changing cultural attitudes toward babies and children, scientific advances in the understanding of newborn infants, and technologic breakthroughs resulting in the ability to provide appropriate interventions.[2] Neonatal physicians and nurses have both pioneered this work,[3] and improved it, by recognizing that specialized knowledge and skills are essential for its success.

In 1970, the American Academy of Pediatrics (AAP) added neonatology as a medical subspecialty with board certification, and in 1975 the Committee on Perinatal Health published the first guidelines for regional perinatal centers.[4] The American Board of Physical Therapy Residency and Fellowship Education (ABPTRFE) has accredited three Neonatal Physical Therapy Fellowships to date in the United States to recognize advanced training and education in the treatment of fragile infants.

The success of neonatology has not been without its pitfalls; many untested practices, initially assumed beneficial or at least benign, for newborn infants have resulted in disastrous outcomes.[2] This has led to a staunch commitment to evidence-based practice that is at the forefront of current neonatology practice. Neonatologists have been relentless in their efforts to improve and perfect care for their tiny patients. Modern initiatives include the expansion of newborn screening[5] as well as a variety of clinical trials on newborn care practices. A search for trials currently enrolling newborns yields 1,589 studies on the ClinicalTrials.gov web site.[6]

Today more babies survive because of the highly specialized and technologic care they receive in neonatal intensive care units (NICUs) across the country; however, it is not without comorbidities such as cerebral palsy (CP), sensory impairments, and intellectual, learning, and social/emotional challenges.[7] Neonatal intensive care, despite being lifesaving, may also be the source of toxic stress for these tiny babies and may unintentionally contribute to long-term neurodevelopmental problems.[8] Neuroprotective, family-centered developmental care is a new concept in the care of sick babies. It is an amalgamation of the theories of trauma-informed care, family-centered care, and developmental care. Trauma-informed care recognizes that traumatic events (like parental separation, painful procedures, disrupted sleep, and the stress of a hostile environment, such as bright lighting, loud noises, and abrupt handling) can result in long-term physical and psychological effects.[9] Trauma-informed care embraces family-centered care. Both approaches seek to support families in assuming parenting roles and infant–parent bonding. Neonatal intensive care continues to evolve because of ongoing research efforts and data collection coordinated across many sites.[10]

It is essential to have physical therapists (PTs) trained in the subspecialty of neonatology in order to collaborate with neonatologists, neonatal nurses, and families to provide the best care for these vulnerable infants, maximizing their developmental potential and minimizing the risk of iatrogenic consequences of NICU care. This chapter provides an overview of the theoretical, developmental, and medical frameworks that guide therapy in the NICU and describes physical therapy examination and interventions, transition to home, and neonatal follow-up for the NICU graduate.

» Levels of newborn intensive care and the role of the physical therapist

The regionalization of neonatal intensive care and consistent definitions and levels of neonatal care were first proposed in the 1970s with the goal to improve neonatal outcomes. Having well-defined and nationally consistent definitions and standards of care created a common language for the public, insurance companies, and medical professionals to use to compare outcomes, resources, and costs and paved the way for comprehensive benchmarking in neonatology. Since 1976 these definitions of level of neonatal care have been revised twice based on data collected from the NICUs. The most recent survey concerned trends toward the deregionalization of care. It showed a decrease in the percentage of births of very low birth weight (VLBW) infants at level III centers and an increased

mortality for VLBW infants born at level II centers. The levels of neonatal care have been revised based on these new data and include capabilities and required providers for each level (Table 4.1).[11]

- Level I: Well newborn nursery
- Level II: Special care nursery
- Level III: NICU
- Level IV: Regional NICU

These guidelines do not specify therapists with neonatal training and expertise as necessary for the provision of care in level III and IV NICUs. The subspecialty of neonatal therapy needs more research demonstrating the efficacy of therapy during neonatal intensive care. It is imperative that

TABLE 4.1.	Levels of Neonatal Care
Level I	Well newborn nursery; provides
	• Neonatal resuscitation at delivery
	• Postnatal care and evaluation for healthy term newborns
	• Stabilization and care for infants born 35–37 wk gestation who remain stable
	• Stabilization of ill infants and infants <35 wk gestation prior to transfer
Level II	Special care nursery; in addition to Level I capabilities provides
	• Care for infants convalescing after intensive care
	• Mechanical ventilation or CPAP for <24 hr
	• Care for infants born ≥32 wk gestation and ≥1,500 g who are not anticipated to need subspecialty care urgently
	• Stabilization of infants born <35 wk gestation and <1,500 g prior to transfer
Level III	Neonatal Intensive Care; in addition to Level II capabilities provides
	• Sustained life support using full range of respiratory supports including conventional and high-frequency ventilation, and inhaled nitric oxide
	• Comprehensive care for infants with critical illness and/or born <1,500 g and <32 wk gestational age
	• Ready access to pediatric medical and surgical specialists, pediatric anesthesiologists, and ophthalmologists
	• Urgently available advanced imaging and interpretation (CT, MRI, and echocardiography)
Level IV	Regional Neonatal Intensive Care; in addition to Level III capabilities provides
	• Surgery for complex congenital or acquired conditions
	• Full range of pediatric medical and surgical subspecialists, and pediatric anesthesiologists maintained on site
	• Outreach education and facilitation of transfers into center

CPAP, continuous positive airway pressure; CT, computed tomography; MRI, magnetic resonance imaging.

neonatal PTs are recognized and employed as practitioners of choice for this population of critically ill infants in order to provide the best care for these infants.

>> Roles and competencies of the therapist in the neonatal intensive care unit

The role of the therapist working in the NICU is very different from that of other areas of physical therapy practice. The neonatal therapist provides consultation, diagnosis, intervention, and family support to extremely fragile infants and families within a very stressful and fast-paced intensive care environment. In addition to understanding a wide range of neonatal conditions, medical interventions, and their potential to impact future development, the neonatal therapist must be a careful observer, good collaborator, and effective communicator.[2,12-14] PTs have a special role to play as part of the NICU team owing to their expertise in movement, postural control, and neurodevelopment. However, the neonatal therapist must also have specialized knowledge and skills to work with very vulnerable infants and their families (Table 4.2). The ability to make decisions quickly in terms of an infant's stability and need for external supports is necessary, as an infant's status can change rapidly. In this environment, interventions that might otherwise be considered benign may have serious immediate and far-reaching consequences.[2,13,14]

Therapy in the NICU is considered to be an advanced level of pediatric physical therapy practice[2,14-16] that needs to be achieved through education and mentored clinical practice. The American Physical Therapy Association (APTA) has established guidelines for therapists practicing in the NICU,[14,17] which include specific roles, competencies, knowledge areas, and precepted clinical training. The clinical practice guidelines were originally published in 1989[18] and updated in 1999[19] and again in 2009.[15] The most recent version of the guidelines is divided into two sections: Part I presents clinical training modules, clinical training competencies, and decision-making algorithms, whereas Part II discusses frameworks and evidence from the literature that support practice of therapists in the NICU. Physical therapy neonatal fellowship programs have been developed to provide the advanced knowledge and mentored practice required to develop highly skilled individuals who provide evidence-based family-centered developmental interventions and to foster research in the setting of the NICU.

An evidence-based clinical pathway developed for neonatal PTs has also been published. The Infant Care Path for Physical Therapy in the NICU addresses observation and assessment, intervention, family support and education, and teamwork among the various disciplines that provide care to high-risk infants and their families in the NICU.[20-25] The written pathway provides a framework and knowledge that neonatal PTs can use to further develop a research-based practice. Although the pathway is a useful tool, neonatal

TABLE 4.2.	Areas of Knowledge for Neonatal Therapists

- Typical and atypical development
- Fetal and newborn development
- Development and interaction of sensory systems in preterm and full-term neonates
- Medical conditions of preterm and full-term neonates and interventions
- General function and safety regarding lines and medical equipment
- Neonatal preterm and full-term behaviors and social development
- Family dynamics, grief/loss process, attachment, parenting in the NICU
- Ecology and culture of the NICU
- The physical environment of the NICU and the effects on high-risk neonates
- Theoretical frameworks supporting care in the NICU
- Neonatal practice guidelines
- Description, administration, psychometric properties, and interpretation of results of neonatal assessments
- Risk factors associated with developmental outcome
- Evidence-based practices for positioning and intervention with high-risk infants
- Teaching strategies for families and caregivers
- Safety regarding car seats and infant positioning equipment
- Early intervention, community resources, neonatal developmental follow-up programs

NICU, neonatal intensive care unit.

therapists should individualize examination and interventions specific to the infant, family, and NICU environment.

>> Theoretical frameworks to guide therapy

Dynamic Systems Theory

Dynamic systems theory describes a model of human development in which behaviors emerge because of the interaction of many subsystems.[26-30] This framework can be used to evaluate and establish care for the high-risk infant in the NICU[16] (Fig. 4.1). The interaction of multiple subsystems within the infant as well as the interaction of the infant and the environment influence the health and development of the individual infant. The infant subsystems include body structure, physiology, and behavior. The environment includes the physical environment of the nursery, multiple caregivers and support personnel, and family. Changes to the intrinsic systems or the environment can have either positive or negative effects. These changes can produce stability to support function or interfere to cause disorganization and potentially maladaptive behaviors. A small change in one system component can have a large effect on another system and ultimately affect function.[16,26,31,32]

The therapist must understand the history, current status of the infant's systems, and the environment, taking into consideration the effect caregiving/therapy will have on that particular infant.[15,27] The therapist must support the

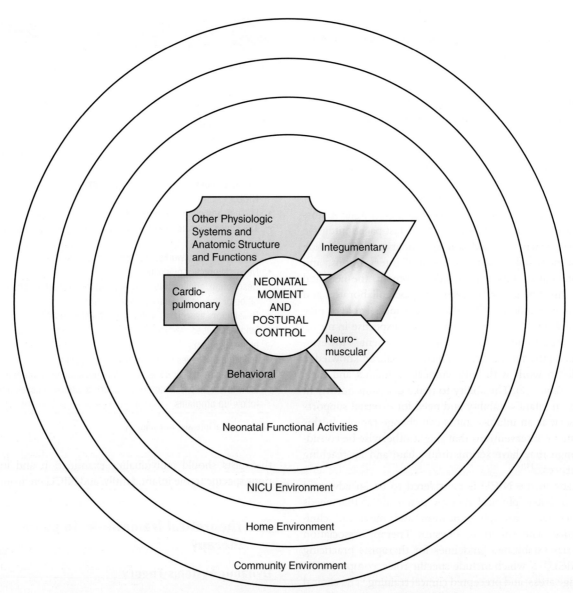

FIGURE 4.1. Dynamic systems theory in the neonatal intensive care unit (NICU). (Reprinted with permission from Sweeney JK, Heriza CB, Reilly MA, et al. Practice guidelines for the physical therapist in the NICU. *Pediatr Phys Ther.* 1999;11(3):120.)

interactions that allow functional behaviors to develop, decrease infant stress, and understand the implications of the environment. At the same time, the therapist must assist the family and other caregivers in recognizing how they too can be supportive to the infant's health and development. The therapist needs to be aware of transitional periods when developmental interventions can be safely implemented and guide families to utilize these same strategies.

Neuronal Group Selection Theory

A theoretical concept of how the nervous system becomes organized, stores information, and creates new behavioral patterns was developed by Gerald Edelman.[33,34] According to this theory, called Neuronal Group Selection Theory (NGST), the brain is dynamically organized into populations

of cells containing individually variable networks. The structures and function of these networks are selected by evolution, the environment, and behavior. The units of selection are composed of hundreds to thousands of strongly interconnected neurons that work as functional units and are referred to as neuronal groups.[35]

NGST, like dynamic systems theory, is grounded in the idea that motor development is nonlinear, has phases of transition, and is affected by both internal and external factors.[35] However, in NGST, genetic factors play as prominent a role in shaping the nervous system as experience. The interaction of genetic and epigenetic factors in the context of specific environment and activity results in individual differences between brains within a species. This interplay also allows for the brain to change over time on the basis of the afferent signals it receives.[33]

There are three basic tenets of NGST that describe how the anatomy of the brain is formed and is shaped during development, how experience selects and strengthens patterns of responses, and how resulting brain maps give rise to uniquely individual behavior.[36]

Developmental selection, in which the characteristic neuroanatomy of brain formation occurs, is the first tenet of Edelman's theory.[36] The genetic code and cellular behavior (division, migration, death) establish the areas of the brain but not specific wiring. Neurons branch in different directions, creating immense, diverse, and variable neural circuits. The neurons compete to form synapses, and these synaptic connections are strengthened or weakened on the basis of afferent information from self-generated variable movements during fetal and early postnatal life.[37] General movements of the fetus and newborn as described by Prechtl[38] illustrate the innate movements of this first phase of variability. The connections that are strengthened by these movements result in a primary neuronal repertoire of behaviors specific and unique to the species. Kicking and stepping, hand to mouth, sucking, visual orientation and following, and projection of the arms toward objects are examples of primary motor repertoires.[38] Overproduction of early synaptic connections formed by self-generated activity and pruning of unexercised connections lead to the individual variability within species-specific behaviors.

Edelman's[36] second tenet involves the development of a secondary repertoire of functional circuits through experiential selection. As the infant interacts with new environmental situations after birth, connections are formed and strengthened. Secondary repertoires of functional connections that meet environmental constraints and support successful, goal-directed movements arise from the neuronal groups of the primary repertoires through experience, repetition, and exploration.[39] The secondary repertoires contain the motor synergies necessary for skilled functional movement as well as memory and other functions. During this phase of secondary variability, the individual explores a variety of movements, and sensory feedback from this exploration shapes the selection of effective strategies. This process continues throughout life, with changing environmental constraints and functional needs.[40-43]

The third tenet of NGST describes how the first two processes interact to form neural maps that connect neuronal groups throughout the nervous system. Massive parallel and reciprocal connections between neuronal maps produce movements that are precisely adapted to the contextual demands and the individual's nervous system's capacity to receive sensory inputs and to select responses. In order for the individual to be able to adapt or respond to environmental demands and internal changes such as change in body structure with growth, there need to be repertoires of variable actions. The final motor strategy is based on demands of the task, the environment, and past experience with similar tasks that has strengthened or weakened the tendencies to select particular neuronal groups from particular neuronal maps.[36]

Higher-order dynamic structures called global maps result from these selections and link sensory and motor maps. These global maps are important for development and learning as they allow connections between local maps and motor behavior, new sensory inputs, and greater neural processing. Global maps continue to be modified over the individual's lifetime.[43]

Events such as premature birth can alter the process of brain development. Preterm infants not only have less mature nervous systems but are faced with different environmental constraints. Instead of the protective environment of the uterus, the NICU environment involves equipment for medical support and monitoring, gravitational forces, the loss of amniotic fluid support for posture and movement, stressful and painful stimuli, decreased nurturing touch, loud noises, bright lighting, and unpredictable patterns of handling.[17] According to Edelman's theory,[33] the processes of brain development are modified when placed under unusual sensory circumstances. Under these conditions, there may be preservation of cells that would otherwise be eliminated, elimination of cells that would otherwise be preserved, modification of neuronal pruning, and changes in connectivity. Neuronal changes in preterm infants have been reported by Als et al. in their study[44] comparing infants receiving Newborn Individualized Developmental Care and Assessment Program (NIDCAP) intervention with infants receiving standard NICU care. The infant's health status, growth, neurobehavior, brain structure by magnetic resonance imaging (MRI), and neurophysiology by electroencephalography (EEG) were assessed at 2 weeks and 9 months. The authors reported that the infants receiving NIDCAP care had better neurobehavioral function and more mature fiber structure in the cortex of the brain.[44]

Neonatal PTs need to consider the impact of the NICU environment and caregiving practices on the immature and developing brain. The formation of brain structure and function may be affected by these early and atypical sensory and motor experiences. Each infant has different genetic, maturational, and intra- and extrauterine environmental experiences, and the effect of the NICU environment and practices may have a different influence on brain development and function. Therefore, the effect of physical therapy assessment and intervention on brain architecture and maturation must be considered and adapted to meet the needs of the individual infant.

International Classification of Functioning, Disability, and Health

Although the NICU is a unique setting for physical therapy practice, the World Health Organization (WHO)'s International Classification of Functioning, Disability, and Health (ICF)[45] model can be applied to guide examination and intervention.[17] The pediatric PT working with high-risk infants in this environment can use the framework as a guide in addressing functional and structural integrity of body parts and systems, promoting the development of postural and motor activities, and promoting appropriate interaction between the infant, the physical environment, and the family, NICU staff, and consultants. As with a child of any age, the contextual factors of the individual infant, family, and environment must be addressed in order to provide effective intervention. For example, the functional goal for an infant may be to socially interact with family while being held. After a thorough examination, the therapist needs to consider what components are required for this activity to be successful for the infant and family as well as those components that may interfere. The therapist may assist the family in positioning the infant in optimal alignment to support physiologic functions such as respiration and in swaddling to maintain the posture, and may assist the infant in bringing hands to face for calming and behavioral organization; the therapist may also dim the lights, reduce the sound in the area to decrease stress and promote arousal, and support the family in recognizing the infant's cues for interaction. In addition, the therapist, family, and NICU staff can work together to find the most optimal times for the infant to be successful in these interactions. Throughout an infant's NICU course the PT can address goals to promote activity and participation by supporting body structures and functions, family and caregiver education, and addressing environmental and other contextual factors. Atkinson and Nixon-Cave[46] have published a clinical reflection tool to assist in translating the ICF into practice that can be applied to infants and families in the NICU.

Synactive Theory

The synactive theory of infant development, proposed by psychologist Heidelise Als,[47] is a model to understand and interpret the behavior of preterm infants and is similar to the dynamic systems approach in that multiple influences contribute and mutually influence the baby's functioning. The fetus from conception onward is thought to be organizing five distinct but interrelated subsystems: autonomic (governing basic physiologic functioning, e.g., heart rate [HR], respiratory rate [RR], visceral functions); motor (governing postures and movements); state (governing ranges of consciousness from sleep to wakefulness); attention/interaction (governing the ability to attend to and interact with caregivers); and self-regulatory (governing the ability to maintain balanced, relaxed, and integrated functioning of all four subsystems). These subsystems continually react and influence each other, thus the term *synactive*.[48-50] Babies born at term have completed the maturation of these subsystems to the degree that, in general, they are able to demonstrate brief periods of social interaction with a caregiver while maintaining stability in the physiologic, motoric, and state subsystems (Fig. 4.2). They can also utilize strategies

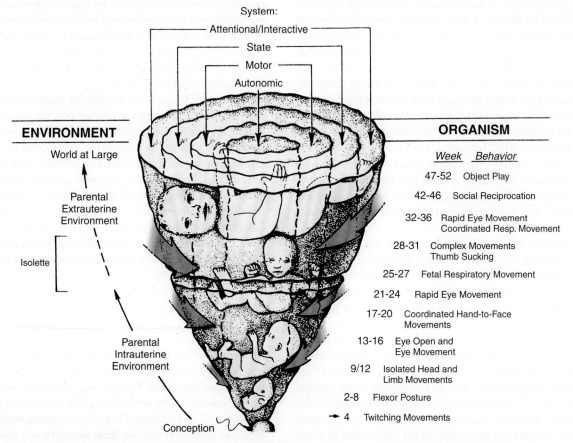

FIGURE 4.2. Model of the synactive organization of behavioral development. (Reprinted with permission from Als H. Toward a synactive theory of development: promise for the assessment and support of infant individuality. *Infant Ment Health J.* 1982;3(4):234.)

to regulate the various subsystems when the environment poses a threat to their stability; for example, when eye contact with a parent becomes too intense, a term infant may yawn, look away briefly, stretch, tuck head to trunk, and bring hands together (strategies represented by the attention/interaction and motor subsystems) before returning to gaze again at a parent's face.

In babies born before term, the maturation of the five subsystems is interrupted. In addition, babies born before term have lost the uterine supports for these subsystems (autonomic supports like temperature regulation, placental nutrition delivery, waste removal, oxygen delivery, and carbon dioxide removal; motoric supports like the containment of the uterine wall and the buoyancy of the amniotic fluid; state supports like the diurnal cycles of the mother's sleep–wake cycle; and attention/interaction supports like diminished visual and auditory input). Babies born before term are required to complete the maturation of each subsystem while also negotiating more independent functioning, such as breathing, feeding, eliminating wastes, maintaining postures, and moving against gravity and while also enduring bright lighting, harsh noises, frequent handling, and multimodal stimulation. The preterm baby is adapted for functioning in the womb, but is required to function outside the womb at a crucial time in development and, therefore, faces a very challenging existence.[47-51]

Developmental Care

Applying this synactive theory of infant development through systematic serial observations of the baby is a very helpful way to identify the baby's areas of success at coping and areas of vulnerability. It is important to communicate these strengths and vulnerabilities to the parents and caregivers and to identify strategies to support the baby receiving this necessary intensive care.[47-49,51-53] The process of systematic serial observations has led to a broad array of interventions to minimize the stress of the NICU for the infant and to individualize the caregiving to the infant's tolerance. These interventions include strategies to decrease noise and light levels, minimize handling of the infant, protect infant sleep states, promote understanding of infant behavioral cues, and promote relationship-based caregiving.[54] This approach to newborn intensive care is called NIDCAP.[52] Ideally, NIDCAP observations are scheduled every 7 to 10 days and include viewing the baby at a baseline for 10 to 20 minutes before nursing care or procedure, throughout the care session or procedure, and after the session or procedure until the baby returns to baseline functioning[52,55] (Fig. 4.3). During this time, the observer is watching for signs of stability and stress from each subsystem (Table 4.3) while recording environmental events and caretaking tasks. The infant's strategies for self-regulation, whether successful or unsuccessful, are then noted, and recommendations to support the infant's attempts at organizing and self-soothing are made as well as recommendations for environmental modification, caregiving, and parental involvement.[47,48,50-53] Formal training

through the NIDCAP regional training centers is required for reliability and certification in NIDCAP. However, using the principles and applying the synactive model to understand a baby's behavior is a helpful way to guide caregivers in developmentally supportive interventions through observations of nursing care.

The synactive model of preterm behavior identifies the autonomic subsystem and the motoric subsystem as the two core subsystems on which the rest of the infant's functioning is based (Fig. 4.4). Together, these two subsystems are the basis for the baby to achieve higher functioning like waking (state subsystem) and gazing at a parent's face (attention/interaction subsystem). A therapist can recommend and intervene to support the motor system through positioning and containment, and in so doing can support the autonomic subsystem as well as the state and interactional subsystems as each system continually interacts and influences the others.[48,49,51,56] The systematic individualization of caring for an infant is the root of developmentally supportive care.[54,57] The knowledge and understanding of how one baby differs from another can only be gleaned by skilled observation of the infant in interaction with the environment. Using this individualized knowledge of the baby's strengths and vulnerabilities to guide the provision of care has been shown to result in short-term benefits to the baby such as shorter hospitalization resulting in less costly care, decreased use of ventilator, earlier attainment of oral feeds, and improved growth. Long-term benefits include improved neurobehavioral functioning and enhanced brain structure in later infancy, advantages in expressive language and neurologic organization and function at 3 years, and improved attention and visual/spatial perception at 8 years.[44,50,51,53-55,56,58-61] Critics of the research on developmental care point out that studies have shown conflicting results, have utilized small sample sizes, and have demonstrated outcomes that may not be clinically significant. Some studies also have serious methodologic flaws in the designs, such as neglecting to blind the outcome assessors and allowing the control and experimental groups to receive the same interventions. The critics of developmental care have not found harmful effects to result from the application of the developmental care philosophy in the NICU, but question whether the benefits are real.[62,63] It is not prudent to implement a philosophy because it does no harm if there are no substantial benefits, as this may detract from other approaches that may prove truly beneficial. Given the abstract nature of the developmental care philosophy and relationship-based caregiving, it is no surprise that it is difficult to study, let alone to teach and implement. During NIDCAP observations, the authors have observed infants becoming progressively exhausted, limp, and passive during routine care, as their attempts to organize are continually thwarted by the noncontingent responses of their caregivers. In contrast, infants have been observed to maintain behavioral and physiologic stability when their caregivers are attentive and responsive to their cues. In addition, research on some specific techniques of supporting a baby during care (e.g., facilitated tucking and nonnutritive sucking [NNS]) has

OBSERVATION SHEET Name: ______________ Date: ______________ Sheet Number ______________

	Time:	0-2	3-4	5-6	7-8	9-10
Resp:	Regular					
	Irregular					
	Slow					
	Fast					
	Pause					
Color:	Jaundice					
	Pink					
	Pale					
	Webb					
	Red					
	Dusky					
	Blue					
	Tremor					
	Startle					
	Twitch Face					
	Twitch Body					
	Twitch Extremities					
Visceral/ Resp:	Spit up					
	Gag					
	Burp					
	Hiccough					
	BM Grunt					
	Sounds					
	Sigh					
	Gasp					
Motor:	Flaccid Arm(s)					
	Flaccid leg(s)					
	Flexed/ Tucked Arms Act.					
	Flexed/ Tucked Arms Post.					
	Flexed/ Tucked Legs Act.					
	Flexed/ Tucked Legs Post.					
	Extend Arms Act.					
	Extend Arms Post.					
	Extend Legs Act.					
	Extend Legs Post.					
	Smooth Mvmt. Arms					
	Smooth Mvmt. Legs					
	Smooth Mvmt. Trunk					
	Stretch/Drown					
	Diffuse Squirm					
	Arch					
	Tuck Trunk					
	Leg Brace					
Face:	Tongue Extension					
	Hand on Face					
	Gape Face					
	Grimace					
	Smile					

	Time:	0-2	3-4	5-6	7-8	9-10
State:	1A					
	1B					
	2A					
	2B					
	3A					
	3B					
	4A					
	4B					
	5A					
	5B					
	6A					
	6B					
	AA					
Face (cont.):	Mouthing					
	Suck Search					
	Sucking					
Extrem.:	Finger Splay					
	Airplane					
	Salute					
	Sitting On Air					
	Hand Clasp					
	Foot Clasp					
	Hand to Mouth					
	Grasping					
	Holding On					
	Fisting					
Attention:	Fuss					
	Yawn					
	Sneeze					
	Face Open					
	Eye Floating					
	Avert					
	Frown					
	Ooh Face					
	Locking					
	Cooing					
	Speech Mvmt.					
Posture:	(Prone, Supine, Side)					
Head:	(Right, Left, Middle)					
Location:	(Crib, Isolette, Held)					
Manipulation:						
	Heart Rate					
	Respiration Rate					
	$TcPO_2$					

FIGURE 4.3. Newborn Individualized Developmental Care and Assessment Program (NIDCAP) observation sheet. (Reprinted with permission from Als H. Reading the premature infant. In: Goldson E, ed. *Nurturing the Premature Infant: Developmental Intervention in the Neonatal Intensive Care Nursery*. Oxford University Press; 1999:37.)

shown significant positive results.[64-72] It is not surprising that preterm infants would also need extra and special supports to cope with intensive care, given the emotional dependency that characterizes the infant and toddler periods.

Trauma-Informed Care

Trauma-informed care is an approach in mental health that recognizes that traumatic events such as abuse or neglect can have long-term physical and psychological effects and that medical care can trigger memories of past traumas in trauma survivors. Practitioners of trauma-informed care strive to build trust and limit distress for their patients.[73] Mary Coughlin[74] has applied this approach to the NICU, recognizing that the typical experiences for babies undergoing NICU care include separation from parents, overstimulating environments with disrupted sleep, frequent handling, and noxious procedures, all of which can be considered traumatic stress.

TABLE 4.3. Signs of Stability and Stress in the Preterm Infant		
System	Signs of Stability	Signs of Stress
Autonomic	Smooth, regular respirations	Respiratory pauses, tachypnea, gasping
	Pink, stable coloring	Paling, perioral duskiness, mottled, cyanotic, gray, flushed, ruddy
	Stable digestion	Hiccups, gagging, grunting, emesis, tremors, startles, twitches, cough, sneeze, yawn, sigh, gasp
Motor	Smooth, controlled posture and muscle tone	Fluctuating muscle tone
	Smooth movements of extremities and head	Flaccidity of trunk, extremities, and face
	Hand/foot clasp, leg brace, finger fold, hand to mouth, grasp, suck, tuck, hand hold	Hypertonicity of trunk and extremities
		Frantic diffuse activity
State	Clear, well-defined sleep states	Diffuse sleep with twitches, jerky movement, irregular breathing, whimpering sounds, grimacing, and fussing
	Focused alertness with animated facial expression	Diffuse wakeful periods with eye floating, glassy-eyed, strained appearance, staring, gaze aversion, panicked, dull look, weak cry

Adapted from Als H. Toward a synactive theory of development: promise for the assessment and support of infant individuality. *Infant Ment Health J*. 1982;3(4):237–238.

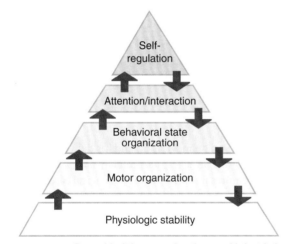

FIGURE 4.4. Pyramid of the synactive theory of infant behavioral organization with physiologic stability at the foundation. (Used with permission from Sweeney JK, Swanson MW. Low birth weight infants: neonatal care and follow-up. In: Umphred DA, ed. *Neurological Rehabilitation*. 4th ed. Mosby; 2001:205.)

Babies are not the only people who can be exposed to trauma from the NICU environment. Parents and families as well as NICU staff can be affected and can experience posttraumatic stress symptoms, or vicarious traumatization, and compassion fatigue/burnout, respectively.[75] Trauma-informed care practices should be broadly applied for all those who experience the NICU environment in order to create and support a true healing environment in the NICU.[8]

Establishing a true healing environment is a central goal of trauma-informed care. Parental presence, holding, and skin-to-skin contact are important in mitigating the inappropriate and harsh sensory inputs of the NICU. Modifications to the environment to promote a more soothing atmosphere are another important way to contribute to a healing environment. Additional strategies of trauma-informed care include preventing pain and stress, protecting sleep, and promoting activities of daily living (ADLs). A NICU baby's "ADLs" are essentially the care tasks the baby requires, including repositioning, diaper changes, bathing, and skin care. These early care tasks serve as the baby's social and emotional interface with the world and the way the baby learns to trust that his or her needs will be met.[9]

These strategies are seen not only as promoting a healing environment but also as specifically protective to the infants' developing brain. The need for neuroprotection grows out of the acknowledgment of the wide-ranging scope of adverse outcomes for babies who require intensive care.[7] Stress response hormones have prolonged effects on the infant and can be disruptive for brain and organ development. The minimization of trauma and stress for the infant patient protects infant growth and development. The stress response can be mitigated through the presence and involvement of the parents and family,[9] which is also a central practice of family-centered care.

Family-Centered Care

Family-centered care is a philosophy of patient care delivery for the maternal–child health division based on respect, collaboration, and support between health care professionals and patients' families. It is a philosophy that recognizes the family (defined as parents, children, and significant others) as the constant in the child's life and strives to include the family as partners in choosing and implementing the plan of care for the child. Family-centered care also acknowledges that hospitalization is stressful for families and can potentially alter the integration of the child into the family and the development of the parental role.[9,76] In order to provide family-centered care in an NICU, a clinician must be knowledgeable about, and sensitive to, both the psychological tasks of pregnancy and the grief process.

Psychological Tasks of Pregnancy

In American culture, pregnancy is typically and naively regarded as a happy time of anticipation, and although that may be partially true, pregnancy is also a time of psychological turmoil. The 40 weeks of pregnancy provide a physical as well as a psychological preparatory period for the expectant parents. When this period is shortened, the baby and the parents may suffer from the incompletion of the pregnancy.[77-80] Bibring[81,82] has identified three psychological tasks of pregnancy, correlating with the three trimesters.[79,81] In the first trimester, parents accept the overwhelming news that their lives have begun a new phase of responsibility for a child (first task). This period is characterized by euphoria, feelings of helplessness and inadequacy, evaluating one's parents' childrearing practices, as well as ambivalence, and fantasies of the perfect babies and parents.[79,83-85]

During the second trimester, the mother-to-be is confronted with the separateness of the baby as she begins to feel the fetal movements (second task). Although she feels a personal closeness to the baby, the mother's bodily changes and the baby's burgeoning movements make the individuality of the baby more real and apparent. During this time, the mother continues to question herself about her adequacy as a parent. Concerns regarding the health and the potential to inflict harm on the fetus are prominent. Ambivalence toward the baby is still very much present for both parents, with fathers also struggling with feelings of resentment and rivalry.[78,80,83-85]

In the third trimester, the baby begins to be personified as names are chosen and rooms painted. In addition, the expectant mother recognizes patterns in fetal behavior and assigns a temperament or a gender based on this behavior. The baby's individuality, revealed in differing responses to the mother's music, food, or other environmental conditions, confirms competence and demonstrates to the parents the ability to handle the rigors of labor and delivery.[78] Simultaneously, the mother-to-be is physically becoming increasingly uncomfortable. She cannot get a break from being pregnant and this physical state leads to the third psychological task: being ready to give up the fetus.[79-81]

A full-term birth prepares the mother to cope with the shock of the separation of the baby from her body and both parents to interact and bond with a particular baby. Parents who give birth prematurely are psychologically ill-prepared,[78] just as their babies are physically ill-prepared for independent living.[78] In addition, when a pregnancy or birth deviates from the expected, parents feel guilty about failing to complete the pregnancy or about any complications the baby experiences.[79,86] In the NICU, the parental psychological focus can become the uncertainty and unpredictability of the situation, which can distract from their ability to prepare for a new family member and assume parenting roles.[85]

When babies are hospitalized at the critical time when parents should be establishing relationships with their newborns and learning parental roles, it is especially stressful.[87] The effects of this stress can continue for months after the NICU experience has ended and can pose severe threats to the parents individually and as a couple.[88] Indeed, the experience of NICU care is a stressor significant enough to cause

symptoms of posttraumatic stress disorder in the parents and has been reported in the literature.[88-93] Families that develop a positive outlook about the experience have children who develop better in the years after birth. Likewise, poor coping can have lasting detrimental effects on the child's development.[94,95] It is important that clinicians working in the NICU recognize the stress families experience and support their individual coping styles. To do this, a clinician must understand the coping and grieving processes.

Coping and Grieving

Both coping and grieving have been described as a linear progression through distinct stages (e.g., shock, denial, anger, guilt, adjustment, and acceptance). However, this linear progression has not been validated empirically.[93,95] It is more helpful to understand grief and coping as ongoing processes involving circular progressions where previous issues and losses are resurrected and revisited.[94,96] The beneficial effects of plain old social support cannot be underestimated in the NICU setting. Approaching families with stereotyped expectations of a rigid time frame regarding their grieving will result in the family feeling judged and will prevent the development of supportive relationships between families and staff, to the ultimate detriment of the baby.[94]

Providing Family-Centered Care in the NICU

The shock of a pregnancy, labor, and/or delivery gone awry, whether resulting in a fragile preterm baby or a full-term baby who requires intensive medical/surgical care, can linger with parents indeterminately. Parents of babies in an NICU are in crisis and should be cared for sensitively. It is important to understand family background. Previous losses because of death, infertility, or miscarriage can be resurrected in the NICU. Current stressors can also include a history of assistive reproductive technology, financial situation, current work and/or school responsibilities, and current relational situations. For these reasons it is essential to read the social work consults. The NICU therapist should not ignore this social history because it "does not change what I do with the baby." Rather, this background knowledge should guide how the therapist interacts with the family.

Every family in the NICU is grieving something, maybe the loss of the expected labor/delivery or the loss of the perfect child. This grief will resurrect past losses and can limit the parents' availability to establish an emotional bond with their infant. In addition, the interactional deprivation imposed by the intensive care the baby requires can prevent families from knowing and connecting with their infant. The high-tech, crisis-prone NICU environment shocks and intimidates families. The families must ask permission to enter the unit as well as to touch or hold their infant, which creates a sense of lost ownership of their infant. Families may not want to risk emotional involvement with their fragile newborn who may later die.

Developmental care of an infant grows out of establishing a supportive and nurturing relationship with the infant. Likewise, family-centered care grows out of establishing a supportive and empowering relationship with the family. An important goal of family-centered care includes facilitating the bonding process between the infant and the family and assisting the family in establishing emotional ties with their infant.[80,97] To be effective in this goal, therapists must be mindful of their own attitudes and nonverbal behaviors and must congruently communicate nonjudgmental acceptance of the family's emotions, coping methods, and pace. Therapists are responsible for crafting the relationship with the family by supporting and empathizing with their emotions while reflecting on the strengths they observe in the family and the infant. Some suggestions to accomplish this include using the baby's name during conversation; commenting on the baby's accomplishments, strengths, attractiveness; as well as the positive interactions between the baby and the family. The NICU therapist should emphasize the parents' importance to the infant; point out the baby's preference for the parents; and compliment the parents' competence with tasks related to the infant's care.[46,97]

A family's human tendency to maintain hope for the future, that the professionals may be wrong, and that miracles can occur should be preserved. Hope is a motivating emotion, providing the energy to cope, work, strive, and stay involved with the infant. It sustains the impetus to maintain the emotional bond to the baby through visiting and interacting. Hope should not be destroyed, but neither should it be falsely fed with unrealistic expectations. Families in crisis with babies in an NICU deserve to hear congruent information from the medical team and the therapy team. This requires sensitivity, diplomacy, and good communication skills.[80]

» Developmental foundations to guide therapy

Embryogenesis and Neonatal Development

In this section, embryogenesis and the current understanding of muscle tone and sensory responses in the second half of gestation are discussed. The evolution of primitive reflexes is left out as it would not be prudent for a therapist today to try to elicit these reactions in a preterm infant for any reason, as it may cause unnecessary stress for the preterm infant. In addition, there is no benefit to a preterm infant to assess his or her muscle tone or sensory reactions solely to determine whether development is occurring appropriately. Rather, this information is included here to provide the neonatal therapist with an understanding of the preterm infant's development and struggle with the intrusiveness of the extrauterine environment at a critical time in his or her development.

Embryogenesis is a remarkable series of events. In 266 days, a 0.1-mm single large cell at fertilization increases in length by a factor of 5,000, in surface area by a factor of 61 million, and in weight by a factor of 6 billion. During the pre-embryonic period, the first 2 weeks after fertilization of the oocyte by the sperm, cell division in the zygote forms three primary germ layers whose segmentation and axis formation are essential to the development of the human baby.[98] The ectoderm evolves into the skin, spinal cord, and teeth; the mesoderm into the blood vessels, muscles, and bone; and the endoderm into the digestive system, lungs, and urinary tract.[99] During the embryonic period (weeks 3 through 8), the mass of cells divides and differentiates into the more than 200 different cell types comprising the various organs of the body.[98] This is a result of amazing and complex processes that are precisely timed and interwoven. In the embryonic period, the cells initially are homogeneous, but increasing differentiation determines an exact biologic function for each cell. By the end of this period, the embryo has a heterogeneous structure. Any misstep in this process can result in demise or a major morphologic malformation in the embryo.[99] The nervous system, the first organ to initiate development and the last to complete development continuing well after birth, is very susceptible to insult. Other systems have shorter critical periods where an interruption or insult can cause a congenital anomaly[98] (see Fig. 4.5 for timing of major/minor anomalies).

In the first week after fertilization, the fertilized egg travels from the fallopian tube and reaches the uterus. In the second week, the fertilized egg, having undergone several mitotic cell divisions to reach the blastocyst stage, implants into the rich vascular wall of the uterus and by the end of the second week forms a primitive placenta. By the end of the third week, the embryo's blood is circulating in a U-shaped tube that later fuses to a single tube and undergoes partitioning into four chambers during weeks 4 to 7. In the fourth week, the embryo is now less than half a centimeter long. In 35 days, a single cell has grown and been transformed into more than 10,000 different cells. The changes are swift and the process so precise and predictable that the timing of a congenital defect can be pinpointed.[99] In addition, an ultrasound during the embryonic period can be used to date the pregnancy within 7 days.[100]

During the fetal period, weeks 9 through 36, the established organs and body parts of the embryo become refined and enlarged. The placenta serves as a barrier, removes wastes, and provides nutrition for the growing fetus, fulfilling the function of the fetal lungs, kidneys, intestines, and liver. In the third month, unbeknownst to the mother, the fetus is quite active, kicking and turning in its 8 oz of amniotic fluid.[99,101] All movement patterns present in a term newborn have been initiated by 15 weeks' gestation, including sucking, swallowing, breathing, and grasping the umbilical cord. Fetal responses to extrauterine stimuli (e.g., turning to auditory or visual stimulation, HR changes to environmental stimulation, and habituation to repeated stimuli) have been documented for decades.[102-104] Fetal activity also demonstrates cyclic fluctuations and circadian rhythms.[104]

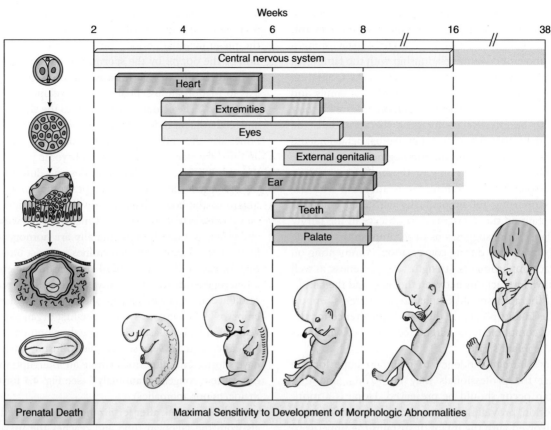

FIGURE 4.5. Embryogenesis and fetal development.(Modified from Rubin E, Gorstein F, Schwarting R, et al. *Pathology.* 4th ed. Lippincott Williams & Wilkins; 2005.)

The Competence of the Term Newborn

Before the 1900s, there were no formal structured examinations for the newborn; the newborn was perceived as disorganized, unstructured, and lacking in sensory and motor capacities. In the early 1900s, under the prevailing Sherrington reflex model, newborn reflexes were investigated and a standard neurologic test for newborns was published. In the mid-1900s, the reflex model was expanded to include generalized motor functioning. Researchers looked at infants' active and passive muscle tone and considered infants able to modulate their behavior. Prechtl and Beintema[105] introduced the concept of infant state as distinct organizations of the brain and associated physiology, affecting how an infant responded to a stimulus. The infant was seen as actively generating responses and modulating performances. In the latter half of the 20th century, more complex infant functioning was appreciated. Infants demonstrated preferential gaze, sound discrimination, affective behaviors, coordination of movements and speech, and differing cries and were considered "social beings."[106] With this newfound appreciation, the infant was perceived as "competent," no longer a passive recipient or blank slate on which the environment and the baby's caregivers could write.[106,107] Comparetti[102] wrote of fetal competencies for induction and participation in labor/delivery (automatic walking and positive support to locate and engage the baby's head in the birth canal and collaborate in the expulsion process from the womb) and for survival

(rooting and sucking for feeding). Brazelton saw the baby as an active participant in the social tasks of eliciting caregiving and initiating the bonding process, organizing her own autonomic and state responses in order to modify the stimulation from the environment while maintaining her own stability.[78]

Likewise, Heidelise Als[47-52] has written numerous articles portraying the preterm infant as striving to initiate and maintain his or her own stability while completing the maturation of organ systems in the high-stress environment of intensive care. Dr. Als has passionately worked to teach caregivers to recognize the attempts of the preterm infant to self-regulate, to support these efforts so that the baby not only succeeds at self-regulation but learns to trust his or her caregivers and him- or herself.

The neonatal competencies of a term baby allowing survival can be grouped into four categories: physiologic, sensorimotor, affective/communication, and complex. Physiologic competencies include the functional maturity and capability of all organ systems to allow breathing, feeding, and growing. Sensorimotor competencies include rooting, sucking, grasping, clearing the airway in prone, and horizontal and vertical tracking.[108] Affective/communication competencies include crying, self-consoling, eye contact, facial animation, and eye aversion. Complex competencies include the newborn's auditory preferences (mother's voice), taste preferences (mother's breast milk), visual preferences (faces), and imitative capacities (sticking tongue out).[109]

Brazelton[11,78] has characterized the newborn as being on a mission to get the parents to care for him or her. The healthy term newborn is a full partner in the work of establishing a bond with the caregiver. Contrast this with the preterm infant, who is a weak partner in this task. A preterm infant is perceived as small and unattractive and is less responsive and more difficult to calm; his or her cry elicits negative emotions in the caregiver. Mothers of preterm infants experience less synchronous interactions, play fewer games, work harder to engage, and derive less gratification from their infants.[110] Thus, the bonding process is at risk between a preterm infant and his or her family.

A Competent Feeder

Feeding has been described as the infant's "primary work,"[12] and the coordination of sucking, swallowing, and breathing requires considerable skill as well as energy.[111] Nevertheless, every day, term newborn infants feed successfully. It is a typical and basic competency of a newborn term baby, who plays a very active role in the whole process, from waking and crying to communicate hunger, rooting to find the feeding source, pacing and coordinating sucking with swallowing and breathing, digesting and eliminating a volume of food, to gaining weight and growing. In a preterm or sick full-term baby, failure with feeding can occur in any one or more of these areas. Sick or preterm babies may have learned an oral aversion as a result of their NICU care. A sick or preterm infant may lack the balance of flexion/extension to attain the appropriate alignment of neck extension and chin tuck to assist sucking and swallowing and breathing, or residual lung disease may cause the infant to breathe too fast to allow time for sucking and swallowing. A preterm baby may not self-regulate physiologic capacities so that the baby is calm and awake and can self-soothe when the environment produces a stressor. A preterm infant may experience periodic apnea, or bradycardia and be unable to manage the coordination of sucking, swallowing, and breathing without becoming physiologically unstable. Other potential obstacles to feeding involve immaturity or problems of the gastrointestinal (GI) tract including reflux and malabsorption.[111] Feeding is one of the primary functional tasks of a newborn infant and generally a requirement for discharge to home. Feeding problems not only delay hospital discharge but can also be a major source of frustration and feelings of failure for parents and caregivers. Feeding interventions for babies in the NICU are beyond the scope of this chapter.

Evolution of Tone, Reflexes, and Musculoskeletal Development

Owing to the increasing sophistication of technology, younger preterm infants, just beyond the halfway mark of gestation, are surviving.[112] The preterm age of viability is now 23 to 24 weeks' gestation. A therapist working in an NICU must be intimately acquainted with fetal development in the last half of gestation in order to understand the behavior of the preterm infant and to intervene with and assess her. Suzanne

Saint-Anne Dargassies[113] in 1955 studied 40 nonviable and previable fetuses from 20 to 27 weeks' gestation to determine the neurologic characteristics of fetal maturation. (At that time, the viability threshold was 27 weeks' gestation, and Dargassies studied these premature infants before they died.) She found that periods of 1 week were long enough to distinguish one stage from another, until 26 weeks, and then the rate of change slowed down. Dargassies observed spontaneous facial activity (excluding tongue and lips) very early; distal responses were manifest before proximal; gallant reflex (trunk incurvation) was completely present at 20 weeks; and active movements, elicited movements, and primary reflexes improved slowly in quality, duration, and completeness. She saw a complete lack of passive muscle tone in extremities and trunk, although this was hard to investigate because of "edema, sclerema, and death agony,"[113] and she observed babies from 21 weeks responding differently to tactile and painful stimuli.[113]

Dargassies[113] also studied 100 viable preterm infants from 28 to 41 weeks' gestation and observed maturational stages in 2-week segments during this time period. She created "maturative" criteria for infants at 28, 30, 32, 35, and 37 weeks and analyzed differences between term newborns and former preterms at 40 weeks' gestation. According to Dipietro,[103] the period between 28 and 32 weeks' gestation is a transitional one for a fetus. HR, activity, state organization, responses to vibroacoustic stimulation, and the coupling between fetal activity and HR are variable with peaks and plateaus in presentation. By gestational weeks 31 to 32, the variability has stabilized and the rate of development has slowed so that a baby at 32 weeks' gestation will demonstrate less startle responses, increasing periods of quiescence, increasing state organization, mature levels of vibroacoustic responsiveness, and increasing abilities to habituate to stimuli. These patterns continue to mature through term age; however, a 32-week fetus behaves more like a term infant than a younger fetus. This transitional period parallels the period of rapid increases in neural development and myelination, including cortical vagal responses and sulcation.[103]

Allen and Capute[112] studied 42 preterm infants, none of whom developed CP, from 24 to 32 weeks' gestation with weekly neurodevelopmental examinations, and found that flexor tone, recoil, and hyperreflexia appeared 2 to 3 weeks earlier in the lower extremities (33 to 35 weeks) than in the upper extremities (35 to 37 weeks). Trunk tone (measured on ventral suspension) was manifest at 36 to 40 weeks. Neck tone was poor, with greater than one-half the babies at term-corrected age continuing with a head lag in pull-to-sit. Primitive reflexes and deep tendon reflexes (DTRs) appeared in lower extremities before upper extremities. (Presence of asymmetric tonic neck reflex [ATNR] was detected in lower extremities first at 31 weeks and in upper extremities at 34 weeks.) They found that the evolution of tone, DTRs, and primitive and pathologic reflexes proceeded in an orderly sequential pattern (i.e., lower extremities to upper extremities and distal to proximal).[112]

Preterm infants, in addition to the previously described hypotonia, also have a decreased ratio of type I (slow twitch) muscle fibers to type II (fast twitch) compared with infants at term. This results in muscular fatigue (particularly respiratory muscles) in preterm infants. Preterm infants also demonstrate incomplete ossification of bones, ligamentous laxity, and connective tissue elasticity compared with term infants. The combination of these unique characteristics of preterm infants places them at the mercy of gravity and the surfaces on which they lie. Just as fetal movements, or lack thereof, are thought to contribute to the shaping of joints, skulls, and spinal curves of babies in utero, preterm infants can fall victim to positionally induced deformities in the NICU. These include skull-shaping abnormalities like dolichocephaly (increased anterior–posterior diameter of the head) and plagiocephaly (flattening of posterior–lateral skull because of preferred head and neck rotation to one side), as well as extremity misalignment.[114] Research comparing former preterm infants at term age (37 to 42 gestational weeks) and term newborns has demonstrated differences in tone and reactivity in the two groups. Unlike infants born at term, preterm infants miss the experience of a crowded uterus to limit their range of active movement and to support the development of flexor tone. In contrast to term infants who are tucked and contained in utero, preterm infants experience gravity, as well as intravenous lines, support boards, and other restraints, during this period of maturational-related hypotonia. For these reasons, at term age, a former preterm infant and a term newborn will demonstrate differences in muscle tone. Former preterm infants at term age demonstrate less flexor tone of extremities and poorer flexor/extensor balance of head and neck, and in addition have greater range of motion in French angles, as well as greater active range of motion, than their term newborn counterparts.[115,116] Former preterm infants at term age are more reactive, demonstrating more startles, tremors, brisk reflexes, and a shorter attention span than their term counterparts.[113,116] Former preterms may also demonstrate toe walking during automatic walking, while their full-term counterparts demonstrate heel–toe walking.[113]

In addition, brain development of former preterm infants at term-corrected age differs from brain development of babies born at term. Newborn term infants show better behavioral functioning of autonomic, motoric, state, and attention/interactional subsystems, as well as higher amplitudes in EEG and photic-evoked responses and increased gray/white matter differentiation and myelination, than healthy former preterm infants at term age. Some of these differences may be explained by the cumulative complications of preterm birth; however, the developmentally inappropriate sensory stimulation of an NICU may also affect preterm brain development.[117-119]

Evolution of Sensory Responses

Research demonstrates neurosensory development in animals to follow a sequential pattern, first touch, then movement, smell and taste, hearing, and lastly sight. Stimulation of a particular system during development can be essential for the development of that system. However, if the stimulus is too intense or is atypically timed, it can interfere with the development of that and other sensory systems.[120] Preterm infants are forced to complete the development and maturation of their sensory systems while in an intensive care environment. The effects of this environment on the developing brain are not fully understood and are only beginning to be studied.

Tactile System

Four different sensory abilities comprise the tactile system: touch, temperature, pain, and proprioception. The first three sensory receptors are housed in the skin, and the last is composed of receptors from not only the skin but also the joints and muscles. The skin is the largest organ, and therefore touch is the largest sensory system as well as the first to develop.[121,122]

THE PROBLEM OF PAIN It is now well recognized that newborn infants (preterm and full term) detect, process, and respond to painful stimulation.[123,124] However, describing and measuring pain and stress in preterm and critically ill infants remains a challenge. There are many inconsistencies across disciplines, NICUs, and countries worldwide in both evaluation and management of pain in neonates and infants in the NICU despite advances in neonatal care.[125-127] The WHO[128] has recognized pain as a public health concern as more and more evidence of short- and long-term neurodevelopmental consequences of unmanaged or undermanaged pain has emerged.[129-132]

Infants in the NICU experience not only painful, skin-breaking procedures such as blood draws, line placement, or surgeries but also pain and discomfort from insertion and manipulation of feeding and breathing tubes, suctioning of endotracheal tubes, and leads and monitoring devices necessary for supporting life in the extrauterine world. Roofthooft et al.[133] reported that high-risk infants are exposed to greater than 10 invasive procedures per day. This is all occurring at a vulnerable time of rapid brain development and programming of stress systems through the hypothalamus–pituitary–adrenal (HPA) axis.[134] During this critical phase of nervous system development, there is heightened neuronal activation to sensation[135] with decreased descending inhibitory inputs,[136] placing infants at increased risk for structural and functional dysmaturation of the nervous system.

The nociceptive pathway develops in stages starting very early in gestation at 7 weeks and continues throughout gestation,[137,138] with maturation of the primary somatosensory cortex beyond 40 weeks' gestation.[139] Myelination of the ascending nociceptive pathways begins around week 25 and is complete by week 30. However, the inhibitory functions of the descending, pain-modulating pathways develop later and are not fully mature until 48 weeks' postmenstrual age (PMA). Pain neurotransmitters such as substance P are plentiful early on, whereas pain modulators such as dopamine and serotonin are not as available for pain modulation until after 40 weeks.[140,141]

The immaturity of the developing nervous system increases the vulnerability of the preterm infant to painful experiences. Fitzgerald and colleagues have demonstrated that preterm infants have large cutaneous receptor fields with heightened sensitivity to tissue injury.[142-144] Discrimination between noxious and nonnoxious stimulation is decreased in the preterm neonate because of transient overlapping between axon terminals in the spinal cord, low threshold tactile inputs,[145] and the underdeveloped inhibitory function through descending pathways.[141,146] Painful and seemingly innocuous touch may have similar reactions and the response may last longer in preterm infants. The NICU environment of care also is another source of stress subjecting the immature preterm systems to increased levels of sound, bright lights, and frequent, unexpected touch and handling.

An Oxford research team demonstrated in 2015[147] that infants have similar pain responses as seen in adults. Using functional MRI, 18 out of 20 regions in the brain active in adults experiencing pain are also active in infants. Neonates experience pain more intensely than adults, demonstrating the same pain response to a stimulus at one-quarter the strength. Preterm infants have 30% to 50% lower pain threshold than adults and a lower pain tolerance than older infants and children.

Preterm infants are being cared for in the NICU and experiencing painful procedures during the time period when rapid brain growth and organization typically occur in the protective environment of the uterus. This is a critical period for brain development with increased sensitivity and vulnerability of the developing brain to external, adverse stimulation. During this time, processes of neuronal projection and cell migration, oligodendroglial maturation, differentiation of subplate neurons, formation of synapses, cerebellar neuronal proliferation and migration, and major axonal development in the cerebrum are occurring.[148,149] Exposure to repeated stress and pain may disrupt these processes by setting off inflammatory, exocytotoxic cascades and oxidative stress with resulting cell death, decreased differentiation of cells, decreased connectivity, and atypical structural development of white and gray matter. Smith et al.[150] reported decreased frontal and parietal brain width, altered diffusion

measures, and functional connectivity in the temporal lobes. Infants with the greatest number of painful procedures in the neonatal period demonstrate decreased postnatal growth and altered brain development with decreased volumes of white and gray matter[146,151] and decreased cerebellar size.[152-154] Zwicker et al.[155] reported impaired corticospinal tract development associated with exposure to pain and stress. Multiple painful procedures in early infancy may result in altered programming of the HPA axis, resulting in decreased cortisol levels.[134,156]

Differences in somatosensory processing, stress responses, and neurodevelopment have been associated with exposure to pain and stress in the NICU. Studies of children who experienced repeated pain-related stressful events and surgical procedures in the neonatal period have shown differences in sensitivity and response to pain.[129,134,156,157] Altered pain sensitivity such as hyposensitivity to acute pain and hypersensitivity to prolonged pain in later life has been documented in follow-up studies.[156] Cognitive and motor delays,[130,131,154] visual–perceptual difficulties,[158] and behavior and attention problems in the toddler period continuing into school age[132,159-161] have also been found to be associated with pain and pain-related stress experienced in the NICU.

Given the potential deleterious effects of pain on the immature, developing nervous system, recognition and prevention of pain and pain-related stress are essential. The AAP has published guidelines for the assessment and management of pain in neonates.[162] Measurement of pain should be performed before, during, and after any painful or stressful procedure. Although the gold standard of pain assessment in older children and adults is patient report of pain, assessment of infants in the NICU is challenging because of their inability to verbalize their discomfort. Comprehensive, valid, and reliable pain assessment requires the identification of multiple responses, both physiologic and behavioral.[162-166] Indicators of pain in infants include physiologic responses such as changes in HR, RR, oxygen saturation, color, intracranial pressure, and blood pressure (BP) as well as specific behavioral and movement responses (Table 4.4).[167] Expression of

TABLE 4.4.	Commonly Used Neonatal Pain Assessment Tools		
Pain Assessment Tool	**Pain Characteristics Assessed**		**Intended Use**
Crying, Requires oxygen administration, Increased vital signs, Expression, Sleeplessness (CRIES)	Crying, requires O_2 to maintain saturations $\geq$ 95%, increased blood pressure, increased heart rate, expression, sleep state, alertness		Acute pain Postoperative pain
Premature Infant Pain Profile (PIPP)	Gestational age, behavioral state, maximum heart rate, percent decrease in O_2 saturation, brow bulge, eye squeeze, nasolabial furrow		Acute pain
Neonatal Facial Coding Scale (NFCS)	Brow lowering, eye squeeze, nasolabial furrowing, lip opening, square mouth shape, taut tongue, chin quiver, lip pursing		Acute pain Prolonged pain Postoperative pain
Neonatal Infant Pain Scale (NIPS)	Facial expression, crying, breathing pattern, arm movements, leg movements, state of arousal		Acute pain Postoperative pain

Adapted from AAP Committee on Fetus and Newborn, and Section on Anesthesiology and Pain Medicine. Prevention and management of procedural pain in the neonate: an update. *Pediatrics*. 2016;137(2):e20154271.

behavioral signs of pain and stress varies among individual infants and is influenced by factors such as gestational age (GA), postnatal age, illness, parent absence or presence, and length of NICU hospitalization. The extent and timing preceding interventions or procedures also influence response to pain and stress.[134] A large number of pain assessments have been developed in an effort to measure pain in preterm and critically ill infants (Table 4.5) for commonly used pain scales. However, the majority of pain scales only measure acute, procedural, or postoperative pain. There are few good measurements at this time for chronic or continuous pain.[127,168,169]

Management of pain in high-risk infants starts with minimizing the number of painful procedures to the greatest

TABLE 4.5.	State-Related Behaviors	

Sleep State	Behaviors
State 1A	Infant in deep sleep with obligatory regular breathing or breathing in synchrony with only the respirator; eyes closed; no eye movements under closed lids; quiet facial expression; no spontaneous activity; typically pale color
State 1B	Infant in deep sleep with predominately modulated regular breathing; eyes closed; no eye movement under closed lids; relaxed facial expression; no spontaneous activity except isolated startles
State 2A	Light sleep with eyes closed; rapid eye movements can be seen under closed lids; low-amplitude activity level with diffuse and disorganized movements; respirations are irregular and there are many sucking and mouthing movements, whimpers; facial, body, and extremity twitchings, much grimacing; the impression of a "noisy" state is given. Color is typically poor.
State 2B	Light sleep with eyes closed; rapid eye movements can be seen under closed lids; low activity level with movements and dampened startles; movements are likely to be of lower amplitude and more monitored than in state 1; infant responds to various internal stimuli with dampened startle. Respirations are more regular; mild sucking and mouthing movements can occur off and on; one or two whimpers may be observed, as well as infrequent sighs or smiles.
Transitional (Drowsy) States	
State 3A	Drowsy or semidozing; eyes may be open or closed; eyelids fluttering or exaggerated blinking; if eyes are open, glassy veiled look; activity level variable with or without interspersed startles from time to time; diffuse movement; fussing and/or much discharge of vocalization, whimpers; facial grimace
State 3B	Drowsy, same as above but with less discharge of vocalization, whimpers, facial grimace, etc.
Awake States[a]	
State 4AL	Awake and quiet, minimal noisy activity, eyes half open or open but with glazed or dull look, giving the impression of little involvement and distance, or focused yet seeming to look through rather than at object or examiner, or the infant is clearly awake and reactive but has eyes closed intermittently
State 4AH	Awake and quiet; minimal motor activity; eyes wide open, "hyperalert" or giving the impression of panic or fear; may appear to be hooked by the stimulus; seems to have difficulty in modulating or breaking the intensity of the fixation to the object or moving away from it
State 4B	Alert with bright shiny animated facial expression; seems to focus attention on source of stimulation and appears to process information actively and with modulation; motor activity is at a minimum.
Active States	
State 5A	Eyes may or may not be open, but infant is clearly aroused as is dictated by motor arousal, tonus, and distressed facial expression, grimacing, or other signs of discomfort. Fussing, if present, is diffuse or strained.
State 5B	Eyes may or may not be open but infant is clearly awake and aroused, with considerable, yet well-defined, motor activity. Infant may also be clearly fussing but not crying robustly.
Crying States	
State 6A	Intense crying, as indicated by intense grimace and cry face, yet cry sound may be very strained or weak or absent; intensity of upset is greater than fussing.
State 6B	Rhythmic, intense, lusty crying that is robust, vigorous, and strong in sound.

[a]For 4A, two types of diffuse alertness are distinguished, 4AL and 4AH. L or H is marked instead of a check mark.

These are subgrouped into the states themselves and specific, typically attention-related behaviors. Various configurations of behaviors encompassing eye movements, eye opening and facial expressions, gross body movements, respirations, and tonus aspects are used in specific temporal relationships to one another to determine at what level of consciousness an infant is at a particular time. It is possible to make meaningful, systematic distinctions between dynamic transformations of various behavioral configurations that appear to correspond to varying states of availability and conscious responsiveness. The following spectrum of observable states is suggested: states labeled as A are "noisy," unclean, and diffuse; states labeled as B are clean, well-defined states.

AA: Should the infant move into prolonged respiratory pause (e.g., beyond 8 seconds), AA should be marked. The infant has removed him- or herself from the state continuum.

More than one box per 2-minute time block can be marked, depending on the fluctuation and behavior the infant shows. Operationally, typically a 2- to 3-second duration of a behavioral configuration is necessary to be registered as a distinct state; however, even briefer excursions, especially into states 4 and 6, can be recorded reliably.

Reprinted with permission from Als H. Reading the premature infant. In: Goldson E, ed. *Nurturing the Premature Infant: Developmental Intervention in the Neonatal Intensive Care Nursery.* New York, NY: Oxford University Press; 1999:82–84.

extent possible. When painful and stressful interventions are necessary, nonpharmacologic and pharmacologic therapies are implemented. Preplanning and preemptive implementation of strategies to minimize pain and stress is an essential part of caregiving for the high-risk infant in the NICU. Nonpharmacologic interventions are the foundation of pain management in the NICU and should be implemented consistently for any painful procedure or noxious touch.[125,162] Nonpharmacologic interventions include NNS, breast milk/ breastfeeding, sucrose, facilitated tucking, swaddling, and kangaroo care or skin-to-skin holding.[170,171] Parent presence has also been shown to lessen or alleviate pain in infants.[172] However, these strategies should not substitute for pharmacologic therapy, which should be utilized in addition to nonpharmacologic pain supports for prolonged or moderate to severe pain in the infant. Careful consideration of analgesics is necessary because of concern for potential side effects, adverse events, and neurodevelopmental impairments.[173] Pharmacologic therapy should be administered in a stepwise approach with careful monitoring of infant response. In addition to nonpharmacologic and pharmacologic interventions, environmental strategies reduce pain and stress indirectly by reducing the level of noxious stimuli present to the infant. Environmental strategies include dimming the lights or shading the eyes of the infant and reducing the noise around the infant's bed space by keeping pagers on vibrate mode, silencing alarms, shutting drawers and porthole doors softly, and talking in soft voices away from the bedside. Other environmental strategies include reducing frequency of handling and painful procedures.[64]

PTs working in the NICU need to be familiar with physiologic and behavioral assessment of pain in young infants, as well as environmental and nonpharmacologic strategies to reduce pain. They also need to be vigilant in anticipating the potential for pain for babies in the NICU and to advocate for early and aggressive intervention to minimize pain for these infants.[21,167]

Vestibular System

The sensory end organs of the vestibular system, the three semicircular canals, and the otolith are housed inside the skull cavity (vestibule), which also contains the hearing sense organ, the cochlea. Both the hearing and the vestibular systems convert stimuli into electrical signals via the cilia. In the vestibular system, these signals are carried by the vestibular nerve to the brainstem and relayed to a variety of areas so that information regarding the baby's position in space can be interpreted, integrated, and used to guide movement and function.[122]

The vestibular system is one of the first to develop in utero, and the vestibular nerve is the first fiber tract to begin myelination at the end of the first trimester. By 20 weeks' gestation, this nerve has reached its full-size shape, and the other vestibular tracts have begun to myelinate.[122] The vestibular system is thought to be responsible for the fetus orienting to the head-down position prior to birth. The vestibular system is mature in the full-term newborn,[174] but modifications and growth in the synapses and dendrites of the vestibular pathways continue until puberty as the child learns to move and adapts to his or her changing body size and shape.[122]

The womb provides almost constant vestibular stimulation to the developing fetus, some contingent (fetal movement) and some noncontingent (maternal movements).[122,175] The preterm baby in an NICU experiences primarily immobilization and therefore reduced vestibular stimulation. The consequences of the constant vestibular stimulation a term baby experiences in utero and the lack of such with a preterm baby are unclear and there is little information to guide interventions with the vestibular system. Research on vestibular stimulation on the preterm infant is often carried out with other modes of stimulation, making it difficult to understand the effects of pure vestibular stimulation. Vestibular stimulation is known to enhance behavioral states; for example, slow rhythmic rocking is soothing and promotes quiet sleep, and fast arrhythmic vestibular stimulation increases activity and agitation.[12] Vestibular stimulation has not been demonstrated to affect feeding, weight gain, length of stay, or neurodevelopmental outcomes in hospitalized infants.[62] More research is needed in this area; however, gentle vestibular stimulation within the infant's tolerance levels and for a developmentally appropriate reason may be implemented in the NICU.[175]

Olfactory and Gustatory Development

Taste and smell are both chemical senses, initiated in response to specific molecules in the immediate environment and transmitted into electrical signals by neurons. Olfactory development begins at 5 weeks' gestation with the appearance of the nasal pit. At 8 weeks, the neurons in the olfactory bulb begin to develop and are mature by 20 weeks. By 11 weeks, the nostrils are replete with olfactory epithelia. The ability to smell begins at 28 weeks when the biochemical development of olfactory epithelia and neurons is completed.

Taste buds begin to mature at approximately 13 weeks when the fetus begins to suck and swallow. At term age, approximately 7,000 taste buds are present over the perimeter of the tongue, soft palate, and upper throat.[122] Sucking and swallowing amniotic fluid stimulate the taste buds and influence their synaptic connections. The amniotic fluid is constantly changing, reflecting the mix of the maternal diet with the fetus' urination. The fetus experiences a variety of tastes and smells while in utero. Likewise, breast milk is flavored by maternal diet and the newborn is able to recognize the mother's breast milk, as its smell and taste are familiar. From 24 weeks until term, a fetus swallows approximately 1 L of amniotic fluid per day. Contrast this with the experiences of the preterm baby, who frequently has an orogastric tube and/or endotracheal tube in the mouth, tape on the face, and the taste of a rubber glove, medications, or vitamins in the mouth. In addition, the preterm infant does not get this constant swallowing practice, making the necessary coordination of sucking, swallowing, and breathing a challenge.[122]

Auditory System

By 24 weeks' gestation, the development of the cochlea and peripheral sensory end organs is complete, and the first blink/startle responses to vibroacoustic stimulation can be elicited. By 28 weeks, these responses are consistent; the hearing threshold is approximately 40 dB and decreases to 13.5 dB (approximating the adult levels) by 42 weeks, demonstrating the continuing maturation of the auditory pathways. A preterm infant in the NICU is subjected to the noise of an NICU during the normal development and maturation of hearing. Exposure to this NICU noise may cause cochlear damage as well as cause sleep disturbances and disrupt the growth and development of the baby.[119,176] The bubbling of water inside a ventilator tubing or tapping on the outside of the incubator can result in noise that is 70 to 80 dB inside an incubator, whereas closing the porthole doors or the drawers under the incubator or dropping the head of the mattress can result in 90 to 120 dB noise.[176] Incubator covers reduce only the noise of objects striking the incubator. However, most noise in an incubator comes from the motor, drawer and door closures, and the infant's own crying.[177] Other common NICU sounds include alarms, overhead pagers, telephones, traffic, and conversations. In one study, peak noise was in the 65- to 75-dB range, and most noise was due to human activity.[178] Normal conversation is typically in the 60-dB range, and whispering is between 20 and 30 dB.[176]

Contrast this with the sounds of pregnancy inside the womb (i.e., muffled maternal speech, maternal HR, and GI sounds), which are structured or patterned but not continuous or fixed. These sounds may also be contingent on maternal or fetal behavior and typically affect more than one sensory organ.[108] Background noise in the human uterus allows low frequencies of maternal speech to be discriminated. In utero, the maternal tissues attenuate sound frequencies greater than 250 Hz and thus shield the developing fetus. The sound environment of an NICU has levels of low- and high-frequency sound, and this may diminish the babies' exposure to maternal speech. The NICU provides a very different auditory sensory experience for the developing baby than the womb.

The AAP[176] recommends that noise levels in an NICU should not exceed 45 dB; in order to accomplish this, staff must be cooperative and NICU design and construction must support this. In addition to strategies to reduce noise from human or mechanical sources, new alternatives to the crowded and noisy state of current NICU designs have been suggested by Evans, Philbin,[179-181] and White.[182]

Visual System

Vision is the most complex human sense and the least mature at term birth. By 23 to 24 weeks' gestation, the major eye structures and the visual pathways are in place; however, the eyelids are fused, the optic media is cloudy, and there are remnants of embryonic tissue in the eye globe.

A few immature photoreceptor cells occupy the retina, and retinal blood vessels in the posterior retina have begun to develop. From 24 weeks to term, the retina and visual cortex undergo extensive maturation and differentiation. At 24 to 28 weeks, the eyelids separate. However, the pupillary reflex is absent; the lid will tighten to bright light, but this fatigues easily. By 34 weeks, the pupillary reflex is present, and bright light causes lid closure without fatigue. Brief eye opening and fixation on a high-contrast form under low illumination may occur. Morante et al.[183] found that most 32-week gestation premature infants could perceive 1/2-inch stripes at 12 inches, and by 35 to 36 weeks most could perceive 1/4-inch stripes. At term, most infants could distinguish 1/8-inch stripes. Also, pattern preference matured from 34 weeks on as well. Unlike Saint-Anne Dargassies,[113] Morante et al.[183] found that former premature infants at 40 weeks did less well with visual acuity and pattern preference than term newborns. By 36 weeks, the infant will orient toward a soft light and demonstrate saccadic visual following horizontally and vertically. At term, infants see with acuity estimates of 20/400. They are farsighted with poor focusing for objects up close.[108]

Typically, visual maturation occurs in a dark womb and does not require light exposure. However, infants born prematurely are subjected to the harsh bright lighting of the NICU, which produces phototoxic effects in animals and can potentially impact brain development. Bilirubin lights to treat hyperbilirubinemia can produce light equivalent to greater than 10,000 foot-candles. Because of their visual immaturity, preterm infants should be shielded from ambient and supplementary light sources. Five foot-candles is desirable to encourage spontaneous eye opening. Although preterm infants will attend to black-and-white patterns, this can be stressful for them. Prolonged attention to black-and-white patterns has been associated with lower IQ in childhood. Visual stimulation may also interfere with typical auditory dominance, resulting in decreased attending to speech and may disrupt the emergence of hand regard and visually directed reaching.[12,108,122]

Evolution of State Differentiation

True behavioral states in terms of a set of characteristic variables linked together may not be present in infants less than 36 to 37 weeks' GA,[110,184] and preterm infants younger than 36 weeks do not possess a full capacity for control over states of arousal.[12] Brazelton and Nugent[185] define six states in their newborn assessment and pay close attention to the range, variety, and duration of the states a baby exhibits during an assessment (see Table 4.5). Als[186] modifies these states for preterm infants, describing them as less well organized and less clearly defined than states a healthy term baby demonstrates. In preterm infants, sleep states predominate, and wakeful periods emerge for brief periods around 28 weeks and become more numerous at 30 weeks.[113] Preterm infant sleep states are disorganized with more motoric responses during sleep. Wakeful periods in preterm infants are brief and sporadic. The proportions of sleep and wake periods change as babies mature. Quiet alert times appear in preterm infants who are close to term age and have a degree of physiologic and motoric stability. Because the state system is foundational for attending and interacting, it is important to be familiar with and to assess the range and robustness of states available to an infant, as well as the ease of transition between states.[186]

» Medical foundations to guide therapy

Language of the NICU

The language of the NICU also reflects the crisis-driven nature of the intensive care required by these critically ill infants. Many complex procedures and diagnoses are referred to by acronyms, and the language can be intimidating for those who do not know what the terms mean. There is a list of commonly used abbreviations in the Appendix at the end of this chapter. In addition, a few key terms will be defined below.

GA refers to the time between the first day of the last menstrual period and the day of delivery.[187] Term gestation is 37 to 41 6/7 weeks, and a baby born before 37 weeks is considered preterm. A baby born at 42 weeks or more is considered postterm.[188] Chronologic age (CA) is defined as the age the baby is based on his or her birthday.

Post Menstrual Age (PMA) is described in weeks beginning the day after birth. It is GA plus CA in weeks. A preterm infant who was born at 24 weeks GA, at 10 weeks CA would be 34 weeks PMA. PMA is the preferred terminology to describe the age of preterm infants during their neonatal hospital admission.[189]

Corrected age should be used for children born preterm who are post-NICU discharge. The general recommendation is for age correction to be used only up to three years of age.[189] Correcting a baby's age is an important skill to understand and to teach to parents. The 40 weeks of gestation are so critical to development that it is unfair to ignore the time lost in utero when a preterm birth occurs. It is important that both the therapist and the family develop expectations for a baby that are based on corrected age and not CA.

AGA, SGA, and LGA are acronyms for appropriate for gestational age, small for gestational age, and large for gestational age, respectively. These terms refer to the weight of the baby at birth. AGA refers to an infant whose weight at birth falls within the 10th and 90th percentiles for age. A baby born 12 weeks early can be AGA, or a baby born at term can be AGA if the weight is within two standard deviations of the mean (10th to 90th percentiles) for babies born at that GA. A baby who is SGA has a weight that is below the 10th percentile (or below two standard deviations from the mean) for age, and a baby who is LGA weighs above the 90th percentile (or above two standard deviations from the

mean) for his or her age at birth (Fig. 4.6). SGA infants can also be called IUGR, or intrauterine growth restricted. The etiology for this may be a chromosomal abnormality in the baby, congenital malformation, or congenital infection.[101] LGA may be due to large parents, maternal diabetes, or postmaturity (>42 weeks' gestation), or the baby may have other genetic syndromes. Babies born LGA are at risk for birth trauma, especially brachial plexus injury or perinatal depression. They may also be more likely to have hyperinsulinism or polycythemia.[188]

Research correlating birth weight with outcome is common and has led to additional acronyms referring to weight such as normal birth weight (NBW), low birth weight (LBW), moderately low birth weight (MLBW), VLBW, and extremely low birth weight (ELBW) (Table 4.6). NBW is 2,500 to 3,999 g (5 lb 8 oz to 8 lb 13 oz). LBW is defined as less than 2,500 g (5 lb 8 oz). MLBW is defined as 1,500 to 2,500 g (3 lb 5 oz to 5 lb 8 oz). VLBW is defined as less than 1,500 g (3 lb 5 oz). ELBW is less than 1,000 g (2 lb 3 oz). Infants less than 750 g (1 lb 10 oz) are micropreemies, and infants weighing more than 4,000 g (8 lb 13 oz) have macrosomia.[12,188]

The medical chart may describe the mother as a 32-year-old G5 P1223. G stands for gravida and P for para. These terms describe the number of maternal pregnancies and pregnancy outcomes, respectively. The mnemonic "**F**lorida **P**ower **A**nd **L**ight" can be used to remember what the numbers following P mean. The first number stands for number of **F**ull-term births, the second for number of **P**reterm births, the third for number of **A**bortions (whether spontaneous or therapeutic), and the fourth for number of **L**iving children. In the case of G5 P1223, the mother had five pregnancies; one full-term infant, two preterm babies, two abortions, and a total of three living children. When only a single number follows the P, it represents the number of living children.

A scoring system to evaluate the physical condition of newborn infants after delivery was developed by Virginia Apgar[190] in 1953, and the name Apgar has evolved into an acronym for this scale. A is for appearance, P is for pulse, G is for grimace, A is for activity, and R is for respiration (Table 4.7). These scores are generally assigned for the first and fifth minute of life if the baby does not require extensive resuscitation. Should the score reflect apnea or bradycardia with an Apgar score of less than 6, resuscitation is begun. A score in the range of 3 to 4 indicates the need for bag and mask ventilation; a score of 5 to 7 requires blow-by oxygen; and a score of 8 to 10 is considered typical for term newborns and the infant does not require resuscitation.[191] An example of an Apgar score as recorded in the medical history is 8195. The Apgar score after 1 minute indicates the infant's changing condition and whether resuscitative efforts are adequate or need to be increased. For infants who require extensive resuscitation, Apgar scores may be taken every 5 minutes until the score is greater than 6 (i.e., 0105210515620).[191,192]

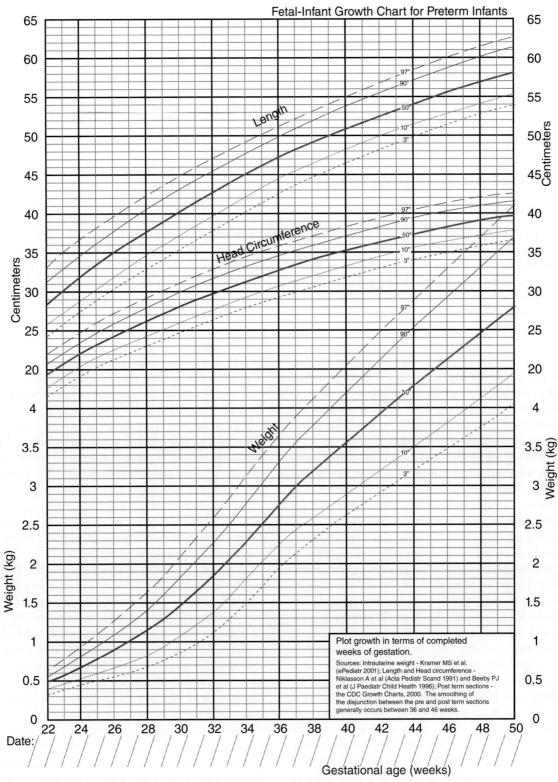

FIGURE 4.6. Fenton preterm growth charts (boys and girls). (Fenton TR, Kim JH. A systematic review and meta-analysis to revise the Fenton growth chart for preterm infants. *BMC Pediatr.* 2013;13:59. https://doi.org/10.1186/1471-2431-13-59)

TABLE 4.6.	Acronyms Regarding Birth Weight	
NBW	Normal Birth Weight	2,500–3,999 g (5 lb 8 oz–8 lb 13 oz)
LBW	Low Birth Weight	<2,500 g (5 lb 8 oz)
MLBW	Moderately Low Birth Weight	1,500–2,500 g (3 lb 5 oz–5 lb 8 oz)
VLBW	Very Low Birth Weight	<1,500 g (3 lb 5 oz)
ELBW	Extremely Low Birth Weight	<1,000 g (1 lb 10 oz)
Micropreemies		<750 g (1 lb 10 oz)
Macrosomia		>4,000 g (8 lb 13 oz)

TABLE 4.7.	Apgar Score			
		Score		
Sign	0	1		2
Heart rate	Absent	<100 bpm		100–140 bpm
Respiratory effort	Absent	Slow, shallow		Good, crying irregular
Reflex irritability	No response	Grimace		Cough or sneeze
Muscle tone	Flaccid	Some flexion		Active motion of extremities
Color	Blue	Pink body, blue extremities		All pink

From Apgar V. A proposal for a new method of evaluation of the newborn infant. *Anesth Analg.* 1953;32(4):260–267.

Environmental Aspects of Intensive Care: Equipment and Technologic Supports

The NICU is built around the highly technical supports that can sustain an infant's life. This technology has exploded in the latter half of the 20th century, allowing more babies to survive. This technology also influences the climate, culture, and workspace of the NICU and can give the NICU a much cluttered, very cold, and metallic appearance. Equipment commonly found in the NICU to support a baby is listed in Table 4.8 (Figs. 4.7 and 4.8).

The primary objective of assisted ventilatory support in high-risk infants is to optimize the infant's cardiopulmonary status while minimizing trauma to the airways and lungs.

TABLE 4.8.	Common Medical Equipment in the NICU
Radiant warmer	Open bed with low, adjustable Plexiglas side rails on a height- and angle-adjustable table with overhead heat source, temperature monitor, and procedure lights
Isolette	Enclosed incubator. Clear plastic unit or box enclosing the mattress with heat and humidity control. Access to infant is through side port holes or side opening.
Open crib	Small bassinet-style bed or small metal crib without a heat source
Bag and mask	Ventilating system consisting of self-inflating bag with reservoir, flow meter, pressure manometer connected to a mask that fits over the infant's nose and mouth
Nasal cannula	Humidified gas delivered via flexible tubing with small prongs that fit into the nares
HFNC	Humidified gas (may be highly humidified) delivered at high-flow rates via a nasal cannula
CPAP	Continuous or variable flow of warmed humidified gas at a set pressure generated by a CPAP unit or mechanical ventilator and delivered by mask
HHHNC	Highly humidified, high-flow system of delivering gas via nasal prongs
CMV	Conventional mechanical ventilation. Neonatal standard mechanical ventilators with ability to provide precise control of gas delivery and ventilator support in a variety of options, including pressure-limited time-cycled, volume-cycled, pressure support ventilation
HFJV	High-frequency jet ventilation delivers short pulses of heated, pressurized gas directly into the upper airway through a jet injector.

(continued)

TABLE 4.8.	Common Medical Equipment in the NICU (*continued*)
HFOV	High-frequency oscillating ventilator has a piston pump or vibrating diaphragm that produces a sinusoidal pressure wave that is transmitted through the airways to the alveoli.
iNO	Nitric oxide is an inspired gas delivered in combination with mechanical ventilation that acts as a vasodilator and vascular smooth muscle relaxant.
ECMO	Extracorporeal membrane oxygenation is a heart-and-lung bypass procedure that involves draining venous blood, supplementing it with O_2, and removing CO_2 by means of a membrane oxygenator and returning the blood to either venous or arterial circulations.
Vital signs monitor	Unit that displays monitoring of HR, RR, BP, and Sa_{O_2}
Pulse oximeter	Measures oxygen concentration in the peripheral circulation with a bandage-type light sensor attached to the infant's arm or leg, which provides a pulse-by-pulse readout of percent oxygen saturation on the screen of the monitor
Transcutaneous oxygen and carbon dioxide monitor	Noninvasive method for monitoring concentrations of O_2 and CO_2 through the skin
Infusion pumps	Electric infusion pump that controls the flow and rate of fluids, intralipids, and transpyloric feedings
Phototherapy	Fiberoptic or overhead bank or spot lights or fiberoptic blanket used to reduce hyperbilirubinemia
Gavage tube	Oral or nasogastric tube used for feeding directly into the stomach. Transpyloric tubes are used for infants who cannot tolerate oral or nasal tubes, have severe GER, or are at risk for aspiration.
PIV	Peripheral intravenous line, which may be used for fluids, nutrition, or antibiotics
CVL	Central venous line used for prolonged parental feeding or antibiotics, or to draw blood
PICC	Percutaneously inserted central catheter. Long, flexible catheter inserted through a peripheral antecubital vein and threaded centrally to the superior vena cava. PICC lines are used for prolonged parental feeding or antibiotics or to draw blood.
UA	Umbilical arterial line inserted through the umbilical artery into the abdominal aorta and used for the first 5–7 day in 2 spots of life for monitoring arterial blood gases, infusion of fluids, and continuous blood pressure monitoring
UV	Umbilical venous line inserted into umbilical vein and used for the first 7–14 day in 2 spots of life and as the initial venous access, to infuse vasopressors, and for exchange transfusions, monitoring of central venous pressure, and infusion of fluids

BP, blood pressure; CPAP, continuous positive airway pressure; GER, gastroesophageal reflux; HR, heart rate; NICU, neonatal intensive care unit; RR, respiratory rate.

This is done by working to improve gas exchange at the lowest amount of inspired oxygen concentration (Fio_2) and the lowest pressures and tidal volume. The individual infant's condition will dictate how ventilatory support is provided.[193]

Continuous positive airway pressure (CPAP) provides a continuous flow of warmed, humidified gas at a set pressure

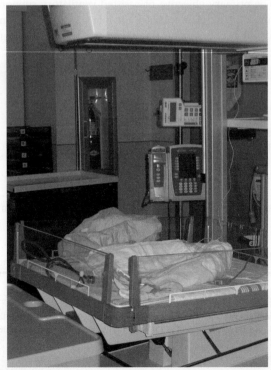

FIGURE 4.7. Radiant warmer bed setup for an admission to the neonatal intensive care unit (NICU).

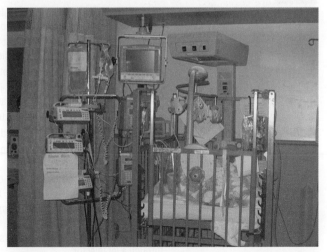

FIGURE 4.8. Crib with radiant warmer, infusion pumps, and monitor.

to maintain an elevated end-expiratory lung volume while the infant breathes spontaneously.[193-196] CPAP can be delivered by mask, nasal prongs, or less frequently through an endotracheal tube.

The gas mixture delivered via CPAP can be either continuous flow or variable flow. In continuous flow, the system provides a noninterrupted supply of gas to the infant. Bubble or water-seal CPAP is a type of continuous flow. The blended gas is delivered to the infant after being heated and humidified. The distal end of the tubing is immersed in sterile water or acetic acid to a specific level to provide the desired amount of CPAP.[195] Bubble CPAP can generate vibrations in the infant's chest at frequencies similar to those used in high-frequency ventilation (HFV).[197] Variable flow nasal CPAP (NCPAP) uses injector jets to deliver gas at a constant pressure through nasal prongs into each naris. The flow is able to change so that the infant does not have to exhale against the CPAP.[195]

CPAP is used to prevent alveolar and airway collapse and to reduce the barotrauma caused by mechanical ventilation. Indications for CPAP include the early treatment of respiratory distress syndrome (RDS), moderately frequent apneic spells, recent extubation, weaning chronically ventilator-dependent infants, and early treatment to prevent atelectasis in premature infants with minimal respiratory distress and minimal need for supplemental oxygen. Negative aspects of NCPAP include gastric distension with high flows and excoriation or breakdown of the nasal septum when nasal prongs are used.[194-196]

The most common approach in the United States for treating respiratory failure in the NICU is with positive-pressure ventilation.[198,199] The two types of positive-pressure mechanical ventilators are volume controlled or pressure limited. Volume-controlled ventilators deliver the same tidal volume of gas with each breath regardless of how much pressure is needed. Although rarely used with newborn infants, volume ventilators designed specifically for neonates can be used in the presence of rapidly changing lung compliance.[193] Pressure-limited ventilators deliver gas until a preset limiting pressure is reached. The peak pressure delivered to the airway is constant, but the tidal volume with each breath is variable. Synchronized intermittent mandatory ventilation (SIMV), assist/control, and pressure support are adaptations of conventional pressure-limited ventilators and are also used in the NICU.

HFV utilizes extremely rapid ventilatory rates to deliver tidal volumes equal to or smaller than anatomic dead space. Continuous pressures are applied to maintain an elevated lung volume with superimposed tidal volumes provided at a rapid rate. The advantages of HFV over conventional ventilation are to provide adequate gas exchange at lower proximal airway pressures in lungs already damaged by barotrauma and volutrauma and to preserve normal lung structure in the relatively uninjured lung.[200-203]

The three types of HFV used in the NICU are high-frequency positive-pressure ventilation (HFPPV), high-frequency jet ventilation (HFJV), and high-frequency oscillating ventilation (HFOV).[200,203] HFPPV is produced by conventional ventilators or modified conventional ventilators set at a high rate.[202] HFJV delivers short pulses of heated, pressurized gas directly into the upper airway through a narrow cannula or jet injector.[202-204] The HFJV can maintain oxygenation and ventilation to wide ranges of lung compliance and patient size. HFOV has a piston pump or vibrating diaphragm that produces a sinusoidal pressure wave that is transmitted through the airways to the alveoli.[202,203] Small tidal volumes are superimposed over a constant airway pressure at a high RR.[205]

HFV is used primarily for infants who are failing conventional ventilation.[192,200] Although outcome studies have been unable to demonstrate clear benefits of HFV over conventional mechanical ventilation (CMV), clinically HFV has been helpful in air leak syndromes, pulmonary interstitial emphysema (PIE), pre-/postcongenital diaphragmatic hernia (CDH) repair, meconium aspiration syndrome (MAS), and some forms of pulmonary hypoplasia.[202,203,205] HFV can also be used as a bridge to extracorporeal membrane oxygenation (ECMO) for infants with severe respiratory failure and may eliminate the need for ECMO in some infants.[189] Neonatal RDS is the most common lung disease treated with HFV in the NICU. HFJV has been shown to be most successful in the treatment of air leak syndromes, whereas HFOV has shown better outcomes for infants with CDH, RDS, and persistent pulmonary hypertension of the newborn (PPHN).[202] The most serious side effect of HFV is an increase in long-term neurologic injury because of early periventricular leukomalacia (PVL) or severe intraventricular hemorrhage (IVH).[203] Some studies have found increased severe IVH in very premature infants treated with HFV versus CMV.[203,206] Other studies found no difference when other confounding variables were taken into consideration such as GA, type of delivery, early large patent ductus arteriosus (PDA), and decreased superior vena cava blood flow (Fig. 4.9).[193,207]

Another form of ventilatory support that is beginning to be used with greater frequency in the NICU is high-flow

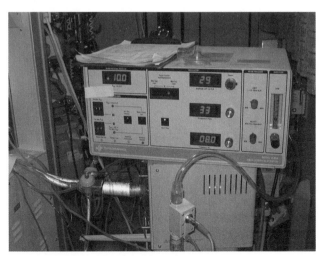

FIGURE 4.9. High-flow oscillating ventilator.

nasal cannula (HFNC). Studies have shown the HFNC to be as effective as NCPAP in providing positive end-distending pressure to the lungs of some infants with mild respiratory disease.

The advantage of nasal cannula over NCPAP is less irritation to the nasal spectrum.[208-210] The nasal cannula allows for greater comfort on the part of the infant and greater ease for the family or nurses to hold and care for the infant than mask or nasal prongs. Highly humidified HFNC is also used to provide higher flows of gas without the usual negative side effects of nasal cannula (i.e., drying, bleeding, or nasal septal breakdown because of the addition of high humidity).[211-215]

In December 1999, the U.S. Food and Drug Administration approved the use of inhaled nitric oxide (iNO) for the treatment of near-term and term infants with hypoxic respiratory failure. PPHN, RDS, aspiration syndromes, pneumonia, sepsis, and CDH are conditions that can cause hypoxic respiratory failure. The primary actions of nitric oxide are vasodilation and the relaxation of vascular smooth muscle, which increases blood flow to alveoli, improving oxygen and carbon dioxide exchange. Nitric oxide is a short-lived molecule, so that it affects the pulmonary vascular smooth muscle without affecting systemic vasculature. Airway smooth muscle is also affected by nitric oxide, and the combined action of airway and vascular smooth muscle relaxation has been effective in the treatment of infants with ventilation–perfusion abnormalities (Fig. 4.10).[216,217]

Infants in the first week of life, who are 34 weeks or greater GA with progressive hypoxic respiratory failure, meet the criteria for use of iNO as an adjunct to therapeutic interventions. The degree of illness and/or the modalities tried prior to the initiation of nitric oxide have not been clearly delineated. Nitric oxide is contraindicated for infants with congenital heart disease whose cardiopulmonary function depends on a right-to-left shunt or who have severe left heart failure.[218] Although iNO has not been effective in treating infants with CDH, multicenter clinical trials have shown that iNO improves oxygenation and the outcome of near-term

and term infants with hypoxic respiratory failure because of other conditions such as PPHN. Studies have also shown that iNO reduces the need for ECMO without increasing neurodevelopmental, behavioral, or medical abnormalities.[219-222]

The use of iNO in preterm infants is controversial, and there is no consensus on the timing for initiation, dosage, and length of time for iNO therapy with infants less than 34 weeks. In two studies of infants less than 32 weeks GA and body weight less than 1,250 g requiring mechanical ventilation, those who received iNO demonstrated decreased incidence of bronchopulmonary dysplasia (BPD), less severe lung disease, decreased length of time requiring supplemental oxygen, decreased incidence of death, and no increased risk of brain injury. The benefits of iNO may be due to decreased airway resistance, which results in decreased need for supplemental oxygen, mechanical ventilation, and oxidative stress.[223,224]

ECMO is similar to a heart–lung bypass machine and provides rest and support for the baby's heart and lungs. ECMO is utilized with patients with cardiac and pulmonary dysfunction whose hypoxia is refractory to conventional therapies such as CMV and HFV. In the last decade, the use of surfactant, iNO, and HFV has replaced ECMO for patients with RDS, MAS, or pulmonary hypertension (PH). ECMO continues to be implemented with patients with CDH, PPHN, and sepsis (Fig. 4.11).[225-229]

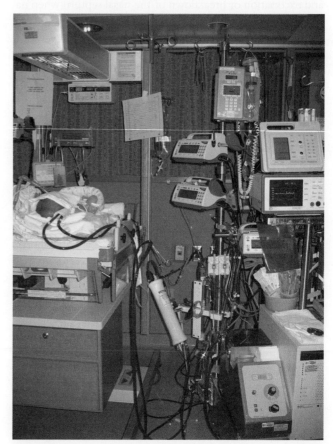

FIGURE 4.11. Infant on extracorporeal membrane oxygenation (ECMO).

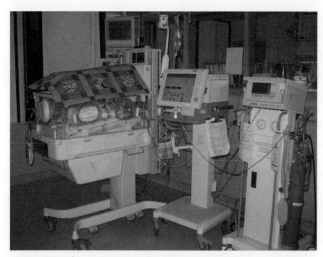

FIGURE 4.10. Conventional ventilator with nitric oxide tank.

To initiate ECMO, catheters are inserted into the right side of the baby's neck and threaded to the heart in a process called "cannulation." The baby's unoxygenated blood drains via gravity (therefore, the baby's bed is elevated) through the catheters to the ECMO pump. The ECMO pump pushes the baby's blood through the ECMO circuit, where a membrane oxygenator acts as an artificial lung, removing carbon dioxide and providing oxygen to the blood. The oxygenated blood is then returned through the catheter into the baby. Babies receiving ECMO are sedated, paralyzed, and given pain medication. They are generally positioned in supine with their heads rotated to the left to allow access to the right neck vessels. These infants also are on large amounts of heparin, in order to prevent the blood from clotting when it contacts the catheters and the ECMO circuit.[230] The heparin, used to prevent clot formation, may cause the baby to bleed, the most significant complication of ECMO. Babies receive daily head ultrasounds to assess whether an intracranial hemorrhage (ICH) has occurred. If present, ICH may be the reason to discontinue ECMO.[231] Babies who have received ECMO are at risk for developing atypical postures, tone, and movement patterns and require close developmental follow-up.[225-229] Babies post-ECMO frequently demonstrate difficulties with oral feeding. Other neurodevelopmental morbidity includes seizures, hearing loss, hyperactivity, behavioral problems, CP, school failure, and developmental delay.[231] Although patients present with a variety of primary diagnoses requiring ECMO, after ECMO these infants demonstrate similar functional and neurodevelopmental outcomes, with the exception of babies with CDH. Infants with CDH have lower survival rates and higher morbidity, particularly in respiratory and digestive function, than other infants after ECMO.[227,232]

Medical Issues of Prematurity

Infants born prematurely are some of the most fragile in the NICU. They are at risk for multiple medical complications because of the immaturity of their body structures and organs, possible exposure to infections and teratogens, and the effects of the medical strategies and the technology required for minimizing illness and sustaining life. In this section, several of the more common medical conditions encountered in the NICU and the medical interventions used to treat them are discussed. The information provided is only a brief overview, and the reader is advised to consult neonatal medical texts, care manuals, and the original references cited at the end of this chapter for more in-depth detail.

Respiratory Distress Syndrome

RDS occurs as a result of pulmonary immaturity and inadequate pulmonary surfactant. Premature infants are predisposed to developing RDS owing to structural and physiologic immaturities, including poor alveolar capillary development, lack of type II alveolar cells, and insufficient production of surfactant. Surfactant is a substance produced by type II alveolar cells and lines the alveoli and small bronchioles. Decreased surfactant leads to respiratory failure because of increased alveolar surface tension, alveolar collapse, diffuse atelectasis, and decreased lung compliance. The preterm infant is further compromised by increased compliance of the chest wall because of the cartilaginous composition of the ribs, decreased number of type I fatigue-resistant muscle fibers in the diaphragm and intercostal muscles, and instability of neural control of breathing.[233-235]

Identification of RDS is made by prenatal risk factors, assessment of fetal lung immaturity, and postnatal clinical signs. Factors that affect lung maturity and increase predisposition for RDS include prematurity (GA < 34 weeks), maternal diabetes (insulin appears to interfere with surfactant production), genetic factors (Caucasian race, siblings with history of RDS, and male gender), and thoracic malformations with lung hypoplasia.[236] Antenatal steroids are often used to accelerate lung maturity in the fetus and stimulate the production of surfactant. The National Institutes of Health (NIH)[237] in 2000 recommended that antenatal steroids be given to all pregnant women at 24 to 34 weeks' gestation who are at risk for preterm delivery within 7 days; however, there is a lack of consensus for the type of steroid used and the method of dosing. Although a number of studies of antenatal steroid therapy have demonstrated increased surfactant production, decreased length of time on mechanical ventilation, and decreased incidence of IVH,[238] others have shown decreased fetal growth, increased mortality, and poor neurobehavioral outcomes.[239-243]

The diagnosis of RDS is based on history, clinical presentation, blood gas studies, and chest radiography. RDS can develop immediately after birth or within the first hours of life, depending on lung immaturity and perinatal events. Clinical signs of RDS include increased RR, expiratory grunting, sternal and intercostal retractions, nasal flaring, cyanosis, decreased air entry on auscultation, hypoxia, and hypercarbia. The lungs on chest radiography have a reticulogranular or "ground glass" appearance.[236]

Interventions for the premature infant with RDS depend on the severity of the disorder and include oxygen supplementation, assisted ventilation, and surfactant administration. Administration of prophylactic surfactant to intubated infants less than 30 weeks GA has been associated with initial improvement in respiratory status and a decrease in the incidence of RDS, pneumothorax, BPD, and IVH.[244] Current practice is moving away from prophylactic surfactant administration for infants who otherwise do not need to be intubated.[245-247] The Texas Neonatal Research Group[248] recommends that infants greater than or equal to 1,250 g with mild to moderate RDS should not be electively intubated solely for the administration of surfactant.

Assisted mechanical ventilation has typically been the intervention of choice for infants with RDS. However, mechanical ventilation can cause airway damage in the form of barotrauma and volutrauma. HFV has been suggested as an alternative to conventional ventilation in order to decrease lung injury.[200-203] Positive-pressure ventilation via nasal or nasal–pharyngeal prongs to address respiratory needs while limiting barotrauma from intubation has also been advocated.[197] Studies have shown the combination of early surfactant administration and NCPAP to improve the clinical course of RDS and decrease the need for mechanical ventilation.[249] According to Honrubia and Stark,[236] the use of CPAP with infants with RDS appears to prevent atelectasis, minimize lung injury, and preserve the functional properties of surfactant. The decision of which form of respiratory intervention to use is based on the individual infant's clinical signs and chest radiography.

The prognosis of infants with RDS varies with the severity of the original lung involvement. Infants who do not require mechanical ventilation are more likely to have resolution of RDS with little or no long-term sequelae. However, the very immature ELBW infants may progress to chronic lung disease (CLD) or BPD owing to prolonged mechanical ventilation and the associated damage to the lungs. Infants with severe RDS are also at increased risk for ICH, retinopathy of prematurity (ROP), and necrotizing enterocolitis (NEC).[235]

In the acute stage of RDS, the infant is considered to be medically unstable and at risk for complications such as apnea, bradycardia, BP variability, and IVH. Minimal environmental stimulation in the form of sound, light, and handling is often recommended to decrease infant stress. The PT may perform observational evaluation of the infant using the NIDCAP to provide information to guide the delivery of care. Using this information, the therapist collaborates with the medical team and parents to develop a care plan to support overall growth and development. Suggestions for caregiving may include positioning, comfort, and protective measures.

Patent Ductus Arteriosus

The ductus arteriosus is a structure in the developing fetal heart that allows blood to bypass circulation to the lungs (Fig. 4.12). Because the fetus does not require the lungs to oxygenate blood, the flow from the right ventricle is shunted from the left pulmonary artery to the aorta. The ductus arteriosus typically closes within 10 to 15 hours after birth by constriction of medial smooth muscle. Anatomic closure is complete by 2 to 3 weeks of age, and factors that precipitate closure include oxygen, prostaglandin E_2 levels, and maturity.[250]

Oxygen appears to be the strongest stimulus for closure of the ductus.[251] The responsiveness of the smooth muscle to oxygen is related to GA. The premature infant has less of a response to oxygen in the environment because of decreased sensitivity to oxygen-induced muscle contractions and high levels of prostaglandin E_2.[252] When the ductus fails to close, it is termed PDA. In premature infants, the pulmonary vascular smooth muscle is not well developed, and there is a more rapid fall in pulmonary vascular resistance (PVR) than in full-term infants. The blood from the left side of the heart is shunted through the ductus to the right side, resulting in

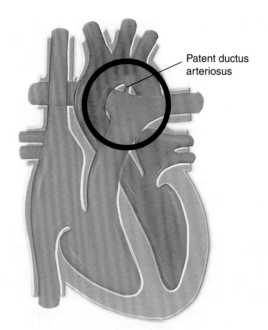

FIGURE 4.12. Illustration of patent ductus arteriosus. (From the Anatomical Chart Company.)

hypotension and poor perfusion, and can cause congestive heart failure from cardiovascular overload. Low mean BP, metabolic acidosis, decreased urine output, and worsening jaundice because of poor organ perfusion are systemic consequences of left-to-right shunting.

The clinical signs of PDA include murmur, increased HR, and respiratory distress. Other symptoms associated with PDA are failure to gain weight, sepsis, congestive heart failure, and pulmonary edema. Diagnosis is made by chest radiography and echocardiography. Treatment is determined by the size of the PDA and clinical presentation. Initially, the PDA is treated with increased ventilatory support, fluid restriction, and diuretic therapy.[252] In symptomatic infants, indomethacin is used for nonsurgical PDA closure and is effective in approximately 80% of cases.[253,254] The use of indomethacin for prophylaxis in nonsymptomatic infants is controversial as side effects from the medication can occur. Symptomatic infants with a PDA that does not close after the second indomethacin treatment or infants for whom indomethacin is contraindicated undergo surgical ligation after echocardiographic documentation of the PDA.

Hyperbilirubinemia

Physiologic jaundice or hyperbilirubinemia is the accumulation of excessive amounts of bilirubin in the blood. Bilirubin is one of the breakdown products of hemoglobin from red blood cells. Hyperbilirubinemia commonly occurs in premature infants owing to immature hepatic function, increased hemolysis of red blood cells from birth injuries, and possible polycythemia (Fig. 4.13).

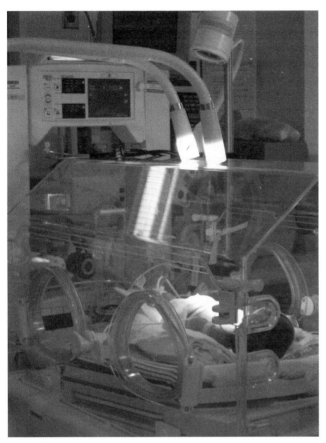

FIGURE 4.13. Phototherapy for hyperbilirubinemia. Note the motor stress signs demonstrated by the infant because of lack of boundaries.

The primary concern in the treatment of hyperbilirubinemia is the prevention of kernicterus or the deposition of unconjugated bilirubin in the brain causing neuronal injury. The areas of the brain most commonly affected are the basal ganglia, cranial nerve nuclei, other brainstem nuclei, cerebellar nuclei, hippocampus, and anterior horn cells of the spinal cord.[255,256] Infants with chronic bilirubin encephalopathy can present with athetosis, partial or complete sensorineural hearing loss, limitation of upward gaze, dental dysplasia, and mild mental retardation. Kernicterus has become rare in preterm infants, but does still occur. Recent studies have shown an association between neurodevelopmental impairment and modest elevations in total serum bilirubin in ELBW infants.[257]

Premature infants are more susceptible to anoxia, hypercarbia, and sepsis, which open the blood–brain barrier, leading to deposition of bilirubin in neural tissue. Bilirubin toxicity in LBW infants may be more a reflection of their overall clinical status than a function of actual bilirubin levels.[255,258]

Hyperbilirubinemia is diagnosed by serum blood levels of bilirubin and treated with phototherapy or exchange transfusion. There are no consensus guidelines for the treatment of infants less than 35 weeks GA with phototherapy or exchange transfusion. Generally, if phototherapy is not effective in reducing serum bilirubin levels or if there is a rapidly increasing bilirubin level, exchange transfusion is done.[259] Phototherapy is used to reduce serum bilirubin levels and is administered by fiberoptic blankets and bank or spot lights. Infants under phototherapy lights are naked except for a diaper and eye patches to protect their eyes in order to provide light exposure to the greatest surface area of skin. Exchange transfusion removes partially hemolyzed and antibody-coated red blood cells and replaces them with donor red blood cells lacking the sensitizing antigen. Bilirubin is removed from the plasma, and extravascular bilirubin binds to the albumin in the exchanged blood. The infant continues under phototherapy after the exchange transfusion.[255,260] Complications of exchange transfusion include hypocalcemia (which can cause cardiac arrhythmias), hypoglycemia, acid–base imbalance, hyperkalemia, cardiovascular problems including perforation of vessels, embolization, vasospasm, thrombosis, infarction, volume overload and cardiac arrest, thrombocytopenia, infection, hemolysis, graft-versus-host disease, hypothermia, hyperthermia, and NEC.[255,256,260] There has been a dramatic decrease in the number of exchange transfusions performed on preterm infants because of more effective phototherapy and prevention of Rh hemolytic disease with Rh (D) immunoglobulin.[259]

Hyperbilirubinemia tends to decrease levels of arousal and activity. The infant may present with lethargy, hypotonia, and poor sucking ability.[259] Paludetto et al.[260] and Mansi et al.[261] found that infants with moderate levels of hyperbilirubinemia demonstrate transient alterations in visual, auditory, social–interactive, and neuromotor capabilities. These findings are important considerations when performing a developmental assessment on an infant with increased levels of bilirubin.[12] Other issues to consider when assessing and planning treatment are the limitations imposed by phototherapy. When receiving phototherapy, the infant is generally positioned so that there is maximal exposure of body surfaces to the lights, limiting how some of the positioning devices and strategies are used for nesting and containment. The therapist will need to assist caregivers in creative ways to promote developmentally supportive postures and comfort without compromising the effectiveness of the phototherapy. Infants under the phototherapy lights need to have their eyes shielded to protect them from damage and to avoid any stress the bright lights may cause. Care must be taken to position eye shields so they are not too tight or too loose as either case can be extremely noxious to the sensitive, high-risk infant.

Gastroesophageal Reflux

Gastroesophageal reflux (GER) has been defined as the involuntary movement of gastric contents in a retrograde fashion into the esophagus and above. The stomach contents that reflux can include acidic or alkaline gastric fluids, semisolids, feedings, enzymes, bile salts, or even air from crying or distended stomach that can move up to any portion of the esophagus, nasopharynx, oropharynx, or into the airway.[262-267]

All infants have some degree of reflux that is considered to be physiologic or asymptomatic if the infant is thriving well and the reflux resolves with maturation. Infants with asymptomatic GER may demonstrate small episodes of emesis; other infants may reswallow the refluxate without emesis. Infants with physiologic GER tend to grow and gain weight appropriately.[268] More frequent episodes of GER (pathologic GER) are referred to as GER disease or GERD and can burn the lining of the esophagus, resulting in inflammation, dysmotility, and pain.[268] These symptoms can lead to poor oral feeding patterns, oral aversion, and excessive crying because of pain. Blood loss in the emesis can lead to iron deficiency anemia. The result of severe reflux can be poor oral intake, poor weight gain, and malnutrition leading to failure to thrive.[269] Additional symptoms of GERD include apnea, aspiration, recurrent pneumonia, CLD, or larger airway inflammation.[270]

The most common mechanism of GER is relaxation of the lower esophageal sphincter (LES).[263] In addition, premature infants have shorter esophageal length and intra-abdominal LES as well as smaller stomach capacity.[271,272] Risk factors that have been identified for neonatal GER include prematurity, birth asphyxia, perinatal stress, neonatal stress, delayed gastric emptying, congenital anomalies of the upper GI tract, acquired problems of the upper intestinal tract, diaphragmatic defects, respiratory disease, neurodevelopmental delays, ECMO, abdominal surgery, and medications. Acidic fluids can cause esophageal inflammation and further aggravate reflux. Higher risk for GER is associated with premature, stressed infants as well as those with CLD and congenital anomalies. Tone of the abdominal wall muscles, diaphragmatic activity, esophageal dysmotility, LES tone, and the physiologic immaturity of digestive function may be related to the increased incidence in these neonates.[267] Studies have demonstrated increased episodes of reflux with the presence of a nasogastric tube as it is an irritant and maintains the patency of the LES.[273-275]

The relationship between apnea, bradycardia, and GER is controversial. Apnea and bradycardia occur frequently in preterm infants during and after feeding when GER is also frequently observed.[273] These apnea and bradycardia events may be related to GER owing to refluxate moving up into the esophagus, blocking the airway and causing obstructive apnea and subsequent bradycardia. Another proposed mechanism of apnea and bradycardia is due to the laryngeal reflex mechanism and laryngospasm.[276] However, research studies have not demonstrated a temporal relationship between GER events and apnea or bradycardia.[273,277,278] DiFiore et al.[277] suggested that apnea and GER may be observed to occur together owing to common risk factors.

Diagnosis of GER in neonates is by history, clinical evaluation, and studies including esophageal pH probe, esophagram, fluoroscopy or upper GI series, gastric scintigraphy or milk scan, esophageal manometry, and endoscopy. History and clinical evaluation are important to rule out other conditions.[279] It is important to also identify whether the reflux is physiologic or pathologic, factors that make reflux worse, the mechanism of reflux, and the presence of complications caused by the reflux.

Nonpharmacologic management of GER in infancy often includes altering the type and delivery of feedings, positioning, and elevation of the head of the bed. Changes in the timing, volume, composition, and viscosity of feedings may assist in decreasing GER. The method of feeding (continuous vs. bolus) and feeding beyond the stomach can also reduce the frequency of regurgitation. Continuous jejunal or duodenal feeding also reduces the risk of aspiration. However, there is also the risk of increased GER events because of the use of chronic nasogastric or nasojejunal feeding tubes.[273]

Positioning the infant in supine, right side-lying, and infant seats have been associated with exacerbation of reflux. Prone, elevation of the head of the bed to 30 degrees, and left side-lying have been shown to decrease episodes of reflux.[279-282] Omari et al.[283] found that in healthy preterm infants, right side-lying is associated with increased transient LES relaxation and increased GER while at the same time increasing gastric emptying. Decreased gastric residuals have been reported in prone and right side-lying as compared with supine and left side-lying.[284,285] Chen et al.[284] suggested that preterm infants be positioned prone for the first 30 minutes postprandial and then change position to supine on the basis of behavioral cues. Van Wijk et al.[286] recommended repositioning from prone to left lateral position after first postprandial hour to decrease reflux. As both prone and lateral positioning have been associated with sudden infant death syndrome (SIDS), these positions are utilized with infants who receive cardiorespiratory monitoring.

Pharmacologic therapy is often initiated in the treatment of infants with GERD. The medications most often prescribed are antacids, histamine-2 receptor agonists, proton pump inhibitors, and prokinetics. These agents are used to neutralize or suppress acid and to promote gastric and/or esophageal motility.[287,288]

Surgery for pathologic GER may be considered for infants who have failed other management of GER and those with pulmonary symptoms from aspiration.[288] The most common antireflux surgical procedure is a fundoplication.[289] Partial or complete wrapping of the upper stomach or fundus around the esophagus is done to create a valve mechanism decreasing retrograde movement of stomach contents and promoting gastric emptying. Fundoplication is often performed in conjunction with feeding gastrostomy for infants requiring long-term tube feedings.[290]

Infants with GER and associated esophagitis may demonstrate pain behaviors that impact behavioral state organization and their ability to participate in activities with family and caregivers. Motor patterns observed may be of increased extension or arching of the head and trunk. Increased muscle tone may be noted in the extremities. Although the medical issues of GER need to be addressed primarily, the therapist in the NICU may be called upon to assist with positioning to minimize reflux and promote comfort. Ongoing neurodevelopmental assessments are required to determine the effect of reflux on behavior and how to adapt interventions to promote appropriate developmental competencies.

Necrotizing Enterocolitis

With an incidence of 1 to 3 per 1,000 live births, NEC is one of the most common GI emergencies in the newborn infant.[291,292] Almost all NEC cases develop in preterm infants who have received enteral feedings,[293-295] and approximately 1% to 7.7% of NICU admissions are due to NEC.[293,294] NEC results from ischemic necrosis of the intestinal mucosa, resulting in intestinal infarction. Although a portion of the terminal ileum and colon are affected in the majority of cases, NEC can affect the entire GI tract in severe cases.[291,293,296,297] Preterm infants are at the highest risk for NEC, and the incidence of NEC is inversely related to GA and birth weight.[291,298-300] Only 13% of NEC cases are reported in term infants, and these babies typically have an underlying condition predisposing them to the disease, such as congenital heart disease, respiratory disease, sepsis, seizures, perinatal asphyxia, hypoglycemia, or intrauterine growth retardation.[291-304]

The etiology and pathogenesis of NEC remain unclear; it seems to be the result of multiple factors in a vulnerable baby. Prematurity and milk feeding are established risk factors in epidemiologic studies of NEC, although microbial bowel overgrowth, circulatory instability of the GI tract, and medications increasing intestinal mucosal injury or bacterial overgrowth are additional risk factors.[293,305-308]

NEC causes acute illness in the short term and is associated with long-term neurodevelopmental impairments in survivors, including CP, visual deficits, and intellectual challenges.[293,309] Male and female newborns are equally affected.[291,310] Although early detection and aggressive management have improved outcomes of survivors, overall mortality rates of 15% to 30% have been reported in the literature.[291,306,311] Mortality rates for babies with NEC are inversely related to birth weight and are higher for babies who require surgery.[291,311-316]

A baby developing NEC will present with both systemic signs and abdominal signs. Systemic signs include apnea, respiratory failure, lethargy, poor feeding, temperature instability, and hypotension. Abdominal signs include changes in feeding tolerance such as abdominal distension, tenderness, gastric residuals, vomiting of bile and/or blood, and/or bloody stools.[291,317-322] As NEC progresses, the infant may develop intestinal hemorrhage, gangrene, submucosal gas, and in some cases perforation of the intestines, sepsis, and shock.

The most important factor in determining outcome appears to be early diagnosis and treatment. Diagnosis is made by physical examination and can be confirmed by abdominal X-ray with the presence of pneumatosis intestinalis (bubbles of gas observed in the intestinal wall); however, there is evidence to suggest that radiologic findings can vary by GA and may not be helpful in preterm infants.[291] Medical treatment is typically initiated in the absence of radiologic confirmation if clinical suspicion is high. The most commonly used uniform criteria for defining NEC is Bell's staging criteria originally published in 1978 and is based on systemic, intestinal, and radiographic findings; Bell's staging criteria have been modified to describe mildly and moderately ill babies in each of the three categories outlined[312]:

- Stage I: Suspected NEC; infant demonstrates nonspecific systemic signs (temperature instability, apnea, and lethargy); abdominal signs such as abdominal distension, gastric residuals, emesis, and heme-positive stools; radiographic findings are normal or show mild bowel dilation.
- Stage II: Proven NEC; infant demonstrates symptoms of stage I plus absent bowel sounds and pneumatosis on abdominal radiography.
- Stage III: Advanced NEC; critically ill infant displaying, in addition to symptoms of stages I and II, hypotension, bradycardia, severe apnea, abdominal tenderness, acidosis, neutropenia, and disseminated intravascular coagulation. The infant may or may not show findings consistent with bowel perforation on abdominal radiography.[291,296,320,323-325]

Medical management is begun immediately when NEC is suspected and includes supportive care, such as bowel rest, discontinuation of enteral feeds, gastric suction to decompress the bowel, total parenteral nutrition, fluid replacement, antibiotics, close monitoring of laboratory values and GI tract (the latter by abdominal X-ray or ultrasound), and mechanical ventilation, if needed, to support the infant. Typically, abdominal radiographs are taken every 6 to 8 hours to detect progression of intestinal obstruction or possible perforation.

When NEC has been proven by changes on radiography, a pediatric surgeon is consulted to provide recommendations regarding the necessity for and timing of surgery. The goal of surgery is to conserve bowel length while not jeopardizing the baby. Surgical procedures include exploratory laparotomy and resection of necrotic bowel or primary peritoneal drainage (PPD). There is no hard evidence to recommend one procedure over the other, although PPD can be performed at the bedside under local anesthesia, will not require a reanastomosis surgery, and therefore may be preferred. Laparotomy typically entails resecting the involved portion of bowel, placing an ostomy and mucous fistula; less typically, if the affected bowel is short enough, the affected portion of the bowel can be resected and a primary anastomosis performed[293,307,323,326-332] (Fig. 4.14).

Complications of NEC include sepsis, meningitis, abscess, hypotension, shock, respiratory failure, and disseminated intravascular coagulation acutely and in the long term, intestinal narrowing (stricture formation), and short bowel syndrome. Strictures requiring surgical resection are reported to occur in 9% to 36% of babies with NEC, whereas

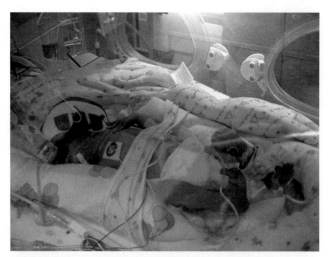

FIGURE 4.14. Infant with necrotizing enterocolitis with ostomy.

short bowel syndrome is reported to occur in 9% of infants who have received surgery for NEC. Short bowel syndrome results in chronic intestinal malabsorption and dependence on total parenteral nutrition. Babies with short bowel syndrome are at risk for sepsis, cholestasis, and liver failure and may require eventual intestinal and hepatic organ transplantation.[307,324,333-336] Babies with NEC can endure long hospitalizations to manage these complications.

A spontaneous and isolated intestinal perforation in the newborn can also occur and needs to be differentiated from NEC. Spontaneous isolated intestinal perforations usually occur in preterm infants weighing less than 1,500 g at birth. The perforation typically happens at the terminal ileum but can also occur in the jejunum or colon in the first 10 days of life. Risk factors for this include chorioamnionitis, maternal exposure to antibiotics before or at delivery,[336,337] and early administration of glucocorticoids.[336-340] Unlike NEC, a spontaneous intestinal perforation has an area of focal hemorrhagic necrosis with normal-appearing bowel proximal and distal to the perforation and can be differentiated from NEC by presentation (hypotension and abdominal distension in the first 10 days of life with bluish discoloration of abdominal wall, radiographs showing pneumoperitoneum in the absence of pneumatosis intestinalis, and portal venous air). Initial management is similar to supportive care for NEC. Surgery is required and like NEC can be either an exploratory laparotomy with bowel resection or PPD. There are no randomized controlled trials (RCTs) to recommend one procedure over another; however, babies receiving PPD are less likely to need an exploratory laparotomy. The drain is left in till drainage ceases; patency of the GI tract can be confirmed via a contrast study or feeding can be started after bowel function has returned.[331-341]

The incidence of problems with growth and neurodevelopmental outcome of infants with NEC has been reported in comparison studies with other VLBW infants.[309,318,320,333,342] No growth or neurodevelopmental differences have been found in infants treated medically for NEC; however, in the population of infants treated surgically for NEC, significant differences in growth and neurodevelopmental functioning have been reported.[291,343,344] Infants with stages II and III NEC are reported to have lower head circumference and body length at 12 months and lower weight at 12 to 20 months than age-matched peers without NEC.[342] Neurodevelopmental outcome assessments performed on VLBW infants with stages II and III NEC and age-matched infants without NEC at 12 and 20 months corrected age demonstrate significantly lower general developmental quotients in infants with NEC at both 12 and 20 months. There is a higher incidence of severe psychomotor retardation in infants with stage III NEC and multiple organ involvement.[312,342] Neurodevelopmental outcome may be better for babies with isolated perforation compared with NEC; however, the former babies appear to have a greater risk of developing ROP and PVL than infants without spontaneous perforation.[338,345-347]

Infants in the acute stages of NEC are critically ill and require constant monitoring by physicians and nurses. Therapists, more than any other professionals in the NICU, are continually thinking how the present moment will affect the baby's current and future development. Therapists can advocate for the protection of the infant during the acute illness by minimizing environmental stimulation and handling, as well as careful attention to positioning with extra support for limbs with arterial or venous lines. The therapist should work in coordination with the medical team and family to assess the infant for signs of stress and comfort. Using this information, recommendations for individualized care can be made. As these infants are at risk for significant developmental delays, it is important that developmental intervention and developmental follow-up continue as their medical status improves and after discharge.

Germinal Matrix-Intraventricular Hemorrhage

Germinal matrix-intraventricular hemorrhage (GM-IVH) is the most common type of brain lesion found in premature infants, occurring most frequently in infants less than 1,500 g and at less than 32 weeks' gestation. The incidence of GM-IVH is inversely related to GA, with the extremely premature being at greatest risk.[149,348-356] The hemorrhage typically originates in the subependymal layer of the germinal matrix and extends into the intraventricular space between the lateral ventricles (Fig. 4.15). During fetal development, this is the site of neuronal proliferation as neuroblasts divide and migrate to the cerebral parenchyma. The neuronal proliferation is complete by 20 weeks, whereas glial cell proliferation continues until approximately 32 weeks' gestation. The matrix decreases in size from 33 to 34 weeks and nearly complete involution occurs by 36 weeks' gestation.[149,348-350,356,357] These developmental changes in the brain influence the area and extent of the hemorrhage in the neonate.

A fragile and primitive capillary network supplies blood to this very metabolically active area. It is within this capillary

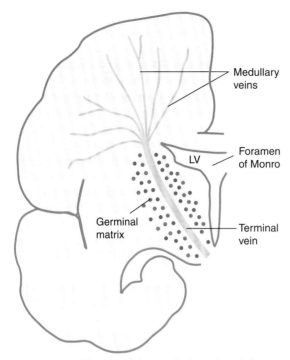

FIGURE 4.15. Diagram of the germinal matrix and the venous drainage of cerebral white matter. LV, lateral ventricular. (Reprinted with permission from Volpe JJ. *Neurology of the Newborn.* 4th ed. Saunders; 2001:432.)

TABLE 4.9.	Grading of Germinal Matrix-Intraventricular Hemorrhage (GM-IVH)	
Grade	Characteristic
I	GM with absent or minimal IVH
II	IVH occupying 10%–15% of the intraventricular area
III	IVH occupying >50% of ventricular area with ventricular distension
Periventricular hemorrhagic infarction	Intraparenchymal venous hemorrhage

Adapted with permission from Volpe JJ. *Neurology of the Newborn.* 4th ed. Philadelphia, PA: Saunders; 2001.

network that periventricular hemorrhage–intraventricular hemorrhage (PVH-IVH) occurs. IVH is thought to be due to hypoxia and/or capillary bleeding resulting from the loss of cerebral autoregulation and an abrupt alteration in blood flow.[149,348,356,358,359] The alteration of cerebral circulation from autoregulation to pressure-passive circulation has been shown to be an important factor in the development of PVH-IVH. Hemorrhage can occur when the pressure-passive circulating pattern is compromised by fluctuations in cerebral blood flow and pressure. Factors associated with the loss of autoregulation are younger GA, ELBW, birth events, asynchrony of spontaneous and mechanical breaths, pneumothorax, rapid volume expansion, seizures, changes in pH, $Paco_2$, Pao_2, metabolic imbalances, tracheal suctioning, and noxious procedures of caregiving.[149,348,356,360-366]

IVHs are diagnosed by cranial ultrasound and classified according to severity.[350,356,367] A four-level grading system was developed by Papile et al.[355] and is still used by many neonatologists, neurologists, and radiologists. Volpe developed a different grading system in 1995 on the basis of neuropathologic and imaging studies. This scale uses three levels to grade IVHs. Grade I is a germinal matrix hemorrhage with no or minimal IVH. Grade II is an IVH occupying 10% to 15% of the intraventricular area without distension of the ventricles. Grade III is an IVH occupying greater than 50% of ventricular area and usually distends the lateral ventricle (Table 4.9).[149,348]

The neuropathologic complications of IVH include germinal matrix destruction, periventricular hemorrhagic

infarction (PHI), and posthemorrhagic ventricular dilation (PVHD).[149,348,353,359] PVL is frequently seen in infants with IVH but is not caused by the hemorrhage itself.[348,353,356,368] Germinal matrix destruction and destruction of glial precursor cells is the result of germinal matrix hemorrhage. Destruction of glial precursor cells may negatively influence future development. Neurodevelopmental outcomes for infants with IVH are related to the severity of the hemorrhage. Vohr et al.[359] found that the LBW infants with IVH were more likely to develop CP. Spastic diplegic CP is most commonly associated with IVH because of the anatomic location of the corticospinal tracts.[149,357,358]

PHI was previously considered to be an extension of a large parenchymal hemorrhage or what Papile described as grade IV IVH. Neuropathologic and ultrasound studies have shown that the lesion represents a hemorrhagic venous infarction.[348,359,369] PHIs are generally large unilateral or asymmetric lesions dorsolateral to the lateral ventricle. This lesion is thought to be caused by obstruction of the terminal vein by a large IVH.[149,348,370] PHI generally occurs on the side of the larger IVH, and there is generally markedly decreased or absent flow in the terminal vein on that side. Studies have also described the lesion in the distribution of the medullary veins that drain into the terminal vein. Necrosis in this area can develop over time into a single large porencephalic cyst.[348] In the neonatal period, PHI is highly associated with an increased mortality rate as compared with IVH alone. Developmental outcomes associated with PHI are spastic hemiparesis, asymmetric quadriparesis, and cognitive deficits. The lower and upper extremities are equally affected in children with a history of PHI. Lesions because of extensive PHI cause more severe cognitive as well as motor deficits.[149,359]

PVD may occur days to weeks after the original IVH. The progressive ventricular dilation is due to a process that prevents the resorption of cerebrospinal fluid (CSF) and/or obstruction of CSF drainage because of a particulate clot. The injury to the brain from PVD is most likely because of hypoxia–ischemia and distension of the ventricle into the surrounding white matter, which may be more susceptible to additional injury after the effects of the initial hemorrhage.[149] The result of PVD is typically a bilateral cerebral white matter injury.[371] As there is a high incidence of arrest in the progression of ventriculomegaly without intervention, PVD is initially managed with close surveillance of ventricular size, head circumference, and clinical condition. Persistent slow ventricular dilation is treated with serial lumbar punctures to remove large volumes of CSF. Medications such as acetazolamide and furosemide can be used to decrease CSF production.[149,359] Rapidly progressive ventricular dilation with moderate to severe dilation, progressive head growth, and increasing intracranial pressure are managed initially with serial lumbar punctures followed by ventricular drainage of CSF with an external ventricular catheter or tunneled ventricular catheter that is connected to a subcutaneous reservoir.[149,359] Ventricular drainage is generally a temporary measure until a ventriculoperitoneal shunt can be placed. This type of shunt diverts CSF from the lateral ventricles into the peritoneal cavity.[149]

PVD occurs at a higher incidence in the extremely premature infant with ELBW as this is the population that is at greater risk for more severe IVH. With each additional week of gestation, the occurrence of PVD decreases. There is an increase in the incidence of PVD with each increase in the grade of IVH.[372] Murphy et al. found that the grade of IVH and need for inotropic support, such as dopamine or dobutamine, were significantly related to PVD requiring surgical intervention. PVD has been associated with neuromotor impairments and pronounced disability.[373-376] Krishnamoorthy et al.[367] demonstrated in their study that ventriculomegaly is an important antecedent of neuromotor sequelae and children with ventriculomegaly had a five times greater risk of developing CP independent of the grade of IVH.

Although the incidence of IVH and PHI has decreased in recent years because of improvements in prenatal and postnatal preventative care, these lesions are still major factors for neurodevelopmental disability in ELBW infants.[149,353,372,377-383] The primary goal of prenatal management is to prevent or delay premature birth. Other strategies focus on providing support during labor and delivery, resuscitation, and plan for neonatal care. Because RDS is highly associated with IVH and PHI, treatments to decrease RDS such as the administration of prenatal steroids are utilized. Postnatal treatment focuses on preventing hypoxia or fluctuations in systemic and blood cerebral pressure. In addition to providing optimal respiratory and medical support, the principles of individualized developmentally supportive care are instituted to minimize stress during caregiving, decrease the potential for loss of physiologic stability, and decrease the risk of IVH.[49,358,381,382]

Periventricular Leukomalacia

PVL refers to specific areas of white matter necrosis adjacent to the external angles of the lateral ventricles. These areas involve the frontal horn and body, and optic and acoustic radiations. The incidence of PVL occurs most prominently in infants of less than 32 weeks' gestation who have survived more than a few days of postnatal life and have cardiorespiratory compromise.[149,348,383,384] Premature infants of younger GAs are at the greatest risk for white matter injury because these areas are poorly vascularized in the immature brain and contain precursors for oligodendrocytes, which are extremely sensitive to ischemia and infection.[348,149,357,383-385]

Focal periventricular necrosis and more diffuse white matter cerebral injury are the pathologic features of PVL. Focal necrosis is related to severe ischemia and occurs most often in infants at greater than 26 weeks' gestation.[149,348,370,384] The two main sites of focal injury are near the trigone of the lateral ventricles and the border zones between the terminal arbors of the middle cerebral artery and the posterior cerebral artery or the anterior cerebral artery. Diffuse white matter injury is most apparent in infants at less than 26 weeks' gestation who develop atrophy, ventriculomegaly, and cortical underdevelopment with loss of oligodendrocytes and impairment in myelination.[149,348,370,384]

Areas of increased echodensity detected by cranial ultrasound are generally the first evidence of PVL. These echodensities represent areas of focal cellular necrosis because of axonal degeneration. Although echodensities may be transient or radiographic "flares" in some infants, other infants will demonstrate the characteristic evolution of focal PVL with the formation of cavitations that evolve into multiple cysts. This process occurs over the course of 1 to 3 weeks,[149,348,358,384] and the diagnosis of PVL will be dependent on the timing and number of cranial ultrasounds performed on the infant. More diffuse lesions less commonly undergo cystic changes and may go undetected by cranial ultrasound. MRI allows for better definition of brain structures and has been used to document diffuse white matter injury.[370]

The pathogenesis of the white matter destruction seen in PVL has been attributed to the interrelated factors associated with immature circulation and vascular structures of the preterm infant, impaired cerebral autoregulation, and the intrinsic vulnerability of the immature cerebral white matter neuroglia to ischemia–reperfusion.[348,149,368,370,384,386,387] Perinatal infection and the inflammatory response, including the release of proinflammatory cytokines, have also been shown to play an important role in the pathogenesis of PVL.[348,356,384,387-391] The effect of medications and other therapies used to treat complications of prematurity has been implicated in the pathogenesis of white matter injury.[392]

There is a strong association with mortality and long-term morbidity in infants with PVL. Death in infants with PVL in the neonatal period is usually attributed to the original insult, whether hypoxic, hemorrhagic, or infectious, rather than from PVL. Infants with PVL who survive the neonatal period are at high risk for neurodevelopment problems that affect motor, cognitive, and visual function.[271,362,380,384,389,390,393] Spastic diplegia, with or without hydrocephalus, is the most prominent long-term sequela of PVL. Han et al.[380] found that the presence of PVL was the "strongest and most independent risk factor" for the development of CP. The clinical presentation is one of motor disturbance in the lower extremities greater than the upper extremities owing to the anatomic

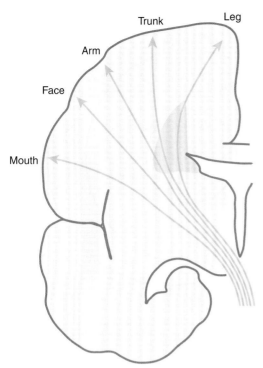

FIGURE 4.16. Illustrations of the periventricular area and motor tracts. (Reprinted with permission from Volpe JJ. *Neurology of the Newborn.* 4th ed. Saunders; 2001:432.)

location of the descending motor tracts (Fig. 4.16). In larger lesions extending further into the periventricular white matter, the upper extremities and cognitive functions will be more affected. Motor tracts associated with visual, auditory, and somesthetic functions can also be involved.[384,389,390] Extremely premature infants have been found to be at greatest risk for global motor and cognitive impairments.[350,351,368,394]

As with other injuries to the neonatal brain, the primary focus is prevention of prematurity, infection, hypotension, and other associated factors. The initial management after the diagnosis of PVL is treating the primary cause and complications of the insult along with preventing further hypoxic–ischemic damage. Management strategies to prevent or minimize hypoxia, hypotension, acidosis, apnea, bradycardia, and infection are implemented. Developmental care strategies can be implemented to decrease stress and promote development. Serial cranial ultrasounds are done to monitor PVL, possible progression, and hydrocephalus.

Retinopathy of Prematurity

Retinopathy is a neurovascular disease of the immature retina. Infants at the highest risk are those born extremely preterm because of the vasculogenesis and angiogenesis that typically occur between 16 and 40 weeks' gestation.[395,396] The incidence and severity of ROP is closely correlated with lower weight and GA at birth. Extreme prematurity, prolonged invasive ventilator support, and oxygen exposure are risk factors for ROP.[397]

The onset of retinopathy is marked by an alteration in the normal development of blood vessels in the eye, which occurs in two stages.[398,399] In the first stage, there is cessation of normal vascularization and obliteration of immature vessels of the retina because of hyperoxia, hypoxia, or hypotension. Hyperoxia leads to marked decrease in vascular endothelial growth factor (VEGF)[399] and insulin-like growth factor (IGF-1),[400] which then leads to cessation of retinal blood vessel growth. Stage two is marked by the release of increased vascular growth factors from the ischemic, hypoxic retina, which stimulates new blood vessel growth (neovascularization) through the retina and into the vitreous humor. These blood vessels are atypical in structure, inadequately perfuse the retina, and are prone to hemorrhage and edema, which leads to the formation of fibrous scar formation. Progressive traction of the scar tissue and the atypical blood vessels lead to retinal detachment.[399]

ROP is classified by the location, stage, and extent of the pathophysiologic process using the International Classification of Retinopathy of Prematurity (ICROP) guidelines.[401] The location of involvement is described using retinal zones and extent of disease in clock hours (Fig. 4.17). The degree of vasculopathy is classified in stages of severity. Stages one through three represent increasing abnormal growth and formation of a demarcation ridge between the posterior vascularized and anterior avascularized retina. In stage three these atypical vessels grow into the vitreous. In stage four there is partial retinal detachment and stage five represents total retinal detachment. Plus disease refers to significant vascular tortuosity and venous engorgement. Pre-plus disease refers to a less severe form of vascular tortuosity and dilation. Threshold disease is present when there is greater than five contiguous or eight cumulative clock hours of stage three growth in zone I or II. Prethreshold disease is the point where ROP may progress to advanced disease and is subdivided into type one (high risk requiring treatment) or type two (lower risk requiring close monitoring).[402] The Early Treatment for Retinopathy of Prematurity (ENTROP) study[402] reclassified type one ROP to also include a more severe form of ROP seen in ELBW infants (aggressive, posterior ROP), which involves very central (zone 1) neovascularization with plus disease.

Ophthalmologists examine and closely monitor infants as to the stage, zone, and monitor on a schedule based on GA, comorbidities, and disease severity starting at 31 weeks PMA. The AAP[403] has developed guidelines for ROP screening examinations for preterm infants. According to these guidelines, infants with a birth weight less than 1,500 g or GA less than 30 weeks, as well as infants with birth weight between 1,500 and 2,000 g or GA greater than 30 weeks with complicated clinical course including mechanical ventilation and supplemental oxygen, should be screened for ROP. Early detection allows for early intervention as indicated and preservation of vision to a greater extent. After the acute process has resolved, infants are scheduled for follow-up based on the severity of the initial disease. Close observation of the retina is required for infants who had retinal interventions/ablation.[404]

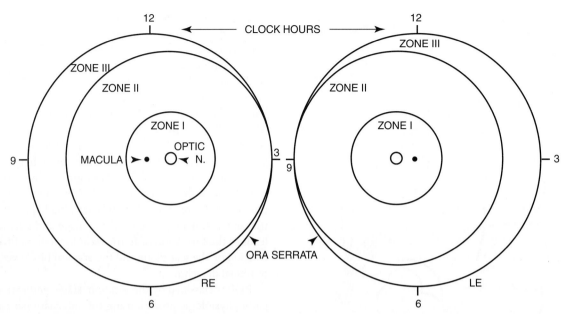

FIGURE 4.17. Schematic of the left and right eye showing the clock hours and the stages and zones of retinopathy of prematurity (ROP). (Reprinted with permission from Committee for Classification of ROP. An International Classification of Retinopathy of Prematurity. *Arch Ophthalmol.* 1989;102(8):1131.)

Outcomes vary with the severity of the disease. Infants who develop mild ROP have a slightly increased incidence of myopia/hyperopia, strabismus, and amblyopia compared to full-term infants. However, infants who develop type 1 ROP and require retinal ablation are at increased risk for severe myopia, glaucoma, and associated sequelae.[404] Infants who develop residual scarring are at risk for retinal detachment and loss of visual acuity later in life.[405]

Chorioamnionitis

Cervicovaginal bacteria that invade the amniotic cavity and cause an inflammatory response in the membranes of the developing fetus cause chorioamnionitis. Chorioamnionitis is the most common cause of preterm labor. Most infants are not septic at birth as the placenta provides an efficient barrier. However, in cases where there is a fetal inflammatory response in addition to the maternal inflammatory response, babies may be more at risk for BPD, NEC, abnormalities on cranial ultrasound, and long-term neurologic impairment.[406] In addition, there has been evidence of an association between maternal intrauterine infection and the occurrence of fetal brain damage with subsequent neurologic deficits, with the strongest association between chorioamnionitis and PVL.[391,407]

Metabolic Bone Disease of Prematurity

The third trimester of fetal development is very important for bone formation. The essential nutrients for this process are provided most efficiently by the placenta when a baby is in utero. Approximately 80% of bone is produced between 24 and 40 weeks' gestation as the fetus accretes large amounts of calcium, phosphorus, and magnesium.[408-414] There is also mechanical stimulation to the bones as the fetus actively moves within the fluid-filled environment and pushes against the uterine wall. In addition, further mechanical loading of the skeletal system occurs during the third trimester as the infant is gaining muscle mass and being compressed by the cramped uterine space.[409-412] Prematurely born infants miss out on a portion or all of this period of bone formation and mineral accretion.

Metabolic bone disease of prematurity is defined as "postnatal bone mineralization that is less than intrauterine bone density at a comparable gestational age."[415] Preterm babies in the NICU are at risk for metabolic bone disease of prematurity, which has implications for their future growth[416] as well as putting them in danger of fractures in the present.[417] Risk factors that contribute to metabolic bone disease of prematurity include:

- Nutritional practices such as feeding restrictions, prolonged use of hyperalimentation, or the use of unfortified breast milk.
- Drugs such as corticosteroids and diuretics that cause increased mineral excretion.[410-414]
- Vitamin D deficiency, which is exacerbated by diseases that contribute to malabsorption such as cholestasis and NEC.
- A lack of mechanical stimulation, which can be intensified by sedatives, paralytics,[416] and supports for intravenous lines that immobilize tiny limbs.

Infants with metabolic bone disease of prematurity have fragile bones at high risk for fractures and positional deformities such as dolichocephaly and respiratory morbidities.[416]

Metabolic bone disease of prematurity can be challenging to diagnose as it may be asymptomatic until fractures occur or signs of rickets appear. Biochemical markers can be difficult to interpret, markers of bone formation lack sensitivity and specificity, and X-rays do not demonstrate osteopenia until significant demineralization has occurred.[416] Osteopenia can go unrecognized until a fracture occurs; there have been reports in the literature of fractures in preterm infants temporally associated with intravenous line placement.[418] Babies in the authors' NICU have also developed fractures that have been temporally associated with immunizations, intravenous line placement, heel sticks, and restraints used during a medical procedure. These developments have compelled the authors to advocate safe handling for all infants, especially replacing twisting and pulling limbs during line placement with repositioning the baby in order to allow the baby's limbs to maintain as neutral an alignment as possible. Other safe handling techniques include lifting an infant by placing one hand under the head and the other under the buttocks rather than picking up under the axilla or around the rib cage, and sliding your hand under the buttocks to lift for a diaper change, rather than grasping around the infant's ankles and lifting.[419]

The incidence of metabolic bone disease of prematurity is inversely related to GA and birth weight. ELBW infants (<1,000 g) have an incidence of osteopenia of 50% to 60%; VLBW infants (<1,500 g) have an incidence of osteopenia of 23%.[417] Fractures are reported in approximately 10% of VLBW infants at 36 to 40 weeks' PMA.[417] In the NICU, the prevention and treatment of bone disease in premature infants is aggressively managed through nutritional management. The medical staff carefully monitors the vitamins and minerals the infant receives through parenteral nutrition, human milk fortifiers, and/or preterm formula.[391-414] Even with carefully managed nutritional programs, cases of metabolic bone disease of prematurity still occur. Studies on the use of passive range of motion to promote bone formation in preterm infants have been reported in the literature[343,420-422]; however, these studies have small numbers of subjects and do not address the physiologic stress that handling can induce in this very fragile population. A Cochrane review[423] of eight trials to determine the effect of physical activity programs on bone mineralization, fractures, and growth in preterm infants did not recommend it on the basis of the current evidence and cited the need for further studies with infants at high risk for metabolic bone disease of prematurity that address adverse events, long-term outcomes, as well as the contributions of nutrition.[423] Care must be taken when handling premature, VLBW infants in terms of their physiologic vulnerabilities as well as the increased risk of fracturing bone. In addition, attention should be paid to cranial molding with the use of positioning devices, varying postures, and including supine positions with head midline. The neonatal therapist should be advocating positioning and supports for infants that do not restrict movement and facilitate active movement. Intravenous lines for medications and endotracheal tubes providing respiratory support do need to be protected; however, babies should be allowed to initiate movement, which will allow opportunities for muscle strengthening and may contribute to bone strength.

Bronchopulmonary Dysplasia

BPD is the most common chronic lung disease of infancy (CLDI) associated with prematurity. CLDI is used often synonymously with BPD. The incidence is closely and inversely related to birth weight and GA, occurring in approximately 45% of infants born at or less than 29 weeks GA.[424,425] Advances in neonatal care have led to decreased mortality rates of extremely premature infants; however, with improved survival, the incidence of BPD has not changed.[425]

Northway and colleagues[426] first described BPD in 1967 as a severe chronic disease affecting both airway and lung parenchyma of moderately preterm infants (mean GA of 34 weeks PMA) because of injury caused by mechanical ventilation and oxygen therapy. The disease was characterized by airway injury and inflammatory response, lung parenchymal fibrosis and cellular hypoplasia, and areas of hyperinflation and atelectasis resulting in thickened and hyperreactive airways, decreased lung compliance because of fibrosis, increased airway resistance, impaired gas exchange with ventilation–perfusion mismatch, and air trapping.[426] Diagnosis was made based on need for supplemental oxygen at 36 weeks PMA and radiographic changes. The clinical presentation and definition have changed over time related to BPD now occurring primarily in very or extremely preterm infants.[427-429] Preterm infants with the "new" BPD present with less fibrosis and more uniform patterns of inflation; however, decreased alveolar formation and lung vascularization are still major factors in the disease process. Fewer and larger simplified alveoli, arrested alveolar capillary development, increased interstitial fibrosis, and abnormal pulmonary vasculature characterize the new form of lung disease.[430]

Because of changes in care practices, survival of extremely preterm infants, and the presentation of BPD, the understanding of the pathogenesis and definition has continued to evolve. The definition has been modified multiple times in order to reflect changes in patient population and to better predict respiratory outcomes. The current consensus definition was developed in 2001 by a workgroup at the National Institutes of Child Health and Human Development (NICHD)/National Heart, Lung, and Blood Institute (NHLBI) workshop who proposed a severity-based definition of BPD, with classification of mild, moderate, and severe disease.[427] Research based on recommendations for revision of the definition of BPD based on criteria to better reflect the phenotypes of BPD and current respiratory care practices as well as predict outcomes is ongoing at this time.[431-434]

Northway et al.[426] originally proposed four major factors in pathogenesis: lung immaturity, respiratory failure, oxygen supplementation, and positive-pressure ventilation. Research has supported these findings and additional factors have been identified including inflammation, aberrations in lung growth and signaling pathways, derangements in transcription factors and growth factors, oxidative lung injury, and genetics.[435-438]

One of the greatest contributing factors to the development of BPD is the immaturity of the infant's lungs. Extremely premature birth occurs in the late canalicular or early saccular stage of parenchymal development when the underdeveloped lung is very vulnerable to injury because of multiple factors including postnatal infections, mechanical trauma from positive-pressure ventilation, oxygen toxicity, and pulmonary edema because of increased pulmonary blood flow from PDA. Injury at this early stage of lung development can interfere with the development of alveoli and pulmonary microvasculature.[427,439-441] The structural and functional lung alterations characteristic of BPD are a result of injury, processes that occur in response to the injury, and the ongoing lung development.[429,442]

Prenatal as well postnatal factors may play a role in the development of BPD. Preeclampsia has been implicated as a risk factor for the development of BPD because of the factors related to the development of the condition and the resultant effects on the infant such as oxidative stress, IUGR, and preterm birth.[443,444] Fetal growth restriction has been shown to be highly predictive for BPD most likely because of impaired alveolar and vascular growth.[445,446] In addition, intrauterine infection or colonization such as chorioamnionitis, one of the leading causes of preterm birth, may contribute to the development of BPD. The inflammatory process because of infection has been linked to the development of BPD.[441,447] Studies have shown that *Chlamydia trachomatis* and cytomegalovirus can cause slowly developing pneumonitis. Chorioamnionitis may increase the inflammatory response in premature lungs to injury caused by mechanical ventilation.[427,447-449] Postnatal contributing factors for BPD include hyperoxia and hypoxia, early fluid overload and persistent left-to-right shunting through a PDA, undernutrition, familial airway hyperreactivity, genetic influences, and decreased surfactant synthesis and infections such as adenovirus and cytomegalovirus.[450-452] Gender has also been found to be associated with susceptibility of preterm infants to BPD and severity of the disease.[450] Surfactant is synthesized later in gestation in the male fetal lung compared to the females, increasing the risk for acute respiratory distress.[448,453,454]

The most optimal method for prenatal prevention of BPD is the prevention of preterm birth. When premature delivery is inevitable, administration of prenatal steroids and gentle resuscitation with low levels of supplemental oxygen is recommended.[426,439,455] Postnatal medical treatment strategies are aimed at preventing or limiting the factors that set off the chain of pathogenic sequelae. Respiratory support is used only when necessary and at the lowest peak airway pressure needed to maintain adequate ventilation and decrease barotrauma.[456] Various modes of invasive and noninvasive respiratory support have been implemented in an attempt to decrease trauma to the lungs.[439] Volume-targeted ventilation has been shown to decrease the incidence of BPD.[457] Careful fluid and nutrition management is used to provide hydration without overload and to promote growth.[450] Diuretic treatment is used to prevent cor pulmonale, congestive heart failure, and pulmonary edema.[439] Other treatments include infection control with careful monitoring and treatment of bacterial and fungal infections, and bronchodilator therapy is also used to decrease bronchospasm.[456] Corticosteroid treatment has been found to decrease bronchospasm and the inflammatory response; however, early use of inhaled corticosteroids has been associated with neurodevelopmental delay and CP.[451,457] A meta-analysis by Doyle and colleagues[458] demonstrated that corticosteroid treatment after 1 week of age for infants with high risk of developing BPD may have benefit. The exact timing and prescription for postnatal corticosteroids continues to be evaluated. Strategies that may be used in the future to prevent the development of BPD in preterm infants include antioxidant, liquid ventilation, and stem cell therapies.[450,451,456,459,460]

Complications associated with BPD are systemic hypertension, metabolic imbalance, hearing loss, ROP, nephrocalcinosis, osteoporosis, GER, and early growth failure.[385,392,394] The same intrinsic and extrinsic risk factors that contribute to the development of BPD also appear to impair the developing pulmonary vasculature, resulting in significant pulmonary vascular disease (PVD). Severe PVD leads to the development of PH.[461] Rates of morbidity and mortality are high for infants with BPD and PH.[461,462]

Impairments in lung growth and function continue into adolescence and early adulthood.[440,463,464] Balinotti et al.[440] reported impairment of alveolar development in infants and toddlers with BPD. Increased respiratory illness, respiratory symptoms (cough, wheeze, asthma), increased risk of hospitalization,[465] impaired pulmonary function tests, and compromised exercise capacity have been documented in preschool and school-age children, adolescents, and young adults who had CLDI.[433,464,466,467]

Developmental outcomes reported in the literature include increased incidence of attention deficits, cognitive deficits, language delays, developmental coordination disorder, and visual-motor functioning in infants with BPD.[149,350,351,464,468-476]

Preterm infants diagnosed with BPD appear to be at greater risk for adverse neurodevelopmental outcome than preterm infants without BPD.[457,471,477] Singer et al.[471] found BPD to be a significant independent predictor of poor developmental outcome at 3 years of age. Severity of BPD, based on the NIH consensus definition, has been shown to have an independent adverse relationship with poorer cognitive, motor, behavioral, social-emotional, and language outcomes and CP.[468,475,476,478,479] The incidence of CP has been shown to increase with severity of BPD.[468,470,476] Severity of CP, defined as higher Gross Motor Function Classification Score (GMFCS)[480] and greater distribution of involvement (diplegia and quadriplegia), was found to occur at higher rates with increasing severity of BPD.[481] Van Marter et al.[481] reported that BPD with requirement for mechanical ventilation and supplemental oxygen at 36 weeks PMA was a strong predictor for diplegia and quadriplegia; however, BPD without mechanical ventilation requirement at

36 weeks PMA was not significantly associated with any form of CP. Non-CP motor impairments also occur at a higher incidence in children with BPD when compared to children without BPD. Poorer fine and gross motor performance, developmental coordination disorder, and neurosensory impairments are all reported at higher rates in children with BPD.[464] Access to occupational and physical therapy is reported to be higher in children with BPD.[469]

The Baby Who Requires Surgery

This section includes some of the more common fetal malformations that require surgical intervention in infancy, including CDH, omphalocele, gastroschisis, and tracheal esophageal fistula (TEF). Lastly, a brief review of fetal surgical interventions is included.

Congenital Diaphragmatic Hernia

CDH is a defect in the formation of the respiratory diaphragm during embryogenesis and is estimated to occur in 1/3,000 live births.[482] During the 3rd to 16th weeks of gestation, when lung bronchi and pulmonary arteries are undergoing critical development, the pleuroperitoneal cavity fails to close. The defect then allows the developing abdominal viscera (bowel, stomach, liver) to protrude through the opening in the diaphragm into the hemithorax. The viscera compresses the developing lung on the ipsilateral side, resulting in decreased bronchial branching and lung mass (pulmonary hypoplasia)[483]; the contralateral lung may be affected as well if the herniated bowel causes a mediastinal shift, placing pressure on the contralateral lung.[484] Compression of the lung promotes overmuscularization of the pulmonary arterial tree leading to PH.[483] The effects are most severe on the ipsilateral side of the diaphragmatic defect.[483]

Because of the left hemidiaphragm being larger and closing later than the right, the defect occurs more frequently on the left. Approximately 75% of all cases of CDH occur on the left, whereas right-sided CDHs occur in 25% of cases and bilateral herniation is rare.[485] Pulmonary hypoplasia and PH caused by CDH can vary in severity and is responsible for the high neonatal mortality and long-term morbidity associated with CDH.[486]

Fifty to 60% of CDH cases are considered "isolated" or without associated anomalies. Pulmonary hypoplasia, intestinal malrotation, and cardiac dextroposition are considered part of the CDH sequence and are not associated anomalies. The other 40% to 50% of babies with CDH can have structural malformations (esophageal atresia [EA], omphalocele, and cleft palate), and chromosomal anomalies such as trisomies 18, 13, and 21.[487,488] The majority of still-born infants with CDH have associated anomalies such as neural tube defects and cardiac anomalies.[489-491]

In the majority of cases, the diagnosis of CDH is made by prenatal ultrasound, demonstrating the presence of abdominal contents in the pleuroperitoneal cavity and a mediastinal shift.[487,492] Prenatal diagnosis is improved by advancing GA and the presence of associated abnormalities. Mean age at prenatal diagnosis is 22 to 24 weeks.[493] Once the prenatal diagnosis of CDH is made, mothers are counseled to deliver in a perinatal center with neonatal specialists, neonatal/pediatric surgeons, and ECMO capabilities.[484] Further imaging with MRI and fetal echocardiography is used to determine the prognostic likelihood of survival and need for ECMO support after delivery. Using imaging, the lung area to head circumference ratio (LHR) is measured to determine fetal lung size. This is calculated by measuring the contralateral lung at the level of the atria and dividing it by the fetal head circumference.[492] Using MRI, the herniated-liver-to-thoracic-volume ratio is also determined. These two indices can predict severity of pulmonary hypoplasia and neonatal survival. The absence of liver herniation is the most reliable prenatal prognosticator of postnatal survival.[494] The baby is monitored closely during pregnancy, labor, and delivery.[492] These prenatal prediction tools can also identify fetuses that may benefit from fetal surgical intervention.[495] Studies looking at preferred GA for delivery related to prognosis have not clearly established improvement in morbidity or mortality with preterm delivery.[496-498] Therefore, the goal is to schedule delivery around 39 weeks GA at a specialized pediatric center with NICU services.[499]

After birth, the surgical repair is delayed until after the baby's pulmonary status and pulmonary artery hypertension have stabilized, which can take hours, days, or even weeks. Initial management involves intubation to prevent acidosis and hypoxia, which can increase the risk of PH, gentle ventilation to prevent the risk of barotrauma to hypoplastic lungs, and stomach decompression to avoid further lung compression. Medications to support BP are administered to prevent right-to-left shunting. If the baby does not respond to the maximum conventional ventilatory therapy, they may be placed on ECMO. Infants with CDH, whether they receive ECMO therapy or not, often experience long hospital admissions because of high level of respiratory support for pulmonary hypoplasia and treatment of PH and cardiac dysfunction.[484,492]

After surgical repair of the CDH, babies may remain critically ill because of hypoxic respiratory failure and associated PH and cardiac dysfunction.[500] Hypoplastic lungs have increased vulnerability for additional injury because of mechanical ventilation leading to the development of CLD. Babies with CDH often have other organ involvement that further complicates and extends their hospital course. Prognosis for survival is worse for babies with an abnormal karyotype, severe associated anomalies, right-sided defect, liver herniation, and lower lung volumes.

Children with CDH require ongoing medical and surgical follow-up after discharge from the NICU. There is a risk of reherniation requiring additional surgery to repair the defect, which can occur in as many of 50% of children with CDH.[501] Close neurodevelopmental follow-up is also necessary as there is a high incidence of sensorineural hearing loss, GER, failure to thrive, feeding problems, seizures, and developmental delay in these infants.[487,492] Recent studies have demonstrated increased risk for cognitive impairment, behavioral difficulties, attention deficit disorder, and autism.[500,502-504] In addition to evaluation and treatment for developmental delays, PTs working with infants and children with CDH also need to be assessing for musculoskeletal impairments such as chest wall defects, scoliosis because of vertebral anomalies, and trunk asymmetry because of unilateral defect, pulmonary hypoplasia, and scarring from surgical repair.[500,505-507]

Omphalocele

Defects occurring in the anterior abdominal wall of the fetus are reported to occur in 1/2,000 live births. The two most common abdominal wall defects, omphalocele and gastroschisis, are described below.[508]

An omphalocele is a midline abdominal wall defect at the base of the umbilical cord with herniation or protrusion of abdominal contents, such as bowel, stomach, and liver, into a sac consisting of amnion, Wharton's jelly, and peritoneum. The prevalence is 2 per 10,000 births and occurs more commonly in mothers <20 or >40 years of age.[508-510] Omphalocele occurs more frequently with fetal aneuploidy and structural anomalies.[508,511] Reported associated syndromes include trisomy 13, 15, 16, 18, and 21, Beckwith–Wiedemann syndrome, Pentalogy of Cantrell, and OEIS syndrome (omphalocele, exstrophy of the bladder, imperforate anus, spinal defects).[509,512,513] Reported associated structural anomalies include congenital heart defects, diaphragmatic and upper midline defects, malrotation of the intestines, intestinal atresia, and genitourinary anomalies.[511,512]

The exact pathogenesis of omphalocele has not been definitively identified. Herniation of the abdominal contents occurs typically around the 6th week of gestation when the abdomen becomes too small for the developing contents. A temporary physiologic herniation of the intestines and other organs into the base of the umbilical stalk occurs. Full reduction of the physiologic hernia typically occurs by week 12 with the abdominal contents returning into the embryologic abdominal cavity. If the abdominal contents fail to migrate back into the embryonic abdominal cavity, an omphalocele is formed.[514] If the abdominal wall fails to close, the liver may also herniate into the base of the umbilicus resulting in a giant omphalocele. Babies with giant omphalocele, containing >75% of the liver, are more likely to have chromosomal anomalies.[515]

Prenatal diagnosis is often made after positive maternal serum alfa-fetoprotein screen and/or by ultrasound. Diagnosis of non–liver-containing omphalocele can be made by 12 weeks GA. Liver-containing or giant omphalocele can be diagnosed as early as 9 to 10 weeks GA.[516,517] Because chromosomal abnormalities and structural anomalies are commonly present in babies with omphalocele, the obstetric workup typically includes a fetal karyotype, echocardiogram,

and MRI. After prenatal diagnosis, the family is usually referred to pediatric surgeons, neonatologists, genetic counselors, maternal–fetal medicine specialists, and social work and other specialists based on the presence of structural anomalies. Serial ultrasounds are performed to monitor the baby along with routine prenatal care. Delivery at a specialized tertiary care center is recommended.[516]

All infants with omphalocele require surgical management. The size of the omphalocele determines either primary repair or if delayed primary closure is indicated. Babies with defects <2 cm have a primary direct closure. Babies with defects from 2 to 9 cm undergo a staged closure with a silo compression dressing. Babies with defects >10 cm receive the topical application of an eschar-inducing agent to promote epithelialization and a planned surgical closure in the following weeks to years.[518,519] Infants with very large, liver-containing, omphaloceles may have increased morbidity because of pulmonary hypoplasia and abdominal competition. These infants may also require multiple reconstructive surgeries.

Survival rate for infants with isolated omphalocele is around 90%.[509] There is greater morbidity and mortality for infants with giant omphalocele and/or multiple congenital anomalies. Feeding intolerance can result in prolonged use of total parenteral nutrition and long hospitalizations. In addition, the other anomalies associated with omphalocele have a major impact on the developmental outcome of the baby. Neurodevelopmental studies report delayed motor development as high as 80% in children with giant omphalocele.[513] Danzer et al.[520,521] report neurologic impairments in more than 50% of their cohort with findings of hypotonia and motor dysfunction associated with delayed staged closure. A significant rate of autism spectrum disorder with delays in cognitive and language has been reported in children with giant omphalocele.[522]

Gastroschisis

Unlike omphalocele, a gastroschisis is a full-thickness abdominal wall defect, usually to the right of the umbilicus, with extrusion of the intestines, and occasionally stomach, into the amniotic space.[523] Gastroschisis does not involve the umbilicus and the abdominal contents are not covered by amnion. Although the exact mechanism for the defect is unknown, gastroschisis appears to be caused by abnormal closure of the anterior body wall during the 4th week of gestation when the lateral folds of the body wall should meet at the umbilicus and close the abdominal cavity; a defect in the abdominal wall occurs, allowing the abdominal contents to leak out of the abdominal cavity.[514,524,525] Gastroschisis is classified as simple or complex based on the absence or presence of intestinal atresia, stenosis, perforation, necrosis, malrotation, or volvulus. Gastroschisis is an isolated defect, often associated with prematurity and growth restriction/LBW. Gastroschisis has a higher prevalence in younger (<20 years) primigravida mothers possibly related to lifestyle and environmental factors.[508,511,526,527] The incidence of gastroschisis is reported to be 3–4/10,000 with prevalence increasing worldwide.[508,528]

Diagnosis of gastroschisis is made by prenatal ultrasound and maternal serum alfa-fetoprotein assessment. A pregnancy with a diagnosis of gastroschisis is followed closely with serial ultrasounds every 2 to 4 weeks. Poor intrauterine growth is a poor prognostic feature.[529] Because there is an increased risk of third-trimester fetal demise, nonstress tests, biophysical profiles, and amniotic fluid indices are followed closely after 30 weeks.[530,531]

As with omphalocele, best practice includes coordinating the delivery at a tertiary care center with pediatric surgeons. Depending on presentation on delivery, the baby can have primary fascial closure shortly after birth or a staged procedure with placement of intestines in a prosthetic silo to allow for gradual visceral reduction with delayed closure.[523,532]

Survival for infants with gastroschisis is greater than 90%. Neonatal hospitalization is frequently prolonged because of difficulties tolerating enteral feeding and poor growth. Good outcomes have been reported for children with simple gastroschisis with neurodevelopmental outcomes and intellectual abilities in the normal range.[531] However, these children demonstrated decreased working memory index and were at increased risk for behavioral problems. Children with complex gastroschisis have increased risk of short bowel syndrome, poor growth, and neurodevelopmental delays.[533] Poorer outcomes and neuromotor impairment have also been associated with lower GA at birth, SGA at birth, multiple surgical interventions, and prolonged hospital stay.[533,534] Impairments in verbal intelligence, attention, response inhibition, and fine motor skills have been reported in school-age children born with gastroschisis.[535]

Tracheal Esophageal Fistula

Between the third and the sixth weeks of gestation, the primitive foregut is in the process of separating into the respiratory and alimentary tracts.[536] A defect in the lateral septation of the foregut into the esophagus and trachea causes a TEF.[537-539] TEF is the most common congenital anomaly of the respiratory tract with an incidence of 1 per 3,500 live births.[537-542] Ninety-five percent of TEFs occur with EA; TEF is classified according to the anatomic configuration and is most commonly present (84%) as a proximal esophageal pouch and a distal TEF (type C) (Fig. 4.18).[537,540,542,543]

Many babies with TEF are not diagnosed prenatally. Babies with EA may present with polyhydramnios in utero[537,544] or present immediately after birth with an accumulation of oral secretions (because of ineffective swallowing), respiratory difficulties, and coughing, choking, and cyanosis with feeds. The medical staff is unable to pass a tube through the nose and into the stomach, and a radiograph may show the tube coiled in the upper esophageal pouch.

The rare TEF without EA (H type) is difficult to diagnose. Unlike babies with EA, babies with H type TEF may be asymptomatic at birth, or they may cough or choke with feeds. Diagnosis of an isolated TEF can be made on upper GI series where the contrast dye is pulled superiorly during the study or by use of 3D computed tomography (CT) scanning.[517,525-549] About half of babies with TEF also have other associated anomalies, often as part of the VACTERL association (vertebral anomalies, anal atresia, congenital heart defects, TEF, EA, renal abnormalities, limb deformities).[538,550]

Treatment of TEF/EA requires surgical ligation of the fistula and anastomosis of the esophagus; however, if the distance separating the two ends of the esophagus is great, a staged repair, including elongation of the esophagus, circular myotomies of the existing esophagus, or replacing the missing esophagus with a portion of the small or large intestine, is required.[537,551-563] A gastrostomy tube is placed to allow feeding while the baby heals from surgery. Treatment of isolated TEF is less difficult; the fistula can be ligated and prognosis is good.[537,563-565]

Prognosis of TEF/EA is less assured and depends on the presence of other associated anomalies as well as the distance between the two esophageal pouches. Both short- and long-term complications of TEF/EA occur more commonly. Short-term complications include anastomotic leak, esophageal strictures, tracheomalacia, and disturbed peristalsis.

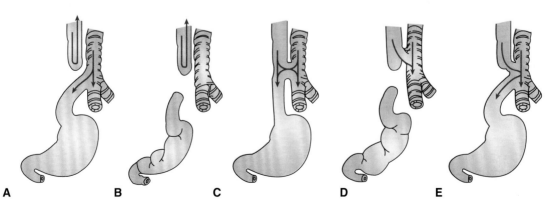

FIGURE 4.18. Esophageal atresia and tracheoesophageal fistula. **A:** EA with distal TEF. **B:** EA. **C:** TEF. **D:** EA with proximal TEF. **E:** EA with double TEF. (From Pillitteri A. *Maternal and Child Nursing.* 4th ed. Philadelphia, PA: Lippincott Williams & Wilkins; 2003.)

Long-term complications include motility disorders, respiratory function abnormalities, and in some cases esophageal squamous cell cancer.[537,550,566-572] Long-term neurodevelopmental delays in language and cognitive and motor delay have been reported.[573,574] The rates also vary according to severity of TEF/EA, other anomalies, GA at birth, surgical interventions, and length of NICU stay.[573]

Fetal Surgery

The clinical application of fetal surgery was first pioneered by Harrison and colleagues at the University of San Francisco in the late 1970s.[575,576] Fetal surgery grew out of the understanding of the progression of an untreated condition and the belief that prenatal intervention could ameliorate damage to developing organs.[577-579] Advances in high-resolution imaging and surgical techniques along with animal model experimentation and clinical practice have led to improved fetal interventions.[580] There are a number of fetal anatomic anomalies that can now be treated with fetal surgery. These include monochorionic twin gestation complications (twin-to-twin transfusion syndrome, acardiac twin, isolated IGR), CDH (intratracheal balloon placement), constrictive amniotic bands, lower urinary tract obstruction, and myelomeningocele.[581]

Although there has been progress in fetal surgical techniques, these procedures are not without risks for the fetus and mother. Risks for the fetus include preterm delivery and its sequalae. Maternal risk factors include preterm labor and delivery, pulmonary edema, placental abruption, hemorrhage, chorioamniotic separation, chorioamnionitis and sepsis, anesthesia risks, and a large uterine incision that may impact future pregnancies and requires cesarean section for delivery.[582] Because of these risk factors, specific criteria for fetal surgery were established by the International Fetal Medicine and Surgery Society (IFMSS) in 1982[583] to protect members of the maternal–fetal dyad. These prerequisites, with minor modifications over time, continue to be applied to maternal–fetal surgical practice. The requirements are (1) the ability to establish accurate prenatal diagnosis; (2) a well-defined natural history of the disorder; (3) the presence of a correctable lesion that, if untreated, will lead to fetal demise, irreversible organ dysfunction before birth, or severe postnatal morbidity; (4) the absence of severe associated anomalies; (5) an acceptable risk-to-benefit ratio for both mother and fetus.[584] Contraindications for maternal–fetal surgery include the identification of complex chromosomal or associated anatomic anomalies, or maternal risk factors such as placentomegaly, short cervix or other predispositions for preterm delivery, and maternal mirror syndrome.[584,585] The IFMSS also mandates that diagnosis, selection, and treatment be done within a strict protocol by a trained multidisciplinary team.[583] Fetal diagnosis and treatment centers should include highly specialized pediatric surgery, obstetrics, radiology, pediatric anesthesia, obstetric anesthesia, cardiology, neonatology,

neonatal nursing, operating room nursing, social work, genetic councilors, bioethicist, and other case-specific relevant pediatric surgical specialties.[575,586,587]

There have been substantial advances in maternal–fetal surgery since the establishment of the IFMSS because of improvements in prenatal diagnosis, selection process for intervention, and treatment of fetuses with anatomic malformations. For the management of select anomalies, fetal surgical surgery offers validated and accepted treatments.[588] There continues to be ongoing work to develop less-invasive and safer techniques for both mother and fetus. Fetoscopic interventions have been successfully used for specific anomalies and continue to evolve and be refined. Further research is still required to advance the practice of maternal–fetal surgery. In addition to ongoing development of interventions for structural malformations, cellular and genetic disorders may be treated in the future using stem cell and gene therapies early in fetal development.[589,590]

The Baby with Neurologic Issues

The Baby with Asphyxia

Perinatal asphyxia is a result of a lack of oxygen (hypoxia) and/or a lack of perfusion (ischemia) to various organs.[591] The incidence of asphyxia is 2 to 6 per 1,000 births.[376] It is more frequent in preterm infants (60% in VLBW births), where it is usually associated with PVH/IVH,[407] and accounts for 20% of perinatal deaths. Asphyxia is more likely to occur in term infants of diabetic or toxemic mothers and is also associated with IUGR and breech presentation. Ninety percent of asphyxiated births are estimated to occur as a result of placental insufficiency during the antepartum or intrapartum periods.[591] However, cardiopulmonary anomalies of the fetus are also a risk factor for asphyxia.[407] All babies experience hypoxia during normal labor but not to a degree that is damaging. An umbilical cord or fetal scalp pH less than 7.0 may indicate substantial intrauterine asphyxia. Other supporting evidence includes the presence of meconium staining, abnormalities in fetal HR and rhythm, and an Apgar score of less than or equal to 3 for greater than 5 minutes. The organs most susceptible to damage during asphyxia are the kidneys, brain, heart, and lungs, with the most important consequence of perinatal asphyxia being hypoxic–ischemic encephalopathy (HIE).[591] There must be evidence of hypoxia and ischemia to make the diagnosis of HIE, and there may also be an underlying neurologic disturbance predisposing the baby to a hypoxic–ischemic event.[592]

HIE can range from mild to severe. Ten percent to 20% of term asphyxiated infants die, and the remainder who survive have a good chance of developing normally even in the presence of seizures in the neonatal period. However, there is a small group of severely asphyxiated infants who, having escaped death, will develop major neurologic sequelae, including CP, mental retardation, seizure disorder,[591] cortical blindness, hearing impairment, and microcephaly.[376] A baby who has been asphyxiated may develop any of the following five neurologic lesions:

1. Focal or multifocal cortical necrosis
2. Watershed infarcts (occurring in the boundary zones between cerebral and cerebellar arteries where blood flow is reduced with hypotension or hypoperfusion)
3. Selective neuronal necrosis (brainstem nuclei or Purkinje cells in the cerebellum)
4. Status marmoratus (necrosis of the thalamic nuclei and basal ganglia with myelination of astrocytic processes vs. neurons)
5. PVL[376,407,591]

More extensive lesions occur with more severe asphyxia. Partial episodes of asphyxia result in diffuse cerebral necrosis, whereas total asphyxia spares the cortex and affects the brainstem, thalamus, and basal ganglia. The Sarnat clinical stages (Table 4.10) are used to estimate the severity of asphyxiation in infants greater than 36 weeks' gestation and are based on clinical presentation and duration of symptoms.[591] Asphyxiation in a preterm infant is more difficult to recognize owing to the brain immaturity, hypotonia, and immature reflexes. Premature infants may be protected from HIE by their immaturity, as the more mature the organism at the time of the asphyxia, the shorter the duration needed to cause brain damage.[407] The most effective intervention is prevention of asphyxia by establishing ventilation and perfusion and minimizing hypotension and hypoxia. Babies should be handled with care with the intention to minimize stress and to avoid fluctuations in BP and sensory overload and to teach parents to do the same (Table 4.10).[376]

The Baby with Seizures

Seizures in the neonatal period are difficult to recognize and diagnose because the perinatal brain is functionally and morphologically immature. The electrical discharge

TABLE 4.10.	Sarnat and Sarnat Stages[a] of Hypoxic–Ischemic Encephalopathy		
Stage	**Stage 1 (Mild)**	**Stage 2 (Moderate)**	**Stage 3 (Severe)**
Level of consciousness	Hyperalert: irritable	Lethargic or obtunded	Stuporous, comatose
Neuromuscular control	Uninhibited, overreactive	Diminished spontaneous movement	Diminished or absent spontaneous movement
Muscle tone	Normal	Mild hypotonia	Flaccid
Posture	Mild distal flexion	Strong distal flexion	Intermittent decerebration
Stretch reflexes	Overactive	Overactive, disinhibited	Decreased or absent
Segmental myoclonus	Present or absent	Present	Absent
Complex reflexes	Normal	Suppressed	Absent
Suck	Weak	Weak or absent	Absent
Moro	Strong, low threshold	Weak, incomplete high threshold	Absent
Oculovestibular	Normal	Overactive	Weak or absent
Tonic neck	Slight	Strong	Absent
Autonomic function	Generalized sympathetic	Generalized parasympathetic	Both systems depressed
Pupils	Mydriasis	Miosis	Midposition, often use poor light reflex
Respirations	Spontaneous	Spontaneous; occasional apnea	Periodic; apnea
Heart rate	Tachycardia	Bradycardia	Variable
Bronchial and salivary secretions	Sparse	Profuse	Variable
Gastrointestinal motility	Normal or decreased	Increased diarrhea	Variable
Seizures	None	Common focal or multifocal (6–24 hr of age)	Uncommon (excluding decerebration)
Electroencephalographic findings	Normal (awake)	Early: generalized low voltage, slowing (continuous delta and theta) Later: periodic pattern (awake): seizures focal or multifocal; 1.0–1.5 Hz spike and wave	Early: periodic pattern with isopotential pH Later: totally isopotential
Duration of symptoms	<24 hr	2–14 d	Hours to weeks
Outcome	About 100% normal	80% normal; abnormal if symptoms more than 5–7 d	About 50% die; remainder with severe sequelae

[a]The stages in this table are a continuum reflecting the spectrum of clinical states of infants over 36 weeks' gestational age.
From Sarnat HB, Sarnat MS. Neonatal encephalopathy following fetal distress: a clinical and electroencephalographic study. *Arch Neurol.* 1976;33:696.

underlying a seizure depends on synaptic connections, axonal/dendritic arborization, and myelination, making the well-organized motoric patterns of a seizure in an older infant unlikely in a newborn.[593] The expression of a seizure in a newborn generally manifests as chewing, lip smacking, sucking, apnea, and gaze abnormalities, probably because of the relative maturity of the limbic structures and their connections to the brainstem.[594] There are five types of seizure patterns:

1. Subtle seizures are the most common in term and preterm infants, comprising about 50% of all seizures in this population. They occur most commonly with other seizures. They may not demonstrate EEG correlation and may be refractory to anticonvulsant treatment. They include tonic horizontal deviation of the eyes, oral/buccal/lingual movements, swimming/bicycling movements, apnea, and other autonomic phenomena.[593,594]
2. Focal clonic seizures are characterized by localized clonic jerking with a fast contraction phase and a slower relaxation phase not associated with loss of consciousness. They are usually because of metabolic disturbances, an underlying structural lesion in the contralateral cerebral hemisphere, or focal traumatic injury and have a good prognostic outcome.[593,594]
3. Multifocal clonic seizures consist of random clonic movement of a limb that migrates to other limbs. This is rare in a newborn because of the immaturity of the newborn brain to propagate the discharge throughout the brain.[593,594]
4. Tonic seizures can be focal or generalized and resemble the decerebrate or decorticate posturing of older children involving tonic flexion or extension of the neck, trunk, and upper extremities with tonic lower extremity extension. Prognosis can vary, but in general is poor.[593,594]
5. Myoclonic seizures are characterized by twitching of one or several body parts and can include the head and trunk as well. They are distinguished from clonic seizures by their speed and irregular pattern. They are associated with diffuse central nervous system (CNS) pathology and carry a poor prognosis.[593,594]

The underlying etiologies of a seizure in a newborn can include CNS trauma, metabolic abnormalities, infection, brain malformation, drugs, polycythemia, and focal infarct and is unknown in 3% to 25% of cases. Recurrent or continuous seizures can cause biochemical effects leading to brain damage. The goal of medical intervention is to identify and treat the underlying cause of the seizure in addition to controlling the seizure through the administration of anticonvulsants. Prognosis depends on the precipitating condition as well as the duration of the seizures and the presence of tonic or myoclonic seizure patterns. Fifteen percent of babies die, 30% have long-term neurologic sequelae, and 55% have a normal outcome.[593,594]

Medical Issues of the Late Preterm Infant

The late preterm infant is born between 34 and 36 and 6/7 weeks GA and is formerly known as the "near-term" infant, a term that implies similar needs and care to the term infant. However, it has been recognized that these infants are more vulnerable and have needs more similar to preterm infants. Late preterm births have risen in incidence over the past three decades in the United States, related both to an increase in medically indicated births and an increase in multiple deliveries as part of the use of assisted reproductive technology.[595-600] Late preterm births account for over 250,000 births per year.[595] The following section describes the medical issues of the late preterm infant.

The late preterm infant has higher morbidity, higher rates of hospital readmission through the first year, and may be at increased risk for long-term neurodevelopmental impairment compared with the term counterpart.[595,601-605] The multiple vulnerabilities are a result of the late preterm infant's overall immaturity. For example, terminal respiratory sacs and lung alveoli continue to mature through the 36th gestational week. The surfactant surge, typically occurring at 34 weeks, responsible for assisting this pulmonary maturation may be missed by the infant born in the late preterm period. The respiratory morbidities of the late preterm infant include transient tachypnea, persistent PH, RDS, pneumonia, and respiratory failure requiring mechanical ventilation.[595,604,606-608] For each advancing week of gestation, an infant's need for respiratory intervention and vulnerability for respiratory morbidities decreases.[595,601,604,607] Another example of the late preterm infant's immaturity contributing to vulnerability is the interplay of the underdeveloped hepatic bilirubin conjugation pathways, poor feeding and swallowing coordination, and not fully formed blood–brain barrier. These multiple immaturities increase the risk of prolonged jaundice and bilirubin-induced brain injury in the late preterm infant.[595,601,604,609,610] In addition, late preterm infants have less adipose tissue, larger surface area–to–weight ratio, and are less capable of generating heat, leading to hypothermia. Apnea and bradycardia are more common in the late preterm infant as well.[595,601,609-614] There is some evidence that long-term neurodevelopmental outcome can be affected in this population, with some researchers reporting increased incidences of both CP and intellectual disability,[595,614-619] although others have not reported this.[595,620]

Medical Issues of the Term Infant

Although prematurity and its associated complications represent the concerns of a large number of infants in the NICU, there are a number of conditions that can cause full-term infants to require intensive care management. These infants are often very critically ill, have extended hospitalizations, and benefit from neonatal physical therapy services. A number of these more common conditions and related interventions are discussed in this section.

Meconium Aspiration Syndrome

In the presence of acute or chronic hypoxia, the fetus may pass meconium into the amniotic fluid prior to delivery. The act of gasping for the first breath may cause the infant to aspirate the meconium-stained amniotic fluid in the lungs where particles of meconium can obstruct the airways, interfere with gas exchange, and result in respiratory distress, with varying degrees of severity from mild respiratory distress to life-threatening respiratory failure requiring resuscitation.[621-624] Meconium staining is reported to occur in approximately 9% of births.[621-624]

MAS is presumed in newborn infants who, after being born through meconium-stained fluid, demonstrate respiratory distress that cannot be explained by another mechanism.[621,625] Approximately 2% to 10% of infants born through meconium-stained amniotic fluid demonstrate MAS.[621-623] The risk of meconium aspiration is largest in postmature infants as well as SGA infants.[621,626-629] Owing to changes in obstetric care in recent years in the United States, specifically a reduction in postmature births and monitoring of fetal well-being during labor, the incidence of MAS has declined.[621,628-631] Conditions of prolonged fetal compromise such as hypoxia, predating labor, and intrauterine infection have been associated with meconium aspiration and may lead to acute asphyxia during labor. Twenty percent to 33% of babies with MAS are depressed at birth and require resuscitation.[621,628,631-636] The meconium can have a direct toxic effect on the lung owing to chemical pneumonitis, infection, inflammation, and inactivation of surfactant or it can occlude the airway, trapping air distally in the lungs leading to lung distension, alveolar rupture, and pneumothorax.[621,636-639] Vasoconstriction of the pulmonary vessels in response to hypoxemia can contribute to the development of PPHN, a secondary effect of MAS.[624,633]

In the neonatal period, respiratory effects of meconium aspiration include marked tachypnea, cyanosis, use of accessory muscles for breathing, intercostal and subxiphoid retractions, barrel-chested appearance, and paradoxical breathing patterns with grunting and nasal flaring.[621] A subset of affected infants can be asymptomatic at birth and develop worsening respiratory distress as the meconium moves distally into smaller airways. Initial management of infants in the delivery room includes direct laryngoscopy to suction the hypopharynx and to intubate and suction the trachea before providing positive-pressure ventilation. Infants with MAS may require supplemental oxygen or, if disease is severe, mechanical ventilation. In cases where the respiratory compromise progresses, management may require HFV, surfactant therapy, and nitric oxide.[621,628,640] Severely ill infants with meconium aspiration, PPHN, and respiratory failure that is not responsive to the above measures may require ECMO.[624] Infants with associated PPHN will have right-to-left shunting and a difference in pre- and postductal oxygenation saturations. Long-term pulmonary morbidity is common in babies with MAS and has been reported to include symptomatic coughing and wheezing consistent with reactive airway disease requiring bronchodilator therapy, airway obstruction, and persistent hyperinflation on pulmonary function tests up to 11 years of age.[322,624,628] Neurodevelopmental outcome varies and depends on the injury to the CNS because of asphyxia.[322,624,641]

Persistent Pulmonary Hypertension of the Newborn

PPHN is most commonly seen in term or postterm infants as the result of disruption in the typical transition from fetal to neonatal circulation. If PVR fails to drop after birth, the right-to-left shunting at the foramen ovale and ductus arteriosus that characterizes typical fetal circulation continues and results in severe hypoxemia. Hypoxia and alveolar atelectasis lead to pulmonary vasoconstriction and maintenance of PH.[642,643]

The PVR can fail to drop owing to three types of abnormalities of the pulmonary vasculature. The pulmonary vasculature can be underdeveloped, with decreased cross-sectional area and result in a fixed elevation of PVR. This is the typical pathophysiology of PPHN in a diagnosis associated with lung hypoplasia, such as CDH. Secondly, pulmonary vasculature can develop with an abnormally thick and extensive muscle layer. Remodeling of the pulmonary vasculature typically occurs in 10 to 14 days after birth, at which time the PVR drops. This abnormality of pulmonary vasculature may have a genetic predisposition, be triggered by the use of nonsteroidal anti-inflammatory drugs during pregnancy or be associated with MAS. Lastly, a normally developed vascular bed may fail to dilate after birth because of adverse perinatal conditions such as a bacterial infection or perinatal depression.[643-647] PPHN has also been associated with maternal factors, including diabetes, or urinary tract infection. Perinatal asphyxia is the diagnosis most commonly associated with PPHN.[643,648]

PPHN is suspected in any infant with severe hypoxemia that is not responsive to the administration of 100% oxygen or positive-pressure respiratory support such as CPAP or ventilation. PPHN is diagnosed by echocardiograph that shows normal heart structural anatomy with evidence of PH and right-to-left shunting through the ductus arteriosus and/or foramen ovale. PPHN is a medical emergency, and diagnosis and treatment need to be made promptly. Goals of treatment are to ensure adequate tissue oxygenation while promoting a decline in PVR. Interventions include supplemental oxygen, vasodilators, intubation and mechanical ventilation, iNO, ECMO, correction of metabolic acidosis, hemodynamic support, and correction of metabolic abnormalities and polycythemia.[642,643,648-650] Because agitation can cause a release of catecholamines that increase PVR, these babies may need to be sedated and pharmacologically paralyzed.[643]

The prognosis for infants with PPHN has improved significantly with improved delivery of mechanical ventilation, iNO, and ECMO. However, survivors are at risk for CLD, ICH, neurodevelopmental delays, and sensorineural hearing impairment.[648] Significant impairments have been found in survivors of moderately severe and severe PPHN in motor, cognitive, and hearing function.[221,643,650-656]

Therapists working with infants with PPHN need to be aware of potential cardiopulmonary compromise and support development without increasing infant stress and agitation. Family and other caregivers should be provided with suggestions to promote motor, social, and feeding skills while maintaining physiologic stability.[12] Therapists also need to be aware of associated sensory and neurodevelopmental risks and provide appropriate screening, family education, and follow-up services.

Fetal Alcohol Spectrum Disorder

Alcohol is a known teratogen throughout gestation, and because no safe threshold level has been established for alcohol ingestion during pregnancy, abstinence is recommended.[657] Current research has found that exposure of the fetus to alcohol can result in a variety of adverse outcomes, including growth abnormalities, CNS abnormalities, facial dysmorphisms, and congenital organ malformations.[149,658-660] The term *fetal alcohol spectrum disorder* (FASD) has been advocated for use as a result of the range of outcomes.[149,661-663] Reports of alcohol use (10.8%), including binge drinking (3.7%) and heavy drinking (1%), have been made by pregnant women from 15 to 44 years of age.[660,664] The prevalence of FASD is reported to be 0.3 to 1.5 cases per 1,000 live births, with highest rates reported among blacks, American Indians, and Alaskan Natives.

The most severe form of FASD is fetal alcohol syndrome (FAS). The criteria for FAS include poor growth, CNS abnormalities, and distinct facial dysmorphisms, with or without confirmed alcohol ingestion[149,658-660,665-669] (Table 4.11). First described in detail by Jones and Smith in 1973,[665] FAS is one of the most common causes of intellectual disability worldwide. The effects of alcohol exposure are related to the amount, timing, and pattern of maternal alcohol consumption, as well as the individual rate of maternal metabolism of alcohol.[660,670-673]

Newborns exposed in utero to alcohol can demonstrate acute withdrawal symptoms, characteristics of FAS, or appear normal.[660] Heavy alcohol consumption around the time of conception and during the first trimester has been associated with alcohol-related birth defects, facial dysmorphology, and growth deficiencies,[657,660,674,675] whereas moderate consumption did not affect IQ at 8 years.[660,676] Exposure to alcohol during the second trimester has been associated with growth disturbances and learning deficits; exposure during the third trimester has been associated with deficits in longitudinal growth.[148,657,662] The hallmark of fetal alcohol exposure is severe growth retardation (length more affected than weight). Growth deficiencies continue postnatally, but weight is more affected than length.[148,666]

The most serious feature of FAS is disturbance of CNS development. Disorders of neuronal proliferation, migration,

TABLE 4.11.	Features of Fetal Alcohol Syndrome
Physical Features	**Neurodevelopmental Concerns**
Prenatal growth deficiencies/IUGR	Developmental delay
Postnatal growth deficiencies	Impaired cognitive function
Microcephaly	Speech impairments
Short palpebral fissures	Conductive hearing loss
Epicanthal folds	Sensorineural hearing loss
Midline facial hypoplasia	Behavioral issues
Short upturned nose	Mental retardation
Hypoplastic long or smooth philtrum	
Thin vermilion of upper lip	
Ear abnormalities	
Optic nerve hypoplasia	
Cardiac defects (ASD, VSD)	
Hydronephrosis	
External genitalia anomalies	
Abnormal palmar creases	
Joint abnormalities (hands, fingers, toes)	
Cutaneous hemangioma	

ASD, atrial septal defect; IUGR, intrauterine growth restriction; VSD, ventral septal defect.

and midline prosencephalic formation occur as a result of the teratogenic effects of alcohol during the first two trimesters of pregnancy.[148] Microcephaly is present in almost all cases, with delayed neurologic development also present in a majority of cases of children with FAS. Kartin and associates[676] found lower-than-average developmental performance in preschool children exposed to alcohol and drugs prenatally. In addition to decreased intellectual functioning, hyperactivity, distractibility, decreased attention span, impaired speech and language development, and impaired visual memory affect functioning in school. Long-term effects on psychosocial function have also been reported.[148,660,661,663,669,676-680]

FAS may be difficult to recognize in the neonatal period and may be mistaken for other syndromes. Infants may have no signs of withdrawal if exposed to even moderate amounts of alcohol. Withdrawal signs of jitteriness, sleep disturbance, tremors, hypotonia, or GI symptoms may be seen in some infants exposed to very high levels of alcohol.[148,680,681] The infant may have been exposed to other substances in addition to alcohol and demonstrate more severe withdrawal symptoms because of these substances. Because facial and physical features of FAS may be subtle and the infant may not demonstrate signs of withdrawal, the diagnosis of FAS may not be made until later in the preschool or school-age years when inattention, hyperactivity, and learning problems are more apparent.[663,681,682] Children with late diagnosis may miss out on early intervention and other services that can address growth and developmental needs. Infants with known prenatal exposure to alcohol or suspected FAS should be referred for developmental follow-up services upon discharge from the hospital.[660,669]

Neonatal Abstinence Syndrome

Neonatal abstinence syndrome (NAS) is a neonatal withdrawal syndrome and refers to a constellation of specific signs and symptoms exhibited by neonates with prolonged in utero exposure to illicit or prescribed drugs.[683] The terminology was originally used to describe infants with prenatal opioid exposure; however, the term is also used to describe symptoms related to exposure to other drugs.[684] NAS is more common in infants with mothers with opioid dependence. Neonatal opioid withdrawal syndrome (NOWS) is a term used in NAS literature to describe the effects of prolonged maternal opioid use during pregnancy.[683,684] NAS can result in substantial infant morbidities during the first weeks to months of life and require prolonged hospitalization.[683,685] In this section, NAS related to in utero opioid exposure will be discussed.

The incidence of NAS has increased over the last two decades with the overall rise in opioid use and use of opioids in pregnancy.[683,686] Opioids including illegal drugs such as heroin, synthetic drugs such as fentanyl, and prescribed pain relievers such as oxycodone, hydrocodone, and morphine are of the same drug class with similar composition.[687] There has been up to sevenfold increase in NAS incidence in the United States between 2000 and 2014, with NAS accounting for 3% of all NICU admissions and increases in health care costs.[688-692] There has also been a disproportionate shift in incidence to rural areas of the country.[689]

Predication as to which infants with prenatal opioid exposure will develop clinical signs of withdrawal is difficult. Biomarkers for certain drugs are not always present and the presentation in the infant does not always correlate with maternal dosage.[684] Signs and symptoms of NAS are not seen in all opioid-exposed infants. For those infants who do exhibit withdrawal, the presentation is variable and lies along a continuum of signs of withdrawal. The degree to which the fetus is affected by substance exposure is multifactorial including biodisposition (the absorption, metabolism, and distribution) of the substance by the placenta, as well as maternal and infant characteristics. Maternal factors related to severity of NAS include the drug class and clearance from the body, dosage, most recent use, and body habitus. Infant factors include GA, birth weight, and metabolism.[683,684,687] Term infants demonstrate more severe withdrawal symptoms than preterm infants. There are several potential explanations for this including a lack of recognition of preterm withdrawal symptoms.[693,694] There is also longer exposure to the drug and greater storage of drugs in fat, leading to increased dependency on these substances with increasing GA.[688]

NAS occurs with the abrupt drug discontinuation to the infant at the time of delivery, resulting in excessive release of noradrenaline in the neonate. This results in hyperactivity of the autonomic nervous system, CNS, and the GI tract as these locations have the highest concentration of opioid receptors.[683,686] This clinical presentation of symptoms can develop during the first 24 to 48 hours of life; however, onset can range from birth to the end of the second week or longer. Acute and subacute phases of NAS can last up to 12 months.[688] The clinical features of opioid withdrawal include autonomic instability, neurologic excitability, and GI dysfunction, leading to neurobehavioral dysregulation, impacting the autonomic, motor, state, and self-regulatory system function.[683,685,686] The specific symptoms include increased irritability and high-pitch cry, poor state control, increased wakefulness, hypertonicity, tremors and jitteriness, seizures, failure to thrive, poor oral feeding, uncoordinated and constant sucking, vomiting, diarrhea, skin breakdown, and autonomic symptoms such as hiccups, gagging, color changes, diaphoresis, tachypnea, and fever.[685,695]

Infants at risk for the development of NAS should be closely monitored for signs and symptoms. AAP recommends close monitoring of opioid-exposed infants for 3 to 7 days after birth.[683] Studies estimate that 55% to 94% of opioid-dependent mothers will develop signs of NAS, and of this group, 50% to 75% will require treatment.[683] The diagnosis of NAS is based on scoring systems that combine objective data (vital signs) and subjective assessment (irritability, hypertonia, feeding coordination) to measure the clinical signs and symptoms.[684] The Modified Finnegan Neonatal Abstinence Scoring Tool (M-FNAST) is recommended by the AAP and is the most commonly utilized to assess infants with NAS.[696,697] The NICU Network Neurobehavioral Scale incorporates features of the Finnegan scale and also assesses maturity, behavioral control, and self-regulation.[698] An alternative program for evaluation and treatment of infants with NAS—the Eat, Sleep, Console method—has been shown to lessen the amount of medication required for treatment and shorten hospital stays.[699]

The first line of intervention is nonpharmacologic, developmentally supportive care. Interventions include environmental modifications (decreasing external stimulation of sound and light) and supporting self-regulation with swaddling/containment, holding/kangaroo mother care, rocking, and nutritive sucking and NNS.[148,693,700-702] There is increasing recognition of the benefits of close parental contact and rooming in of parents with their babies.[685,695] The decision to start pharmacologic intervention is based on objective measurement of symptoms recorded using a neonatal abstinence score. NAS scoring is used to determine the need to increase or wean medication.[683,693,700,701] The article by McCarty et al.[695] is an excellent summary of assessment and management in the infant with NAS.

Infants with NAS may have lower birth weight, height, and head circumference. They can exhibit depressed or inconsistent interactive behaviors and have poor self-calming, which can impact development. In addition, treatment of NAS may require weeks to months of hospitalization, which can interfere with maternal bonding and overall development.[148,684,701,702-704] Developmental follow-up studies of infants with NAS have found a higher incidence of hyperactivity, learning and behavior disorders, and poor social adjustment.[684,685,704] Adverse visual outcomes have been increasingly reported in follow-up studies of infants with prenatal opioid exposure.[684] Kartin et al.[676] reported that the developmental performance of preschool children with prenatal alcohol and drug exposure was lower than expected for age. It is unclear to what extent environmental factors such as maternal characteristics, tobacco use, polydrug use, poverty, and social factors associated with substance abuse are responsible for these outcomes versus prenatal substance exposure.[148,684,685,704] Although it is difficult to make a direct link between neonatal substance exposure and developmental outcomes, these children and their families are clearly at risk for social, behavioral, and developmental problems. Therefore, close follow-up and maternal–child services including early intervention are warranted.

» Physical therapy examination and intervention

Chart Review

A complete history should include information from the medical chart, nursing and physician staff, and the family. Pertinent information from the medical chart includes prenatal history, birth history, history of the present illness, and family social history. Prenatal history consists of maternal age, circumstances regarding conception (the use of assistive reproductive technology), prenatal care and test results, complications during pregnancy, infections, illnesses, medications and/or drug use and interventions such as fetal/maternal surgery, maternal past medical history, and presence/treatment of preterm labor. Birth history includes GA at delivery, mode of delivery (spontaneous or induced vaginal delivery, with or without vacuum or forceps assist, or cesarean section), weight, length, head circumference, Apgar scores (see Table 4.7), infant's clinical presentation at delivery, resuscitative efforts, and infant's need for ongoing interventions in the delivery room.

History of present illness includes an in-depth review of medical status by systems. A baby may require newborn intensive care for a variety of reasons. The systems listed in the medical chart may vary somewhat between babies on the unit, based on the baby's diagnosis and medical issues. In general, every chart will include the following systems: fluids, electrolytes, and nutrition also called "FEN"; Respiratory; and Cardiac. Other systems that may be included based on the baby's needs include Neurologic, GI, Genitourinary, and Endocrine.

In reviewing the chart, the therapist should attend to respiratory requirements since birth, current respiratory support, and modifications required during nursing care or feeding sessions. The therapist should note the frequency and severity of episodes of apnea, bradycardia, and oxygen desaturation, as well as interventions required to assist the baby's return to baseline. Babies with respiratory compromise, like BPD, are known for their ability to decompensate, have cyanotic episodes or "spells,"[442] and may require medical intervention to recover physiologic stability. The baby's cardiovascular health impacts the baby's other organ systems, in particular the CNS, respiratory system, and GI system, and should be noted. The baby's nutritional course since birth provides a window into the baby's overall health, functioning, and ability to grow. Feeding tolerance and schedules may also influence the scheduling of the PT evaluation.

For babies with a history of surgery, the PT must pay particular attention to the indications for surgery, the surgical procedure, the outcome of the surgery, and any precautions or contraindications. Surgery can produce scarring that can affect an infant's posture and mobility. Likewise, the baby's medications can affect alerting and interaction. Infants who require sedatives or narcotics for medical management or pain relief postsurgery may display signs and symptoms of withdrawal during weaning. The infant's tolerance to weaning from sedation or withdrawal from substance exposure will be recorded in neonatal abstinence scores. Babies undergoing intensive care may have infections, metabolic issues, hyperbilirubinemia, genetic syndromes, and congenital malformations. All can affect the baby's current level of functioning and future risk.

Consultation by specialists is also important to review. Particular attention should be paid to the neurology consultation, any neuroradiographic studies (cranial ultrasound, MRI, CT scan), and EEGs. The area and size of lesion(s) are important as well as the clinical findings. Medical/surgical interventions such as medications, CSF tapping, and shunting or ventriculostomy should be noted. Medications such as anticonvulsants can decrease arousal and muscle tone as they can impact the baby's performance during the evaluation. The therapist should be aware of the prognosis made by the neurologist, if that prognosis has been discussed with the family, and the family's response to that discussion.

The PT begins with a thorough chart review as detailed earlier. Information regarding family psychosocial history and concerns should also be reviewed and discussed with the social worker if appropriate. Chart reviews are essential; however, sometimes the most up-to-date information about the infant will come from the baby's bedside nurse.

Nursing Interview

After a thorough review of the chart, the therapist should interview nursing staff about the overall status of the infant, as the bedside nurse will be aware of the most current changes in the medical plan for the infant. The nurse can provide vital information about the events of the infant's day as this may affect the baby's energy level, alertness, and tolerance for the evaluation. The nursing interview is influenced by the baby's history and need for intensive care. For example, for a baby with CLD/BPD, it is imperative to interview the infant's nurse as to which activities the infant tolerates and which activities cause the baby distress, especially distress that may cause the baby to enter a cycle of respiratory instability. If the infant has seizures, the therapist should inquire as to the typical presentation of seizure activity and whether there are triggers for seizures. Other important information includes timing of administration of seizure medication, presence and quality of awake states, observed active movement, and atypical posturing.

For babies who are recovering from surgery, the interview should include questions about the baby's pain management. Does the nurse think the baby's current pain management is adequate for the baby at rest and during nursing care? A baby who requires surgical intervention may also need technologic supports such as mechanical ventilation, chest tubes, drains, or gastric suctioning devices. These supports add to the baby's discomfort as well as limit positioning and handling for nursing care.

For all babies, it is important to know the individual infant's baseline physiologic parameters and recognize that these may differ from age norms. Other pertinent information includes changes in status leading to changes in medical care, tolerance to nursing care, care procedures that lead to infant distress, and the infant's preferred comfort measures.

If the family members are present, the therapist can begin to establish a relationship with them by initiating a dialogue about their baby. Goals of the family interview include ascertaining their understanding of their infant's medical condition and prognosis, their interpretation of the infant's behaviors, and their comfort in interacting with their baby. A discussion with the family members as to their concerns for their infant is a helpful starting point in developing a relationship with the family and planning therapy interventions, including family education.

During this initial visit to the infant's bedside, the therapist should be observing the bedside environment and noting levels of light, sound, proximity to high-traffic areas, and how the baby is responding to the NICU environment.

Clinical Decisions

Based on the above information, the therapist then needs to decide if the infant can withstand an evaluation that involves handling. PTs strive to practice under the principle of beneficence—"above all, do no harm" to patients. When working with the population of high-risk infants, the potential is always present to harm a baby with any intervention, even examination. A skilled therapist will collaborate with nursing staff to understand the baby's current medical status, tolerance to handling, and previous events of the day before undertaking any direct interaction with the baby. Careful

and skilled observations of the baby's physiologic status allow the therapist to decide on the competence of the infant to withstand an examination as well as when to terminate or proceed with handling an infant. The infant should also be evaluated before, during, and after any examination or intervention for signs of pain using the neonatal pain assessment approved by the medical facility.

Observational Assessments

If the results of this preliminary gathering of information show that the baby is easily stressed by the routines of the day and/or if the baby is very preterm (<34 weeks PMA), the best approach may be observational. Infants recovering from medical conditions such as MAS or PPHN may not tolerate a hands-on examination if they are still critically ill and require large amounts of medical support to promote physiologic function. Infants exposed to prenatal infections may also be very ill and unable to tolerate handling. Although withdrawing from substance exposure, infants may not be able to tolerate the stimulation of handling as well.

An observational approach is based on the principles of the NIDCAP.[52] With an observational approach, the therapist observes the infant both at rest and during care activities with nursing or other health care professionals. The therapist needs to observe baseline HR, RR and respiratory pattern, and oxygen saturation. Posture, movements, and muscle tone are noted as well as the baby's state and interaction with the environment. Signs of stress or readiness for interaction are noted. All of the above is then observed when the baby is participating in medical or nursing care activities. Finally, the above is observed when care is over and the baby is recovering. The observations are reviewed to determine how the baby is participating in care activities, noting the baby's strengths and vulnerabilities.

During an observation, a baby may demonstrate sensitivity to environmental sounds. The therapist would then recommend strategies to minimize sounds such as encouraging staff to refrain from writing upon or placing objects on top of the isolette, quietly closing porthole and bedside cart drawers, keeping pagers on vibrate mode, and keeping voices low and conversations at the bedside to a minimum. Other strategies include posting signs (Fig. 4.19) to keep noise down to promote a healing environment, so that all staff and visitors are aware of the need to keep noise to a minimum. If these measures are not sufficient, the baby's bed may need to be moved to a quieter space away from a sink, a trashcan, or a heavily traveled corridor. Similarly, if a baby is sensitive to light, discussing strategies for shielding the baby's eyes with family and caregivers is important. Overhead lights can be dimmed, and the isolette can be covered. A baby can also be shielded from bright lighting by shading the infant's eyes with a cupped hand, propping a blanket like a tent to shade the face, or draping a sheet over the crib. The physical environment of the NICU should be adapted with individual lighting for each bed space.[705] Overhead lighting can be

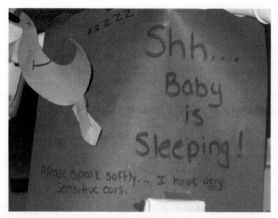

FIGURE 4.19. Signs such as this are used to alert staff and visitors that the infant is sensitive to sound.

turned off and more peripheral lighting over sinks or bedside carts can be used to create a dimly lit space near the baby.

A baby may also demonstrate frequent physiologic and motoric stress signs at rest as well as during intervention (see Table 4.3). In order to assist the autonomic and the motor subsystems, the baby may benefit from containment with positioning aids. Commercially made products or blanket rolls can be used to provide a nest that simulates the enclosed environment of the womb (Fig. 4.20).

During an observation, a baby may demonstrate unsuccessful attempts to self-calm. If the baby is unsuccessful at calming, he or she may become exhausted, limp, and

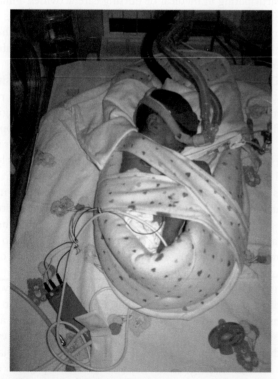

FIGURE 4.20. Infant positioned in a nest made from a Children's Medical Ventures Snuggle Up.

physiologically compromised by the end of the caregiving episode. Suggestions for providing assistance for the baby's self-calming strategies include offering a pacifier, containing hands near face/mouth, and positioning legs in a tucked position near the baby's trunk. Caregiving may need to be provided at the infant's tolerance, allowing the infant frequent breaks to rest after particularly disorganizing aspects of care (e.g., diaper change or suctioning). During the rest break, the baby should be contained. A therapist places her open hands on top of the baby and contains the baby's limbs close to midline, facilitating a tucked position. A blanket wrap can also be used to swaddle the infant and prevent the infant from exhaustion.[67,706-708] At this stage in the infant's hospital course, the therapist is consulting with the nursing staff and the family to make suggestions for positional and environmental modifications to promote comfort, physiologic function, and, if possible, positional alignment for future developmental tasks.

Infants withdrawing from prenatal substance exposure often require long hospital stays and present with unique needs. Generally older and more physiologically stable, it is not uncommon for these infants to demonstrate poor behavioral organization, extended deep sleep, agitated sleep, vacillation between sleep and crying states, and panicked awakening.[709] The examination should include all the elements previously discussed and evaluation of neonatal abstinence scores. Initially, recommendations for environmental modifications in order to decrease environmental stress as well as caregiving recommendations to streamline and organize care to avoid overstimulation are essential. Assessing and promoting the baby's attempts at self-regulatory behaviors are also important. The infant may only tolerate comfort measures, particularly early in his or her withdrawal.

As the infant demonstrates improving stability, the therapist should continue to weigh the inherent potential costs to the infant with an examination that involves handling.

Neuromotor Assessment

One way to further assess a baby's readiness for an assessment that involves handling and position changes is habituation items.[710,711] When the baby is in a sleep state, serial responses to repeated light (flashlight across the eyes) and sound (a soft rattle) are used to assess the baby's ability to filter repetitive stimuli. This provides information regarding the stability of the sleep state and also gives the therapist a chance to determine the readiness for handling. If the baby becomes overly stressed and loses physiologic stability, the therapist can end the evaluation session and provide supports for regulation. However, if the baby is able to transition to an alert state and maintain physiologic stability, the therapist can proceed slowly with examination items that require gentle handling. The authors do not recommend one standardized assessment tool. See Table 4.12 for a variety of standardized neonatal assessments. Throughout the examination, the therapist needs to assess the baby's state control (i.e., the

TABLE 4.12.	Standardized Neonatal Assessment Tools			

Name/Author	Purpose	Description	Training
Neurologic Assessment of Preterm and Full-Term Infants (Hammersmith Neonatal Neurological Examination HNNE) Authors: Dubowitz V Dubowitz L[710,711]	To record the functional state of the nervous system and to document preterm infant neurologic maturation and recovery from perinatal insult Age: Preterm and full-term infants	Assessment of behavioral state, neurobehavior, posture, movement, muscle tone, and reflexes with passive manipulation Emphasis on patterns of responses. Test cannot be quantified or compared with normative expectations for age over time. Time to administer: 15 min	Requires minimal training or experience Items within the area of expertise of developmental therapists
Neurobehavioral Assessment of the Preterm Infant (NAPI) Authors: Korner AF Thom VA[814,815]	To assess infant maturity, monitor progress, and detect lags in development and neurologically suspect performance Age: 32–42 wk PCA	Assessment of state, behavior, reflexes, motor patterns, and tone Most items overlap with other assessments and must be administered from rousing to soothing to alerting. Time to administer: 45 min	To be used by any professional caring for or studying preterm infants in the intensive or intermediate care nursery
Neonatal Behavioral Assessment Scale (NBAS) Author: Brazelton TB Nugent J[185,715]	To assess the infant's contributions to the interactional process. Age: 36–44 wk gestation	Consists of 28 behavioral items and 18 reflex items Sequence of administration is flexible, and examiner seeks to elicit the infant's best performance Time to administer: 30–45 min and scored in 15–20 min	Requires training for reliability in administration and scoring[816] Trainees complete a four-phase process consisting of self-study, skill test, and practice (on 25 babies) before completing certification session.
Assessment of Preterm Infant Behavior (APIB) Authors: Als H Lester BM Tronick EZ Brazelton TB[817,818]	To assess the individual behavioral organizational repertoire of the preterm infant Age: Preterm infants	Based on the Brazelton's NBAS but focusing on the preterm infant Looks at the preterm infant's physiologic, motor, state, attentional–interactive, and regulatory systems Time to administer: 30–45 min. Scoring is labor intensive.	Requires extensive training in the assessment as well as human development
NICU Network Neurobehavioral Scale (NNNS) Authors: Lester BM Tronick EZ[106,698]	To assess neurologic integrity and behavioral functioning of infants at high risk Stress scale to document signs of withdrawal Age: 34–46 wk PCA Can be used in term, healthy infants, and high-risk infants (substance exposures and preterm infants) Infants <33 wk use just observational items.	Draws on NBAS, NAPI, APIB, Neurologic Examination of the Full-term Newborn Infant, and the Neurologic Examination of the Maturity of Newborn Infants Items are grouped in packages, which are presented depending on infant state in a prescribed sequence. Can be modified for the very preterm, physiologically unstable infant Time to administer: 30 min	Requires certification through 2- or 5-d training programs with certified trainers along with practice administering the test to infants in own facility Amount of practice depends on experience, comfort handling infants, and clinical acumen.
Assessment of General Movements (GMA) Author: Einspieler C Pretchl HF Bos AF Ferrari F Cioni G[777,778]	To assess for early signs of brain dysfunction using qualitative measure Age: 36 wk PCA to 4 mo Can be used with both preterm and full-term infants.	Infants are videotaped, and observational analysis of movements in terms of variety, fluidity, elegance, and complexity is performed. Video recording and analysis should be done longitudinally. Time: 1 hr initial videotape and 15-min follow-up tapes plus time for analysis	Two-day training required for basic principles Practice of 100 recordings required to become a skilled observer Training videotape available, which demonstrates qualitative aspects of movement.[819]
Test of Infant Motor Performance (TIMP) Authors: Campbell SK Girolami GO Oston E Lenke M[820]	To identify motor delay in infants before 4 mo corrected age Age: 34 wk gestation to 4 mo postterm	Consists of 13 observed items focusing on midline alignment, selective control, and quality of movement; 29 elicited items focusing on antigravity postural control elicited by handling typically experienced by an infant	Workshops or self-study instructional CD[493,821]

(continued)

TABLE 4.12.	Standardized Neonatal Assessment Tools (*continued*)			
Name/Author	**Purpose**	**Description**	**Training**
Alberta Infant Motor Scale (AIMS) Authors: Piper M Darrah J[822]	To identify motor delays, monitor individual development, and evaluate intervention. Age: 0–18 mo	Observational assessment of 58 transitional gross motor patterns and postures in supine, prone, sitting, and standing	No training requirements specified To be used by any professional with a background in infant motor development
Hammersmith Infant Neurological Examination[710,711] Dubowitz V Dubowitz L	Based on the same principles as the Hammersmith Neonatal Neurological Examination; Assists in early diagnosis and prognosis of infants at risk for cerebral palsy Age: 2–24 mo	Twenty-six items assess cranial nerve function, movements, reflexes, and protective reactions and behavior. Also some developmental items related to gross and fine motor function Time to administer: 15 min	Training associated with the American Academy of Cerebral Palsy and Developmental Medicine (AACPDM) annual meeting and Implementation of Early Detection and Intervention for Cerebral Palsy Conference[823]

PCA, postconceptual age.

ability to maintain organized sleep states and demonstrate a range of states; see Table 4.5 for state-related behaviors). The baby's physiologic responses (HR, BP, RR) should be closely monitored throughout the session.

The evaluation of the infant who is able to tolerate handling should begin with an observation of the type of respiratory support, presence of central or peripheral lines, and presence of feeding tubes, as these are not only indications of the fragility of the infant but may also limit the infant's positioning and active movement. The therapist should assess the baby for edema, skin integrity issues, and surgical incisions for extent of healing and presence of scar tissue. Healing can be compromised by iatrogenic infections and antibiotic-resistant bacteria prevalent in medical settings and can significantly prolong a baby's hospitalization. Prolonged illness, immobilization, and hospitalization can interfere with the baby's acquisition of developmental milestones as well as with socialization and bonding with family and puts the baby at greater risk for delays. Living in a crisis-prone environment disadvantages children who "grow old in the NICU" as they experience multiple caregivers, limited interactions with family, and limited opportunities to move, practice developmental activities, and have typical sensory experiences. In addition, NICU staff may feel challenged to provide the appropriate stimulation for older infants in the newborn intensive care setting.[712]

The infant with respiratory compromise such as BPD/CLD may frequently demonstrate tachypnea, which is defined as an RR greater than 60 breaths per minute. These babies often exhibit paradoxical breathing and recruit accessory respiratory muscles rather than utilizing the typical pattern of abdominal breathing. The baby should be carefully assessed throughout the evaluation for signs of respiratory distress, including retractions of the chest wall, nasal flaring, grunting, and stridor.

If the baby is able to withstand touch and gentle handling, an evaluation involving changes in position and elicited items

in order to assess the baby's muscle strength and tone may be initiated. Some babies' participation in a neuromotor assessment may be limited because of medical interventions like invasive respiratory supports or umbilical lines. A neuromotor examination, to be accurate, requires a baby to be in a calm, awake state as other states (sleep, crying) can affect muscle tone, range of motion, and active movement.[710,711] Infants who have sustained a neurologic insult may present with atypical states that lack variety, lack smooth transitions, and limit interaction. For example, the infant may only display a sleep state or irritable wakeful state. Completing a neurologic examination in either of these two states would limit the accuracy; however, the therapist can still obtain useful information by observing active movement of trunk and extremities. Active movement should be observed for symmetry, smoothness, variety, complexity, and isolation. The infant should be reassessed in a serial fashion for changes in behavioral state organization and neuromotor status. When appropriate, a neurologic examination including reflexes, range of motion, and muscle tone should be completed. There are some babies who present with symmetric active movement but may demonstrate asymmetries in elicited responses. Examples include a brisk gallant response, stronger palmar/plantar grasp reflex on one side, and/or asymmetric French angles (see Fig. 4.21). These may be subtle signs and should be monitored as they have been predictive of neuromotor outcomes.[595]

It is generally safe to initiate a neuromotor examination on an infant who is medically stable, on room air, and in an open crib. However, this portion of the examination can be most stressful to the infant; therefore, the therapist should proceed with caution while maintaining vigilance for signs of tolerance or fatigue.

Prior to the initiation of a neuromotor examination, the therapist should consider which test items may be unduly stressful for the infant and modify the examination accordingly. Modified hands-on examination may include diaper

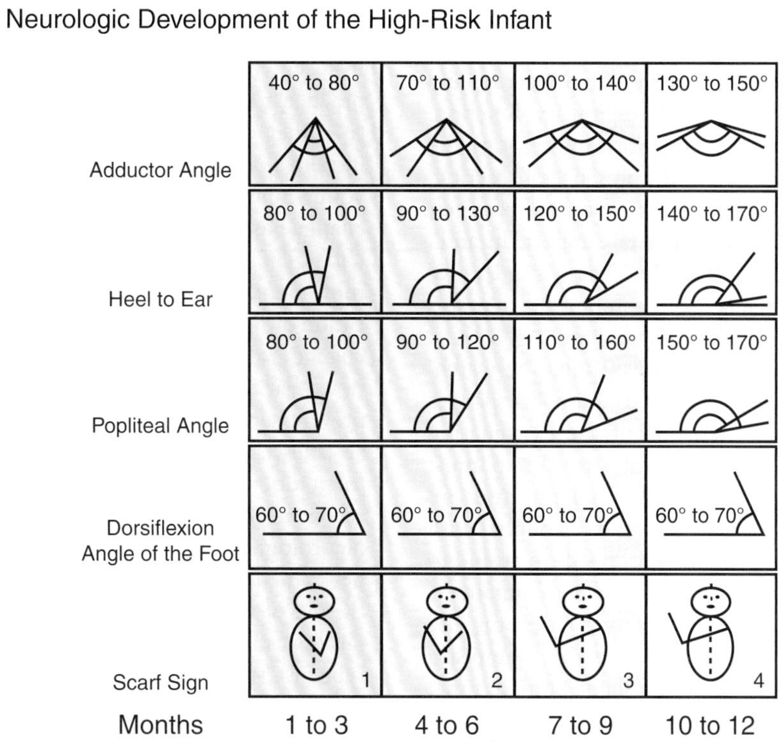

Neurologic Development of the High-Risk Infant

FIGURE 4.21. Symmetric active movement demonstrating asymmetries in elicited responses, as seen in these French angles.[713] (Reprinted with permission from Ellison PH. Neurologic development of the high-risk infant. *Clin Perinatol.* 11(1):45 and adapted from Amiel-Tison C. A method for neurological evaluation within the first year of life. *Curr Probl Pediatr.* 1976;7(1):45.)

change, repositioning, gentle facilitation of active movement, observation of general movements, recoil responses in the extremities, scarf sign, grasp reflex, and self-regulatory strategies.[21] The therapist should pay close attention to the baby's physiologic responses and tolerance to handling. Throughout the examination, the therapist must monitor the baby's work of breathing and oxygen saturation. Infants with BPD and respiratory compromise have limited respiratory reserve, and a noxious test item may cause the infant to start a cycle of respiratory distress and compromise that requires medical intervention. Increased energy costs and fatigue because of a neuromotor examination can occur in an infant without severe respiratory decompensation as well and should be conducted slowly and with careful monitoring of an infant's responses and tolerance.

A baseline neuromotor examination includes observation of:

- posture at rest,
- quality and quantity of active movements,
- palmar and plantar grasp reflexes,
- flexor recoil,
- traction responses,
- passive range of motion, and
- French angles (adductor, popliteal, heel to ear, dorsiflexion, and scarf sign angles)[713,714] (Fig. 4.21).

If the baby is tolerating these procedures, the therapist can move on to more intensive handling items, such as pull-to-sit, slip through, ventral suspension, and position changes to prone, side-lying, and sitting. The neurodevelopmental examination should be completed as the infant's tolerance allows. Many infants in the NICU may have decreased tolerance for developmental activities. A therapist may need to modify test items and test flow of a standardized assessment tool in order to accommodate the infant's level of tolerance. Breathing is always a baby's first priority and everything else is secondary. The therapist may need to start with modified hands-on examination and then perform full hands-on assessment when the baby is able to tolerate the handling and length of time needed to complete a standardized test.[13,17,21] A posture and musculoskeletal examination of the baby provides information relevant to the baby's respiratory function as well as neuromotor development. Many high-risk infants may have fragile bones, as discussed in "Metabolic Bone Disease of Prematurity" section. The baby with BPD or other respiratory compromise may develop compensatory motor patterns to assist respiration by opening up the airway and chest and recruiting accessory muscles. Typical posture seen in babies with respiratory compromise like CLD/BPD is hyperextension of the head and neck, shoulder elevation and retraction, trunk extension, and anterior pelvic tilt. These postures can interfere not only with the development of efficient respiratory function but also with the infant's ability to develop self-calming, feeding, and fine and gross motor skills. Integumentary examination should include the presence and integrity of scars on the trunk, specifically from PDA ligation, chest tubes, and abdominal surgery. These scars can cause limitations in trunk range of motion and lead to asymmetric trunk postures. Skin color and temperature indicate perfusion to the trunk and extremities.

The examination should also include the impact of any surgical intervention on the infant's respiratory function. The rate and the pattern of the baby's breathing should be examined as it may be influenced by the presence of scarring, thoracic and abdominal pressure changes, anatomic changes, pain, edema, and lack of musculoskeletal support. In addition, the above may also affect the baby's passive and active range of motion. For these infants, it is important to assess their developmental skills in an ongoing fashion.

During this examination, the therapist should be watching for an optimal time to elicit visual and auditory responses from the infant. This sensory portion of the examination should also be administered from least stressful to most stressful and unimodal to multimodal stimulation (i.e., inanimate object, blank face, animated face, face coupled with speech).[715] During this time, the therapist needs to attend to the baby's responses and the baby's strategies to maintain organization in autonomic, state, and motor subsystems and calming strategies. The examination allows the therapist a window into the baby's functioning at a single point in time; however, the baby's responses are based on the level of maturity as well as contextual factors. Therefore, it is wise to reexamine infants over time to gain an accurate picture of their function. It is important to be observant of the infant's cardiopulmonary status and behavioral cues when handling the infant and to help the family to understand that the infant may not be able to tolerate as much activity as other infants his or her age.

The therapist uses the information from the history, observation, and hands-on examination to determine the baby's strengths and needs and the family's strengths, needs, and expectations. Clinical decision making with regard to the priority of identified needs is essential. A plan of care is developed using interventions that challenge the baby within his or her range of tolerance. Ideal recommendations challenge the baby appropriately and support the family and caregivers throughout the week. For instance, a baby may have shown excessive extensor posturing and tight scapulohumeral and neck extensor musculature. The therapist would then recommend ways to incorporate flexion activities into daily routines and interactions with family and to avoid activities that promote excessive extension. As the baby develops and changes, recommendations require updating.

Physical therapy intervention is then based on the individual infant's strengths and concerns. The concerns are prioritized according to the infant's medical status and immediate needs in the NICU environment. Owing to the nature of the illness and intensive care these babies require, they often demonstrate developmental delays and changes in medical status. The NICU therapist's role may change from primarily consultative for infants who need assistance to tolerate nursing care to more traditional "hands-on" physical therapy interventions during the course of the infant's hospitalization.

Early Detection of Cerebral Palsy

In recent years, there has been a change in philosophy and practice from waiting to diagnose CP at 2 years or older to earlier diagnosis prior to 6 months and the use of an interim diagnosis of "high risk for cerebral palsy" for very young infants where clinical suspicion for CP is high.[716] This change has been driven in part by the proven success of Prechtl's general movements assessment (GMA) in assessing the movements of preterm and term-age infants and the identification of fidgety movements at 3 months corrected age. The change is also driven by the desire to provide earlier interventions that take advantage of the infant's neuroplasticity and prevent secondary impairments. In addition, earlier diagnosis is less stressful for parents. The guidelines for the implementation of early CP diagnosis in neonatal follow-up clinics recommend the use of the GMA, the Hammersmith Infant Neurological Examination (HINE), the test of infant motor performance (TIMP), and neuroimaging to detect CP. With the use of the "high risk of cerebral palsy" diagnosis, neonatal PTs can provide interventions specifically targeted to the type of CP and these targeted interventions can be provided earlier, taking advantage of the neuroplasticity of the infant brain to promote connections.[716] These interventions will be discussed in more detail later.

Physical Therapy Interventions

PT interventions should be based on the information synthesized from the examination. For every baby in the NICU, the therapist wants to teach the parents how to read and respond appropriately to their infant as well as more specific activities to encourage development. This section will provide an overview of considerations for timing of interventions, environmental and caregiving recommendations, parent/caregiver education, positioning, hydrotherapy, kangaroo care, scar massage, and interventions for babies at high risk for CP.

The baby's sleep is very important, and physical therapy interventions should not interrupt it. Infants in the NICU may demonstrate episodes of irritability and restlessness owing to discomfort and/or hypoxemia. They may also have difficulty sleeping because of environmental or caregiving disturbances. When scheduling physical therapy, other procedures and events in the infant's day need to be considered in order to avoid undue stress and fatigue on the infant. The baby is always the boss and his or her reserve capacity and tolerance for activity guide physical therapy interventions in the NICU.

A skilled therapist will recommend developmental activities that promote motor skills and postural control and that can be built into the baby's routines such as feeding, burping, diaper changes, and bathing.[21] Appropriate positions/activities for play and interaction, along with precautions based on the baby's cues, can be provided to the infant's family and care providers. For infants who require long-term intubation, neonatal PTs need to collaborate with other members of the care team to find creative ways to safely provide opportunities for supported upright and prone positions that can be integrated into daily routines and developmental play activities. Shephard et al.[717] found improved neurodevelopmental outcomes and decreased readmission rates with a comprehensive interdisciplinary approach to the management of infants with BPD.

Environmental and Caregiving Recommendations

The NICU environment is notoriously harsh and intrusive for babies. In its effort to save babies' lives, the NICU provides bright lighting, so that caregivers can observe their tiny patients, and continual background noise from high-technology devices, with loud noises such as alarms peaking abruptly. Babies also experience frequent handling and painful procedures. The neonatal therapist must be vigilant for the ways the environment is stressful for each infant. Environmental modifications include recommendations to provide appropriate lighting to encourage infant alerting, opportunities for infants to hear speech, particularly that of their parents, as well as opportunities for pleasurable touch. Therapists should advocate for consistent use of nonpharmacologic pain supports during any routine and nonroutine noxious procedures. The sickest and most vulnerable infants in the NICU may only display minimal or no responses to painful experiences, tricking their caregivers into believing it does not affect them. However, research has provided sobering accounts of the short- and long-term effects of painful procedures for this population, as well as gaps in knowledge and practice regarding pain management in the NICU.[132,718,719] Neonatal therapists should not be naïve about the exposure to and the effects of pain for babies in the NICU.

The baby may also benefit from altering the pace of caregiving. Many infants require a rest break to regain physiologic stability during the course of nursing care or a medical procedure. Therapists can also advocate for a second caregiver to monitor the infant's tolerance, call for rest breaks, and provide facilitated tucking and containment to support the baby until they regain physiologic stability. In addition, therapists can teach parents to be this second caregiver. Nursing education can promote a culture of fast, efficient autonomous practice among nurses but babies in the NICU benefit from care that is provided in response to their cues.

Recommendations for environmental modifications and caregiving help to decrease a baby's stress and energy expenditure and promote sleep. Many babies spend months in the NICU, and it is imperative that their environment and caregiving practices promote an environment that fosters healing and recovery and protects their sleep. Kangaroo care is one such recommendation that accomplishes the above.

Kangaroo Care

Kangaroo care was a serendipitous discovery in Bogota, Columbia, during a time when there was limited availability of incubators.[720] Naked, diapered babies were placed on their mother's bare chests, skin to skin, and covered with a blanket.[721] Despite not being placed in an incubator, babies maintained their temperatures, demonstrated good stable vital signs, and gained weight. Since then, kangaroo care, also known as skin-to-skin holding, has been researched and proven to benefit both babies and their caregivers and has gained wider acceptance in the United States for use in the NICU.

Research has demonstrated many varied benefits in addition to the improved physiologic parameters for infants as stated earlier. Other benefits include increased maternal milk production and breastfeeding, opportunities for positive interactions with the infant, analgesic effects during painful procedures on infants, and decreased length of hospitalization.[722-731] Feldman and associates[731] found the parents of premature infants who used skin-to-skin holding to be more sensitive to their infant's cues and to provide a better home environment after discharge. The infants in this study also had improved neurodevelopmental assessments at 6 months as compared with peers who received no skin-to-skin holding. More recently, Feldman et al.[732] have published a 10-year follow-up of this trial and found significant differences at 5 and 10 years between the two groups. Children who had received kangaroo care had attenuated stress responses, improved respiratory sinus arrhythmia, better organized sleep, and better cognitive control and mother–child reciprocity than the control group.[732]

The initiation of skin-to-skin holding will vary between institutions and is typically based on GA, weight, and the acuity of the infant. Early in the infant's admission, the PT can help to educate the family as to the benefits of skin-to-skin holding and then encourage the family to engage in the intervention as soon as the medical team approves the practice. The PT can also assist with optimal positioning to promote comfort, physiologic stability, and behavioral organization during skin-to-skin holding.

Parent Education

The therapist must assess the best learning style for the parent and provide parent education to support independence with developmental interventions during hospitalization and after transition to home.[733,734] Parent education is a focus of any neonatal physical therapy plan of care. Scales et al.[733] found that parents receiving early intervention services reported parent education on ways to support infant motor development to be more effective than direct physical therapy services. Dusing[734] found a combination of approaches to parent education to be most effective, including demonstrations, observations of assessment, written materials, and opportunities to ask questions. In order to be effective, parent education should be started early during the admission, occur regularly throughout the hospitalization, and be interdisciplinary.[735]

In order for parents to perform the challenging role of parenting, they need to understand the behaviors of a preterm baby, as well as the course of typical development and what to expect in the future. Parents need to be able to "read" their infants and respond supportively to them. Parents have benefited in the short and long term from gaining awareness of their baby's interactive and developmental capabilities and responding appropriately to them.[736-739] This supports parents' confidence and competence and facilitates their relationship with their baby. An NICU therapist is in a unique role to assist parents in parenting their infants.

The therapist can start the dialogue with the parents by asking, "How do you think your baby is doing?" and then listen to hear their concerns and their interpretations of the baby's behavior. This interaction will give the therapist a window into the parents' understanding of their baby. The therapist can invite the parents to watch the baby together, and the therapist can use that opportunity to point out the baby's unique capabilities, strategies of self-regulation, and sensitivities and vulnerabilities to the environment and medical care. Therapists can educate parents about the early development of the infant's tactile system and the importance of pleasurable touch in contrast to medical touch (abrupt, disorganizing, on/off touch) that accompanies intensive medical care. Many parents can be intimidated to touch or hold their baby and underestimate the comfort they can bring to their infant and the importance of their role when their baby requires life-saving medical care. Parental presence and holding the infant bring a familiar comfort for the infant that contrasts with the harsh and unfamiliar experiences of the NICU environment.

NICU therapists can educate parents on the typical order of preterm sensory development and coach them in how best to bond and interact with their preterm infants. Olfactory and auditory competence develops before vision.[740] Many parents are eager for direct eye contact with their infant and don't realize that their preterm baby recognizes them by their scent or their voices and may not be ready yet for eye contact and face-to-face interaction. The therapist can collaborate on a developmental care plan with the parents and through that dialogue both assess the parents' knowledge and perceptions and educate them as well. By asking the parents to name their baby's strengths, struggles with NICU care or environment, preferred comfort measures, and recommendations to support the baby, the therapist can further sharpen the parents' observations. Because therapists have an intimate knowledge of prenatal and postnatal motor and sensory development, the therapist can guide the parent with the appropriate activities for babies throughout the NICU stay.

Neonatal therapists are the best teachers to support infant motor development as well. Babies requiring NICU care can experience immobilization and altered positions. Teaching families optimal positioning and the importance of allowing active movement while supervising the baby in order to protect essential medical interventions like breathing and feeding tubes is important. Teaching parents how to handle and position the baby to facilitate a balance of flexion and extension as well as to protect the baby from iatrogenic consequences of NICU care is also essential.[114] Byrne et al.[741] found that both direct and video teaching were more effective than written instructions for teaching handling techniques.

For additional ideas regarding parent teaching strategies, see Lowman et al.'s[738] article on using developmental assessments in the NICU to empower families. Parenting is a challenging job at any stage of a child's development, but especially in infancy when children are not capable of articulating their needs and desires. Parental education should occur throughout hospital admission and be finalized as discharge approaches. It is important that parents feel comfortable with developmental interventions in order for continued participation in these activities at home.[733,735]

Positioning for Comfort and Development

Preterm infants are more likely to experience muscular fatigue, particularly in the respiratory muscles.[114] Because of the combination of hypotonia, gravitational forces, and loss of uterine constraints, the infant develops extended postures that can lead to discomfort and an imbalance of flexion and extension. Optimal positioning supports the respiratory and musculoskeletal systems and promotes infant comfort. Optimal alignment includes a neutral head and neck position with a chin tuck, scapular protraction to promote upper extremity flexion and hands midline (Fig. 4.22), flexion of the trunk with posterior pelvic tilt, and flexion of lower extremities with neutral abduction/adduction and rotation of the hips. Supports to assist the infant in maintaining an optimal position can be fabricated using blanket rolls or commercially available devices.

The preterm infant needs to have regular positional changes in order to promote comfort, prevent skin breakdown, promote the development of the musculoskeletal system, promote gas exchange in all lung fields, and maintain

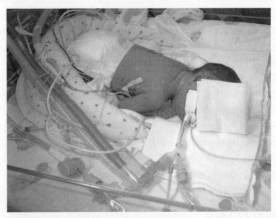

FIGURE 4.22. Infant positioned in prone position using anterior, midline roll under chest. The nest helps to promote flexion of the trunk, arms, and legs.

head shape.[114,742-745] When medically tolerated, preterm infants benefit from prone positioning. Studies have shown that the prone position improves oxygenation and ventilation, decreases GER, improves cerebral venous return, lowers intracranial pressure, and promotes sleep states and self-regulation.[746-751] Grenier et al.[751] have found that infants placed in prone have the fewest stress behaviors compared with infants placed in either side-lying or supine. However, some nurseries have policies discouraging prone for babies who have umbilical lines or who are intubated. It is best to know the nursery policy on prone positioning before recommending prone placement for an infant.

An unsupported prone position promotes shoulder retraction, neck hyperextension, truncal flattening, and hip abduction/external rotation. This position is uncomfortable and if left uncorrected can interfere with future motor development.[114,655] Infants placed in prone should have a ventral support under their chests to raise their chests from the surface and allow shoulder protraction and a more neutral neck alignment. A roll should be placed under the infant's hips to promote lower extremity flexion and a larger roll around the infant's sides and feet to provide boundaries.

Infants supported in side-lying also demonstrate decreased stress behaviors compared with supine. Other optimal effects of side-lying are symmetry and midline orientation of trunk and extremities, which promotes hands to mouth. In addition, in side-lying the respiratory diaphragm is in a gravity-eliminated plane, which lessens the work of breathing.[235,263,746] Blanket rolls are necessary to support infants placed in side-lying in order for side-lying to be beneficial to the infant. Unsupported side-lying has the potential to be stressful for the baby and provides the least amount of postural support, making the preterm infant maintain body postures and self-organization on his or her own.[235,746,751] In an effort to seek boundaries for postural control, a preterm baby is more likely to extend the neck and trunk to end ranges. These hyperextended postures are counterproductive, as tucking, flexion, and hands to face are the postures that promote comfort, calming, and self-regulation.[751]

Although left side-lying has been shown to improve reflux symptoms in adults, it has inconsistent effects on reflux symptoms in infants. In addition, a side-lying sleep position puts an infant at increased risk for SIDS.[752]

Supine allows for maximal observation and access to the infant by caregivers. However, when compared with prone or side-lying, supine poses the most challenges for the infant. In supine, the forces of gravity pull the baby into neck extension, trunk extension, scapular retraction, anterior pelvic tilt, external hip rotation, and abduction. This position does not promote calming and self-regulation. In supine, infants have shorter sleep periods; labored, less-coordinated breathing; and more episodes of GER.[753-755] Supine is the most challenging position for the preterm infant; infants should be supported with rolls to promote symmetric midline postures with head and trunk in midline, hands near mouth or

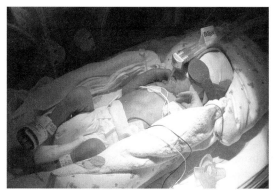

FIGURE 4.23. An infant positioned in the supine position using a nest made from a Philips Children's Medical Ventures Snuggle Up around the legs and trunk, and a Frederick T frog positioning aid around the head and neck to promote midline flexion.

face, and legs tucked close to the body with neutral hip position (Fig. 4.23). Benefits of supported supine include the unique potential for weight bearing on the posterior skull, an antidote to dolichocephaly. For the older baby, supine allows increased visual exploration of the environment and face-to-face interaction. For the micropreemie during the first few days of life, supine prevents obstruction of cerebral venous drainage and increased cerebral blood flow.[756] In 1992, the AAP[757] initiated the "Back-to-Sleep" program, which advocates supine sleeping to prevent SIDS. Preterm infants are more at risk for SIDS and should be transitioned to supine sleeping at 32 weeks PMA in order to be acclimated to supine sleeping by discharge.[757]

The very medically fragile infant may be limited in positioning options owing to technologic supports and medical conditions. Under these circumstances, the neonatal therapist strives to attain the most optimal alignment available. The goal is to promote physiologic stability and infant comfort rather than perfect biomechanical alignment. As the infant's condition improves, tolerance to positioning in better alignment and other positions is assessed.

The musculoskeletal consequences of poor alignment over time in a preterm baby include tightness of neck extensors, scapular retractors, low back extensors, and hip abductors. Tight muscles predispose the infant to reinforce certain motor patterns while inhibiting others. The repetitive use of these motor patterns can cause the formation of dominant cerebral motor pathways and the regression of the less frequently used patterns. These muscle imbalances, poor alignment, and dominant motor pathways can prevent the acquisition of important developmental skills. Basic motor milestones, such as midline head control with chin tuck, eye–hand regard, reaching, weight shifting, and rolling, are challenging for these infants.[746,758,759] Fine and gross motor delays interfere with play and exploration and delay cognitive development.[758] Research has demonstrated the persistence of an out-toeing gait in children as old as 4 to 6 years and the persistence of toe walking up to 18 months in former preterm infants.[114,760,761]

Positioning can also affect cranial molding and head shape. The skulls of preterm infants are softer and thinner than those of full-term infants, putting them at increased risk for cranial deformations.[762-764] Head shaping can affect parental perceptions of infant attractiveness and can interfere with the attachment process.[765,766] When a preterm infant is positioned in supine and is unable to sustain a midline head position, the baby's skull can be misshapen by the mattress. This head shape with elongated anterior–posterior diameter and shortened medial lateral diameter is known as dolichocephaly and can interfere with the development of midline position of the head in supine. Plagiocephaly or unilateral posterolateral head flattening can occur from prolonged supine positioning with a head preference and lack of head turning to the opposite side. Torticollis, unilateral shortening of the sternocleidomastoid muscle (SCM), can develop as a result of plagiocephaly and is characterized by ipsilateral head tilt and contralateral head rotation. Torticollis may influence the posture of not only the infant's head but also his or her trunk and may delay motor skill acquisition as well as prevent the development of binocular vision and visual convergence. To prevent cranial deformities and torticollis, commercially available gel pillows to disperse pressure across the skull can be used.[744,767-770] In addition, regular changes in the head position throughout the day and midline alignment of the head in supine can help to minimize cranial deformities and torticollis.

Scar Massage

Infants after surgery may benefit from scar massage to improve the flexibility of scar tissue and thereby improve the flexibility and alignment of the trunk and limbs. Specific treatment strategies are discussed in detail in the care path developed by Byrne and Garber.[22] It is not uncommon for babies who have required surgical intervention to their thoracic or abdominal areas to develop asymmetric postures. This may be due to the underlying anatomic lesion or result from postsurgical scarring and limitations to positioning. Positioning programs should be created and caregivers can be shown techniques to incorporate mobilization into daily routines.

Infant Hydrotherapy

Jane Sweeney[771] first piloted hydrotherapy with infants in an NICU setting in 1983. Since then, others have studied it as well and found it to be beneficial for reduction of infant pain and stress, improved weight gain, and the promotion of sleep.[771-775] Because babies are undressed and immersed in water, the risk for heat loss is increased and care must be taken with water temperature and timing to maintain infant temperature. In addition, depending on the acuity of the NICU, only a small subset of infants may meet criteria for infant hydrotherapy. Nevertheless, it is a treatment that can bring a pleasant and positive experience for an infant who is experiencing the stress of newborn intensive care. Medically

stable infants are swaddled and immersed in 37°C to 38°C water for 10 to 15 minutes. Based on infant tolerance and response, the infant may be unswaddled and pelvic and trunk movements emphasizing flexion and rotation as well as sliding the baby through the water may occur.[771-775]

Instituting a hydrotherapy program in an NICU requires methodical planning as well as collaboration with other NICU staff to determine exclusion criteria and definition of medically stable infant.

Early Interventions for Cerebral Palsy

With the change in practice to earlier identification of babies with, or at high risk for, CP, the neonatal therapist must be ready to support the young infant's motor development with the most up-to-date therapies. Earlier identification of CP promotes the early implementation of targeted, evidence-based interventions to maximize the baby's neuroplasticity. Interventions for infants with CP should be informed by the infant's type and topography of CP and individualized to the infant's clinical presentation.[776] Novak et al.[716] have published a table with clinical signs in infancy indicating motor type and lesion topography for five types of CP. The table includes descriptors from Prechtl's GMA,[777,778] MRI findings, HINE scores, and motor behavior (Table 4.13).

CP is associated with a myriad of comorbidities in addition to motor impairments. These comorbidities in decreasing order of frequency include pain, intellectual disability, hip displacement, impairments in expressive language, seizure disorder, behavior problems, incontinence, sleep disorders, blindness, feeding disorders, and deafness.[779] Goals for early interventions for CP are threefold: (1) Maximize the infant's activity-dependent neuroplasticity by establishing neural pathways and promoting motor function as well as learning, (2) minimize the development of secondary impairments such as muscle weakness and shortening, and (3) promote caregiver coping and mental health that reinforces engagement and therefore provides a positive environment for the child.[779] Although the research is limited, experts are agreeing that in order to be effective, motor interventions should be based on the principles of motor learning, particularly repeated, task-specific training, and should elicit the baby's self-generated active movements in functional activities. Environmental enrichment and caregiver involvement are also essential.[776,779,780]

Some motor interventions have supporting evidence in the literature. For example, babies with asymmetries in tone and movements of upper extremities may benefit from baby constraint-induced movement therapy (CIMT). Baby CIMT is an application of the principles of constraint-induced movement training where a removable restraint, such as a sock or a mitten, is placed on the less affected hand. In infants, where motor skills are developing in all limbs, the restraint is used for short periods daily (30 minutes) during a time when the baby is awake, well-rested, calm, and well-positioned in an infant seat or high chair with small

TABLE 4.13.	Clinical Signs of Cerebral Palsy Motor Type/Typography in Infant Period				
	Spastic Hemiplegia	Spastic Diplegia	Spastic Quadriplegia	Dyskinesia	Ataxia
General Movements Assessment at Preterm or Term Age					
	Poor Repertoire or Cramped Synchronized Movements	Cramped Synchronized Movements	Cramped Synchronized Movements of early onset and long duration	Poor Repertoire Movements	Unknown
General Movements Assessment at 52–60 wk PMA					
	Absent Fidgety plus asymmetry in segmental movements	Absent Fidgety	Absent Fidgety	Absent Fidgety plus circular arm movements and finger spreading	
Magnetic Resonance Imaging					
	Focal vascular insults; malformations; grade IV unilateral hemorrhage w/porencephaly; parietal white matter lesions involving the trigone; middle cerebral artery stroke	B white matter injury; cystic PVL; moderate to severe white matter injury	Gray matter injury; malformations; cystic PVL; severe white matter injury	Gray matter injury (thalamic and lentiform nuclei)	Normal imaging; malformations; cerebellar injury
Hammersmith Infant Neurological Examination Scores					
	50–73	<50	<50 <40 GMFCS Level IV–V	<50	Unknown
Motor Tests					
	Asymmetric hand preference; inability to transition out of floor sitting; cruising/stepping with same leg leading; decreased variability in movements	Hand function exceeds lower limb function; dislikes floor sitting; weight bearing on toes; decreased variability in movements	Head lag; persistent rounded back in supported sitting; hands fisted B; slow reach and grasp B; decreased variability in movements	Voluntary movements elicit twisting arm or neck postures; difficulty with midline hand use; switches hands during reaching; slow initiation of movements; voluntary movements and emotion worsen postures; decreased variability in movements	Nonspecific

GMFCS, Gross Motor Function Classification Score; PVL, periventricular leukomalacia.

Adapted from Novak I, Morgan C, Adde L. et al (738) Early Accurate Diagnosis and Early Intervention in Cerebral Palsy. Advances in Diagnosis and Treatment. *2017 Jama Pediatrics*. July 17,2017:e 1-11.

pillows for additional stability as needed. When the baby can sit independently, then floor sitting is used. The caregiver is in front of the baby and presents toys that are of interest and match the baby's ability. Toy selection and presentation is critical for the success of this intervention. Toys are placed within reach, to encourage self-initiated reaching and touching. When the baby is ready for grasping, a variety of easy-to-grasp toys are positioned near the hand so the baby can practice a variety of grasping patterns. Then smaller objects are presented so the baby can further refine the grasping and manipulating objects.[781] Baby CIMT in 3- to 8-month-old infants has been shown to improve the affected hand use at 18 and 24 months, compared to infant massage.[782,783] The use of "sticky mittens" during reaching training is also being investigated but has not been trialed in infants with CP or at high risk for CP diagnosis.[784-787] The implementation of all these interventions is based on providing repeated opportunities for the infant's self-initiated motor activity in order to promote activity-dependent reorganization of the corticospinal tract during its critical period of development.[788-790]

Neonatal therapists need to be creative and proactive in protecting and encouraging an infant's active movements. The culture of neonatal intensive care is to prioritize the integrity of medical interventions and respiratory support as these are in place to preserve the infant's life. Healthy babies move and infant movement is an expression of wellness. Nurses and parents need to hear that and be taught to unswaddle their babies to allow self-initiated movements while supervising the baby to prevent the accidental removal of lines or tubes. Supporting a weak infant's movements through a variety of positions, positioning rolls, slings, and springs like those used for infants with neuromotor diseases, and tethering toys to active limbs to provide the experience of causality, are ways to encourage self-generated movements. These ideas for play should be communicated to families and nurses so that opportunities for self-initiated movements can occur on a daily basis when the baby is awake. Activity gyms can be left at the bedside with instructions for positioning options that will support the infant's spontaneous movements and provide repeated daily incentives for movement and play.

» Transition to home

Normally, discharge planning begins on the first day of hospital admission; however, when caring for medically fragile high-risk infants whose survival is not certain, this may be premature. The exact date of discharge may not be predictable, but when an infant begins to demonstrate more consistent physiologic stability, steps can be initiated toward a discharge plan. Infants leaving the NICU often require unique long-term health care follow-up, and their families require time to learn their care. Current trends in health care for early discharge mean that families are required to care for younger, less stable infants, and therefore families should be included in the discharge process as soon as possible.

A good discharge plan is individually tailored to both the infant and his or her family with clearly identified goals. These goals should be communicated to the family and the medical team so as to eliminate duplication and fragmentation of family education and follow-up care, to prevent delays in access to health care, to establish links to resources for health and development in the community, and to promote success of the infant and family at home.[791-794] The medical team needs to assess the particular strengths and needs of the infant's family, including caretaking capabilities, resource requirements, social supports, and home physical facilities. The AAP[791] recommends that at least two family caregivers are able, available, and committed to learning and providing for the infant(s). Increased risk of attachment disturbances and abuse has been identified for children born prematurely and children with prenatal substance exposure. Family issues that put an infant at risk are lower education level, lack of social support, marital instability, fewer prenatal care visits, substance use, and fewer family visits during hospitalization. Active parent involvement and preparation for posthospital care demonstrate a family's readiness to care for the infant at home.[791,793]

Elements commonly identified as medical requirements for discharge from the NICU include sustained pattern of weight gain, maintenance of normal body temperature in an open environment, a successful mode of feeding (oral or tube feeding), and no episodes of apnea and bradycardia for 5 days.[791,793] Some level II and level III nurseries may have discharge requirements based on GA and weight. Feedings and medications need to be streamlined for home routines. Discharge teaching needs to be initiated early to allow the family time to process information and demonstrate proficiency. Families should be provided with blocks of time to provide care for their infant, and "rooming in" (where the parents spend the night in the hospital acting as sole caretakers for their infant) prior to discharge is recommended.[791,793]

The physical therapy regimen should also be modified for home implementation so that parents are able to carry out all of the infant's care without undue exhaustion. The therapist can assist the family in transition to the home environment in terms of positioning and providing appropriate sensory experiences and developmental activities. Positioning supports are common in the NICU; however, the AAP[757] has strongly recommended that the infants should be positioned on their backs for sleeping, and the sleep environment should be free of soft or loose bedding materials and stuffed toys or animals that could obstruct infant airways. The therapist can develop a plan to wean the infant off positioning supports and transition to back sleeping as necessary.[795] Positioning supports can be utilized and may be very important for some infants for play and activities while awake. Blanket rolls may be positioned behind the infant's shoulders and along the thighs while he or she is seated in an infant seat to promote symmetry and hands-to-midline. It is important that the therapist educate the family in safe prone positioning for play when the infant is awake as this may be forgotten in light of the back-to-sleep recommendations. Supervised prone play while the infant is awake offers opportunities to strengthen shoulder, neck, and trunk musculature in preparation for future gross motor skills.

Infants who have required intensive care may continue to have sensitivities to light and sound after discharge to home. In order to help the infant transition successfully to the home environment, the therapist can help the parents to identify the infant's vulnerabilities and make home modifications and recommendations for appropriate settings. The parents may need to dim or shade bright lights and minimize sound around the infant in order to support regulation and to promote arousal and interaction. The therapist needs to role-model problem solving and ongoing adaptations to the infant's changing cues.

Developmental activities will also change over time as the infant matures. Parents will need to continue to correct the infant's age for prematurity in order to have an accurate framework of expectations, for instance, if the infant's CA at discharge is 4 months, but the adjusted age is 1 month. Toys and play experiences should be targeted at the adjusted age. Activity recommendations should be specific to each infant; however, there are common elements for most babies in early infancy. Many babies who have had high-tech respiratory support, increased work of breathing, and GER; babies who have required supine positioning owing to medical status; and preterm infants who missed out on the cramping and crowding of the uterine experience may have difficulty initiating flexion of head, trunk, and limbs. Families should be educated in positioning and techniques to facilitate flexion within the infant's tolerance. For example, the parent places the infant on his or her lap, cradled by the thighs, to promote head midline, chin tuck, and shoulder protraction. The infant should be positioned so that his or her legs are flexed against the parent's abdomen. In this position, the infant can gaze at the parent's face to promote downward convergent gaze and chin tuck (Fig. 4.24). Other activities that fit into families' daily routines can also be provided. For infants whose age or adjusted age is at term or near term, activities should promote symmetry, flexion, and midline orientation.

In addition to providing families with home programs, referrals should be made to community resources such as

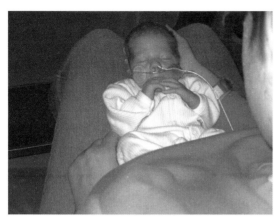

FIGURE 4.24. Interaction with an infant in the supine position on the parent's lap.

early intervention. Early intervention services are programs throughout the United States and its territories funded by federal and local governments that are mandated by the Individuals with Disabilities Education Act (IDEA). Early intervention services provide developmental services for children and their families. These programs can provide a variety of therapy and educational services for infants at risk for developmental delays or documented delays and their families. However, the period between referral to the program and initiation of services can be 45 days or longer.[796] Therefore, it may be necessary to set up interim services provided by outpatient or private home-based therapists until early intervention services can start. Interim services are particularly necessary when a child may need frequent monitoring of a splint or peripheral nerve injury such as brachial plexus injury.

» Neonatal follow-up services

Infants who have required neonatal intensive care are at high risk for both major and minor disabilities. Forty-eight percent of high-risk infants demonstrate transient neurologic abnormalities consisting of hypotonia or hypertonia, and 10% go on to demonstrate major neurologic sequelae such as CP, hydrocephalus, blindness, seizure disorder, and hearing impairment.[375,391,797-802] Minor neurodevelopmental and neurobehavioral impairments include IQ significantly lower than full-term siblings, "temperament problems, language delays, fine motor deficits, visual-motor deficits, sensory integration dysfunction, social incompetence, emotional immaturity, attention deficits, learning disorders, and ultimately diminished school performance."[803] These impairments are prevalent among survivors and become increasingly more apparent with age.[65,350,366,394,802-808] In addition, LBW infants and critically ill term and near-term infants who required intensive care have long-term health issues such as frequent rehospitalization, shunt complications, orthopedic and eye surgeries, CLD, and failure to thrive.[391,463,797,805,809,810] For these reasons, NICU graduates require specialized long-term

follow-up services. The AAP recommends follow-up services for these developmental concerns as well as for organized postdischarge tracking and to provide information regarding outcomes for this population.[791,798] Most NICUs are associated with neonatal follow-up programs to monitor the outcomes for these high-risk neonates and to determine the effects of NICU interventions on outcomes. In addition, these programs maintain outcome databases, conduct single-center studies, and participate in larger multicentered studies. Tracking information includes growth parameters over time (head circumference, height, and weight), feeding and nutrition, medication use, illnesses and hospitalizations, pain, home technology use (oxygen, apnea monitor, feeding tube/pump), sleep position and sleep patterns, car seat use, follow-up with other specialists, home environment, caretaking plan, parental concerns, and medical and neurologic examinations. Standardized developmental assessments are administered as part of the follow-up program. There are many from which to choose; the *Bayley Scales of Infant and Toddler Development Edition III (BSID III)* is the recognized standard for measuring infant development between 0 and 42 months. Many follow-up programs will administer the BSID III in conjunction with other domain-specific assessments for social and emotional development, gross and fine motor development, language and behavior development, and family function.[798,797] Babies should be seen in the follow-up program (not to be confused with the first pediatrician visit, which should occur the first week from discharge) at 3 months adjusted age unless the discharge team, PT, community pediatrician, home-visiting nurse, or caregiver has concerns warranting earlier follow-up. Generally, babies who are discharged with technologic supports such as tracheostomy, supplemental oxygen, apnea monitor, and feeding tube are seen within the first month after discharge. The babies return for neonatal follow-up every 3 months for the first year, every 6 months in the second year, and yearly from 3 years adjusted age to school age. However, this schedule can change to more frequent follow-up if more specific concerns are being monitored. For infants who are followed as part of a study, the frequency may be determined as per the protocol for that particular study.

The follow-up team is usually composed of professionals from many disciplines and can include a developmental pediatrician, neonatologist, pediatric nurse practitioner, social worker, psychologist, nutritionist, and physical, occupational, and speech therapists. Administrative support staff includes a clinic coordinator, data manager, and secretary. Owing to the multidisciplinary nature of the follow-up clinic, the visits are highly coordinated for efficiency and to address the needs of the high-risk infants and their families. Families often perceive the clinic staff as "experts" in the care of their babies and will utilize them as a resource and to confirm recommendations made by outside health care providers. Some members of the follow-up team may also have provided care for the infant and his or her family during hospitalization in the NICU, which may provide the family with a level of comfort and familiarity. In this way, the family's needs identified during the hospitalization can be more effectively followed, and the family may also feel more at ease to discuss new concerns. The social worker can identify and address financial issues and social risk factors such as poverty, housing, substance abuse, and lack of education, which can pose additional risks for the health and development of the infant. Studies have shown that environmental factors such as maternal years of education and socioeconomic status can mitigate or exacerbate the biologic risk factors typically associated with neonatal intensive care.[65,366,811-813]

PTs bring a unique strength to the follow-up of high-risk infants as their background in kinesiology and development allows them to examine the qualitative aspects of infant movement. Understanding the fundamental components of a movement pattern allows the therapist to determine whether the infant is developing a balanced repertoire of movement patterns needed for the progression of development or is reusing the same maladaptive patterns that prevent this progression. It is helpful for PTs to take part in a neonatal follow-up clinic for their own understanding of development and long-term outcomes of high-risk infants. It is important that therapists observe the changes in infants over time as some of the "red flags" seen in the NICU may be transient and may be replaced by more typical movement patterns as the infant develops. It is also a good learning experience, albeit sad, to see babies who have seemingly left the NICU unscathed only to return to a follow-up clinic with atypical neurodevelopmental assessments. Although this is sobering, it can serve to challenge the therapist to seek out other assessment tools and look more closely for subtleties in infant performance. While participating in a follow-up clinic, therapists may also see the responsiveness or limitations of community resources and perhaps learn of new resources that may prove to be effective. In addition, therapists participating in neonatal follow-up programs have the opportunity to see family resilience and the challenges a family may face on the journey that began in the NICU. The experiences of neonatal follow-up care provide the therapist caring for infants in the NICU with a wealth of information, which should be used when intervening with infants in the NICU, providing discharge recommendations, and communicating with families regarding future outcomes.

Summary

The last century has seen the evolution of the subspecialty of neonatology, and as this practice has changed over time, so too has the role of the PT in the NICU. The increasing understanding of preterm infant development and the effects of the environment, neonatal care, and family involvement on the evolving infant systems have led to a unique and specialized opportunity for PTs to act as developmental specialists within the setting of the NICU. In order to effectively and appropriately fulfill this need, therapists

require in-depth understanding and knowledge of medical conditions and interventions; fetal and infant behavior and development; family stresses related to pregnancy, child birth, and transition to parenthood within the NICU; risk factors; and long-term outcomes. In addition, the therapist needs to have a mentored practice within the NICU setting and participate in a neonatal follow-up program. It is also important that the PT be an integrated member of the team providing care for the high-risk baby and his or her family. The PT must take the initiative to keep abreast of the rapidly changing technology and management and their effects on infant health and development. This requires keeping current with both physical therapy and neonatal literature.

The therapist practicing in the NICU requires the advanced knowledge and skills as outlined previously and the time, training, and mentoring to achieve the highest level of practice that their infants deserve. To be a PT in the NICU is a meaningful and rewarding role and is well worth the time and training.

CASE STUDIES

KAYLA

Kayla was born at 23 3/7 weeks' gestation with a birth weight of 570 g (1 lb 4 oz) (Fig. 4.25) to a married 30-year-old G2P2 mother who had good prenatal care. Maternal complications included group B *Streptococcus*, bleeding at 22 weeks, and preterm labor at 23 3/7 weeks, at which time she was dilated and contracting. The infant was born via vaginal breech delivery with Apgar scores of 4 at 1 minute and 7 at 5 minutes. Resuscitative efforts in the delivery room included intubation, positive-pressure ventilation, and surfactant. Kayla was transported to the NICU, where she was placed on conventional ventilator, and umbilical artery and umbilical vein lines were placed. Phototherapy was initiated because of bruising.

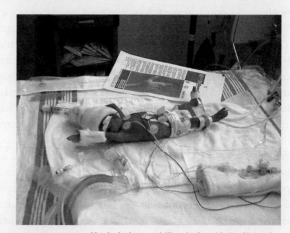

FIGURE 4.25. Kayla being stabilized after birth. Note the size of the infant versus the size of the glove wrapper.

Because of worsening respiratory status, Kayla was placed on HFOV, which she received for 33 days before she was able to wean to CMV. She was able to be extubated and placed on CPAP after 2 months on the conventional ventilator. After 2 weeks on CPAP, Kayla was weaned to a nasal cannula, but had to be reintubated and placed on mechanical ventilation 2 weeks later because of sepsis. Kayla was extubated and placed on nasal cannula 2 weeks later. She was finally weaned off all respiratory support at 143 days of life.

Kayla's hospital course was complicated by severe BPD, PIE, large PDA requiring surgical ligation, hyperbilirubinemia, mild supravalvular pulmonic stenosis, and multiple bouts of sepsis, including meningitis, *Pseudomonas tracheitis*, methicillin-resistant *Staphylococcus aureus* (MRSA), and pneumonia.

Pain Management

Pain management was initiated on Kayla's first day of life with the administration of morphine. She continued to receive morphine until day of life 34 when a tapered wean was completed. Morphine was restarted on day of life 120 when she required reintubation and mechanical ventilation. Kayla was weaned off morphine slowly beginning day of life 133 and ending on day of life 143. She tolerated this weaning process well, and neonatal abstinence scores were followed closely for any adverse response to withdrawal. Throughout her hospitalization, Kayla was assessed for pain by all staff. Pain assessments were also performed by the PT and documented in the chart after each interaction with the therapist.

Physical Therapy Services

Kayla was referred for physical therapy services at 2 weeks of life (25 weeks' postconceptional age). The PT reviewed Kayla's history by thoroughly reading her medical chart and discussing Kayla's status with her nurse. Kayla's nurse reported that she was very restless and became irritable with hands-on care. The PT observed Kayla in her isolette before, during, and after caregiving activities. At this time Kayla was intubated, requiring HFOV, and was under phototherapy. She demonstrated increased extensor posturing of her head, trunk, and extremities and jerky restless movements prior to care. Sensitivity to sound and light was also noted. Kayla had very low tolerance to handling and position changes during care. Her stress signs included color changes, increased HR, oxygen desaturation, and motor stress signs of arching of head and trunk and extension of extremities. Kayla was unable to effectively utilize any self-calming behaviors and was difficult to calm with external supports. She did respond to facilitated tucking and firm touch when provided long enough for her to relax and settle into the position. After care she was pale and exhausted.

Physical Therapy Goals

Physical therapy goals at this time were as follows:

1. To decrease environmental stress
2. To promote calming behaviors
3. To promote flexed postures for calming and optimal body alignment for musculoskeletal development

4. To assist family and caregivers in identifying and responding to Kayla's cues
5. To provide education to the family regarding developmentally supportive care

Suggestions included:

1. Minimizing environmental stimulation by covering her isolette and shading her eyes from bright lights, alerting people to keep noise levels down around her bedside with a sign, and education
2. Pacing care activities, providing rest breaks with facilitated tucking, using slow movements, and firm touch
3. Positioning in flexion in a deep nest and varying positions between prone, side-lying, and supine as tolerated
4. Allowing for hands to head and grasping, and offering the pacifier for self-calming

Kayla's mother visited every day and the PT was able to meet with her to discuss Kayla's status and suggestions to support her development. Together, they looked at Kayla's cues and discussed strategies for calming and bonding. Kayla's father visited in the evening, and her mother shared the suggestions for developmentally supportive care with him.

For the next 2 months Kayla continued to be an extremely fragile, critically ill infant with high respiratory requirements, surgical ligation of her PDA, and episodes of sepsis. PTs continued to observe Kayla and adjust her developmental care plan as appropriate. At 10 weeks of age (33 weeks' postconceptual age [PCA]), Kayla was able to wean from HFOV to the conventional ventilator. She continued to have low tolerance for handling, but was easier to console with the pacifier and firm touch/containment in flexion. She also demonstrated attempts at self-calming with hand-to-head, grasping, and foot-bracing behaviors. The PT continued to work with the nursing staff and Kayla's family to develop care plans to promote self-calming, optimal positioning, and tolerance to caregiving activities. At this time Kayla's parents were practicing kangaroo care and holding Kayla daily (Fig. 4.26). The PT was able to provide suggestions for positioning Kayla during kangaroo care.

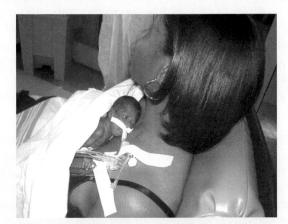

FIGURE 4.26. Kayla and her mother practicing kangaroo care, or skin-to-skin holding.

Kayla made slow improvements medically, and at 36 weeks' PCA she still required mechanical ventilation. Her tolerance to handling and position changes was improving. She was able to maintain a quiet, alert state using her pacifier and containment for support. Even with external supports she had limited tolerance for visual or social stimulation. Kayla was very sensitive to light and sound in the environment. Physical therapy examination revealed increased flexor posturing in her lower extremities, with full passive range of motion. She held her upper extremities in scapular retraction, shoulder abduction, and external rotation. Kayla had antigravity movement of her extremities through limited range of motion with jerky, tremulous quality of movement. She still frequently moved into extension rather than flexion. Despite the use of a gel pillow, the time spent on HFOV had left Kayla with flattening of the lateral sides of her head, or dolichocephaly. She held her head in extension with shortening of her capital and neck extensors. Tightness in her thoracic, lumbar, and sacral areas was also noted. Goals for Kayla included

1. Maintaining a quiet alert state for increasing duration of time
2. Improved ability to self-calm
3. Neutral head alignment with decreased tightness in cervical spine
4. Increased flexibility in lumbosacral spine
5. Decreased tightness in scapulae and shoulders
6. Increased antigravity flexion movement
7. An additional goal was for Kayla's family and caregivers to be independent in positioning and developmentally supportive activities.

The therapist continued to work with Kayla's family and nurses in reading her cues and progressing handling and social interactions to her tolerance. The therapist also provided positioning suggestions to promote midline alignment, flexion, and shoulder protraction. Gentle mobilization to her spine was provided, starting in the lumbosacral area and slowly moving proximally over the course of several weeks, based on Kayla's response.

Over the next month, Kayla was weaned off the ventilator to CPAP and then to nasal cannula. She had one setback in her respiratory stability because of sepsis, but was able to be weaned off all support by 43 weeks' PCA. The therapist continued to work on the previously stated goals until time of discharge to home. Concerns at the time of discharge included

1. Sensitivity to light and sound
2. Limited tolerance to handling
3. Limited range of motion in cervical spine and shoulders
4. Delayed postural responses

Her strengths were robust and defined behavioral states, improved ability to self-calm, and greater availability for social interactions. She was able to visually fix on an object and track it to the left and right. Her parents were able to read Kayla's behavioral cues and respond appropriately. Suggestions for home were provided to her parents, who were able to demonstrate independence in performing these activities. Kayla was discharged to home at 45 weeks' PCA without any respiratory support and

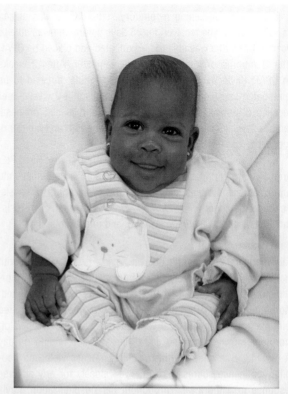

FIGURE 4.27. Kayla at 7.5 months chronologic age, or 3.25 months adjusted age.

taking all feedings by bottle. Follow-up services included ophthalmology, special babies clinic (neonatal follow-up), cardiology, and early intervention services (Fig. 4.27).

BABY BOY

History

Baby boy was born at community hospital by spontaneous vaginal delivery to a 22-year-old G1 mother at 26 weeks 1 day gestation. Maternal medical and surgical history was unremarkable. Pregnancy history was significant for advanced cervical dilation, nephrolithiasis, gestational diabetes, and yeast infection. Mom went into preterm labor and received two courses of betamethasone and magnesium for neuroprotection. Baby required CPAP at birth and was admitted to the NICU.

Baby was in the community NICU for approximately 1 month and was then transferred to tertiary care NICU at 30 weeks 1 day PMA for continued treatment of sepsis, meningitis, and management of cerebral abscesses under the care of the neurosurgical team. The baby was treated in the tertiary care NICU for approximately 4 months and then in the NICU step-down unit for 2.5 weeks prior to discharge home at 50 weeks 1 day PMA.

Physical Therapy Course

Initial physical therapy examination was done at 31 weeks 4 days in the tertiary care NICU. The baby was observed during routine nursing care. Autonomic instability (desaturations, color changes, increased work of breathing [WOB]), motoric stress (tremulous and limp), and diffuse awake calm state were noted.

PT was planned for one to two times/week. Interventions were ongoing assessment, positioning, environmental modifications, facilitation of self-regulation, parent education, progression of activities as medical status allows, and assistance with discharge planning.

Short-term PT goals: time frame: 6 to 8 weeks

1. Baby will demonstrate regular RR for 60 to 90 seconds during nursing care session.
2. Baby will utilize NNS on binky for self-regulation for 20 to 30 seconds during nursing care session.
3. Baby will demonstrate stable vital signs during nursing care session.

Long-term PT goals: time frame: during hospitalization

1. Baby's developmental potential will be maximized.
2. Baby will demonstrate age-appropriate passive range of motion (ROM) and strength of limbs.
3. Baby will demonstrate no skin breakdown.
4. Baby will demonstrate rounded head shape and no head preference.

Recommendations:

1. Keep lighting dim at bed space to encourage alert periods.
2. Keep noise to a minimum at bed space to promote infant regulation.
3. Encourage family to do kangaroo skin-to-skin holding and to be involved with infant care tasks.
4. Offer baby pacifier during nursing care sessions and feedings to promote development of NNS for self-regulation.
5. Vary infant position to promote muscle strengthening.
6. Keep baby's head in midline in supine to promote head shaping and prevent dolichocephaly.
7. Use rolls under shoulders to promote midline hand contact and hands to face when baby is in supine.
8. Use caution with positioning devices in order to promote infant active ROM and not restrict movements.

Outcome Measures:

31 weeks 4 days PMA: Prechtl's GMA Poor Repertoire movements—These types of movements are a nonspecific finding that is of low clinical value, as the vast majority of infants with this finding develop normally.

34 weeks 4 days PMA: Prechtl's GMA Cramped Synchronized Movements—This finding is abnormal and indicates a need for very close follow-up, as having cramped synchronized movements indicates a much higher risk for CP. It is important to note that these movements do not have definitive negative implications for later movement, as there are false-positive results. For this reason, neurodevelopmental follow-up is critical to further delineate risk and provide any necessary intervention.

Physical Therapy Reevaluation at PMA 39 weeks 1 day: noted persistent right-handed fisting during reevaluation session

Short-term PT goals: time frame: 6 to 8 weeks

1. Baby will follow toy or face in 160-degree arc horizontally in supine with active head turning.
2. Baby will independently clear airway in prone twice per session.
3. Baby will sustain neutral head position in supported sitting for 12 to 15 seconds.
4. Baby's family will be independent with three developmentally supportive activities.
5. Baby's plagiocephaly score will improve by 5% by caliper measurements.

Increase Physical Therapy to two times/week; Occupational Therapy consult recommended
Recommendations:

1. Vary infant position (B side-lying, supine and infant seating) during day to promote motor development.
2. Place infant in prone when awake and supervised to promote neck and shoulder girdle strengthening and promote motor development.
3. Hold at shoulder to promote neck strengthening and motor development.
4. Offer pacifier and containment to encourage flexion during nursing care sessions.
5. Approach from left side of crib to promote head turning to left and to promote head shaping.
6. Encourage parent involvement at bedside and kangaroo skin-to-skin holding.
7. Consider turning crib to promote interaction to left of infant.

Outcome Measures: Plagiocephaly Assessment

Cephalic index = 85.6%
Cranial width (M/L) = 105 mm
Cranial length (A/P) = 123 mm
Cranial vault asymmetry index = 5.6 mild
Diagonal A = 124 mm
Diagonal B = 117 mm
Head circumference = not measured
Narrative description = mild R plagiocephaly

Physical Therapy Reevaluation after G tube placement at 47.6 weeks PMA
Short-term PT goals: time frame: 6 to 8 weeks

1. Baby will track toy or face in 160-degree arc with active head turning in supported sitting.
2. Baby will kick lower extremities (LE's) in three consecutive cycles 1/3 trials in side-lying.
3. Baby will sustain head extension in prone on forearms for 8 to 10 seconds.
4. Baby will demonstrate mutual fingering in supine three times per session.

Long-term PT goals: time frame: during hospitalization

5. Baby's developmental potential will be maximized.
6. Baby will demonstrate age-appropriate passive ROM and strength of limbs.

7. Baby will demonstrate no skin breakdown.
8. Baby will improve R plagiocephaly by 2 to 4 mm when measured by calipers.
9. Baby's family will be independent with three developmentally supportive activities.

Occupational Therapy increased frequency to two times/week

Discharge to home at 50 weeks 1 day PMA. Set up with outpatient PT once/week in addition to early intervention and neonatal follow-up services.

REFERENCES

1. Prescott S, Hebman MC. Premature infant care in the early 20th century. *J Obstet Gynecol Neonatal Nurs.* 2017;46:637-646.
2. Robertson AF, Baker JP. Lessons from the past. *Semin Fetal Neonatal Med.* 2005;(10):23-30.
3. Avery ME. Neonatology. *Pediatrics.* 1998;2(1):270-271.
4. Nelson NM. A decimillennium in neonatology. *J Pediatr.* 2000;(137):731-735.
5. Kronn D. Navigating newborn screening in the NICU: a user's guide. *NeoReviews.* 2019;20(5):e280-e291.
6. U.S. National Library of Medicine. Accessed July 10, 2019. https://clinicaltrials.gov/ct2/results?term=newborn&Search=Apply&recrs=a&recrs=f&age_v=&gndr=&type=&rslt=
7. Miletta I, Martel M-J, Ribeiro da Silva M, McNeil MC. Guidelines for the institutional implementation of developmental neuroprotective care in the neonatal intensive care unit. Part A: background & rationale. *Can J Nurs Res.* 2017;49(2):46-62.
8. Bruton C, Meckley J, Nelson L. NICU Nurses and Families Partnering to provide neuroprotective, family-centered, developmental care. *Neonatal Netw.* 2018;37(6):351-357.
9. Eliades C. Mitigating infant medical trauma in the NICU: skin to skin contact as a trauma-informed, age–appropriate best practice. *Neonatal Netw.* 2018;37(6):343-350.
10. Higgins RD, Shankaran S. The neonatal research network: history since 2003, future directions and challenges. *Semin Perinatol.* 2016;40:337-340.
11. Committee on Fetus and Newborn. Policy Statement. Levels of neonatal care. *Pediatrics.* 2012;130(3):587-597.
12. Vergara ER, Bigsby R. *Developmental and Therapeutic Interventions in the NICU.* Paul H Brookes Publishing Co; 2004.
13. Sweeney JK. Assessment of the special care nursery environment: effects on the high-risk infant. In: Wilhelm IJ, ed. *Physical Therapy Assessment in Early Infancy.* Church Livingstone; 1993.
14. Sweeney JK, Swanson MW. Low birth weight infants: neonatal care and follow-up. In: Umphred DA, ed. *Neurological Rehabilitation.* 4th ed. Mosby; 2001.
15. Sweeney JK, Heriza CB, Blanchard Y. Neonatal physical therapy. Part I: clinical competencies and neonatal intensive care unit clinical training models. *Pediatr Phys Ther.* 2009;21:296-307.
16. Campbell SK. *Decision Making in Pediatric Neurologic Physical Therapy.* Churchill Livingstone; 1999.
17. Sweeney JK, Heriza CB, Blanchard Y, et al. Neonatal physical therapy. Part II: practice frameworks and evidence-based practice guidelines. *Pediatr Phys Ther.* 2010;22:2-16.
18. Scull S, Deitz J. Competencies for physical therapists in the neonatal intensive care unit (NICU). *Pediatr Phys Ther.* 1989;1:11-14.
19. Sweeney JK, Heriza CB, Reilly MA, et al. Practice guidelines for the physical therapist in the neonatal intensive care unit (NICU). *Pediatr Phys Ther.* 1999;11:119-132.
20. Campbell SK. Use of care paths to improve patient management. *Phys Occupat Ther Pediatr.* 2013;33(1):27-38.
21. Byrne E, Campbell SK. Physical therapy observation and assessment in the neonatal intensive care unit (NICU). *Phys Occupat Ther Pediatr.* 2013;33(1):39-74.
22. Byrne E, Garber J. Physical therapy intervention in the neonatal intensive care unit. *Phys Occupat Ther Pediatr.* 2013;33(1):75-110.
23. Garber J. Oral-motor function and feeding intervention. *Phys Occupat Ther Pediatr.* 2013;33(1):111-138.
24. Goldstein LA. Family support and education. *Phys Occupat Ther Pediatr.* 2013;33(1):139-161.
25. Barbosa VM. Teamwork in the neonatal intensive care unit. *Phys Occupat Ther Pediatr.* 2013;33(1):5-26.
26. Kamm K, Thelen E, Jenson JL. A dynamical systems approach to motor development. *Phys Ther.* 1990;70(12):763-775.
27. Heriza CB. Implications of dynamic systems approach to understanding infant kicking behavior. *Phys Ther.* 1991;71(3):222-234.
28. Heriza CB. Motor development: traditional and contemporary theories. Contemporary management of motor control problems. In: *Proceedings of the II Step Conference.* Foundation of Physical Therapy; 1991.
29. Lockman JS, Thelen E. Developmental biodynamics: brain, body, behavior connections. *Child Dev.* 1993;64:953.
30. Thelen E. Motor development: a new synthesis. *Am Psychol.* 1995;50(2):79-90.
31. Guiliani CA. Theories of motor control: new concepts for physical therapy. Contemporary management of motor control problems. In: Proceedings of the II Step Conference.
32. Horak FB. Assumptions underlying motor control for neurologic rehabilitation. Contemporary management of motor control problems. In: *Proceedings of the II Step Conference.* Foundation for Physical Therapy; 1991.
33. Edelman GM. *Neural Darwinism: Theory of Neuronal Group Selection.* Oxford University Press; 1989.
34. Edelman GM. *Bright Air, Brilliant Fire: On the Matter of the Mind.* Basic Books Inc; 1992.
35. Hadders Algra M. The neuronal group selection theory: a framework to explain variation in normal development. *Dev Med Child Neurol.* 2000;42:566-572.
36. Edelman GM. Neural Darwinism: selection and re-entrant signalling in higher brain function. *Neuron.* 1993;10:115-125.
37. Hadders Algra M. The neuronal group selection theory: promising principles for understanding and treating developmental motor disorders. *Dev Med Child Neurol.* 2000;42:707-715.
38. Prechtl HFM. Developmental neurology of the fetus. *Bailliere's Clin Obstetr Gynecol.* 1988;2(1):21-36.
39. Sporns O, Edelman GM. Solving Bernstein's problem: a proposal for the development of coordinated movements by selection. *Child Dev.* 1993;64:960-981.
40. Hadders Algra M. Variation and variability: key words in human motor development. *Phys Ther.* 2010;90:1823-1837.
41. Smith LB, Thelan E. Development as a dynamic system. *Trends Cogn Sci.* 2003;7(8):343-348.
42. Adolph KE. Learning in the development of locomotion. *Monogr Soc Res Child Dev.* 1997;62(1-4):1-158.
43. Campbell SK. The child's development of functional movement. In: Campbell SK, Palisano RJ, Orlin MN, eds. *Physical Therapy for Children.* 4th ed. Elsevier Saunders; 2012.
44. Als H, Duffy FH, McAnulty GB, et al. Early experience alters brain function and structure. *Pediatrics.* 2004;11(4):846-857.
45. World Health Organization. *International Classification of Functioning, Disability and Handicaps.* World Health Organization; 2001.
46. Atkinson HL, Nixon-Cave K. A tool for clinical reasoning and reflection using the International Classification of Functioning, Disability, and Health (ICF) framework and patient management model. *Phys Ther.* 2011;91(3):416-430.
47. Als H. Toward a synactive theory of development: promise for the assessment and support of infant individuality. *Infant Ment Health J.* 1982;3(4):229-243.

48. Als H. Infant individuality: assessing patterns of very early development. In: Call J, Galenson E, Tyson RL, eds. *Frontiers of Infant Psychiatry*. Basic Books; 1983.

49. Als H. A synactive model of neonatal behavioral organization: framework for the assessment of neurobehavioral development in the premature infant and for support of infants and parents in the neonatal intensive care environment. *Phys Occup Ther Pediatr*. 1986;6:3-55.

50. Als H, Lawhon G, Brown E, et al. Individualized behavioral and environmental care for the very low birth weight preterm infant at high risk for bronchopulmonary dysplasia: neonatal intensive care unit and developmental outcome. *Pediatrics*. 1986;78(6):1123-1132.

51. Als H, Lester BM, Brazelton TB. Dynamics of the behavioral organization of the premature infant: a theoretical perspective. In: Field TM, Sostek AM, Goldberg S, et al., eds. *Infants Born at Risk*. Spectrum; 1979.

52. Als H. *Manual for the Naturalistic Observation of Newborn Behavior: Newborn Individualized Developmental Care and Assessment Program (NIDCAP)*. National NIDCAP Training Center; 1995.

53. Lawhon G, Melzar A. Developmental care of the very low birth weight infant. *J Perinatal Neonatal Nurs*. 1988;2(1):56-65.

54. Bowden VR, Greenberg CS, Donaldson NE. Developmental care of the newborn. *Online J Clin Innovations*. 2000;3(7):1-77.

55. Gilkerson L, Als H. Role of reflective process in the implementation of developmentally supportive care in the newborn intensive care nursery. *Infants Young Child*. 1995;7(4):20-28.

56. Johnson B. Family centered care: four decades of progress. *Fam Syst Health*. 2000;18(2):137.

57. Chappel J. *Advancing Clinical Practice and Perspectives of Developmental Care in the NICU*. NICU; 2004.

58. Als H, Lawhon G, Duffy FH, et al. Individualized developmental care for the very low-birth-weight preterm infant. *JAMA*. 1994;272(11):853-858.

59. Becker PT, Grunwald PC, Moorman J, et al. Outcomes of developmentally supportive nursing care for very low birth weight infants. *Nurs Res*. 1991;40:150-155.

60. Becker PT, Grunwald PC, Moorman J, et al. Effects of developmental care on behavioral organization in very-low-birth-weight infants. *Nurs Res*. 1993;42(4):214-220.

61. Buehler DM, Als H, Duffy FH, et al. Effectiveness of individualized developmental care for low-risk preterm infants: behavioral and electrophysiologic evidence. *Pediatrics*. 1995;96(5):923-932.

62. Symington A, Pinelli J. Distilling the evidence on developmental care: a systematic review. *Adv Neonatal Care*. 2002;2(4):198-221.

63. Symington A, Pinelli J. Developmental care for promoting development and preventing morbidity in preterm infants (Cochrane Review). *Cochrane Database Syst Rev*. 2002;4.

64. Franck LS, Lawhon G. Environmental and behavioral strategies to prevent and manage neonatal pain. *Semin Perinatol*. 1998;22(5):434-443.

65. Hill S, Engle S, Jorgensen J, et al. Effects of facilitated tucking during routine care of infants born preterm. *Pediatr Phys Ther*. 2005;17:158-163.

66. Ward-Larson C, Horn RA, Gosnell F. The efficacy of facilitated tucking for relieving procedural pain of endotracheal suctioning in very low birth weight infants. *Am J Matern Child Nurs*. 2004;29(3):151-156.

67. Taquino L, Blackburn S. The effects of containment during suctioning and heelstick on physiological and behavioral responses of preterm infants. *Neonatal Nurs*. 1994;13(7):55.

68. Corff KE, Seideman R, Venkataraman PS, et al. Facilitated tucking: a nonpharmacologic comfort measure for pain in preterm neonates. *J Gynecol Neonatal Nurs*. 1995;24(2):143-147.

69. Corff KE. An effective comfort measure for minor pain and stress in preterm infants: facilitated tucking. *Neonatal Netw*. 1993;12(8):74.

70. Corbo MG, Mansi G, Stagni A, et al. Nonnutritive sucking during heelstick procedures decreases behavioral distress in the newborn infant. *Biol Neonate*. 2000;77:162-167.

71. Field T, Goldson E. Pacifying effects of nonnutritive sucking on term and preterm neonates during heelstick procedures. *Pediatrics*. 1984;74(6):1012-1015.

72. Pinelli J, Symington A. How rewarding can a pacifier be? A systematic review of nonnutritive sucking in preterm infants. *Neonatal Netw*. 2000;19(8):41-48.

73. Reeves E. A synthesis of the literature on trauma-informed care. *Issues Ment Health Nurs*. 2015;36(9):698-709.

74. Coughlin ME. *Trauma-Informed Care in the NICU. Evidence-Based Practice Guidelines for Neonatal Clinicians*. Springer Publishing Co; 2017.

75. Discenza D. "Mental Health" in the NICU: time to catch up and provide Trauma-informed care for families and pros. *Neonatal Netw*. 2017;36(5):318-320.

76. Galvin E, Boyers L, Schwartz PK, et al. Challenging the precepts of family-centered care: testing a philosophy. *Pediatr Nurs*. 2000;26(6):625-632.

77. Harrison H. The principles of family-centered neonatal care. *Pediatrics*. 1993;92(5):643-650.

78. Brazelton TB, Cramer BG. *The Earliest Relationship*. Addison-Wesley Publishing Company Inc.; 1990.

79. Lawhon G. Management of stress in premature infants. In: Angelini DJ, Whelan Knapp CM, Gibes RM, eds. *Perinatal-Neonatal Nursing: A Clinical Handbook*. Blackwell Scientific Publications; 1986.

80. Mercer RT. *Nursing Care for Parents at Risk*. Charles B Slack Inc; 1977.

81. Bibring GL. Some considerations of the psychological process in pregnancy. *Psychoanal Study Child*. 1959;14:113-121.

82. Bibring GL, Dwyer TF, Huntington DS, et al. A study of the psychological processes in pregnancy and of the earliest mother-child relationship. *Psychoanal Study Child*. 1961;16:9-24.

83. Cowan CP, Cowan PA. *When Partners Become Parents: The Big Life Change for Couples*. Lawrence Erlbaum Associates Publishers; 1999.

84. Cowan CP, Cowan PA. Interventions to ease the transition to parenthood. *Fam Relations*. 1995;44:412-423.

85. Cowan CP, Cowan PA, Heming G, et al. Transitions to parenthood his, hers, and theirs. *J Fam Issues*. 1985;6(4):451-481.

86. Stainton MC, McNeil D, Harvey S. Maternal tasks of uncertain motherhood. *Matern Child Nurs J*. 1992;20(3,4):113-231.

87. Miles MS, Brunssen SH. Psychometric properties of the parental stressor scale: infant hospitalization. *Adv Neonatal Care*. 2003;3(4):189-196.

88. Melnyk BM, Alpert-Gillis LJ, Hensel PB, et al. Helping mothers cope with a critically ill child: a pilot test of the COPE intervention. *Res Nurs Health*. 1997;20:3-14.

89. *Diagnostic and Statistical Manual of Mental Disorders*. 4th ed. American Psychiatric Association; 1994.

90. Jotzo M, Poets CF. Helping parents cope with the trauma of premature birth: an evaluation of a trauma-preventive psychological intervention. *Pediatrics*. 2005;115(4):915-919.

91. Holditch-Davis D, Bartlett TR, Blickman AL, et al. Posttraumatic stress symptoms in mothers of premature infants. *J Obstet Gynecol Neonatal Nurs*. 2003;32(2):161-171.

92. Peebles-Kleiger MJ. Pediatric and neonatal intensive care hospitalization as traumatic stressor: implications for intervention. *Bull Menninger Clin*. 2000;64(2):257-280.

93. DeMier RL, Hynan MT, Harris HB, et al. Perinatal stressors as predictors of symptoms of posttraumatic stress in mothers of infants at high risk. *J Perinatal*. 1996;16(4):276-280.

94. Affleck G, Tennen H. The effect of newborn intensive care on parents' psychological well-being. *Child Health Care*. 1991;20(1):6-14.

95. Sydnor-Greenberg N, Dokken D, Ahmann E. Coping and caring in different ways: understanding and meaningful involvement. *Pediatr Nurs*. 2000;26(2):185-190.

96. Clubb RL. Chronic sorrow: adaptation patterns of parents with chronically ill children. *Pediatr Nurs*. 1991;17(5):461-466.

97. Pohlman S. Fathers role in the NICU care: evidence-based practice. In: Kenner C, McGrath JM, eds. *Developmental Care of Newborns and Infants: A Guide for Health Professionals*. Mosby; 2004.

98. Kaplan S, Bolender DL. Embryology. In: Polin RA, Fox WW, Abman SH, eds. *Fetal and Neonatal Physiology*. 2nd ed. WB Saunders Co; 1998.

99. Graham EM, Morgan MA. Growth before term. In: Batshaw MA, ed. *Children with Disabilities*. 4th ed. Paul Brooks Publishing Company; 1997.

100. MacKenzie AP, Stephenson CD, Funai AF. *Prenatal assessment of gestational age*. Accessed April 2013. http://www.uptodate.com/contents/prenatal-assessment-of-gestational-age?detectedLanguage=en&source=search_result&search=prenatal+assessment+of+gestational+age&selectedTitle=1%7E150&provider=noProvider

101. Wilkens-Haug L, Heffner LJ. Fetal assessment and prenatal diagnosis. In: Cloherty JP, Eichenwald EC, Stark AR, eds. *Manual of Neonatal Care*. 5th ed. Lippincott Williams & Wilkins; 2004.

102. Comparetti AM. Pattern analysis of normal and abnormal development: the fetus, the newborn, the child. In: Slaton DS, ed. *Development of Movement in Infancy*. UNC; 1980.

103. Dipietro JA. Fetal neurobehavioral assessment. In: Singer LT, Zeskind PS, eds. *Biobehavioral Assessment of the Infant*. The Guilford Press; 2001.

104. Rivkees SA, Mirmiran M, Ariagno RL. Circadian rhythms in infants. *NeoReviews*. 2003;4(11):298-303.

105. Prechtl H, Beintema D. *The Neurological Examination of the Newborn Infant. Clinics in Developmental Medicine, 12*. Heinemann Educational Books; 1964.

106. Lester BM, Tronick EZ. History and description of the neonatal intensive care unit network neuro-behavioral scale. *Pediatrics*. 2004;113(3):634-640.

107. Friedrich O. *What do babies know? TIME*. Accessed August 15, 1983. http://content.time.com/time/magazine/article/0,9171,1580382,00.html

108. Glass P. Development of the visual system and implications for early intervention. *Infants Young Child*. 2002;15(1):1-10.

109. Morrissey K. *Seminar in Pediatric Physical Therapy: Infant Development and Therapeutic Interventions*. Fall Semester 1994. Hahnemann University Program in Pediatric Physical Therapy.

110. Yoos L. Applying research in practice: parenting the premature infant. *Appl Nurs Res*. 1989;2(1):30-34.

111. Hunter JG. Neonatal intensive care unit. In: Case-Smith J, ed. *Occupational Therapy for Children*. 4th ed. Mosby; 2001.

112. Allen MC, Capute AJ. Tone and reflex development before term. *Pediatrics*. 1990;85:393-399.

113. Dargassies SSA. *Neurological Development in the Full-Term and Premature Neonate*. Exerpta Medica; 1977.

114. Sweeney JK, Gutierrez T. Musculoskeletal implications of preterm infant positioning in the NICU. *J Perinatal Neonatal Nurs*. 2002;16(1):58-70.

115. Palmer PG, Dubowitz LMS, Verghote M, et al. Neurological and neurobehavioral differences between preterm infants at term and full-term newborn infants. *Neuropediatrics*. 1982;13:183-189.

116. Mercuri E, Guzzetta A, Laroche S, et al. Neurologic examination of preterm infants at term age: comparison with term infants. *J Pediatr*. 2003;142:647-655.

117. Duffy FH, Als H, McNulty, GB. Behavioral and electrophysiological evidence for gestational age effects in healthy preterm and full-term infants studied two weeks after expected due date. *Child Dev*. 1990;61:1271-1286.

118. Huppi PS, Schuknecht B, Boesch C, et al. Structural and neurobehavioral delay in postnatal brain development of preterm infants. *Pediatr Res*. 1996;39(5):895-901.

119. Mouradian LE, Als H, Coster WJ. Neurobehavioral functioning of healthy preterm infants of varying gestational ages. *Dev Behav Pediatr*. 2000;21(6):408-416.

120. Graven SN. Sound and the developing infant in the NICU: conclusions and recommendations for care. *J Perinatol*. 2000;20:S88-S93.

121. McGrath JM. Neurologic development. In: Kenner C, McGrath JM, eds. *Developmental Care of Newborns and Infants: A Guide for Health Professionals*. Mosby; 2004.

122. Lutes LM, Graves CD, Jorgensen KM. The NICU experience and its relationship to sensory integration. In: Kenner C, McGrath JM, eds. *Developmental Care of Newborns and Infants. A Guide for Health Professionals*. Elsevier; 2004.

123. Anand KJ, Hickey PK. Pain and its effects in the human neonate and fetus. *N Engl J Med*. 1987;317:1321-1329.

124. Anand KJ, Carr DB. The neuroanatomy, neurophysiology, and neurochemistry of pain, stress, and analgesia in newborns and children. *Pediatr Clin North Am*. 1989;36:795-822.

125. Carbajal R, Rousst A, Dana C, et al. Epidemiology and treatment of painful procedures in neonates in intensive care units. *JAMA*. 2008;300(1):60-70.

126. Cruz MP, Fernandes AM, Olivveira CR. Epidemiology of painful procedures performed in neonates: a systematic review of observational studies. *Eur J Pain*. 2016;20(4):489-498. doi:10.1002/ejp.757

127. Perry M, Tan Z, Chen J, et al. Neonatal pain: perceptions and current practice. *Crit Care Nurs Clin N Am*. 2018;30:549-561. doi:10.106/j.cnc.2018.07.013

128. *World Health Organization Guidelines on the Pharmacological Treatment of Persisting Pain in Children with Medical Illnesses*. World Health Organization; 2012.

129. Grunau RE, Holsti L, Haley D, et al. Neonatal procedural pain exposure predicts lower cortisol and behavioral reactivity in preterm infants in the NICU. *Pain*. 2005;113(3):293-300.

130. Grunau RE. Neonatal pain in very preterm infant: long term effects on brain, neurodevelopment, & pain reactivity. *Rambam Maimonides Med J*. 2013;4(4):e0025.

131. Ranger M, Grunau RE. Early repetitive pain in preterm infants in relation to the developing brain. *Pain Manag*. 2014;4(1):57-67.

132. Brummelte S, Grunau RE, Vann C, et al. Procedural pain and brain development in premature newborns. *Ann Neurol*. 2015;71:385-396. doi:10.1002/ana.22267

133. Roofthooft DE, Simons SH, Anad KJ, et al. Eight years later, are we still hurting newborn infants? *Neonatology*. 2014;105(3):218-226.

134. Ranger M, Beggs S, Grunau RE. Developmental aspects of pain. In: Polin RA, Abman SH, Rowitel DH, Benitz WE, eds. *Fetal and Neonatal Physiology*. 5th ed. Elsevier; 2017:1390.e2-1395.e2.

135. Corneilissen L, Fabrizi L, Patten D, et al. Postnatal temporal, spatial and modality tuning of nociceptive cutaneous flexion reflexes in human infants. *PLoS One*. 2013;8:e76470.

136. Heinricher MM, Tavares I, Leith JL, et al. Descending control of nociception: specificity and plasticity. *Brain Res Rev*. 2009;60(10):214-225.

137. Hatfield LA. Neonatal pian: what's age got to do with it? *Surg Neurol Int*. 2014;5(suppl 13):S479-S489.

138. Salihagic Kadic A, Predojevic M. Fetal neurophysiology according to gestational age. *Semin Fetal Neonatal Med*. 2012;17:256-260.

139. Salihagic Kadic A, Predojevic M, Kurjak A. Advances in fetal neurophysiology. In: Pooh RK, Kurjak A, eds. *Fetal Neurology*. Jaypee Brothers; 2009:161-221.

140. Koch SC, Tochiki KK, Hirschberg S, et al. C-fiber activity-dependent maturation of glycinergic inhibition in the spinal dorsal horn of the postnatal rat. *Proc Natl Acad Sci U S A*. 2012;109(30):12201-12206.

141. Bremner LR, Fitzgerald M. Postnatal tuning of cutaneous inhibitory receptive fields in the rat. *J Physiol*. 2008;586:1529-1537.

142. Fitzgerald M, Walker SM. Infant pain management: a developmental neurobiological approach. *Nat Rev Neurol*. 2009;5:35-50.

143. Andrews K, Fitzgerald M. The cutaneous withdrawal reflex in human neonates: sensitization, receptive fields, and the effects of contralateral stimulation. *Pain*. 1994;56:95-101.

144. Jennings E, Fitzgerald M. Postnatal changes in responses of rat dorsal horn cells to afferent stimulation: a fibre-induced sensitization. *J Physiol*. 1998;509(3):859-868.

145. Beggs S, Torsney C, Drew LJ, et al. The postnatal reorganization of primary afferent input and dorsal horn cell receptive fields in

the rat spinal cord is an activity-dependent process. *Eur J Neurosci.* 2002;16:1249-1258.

146. Valeri BO, Holsti L, Linhares BM. Neonatal pain and developmental outcomes in children born preterm: a systematic review. *Clin J Pain.* 2015;31:355-362.

147. Goksan S, Hartley C, Emery F, et al. fMRI reveals neural activity overlap between adult and infant pain. *Elife.* 2015;4:e06356.

148. Volpe JJ. Brain injury in premature infants: a complex amalgam of destructive and developmental disturbances. *Lancet Neurol.* 2009;8:110-124.

149. Volpe JJ. *Neurology of the Newborn.* 4th ed. Saunders; 2001.

150. Smith GC, Gutovich J, Smyser C, et al. Neonatal intensive care unit stress is associated with brain development in preterm infants. *Ann Neurol.* 2011;70:541-549.

151. Vinall J, Miller SP, Chau V, et al. Neonatal pain in relation to postnatal growth in infants born very preterm. *Pain.* 2012;153:1374-1381.

152. Ranger M, Zwicker JG, Chau CMY, et al. Neonatal pain and infection relate to smaller cerebellum in very preterm children at school age. *J Pediatr.* 2015;167:292-298.

153. Zwicker JG, Miller SP, Grunau RE, et al. Smaller cerebellar growth and poorer neurodevelopmental outcomes in very preterm infants exposed to neonatal morphine. *J Pediatr.* 2016;172:81-87.

154. Duerden EG, Grunau RE, Guo R, et al. Early procedural pain is associated with regionally-specific alterations in thalamic development in preterm neonates. *J Neurosci.* 2018;38(4):878-886.

155. Zwicker JG, Grunau RE, Adams E, et al. Score for neonatal acute physiology-II and neonatal pain predict corticospinal tract development in premature newborns. *Pediatr Neurol.* 2013;48:123.e1-129.e1.

156. Schwaller F, Fitzgerald M. The consequences of pain in early life: injury-induced plasticity in developing pain pathways. *Eur J Neurosci.* 2014;39:344-352.

157. Grunau RE, Oberlander TF, Whitfield MF, et al. Demographic and therapeutic determinants of pain reactivity in very low birth weight neonates at 32 weeks' postconceptional age. *Pediatrics.* 2001;107(1):105-112.

158. Doesburg SM, Chau CM, Cheung TP, et al. Neonatal pain-related stress, functional cortical activity and visual-perceptual abilities in school-age children born extremely low gestational age. *Pain.* 2013;154(10):1946-1952.

159. Cong X, Wu J, Vittner D, et al. The impact of cumulative pain/stress on neurobehavioral development of preterm infants in the NICU. *Early Hum Dev.* 2017;108:9-16.

160. Montirosso R, Casini E, Del Prete A, et al. Neonatal developmental care in infant pain management and internalizing behaviours at 18 months in prematurely born children. *Eur J Pain.* 2016;20:1010-1021.

161. Tu MT, Grunau RE, Petrie-Thomas J, et al. Maternal stress and behavior modulate relationships between neonatal stress, attention, and basal cortisol at 8 months in preterm infants. *Dev Psychobiol.* 2007;49:150-164.

162. AAP Committee on Fetus and Section on Anesthesiology and Pain Medicine. Prevention and management of procedural pain in the neonate: an update. *Pediatrics.* 2016;137(2):e20154271. doi:10.1542/peds.2015-4271

163. Johnston CC, Stevens BJ, Yang F, et al. Differential response to pain by very preterm neonates. *Pain.* 1995;61:471-479.

164. Holsti L, Grunau RE, Oberlander TF. Is it painful or not? Discreet validity of the behavioural indicators of infant pain (BIIP) scale. *Clin J Pain.* 2008;24(1):83-88.

165. Relland LM, Gehred A, Maitre NL. Behavioral and physiological signs for pain assessment in preterm and term neonates during nociception-specific response: a systematic review. *Pediatr Neurol.* 2019;90:13-23.

166. Eriksson M, Campbell-Yeo M. Assessment of pain in newborn infants. *Semin Fetal Neonatal Med.* 2019;24:101003.

167. Holsti L, Grunau RE, Oberlander TF, et al. Body movements: an important additional factor in discriminating pain for stress in preterm infants. *Clin J Pain.* 2005;21:491-498.

168. Anand KJS. Defining pain in newborns: need for a uniform taxonomy? *Acta Paediatr.* 2017;106:1438-1444.

169. Anand KJS, Eriksson M, Boyle EM, et al. Assessment of continuous pain in newborns admitted to NICUs in 18 European countries. *Acta Paediatr.* 2017;106:1248-1259.

170. Field T. Preterm newborn pain research review. *Infant Behav Dev.* 2017;49:141-150.

171. Hatfield LA, Murphy N, Karp K, et al. A systematic review of behavioral and environmental interventions for procedural pain management in preterm infants. *J Pediatr Nurs.* 2019;44:22-30.

172. Filippa M, Poisbeau P, Mairesse J, et al. Pain, parental involvement, and oxytocin in the neonatal intensive care unit. *Front Psychol.* 2019;10:715. doi: 10.3389/fpsyg.2019.00715

173. Hall RW, Shbarou RM. Drugs of choice for sedation and analgesia in the neonatal ICU. *Clin Perinatol.* 2009;36(2):215-226.

174. Harrison LH, Lotas MJ, Jorgensen KM. Environmental issues. In: Kenner C, McGrath JM, eds. *Developmental Care of Newborns and Infants: A Guide for Health Professionals.* Elsevier; 2004.

175. Turnage-Carrier CS. Caregiving and the environment. In: Kenner C, McGrath JM, eds. *Developmental Care of Newborns and Infants: A Guide for Health Professionals.* Elsevier; 2004.

176. American Academy of Pediatrics, Committee on Environmental Health. Noise: a hazard for the fetus and newborn. *Pediatrics.* 1997;100(4):724-727.

177. Philbin MK. Planning the acoustic environment of a neonatal intensive care unit. *Clin Perinatol.* 2004;31:331-352.

178. Chang YJ, Lin CH, Lin LH. Noise and related events in a neonatal intensive care unit. *Acta Paediatr.* 2001;42:212-217.

179. Evans JB, Philbin MK. The acoustic environment of hospital nurseries. *J Perinatol.* 2000;20(8):S105-S112.

180. Philbin MK. Some implications of early auditory development for the environment of hospitalized preterm infants. *Neonatal Netw.* 1996;15(7):71-73.

181. Philbin MK, Evans JB. Noise levels, spectra and operational function of an occupied newborn intensive care unit built to meet recommended permissible noise criteria. *J Acoust Soc Am.* 2003;114(4, part 2):2326.

182. White RD. Recommended standards for the newborn ICU design. *J Perinatol.* 2003;23(1):5-21.

183. Morante A, Dubowitz LMS, Levene M, et al. The development of visual function in normal and abnormal preterm and full term infants. *Dev Med Child Neurol.* 1982;24:771-784.

184. Prechtl HFR, Fargel JW, Weinmann HM, et al. Postures and respiration of low-risk pre-term infants. *Dev Med Child Neurol.* 1979;21:3-27.

185. Brazelton TB, Nugent JK. *The Neonatal Behavioral Assessment Scale.* 3rd ed. MacKeith Press; 1995.

186. Als H. Reading the premature infant. In: Goldson E, ed. *Nurturing the Premature Infant Developmental Intervention in the Neonatal Intensive Care Nursery.* Oxford University Press; 1999.

187. Pompa KM, Zaichkin J. The NICU baby. In: Zaichkin J, ed. *Newborn Intensive Care. What Every Parent Needs to Know.* NICU Ink Book Publishers; 2002.

188. Lee KG, Cloherty JP. Identifying the high risk newborn and evaluating gestational age, prematurity, post maturity, large for gestational age, and small for gestational age. In: Cloherty JP, Eichenwald EC, Stark AR, eds. *Manual of Neonatal Care.* 5th ed. Lippincott Williams & Wilkins; 2004.

189. American Academy of Pediatrics Committee on Fetus and Newborn. Age terminology during the perinatal period. *Pediatrics.* 2004;114:1362-1364.

190. Apgar V. A proposal for a new method of evaluation of the newborn infant. *Curr Res Anesth Analg.* 1953;32(4):260-267.

191. American Academy of Pediatrics, Committee on Fetus & Newborn, American College of Obstetricians & Gynecologists. The Apgar score. *Pediatrics.* 2006;117(4):1444-1447.

192. American Academy of Pediatrics Committee on Fetus & Newborn, American College of Obstetricians & Gynecologists & Committee

on Obstetric Practice. The apgar score. *Pediatrics*. 2006;117(4):1444-1447.

193. Eichenwald EC. Mechanical ventilation. In: Cloherty JP, Eichenwald EC, Stark AR, eds. *Manual of Neonatal Care*. 5th ed. Lippincott Williams & Wilkins; 2004.

194. Cameron J, Haines J. Management of respiratory disorders. In: Boxwell G, eds. *Neonatal Intensive Care Nursing*. Routledge; 2000.

195. Wiswell TE, Pinchi S. Continuous positive airway pressure. In: Goldsmith JP, Karotin EH, eds. *Assisted Ventilation of the Neonate*. 4th ed. Saunders; 2003.

196. Czervinske MP. Continuous positive airway pressure. In: Czervinske MP, Barnhart SC, eds. *Perinatal and Pediatric Respiratory Care*. 2nd ed. Saunders; 2003.

197. Lee KS, Dunn MS, Fenwick M. A comparison of underwater bubble continuous positive airway pressure with ventilator derived continuous positive airway pressure in premature infants ready for extubation. *Biol Neonate*. 1998;73(2):69-75.

198. Spitzer AR, Greenspan JS, Fox WW. Positive-pressure ventilation-pressure-limited and time cycled ventilation. In: Goldsmith JP, Karotin EH, eds. *Assisted Ventilation of the Neonate*. 4th ed. Saunders; 2003.

199. Schwartz JE. New technologies applied to management of the respiratory system. In: Kenner C, Lott JW, eds. *Comprehensive Neonatal Nursing: A Physiologic Perspective*. 3rd ed. Saunders; 2003.

200. Meredith KS. High frequency ventilation. In: Czervinske MP, Barnhart SC, eds. *Perinatal and Pediatric Respiratory Care*. 2nd ed. Saunders; 2003.

201. Mammel MC. Mechanical ventilation of the newborn. *Arch Dis Child Fetal Neonatal Ed*. 2000;83(3):F224.

202. Mammel MC. High frequency ventilation. In: Goldsmith JP, Karotin EH, eds. *Assisted Ventilation of the Neonate*. 4th ed. Saunders; 2003.

203. Keszler M, Derand DJ. Neonatal high frequency ventilation: past, present, future. *Clin Perinatol*. 2001;28(3):579-607.

204. MacIntyre NR. High frequency jet ventilation. *Respir Care Clin N Am*. 2001;7(4):599-610.

205. Bouchet JC, Goddard J, Claris O. High frequency oscillatory ventilation. *Anesthesiology*. 2004;100:1007-1012.

206. Moriette G, Paris-Llado J, Walti H, et al. Prospective randomized multicenter comparison of high frequency oscillatory ventilation and conventional ventilation in preterm infants of less than 30 weeks with respiratory distress syndrome. *Pediatrics*. 2001;107(2):363-372.

207. Osborn DA, Evans N. Randomized trial of high frequency oscillatory ventilation versus conventional ventilation: effect on systemic blood flow in very premature infants. *J Pediatr*. 2003;143(2):192-202.

208. Sreenan C, Lemke RP, Hudson-Mason A, et al. High-flow nasal cannulae in the management of apnea of prematurity: a comparison with conventional nasal continuous positive airway pressure. *Pediatrics*. 2001;107(5):1081-1083.

209. Locke RG, Wolfson MR, Shaffer TH, et al. Inadvertent administration of positive-end-distending pressure during nasal cannula flow. *Pediatrics*. 1993;91(1):135-138.

210. Saslow JG, Aghar ZH, Nakhla TA, et al. Work of breathing using high flow nasal cannula in preterm infants. *J Perinatol*. 2006;26(8):476-480.

211. Walsh B. Comparison of Vapotherm 2000i with a bubble humidifier humidifying flow through a nasal cannula. *Respir Care*. 2003;48(18).

212. Kopelman AE, Holbert D. Use of oxygen cannulas in extremely low birthweight infants. *J Perinatol*. 2003;23:94-97.

213. Collins CL, Holberton JR, Barfield C, et al. A randomized controlled trial to compare heated humidified high-flow nasal cannulae with nasal continuous positive airway pressure postextubation in premature infants. *J Pediatr*. 2013;162(5):949-54.e1. doi: 10.1016/j.jpeds.2012.11.016. Epub 2012 Dec 20. PMID: 23260098.

214. Woodhead DD, Lambert DK, Clark JM, et al. Comparing two methods of delivering high-flow gas therapy by nasal cannula following endotracheal extubation: a prospective, randomized, masked, crossover trial. *J Perinatol*. 2006;26(8):481-485.

215. Waugh JB, Granger WM. An evaluation of two new devices for nasal high flow gas therapy. *Respir Care*. 2004;49(8):902-906.

216. Panitch HB, Wolfson MR, Shaffer TH. Epithelial modulation of preterm airway smooth muscle contraction. *J Pediatr*. 1993;74(3):1437-1443.

217. Cullen AB, Wolfson MR, Shaffer TH. The maturation of airway structure and function. *NeoReviews*. 2002;3(7):e125-e130.

218. Williams LJ, Shaffer TH, Greenspan JS. Inhaled nitric oxide therapy in the nearly term or term infant with hypoxic respiratory failure. *Neonatal Netw*. 2004;23(1):5-13.

219. Neonatal Inhaled Nitric Oxide Study Group (NINOS). Inhaled nitric oxide in full-term and nearly term infants with hypoxic respiratory failure. *N Engl J Med*. 1997;336:597-604.

220. Neonatal Inhaled Nitric Oxide Study Group (NINOS). Inhaled nitric oxide in term and nearly term infants: neurodevelopmental follow-up of the neonatal inhaled nitric oxide study group (NINOS). *J Pediatr*. 2000;136(5):611-617.

221. Ellington M, O'Reilly D, Allred EN, et al. Child health status, neurodevelopmental outcome, and parent satisfaction in a randomized, controlled trial of nitric oxide for persistent pulmonary hypertension of the newborn. *Pediatrics*. 2001;107(6):1351-1356.

222. American Academy of Pediatrics, Committee on Fetus and Newborn. Use of inhaled nitric oxide. *Pediatrics*. 2000;106(2, part 1):344-345.

223. Ballard RH, Truog WE, Cnaan A, et al. Inhaled nitric oxide in preterm infants undergoing mechanical ventilation. *N Engl J Med*. 2006;355(4):343-353.

224. Kinsella JP, Cutter GR, Walsh WF, et al. Early inspired nitric oxide therapy in premature newborns with respiratory failure. *N Engl J Med*. 2006;355(4):354-364.

225. Ford JW. Neonatal ECMO: current controversies and trends. *Neonatal Netw*. 2006;25(4):229-238.

226. Rais-Bahrami K, Short BL. The current status of neonatal extracorporeal membrane oxygenation. *Semin Perinatol*. 2000;24(6):406-417.

227. Jaillard S, Pierrat V, Truffert P, et al. Two years follow-up of newborn infants after extracorporeal membrane oxygenation. *Eur J Cardiothorac Surg*. 2000;18(3):328-333.

228. Kim ES, Stolar CJ. ECMO in the newborn. *Am J Perinatol*. 2000;17(7):345-356.

229. Rais-Bahrami K, Wagner AE, Coffman C, et al. Neurodevelopmental outcome in ECMO vs near-miss ECMO patients at 5 years of age. *Clin Pediatr*. 2000;39(3):145-152.

230. Tappero EP. NICU technology. In: Zaichkin J, ed. *Newborn Intensive Care: What Every Parent Needs to Know*. 2nd ed. NICU Ink Book Publishers; 2002.

231. Cooper M, Arnold J. Extracorporeal membrane oxygenation. In: Cloherty JP, Eichenwald EC, Stark AR, eds. *Manual of Neonatal Care*. 5th ed. Lippincott Williams & Wilkins; 2004.

232. Nield TA, Langenbacher D, Poulsen MK, et al. Neurodevelopmental outcome at 3.5 years of age in children treated with extracorporeal life support: relationship to primary diagnosis. *J Pediatr*. 2000;136(3):338-344.

233. Massery M. Chest development as a component of normal motor development: implications for treatment for pediatric physical therapists. *Pediatr Phys Ther*. 1991;3(1):3-8.

234. Make BJ, Hill NS, Goldberg AI, et al. Mechanical ventilation beyond the intensive care unit: report of a consensus conference of the American College of Chest Physicians. *Chest*. 1998;113(5):289S-344S.

235. Vohr BR, Cashore WJ, Bigsby R. Stresses & interventions in the neonatal intensive care unit. In: Levine MD, Carey WB, Crocker AC, eds. *Developmental-Behavioral Pediatrics*. 3rd ed. Saunders; 1999.

236. Honrubia D, Stark AR. Respiratory distress syndrome. In: Cloherty JP, Eichenwald EC, Stark AR, eds. *Manual of Neonatal Care*. 5th ed. Lippincott Williams & Wilkins; 2004.

237. National Institutes of Health. *Report of the Consensus Development Conference on Anti-natal Corticosteroids Revisited: Repeat Courses*. National Institute of Child Health and Human Development; 2000.

238. Baud O. Antenatal glucocorticoid treatment and cystic periventricular leukomalacia in very preterm infants. *N Engl J Med.* 1999;341(16):1190-1196.

239. Banks BA, Cnaan A, Morgan MA, et al. Multiple courses of antenatal corticosteroids and outcome of premature neonates. *Am J Obstet Gynecol.* 1999;181:709-717.

240. Banks BA, Macones G, Cnaan A, et al. Multiple courses of antenatal corticosteroids are associated with early severe lung disease in preterm neonates. *J Perinatol.* 2002;22:101-107.

241. Jobe AH, Ikegami M. Biology of surfactant. *Clin Perinatol.* 2001;28:671-694.

242. Egerman RS, Mercer BM, Doss JL, et al. A randomized controlled trial of oral and intramuscular dexamethasone in the prevention of neonatal respiratory distress syndrome. *Am J Obstet Gynecol.* 1998;179(5):1120-1123.

243. Hack MF, Minisch N, Fanaroff A. Antenatal steroids have not improved the outcomes of surviving extremely low birth weight (ELBW) infants [<750 grams]. *Pediatr Res.* 1998;43(2):214A.

244. Soll RF. Surfactant treatment of the very premature infant. *Biol Neonate.* 1998;74(suppl 1):35-42.

245. Suresh GK. Current surfactant use in premature infants. *Clin Perinatol.* 2001;28:671-694.

246. Escobedo MB, Gunkel JH, Kennedy RA, et al. Texas Neonatal Research Group. Early surfactant for neonates with mild to moderate RDS: a multicenter randomized trial. *J Pediatr.* 2004;144(6):804-808.

247. Jobe AH. Surfactant for RDS: when and why? *J Pediatr.* 2004;144(6):A2.

248. Dani C, Bertini G, Pezzati M, et al. Early extubation and nasal continuous positive airway pressure after surfactant treatment for respiratory distress syndrome among preterm infants <30 weeks gestation. *Pediatrics.* 2004;113(6):e560-e563.

249. Park MK. *Pediatric Cardiology for Practitioners.* 4th ed. Mosby; 2002.

250. Heyman MA, Teitel DF, Liebman J. The heart. In: Klaus MH, Fanaroff AA, eds. *Care of the High-Risk Neonate.* 4th ed. Saunders; 1993.

251. Wechsler SB, Wernovsky G. Cardiac disorders. In: Cloherty JP, Eichenwald EC, Stark AR, eds. *Manual of Neonatal Care.* 5th ed. Lippincott Williams & Wilkins; 2004.

252. Gersony WM, Peckham GJ, Ellison RC, et al. Effects of indomethacine in premature infants with patent ductus arteriosus: results of a national collaborative study. *J Pediatr.* 1984;102(6):895-906.

253. Gersony WM. Patent ductus arteriosus. *Pediatr Clin North Am.* 1986;33(3):545-560.

254. Martin CR, Cloherty JP. Neonatal hyperbilirubinemia. In: Cloherty JR, Eichenwald EC, Stark AR, eds. *Manual of Neonatal Care.* 5th ed. Lippincott Williams & Wilkins; 2004.

255. Dennery PA, Seidman DS, Stevenson DK. Neonatal hyperbilirubinemia. *N Engl J Med.* 2001;334:581-590.

256. Poland RL, Ostrea EM. Neonatal hyperbilirubinemia. In: Klaus MH, Fanaroff AA, eds. *Care of the High Risk Neonate.* Saunders; 1993.

257. Maisels MJ, Watchko JF, Bhutani VK, et al. An approach to the management of hyperbilirubinemia in the preterm infants less than 35 weeks of gestation. *J Perinatol.* 2012;32:660-664.

258. AAP Subcommittee on Neonatal Hyperbilirubinemia. Neonatal jaundice and kernicterus. *Pediatrics.* 2001;108(3):763-765.

259. Patra K, Storfer-Isser A, Siner B, et al. Adverse events associated with neonatal exchange transfusion in the 1990's. *J Pediatr.* 2004;144:626-631.

260. Paludetto R, Mansi G, Raimondi F, et al. Moderate hyperbilirubinemia induces a transient alteration of neonatal behavior. *Pediatrics.* 2002;110(4):e50.

261. Mansi G, De Maio C, Araimo G, et al. "Safe" hyperbilirubinemia is associated with altered neonatal behavior. *Biol Neonate.* 2003;83(1):19-21.

262. Jadcherla SR. Gastroesophageal reflux in the neonate. *Clin Perinatol.* 2002;29(1):135-158.

263. Omari TI. Lower esophageal sphincter function in the neonate. *NeoReviews.* 2006;7(1):e13-e17.

264. Jadcherla SK, Rudolph CD. Gastroesophageal reflux in the preterm neonate. *NeoReviews.* 2005;6:e87-e95.

265. Tipnis NA, Tipnis SM. Controversies in the treatment of gastroesophageal reflux in preterm infants. *Clin Perinatol.* 2009;36:153-164.

266. Noviski N, Yehuda YB, Yorum B, et al. Does the size of nasogastric tube affect gastroesophageal reflux in children. *J Pediatr Gastroenterol Nutr.* 1999;29:448-451.

267. Hammer D. Gastroesophageal reflux and prokinetic agents. *Neonatal Netw.* 2005;24(2):51-58.

268. Sherman PM, Hassell F, Fagundes-Nero U, et al. A global evidence-based consensus on the definition of gastroesophageal reflux in the pediatric patient. *Am J Gastroenterol.* 2009;104:278-298.

269. Menon AP, Schefft GL, Thach BT. Apnea associated with regurgitation in infants. *J Pediatr.* 1985;106(4):625-629.

270. Jadcherla SR. Upstream effect of esophageal distension: effect on airway. *Curr Gastroenterol Rep.* 2006;8(3):190-194.

271. Gupta A, Gulati P, Kim W, et al. Effect of postnatal maturation on the mechanics of esophageal propulsion in preterm human neonates: primary and secondary peristalsis. *Am J Gastroenterol.* 2009;104:411-419.

272. Jadcherla SR. Pathophysiology of aerodigestive pulmonary disorders in the neonate. *Clin Perinatol.* 2012;39:631-654.

273. Peter CS, Sprodowski N, Bohnhorst B, et al. Gastroesophageal reflux and apnea of prematurity. No temporal relationship. *Pediatrics.* 2002;109(8):8-11.

274. Poets CF. Gastroesophageal reflux: a critical review of its role in preterm infants. *Pediatrics.* 2004;113(2):e128-e132.

275. Krishnamoorthy M, Muntz A, Liem T, et al. Diagnosis and treatment of respiratory symptoms of initially unsuspected gastroesophageal reflux in infants. *Am Surg.* 1994;60:783-785.

276. Davies AM, Koenig JS, Thatch BT. Upper airway chemoreflex responses to saline and water in preterm infants. *J Appl Phys.* 1988;64(4):1412-1420.

277. DiFiore J, Arko M, Herynk B, et al. Characterization of cardiorespiratory events following gastroesophageal reflux in preterm infants. *J Perinatol.* 2010;30(10):683-687.

278. Poets CF. Gastroesophageal reflux and apnea of prematurity-coincidence not causation. *Neurology.* 2013;103:103-104.

279. Orenstein SR, Whittington PF. Positioning for prevention of infant gastroesophageal reflux. *J Pediatr.* 1983;103:534-537.

280. Tobin JM, McCloud P, Cameron DJS. Posture and gastroesophageal reflux: a case for left lateral positioning. *Arch Dis Child.* 1997;76:254-258.

281. Ewer AK, James ME, Tobin JM. Prone and lateral position reduce gastroesophageal reflux in premature infants. *Arch Dis Child.* 1999;81:F201-F205.

282. Corvaglia L, Rotatori R, Ferlini M, et al. The effect of body positioning on gastroesophageal reflux in the premature infant: evaluation by combined impedance and pH monitoring. *J Pediatr.* 2007;151:591-596.

283. Omari T, Rommel N, Staunton E, et al. Paradoxical impact of body positioning on gastroesophageal reflux and gastric emptying in the premature infant. *J Pediatr.* 2004;145:194-200.

284. Chen SS, Tzeng YL, Gau BS, et al. Effects of prone and supine positioning on gastric residuals in preterm infants: a time series with cross-over study. *Int J Nurs Stud.* 2013. doi:10.1016/j.ijnurstu.2013.02.009

285. Sangers H, de Jong PM, Mulder SE. Outcomes of gastric residuals whilst feeding preterm infants in various body positions. *J Neonatal Nurs.* 2012. doi:10.1016/j.jnn

286. van Wijk MP, Bennigan MA, Dent J, et al. Effect of body position changes on postprandial gastroesophageal reflux and gastric emptying in the healthy premature neonate. *J Pediatr.* 2007;151:585-590.

287. Malcolm WF, Cotton M. Metoclopramide, H₂ blockers, and proton inhibitors: pharmacology for gastroesophageal reflux in neonates. *Clin Perinatol.* 2012;39:99-109.

288. Czinn SJ, Blanchard S. Gastroesophageal disease in neonates and infants. When and how to treat. *Pediatr Drugs.* 2013;15:19-27.

289. Loots CM, Benniga MA, Omari M. Gastroesophageal reflux in pediatrics (patho) physiology and new insights in diagnosis and treatment. *Minerva Pediatr.* 2012;64(1):104-119.

290. Loots C, van Herwaarden MY, Benniga MA, et al. Gastroesophageal reflux, esophageal function, gastric emptying and the relationship to dysphagia before and after antireflux surgery in children. *J Pediatr.* 2013;162:526-573.

291. Schanler RJ. *Clinical features and diagnosis of necrotizing enterocolitis in newborns.* UpToDate. Accessed May 2013. http://www.uptodate.com/contents/clinical-features-and-diagnosis-of-necrotizing-enterocolitis-in-newborns?source=search_result&search=NEC+totalis&selectedTitle=2%7E150

292. Kosloske AM. Epidemiology of necrotizing enterocolitis. *Acta Paediatr Suppl.* 1994;396:2.

293. Schanler RJ. *Pathology and pathogenesis of necrotizing enterocolitis in newborns.* UpToDate. Accessed May 2013. http://www.uptodate.com/contents/pathology-and-pathogenesis-of-necrotizing-enterocolitis-in-newborns?source=search_result&search=necrotizing+enterocolitis&selectedTitle=4%7E150#references

294. Neu J, Weiss MD. Necrotizing enterocolitis: pathophysiology and prevention. *J Parenteral Enteral Nutr.* 1999;23:S13.

295. Hunter CJ, Upperman JS, Ford HR, et al. Understanding the susceptibility of the premature infant to necrotizing enterocolitis (NEC). *Pediatr Res.* 2008;63:117.

296. Neu J. Necrotizing enterocolitis: the search for a unifying pathogenic theory leading to prevention. *Pediatr Clin North Am.* 1996;43:409.

297. Ballance WA, Dahms BB, Shenker N, et al. Pathology of neonatal necrotizing enterocolitis: a ten-year experience. *J Pediatr.* 1990;117:S6.

298. Horbar JD, Badger GJ, Carpenter JH, et al. Trends in mortality and morbidity for very low birth weight infants, 1991-1999. *Pediatrics.* 2002;110:143.

299. Sankaran K, Puckett B, Lee DS, et al. Variations in incidence of necrotizing enterocolitis in Canadian neonatal intensive care units. *J Pediatr Gastroenterol Nutr.* 2004;39:366.

300. Lee SK, McMillan DD, Ohlsson A, et al. Variations in practice and outcomes in the Canadian NICU network: 1996-1997. *Pediatrics.* 2000;106:1070.

301. Wiswell TE, Robertson CF, Jones TA, et al. Necrotizing enterocolitis in full-term infants. A case-control study. *Am J Dis Child.* 1988;142:532.

302. Polin RA, Pollack PF, Barlow B, et al. Necrotizing enterocolitis in term infants. *J Pediatr.* 1976;89:460.

303. Ostlie DJ, Spilde TL, St. Peter SD, et al. Necrotizing enterocolitis in full-term infants. *J Pediatr Surg.* 2003;38:1039.

304. Lambert DK, Christensen RD, Henry E, et al. Necrotizing enterocolitis in term neonates: data from a multihospital health-care system. *J Perinatol.* 2007;27:437.

305. Kliegman RM, Walker WA, Yolken RH. Necrotizing enterocolitis: research agenda for a disease of unknown etiology and pathogenesis. *Pediatr Res.* 1993;34:701.

306. Holman RC, Stoll BJ, Clarke MJ, et al. The epidemiology of necrotizing enterocolitis infant mortality in the United States. *Am J Public Health.* 1997;87:2026.

307. McAlmon KR. Necrotizing enterocolitis. In: Cloherty JP, Eichenwald EC, Stark AR, eds. *Manual of Neonatal Care.* 5th ed. Lippincott Williams & Wilkins; 2004.

308. Reber KM, Nankervis CA. Necrotizing enterocolitis: preventative strategies. *Clin Perinatol.* 2004;31(1):157-167.

309. Rees CM, Pierro A, Eaton S. Neurodevelopmental outcomes on neonates with medically and surgically treated necrotizing enterocolitis. *Arch Dis Child Fetal Neonatal Ed.* 2007;92:F193-F198.

310. Rees CM, Eaton S, Pierro A. National prospective surveillance study of necrotizing enterocolitis in neonatal intensive care units. *J Pediatr Surg.* 2010;45:1391.

311. Snyder CL, Gittes GK, Murphy JP, et al. Survival after necrotizing enterocolitis in infants weighing less than 1,000 g: 25 years' experience at a single institution. *J Pediatr Surg.* 1997;32:434.

312. Schanler RJ. *Management of necrotizing enterocolitis in newborns.* UpToDate. Accessed May 2013. http://www.uptodate.com/contents/management-of-necrotizing-enterocolitis-in-newborns?source=search_result&search=NEC+totalis&selectedTitle=1%7E150#H20

313. Abdullah F, Zhang Y, Camp M, et al. Necrotizing enterocolitis in 20,822 infants: analysis of medical and surgical treatments. *Clin Pediatr (Phila).* 2010;49:166.

314. Fasoli L, Turi RA, Spitz L, et al. Necrotizing enterocolitis: extent of disease and surgical treatment. *J Pediatr Surg.* 1999;34:1096.

315. Fitzgibbons SC, Ching Y, Yu D, et al. Mortality of necrotizing enterocolitis expressed by birth weight categories. *J Pediatr Surg.* 2009;44:1072.

316. Horwitz JR, Lally KP, Cheu HW, et al. Complications after surgical intervention for necrotizing enterocolitis: a multicenter review. *J Pediatr Surg.* 1995;30:994.

317. Kliegman RM, Fanaroff AA. Necrotizing enterocolitis. *N Engl J Med.* 1984;310:1093.

318. Walsh MC, Kliegman RM, Fanaroff AA. Necrotizing enterocolitis: a practitioner's perspective. *Pediatr Rev.* 1988;9(7):219-226.

319. Yu VY, Tudehope DI, Gill GJ. Neonatal necrotizing enterocolitis: 1. Clinical aspects. *Med J Aust.* 1977;1:685.

320. Kleigman RM, Walsh MC. Neonatal necrotizing enterocolitis: pathogenesis, classification, and spectrum of illness. *Curr Probl Pediatr.* 1987;17:213-288.

321. Kanto WP, Hunter JE, Stoll BJ. Recognition and medical management of necrotizing enterocolitis. *Clin Perinatol.* 1994;21:335-346.

322. Stoll BJ, Kliegman RM. *Necrotizing Enterocolitis. Clinics in Perinatology.* Saunders; 1994.

323. Walsh MC, Kliegman RM. Necrotizing enterocolitis: treatment based on a staging criteria. *Pediatr Clin North Am.* 1986;33:179-201.

324. Kleigman RM. Necrotizing enterocolitis: bridging the basic science with the clinical disease. *J Pediatr.* 1990;117(5):833-835.

325. Bell MJ, Ternberg JL, Feigin RD, et al. Neonatal necrotizing enterocolitis. Therapeutic decisions based upon clinical staging. *Ann Surg.* 1978;187:1.

326. Clark DA, Miller MJ. Intraluminal pathogenesis of necrotizing enterocolitis. *J Pediatr.* 1990;117:S64.

327. Morgan J, Young L, McGuire W. Slow advancement of enteral feed volumes to prevent necrotising enterocolitis in very low birth weight infants. *Cochrane Database Syst Rev.* 2011;CD001241.

328. Morgan J, Young L, McGuire W. Delayed introduction of progressive enteral feeds to prevent necrotising enterocolitis in very low birth weight infants. *Cochrane Database Syst Rev.* 2011;CD001970.

329. La Gamma EF, Browne LE. Feeding practices for infants weighing less than 1500 G at birth and the pathogenesis of necrotizing enterocolitis. *Clin Perinatol.* 1994;21:271.

330. Schanler RJ, Shulman RJ, Lau C, et al. Feeding strategies for premature infants: randomized trial of gastrointestinal priming and tube-feeding method. *Pediatrics.* 1999;103:434.

331. Bombell S, McGuire W. Early trophic feeding for very low birth weight infants. *Cochrane Database Syst Rev.* 2009;CD000504.

332. Caplan M. Is EGF the holy grail for NEC? *J Pediatr.* 2007;150:329.

333. Cikrit D, Mastandrea J, West KW, et al. Necrotizing enterocolitis: factors affecting mortality in 101 surgical cases. *Surgery.* 1984;96:648-665.

334. Salvia G, Guarino A, Terrin G, et al. Neonatal onset intestinal failure: an Italian Multicenter Study. *J Pediatr.* 2008;153:674.

335. Cole CR, Hansen NI, Higgins RD, et al. Bloodstream infections in very low birth weight infants with intestinal failure. *J Pediatr.* 2012;160:54.

336. Kim ES, Brandt ML. *Spontaneous intestinal perforation of the newborn.* Accessed May 2013. http://www.uptodate.com/contents/spontaneous-intestinal-perforation-of-the-newborn?source=search_result&search=spontaneous+infant+performation&selectedTitle=3%7E150

337. Ragouilliaux CJ, Keeney SE, Hawkins HK, et al. Maternal factors in extremely low birth weight infants who develop spontaneous intestinal perforation. *Pediatrics.* 2007;120:e1458.

338. Gordon PV, Young ML, Marshall DD. Focal small bowel perforation: an adverse effect of early postnatal dexamethasone therapy in extremely low birth weight infants. *J Perinatol.* 2001;21:156.

339. Stark AR, Carlo WA, Tyson JE, et al. Adverse effects of early dexamethasone in extremely-low-birth-weight infants. National Institute of Child Health and Human Development Neonatal Research Network. *N Engl J Med.* 2001;344:95.

340. Gordon P, Rutledge J, Sawin R, et al. Early postnatal dexamethasone increases the risk of focal small bowel perforation in extremely low birth weight infants. *J Perinatol.* 1999;19:573.

341. Baird R, Puligandla PS, St. Vil D, et al. The role of laparotomy for intestinal perforation in very low birth weight infants. *J Pediatr Surg.* 2006;41:1522.

342. Sonntag J, Grimner I, Scholtz T, et al. Growth and neurodevelopmental outcome of very low birth weight infants with necrotizing enterocolitis. *Acta Paediatr.* 2004;89:528-532.

343. Hintz SR, Kendrick DE, Stoll BJ, et al. Neurodevelopmental and growth outcomes of extremely low birth weight infants after necrotizing enterocolitis. *Pediatrics.* 2005;115:696.

344. Martin CR, Dammann O, Allred EN, et al. Neurodevelopment of extremely preterm infants who had necrotizing enterocolitis with or without late bacteremia. *J Pediatr.* 2010;157:751.

345. Attridge JT, Herman AC, Gurka MJ, et al. Discharge outcomes of extremely low birth weight infants with spontaneous intestinal perforations. *J Perinatol.* 2006;26:49.

346. Adesanya OA, O'shea TM, Turner CS, et al. Intestinal perforation in very low birth weight infants: growth and neurodevelopment at 1 year of age. *J Perinatol.* 2005;25:583.

347. Roze E, Ta BD, van der Ree MH, et al. Functional impairments at school age of children with necrotizing enterocolitis or spontaneous intestinal perforation. *Pediatr Res.* 2011;70:619.

348. Volpe JJ. Brain injury in the preterm infant. *Clin Perinatol.* 1997;24(3):567-583.

349. Vohr B, Allen WC, Scott DT, et al. Early onset intraventricular hemorrhage in preterm neonates: incidence of neurodevelopmental handicap. *Semin Perinatol.* 1999;23(3):212-217.

350. Vohr B, Wright LL, Dusick AM, et al. Neurodevelopmental and functional outcomes for extremely low birth weight infants in the National Institutes of Child Health and Human Development Neonatal Research Network, 1993–1994. *Pediatrics.* 2000;105(6):1216-1226.

351. Vohr B, Allan WC, Westerveld M, et al. School-age outcomes of very low birth weight infants in the indomethacin intraventricular hemorrhage prevention trial. *Pediatrics.* 2003;111(4):e340-e346.

352. Larroque B, Morret S, Ancel PY, et al. White matter damage and intraventricular hemorrhage in very preterm infants: the EPIPAGE study. *J Pediatr.* 2003;(143):477-483.

353. Vohr B, Ment LR. Intraventricular hemorrhage in the preterm infant. *Early Human Dev.* 1996;44(1):1-16.

354. Lucey JF, Rowan CA, Shiono P, et al. Fetal infants: the fate of 4172 infants with birth weights of 410 to 500 grams-The Vermont Oxford Network experience (1996–2000). *Pediatrics.* 2004;113(4):1559-1566.

355. Papile LA, Burstein J, Burston R. Incidence and evolution of subependymal and intraventricular hemorrhage: a study of infants with birthweights less than 1500 grams. *J Perinatol.* 1978;92:529-534.

356. Papile LA. Periventricular-Intraventricular hemorrhage. In: Fanaroff AA, Martin RJ, eds. *Neonatal-Perinatal Medicine: Diseases of the Fetus and Infant.* 5th ed. Mosby; 1992.

357. Shalik L, Perlman JM. Hemorrhagic-ischemic cerebral injury in the preterm infant: clinical concepts. *Clin Perinatol.* 2002;29:745-763.

358. Cullens V. Brain injury in the premature infant. In: L Boxwell G, ed. *Neonatal Intensive Care Nursing.* Routledge; 2000.

359. Vohr BR, Garcia-Coll C, Mayfield S, et al. Neurologic and developmental status related to the evolution of visual-motor abnormalities from birth to 2 years of age in preterm infants with intraventricular hemorrhage. *J Pediatr.* 1989;115(2):296-302.

360. Bada HS, Korones SB, Perry EH, et al. Frequent handling in the neonatal intensive care unit and intraventricular hemorrhage. *J Pediatr.* 1990;117(1, part 1):126-131.

361. Bada HS, Korones SB, Perry EH, et al. Mean arterial blood pressure changes in premature infants and those at risk for intraventricular hemorrhage. *J Pediatr.* 1990;117(4):607-614.

362. Perlman JM, Thach B. Respiratory origins of fluctuations in arterial blood pressure in premature infants with respiratory distress syndrome. *Pediatrics.* 1988;81(3):399-403.

363. Perlman JM, McMenamin JB, Volpe JJ. Fluctuating cerebral blood velocity in respiratory distress syndrome: relationship to subsequent development of intraventricular hemorrhage. *N Engl J Med.* 1983;309(4):204-209.

364. Fanconi S, Duc G. Intratracheal suctioning in sick preterm infants: prevention of intracranial hemorrhage and cerebral hypofusion by muscle paralysis. *Pediatrics.* 1987;79:583-543.

365. Bregman J, Kimberlin LVS. Developmental outcomes in extremely premature infants. *Pediatr Clin North Am.* 1993;40(5):937-950.

366. Perlman JM. Cognitive and behavioral deficits in premature graduates of intensive care. *Clin Perinatol.* 2002;29(4):779-797.

367. Krishnamoorthy KS, Kuban KC, Leviton A, et al. Periventricular-intraventricular hemorrhage, sonographic localization, phenobarbital, and motor abnormalities in low birth weight infants. *Pediatrics.* 1990;85(6):1027-1033.

368. Zach T, Brown JC. Periventricular leukomalacia. *Emedicine J.* 2003. Accessed January 13, 2021. https://emedicine.medscape.com/article/975728-overview#a0199

369. Shankaran S. Hemorrhagic lesions of the central nervous system. In: Stevenson DK, Benitz WE, Sunshine P, eds. *Fetal and Neonatal Brain Injury.* 3rd ed. Cambridge University Press; 1997.

370. Inder TE, Weels SJ, Mogride NB, et al. Defining the nature of cerebral abnormalities in the premature infant: a qualitative magnetic resonance imaging study. *J Pediatr.* 2003;143(2):171-179.

371. Scher MS. Fetal and neonatal neurologic consultations and identifying brain disorders in the context of fetal-maternal-perinatal disease. *Semin Pediatr Neurol.* 2001;8(2):55-75.

372. Murphy BP, Inder TE, Rooks V, et al. Posthemorrhagic ventricular dilation in the premature infant: natural history and predictors of outcome. *Arch Dis Child.* 2002;87:F37-F41.

373. Anonymous. Randomised trial of early tapping neonatal post hemorrhagic ventricular dilatation results at 30 months. *Arch Dis Child Fetal Neonatal Ed.* 1994;70(2):F129-F136.

374. Allan WC, Sobel DB. Neonatal intensive care neurology. *Semin Pediatr Neurol.* 2004;11(2):119-128.

375. Peterson BS, Vohr B, Staib LH, et al. Regional brain volume abnormalities and longterm cognitive outcome in preterm infants. *JAMA.* 2000;284(15):1939-1947.

376. Blackburn ST. Assessment and management of the neurologic system. In: *Comprehensive Neonatal Nursing: A Physiologic Perspective.* 3rd ed. Saunders; 2003.

377. Jones MW, Bass WT. Perinatal brain injury in the premature infant. *Neonatal Netw.* 2003;22(1):61-67.

378. Schmidt B, Davis P, Moddemann D, et al. Long-term effects of indomethacin prophylaxis in extremely-low-birth-weight infants. *N Engl J Med.* 2001;344(26):1966-1972.

379. Ment LK, Vohr B, Allen W, et al. Change in cognitive function over time in very low-birth-weight infants. *JAMA.* 2003;289(6):705-711.

380. Han TR, Bang MS, Yoon BH, et al. Risk factors for cerebral palsy in preterm infants. *Am J Phys Med Rehabil.* 2002;81:297-303.

381. Westrup B, Bohm B, Lagercrantz H, et al. Preschool outcomes in children born very prematurely. *Acta Paediatr.* 2004;93:498-507.

382. Sizan J, Ratynski N, Boussard C. Humane neonatal care initiative: NIDCAP and family centered neonatal care. Neonatal individualized developmental care and assessment program. *Acta Paediatr.* 1999; 88(10):1172.

383. Zupan V, Gonzalez P, Laaze-Masmonteil T, et al. Periventricular leukomalacia: risk factors revisited. *Dev Med Child Neurol.* 1996;38(12):1061-1067.

384. Volpe JJ. Neurobiology of periventricular leukomalacia in the preterm infant. *Pediatr Res.* 2001;50(5):553-562.

385. Larroque B, Marret S, Ancel P-Y, et al. White matter damage and intraventricular hemorrhage in very preterm infants. The EPIPAGE study. *J Pediatr.* 2003;143:477-503.

386. Blumenthal I. Periventricular leukomalacia: a review. *Eur J Pediatr.* 2004;163:435-442.

387. Batten D, Kirtley X, Swails T. Unexpected versus anticipated cystic periventricular leukomalacia. *Am J Perinatol.* 2003;20(1):33-40.

388. Kadhim H, Tabarki B, Verellen G, et al. Inflammatory cytokines in the pathogenesis of periventricular leukomalacia. *Neurology.* 2001;56:1278-1284.

389. Dammann O, Kuban KC, Leviton A. Perinatal infection, fetal inflammatory response, white matter damage and cognitive limitations in children born preterm. *Ment Retard Dev Disabil Res Rev.* 2002;8(1):46-50.

390. Dammann O, Leviton A. Infection remote from the brain, neonatal white matter damage and cerebral palsy in the preterm infant. *Semin Pediatr Neurol.* 1998;5:190-201.

391. Wilson-Costello D, Borawski E, Freidman H, et al. Perinatal correlates of cerebral palsy and other neurologic impairment among very low birth weight children. *Pediatrics.* 1998;102(2):315-322.

392. Gressens P, Rogido M, Paindaveine S, et al. The impact of neonatal intensive care practices on the developing brain. *J Pediatr.* 2002;140:646-653.

393. Perrott S, Dodds L, Vincer M. A population-based study of prognostic factors in very preterm survivors. *J Perinatol.* 2003;23(2):111-116.

394. Lemons JA, Bauer CR, Oh W, et al. Very low birth weight outcomes of the national institute of child health and human development neonatal research network, January 1995 through December 1996. *Pediatrics.* 2001;107(1):E1-E8.

395. Askin DF, Diehl-Jones W. Retinopathy of prematurity. *Crit Care Nurs Clin N Am.* 2009;337:83-84.

396. Lundgren P, Kistner A, Andersson EM, et al. Low birthweight is a risk factor for severe retinopathy of prematurity depending on gestational age at birth. *PLoS ONE.* 2014;9:e109460.

397. Ortega-Molina JM, Anaya-Alaminos R, Uneros-Fernandez J, et al. Genetic and environmental influences on retinopathy of prematurity. *Mediators Inflamm.* 2015:764159.

398. Smith LE. IGF-1 and retinopathy of prematurity in the preterm infant. *Biol Neonate.* 2005;88:237-244.

399. Chen J, Smith LE. Retinopathy of prematurity. *Angiogenesis.* 2007;10:133-140.

400. Hellstrom A, Ley D, Hansen-Pupp I, et al. Role of insulinlike growth factor 1 in fetal development and in the early postnatal life of premature infants. *Am J Perinatol.* 2016;33:1067-1071.

401. International Committee for Classification of ROP. The International Classification of Retinopathy of Prematurity revisited. *Arch Ophthalmol.* 2005;123:991-999.

402. Early Treatment for Retinopathy of Prematurity Cooperative Group. Revised indications for the treatment of retinopathy of prematurity. Results of the early treatment for retinopathy of prematurity randomized trial. *Arch Ophthalmol.* 2003;121(12):1684-1694.

403. Fierson WM, AAP American Academy of Pediatrics Section on Ophthalmology, AAP American Academy for Pediatric Ophthalmology and Strabismus, AAP American Association of Certified Orthoptists. Screening examination of premature infants for retinopathy of prematurity. *Pediatrics.* 2018;142(6):e20183061.

404. Hwang CK, Hubbard GB, Hutchinson AK, et al. Outcomes after intravitreal bevacizumab versus laser photocoagulation for retinopathy of prematurity: a five year retrospective analysis. *Ophthalmology.* 2015;122(5):1008-1015.

405. Sanghi G. Aggressive posterior retinopathy: risk factors for retinal detachment despite confluence laser photocoagulation. *Am J Ophthalmol.* 2013;151:159-164.

406. Redline RW. Placental pathology. In: Fanaroff AA, Martin RJ, eds. *Neonatal-Perinatal Medicine Diseases of the Fetus and Infant.* 7th ed. Mosby; 2002.

407. Vannucci RC, Palmer C. Hypoxia-ischemia: neuropathology, pathogenesis, and management. In: Fanaroff AA, Martin RJ, eds. *Neonatal-Perinatal Medicine Diseases of the Fetus and Infant.* 7th ed. Mosby; 2002.

408. Demari S. Calcium and phosphorus nutrition in preterm infants. *Acta Paediatr Suppl.* 2005;94(449):87-92.

409. Huttner KM. Metabolic bone disease of prematurity. In: Cloherty JP, Eichenwald EC, Stark AR, eds. *Manual of Neonatal Care.* 5th ed. Lippincott Williams & Wilkins; 2004.

410. Miller M. The bone disease of preterm birth: a biomechanical perspective. *Pediatr Res.* 2003;53(1):10-15.

411. Krug SK. Osteopenia of prematurity. In: Groh-Wargo S, Thompson M, Cox J, eds. *Nutritional Care for High-Risk Newborns Rev.* 3rd ed. Precept Press Inc; 2000.

412. Rauch F, Schoenau E. Skeletal development in premature infants: a review of bone physiology beyond nutritional aspects. *Arch Dis Child Fetal Neonatal Ed.* 2002;86:F82-F85.

413. Rigo J, DeCurtis M, Pieltain C, et al. Bone mineral metabolism in the micropreemie. *Clin Perinatol.* 2000;27:147-170.

414. Rigo J, Senterre J. Nutritional needs of premature infants: current issues. *J Pediatr.* 2006;149(3 suppl):S80-S88.

415. Abrams SA. *Calcium and phosphorus requirements of newborn infants.* UpToDate. Accessed June 2013. http://www.uptodate.com/contents/calcium-and-phosphorus-requirements-of-newborn infants?source=search_result&search=metabolic+bone+disease+o f+prematurity&selectedTitle=1%7E150#H12

416. Fewtrell MS, Cole TJ, Bishop NJ, et al. Neonatal factors predicting childhood height in preterm infants: evidence for a persisting effect of early metabolic bone disease? *J Pediatr.* 2000;137:668-673.

417. Vachharajani AV, Mathur AM, Rao R. Metabolic bone disease of prematurity. *NeoReviews.* 2009;10:e402-e411.

418. Jones S, Bell MJ. Distal radius fracture in a premature infant with osteopenia caused by handling during intravenous cannulation. *Injury.* 2002;33:265-266.

419. *Osteogenesis Imperfecta Foundation.* http://www.oif.org/site/DocServer/Infant_Care_Suggestions_for_Parents.pdf?docID=7213.

420. Eliakim A, Nemet D. Osteopenia of prematurity-the role of exercise in the prevention and treatment. *Pediatr Endocrinol Rev.* 2005;2(4):675-682.

421. Moyer-Mileur LJ, Brunstetter V, McNaught TP, et al. Daily physical activity program increases bone mineralization and growth in preterm very low birth weight infants. *Pediatrics.* 2000;106(5):1088-1092.

422. Litmanovitz I, Dolfin T, Friedland O, et al. Early physical activity intervention prevents decrease of bone strength in very low birth weight infants. *Pediatrics.* 2003;112(1):15-19.

423. Schulzke SM, Trachsel D, Patole SK. Physical activity programs for promoting bone mineralization and growth in preterm infants. *Cochrane Database Syst Rev.* 2007;(2):CD005387.

424. Jenson EA, Schmidt B. Epidemiology of bronchopulmonary dysplasia. *Birth Defects Res A Clin Mol Teratol.* 2014;100:145-157.

425. Stoll BJ, Hansen NJ, Bell EF, et al. Trends in care practices, morbidity, and mortality of extremely preterm neonates, 1993–2012. *JAMA.* 2015;314:1039-1051.

426. Northway WH, Rosan RC, Porter DY. Pulmonary disease following respiratory therapy of hyaline-membrane disease. Bronchopulmonary dysplasia. *N Engl J Med.* 1967;16(276):357-368.

427. Jobe AH, Bancalari E. Bronchopulmonary dysplasia. *Am J Respir Crit Care Med.* 2001;63(7):1723-1729.

428. Voynow JA. "New" bronchopulmonary dysplasia and chronic lung disease. *Padiatr Respir Rev*. 2017;24:17-18.

429. Logan JW, Lynch SK, Curtiss J, et al. Clinical phenotypes and management concepts for severe, established, bronchopulmonary dysplasia. *Paediatr Resp Rev*. 2019;31:58-63.

430. Coalson JJ. Pathology of new bronchopulmonary dysplasia. *Semin Neonatol*. 2003;8(1):73-81.

431. Jensen EA, Wright CJ. Bronchopulmonary dysplasia: the ongoing search for one definition to rule them all. *J Pediatr*. 2018;197:8-10.

432. Jensen EA, Dysart K, Gantz MG. The diagnosis of bronchopulmonary dysplasia in very preterm infants. An evidence-based approach. *Am J Respir Crit Care Med*. 2019;220(6):751-759.

433. Isayama T, Lee SK, Yang J, et al. Revisiting the definition of bronchopulmonary dysplasia. Effect of changing panoply of respiratory support for preterm neonates. *JAMA Pediatr*. 2017;171(3):271-279.

434. Poindexter BB, Feng R, Schmidt B, et al. Comparisons & limitations of current definitions of bronchopulmonary dysplasia for the prematurity and respiratory outcomes program. *Ann Am Thorac Soc*. 2015;12:1822-1830.

435. Van Marter LJ. Epidemiology of bronchopulmonary dysplasia. *Semin Fetal Neonatal Med*. 2009;14:358-366.

436. Thebaud B, Abman SH. Bronchopulmonary dysplasia: where have all the vessels gone? Roles of angiogenic growth factors in chronic lung disease. *Am J Respir Crit Care Med*. 2007;175:978-985.

437. Parker RA, Lindstrom DP, Cotton RB. Evidence from twin study implies possible genetic susceptibility to bronchopulmonary dysplasia. *Semin Perinatol*. 1996;20:206-209.

438. Bhandari V, Bizzaro MS, Shetty A, et al. Familial and genetic susceptibility to major neonatal morbidities in preterm twins. *Pediatrics*. 2006;117:1901-1906.

439. Askin DF, Diehl–Jones W. Pathogenesis and prevention of chronic lung disease in the neonate. *Crit Care Nurs Clin N Am*. 2009;21:11-25.

440. Balinotti JE, Chakr VC, Tiller C. Growth of lung parenchyma in infants and toddlers with chronic lung disease of infancy. *Am J Respir Crit Care Med*. 2010;181:1093-1097.

441. Trembath A, Laughton MM. Predictors of bronchopulmonary dysplasia. *Clin Perinatol*. 2012;39:585-601.

442. Abman S, Bancalari E, Jobe A. The evolution of bronchopulmonary dysplasia after 50 years. Historical perspective. *Am J Resp Crit Care Med*. 2017;195(4):412-424.

443. Rugolo LMSS, Bentin MK, Petean CE. Preeclampsia: effect on the fetus and newborn. *NeoReviews*. 2011;12:e1298-e2206.

444. Taglauer E, Abman SH, Keller RL. Recent advances in antenatal factors predisposing to bronchopulmonary dysplasia. *Semin Perinatol*. 2018;42:413-424.

445. Bose CL, Van Marter LJ, Laughan M, et al. Fetal growth restriction and chronic lung disease among infants born before the 28th week of gestation. *Pediatrics*. 2009;124:e450-e458.

446. Rozance PJ, Seedorf GJ, Brown A, et al. IUGR decreased pulmonary alveolar and vessel growth and causes pulmonary artery endothelial cell dysfunction in vitro in fetal sheep. *Am J Physiol Lung Cell Mol Physiol*. 2011;301:L860-L871.

447. Lahra M. Intrauterine inflammation, neonatal sepsis, and chronic lung disease: a 13–year hospital cohort study. *Pediatrics*. 2009;123(5):1314-1319.

448. Speer CP. Inflammation and bronchopulmonary dysplasia. *Semin Neonatol*. 2003;8(1):29-38.

449. Jobe AH. Effects of chorioamnionitis on the fetal lung. *Clin Perinatol*. 2012;39:441-457.

450. Ali Z, Schmidt P, Dodd J, et al. Bronchopulmonary dysplasia: a review. *Arch Gynecol Obstet*. 2013;288:325–333. https://doi.org/10.1007/s00404-013-2753-8

451. Sosenko IRS, Bancalari E. New developments in the pathogenesis and prevention of bronchopulmonary dysplasia. In: Bancalari E, Polin RA, eds. *The Newborn Lung: Neonatology Questions and Controversies*. 2nd ed. Elsevier Saunders; 2012:217-233.

452. Kelly MS, Benjamin DK, Puopolo KM, et al. Postnatal cytomegalovirus infection and the risk of bronchopulmonary dysplasia. *JAMA Pediatr*. 2015;169(12):e153785.

453. Bancalari E, Abdenocir GE, Feller R, et al. Bronchopulmonary dysplasia: clinical presentation. *J Pediatr*. 1979;95(5 part 2):819-823.

454. Fleisher B, Kulovich M, Hallman M, et al. Lung profile: sex differences in normal pregnancy. *Obstet Gynecol*. 1985;66(3):327-330.

455. Philip AGS. Bronchopulmonary dysplasia: then and now. *Neonatology*. 2012;102:1-8.

456. Kair LR, Leonard DT, Anderson JDM. Bronchopulmonary dysplasia. *Pediatr Rev*. 2012;33(5):255-263.

457. Halliday M, Ehrenkranz RA, Doyle LW. Early (<8 days) postnatal corticosteroids for preventing chronic lung disease in ventilated very low birthweight preterm infants. *Cochrane Database Syst Rev*. 2017;2017:CD002057.

458. Doyle LW, Cheong JLY. Postnatal corticosteroids to prevent or treat bronchopulmonary dysplasia—Who might benefit? *Semin Fetal Neonatal Med*. 2017;22(5):290-295.

459. Thebaud B, Goss KN, Laughon M, et al. Bronchopulmonary dysplasia. *Nat Rev Dis Primers*. 2019;5(1):78.

460. Demauro SB. The impact of bronchopulmonary dysplasia on childhood outcomes. *Clin Perinatol*. 2018;45:439-452.

461. Khemani E, McElhinney DB, Rhein L, et al. Pulmonary artery hypertension in formally premature infants with bronchopulmonary dysplasia: clinical features and outcomes in the surfactant era. *Pediatrics*. 2007;120:1260-1269.

462. Mirza H, Ziegler J, Ford S, et al. Pulmonary hypertension in preterm infants: prevalence and association with BPD. *J Pediatr*. 2014;165:909-914.

463. Korhonen P, Laitmen J, Hyodymaa E, et al. Respiratory outcome in school aged, very-low-birth-weight children in the surfactant era. *Acta Paediatr*. 2004;93:316-321.

464. Cheong JLY, Doyle LW. An update on pulmonary and neurodevelopmental outcomes of bronchopulmonary dysplasia. *Semin Perinatol*. 2018;42:478-484.

465. Kuint J, Lerner-Geva L, Chodick G, et al. Rehospitalization through childhood and adolescence: association with neonatal morbidities in infants of very low birth weight. *J Pediatr*. 2017;188:135.e2-141.e2.

466. Sanchez-Solis M, Perez-Fernandez V, Bosch-Gimenez V, et al. Lung function gain in preterm infants with and without bronchopulmonary dysplasia. *Pediatr Pulm*. 2016;51(9):936-942.

467. Doyle LW, Irving L, Harkerwal A, et al. Airway obstruction in young adults born extremely preterm or extremely low birthweight in the post surfactant era. *Thorax*. 2019;10:1-7.

468. Jeng SF, Hsu CH, Tsai PN, et al. Bronchopulmonary dysplasia predicts adverse developmental and clinical outcomes in very-low-birthweight infants. *Dev Med Child Neurol*. 2008;50:51-57.

469. Short E, Kirchner L, Asaad GR, et al. Developmental sequelae in preterm infants having a diagnosis of bronchopulmonary dysplasia: analysis using a severity-based classification system. *Arch Pediatr Adolesc Med*. 2007;161(11):1082-1087.

470. Ehrenkrantz RA, Walsh MC, Vohr BR, et al. National Institutes of Child Health and Human Development Neonatal Research Network. Validation of the National Institutes of Health consensus definition of bronchopulmonary dysplasia. *Pediatrics*. 2005;116(6):1353-1360.

471. Singer L, Yamashita TS, Lilien L, et al. A longitudinal study of developmental outcome of infants with bronchopulmonary dysplasia and very low birthweight. *Pediatrics*. 1997;100:987-993.

472. Karogianni P, Tsakaidis C, Kyriakidou M, et al. Neuromotor outcomes in infants with bronchopulmonary dysplasia. *Pediatr Neurol*. 2011;44(1):40-46.

473. Majnemer A, Riley P, Shevell M, et al. Severe bronchopulmonary dysplasia increase risk for later neurological and motor sequelae in preterm survivors. *Dev Med Child Neurol*. 2000;42:53-60.

474. Skidmore MD, Rivers A, Hack M. Increased risk of cerebral palsy among very low birthweight infants with chronic lung disease. *Dev Med Child Neurol.* 1990;82:325-332.

475. Kobaly K, Schluchter M, Minich N, et al. Outcomes of extremely low birthweight (<1 kg) and extremely low gestational age (<28 weeks) infants with bronchopulmonary dysplasia: effects of practice changes in 2000 to 2003. *Pediatrics.* 2008;121(1):73-81.

476. Natarajan G, Pappas A, Shankaran S, et al. Outcomes of extremely low birth weight infants with bronchopulmonary dysplasia: impact of the physiologic definition. *Early Hum Dev.* 2012;88:509-515.

477. Morely CJ. Volume limited and volume targeted ventilation. *Clin Perinatol.* 39(3):513-523.

478. Schlapbach LJ, Adams M, Proietti E, et al. Swiss National Network & Follow-up Group. Outcome at 2 years of age in a Swiss national cohort of extremely preterm infants born between 2000 and 2008. *BMC Pediatr.* 2012;12(1):198.

479. Twilhaar ES, Wade RM, Kieviet JF. Cognitive outcomes of children born extremely or very preterm since the 1990's and associated risk factors: a meta analysis and meta regression. *JAMA Pediatr.* 2018;172(4):361-367.

480. Palisano RJ, Hanna SE, Rosenbaum PL, et al. Validation of a model of gross motor function for children with cerebral palsy. *Phys Ther.* 2000;80(10):974-985.

481. Van Marter LJ, Kuban KC, Allred E, et al. Does bronchopulmonary dysplasia contribute to the occurrence of cerebral palsy among infants born before 28 weeks gestation? *Arch Dis Child Fetal Neonatal Ed.* 2011;96:F20-F29.

482. De Buys AS, Dinh-Xuan AT. Congenital diaphragmatic hernia: current status and review of the literature. *Eur J Pediatr.* 2018;53:113-117.

483. Bloss RS, Aranda JV, Beardmore HE. Congenital diaphragmatic hernia: pathophysiology and pharmacologic support. *Surgery.* 1981;89:518.

484. Bianchi DW, Crumbleholme TM, D'Alton ME. Diaphragmatic hernia. In: *Fetology Diagnosis and Management of the Fetal Patient.* McGraw-Hill; 2000.

485. Abramov A, Fan W, Hernan R, et al. Comparative outcomes of right vs left congenital diaphragmatic hernia: a multicentre analysis. *J Pediatr Surg.* 2019. doi:10.1016/j.jpedsurg.2019.09.046

486. Kosinski P, Wielgos M. Congenital diaphragmatic hernia: pathogenesis, prenatal diagnosis and management-literature review. *Ginekol Pol.* 2017;88(1):24-30.

487. Hedrick HL, Adzick NS. *Congenital diaphragmatic hernia in the neonate.* UpToDate. Accessed March 2013. http://www.uptodate.com/contents/congenital-diaphragmatic-hernia-in-the-neonate?source=search_result&search=congenital+diaphragmatic+hernia&selectedTitle=2%7E31

488. Pober BR. Overview of epidemiology, genetics, birth defects, and chromosomal abnormalities associated with CDH. *Am J Med Genet C Semin Med Genet.* 2007;145C(2):158-171.

489. Crane JP. Familial congenital diaphragmatic hernia: prenatal diagnostic approach and analysis of twelve families. *Clin Genet.* 1979;16:244.

490. Puri P, Gorman F. Lethal nonpulmonary anomalies associated with congenital diaphragmatic hernia: implications for early intrauterine surgery. *J Pediatr Surg.* 1984;19:29.

491. Witters I, Legius E, Moerman P, et al. Associated malformations and chromosomal anomalies in 42 cases of prenatally diagnosed diaphragmatic hernia. *Am J Med Genet.* 2001;103:278.

492. Hedrick HL, Adzick NS. *Congenital diaphragmatic hernia: prenatal diagnosis and management.* UpToDate. Accessed March 2013. http://www.uptodate.com/contents/congenital-diaphragmatic-hernia-prenatal-diagnosis-andmanagement?source=search_result&search=cdh&selectedTitle=2%7E11

493. Slavontinek AM. The genetics of common disorders-congenital diaphragmatic hernia. *Eur J Med Genet.* 2014;57(8):418-423.

494. Townsend. Abdomen. In: *Sabiston Textbook of Surgery.* 16th ed. WB Saunders Co; 2001:1478.

495. Jancelewicz T, Brindle ME. Prediction tools in congenital diaphragmatic hernia. *Semin Perinatol.* 2019 (In press). doi:10.1053/j.semperi.2019.07.004

496. Hutcheon J, Butler B, Lisonkova S, et al. Timing of delivery for pregnancies with congenital diaphragmatic hernia. *BJOG.* 2010;117:1658-1662.

497. Odibo AO, Njaf T, Vachharajani A, et al. Predictors of the need for extracorporeal membrane oxygenation and survival in congenital diaphragmatic hernia: a center's 10-year experience. *Prenat Diagn.* 2010;30:518-521.

498. Safavi A, Lin Y, Skarsgard ED, et al. Canadian Pediatric Surgery Network. Perinatal management of congenital diaphragmatic hernia: when and how should babies be delivered? Results from the Canadian Pediatric Surgery Network. *J Pediatr Surg.* 2010;45:2334-2339.

499. Lakshminrusimha S, Vali P. Congenital diaphragmatic hernia: 25 years of shared knowledge; what about survival? *J Pediatr (Rio J).* 2019. doi:10.1016/j.jped.2019.10.002

500. Morini F, Valfre L, Bagolan P. Long-term morbidity of congenital diaphragmatic hernia: a plea for standardization. *Semin Pediatr Surg.* 2017;26:301-310.

501. Lally KP, Paranka MS, Roden J, et al. Congenital diaphragmatic hernia. Stabilization and repair on ECMO. *Ann Surg.* 1992;216(5):569-573.

502. Danzer E, Gerdes M, Bernbaum J, et al. Neurodevelopmental outcome of infants with congenital diaphragmatic hernia prospectively enrolled in an interdisciplinary follow-up program. *J Pediatr Surg.* 2010;45(9):1759-1766.

503. Danzer E, Hoffman C, D'Agostino JA, et al. Neurodevelopmental outcomes at 5 years of age in congenital diaphragmatic hernia. *J Pediatr Surg.* 2017;52:437-443.

504. Bevikacqua F, Morini F, Zaccara A, et al. Neurodevelopmental outcome in congenital diaphragmatic hernia survivors: a role of ventilatory time. *J Pediatr Surf.* 2015;50(3):394-398.

505. Russell KW, Barnhart DC, Rollins MD, et al. Musculoskeletal deformities following repair of large congenital diaphragmatic hernias. *J Pediatr Surg.* 2014;49(6):851-854.

506. Kuklová P, Zemková D, Kyncl M, et al. Large diaphragmatic defect: are skeletal deformities preventable? *Pediatr Surg Int.* 2011;27(12):1343-1349.

507. Lund DP, Mitchell J, Kharasch V, et al. Congenital diaphragmatic hernia: the hidden morbidity. *J Pediatr Surg.* 1994;29(2):258-262.

508. Stallings EB, Isenberg JL, Short TD, et al. Population-based birth defects data in the United States, 2012-2016: a focus on abdominal wall defects. *Birth Defects Res.* 2019;111:1436.

509. Marshall J, Salemi JL, Tanner JP, et al.; National Birth Defects Prevention Network. Prevalence, correlates, and outcomes of Omphalocele in the United States, 1995–2005. *Obstet Gynecol.* 2015;126(2):284-293.

510. Agopian A, Marengo L, Mitchell LE. Descriptive epidemiology of nonsyndromic omphalocele in Texas, 1999–2004. *Am J Med Genet A.* 2009;149A(10):2129-2133.

511. Benjamin B, Wilson GN. Anomalies associated with gastroschisis and omphalocele: analysis of 2825 cases from the Texas birth defects registry. *J Pediatr Surg.* 2014;49(4):514-519.

512. Stoll C, Alembik Y, Dott B, et al. Omphalocele and gastroschisis and associated malformations. *Am J Med Genet A.* 2008;146A(10):1280-1285.

513. Hijkoop A, Peters NC, Lechner RL, et al. Omphalocele: from diagnosis to growth and developmental at 2 years of age. *Arch Dis Child Fetal Neonatal Ed.* 2019;104:F18-F23.

514. Sadler TW. The embryologic origin of ventral body wall defects. *Semin Pediatr Surg.* 2010;19:209-214.

515. Kleinrouweler CE, Kuijper CF, van Zalen-Sprock MM, et al. Characteristics and outcome and the omphalocele circumference/abdominal circumference ratio in prenatally diagnosed fetal omphalocele. *Fetal Diagn Ther.* 2011;30:60-69.

516. Davis AS, Blumenfeld Y, Rubesova E, et al. Challenges of giant omphalocele: form fetal diagnosis to follow-up. *NeoReviews.* 2008;9(8):e338-e346.

517. Gamba P, Midrio P. Abdominal wall defects: prenatal diagnosis, newborn management, and long-term outcomes. *Semin Pediatr Surg.* 2014;23:283-290.

518. Ledbetter DJ. Congenital abdominal wall defects and reconstruction in pediatric surgery. Gastroschisis and omphalocele. Surg Clin N Am. 2012;92:713-727.

519. Pacilli M, Spitz L, Kiely EM, et al. Staged repair of giant omphalocele in the neonatal period. *J Pediatr Surg.* 2005;40:785-788.

520. Danzer E, Gerdes M, D'Agostino JA, et al. Prospective, interdisciplinary follow-up of children with prenatally diagnosed giant omphalocele: short-term neurodevelopmental outcome. *J Pediatr Surg.* 2010;45:718-723.

521. Danzer E, Gerdes M, D'Agostino JA, et al. Patient characteristics are important determinants of neurodevelopmental outcome during infancy in giant omphalocele. *Early Hum Dev.* 2015;91:187-193.

522. Danzer E, Hoffman C, Miller JS, et al. Autism spectrum disorder and neurodevelopmental delays in children with giant omphalocele. *J Pediatr Surg.* 2019;54(9):1771-1777.

523. Skarsgard E. Management of gastroschisis. *Curr Opin Pediatr.* 2016;28(3):363-369.

524. Sadler TW, Feldkamp MC. The embryology of body wall closure: relevance to gastroschisis and other ventral body wall defects. *Am Med Genet C Semin Med Genet.* 2008;148C:180-185.

525. Feldkamp, ML Carey JC, Sadler TW. Development of gastroschisis: review of hypotheses, a novel hypothesis, and implications for research. *Am J Med Genet A.* 2007;143(7):639-652.

526. Anderson JE, Galganski LA, Cheng Y, et al. Epidemiology of gastroschisis: a population-based study in California from 1995 to 2012. *J Pediatr Surg.* 2018;53(12):2399-2403. doi:10.1016/j.jpedsurg.2018.08.035

527. Short TD, Stallings EB, Isenberg J, et al. Gastroschisis trends and ecologic link to opioid prescription rates—United States, 2006-2015. *MMWR Morb Wkly Rep.* 2019;68:31.

528. Friedman AM, Ananth CV, Siddiq Z, et al. Gastroschisis: epidemiology and mode of delivery, 2005-2013. *Am J Obstet Gynecol.* 2016;215(3):348.e1-348.e9.

529. Nicholas SS, Stamilio DM, Dicke JM, et al. Predicting adverse neonatal outcomes in fetuses with abdominal wall defects using prenatal risk factors. *Am J Obstet Gynecol.* 2009;201:383.e1-383.e6.

530. Amin R, Domack A, Bartoletti J, et al. National practice patterns for prenatal monitoring in gastroschisis: gastroschisis outcomes of delivery (GOOD) provider study. *Fetal Diagn Ther.* 2019;45:125-130.

531. Harris EL, Hart SJ, Minutillo C, et al. The long-term neurodevelopmental and psychological outcomes of gastroschisis: a cohort study. *J Pediatr Surg.* 2016;51:549-553.

532. Ledbetter DJ. Gastroschisis and omphalocele. Surg Clin North Am. 2006;86(2):249-260.

533. Tosello B, Guimond F, Faure A, et al. Neurodevelopment and health-related quality of life in infants born with gastroschisis: a 6 year retrospective French study. *Eur J Pediatr Surg.* 2017;27(4):352-360. doi: 10.1055/s-0036-1597268

534. Minutillo C, Rao SC, Pirie S, et al. Growth and developmental outcomes of infants with gastroschisis at one year of age: a retrospective study. *J Pediatr Surg.* 2013;48:1688-1696.

535. Lap CCMM, Bolhuis SW, Van Braeckel KNJA, et al. Functional outcome at school age of children born with gastroschisis. *Early Hum Dev.* 2017;106-107:47-52.

536. West SE. Normal and abnormal structural development of the lung. In: Polin RA, Fox WW, Abman SH, eds. *Fetal and Neonatal Physiology.* 2nd ed. WB Saunders Co; 1998.

537. Oermann CM. *Congenital anomalies of the intrathoracic airways and tracheoesophageal fistula.* UpToDate. Accessed April 2013. http://www.uptodate.com/contents/congenital-anomalies-of-the-intra-thoracic-airways-and-tracheoesophageal-fistula?source=search_result&search=tef&selectedTitle=1%7E62

538. Crisera CA, Grau JB, Maldonado TS, et al. Defective epithelial-mesenchymal interactions dictate the organogenesis of tracheoesophageal fistula. *Pediatr Surg Int.* 2000;16:256.

539. Goyal A, Jones MO, Couriel JM, et al. Oesophageal atresia and tracheo-oesophageal fistula. *Arch Dis Child Fetal Neonatal Ed.* 2006;91:F381.

540. Depaepe A, Dolk H, Lechat MF. The epidemiology of tracheo-oesophageal fistula and oesophageal atresia in Europe. EUROCAT Working Group. *Arch Dis Child.* 1993;68:743.

541. Robb A, Lander A. Oesophageal atresia and tracheo-oesophageal fistula. *Surgery (Oxford).* 2007;25:283. Accessed November 16, 2007. linkinghub.elsevier.com/retrieve/pii/S0263931907001135.

542. Keckler SJ, St. Peter SD, Valusek PA, et al. VACTERL anomalies in patients with esophageal atresia: an updated delineation of the spectrum and review of the literature. *Pediatr Surg Int.* 2007;23:309.

543. Ross AJ. Organogenesis, innervation and histologic development of the gastrointestinal tract. In: Polin RA, Fox WW, Abman SH, eds. *Fetal and Neonatal Physiology.* 2nd ed. WB Saunders Co; 1998.

544. Pretorius DH, Drose JA, Dennis MA, et al. Tracheoesophageal fistula in utero. Twenty-two cases. *J Ultrasound Med.* 1987;6:509.

545. Karnak I, Senocak ME, Hiçsönmez A, et al. The diagnosis and treatment of H-type tracheoesophageal fistula. *J Pediatr Surg.* 1997;32:1670.

546. Laffan EE, Daneman A, Ein SH, et al. Tracheoesophageal fistula without esophageal atresia: are pull-back tube esophagograms needed for diagnosis? *Pediatr Radiol.* 2006;36:1141.

547. Nagata K, Kamio Y, Ichikawa T, et al. Congenital tracheoesophageal fistula successfully diagnosed by CT esophagography. *World J Gastroenterol.* 2006;12:1476.

548. Islam S, Cavanaugh E, Honeke R, et al. Diagnosis of a proximal tracheoesophageal fistula using three-dimensional CT scan: a case report. *J Pediatr Surg.* 2004;39:100.

549. Dogan BE, Fitoz S, Atasoy C, et al. Tracheoesophageal fistula: demonstration of recurrence by three-dimensional computed tomography. *Curr Probl Diagn Radiol.* 2005;34:167.

550. Thigpen TL, Kenner C. Assessment and management of the gastrointestinal system. In: Kenner C, Lott JW, eds. *Comprehensive Neonatal Nursing: A Physiologic Perspective.* 3rd ed. Saunders; 2003.

551. Little DC, Rescorla FJ, Grosfeld JL, et al. Long-term analysis of children with esophageal atresia and tracheoesophageal fistula. *J Pediatr Surg.* 2003;38:852.

552. Orford J, Cass DT, Glasson MJ. Advances in the treatment of oesophageal atresia over three decades: the 1970s and the 1990s. *Pediatr Surg Int.* 2004;20:402.

553. Tsao K, Lee H. Extrapleural thoracoscopic repair of esophageal atresia with tracheoesophageal fistula. *Pediatr Surg Int.* 2005;21:308.

554. Krosnar S, Baxter A. Thoracoscopic repair of esophageal atresia with tracheoesophageal fistula: anesthetic and intensive care management of a series of eight neonates. *Paediatr Anaesth.* 2005;15:541.

555. Rothenberg SS. Thoracoscopic repair of esophageal atresia and tracheo-esophageal fistula. *Semin Pediatr Surg.* 2005;14:2.

556. Meier JD, Sulman CG, Almond PS, et al. Endoscopic management of recurrent congenital tracheoesophageal fistula: a review of techniques and results. *Int J Pediatr Otorhinolaryngol.* 2007;71:691.

557. Holcomb GW 3rd, Rothenberg SS, Bax KM, et al. Thoracoscopic repair of esophageal atresia and tracheoesophageal fistula: a multi-institutional analysis. *Ann Surg.* 2005;242:422.

558. Freire JP, Feijó SM, Miranda L, et al. Tracheo-esophageal fistula: combined surgical and endoscopic approach. *Dis Esophagus.* 2006;19:36.

559. Patkowsk D, Rysiakiewicz K, Jaworski W, et al. Thoracoscopic repair of tracheoesophageal fistula and esophageal atresia. *J Laparoendosc Adv Surg Tech A.* 2009;19(suppl 1):S19.

560. Varjavandi V, Shi E. Early primary repair of long gap esophageal atresia: the VATER operation. *J Pediatr Surg.* 2000;35:1830.

561. Spitz L. Oesophageal atresia treatment: a 21st-century perspective. *J Pediatr Gastroenterol Nutr.* 2011;52(suppl 1):S12.

562. van der Zee DC. Thoracoscopic elongation of the esophagus in long-gap esophageal atresia. *J Pediatr Gastroenterol Nutr.* 2011; 52(suppl 1):S13.

563. LaSalle AJ, Andrassy RJ, Ver Steeg K, et al. Congenital tracheoesophageal fistula without esophageal atresia. *J Thorac Cardiovasc Surg.* 1979;78:583.

564. Ko BA, Frederic R, DiTirro PA, et al. Simplified access for division of the low cervical/high thoracic H-type tracheoesophageal fistula. *J Pediatr Surg.* 2000;35:1621.

565. Teich S, Barton DP, Ginn-Pease ME, et al. Prognostic classification for esophageal atresia and tracheoesophageal fistula: Waterston versus Montreal. *J Pediatr Surg.* 1997;32:1075.

566. Choudhury SR, Ashcraft KW, Sharp RJ, et al. Survival of patients with esophageal atresia: influence of birth weight, cardiac anomaly, and late respiratory complications. *J Pediatr Surg.* 1999;34:70.

567. Konkin DE, O'hali WA, Webber EM, et al. Outcomes in esophageal atresia and tracheoesophageal fistula. *J Pediatr Surg.* 2003;38:1726.

568. Upadhyaya VD, Gangopadhyaya AN, Gupta DK, et al. Prognosis of congenital tracheoesophageal fistula with esophageal atresia on the basis of gap length. *Pediatr Surg Int.* 2007;23:767.

569. Engum SA, Grosfeld JL, West KW, et al. Analysis of morbidity and mortality in 227 cases of esophageal atresia and/or tracheoesophageal fistula over two decades. *Arch Surg.* 1995;130:502.

570. Antoniou D, Soutis M, Christopoulos-Geroulanos G. Anastomotic strictures following esophageal atresia repair: a 20-year experience with endoscopic balloon dilatation. *J Pediatr Gastroenterol Nutr.* 2010;51:464.

571. Michaud L, Gottrand F. Anastomotic strictures: conservative treatment. *J Pediatr Gastroenterol Nutr.* 2011;52(suppl 1):S18.

572. de Lagausie P. GER in oesophageal atresia: surgical options. *J Pediatr Gastroenterol Nutr.* 2011;52(suppl 1):S27.

573. Mawlana W, Zamiara P, Lane H. Neurodevelopment of infants with esophageal atresia and tracheoesophageal fistula. *J Pediatr Surg.* 2018;53:1651-1654.

574. Newton LE, Abdessalam SF, Raynor SC. Neurodevelopmental outcomes of tracheoesophageal fistulas. *J Pediatr Surg.* 2016; 51(5):743-747.

575. Harrison MR, Golbus MS, Filly RA, et al. Management of the fetus with congenital hydronephrosis. *J Pediatr Surg.* 1982;17(6): 728-742.

576. Luks FI. New and/or improved aspects of fetal surgery. *Prenat Diagn.* 2011;31:252-258.

577. DiFiore JW, Fauza DO, Slavin R, et al. Experimental fetal tracheal ligation and congenital diaphragmatic hernia: a pulmonary vascular morphometric analysis. *J Pediatr Surg.* 1995;30(7):917.

578. Bianchi DW, Crumbleholme TM, D'Alton ME. Invasive fetal therapy and fetal surgery. In: *Fetology Diagnosis and Management of the Fetal Patient.* McGraw-Hill; 2000.

579. Deprest JA, Done E, Van Mieghem T, et al. Fetal surgery for anesthesiologists. *Curr Opin Anaesthesiol.* 2008;21:298-307.

580. Baumgarten HD, Flake AW. Fetal surgery. *Pediatr Clin North Am.* 2019;66:295-308.

581. Pedreira DAL. Advances in fetal surgery. *Einstein.* 2016;14(1):110-112.

582. Sacco A, Van der Veekin L, Bagshaw E, et al. Maternal complications following open and fetoscopic fetal surgery: a systematic review and meta-analysis. *Prenat Diagn.* 2019;39(4):251-268. doi: 10.1002/pd.5421

583. International Fetal Medicine and Surgery Society. *1st annual meeting in 1982: consensus statement and registry developed.* Accessed February 23, 2021. https://ifmss.org/about-ifmss/history/

584. Partridge EA, Flake AW. Maternal-fetal surgery for structural malformations. *Best Pract Res Clin Obstet Gynaecol.* 2012;26:669-682.

585. Wenstrom KD, Carr SR. Fetal surgery principles, indications, and evidence. *Obstet Gynecol.* 2014;124(4):817-835.

586. Moon-Grady AJ, Baschat A, Cass D, et al. Fetal treatment 2017: the evolution of fetal therapy centers: a joint opinion from the International Fetal Medicine and Surgical Society (IFMSS) and the North American Fetal Therapy Network (NAFTNet). *Fetal Diagn Ther.* 2017;42(4):241-248. doi: 10.1159/000475929

587. American College of Obstetricians Gynecologists, Committee on Ethics American Academy of Pediatrics, Committee on Bioethics. Maternal-fetal intervention and fetal care centers. *Pediatrics.* 2011;128:e473-478.

588. Farmer DL, Thorn EA, Brock JW 3rd, et al. Management of myelomeningocele study. Full cohort 30-month pediatric outcomes. *Am J Obstet Gynecol.* 2018;218(2):256.e1-256.e13.

589. Codsi EC, Audibert F. Fetal surgery: past, present, and future. *J Obstet Gynaecol Can.* 2019;4(S2):S287-S289.

590. Shieh HF, Tracy SA, Hong CR, et al. Transamnionic stem cell therapy (TRASCET) in a rabbit model of spina bifida. *J Pediatr Surg.* 2019;54:293-296.

591. Aurora S, Snyder EY. Perinatal asphyxia. In: Cloherty JP, Eichenwald EC, Stark AR, eds. *Manual of Neonatal Care.* 5th ed. Lippincott-Raven; 2004.

592. Kuban KCK, Philiano J. Neonatal seizures. In: Fanaroff AA, Martin RJ, eds. *Neonatal-Perinatal Medicine Diseases of the Fetus and Infant.* 4th ed. Mosby; 1998.

593. Yager JY, Vannucci RC. Seizures in neonates. In: Fanaroff AA, Martin RJ, eds. *Neonatal-Perinatal Medicine Diseases of the Fetus and Infant.* 7th ed. Mosby; 2002.

594. du Plessis AJ. Neonatal seizures. In: Cloherty JP, Eichenwald EC, Stark AR, eds. *Manual of Neonatal Care.* 5th ed. Lippincott-Raven; 2004.

595. Lekskulchai R, Cole J. The relationship between the scarf ratio and subsequent motor performance in infants born preterm. *Pediatr Phys Ther.* 2000;12:150-157.

596. Barfield WD, Lee KG. *Late preterm infants.* UpToDate. Accessed May 2013. http://www.uptodate.com/contents/late-preterm-infants?source=search_result&search=late+preterm+infant&selectedTitle=1%7E42

597. Spong CY, Mercer BM, D'Alton M, et al. Timing of indicated late-preterm and early-term birth. *Obstet Gynecol.* 2011;118:323.

598. Hamilton BE, Martin JA, Ventura SJ, et al. Births: final data for 2007. *Natl Vital Stat Rep.* 2010;58:24. Accessed May 2013. http://www.cdc.gov/nchs/data/nvsr/nvsr58_24.pdf

599. Goldenberg RL, Culhane JF, Iams JD, et al. Epidemiology and causes of preterm birth. *Lancet.* 2008;371:75.

600. Schieve LA, Ferre C, Peterson HB, et al. Perinatal outcome among singleton infants conceived through assisted reproductive technology in the United States. *Obstet Gynecol.* 2004;103:1144.

601. Reddy UM, Wapner RJ, Rebar RW, et al. Infertility, assisted reproductive technology, and adverse pregnancy outcomes: executive summary of a National Institute of Child Health and Human Development workshop. *Obstet Gynecol.* 2007;109:967.

602. Wang ML, Dorer DJ, Fleming MP, et al. Clinical outcomes of near-term infants. *Pediatrics.* 2004;114:372.

603. Shapiro-Mendoza CK, Tomashek KM, Kotelchuck M, et al. Effect of late-preterm birth and maternal medical conditions on newborn morbidity risk. *Pediatrics.* 2008;121:e223.

604. Bird TM, Bronstein JM, Hall RW, et al. Late preterm infants: birth outcomes and health care utilization in the first year. *Pediatrics.* 2010;126:e311.

605. Engle WA, Tomashek KM, Wallman C, et al. "Late-preterm" infants: a population at risk. *Pediatrics.* 2007;120:1390.

606. Leone A, Ersfeld P, Adams M, et al. Neonatal morbidity in singleton late preterm infants compared with full-term infants. *Acta Paediatr.* 2012;101:e6.

607. Engle WA, Kominiarek MA. Late preterm infants, early term infants, and timing of elective deliveries. *Clin Perinatol.* 2008;35:325.

608. Consortium on Safe Labor, Hibbard JU, Wilkins I, et al. Respiratory morbidity in late preterm births. *JAMA.* 2010;304:419.

609. Rubaltelli FF, Bonafe L, Tangucci M, et al. Epidemiology of neonatal acute respiratory disorders. A multicenter study on incidence and fatality rates of neonatal acute respiratory disorders according

to gestational age, maternal age, pregnancy complications and type of delivery. Italian Group of Neonatal Pneumology. *Biol Neonate.* 1998;74:7.

610. Escobar GJ, McCormick MC, Zupancic JA, et al. Unstudied infants: outcomes of moderately premature infants in the neonatal intensive care unit. *Arch Dis Child Fetal Neonatal Ed.* 2006;91:F238.

611. Sarici SU, Serdar MA, Korkmaz A, et al. Incidence, course, and prediction of hyperbilirubinemia in near-term and term newborns. *Pediatrics.* 2004;113:775.

612. Hunt CE. Ontogeny of autonomic regulation in late preterm infants born at 34–37 weeks postmenstrual age. *Semin Perinatol.* 2006;30:73.

613. Ramanathan R, Corwin MJ, Hunt CE, et al. Cardiorespiratory events recorded on home monitors: comparison of healthy infants with those at increased risk for SIDS. *JAMA.* 2001;285:2199.

614. Henderson-Smart DJ, Pettigrew AG, Campbell DJ. Clinical apnea and brain-stem neural function in preterm infants. *N Engl J Med.* 1983;308:353.

615. Morse SB, Zheng H, Tang Y, et al. Early school-age outcomes of late preterm infants. *Pediatrics.* 2009;123:e622.

616. Petrini JR, Dias T, McCormick MC, et al. Increased risk of adverse neurological development for late preterm infants. *J Pediatr.* 2009;154:169.

617. Chyi LJ, Lee HC, Hintz SR, et al. School outcomes of late preterm infants: special needs and challenges for infants born at 32 to 36 weeks gestation. *J Pediatr.* 2008;153:25.

618. Talge NM, Holzman C, Wang J, et al. Late-preterm birth and its association with cognitive and socioemotional outcomes at 6 years of age. *Pediatrics.* 2010;126:1124.

619. Moster D, Lie RT, Markestad T. Long-term medical and social consequences of preterm birth. *N Engl J Med.* 2008;359:262.

620. McGowan JE, Alderdice FA, Holmes VA, et al. Early childhood development of late-preterm infants: a systematic review. *Pediatrics.* 2011;127:1111.

621. Gurka MJ, LoCasale-Crouch J, Blackman JA. Long-term cognition, achievement, socioemotional, and behavioral development of healthy late-preterm infants. *Arch Pediatr Adolesc Med.* 2010;164:525.

622. Garcia-Prats JA, Abrams SA. *Clinical features and diagnosis of meconium aspiration syndrome.* UpToDate. Accessed June 2013. http://www.uptodate.com/contents/clinical-features-and-diagnosis-of-meconium-aspiration-syndrome?source=search_result&search=meconium+aspiration&selectedTitle=1%7E36#references

623. Singh BS, Clark RH, Powers RJ, et al. Meconium aspiration syndrome remains a significant problem in the NICU: outcomes and treatment patterns in term neonates admitted for intensive care during a ten-year period. *J Perinatol.* 2009;29:497.

624. Whitfield JM, Charsha DS, Chiruvolu A. Prevention of meconium aspiration syndrome: an update and the Baylor experience. *Proc (Bayl Univ Med Cent).* 2009;22:128.

625. Garcia-Prats JA, Abrams SA. *Prevention and management of meconium aspiration syndrome.* UpToDate. Accessed May 2013. http://www.uptodate.com/contents/prevention-and-management-of-meconium-aspiration-syndrome?source=search_result&search=meconium+aspiration&selectedTitle=2%7E36

626. Fanaroff AA. Meconium aspiration syndrome: historical aspects. *J Perinatol.* 2008;28(suppl 3):S3.

627. Balchin I, Whittaker JC, Lamont RF, et al. Maternal and fetal characteristics associated with meconium-stained amniotic fluid. *Obstet Gynecol.* 2011;117:828.

628. Clausson B, Cnattingius S, Axelsson O. Outcomes of post-term births: the role of fetal growth restriction and malformations. *Obstet Gynecol.* 1999;94:758.

629. Lee JS, Stark AR. Meconium aspiration. In: Cloherty JP, Eichenwald EC, Stark AR, eds. *Manual of Neonatal Care.* 5th ed. Lippincott Williams & Wilkins; 2004.

630. Martin RJ, Fanaroff AA, Klaus MH. Respiratory problems. In: Klaus MH, Fanaroff AA, eds. *Care of the High-Risk Neonate.* 4th ed. Saunders; 1993.

631. Yoder BA, Kirsch EA, Barth WH, et al. Changing obstetric practices associated with decreasing incidence of meconium aspiration syndrome. *Obstet Gynecol.* 2002;99:731.

632. Shankaran S. The postnatal management of the asphyxiated term infant. *Clin Perinatol.* 2002;29(4):675-692.

633. Gelfand SL, Fanaroff JM, Walsh MC. Controversies in the treatment of meconium aspiration syndrome. *Clin Perinatol.* 2004;31:445-452.

634. Dargaville PA, Copnell B, Australian and New Zealand Neonatal Network. The epidemiology of meconium aspiration syndrome: incidence, risk factors, therapies, and outcome. *Pediatrics.* 2006;117:1712.

635. Cleary GM, Wiswell TE. Meconium-stained amniotic fluid and the meconium aspiration syndrome. An update. *Pediatr Clin North Am.* 1998;45:511.

636. Wiswell TE, Tuggle JM, Turner BS. Meconium aspiration syndrome: have we made a difference? *Pediatrics.* 1990;85:715.

637. Wiswell TE, Bent RC. Meconium staining and the meconium aspiration syndrome. Unresolved issues. *Pediatr Clin North Am.* 1993;40:955.

638. Ghidini A, Spong CY. Severe meconium aspiration syndrome is not caused by aspiration of meconium. *Am J Obstet Gynecol.* 2001;185:931.

639. Tran N, Lowe C, Sivieri EM, et al. Sequential effects of acute meconium obstruction on pulmonary function. *Pediatr Res.* 1980;14:34.

640. Tyler DC, Murphy J, Cheney FW. Mechanical and chemical damage to lung tissue caused by meconium aspiration. *Pediatrics.* 1978;62:454.

641. Beligere N, Rao R. Neurodevelopmental outcome of infants with meconium aspiration syndrome: report of a study and literature review. *J Perinatol.* 2008;28(S3):93.

642. Konduri GG. New approaches for persistent pulmonary hypertension of the newborn. *Clin Perinatol.* 2004;31:591-611.

643. Adams JM, Stark AR. *Persistent pulmonary hypertension of the newborn.* UpToDate. Accessed May 2013. http://www.uptodate.com/contents/persistent-pulmonary-hypertension-of-the-newborn?source=search_result&search=pphn+of+newborn&selectedTitle=1%7E46#references

644. Levin DL. Morphologic analysis of the pulmonary vascular bed in congenital left-sided diaphragmatic hernia. *J Pediatr.* 1978;92:805.

645. Geggel RL, Murphy JD, Langleben D, et al. Congenital diaphragmatic hernia: arterial structural changes and persistent pulmonary hypertension after surgical repair. *J Pediatr.* 1985;107:457.

646. Murphy JD, Rabinovitch M, Goldstein JD, et al. The structural basis of persistent pulmonary hypertension of the newborn infant. *J Pediatr.* 1981;98:962.

647. Dhillon R. The management of neonatal pulmonary hypertension. *Arch Dis Child Fetal Neonatal Ed.* 2012;97:F223.

648. VanMarter LJ. Persistent pulmonary hypertension of the newborn. In: Cloherty JP, Eichenwald EC, Stark AR, eds. *Manual of Neonatal Care.* 5th ed. Lippincott Williams & Wilkins; 2004.

649. Lipkin PH, Davidson D, Spivak L, et al. Neurodevelopmental and medical outcomes of persistent pulmonary hypertension of the newborn in term neonates treated with nitric oxide. *J Pediatr.* 2002;140(3):306-310.

650. Walsh MC, Stark ER. Persistent pulmonary hypertension of the newborn. Rational therapy based on pathophysiology. *Clin Perinatol.* 2001;28(3):609-627.

651. Inhaled nitric oxide in term and near-term infants: neurodevelopmental follow-up of the neonatal inhaled nitric oxide study group (NINOS). *J Pediatr.* 2000;136:611.

652. Rosenberg AA, Kennaugh JM, Moreland SG, et al. Longitudinal follow-up of a cohort of newborn infants treated with inhaled nitric oxide for persistent pulmonary hypertension. *J Pediatr.* 1997;131:70.

653. Robertson CM, Finer NN, Sauve RS, et al. Neurodevelopmental outcome after neonatal extracorporeal membrane oxygenation. *CMAJ.* 1995;152:1981.

654. Cohen DA, Nsuami M, Etame RB, et al. A school-based Chlamydia control program using DNA amplification technology. *Pediatrics.* 1998;101:E1.

655. Fligor BJ, Neault MW, Mullen CH, et al. Factors associated with sensorineural hearing loss among survivors of extracorporeal membrane oxygenation therapy. *Pediatrics.* 2005;115:1519.

656. Eriksen V, Nielsen LH, Klokker M, et al. Follow-up of 5- to 11-year-old children treated for persistent pulmonary hypertension of the newborn. *Acta Paediatr.* 2009;98:304.

657. Chang G. *Alcohol intake and pregnancy.* UpToDate. Accessed May 2013. http://www.uptodate.com/contents/alcohol-intake-and-pregnancy?source=search_result&search=alcohol+in+pregnancy&selectedTitle=1%7E150

658. Jones KL. *Smith's Recognizable Patterns of Human Malformation.* 5th ed. Saunders; 1997.

659. AAP Committee on Substance Abuse 1999–2000. Fetal alcohol syndrome & alcohol related neurodevelopmental disorders. *Pediatrics.* 2000;106(2):358-361.

660. *LA Siellski Infant of mothers with substance abuse.* UpToDate. Accessed May 2013. http://www.uptodate.com/contents/infants-of-mothers-with-substance-abuse?source=search_result&search=nas&selectedTitle=2%7E15

661. Jones MW, Bass WT. Fetal alcohol syndrome. *Neonatal Netw.* 2003;22(3):63-70.

662. Day NL, Jasperse D, Richardson G, et al. Prenatal exposure to alcohol: effect of growth & morphologic characteristics. *Pediatrics.* 1989;84(3):536-541.

663. Sokol RJ, Delaney-Black V, Norstrom B. Fetal alcohol spectrum disorder. *JAMA.* 2003;290(22):2996-2999.

664. US Department of Health and Human Services. *Results from the 2010 National Survey on Drug Use and Health: Summary of National Findings. Substance Abuse and Mental Health Services Administration; Center for Behavioral Health Statistics and Quality,* 2010. Accessed October 2012. http://oas.samhsa.gov/NSDUH/2k10NSDUH/2k10Results.htm

665. Jones KL, Smith DW. Recognition of the fetal alcohol syndrome in early infancy. *Lancet.* 1973;2:9.

666. Jobe AR. Alcohol as a fetal neurotoxin. *J Pediatr.* 2004;194(3):338.

667. Mukherjee RAS, Hollins S, Turk J. Fetal alcohol spectrum disorder: an overview. *J R Soc Med.* 2006;99:298-302.

668. Hoyme HE, May PA, Kalberg WO, et al. A practical clinical approach to diagnosis of fetal alcohol spectrum disorders: clarification of the 1996 Institute of Medicine criteria. *Pediatrics.* 2005;115:39.

669. American Academy of Pediatrics. Committee on Substance Abuse and Committee on Children with Disabilities. Fetal alcohol syndrome and alcohol-related neurodevelopmental disorders. *Pediatrics.* 2000;106:358.

670. Warren KR, Li TK. Genetic polymorphisms: impact on the risk of fetal alcohol spectrum disorders. *Birth Defects Res A Clin Mol Teratol.* 2005;73:195.

671. Jacobson SW, Carr LG, Croxford J, et al. Protective effects of the alcohol dehydrogenase-ADH1B allele in children exposed to alcohol during pregnancy. *J Pediatr.* 2006;148:30.

672. McCarver DG, Thomasson HR, Martier SS, et al. Alcohol dehydrogenase-2*3 allele protects against alcohol-related birth defects among African Americans. *J Pharmacol Exp Ther.* 1997;283:1095.

673. Stoler JM, Ryan LM, Holmes LB. Alcohol dehydrogenase 2 genotypes, maternal alcohol use, and infant outcome. *J Pediatr.* 2002;141:780.

674. Feldman HS, Jones KL, Lindsay S, et al. Prenatal alcohol exposure patterns and alcohol-related birth defects and growth deficiencies: a prospective study. *Alcohol Clin Exp Res.* 2012;36:670.

675. Alati R, Macleod J, Hickman M, et al. Intrauterine exposure to alcohol and tobacco use and childhood IQ: findings from a parental-offspring comparison within the Avon Longitudinal Study of Parents and Children. *Pediatr Res.* 2008;64:659.

676. Kartin D, Grant TM, Streissguth AP, et al. Three-year developmental outcomes in children with prenatal alcohol and drug exposure. *Pediatr Phys Ther.* 2002;14(3):145-153.

677. Streissguth AP, Aase JM, Clarren SK, et al. Fetal alcohol syndrome in adolescents and adults. *JAMA.* 1991;265:1961.

678. Spohr HL, Willms J, Steinhausen HC. Prenatal alcohol exposure and long-term developmental consequences. *Lancet.* 1993;341:907.

679. Spohr HL, Willms J, Steinhausen HC. Fetal alcohol spectrum disorders in young adulthood. *J Pediatr.* 2007;150:175.

680. Roussotte F, Soderberg L, Sowell E. Structural, metabolic, and functional brain abnormalities as a result of prenatal exposure to drugs of abuse: evidence from neuroimaging. *Neuropsychol Rev.* 2010;20:376.

681. Gardner J. Fetal alcohol syndrome: recognition and intervention. *J Matern Child Nurs.* 1997;22(6):318-322.

682. Koren G, Nulman I, Chudley AE, et al. Fetal alcohol spectrum disorder. *Can Med Assoc J.* 2003;169(11):1181-1185.

683. Hudak ML, Tran RC, The Committee on Drugs & The Committee on Fetus and Newborn. Neonatal drug withdrawal. *Pediatrics.* 2012;129:e540. doi: 10.1542/peds.2011-3212

684. Coyle MG, Brogly SB, Ahmed MS, et al. Neonatal abstinence syndrome. *Nature Rev.* 2018;4(1):47.

685. Jansson LM, Patrick SW. Neonatal abstinence syndrome. *Pediatr Clin North Am.* 2019;66:353-367.

686. Sanlorenzo LA, Stark AR, Patrick SW. Neonatal abstinence syndrome: an update. *Curr Opin Pediatr.* 2018;30(2):182-186.

687. US Food and Drug Administration. *Opioid medications.* 2018. Accessed February 6, 2020. https://www.fda.gov/Drugs/DrugSafety/InformationbyDrugClass/ucm337066.htm

688. Allocco E, Melker M, Rojas-Miguez F, et al. Comparison of neonatal abstinence syndrome manifestations in preterm versus term opioid-exposed infants. *Adv Neonatal Care.* 2016;16:329-336.

689. Villapiano NG, Winkelman TA, Kozhimannil KB, et al. Rural and urban differences in neonatal abstinence syndrome and maternal opioid use, 2004 to 2013. *JAMA Pediatr.* 2017;171(2):194-196.

690. Patrick SW, Schumacher RE, Benneyworth BD, et al. Neonatal abstinence syn-drome and associated health care expenditures: United States, 2000-2009. *JAMA.* 2012;307:1934-1940.

691. Patrick SW, Davis MM, Lehmann CU, et al. Increasing incidence and geographic distribution of neonatal abstinence syndrome: United States 2009 to 2012. *J Perinatol.* 2015;35:650-655.

692. Winkelman TNA, Villapiano N, Kozhimannil KB, et al. Incidence and costs of neonatal abstinence syndrome among infants with Medicaid: 2004-2014. *Pediatrics.* 2018;141(4).

693. AAP Committee on Drugs. Neonatal drug withdrawal. *Pediatrics.* 1998;10:1079-1088.

694. Sielslki LA. *Neonatal opioid withdrawal (Neonatal Abstinence Syndrome).* UpToDate. http://www.uptodate.com/contents/neonatal-opioid-withdrawal-neonatal-abstinence-sydrome

695. McCarty DB, Peat JR, O'Donnell S, et al. "Choose Physical Therapy" for neonatal abstinence syndrome: clinical management for infants affected by the opioid crisis. *Phys Ther.* 2019;99:771-785.

696. Finnegan LP, Connaughton JF, Kron RE, et al. Neonatal abstinence syndrome: assessment and management. *Addict Dis.* 1975;2(1-2):141-158.

697. Finnegan LP. Neonatal abstinence syndrome: assessment and pharmacotherapy. In: Rubatelli FF, Granati B, eds. *Neonatal Therapy: An Update.* Exerpta Medica; 1986.

698. Lester BM, Tronick EZ. The neonatal intensive care unit network neurobehavioral scale procedures. *Pediatrics.* 2004;113(3):641-667.

699. Grossman MR, Berkwitt AK, Osborn RR, et al. An initiative to improve the quality of care of infants with neonatal abstinence syndrome. *Pediatrics.* 2017;139.

700. Schechner S. Drug abuse and withdrawal. In: Cloherty JP, Eichenwald EC, Stark AR, eds. *Manual of Neonatal Care.* 5th ed. Lippincott Williams & Wilkins; 2004.

701. Johnson K, Gerada C, Greenough A. Treatment of neonatal abstinence syndrome. *Archives of Disease in Childhood - Fetal and Neonatal Edition.* 2003;88:F2-F5.

702. Akera C, Ro S. Medical concerns in the neonatal period. *Clin Fam Pract.* 2003;5(2):265.

703. Fike DL. Assessment and management of the substance-exposed infant. In: Kenner C, Lott JW, eds. *Comprehensive Neonatal Nursing: A Physiologic Perspective*. 3rd ed. Saunders; 2003.

704. D'Apolito K. Substance abuse: infant and childhood outcomes. *J Pediatr Nurs*. 1998;13(5):307-316.

705. White RD, Smith JA, Shepley MM; Committee to Establish Recommended Standards for Newborn ICU Design. Recommended standards for newborn ICU design, eighth edition. *J Perinatol*. 2013;33 Suppl 1:S2-16. Doi: 10.1038/jp.2013.10. PMID: 23536026.

706. Vandenberg KA. Basic principles of developmental caregiving. *Neonatal Netw*. 1997;16(7):69-71.

707. Lawhon G. Providing developmentally supportive care in the neonatal intensive care unit: an evolving challenge. *J Perinatal Neonatal Nurs*. 1997;10(4):48-61.

708. Ohgi S, Akiyama T, Arisawa K, et al. Randomized controlled trial of swaddling versus massage in the management of excessive crying in infants with cerebral injuries. *Arch Dis Child*. 2004;89(3):212-216.

709. Bauer CR. Perinatal effects of prenatal drug exposure. Neonatal aspects. *Clin Perinatol*. 1999;26:87.

710. Dubowitz L, Dubowitz V. *The Neurological Assessment of the Preterm and Full-Term Newborn Infant. Clinics in Developmental Medicine. No. 12*. Lippincott; 1981.

711. Dubowitz L, Dubowitz V, Mercuri E. *The Neurological Assessment of the Preterm and Full-Term Newborn Infant*. 2nd ed. MacKeith; 1999.

712. Jones MW, McMurray JL, Englestad D. The "geriatric" NICU patient. *Neonatal Netw*. 2002;21(6):49-58.

713. Ellison PH. Neurologic development of the high-risk infant. *Clin Perinatol*. 11(1):45.

714. Amiel-Tison C. A method for neurological evaluation within the first year of life. *Curr Probl Pediatr*. 1976;7(1):45.

715. Brazelton TB. *Neonatal Behavioral Assessment Scale*. 2nd ed. JB Lippincott Company; 1984.

716. Novak I, Morgan C, Adde L, et al. Early accurate diagnosis and early intervention in cerebral palsy: advances in diagnosis and treatment. *JAMA Pediatr*. 2017;171(9):919. doi:10.1001/jamapediatrics.2017.3169

717. Shephard EG, Knupp AM, Welty SE. An interdisciplinary bronchopulmonary dysplasia program is associated with improved neurodevelopmental outcomes and fewer rehospitalizations. *J Perinatol*. 2012;32:33-38.

718. Walter-Nicolet E, Calvel L, Gazzo G, et al. Neonatal pain, still searching for the optimal approach. *Curr Pharm Des*. 2017;23:5861-5878.

719. Carter B, Brunkhorst J. Neonatal pain management. *Semin Perinatol*. 2017;41:111-116.

720. Sloan N, Camacho LWI, Rojas EP. Kangaroo mother method: randomized controlled trial of an alternative method of care for stabilized low-birth-weight infants. *Lancet*. 1994;344:782-785.

721. Gale G, VandenBerg KA. Kangaroo care. *Neonatal Netw*. 1998; 17(5):69-71.

722. Gray L, Watt L, Blass EM. Skin-to-skin contact is analgesic in healthy newborns. *Pediatrics*. 2000;105(1):4-19.

723. Acolet D, Sleath K, Whitelaw A. Oxygenation, heart rate and temperature in very low birthweight infants during skin-to-skin contact with their mothers. *Acta Paediatr*. 1989;78:189-193.

724. Fohe K, Kropf S, Avenarius S. Skin-to-skin contact improved gas exchange in premature infants. *J Perinatol*. 2000;20:311-315.

725. Feldman R, Eidelman AI. Skin-to-skin contact (kangaroo care) accelerates autonomic and neurobehavioral maturation in preterm infants. *Dev Med Child Neurol*. 2003;45:274-281.

726. Lundington-Hoe SM, Anderson GC, Swine JY, et al. A randomized control of kangaroo care and cardiorespiratory and thermal effects on healthy preterm infants. *Neonatal Netw*. 2004;23(3):39-48.

727. Johnston CC, Stevens B, Pinelli J, et al. Kangaroo care is effective in diminishing pain response in preterm neonates. *Arch Pediatr Adolesc Med*. 2003;157(11):1084-1088.

728. Bier JA, Ferguson AE, Morales Y, et al. Comparison of skin-to-skin contact with standard contact in low birth weight infants who are breast fed. *Arch Pediatr Adolesc Med*. 1996;150(12):1265-1269.

729. Anderson G. Kangaroo care and breastfeeding for preterm infants. *Breastfeed Abstr*. 1989;9(2):7.

730. Feldman R, Weller A, Sirota L, et al. Testing a family intervention hypothesis: the contribution of mother-infant skin-to-skin contact (kangaroo care) to family interaction, proximity, and touch. *J Fam Psychol*. 2003;17(11):94-107.

731. Feldman R, Eidelman AI, Sirota L, et al. Comparison of skin-to-skin (kangaroo) and traditional care: parenting outcomes and preterm infant development. *Pediatrics*. 2002;110(1):16-26.

732. Feldman R, Rosenthal Z, Eidelman AI. Maternal-preterm skin-to-skin contact enhances child physiologic organization and cognitive control across the first 10 years of life. *Biol Psychiatry*. 2014;75:56-64.

733. Scales LH, McEwen IR, Murray C. Parent's perceived benefits of physical therapists' direct intervention compared with parental instruction in early intervention. *Pediatr Phys Ther*. 2007;19:196-202.

734. Dusing SC, Van Drew C, Brown SE. Instituting parent education practices in the neonatal intensive care unit: an administrative case report of practice evaluation and statewide action. *Phys Ther*. 2012;92(7):967-975.

735. Dusing SC, Muraay T, Stern M. Parent preferences for motor development education in the neonatal intensive care unit. *Pediatr Phys Ther*. 2008;20:363-368.

736. Eiden RD, Reifman A. Effects of Brazelton demonstrations on later parenting: a meta-analysis. *J Pediatr Psychol*. 1996;21(6):857-868.

737. Culp RE, Culp AM, Harmon RJ. A tool for educating parents about their premature infants. *Birth*. 1989;16(1):23-26.

738. Lowman LB, Stone LL, Cole JG. Using developmental assessments in the NICU to empower families. *Neonatal Netw*. 2006;25(3):177-186.

739. Loo KK, Espinosa M, Tyler R, et al. Using knowledge to cope with stress in the NICU: how parents integrate learning to read the physiologic and behavioral cues of the infant. *Neonatal Netw*. 2003;22(1):31-37.

740. McGrath J. Supporting parents in understanding and enhancing preterm infant brain development. *Newborn Infant Nurs Rev*. 2008;8:164-165.

741. Byrne EM, Sweeney JK, Schwartz N, et al. Effects of instruction on parent competency during infant handling in a neonatal intensive care unit. *Pediatr Phys Ther*. 2019;31:43-49.

742. Hemingway M, Oliver S. Water bed therapy and cranial molding of the sick preterm infant. *Neonatal Netw*. 1991;10(3):53-56.

743. Hemingway M, Oliver S. Bilateral head flattening in hospitalized premature infants. *Neonatal Intensive Care*. 2000;13(6):18-22.

744. Hemingway M. Preterm infant positioning. *Neonatal Intensive Care*. 2000;13(6):18-22.

745. Vaivre-Douret L, Ennouri K, Jrad I, et al. Effect of positioning on the incidence of abnormalities of muscle tone in low-risk, preterm infants. *Eur J Pediatr Neurol*. 2004;8:21-34.

746. Hallsworth M. Positioning the pre-term infant. *Clin Neonatal Nurs*. 1995;7(1):18-20.

747. Chang YJ, Anderson GC, Lin CH. Effects of prone and supine positions on sleep state and stress responses in mechanically ventilated preterm infants during the first postnatal week. *J Adv Nurs*. 2002;40(2):161-169.

748. Wolfson MR, Greenspan JS, Deoras KS, et al. Effect of positioning on the mechanical interaction between the rib cage and abdomen in preterm infants. *J Appl Physiol*. 1992;72(3):1032-1038.

749. Bjornson K, Deitz J, Blackburn S, et al. The effect of body position on the oxygen saturation of ventilated preterm infants. *Pediatr Phys Ther*. 1992;4(3):109-115.

750. Goldberg RN, Joshi A, Moscoso P, et al. The effect of head position on intracranial pressure in the neonate. *Crit Care Med*. 1983;11:428-430.

751. Grenier IR, Bigsby R, Vergara ER, et al. Comparison of motor self-regulatory and stress behaviors of preterm infants across body positions. *Am J Occup Ther*. 2003;57(3):289-297.

752. Lightdale JR, Gremse DA; Section on Gastroenterology, Hepatology, and Nutrition. Gastroesophageal reflux: management guidance for the pediatrician. *Pediatrics.* 2013;131(5):e1684-95. Doi: 10.1542/peds.2013-0421. Epub 2013 Apr 29. PMID: 23629618.

753. Hashimoto T, Hiurs K, Endo S, et al. Postural effects on behavioral states of newborn infants: a sleep polygraphic study. *Brain Dev.* 1983;5:286-291.

754. Hadders-Algra M, Prechtl HFR. Developmental course of general movements in early infancy. I. Descriptive analysis of change in form. *Early Hum Dev.* 1992;28:201-213.

755. Adams JA, Zabaleta IA, Sackner MA. Comparison of supine and prone noninvasive measurements of breathing patterns in fullterm newborns. *Pediatr Pulmonol.* 1994;18:8-12.

756. Pellicier A, Gaya F, Madero R, et al. Noninvasive continuous monitoring of the effects of head position on brain hemodynamics in ventilated infants. *Pediatrics.* 2002;109(3):434-440.

757. American Academy of Pediatrics. Task force on sudden infant death syndrome. SIDS and other sleep-related infant deaths: updated 2016 recommendations for a safe infant sleeping environment. *Pediatrics.* 2016;138(5):e20162938.

758. van Heijst JJ, Touwen BCL, Vos JE. Implications of a neural network model of sensori-motor development for the field of developmental neurology. *Early Hum Dev.* 1999;55(1):77-95.

759. de Groot L. Posture and motility in preterm infants. *Dev Med Child Neurol.* 2000;42:65-68.

760. Fay MJ. The positive effects of positioning. *Neonatal Netw.* 1988:23-28.

761. Monterososso L, Kristjanson L, Cole J. Neuromotor development and the physiologic effects of positioning in very low birthweight infants. *J Obstet Gynecol Neonatal Nurs.* 2002;31(2):138-146.

762. Shaw JC. Growth and nutrition of the preterm infant. *Br Med Bull.* 1988;44(4):984-1009.

763. Clarren SK, Smith DW, Hanson JW. Helmet treatment for plagiocephaly and congenital muscular torticollis. *J Pediatr.* 1979;94(1):43-46.

764. Kriewell TJ. Structural, mechanical, and material properties of fetal cranial bone. *Am J Obstet Gynecol.* 1982;143(6):707-714.

765. Budreau GK. The perceived attractiveness of preterm infants with cranial molding. *J Obstet Gynecol Neonatal Nurs.* 1989;18(1):38-44.

766. Budreau GK. Postnatal cranial molding and infant attractiveness: implications for nursing. *Neonatal Netw.* 1987;5(5):13-19.

767. Schwirian PM, Eesley T, Cuellar L. Use of water pillows in reducing head shape distortion in preterm infants. *Res Nurs Health.* 1986;9(3):203-207.

768. Geerdink JJ, Hopkins B, Hoeksma JB. The development of head positioning preference in preterm infants beyond term age. *Dev Psychobiol.* 1994;27(3):253-268.

769. Cartlidge PH, Rutter N. Reduction of head flattening in preterm infants. *Arch Dis Child.* 1988;63(7):755-757.

770. Chan JS, Kelley MC, Khan J. The effects of a pressure relief mattress on postnatal head molding in very low birth weight infants. *Neonatal Netw.* 1993;12(5):19-22.

771. Sweeney JK. Neonatal hydrotherapy: an adjunct to developmental intervention in an intensive care nursery setting. *Phys Occup Ther Pediatr.* 1983:39-52.

772. Zhao S, Xie L, Hu H, et al. A study of neonatal swimming (water therapy) applied in clinical obstetrics. *J Matern Fetal Neonatal Med.* 2005;17(1):59-62.

773. Vignochi C, Teixeira PP, Nader SS. Effect of aquatic physical therapy on pain and state of sleep and wakefulness among stable preterm newborns in neonatal intensive care units. *Rev Bras Fisioter.* 2010;14(3):214-220.

774. Oliveira Tobinaga WC, Lima Marinho C, Abelenda VLB. Short-term effects of hydrokinesiotherapy in hospitalized preterm newborns. *Rehabil Rev Pract.* 2016:8.

775. Novakoski KRM, Valderramas SR, Israel VL, et al. Back to the liquid environment: effects of aquatic physiotherapy intervention performed on preterm infants. *Rev Bras Cineantropom Desempenho Hum.* 2018;20(6):566-575.

776. Spittle AJ, Morgan C, Olsen J, et al. Early diagnosis and treatment of cerebral palsy in children with a history of preterm birth. *Clin Perinatol.* 2018;45:409-420.

777. Einspieler C, Prechtl HFR, Bos AF, et al. *The Qualitative Assessment of General Movements in Preterm, Term, and Young Infants.* Mac Keith; 2004.

778. Einspieler C, Prechtl HFR, Ferrari F, et al. The qualitative assessment of general movements in preterm, term, and young infants-review of the methodology. *Early Hum Dev.* 1997;50:47-60.

779. Novak I. Evidence-based diagnosis, health care, and rehabilitation for children with cerebral palsy. *J Child Neurol.* 2014;29(8):1141-1156.

780. Morgan C, Darrah J, Gordon AM, et al. Effectiveness of motor interventions in infants with cerebral palsy: a systematic review. *Dev Med Child Neurol.* 2016;58:900-909.

781. Eliasson AC, Sjostrand L, Ek L, et al. Efficacy of baby-CIMT: study protocol for a randomised controlled trial on infants below age 12 months, with clinical signs of unilateral CP. *BMC Pediatr.* 2014;14:141.

782. Eliasson AC, Nordstrand L, Ek L, et al. The effectiveness of BABy-CIMT in infants younger than 12 months with clinical signs of unilateral-cerebral palsy: an explorative study with randomized design. *Res Dev Disabil.* 2018;72:191-201.

783. Nordstrand L, Holmefur M, Kits A, Eliasson AC. Improvements in bimanual hand function after baby-CIMT in two-year old children with unilateral cerebral palsy: a retrospective study. *Res Dev Disabil.* 2015;41-42:86-93.

784. Needham A, Barrett T, Peterman K. A pick-me-up for infants' exploratory skills: early simulated experiences reaching for objects using "sticky mittens" enhances young infants' object exploration skills. *Infant Behav Dev.* 2002;25:279-295.

785. Corbettaa D, Williams JL, Haynes JM. Bare fingers, but no obvious influence of "prickly" Velcro! In the absence of parents' encouragement, it is not clear that "sticky mittens" provide an advantage to the process of learning to reach. *Infant Behav Dev.* 2015;42:168-178.

786. Nascimentoa AL, Toledo AM, Merey LF, et al. Brief reaching training with "sticky mittens" in preterm infants: randomized controlled trial. *Hum Mov Sci.* 2019;63:138-147.

787. Williams JL, Corbetta D, Guan Y. Learning to reach with "sticky" or "non-sticky" mittens: a tale of developmental trajectories. *Infant Behav Dev.* 2015;38:82-96.

788. Klepper SE, Krasinski DC, Gilb MC, et al. Comparing unimanual and bimanual training in upper extremity function in children with unilateral cerebral palsy. *Pediatr Phys Ther.* 2017;29:288-306.

789. Friel KM, Chakrabarty S, Martin JH. Pathophysiological mechanisms of impaired limb use and repair strategies for motor systems after unilateral injury of the developing brain. *Dev Med Child Neurol.* 2013;55(suppl 4):27-31.

790. Martin JH, Friel KM, Salimi I, et al. Activity- and use-dependent plasticity of the developing corticospinal system. *Neurosci Biobehav Rev.* 2007;31(8):1125-1135.

791. American Academy of Pediatrics. Committee on Fetus and Newborn. Hospital discharge of the high risk neonate—proposed guidelines. *Pediatrics.* 1998;102(2):411-417.

792. Kenner C, Bagwell GA, Torok LS. Transition to home. In: Kenner C, Lott JW, ed. *Comprehensive Neonatal Nursing: A Physiologic Perspective.* 3rd ed. Saunders, 2003.

793. Zaccagnini L. Discharge planning. In: Cloherty JP, Eichenwald EC, Stark AR, eds. *Manual of Neonatal Care.* 5th ed. Lippincott Williams & Wilkins; 2004.

794. Hack M. The outcomes of neonatal intensive care. In: Klaus MH, Fanaroff AA, eds. *Care of the High-Risk Neonate.* 5th ed. Saunders; 2001.

795. Lockridge T, Taquino LT, Knight A. Back to sleep: is there room in that crib for both AAP recommendations and developmentally supportive care? *Neonatal Netw.* 1999;18(5):29-33.

796. Bailey DB, Hebbeler K, Scarborough A, et al. First experiences with early intervention: a national perspective. *Pediatrics.* 2004;113(4):887-896.

797. Hack MB, Wilson-Costello D, Friedman H, et al. Neurodevelopmental predictors of outcomes of children with birth weight of less than 1000 grams: 1992–1995. *Arch Pediatr Adolesc Med.* 2000;154(7):725-751.

798. Vohr BR, O'Shea M, Wright LL. Longitudinal multicenter follow-up of high-risk infants: why, who, when, and what to assess. *Semin Perinatol.* 2003;27(4):333-342.

799. Vohr B. Overview of infants and children with hearing loss. Part 1. *Ment Retard Dev Disabil Res Rev.* 2003;9(2):62-64.

800. Vohr B. Infants and children with hearing loss—part 2: overview. *Ment Retard Dev Disabil Res Rev.* 2003;9(4):218-219.

801. Bear LM. Early identification of infants at risk for developmental disabilities. *Pediatr Clin North Am.* 2004;51:685-701.

802. Wood NS, Marlow N, Costloe K, et al. Neurologic and developmental disability after extremely premature birth. *N Engl J Med.* 2000;343(6):378-384.

803. Bennett FC. Perspective: low birth weight infants: accomplishments, risks, and interventions. *Infants Young Child.* 2002;15(1):vi-ix.

804. Wolf MJ, Koldewijn K, Beelen A, et al. Neurobehavioral and developmental profile of very low birthweight preterm infants in early infancy. *Acta Paediatr.* 2002;91:930-938.

805. Stewart JE. Follow-up of very-low-birth-weight infants. In: Cloherty JP, Eichenwald EC, Stark AR. *Manual Neonatal Care.* 5th ed. Lippincott Williams & Wilkins; 2004.

806. Davis DW. Cognitive outcomes in school-age children born prematurely. *Neonatal Netw.* 2003;22(3):27-38.

807. Foulder-Hughes LA, Cooke RW. Motor, cognitive, and behavioral disorders in children born very preterm. *Dev Med Child Neurol.* 2003;45(2):97-103.

808. Pinto-Martin J, Whitaker A, Feldman J, et al. Special education services and school performance in a regional cohort of low-birth weight infants at age nine. *Pediatr Perinatal Epidemiol.* 2004;18:120-129.

809. Latal-Hajnal B, von Siebenthal K, Kovari H, et al. Postnatal growth in VLBW infants: significant association with neurodevelopmental outcome. *J Pediatr.* 2003;143(2):163-170.

810. Smith VC, Zupancic JA, McCormick MC, et al. Rehospitalization in the first year of life among infants with bronchopulmonary dysplasia. *J Pediatr.* 2004;144(6):799-803.

811. McCormick MC. The outcomes of very low birth weight infants: are we asking the right questions? *Pediatrics.* 1997;99(6):869-875.

812. Weisglas-Kuperus N, Baerts W, Smrkovsky M, et al. Effects of biological and social development of very low birth weight children. *Pediatrics.* 1993;92(5):658-665.

813. Bayley N. *Bayley Scales of Infant and Toddler Development.* 3rd ed. The Psychological Corporation; 2006.

814. Korner AF, Brown JV, Thom VA, et al. *The Neurological Assessment of the Preterm Infant.* 2nd ed. Child Development Media, Inc.; 2000.

815. Korner AF, Thom VA. *Neurobehavioral Assessment of the Preterm Infant (NAPI).* The Psychological Corporation; 1990.

816. Brazelton Institute at Boston Children's Hospital. http://www .childrenshospital.org/research/centers-departmental-programs/ brazelton-institute

817. Als H, Lester BM, Tronick EZ, et al. Manual for the assessment of preterm infant's behavior (APIB). In: Fitzgerald HE, Lester BM, Yogman MW, eds. *Theory and Research in Behavioural Pediatrics.* Plenum Press; 1982:35-63.

818. Als H, Butler S, Kosta S, et al. the assessment of preterm infant's behavior (APIB): furthering understanding and measurement of neurodevelopmental competence in preterm and full-term infants. *Ment Retard Dev Disabil Res Rev.* 2005;11:94-102.

819. General Movement Trust. Accessed January 25, 2020. http://www .general-movements-trust.info

820. Campbell SK. *The Test of Infant Motor Performance. Test User's Manual Version 5.0.* Infant Motor Performance Scales, LLC, 2005.

821. TIMP. Accessed January 25, 2020. http://thetimp.com

822. Piper MC, Darrah J. *Motor Assessment of the Developing Infant.* WB Saunders; 1994.

823. Hammersmith Neurological Examinations. Accessed January 25, 2020. http://hammersmith-neuro-exam.com

RECOMMENDED READINGS

Bigsby R. Neonatal intensive care unit. In: O'Brien JC, Kuhaneck H, eds. *Case-Smits's Occupational Therapy for Children and Adolescents.* 8th ed. Elsevier Mosby; 2019.

Brazelton TB, Nugent JK. *Neonatal Behavioral Assessment Scale.* 3rd ed. Mac Keith Press; 1995.

Goldson E. *Nurturing the Premature Infant.* Oxford University Press; 1999.

Hansen AR, Eichenwald EC, Stark AR, et al. *Cloherty and Stark's Manual of Neonatal Care.* 8th ed. Wolters Kluwer; 2017.

Kenner C, Altimier LB, Boycova MV, eds. *Comprehensive Neonatal Nursing Care.* 6th ed. Springer Publishing; 2020.

Kenner C, McGrath JM, eds. *Developmental Care of Newborns and Infants: A Guide for Health Professionals.* Elsevier; 2004.

Sweeney JK. Medical and developmental challenges of infants in neonatal intensive care: management and follow-up considerations. In: Lazaro RT, Reina-Guerra SG, Quiben MU, eds. *Unphred's Neurological Rehabilitation.* 7th ed. Elsevier; 2020.

Sweeney JK, Heriza CB, Blanchard Y. Neonatal physical therapy. Part I: clinical competencies and neonatal intensive care unit clinical training models. *Pediatr Phys Ther.* 2009;21:296-307.

Sweeney JK, Heriza CB, Blanchard Y, et al. Neonatal physical therapy. Part II: practice frameworks and evidence-based practice guidelines. *Pediatr Phys Ther.* 2010;22:2-16.

Vergara ER, Bigsby R. *Developmental and Therapeutic Interventions in the NICU.* Paul H. Brookes Publishing Co; 2004.

Volpe's Neurology of the Newborn. *JJ Volpe, Ed. in Chief.* 6th ed. Elsevier; 2018.

Zaichkin J, ed. *Newborn Intensive Care: What Every Parent Needs to Know.* 3rd ed. AAP; 2009.

» Common Abbreviations

A	Apnea
ABG	Arterial blood gas
AGA	Appropriate for gestational age
AOP	Apnea of prematurity
APIB	Assessment of Preterm Infant Behavior
AROM	Artificial rupture of membranes
B	Bradycardia
BAER	Brainstem auditory-evoked response
BPD	Bronchopulmonary dysplasia
BPI	Brachial plexus injury
BW	Birth weight
CDH	Congenital diaphragmatic hernia
CHD	Congenital heart disease
CHD	Congenital hip dysplasia
CLD	Chronic lung disease
CMV	Conventional mechanical ventilation
CMV	Cytomegalovirus
CPAP	Continuous positive airway pressure
CS	Cesarean section
D	Desaturation
DOL	Day of life
ECMO	Extracorporeal membrane oxygenation
EGA	Estimated gestational age
ELBW	Extremely low birth weight
FAS	Fetal alcohol syndrome
FiO_2	Fraction of inspired oxygen
FT	Full term
G	Gravida
GA	Gestational age
GBS	Group B streptococcus
GER	Gastroesophageal reflux
GM	Germinal matrix
GMA	General Movement Assessment
HAL	Hyperalimentation
HC	Head circumference
HFFI	High-frequency flow interruption
HFJV	High-frequency jet ventilation
HFOV	High-frequency oscillatory ventilation
HFV	High-frequency ventilation
HIE	Hypoxic–ischemic encephalopathy
HINE	Hammersmith Infant Neurological Examination
HMD	Hyaline membrane disease
HNNE	Hammersmith Newborn Neurological Examination
HR	Heart rate
ICH	Intracranial hemorrhage
ICN	Intensive care nursery
IDVA	Intravenous drug abuse
IMD	Infant of diabetic mother
IMV	Intermittent mandatory ventilation
iNO	Inspired nitric oxide
IUGR	Intrauterine growth restriction
IVH	Intraventricular hemorrhage
LBW	Low birth weight
LGA	Large for gestational age
MAS	Meconium aspiration syndrome
MCA	Multiple congenital anomalies
MV	Mechanical ventilation
NAPI	Neurobehavioral Assessment of the Preterm Infant
NAS	Neonatal abstinence syndrome/neonatal abstinence scale
NBAS	Neonatal Neurobehavioral Assessment Scale
NC	Nasal cannula
NEC	Necrotizing enterocolitis
NG	Nasogastric
NICU	Neonatal intensive care unit
NIDCAP	Newborn Individualized Developmental Care and Assessment Program
NJ	Nasojejunal
NNNS	Neonatal Intensive Care Network Neurobehavioral Scale
NO	Nitric oxide
NP	Nasal prongs
OC	Open crib
OD	Right eye
OG	Orogastric
OS	Left eye
P	Para
PCA	Postconceptual age
PDA	Patent ductus arteriosus
PEEP	Positive end-expiratory pressure

PHI	Periventricular hemorrhage infarction	RR	Respiratory rate
PIE	Pulmonary interstitial emphysema	Sao_2	Oxygen saturation
PO	By mouth	SGA	Small for gestational age
PPHN	Persistent pulmonary hypertension of the newborn	SIMV	Synchronized intermittent mechanical ventilation
PPV	Positive-pressure ventilation	TORCH	Congenital viral infections (toxoplasmosis, other infections, rubella, cytomegalovirus, herpes)
PROM	Premature rupture of membranes	TPF	Toxoplasmosis fetalis
PT	Preterm	TPN	Total parenteral nutrition
PTL	Preterm labor	TTN	Transient tachypnea of the newborn
PVD	Pulmonary vascular disease	UAC	Umbilical arterial catheter
PVHD	Posthemorrhagic ventricular dilation	US	Ultrasound
PVL	Periventricular leukomalacia	UVC	Umbilical venous catheter
RDS	Respiratory distress syndrome	VLBW	Very low birth weight
ROM	Rupture of membranes		
ROP	Retinopathy of prematurity		

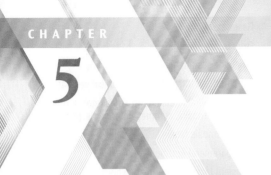

CHAPTER

5

Physical Therapy in the Medical Setting (Acute Care, Inpatient and Outpatient Rehabilitation)

Meg Stanger

≫ Introduction

The practice of physical therapy with children is provided in a variety of settings with a unique perspective of the role of the physical therapist depending on the setting and the circumstances of the child and family. Unlike other patient populations, pediatrics typically involves a parent or guardian who is intimately involved in the care, well-being, and decision making of the patient, namely, the child. And like other patient populations, a variety of professionals and paraprofessionals are frequently involved in the delivery of a variety of services in each setting. This chapter will identify the general role and practice of the physical therapist in the inpatient hospital setting, both acute care and inpatient rehabilitation and the transition to the outpatient setting. A brief overview of the development and philosophies of these practice settings and the unique external factors that influence the delivery of services in these settings will be the focus of this chapter.

≫ The practice environment

In the 1700s and 1800s, early hospitals in the United States were charitable organizations focused on caring for the physically sick as well as protecting the public from those who had either physical or mental illness. Individuals with financial means obtained the services of a physician or nurse in their homes. Families without financial resources or the ability to care for their family members sent them to hospitals where they were isolated from the public, with visitation restricted. This may have helped to curb the spread of disease in the general public but not in the hospital building. Hospitals in the 1800s were overcrowded and offered limited health care. Physicians saw the importance of this separation and isolation but also the opportunity to study, teach medical students, and practice skills on a population brought together in one place—the hospital.[1] A transformation from care to cure had begun.

As with the development of the profession of physical therapy, hospitals were also transformed by wars, epidemics, and federal legislation. The growing need to care for individuals disabled by war or by diseases such as influenza or poliomyelitis led to a greater need for facilities to aid these populations. In the 1900s, the development of private third-party payment systems, the rapid expansion of hospitals, facilitated by the Hill-Burton Hospital Construction Act of 1946, and the passage of Title XVIII of the Social Security Act, Medicare, were major factors that led to the structure and function of hospitals today.

The growth, development, and utilization of hospitals also brought about new issues. With the increasing utilization of hospitals came the need to address issues of infection control, to curb the spread of diseases within the hospital building, the need to protect the information about the people who were admitted to the hospital, and the need to provide a certain level of quality care to all people who received a service from the hospital. These identified factors, as well as others, reflect the growing influence of external agencies and legislation on the delivery of services in the hospital setting.

» The federal government

The Department of Health and Human Services (DHHS) is the government's primary agency that is responsible for protecting the health of all Americans and for providing health services to identified populations. DHHS includes over 300 services or programs covering a variety of topics such as programs to improve maternal and child health, prevention of child abuse and domestic violence, as well as medical and social science research. DHHS manages these activities through operating divisions such as the National Institutes of Health, the Food and Drug Administration, the Center for Disease Control and Prevention, the Centers for Medicare and Medicaid Services, and the Administration for Children and Families, and the National Center for Medical Rehabilitation Research, Office of the Inspector General, to name a few.[2]

In addition, Congress has passed several significant pieces of legislation that influence the delivery of health care. Examples of this legislation include the Patient Self-Determination Act of 1990; the Health Insurance Portability and Accountability Act also known as HIPAA; and the Affordable Care Act. Some legislation is more applicable as the patient/child transitions from the inpatient acute care setting to the inpatient rehabilitation and/or outpatient settings. Examples include the Technology-Related Assistance for Individuals with Disabilities Act of 1988, also referred to as the Tech Act and The Americans with Disabilities Act (ADA). These specific pieces of legislation will be discussed in further detail.

The Patient Self-Determination Act of 1990 requires health care facilities that participate in Medicare and Medicaid to inform adult individuals of their rights to make decisions regarding their health care. Included in this legislation is that health care facilities must periodically review with patients their advanced directives, record those directives, and ensure that they are adhered to without repudiation to the patients for their independent decisions.[3] This Act defines an adult patient as a person 18 years or older. Therefore, any pediatric hospital or rehabilitation facility that provides services to young adults must adhere to these regulations, often thought to pertain to only adult facilities. Patients over 18 years of age have the right to consent to treatment, refuse treatment, and to formulate advance directives in regard to the health care provided. The two most common types of advance directives are a living will and a designated durable power of attorney. One purpose of this law is to address the confusion and ambiguity that may arise when an adult patient becomes incompetent during the hospitalization. Clear written instructions help in the decision-making process in the event of the occurrence of this type of situation. If the patient is under the age of 18 years, a parent or legal guardian must provide the necessary consent for treatment and is responsible for the decisions if a grave situation arises during the hospitalization.

The Health Insurance Portability and Accountability Act of 1996 is a federal law that required the creation of national standards to protect patient health information from being disclosed without the individual's consent of knowledge, to improve the portability of health insurance coverage, and to reduce health care fraud and abuse. The DHHS developed the regulations for this legislation and published what are commonly referred to as The Privacy Rule and The Security Rule.[4] The Privacy Rule protects an individual's identifiable health information that is either held or transferred by a provider. The Privacy Rule determines how, when, and under what circumstances a patient's protected health information (PHI) may be used and disclosed and what must be implemented to de-identify information. Examples of implementation of the Privacy Rule would be limiting who may access a patient's chart, de-identification of the patient, and a signed authorization from the parent to allow a hospital-based therapist to talk with the child's school-based therapist. The Security Rule ensures the safeguarding of electronic health information. Examples range from technology safeguards to protection of computer screens in a public area.

HIPAA applies to all government health plans; managed care plans; and many private health plans; as well as health care providers such as hospitals, ambulatory care centers, home care agencies, and durable medical equipment (DME) suppliers. There have been numerous updates and additions to HIPAA since the original public law of 1996, but the original intent remains unchanged.

The Affordable Care Act (ACA and previously called the Patient Protection and Affordable Care Act) was signed into law by President Obama in 2010. Therefore, it is often also referred to as "Obamacare." The three main goals included in the ACA were to make affordable health insurance available to more people, to expand Medicaid to extend coverage to more Americans, and to support innovation in delivery systems that lowered the cost of health care.[5] The ACA brought many changes to health care, has been controversial, and is frequently challenged in court but currently remains in the forefront of health care.

Some of the protections offered under the ACA include the inability of insurers to refuse applicants based on preexisting conditions or to charge those members higher premiums as well as the need for states to ensure the availability of health insurance for children under their family's plan if they do not have their own coverage. These requirements have allowed families with children with preexisting conditions to change employers and insurances without fear of loss of coverage and for young adults up until 26 years of age to stay on their parent's insurance plan. The ACA also implemented reforms to improve quality of care and reduce health care costs. Examples include bundled payments for an episode of care rather than the traditional fee-for-service previously seen in health care facilities. Hospitals are also subject to reduction in Medicare reimbursements dependent on their prevalence of hospital-acquired conditions (usually related to infection transmission) or for higher readmission rates for patients.

The Technology-Related Assistance for Individuals with Disabilities Act of 1988 is commonly referred to as the Tech Act and was reauthorized several times. The Tech Act recognizes that technological advances would benefit individuals with disabilities and aims to provide states with federal funding to implement technology assistance programs.[6] Assistive technology is defined as "any item, piece of equipment or product system, whether acquired commercially off the shelf, modified, or customized, that is used to increase, maintain, or improve the functional capabilities of individuals with disabilities." Assistive technology ranges from low-tech devices such as walkers or bath seats to high-tech equipment such as powered mobility systems and communication devices with various methods of switch activation. In addition, the law defines assistive technology services as evaluation, selection of the device, and training in the use of the device. The Tech Act was replaced by the Assistance Technology Act of 2004, which required states to assist with alternative financing or loan programs for technology equipment.[6] This act has significant impact as the child transitions from the inpatient setting to outpatient settings and the school environment.

The Americans with Disabilities Act of 1990 (ADA) prohibits discrimination and ensures equal opportunity for individuals with disabilities in employment, public transportation, public accommodations, and telecommunications.[7] The physical therapist working in a rehabilitation or outpatient setting should assist the child and family with the development of goals that will prepare them for transition to an accessible work and living environment as a young adult.

» The state government

Each state has a Physical Therapy Practice Act that governs the role of physical therapists and physical therapist assistants. Physical therapists can release aspects of their interventions to other professionals and caretakers to ensure continuity of care. In the inpatient setting, physical therapists will often instruct nursing personnel in positioning and transfer techniques, range of motion (ROM) exercises, and donning and doffing of orthotic devices to provide continuity of care for the patient.

States also have specific regulations and laws to protect children from physical or sexual abuse or neglect. Physical or sexual abuse and negligent treatment of a child under 18 years of age are clearly defined in the Child Abuse Prevention and Treatment Act of 1974 and were most recently amended in 2019.[8] Regulations vary from state to state but generally require that any case of suspected child abuse or neglect be reported to the appropriate personnel. Physical therapists are mandatory reporters by law. As a mandatory reporter, failure to report a case of suspected child abuse or neglect may result in a fine, imprisonment, and/or suspension or revocation of a physical therapist's professional license. Most facilities provide training at regular intervals in recognizing the signs of physical, emotional, or sexual abuse in children and how to report those suspected cases in the state.

A physical therapist working in an outpatient rehabilitation setting may be the health professional to first see the signs of abuse or neglect. In this setting, the physical therapist will see patterns of attendance and compliance. During routine outpatient treatment interventions, the physical therapist may typically have the child remove an article of clothing or roll up shirt sleeves or pant legs, revealing bruises, burns, or welts. The physical therapist is considered a mandatory reporter and is obligated by law to report such occurrences.

» Reimbursement

Physical therapists also need to be aware of the state's laws that affect reimbursement issues. Reimbursement differs significantly from the inpatient to the outpatient setting. In many states, the third-party payers have not adopted the Diagnostic Related Group (DRG) system for inpatient pediatric rehabilitation that is utilized in the acute care and adult rehabilitation settings. However, prior to a child's admission to a rehabilitation unit a contract for services or individual negotiations that determine a set price/day or length of stay have been determined. This means that the third-party payer will reimburse the facility at a predetermined rate regardless of the individual services provided or adaptive equipment supplied to the child. Most third-party payers will reimburse a medical equipment vendor separately for high-end or high-tech assistive technology items such as wheelchairs and communication devices when the child is receiving services in the outpatient setting.

If an orthotic device or DME is issued to the child while in the inpatient setting, the medical facility is typically responsible for that cost. Outpatient services are typically billed as a fee for service related to the service performed and the time the physical therapist spent with the patient. Payment may be dependent on contractual agreements between a provider or facility and the third-party payer. Physical therapists must have knowledge of billing codes, whether those codes are billed as a timed unit or not, and the billing practices that may be unique to their work setting or state practice act.

>> Infection control and prevention

The hospital setting is a prime place for the spread of germs and infections owing to the number of people who are ill with an infection, people who are ill and have a weakened immune system and are therefore susceptible to exposure, the multitude of people and equipment moving among rooms and patients, and the invasive procedures that may be performed. It is essential that steps are taken to minimize the spread of infections in the hospital setting. The US DHHS, Centers for Disease Control and Prevention (CDC) recommends a two-tiered system for infection prevention, including Standard Precautions and Transmission-Based Precautions.[9]

The CDC publishes guidelines on the standard precautions that should be taken to reduce the risk of transmission of microorganisms from infectious materials that apply to all patients receiving care in a hospital, regardless of the patient's diagnosis or infectious status.[9] These standard precautions include procedures for hand washing; the use of personal protective equipment (PPE) such as gloves, masks, gowns, and eye protection; respiratory/cough etiquette; the use of patient care equipment; procedures for the routine care, cleaning, and disinfection of equipment, furniture, and other environmental surfaces; the use of linens; the handling of blood and procedures to follow if inadvertently exposed to blood or injury caused by sharps (needles, scalpels, or other sharp instruments); and the placement of patients who are infectious. Transmission-based precautions are used in addition to standard precautions for patients with suspected or known infections. Transmission-based precautions will include specific recommendations for PPE, cleaning, and isolation of the patient, depending on the method of spread of the organism. Specific contact, droplet, or airborne precautions will be implemented for the patient depending on the method of spread of the infectious organism. Hospitals typically have color-coded signs with visual cues at the patient's door or bed to guide visitors and health care workers to adhere to the proper transmission precautions (Display 5.1).

Examples of the more common infections encountered in the acute care hospital today are multidrug resistant organisms (MDOs) such as methicillin *Staphylococcus aureus* (MRSA), vancomycin resistant enterococcus (VRE), and the gram negative bacilli (GNB). *Clostridium difficile (C. diff)* is not an MDO but is seen in patients with weakened immune systems in a hospital setting.

Patients with prolonged hospital stays and heavy antimicrobial therapy are at an increased risk for acquiring MRSA. MRSA frequently colonizes in the nose, axilla, groin, and/or wound sites, including burns. The most common mode of transmission is by contact. Droplet/contact precautions are used for patients infected with MRSA. The patient is placed in a private room or with a roommate that is also infected with MRSA. Everyone who enters the room should don a mask. Gloves should be worn if the patient will be touched, and a gown should be worn if there is a possibility of clothing coming in contact with the patient or anything in the patient's room. If the patient must walk in the hallway, he or she must wear a mask, gloves, and a gown. The patient should avoid common areas such as the activity room, cafeteria, or gift shop. Any equipment (e.g., walker, cuff weights) or testing tools (e.g., goniometer, tape measure, stethoscope) used with the infected patient must be disinfected after use.

VRE is a bacterium that colonizes in the gastrointestinal tract. Patients with prolonged hospital stays and antimicrobial therapy are at risk for acquiring VRE. The most common mode of transmission is by contact. Contact precautions are used for patients infected with VRE. The patient is placed in a private room or with a roommate who is also infected with VRE. Everyone who enters the room must wear gloves if the patient will be touched and a gown if there is a possibility of clothing coming in contact with the patient or anything in the patient's room. The patient can walk in the hallway as long as they wear gloves and a gown. Ideally, if physical therapy is provided in the department, it should be at the end of the day and away from other patients. All equipment (e.g., parallel bars, mat table) or testing tools used with the infected patient must be disinfected after use.

GNB are another group of bacteria that are resistant to multiple antibiotics and may result in pneumonia, bloodstream infections, meningitis, or surgical site infections. Examples of GNB are *Klebsiella, Pseudomonas aeruginosa,* and *E. coli.* Use of PPE and cleaning procedures would mimic those described for patients with other MDSs.

C. diff is a bacteria that colonizes in the large bowel or colon. It releases a toxin that causes diarrhea and abdominal pain. Patients who had abdominal surgery or are receiving antibiotics or chemotherapy are at an increased risk for acquiring *C. diff.* The most common mode of transmission is by contact. Contact precautions are used for patients infected with *C. diff*. The difference when treating a patient with *C. diff* is that all handwashing is with soap and water and not the standard hand sanitizer used throughout the facility as part of Standard Precautions. The patient is placed in a private room or with a roommate who is also infected with *C. diff*. Everyone who enters the room must wear gloves if the patient will be touched and a gown if there is a possibility of clothing coming in contact with the patient or anything in the patient's room. If the patient must walk in the hallway, they must wear gloves and a gown. The patient should avoid walking in common areas. As with other infectious diseases, all equipment or testing tools used with the infected patient must be disinfected after use; however, the disinfectant must contain bleach or a sporicidal agent.

The Infection Prevention department of the hospital will also be a source of information in the face of a pandemic. The world at times has had various pandemics, ranging from the yearly flu, or influenza, to a rare event such as COVID-19 or the SARS-2. The infection prevention department will coordinate with senior administrative leadership to develop and disseminate guidelines, policies, and protocols for staff, patients, and visitors to follow. These guidelines are typically based on evidence from organizations such as the Center for Disease Control and World Health Organization and may change quickly as new information is learned regarding a new organism or virus that is the source of the pandemic.

» Accreditation

Most hospitals are voluntarily accredited through an external organization such as The Joint Commission (TJC) and/or the Commission on Accreditation of Rehabilitation Facilities (CARF). A facility with a TJC and/or CARF accreditation has demonstrated that they have met the standards for patient care issued by the accrediting organization that represents a body of their peers. Facilities are accredited for a certain period, typically 2 to 3 years, must regularly submit predetermined data to maintain their accreditation, and must be reaccredited after the 2- to 3-year period. Accreditation standards generally address patient safety, quality of patient care, patient satisfaction, and performance measurement. There is an overlap between the TJC and CARF accreditation purposes and standards, but TJC focuses on accreditation of medically based facilities, whereas CARF focuses on accreditation of the health and human services sector of health care.

The mission of TJC is to continuously improve the safety and quality of care provided to the public through the provision of health care accreditation and related services that support performance improvement in health care organizations.[10] Almost half of the TJC standards are related to patient safety issues, such as staffing levels and competency, medication use, infection control, use of restraints, fire safety, and safety of medical equipment, to name a few. In 2002, TJC issued the first set of national patient safety goals with annual updates. The goals focus on safety issues identified in health care and how to remediate those safety issues. Accredited facilities must adhere to the national goals and are held accountable to demonstrate compliance. Examples of national safety goals include proper patient identification to address the incidence of procedures occurring to the wrong patients, medication safety timely responses to patient alarms, infection prevention, and suicide prevention. Each facility determines their procedures and protocols for adherence to the various standards, including staff education and knowledge of the various procedures. Physical therapists are a very integral part of the delivery of patient care services and must adhere to their facility's standards.

TJC has also taken measures to ensure that medical errors and events are reported and analyzed, new procedures implemented after analysis, and that the information learned is shared with other organizations to improve patient safety nationally. Steps have been taken legislatively to create a nonpunitive environment and limit the damage from civil lawsuits when a health care worker makes a report.

Beginning in 2006, all on-site TJC surveys for accreditation became unannounced, meaning that the surveyors can present themselves at the facility at any time. The surveyors complete much of their survey through a tracer method; they follow identified patients through the patient care process and talk with hospital personnel as the patient moves through the day and scheduled procedures. All hospital personnel, including physical therapists, must be aware of the standards and policies of their facility and be comfortable discussing those procedures with a surveyor. After an accreditation survey, a hospital is provided with a detailed report from the Commission and a score. Joint Commission quality reports contain information on accredited health care organizations and are available to the public.

Another key component of TJC accreditation is the inclusion of performance measures to support quality improvement initiatives among hospitals. The performance measures are referred to as the ORYX initiative (**O**utcome **R**esearch **Y**ields **Ex**cellence). The ORYX performance measures must be data-driven and statistically valid indicators that will provide performance information for the organization. The performance data are available for comparison among other health care organizations and for review by outside stakeholders. Physical therapists need to be aware of their facilities' ORYX initiatives and how their role impacts the data collected and ultimately the facility's performance.

In addition to federal laws and regulations, most rehabilitation hospitals are accredited through an external organization such as TJC and/or the CARF. The mission of CARF is to promote quality, value, and optimal outcomes of services through a consultative accreditation process that centers on enhancing the lives of the persons served.[11] CARF accreditation signifies that the facility has demonstrated a commitment to continually enhance the quality of their services and to focus on the satisfaction of the patients served. Examples of values of quality of service are the inclusion of the patients in the design of their service plans, individualization of services to meet the patient's unique needs, satisfaction of patients/families with the services they have received and utilization of data from a continuous performance improvement system to manage the quality of services delivered to patients.

A key element of CARF's strategic plan is to enhance the use of outcomes management as part of a continuous quality performance improvement system. An outcome management system is utilized to measure the performance of a program, both internally over time and with external peers, and to monitor the results of patient outcomes. The information obtained from outcomes measurement is utilized by the organization to manage and improve their programs and to benchmark their programs with similar programs across the country.

» The acute inpatient hospital setting

In the acute care hospital, there may be a variety of levels of care and specialized units for providing services to a pediatric patient. For a newborn infant, this could be a neonatal intensive care unit (NICU); for a child, a pediatric intensive care unit (PICU) or a cardiac intensive care unit (CICU). For infants and children requiring less critical care, it may be a specialized unit on a floor of the hospital such as an oncology unit, a postsurgical unit, or a general medical unit. The child may be admitted to the hospital through the emergency department or as a planned admission for a predetermined surgical or medical procedure. Many pediatric hospitals are specialized in specific areas of acutely ill children and may have specific designations such as a Level One Trauma Center, or their NICU may be designated as a Level III or IV. These specific levels designate that the hospital has met specific criteria to provide pediatric services to a specific patient population including medical subspecialties, pediatric equipment, a pediatric emergency department and intensive care, and multiple other criteria.

In the inpatient pediatric acute care hospital, the overall goals are to maintain life; to promote health; to maintain, restore, or minimize the loss of function; to minimize the negative aspect of the experience on the patient; and to control pain. There are a variety of reasons a child might be admitted to an acute hospital setting. They can range from a fever, to a femur fracture, to traumatic brain injury (TBI) secondary to a car accident, to treatment for cancer, to the need for an organ transplant. Because of the range of diagnoses, it is difficult to be specific as to what a physical therapist should and should not do. However, there are some general guidelines that apply to the examination and delivery of services that would apply to any pediatric patient in the hospital. The physical therapist should work to minimize the fear and stress of the child. The following are suggestions on how a physical therapist or a physical therapy department might do this during the examination or delivery of services:

A physical therapist should take a few minutes to introduce himself or herself to the child and the parent/guardian, explain why physical therapy has been ordered, and what will be done during the session.

A child may feel more comfortable with his or her parent/guardian in the room during the delivery of service.

A physical therapist should try to achieve goals through age-appropriate activities.

Allow the child to choose or offer a choice of activities.

Try to have the same physical therapist see the child each session.

See if there is a time of the day that is better for the child. For example, the child may routinely take a nap in the afternoon or feel more energetic in the morning. Ask the parents what they feel would be a good time of day for the child to participate in physical therapy.

Repeating some of the same activities each session may give the child a feeling of predictability, which may be comforting and may reduce the child's anxiety (Display 5.2).

Prior to initiating any examination, evaluation, or treatment intervention in the hospital setting, the physical therapist should be aware of lines, tubes, and monitors associated with the child's medical care as well as the specialized equipment unique to that child's diagnosis or condition.

In addition to the vital sign monitors, the child may also have a pulse oximeter. This device monitors the concentration of oxygen attached to hemoglobin in the child's peripheral circulatory system. A sensor is typically attached to the finger or toe of the child, and the alarm will be set to sound if the oxygen level reading goes below a predetermined percentage. The sensor is sensitive to movement, so it is not unusual for the alarm to trigger if the child moves or is moved. If this occurs, observe the child and other monitors to determine the safety of the child. If in doubt, call the child's nurse. Transcutaneous peripheral oxygen and carbon dioxide monitors measure the concentration of oxygen or carbon dioxide through the skin. The readings are more accurate than those from the pulse oximeter but less accurate than blood chemistry.

Intravenous lines, or IVs, can be used to administer medication, fluids, volume expanders, blood products, and parenteral nutrition. A central line is an intravenous line inserted into a larger vein than a regular IV. It is placed in the chest, neck, arm, or groin and is used to deliver medicines or total parenteral nutrition (TPN: nourishment provided by a non-gastrointestinal route). A PICC (peripherally inserted central

DISPLAY 5.2	Point to Remember—Acute Care

The goal of acute care is to medically stabilize the child and then begin the process of rehabilitation, which typically includes some level of mobility.

catheter) line is a type of central line that is inserted in the arm and threaded from there into a larger vein in the body close to the heart.

Children who are medically unstable may require other invasive methods of monitoring, often to attempt to minimize further neurologic damage. Examples include an arterial line, intracranial pressure (ICP) monitor, cerebral oxygenation monitor, and external ventricular drain (EVD). There will be significant limitations on the positions and/or movement that is permitted when a child has these types of lines and monitors. An arterial line is inserted directly into an artery such as the femoral artery to monitor blood pressure; there are often restrictions on movement of the extremity with the arterial line to minimize dislodging or kinking the line. ICP can be monitored through an epidural bolt, a subarachnoid bolt, or the EVD itself. The EVD is inserted directly into the ventricles, typically a lateral ventricle, and monitors the ICP as well as acts as a drain or method of aspirating excessive fluid. ICP is measured in millimeters of Hg and the monitor will sound an alarm when the ICP exceeds a set pressure; ICP often increases if the child is moved or becomes agitated, so the physical therapist must be able to read and understand the monitors. These types of monitors are typically seen with children who have sustained a severe head injury and are typically in the ICU and may also require mechanical ventilation.

The cardiac intensive care incorporates very specialized equipment that requires extensive training by physical therapists before they can safely mobilize these children. This is beyond the scope of this chapter, but examples include the various ventricular assist devices (VAD) or extracorporeal membrane oxygenation (ECMO). A VAD is an external pump that takes over pumping the child's blood and allows the heart to rest and heal or keeps the child alive while waiting for a heart transplant. ECMO is a type of a heart–lung machine that functions like a circuit to oxygenate the blood while the child's heart and lungs are rested or awaiting transplant. Physical therapists will be consulted to provide interventions for these children, so it is vital that the therapist understand the precautions that need to be followed and limitations for each particular child.

Some children in the acute care setting will require mechanical ventilatory support. Often with a severe injury, especially a head injury, the child may require mechanical respiratory support for a certain period. The respiratory support will be provided through an endotracheal tube; if long-term respiratory support is required, the child may eventually require a tracheostomy. Many children receiving ventilatory support owing to a severe injury may also be sedated to allow their neurologic systems to rest and minimize further damage to their brain. The therapist should be aware of the child's ventilator settings, safe range for oxygen saturation, and any movement precautions based on the type of intubation; is the child orally intubated through an endotracheal tube or does the child have a more permanent tracheostomy?

Many children with the multiple lines, tubes, and monitors described in the foregoing will be in the intensive care setting. The existence of these various lines and tubes does not negate the child's ability to participate in physical therapy or to move and engage with the environment. Competence with the lines and tubes is crucial to practice in this setting, as is the ability to read and understand the data displayed on the various monitors and to communicate with the hospital personnel caring for the child.

Examination

An examination is done prior to the initiation of physical therapy services. It consists of history, systems review, and tests and measurements that are appropriate for the individual. A chart review and communication with the child's nurse should be a routine aspect of the physical therapist's examination and treatment process in the hospital. In acute care, the child's status can change quickly. Additional services, medical tests, and other professionals are also involved in the care of the child and are scheduled at various times during the hospital stay. Coordination of care is an important aspect of services in this setting. If possible, the child's parents or guardian should be present during the examination. If they are not available, a timely review of the evaluation with them would be appropriate.

In the hospital the child is typically limited not only by pain, but also by medical procedures that have been implemented during the current admission, such as surgery. Performing a standardized test with the typical tests and measurements used in a physical therapy examination could be time consuming and inappropriate, given the shorter duration in the length of stay and the ability of the acutely ill patient to participate in this environment. However, the physical therapist may consider the use of a standardized test depending on the ability of the child to participate and the value of the results obtained with regard to intervention decisions or outcome management.

There are a variety of standardized tests and measurements that are applicable in the acute care setting. A quick and reliable test may be more appropriate on the basis of the expected decreased endurance of the child in this setting. The Functional Independence Measure for children (WeeFIM II), as described in more detail in the inpatient rehabilitation section of this chapter, is one such standardized test that may be appropriate.[12] This test measures a child's disability and the level of assistance required in daily activities, or burden of care for the caregiver. It can be done at admission and discharge with the scores used as an outcome measurement. In addition, the Functional Reach Test, which is commonly used with the adult population, has also been found to be reliable (interrater [$r = 0.98$], intrarater [$r = 0.83$], and test–retest [$r = 0.75$]) in the pediatric population without disabilities.[13] One study suggested that an alternative measurement of toes to the fingers may improve reliability and decrease sway seen with children of varying ages and heights.[14] This dynamic balance test examines forward weight shift, reaching, and postural control using both feet, as opposed to other one-legged balance tests. Admission and discharge scores of appropriate children could be used to note changes in balance skills. The Timed Up and Go test (TUG) is another quick and practical test of functional mobility. A modified version of this test, which was designed for adults, has been shown to be reliable with children, with and without disabilities, as young as 3 years of age.[15] All children in the study were able to walk independently with orthoses or assistive devices, such as walkers or crutches. Reliability was high, with an intraclass correlation coefficient (ICC) of 0.89 (without disabilities) and 0.99 (with disabilities) within session, and 0.83 for test–retest reliability. The TUG has also been shown to be responsive to change over time, providing another possibility for an outcome measurement.[15]

In addition to mobility and functional skills, the child's level of pain should be measured. A child who has just undergone a surgery, who is undergoing treatment for cancer, or who has sustained a fracture of a bone may be very anxious about the pain he or she expects to feel during the physical therapy session. In an acute care hospital, pain relief may be addressed in a variety of ways, from self-controlled analgesia (PCA; personally administered doses of pain medication into IV lines that are time limited), to pain medication administered through epidural catheters or IV lines, to oral medication. Before beginning physical therapy, the physical therapist should check with the child's nurse to obtain information on what pain medication the child is receiving and the schedule for delivery of the medication. A bolus of pain medication can be given through a PCA system right before physical therapy. Pain medication can be given through an IV line that should take effect within approximately 10 minutes of administration but has a limited duration of approximately 30 minutes. Oral pain medication may take at least 30 minutes before the effects are felt by the patient but generally maintains its analgesic effect for several hours. The physical therapist should try to time the examination or delivery of interventions when the pain medication is most effective.

In the examination of pain, have the child rate his or her pain before, during, and after physical therapy. A number of pain scales have been shown to provide valid self-reports in children[16,17] (Display 5.3). Children over the age of 8 years are usually able to rate their pain using the typical 0 to 10 numbered Visual Analog scale.[16] Younger children are able to rate their pain with a less abstract system than numbers and may benefit from the use of specifically designed pediatric pain scales that feature faces, colors, or "ouchers."[18-21] Specific pain scales have been developed for infants and toddlers who are not yet verbal or cognitively able to understand the abstractness of the pain scales described here. These scales are based on observation of behaviors.

If medically cleared, the physical therapist may have the child actively help with their transitions during physical therapy because, in general, the child may perceive less pain if he or she is in control of the movements. The physical therapist

DISPLAY 5.3	Pediatric Pain Assessments	
Visual Analog Scale[16]	8+ years
Wong-Baker FACES Scale[17]	3+ years
OUCHER[18]	3+ years
Faces Pain Scale Revised[19]	4+ years
Color Analog Scale[21]	5+ years

should reassure the child that the activity will be done slowly, if appropriate, and will be kept within the child's level of pain tolerance.

Part of the examination may also include information gained from diagnostic imaging. Understanding diagnostic imaging and the fundamental relationship to anatomy will aid the physical therapist in understanding the extent of the medical diagnosis, medical interventions, and prognosis of the child. This information will also aid in the evaluation of the child by the physical therapist and assist in the management process and development of a realistic plan of care and appropriate caregiver education.

Evaluation and Plan of Care

Once the examination is complete, the physical therapist evaluates the information and makes a diagnosis on the basis of the information obtained. This diagnosis guides the physical therapist in the selection of interventions, goals, and outcomes for this particular child.

Physical therapy goals in an acute care setting are not the same as those for a rehabilitation hospital or outpatient setting. Physical therapy is not the main reason the child was admitted to the hospital, so generally the goal is to maintain or minimize loss of function during the child's stay. If the child is in need of more intense rehabilitation services, he or she may be transferred to a rehabilitation hospital or referred for outpatient physical therapy services when medically appropriate. The primary goal in the acute care hospital is to promote the optimal amount of independence and mobility given the medical status of the child and to plan for discharge at the onset of the child's admission. Often, the goal is to keep the child as mobile as possible and to prevent or minimize any deterioration in function and impairments. The physical therapist integrates the following five elements of patient management: examination, evaluation, diagnosis, prognosis, and intervention (Display 5.4).

Communication, coordination, and documentation are the most important physical therapy interventions in the acute care setting. A child's status can change quickly. It is important for the physical therapist to review the child's medical record for current up-to-the-minute information on the health status of the child. What is the current medical stability of the patient? What are the current vitals or lab values? This information will aid the determination of the type and intensity of the physical therapy intervention, if appropriate at this time. Lab values, such as hemoglobin, hematocrit, and platelet count (as examples), should be evaluated to determine whether the child can be expected to perform exercise of specific intensities. If any lab values are abnormal for the child's age, the physical therapist should determine the effect the lab value would have on the child's ability to participate in the physical therapy session and alter the intervention as appropriate. Additional questions could include the following: What are the current orders of the physician or specialist? Were any medical tests done recently or anticipated in the next few hours? Are there any restrictions associated with the medical test, such as wearing of a cervical collar until the cervical spine has been cleared by radiograph or bed rest following a lumbar puncture? Were there any recent test results that identified an infection or the presence of an infectious disease? This information can be found documented in the child's medical record, but for the most up-to-date information, it is recommended to talk to the child's primary nurse before beginning physical therapy. The primary nurse will know the status of the child and any anticipated procedures and will help with the coordination of services that are provided. The child may be scheduled for a radiograph within the next 30 minutes or may have just completed a session with the occupational therapist and requires a rest before proceeding with the next service.

Once the documentation has been reviewed and the care coordinated, the child is seen and a systems review is done again to evaluate the current status of the child and to determine whether the anticipated interventions are appropriate and the level of intensity that should be expected. Child and family-related instruction is an important intervention in this environment. Owing to the possible fluctuations in the child's ability to learn and perform motor tasks, the risk of injury, and the rapid recovery that can also be expected, repeated reviews of safety precautions, movement restrictions, use of assistive devices, and the importance of child and caregiver involvement in daily exercises or activities is necessary. The child, as well as the parents, may not be in the optimal state to learn or assimilate new information and apply it consistently. Parents are under considerable stress when their child is hospitalized. Prioritizing and understanding information can be a challenge. Repeated review and positive reinforcement of the rehabilitation

process should be part of every physical therapist's protocol for child and family interaction in the acute care setting (Display 5.5).

Intervention

The interventions used in the acute care setting can include the variety of those provided by physical therapists as listed in the Guide to Physical Therapist Practice.[22] These can range from airway clearance techniques to therapeutic exercise. Intervention may include activities in a physical therapy department where additional equipment is available but will often be carried out bedside in the child's room. If the child is able to leave the unit, physical therapy intervention in the department or gym may provide access to mat tables, parallel bars, modalities, and steps that are not easily accessed on the unit. Exercises using resistance as well as aerobic and endurance training through use of a treadmill or stationary bicycle are also commonly seen in the physical therapy department.

With children who have sustained lower extremity or pelvic fractures or have undergone orthopedic surgery on a leg, the physical therapist is often asked to teach the child to walk with crutches or a walker. As a general guideline, it is recommended that children who are under 6 years old, have coordination difficulties, or are fearful of walking, be taught to ambulate with a walker. The main limitation of using a walker is that it cannot be used on stairs, and a child will ambulate at a slower rate. A young child who is using a walker can be taught to go up and down stairs on his buttocks, or an adult can carry the child if needed. Children who are 6 years old or older and do not have coordination issues are generally taught to use axillary crutches. Crutches can assist a child to negotiate stairs, although it is always recommended to use a railing, if available, with the crutches.

For those children in the ICU setting, early mobilization should be a key goal for all children. There is mounting evidence to show the negative effects of long-term immobility of a child in the ICU, including physical, psychosocial, and cognitive impairments that impact recovery.[23–26] Early mobilization in the ICU is described as a child's active participation in therapeutic activity within 48 to 72 hours of admission or on hemodynamic stability.[27] Key factors for an effective early mobility program include training and competence of the physical therapist, parent education regarding the rationale for early therapy interventions and mobility in the ICU, and strong multidisciplinary communication and teamwork. To mobilize a child with a multitude of lines and tubes to sit at the edge of the bed or begin standing activities is an undertaking that often requires multiple staff members for the child's safety. Often, mobility initiatives will be bundled around care times to optimize the use of staff and to allow the child undisturbed blocks of time to rest. There are studies that support the feasibility and safety of initiation of early mobility programs in a pediatric ICU, but further research is needed to determine the impact on the child's length of stay and ultimate long-term functional outcome.[27–29]

In the acute care setting, the focus on physical therapy may also often be on the prevention of future impairments that impact the child's function and recovery. Examples include monitoring skin integrity as well as development of contractures for those children who are sedated or immobile. Pressure-mapping and the use of special seat cushions or mattresses often serve as viable preventative measures against skin breakdown. The physical therapist may need to utilize prefabricated splints or orthotic devices to minimize contractures that impede recovery or to consult with the medical attendings regarding the use of pharmacologic interventions. Examples would include an orthotic device and or use of a pharmacologic agent such as baclofen to minimize the development of a plantarflexion contracture for a child who sustained a TBI and is beginning to exhibit increased plantar flexor muscle tone and posture.

Transitioning

Once the child is medically stable, the medical staff may consider discharge from the acute care hospital to home or another setting, such as a rehabilitation hospital. When the child is close to being discharged, it is the role of the physical therapist in this setting to provide input on whether further physical therapy services are needed for the child, and if so, whether an in-house rehabilitation facility or an outpatient facility is recommended. Generally, once the child is medically stable, the health care team would decide whether the child's current impairments and functional

---

DISPLAY 5.6 Discharge Criteria

The child is medically stable.
The child's current impairments and functional limitations are adequately managed with the assistance of a knowledgeable caregiver (At home: parent. At a rehabilitation hospital or outpatient clinic: physical therapist).
Follow-up visits have been coordinated and scheduled.

---

limitations require a certain level of professional input to achieve a prior level of functioning or rehabilitation. Can the parents adequately manage the impairments or functional limitations, or do the limitations require the skilled intervention and knowledge of rehabilitation professionals? Is the child appropriate for outpatient services, or is admission to a rehabilitation hospital a safer option? Once these issues have been determined, the case manager is typically responsible for ensuring that all follow-up appointments have been scheduled with the appropriate providers and the family prior to the child's discharge from the acute care hospital (Display 5.6).

The physical therapist plays an important role in the pediatric acute care hospital. The physical therapist can help minimize the effects of the hospitalization and immobilization on the child's motor skills and function during the hospital stay. The primary goal of physical therapy in this setting is to promote recovery and optimal independence, including mobility, given the current medical status of the child. Once the child is medically stable, the physical therapist plays a key role in the recommendation of future physical therapy services, through either the outpatient or the inpatient rehabilitation setting. A physical therapist practicing in the acute care setting must possess knowledge of the various lines, tubes, and monitors; understand how the child with specialized medical equipment and monitors may be mobilized; and have strong communication skills to effectively work as a multidisciplinary team member.

» The inpatient rehabilitation setting

Once the child in an acute care hospital is medically stable, the medical staff may consider discharge from the hospital to home or another setting, such as a rehabilitation hospital. Many general rehabilitation hospitals require that the child be medically stable to maximize participation in rehabilitation. There must be reason to believe that the child has not met his or her full level of independence and has the potential to benefit from rehabilitative services. The child should also be able to tolerate several hours of therapy service a day and have the need for more than one type of rehabilitation service, such as physical therapy, occupational therapy, or speech therapy.

Inpatient rehabilitation provides an intensive comprehensive interdisciplinary approach to the restoration of function for children and adolescents who have sustained injuries or undergone surgical procedures that impact their activity and participation levels compared with their baseline level of function. An inpatient rehabilitation unit can be a freestanding facility or a specialized unit within an acute care hospital. The Centers for Medicare and Medicaid Services (CMS) criteria for admission to an inpatient rehabilitation hospital include a patient who is medically stable and able to tolerate a minimum of 3 hours of rehabilitation therapy a day for at least 5 days per week. CMS classifies payment to inpatient rehabilitation hospitals as inpatient facilities by their compliance with admissions that include 13 diagnostic groupings.[30] The majority of those seen in most pediatric rehabilitation facilities does not fall under the Medicare rulings. Pediatric inpatient rehabilitation hospitals generally follow the CMS criteria for a number of hours of therapy as part of their admission criteria as well as one who is medically stable and has the potential to benefit from interdisciplinary rehabilitation services (Display 5.7).

The multidisciplinary inpatient rehabilitation team includes physicians, nurses trained in rehabilitation, dieticians, occupational therapists, physical therapists, speech pathologists, psychologists, social workers, and orthotists. The team is generally led by a pediatric physiatrist, pediatrician, orthopedist, or neurosurgeon, but this can vary among facilities. Other physician subspecialists will be requested for consultation as needed. The child's family and caregivers are an integral part of the team throughout the rehabilitation process. Multidisciplinary teams will function differently among rehabilitation facilities. Some teams may work as an interdisciplinary team or even a transdisciplinary team at times, whereas in other facilities the team will remain a multidisciplinary team, in which each discipline works separately on its own goals. In the ideal scenario, the team will work as an interdisciplinary team whose members are all aware of and strive toward the same goals.

Weekly multidisciplinary conferences or care-coordination conferences are held in most rehabilitation units. These conferences serve to update the entire team about the child's progress, plans for discharge, teaching and equipment that is needed prior to discharge, and status of caregivers competency with carryover of care at home. Typically, updates are

also provided on the child's functional status. An identified team member, often the physician or the social worker, will meet with the child and/or family to review the conference findings and plan of care.

Certain inpatient rehabilitation units specialize in one type of patient population such as TBI or spinal cord injury and have the appropriate staff to meet the unique needs of patients with these specific diagnoses. Regardless of the specialty, admission to an inpatient rehabilitation unit would be followed by an examination and evaluation of the child.

Examination

When a child is transferred to an inpatient rehabilitation unit, either from another facility or from within an acute care hospital, an initial examination is performed to determine the child's baseline and to develop a plan of care. In an interdisciplinary setting, much of the initial history can be gathered from the child's medical record rather than asking the parent or caregivers the same questions repeatedly. Important information to obtain prior to examining the child include the child's diagnosis and mechanism of injury if pertinent, surgical procedures performed, precautions to be followed owing to infection risk, medical instability and/or surgical procedures, current medications, and level of function prior to the recent admission. If a child has a chronic diagnosis, such as cerebral palsy, past medical and surgical history can provide very pertinent information.

Many children admitted to an inpatient rehabilitation unit present with significant medical issues and/or significant impairment in levels of arousal and alertness. These children may have multiple leads connected to monitors that record their vital signs continuously. They may also have a tracheostomy with or without ventilator support, a gastrostomy tube for nutrition, a peripheral intravenous line, or a central IV line. Safe practice might be to complete the initial examination at the child's bedside and progress to the gym area as appropriate from a patient safety standpoint.

An initial review of systems should include the child's heart rate, oxygen saturation levels, and blood pressure, as appropriate. The integrity of the child's skin should be examined as well as skin color and healing scars. Some children will be transferred to the rehabilitation unit with casts, external fixators, or internal hardware for fracture management; skin color and temperature of the distal casted extremity should be closely monitored. Observation of the child's position is also important—Is the child relaxed in bed? Is the child exhibiting abnormal postures that may indicate underlying abnormal muscle tone or movement disorders? Could these abnormal postures lead to skin breakdown, further joint ROM issues?

The initial examination will vary from child to child but will include muscle performance, both muscle tone and strength as well as voluntary control of movement, ROM, pain, neuromotor development, and gait. A standardized assessment tool to assist with goal development and to

---

DISPLAY 5.7 | **Point to Remember—Admission Criteria for Inpatient Rehabilitation**

Patient is:
   medically stable
   has not reached full potential for independence
   has potential to benefit from therapy services
   able to participate in 3 hours of therapy a day
   in need of more than one rehabilitative service

monitor outcomes will be required in most inpatient rehabilitation facilities that are CARF accredited. In what follows, key components of tests and measures are briefly described and specific references provided to commonly encountered diagnoses on an inpatient pediatric rehabilitation unit.

Children who have sustained a TBI may demonstrate impaired levels of arousal and attention. The level of coma may be monitored using several criterion-based scales; progressing from a lower number to a higher number is indicative of improvement. The Glasgow Coma Scale (GCS) is a standardized tool that evaluates a patient's responses in eye opening, motor activity, and verbal responses.[31] A pediatric version of the GCS, the Pediatric Coma Scale (PCS), has been developed for children 9 to 72 months old with norms for specific age groups.[32]

The Rancho Los Amigos Level of Cognitive Function Scale (Rancho Scale) is frequently used during inpatient rehabilitation to rate cognitive and behavior function and guide interventions.[33] A specific test to assess orientation post TBI has been designed for children, the Children's Orientation and Amnesia Test (COAT),[34] which asks questions that children would know and has been found to be reliable for children 4 to 15 years of age. Other members of the team will complete in-depth examinations to determine communication abilities, ability to attend to tasks and solve problems. This information will be shared at the multidisciplinary meetings to determine consistent methods of communication, behavior management, improving memory, and other aspects that influence the plan of care.

The initial examination should include current assistive and adaptive devices used by the child or the family. These devices will most likely change over the course of the admission and may be a focus of the intervention for some children. Many children with a chronic diagnosis will have assistive devices that they use very well to improve their function and independence. If a surgical procedure has been performed, they may need assistance to use the device again or to progress to another type of assistive device. Parents can provide valuable input on what they may need help with at home and what devices have been tried but found unsuccessful in the past.

Adaptive devices for function at home and school may become a significant focus of the interventions provided during the admission of children with a newly acquired diagnosis. Most children with a new diagnosis, such as a spinal cord injury, will not have adaptive devices at home. The initial examination will need to determine the accessibility of the child's home environment to assist with later determinations of devices to be fabricated or ordered prior to discharge.

Children will often be admitted to the rehab unit with orthotic, protective and/or supportive devices that they received in the acute care setting. Mechanical ventilators, endotracheal tubes, and gastrostomy tubes are frequently encountered on a rehab unit. A review of the medical record and communication with the nursing, respiratory, and/or physician staff will detail the child's ventilator settings, respiratory status, and the child's ability to be weaned from the ventilator for certain periods during the day.

Children who have sustained a traumatic brain injury may be admitted to the unit with orthotic devices or serial casts to maintain or improve their ROM. Children who have had a spinal fusion after a spinal cord injury may wear a thoracic lumbar sacral orthosis (TLSO) to protect the spine until the fusion is stable. Those who have had orthopedic procedures such as a femoral osteotomy or adductor tendon lengthening may also utilize positioning devices, such as abductor wedges. Pressure wraps or pressure garments may be worn continuously or for specific periods during the day in the case of skin grafts secondary to severe burns. Whatever the device, it is important to know if the device can safely be removed for the therapy session, how often and for how long it should be worn, and whether the physical therapist is expected to make recommendations to change or progress the device?

As in the acute care setting, evaluation of pain should also be completed for all children, but specific attention should be given to those children who have had surgery recently, sustained a fracture, or have been admitted with a diagnosis associated with pain such as hemophilia, arthritis, or chronic pain syndrome. A variety of pain scales are available for use with children and adolescents depending on their age and cognitive abilities. Refer to Display 5.3 for a list of common pediatric pain scales. Evaluation of pain in all children during the initial examination should also include questions about pain during activity or movement, waking from sleep secondary to pain, what alleviates the pain, and what medications or other interventions may be currently used for pain management.

The integrity of the skin should be examined in all children, but special attention should be given to those with limited or absent voluntary movement or those with limited or altered sensation, as is seen with a spinal cord injury. As mentioned earlier, the skin of any child wearing orthotic devices or casts should also be inspected for color and integrity. Scar formation in children who have been transferred from a burn unit needs to be examined for continued healing and potential impediment of joint motion. For a child with impaired sensation, such as spinal cord injury, pressure mapping of the wheelchair seat and/or mattress may be imperative to prevent skin breakdown.

Children with a neurologic diagnosis, whether chronic or recently acquired, will exhibit some type of secondary movement disorder. The muscle tone of children with a movement disorder is often affected, resulting in spasticity, dystonia, athetosis, chorea, ataxia, myoclonus, and tremors. Children often exhibit more than one movement disorder. Spasticity and dystonia are frequently seen in children with cerebral palsy or children who have sustained a brain injury. Tremors may be seen in children who have sustained a brain injury or who have a brain tumor. Ataxia is typically seen in children with a brain tumor, after an infectious process or a head injury.

TABLE 5.1.	Ashworth Scales

Ashworth Scale	Modified Ashworth Scale
1 No increase in muscle tone	**0** No increase in muscle tone
2 Slight increase in tone, giving a "catch" affected part is moved in flexion or extension	**1** Slight increase in muscle tone, manifested by a catch and release or by minimal resistance at the end of the ROM
3 More marked increase in tone; passive movements difficult	**1+** Slight increase in muscle tone, manifested by a catch, followed by minimal resistance throughout the remainder of the ROM (less than half)
4 Considerable increase in tone; passive movements difficult	**2** More marked increase in muscle tone through most of the ROM, but affected part(s) move easily
5 Affected part rigid in flexion or extension	**3** Considerable increase in muscle tone, passive movement difficult
	4 Affected part(s) rigid in flexion or extension

From Hass B, Bergstrom E, Jamous A, et al. The inter-rater reliability of the original and of the modified Ashworth scale for the assessment of spasticity in patients with spinal cord injury. *Spinal Cord.* 1996;34:560-564; Clopton N, Dutton J, Featherston T, et al. Interrater and intrarater reliability of the modified Ashworth scale in children with hypertonia. *Pediatr Phys Ther.* 2005;17:268-274.

Spasticity is typically graded clinically using the Ashworth Scale or Modified Ashworth scale[35,36] (Table 5.1). They are both ordinal scales, but the Modified Ashworth includes an additional rating at the lower end of the scale to render the scale more discrete. The scales are not meant to be summed but rather to grade muscle groups individually. Both of these scales require moving a joint passively through the ROM at a standard speed and then rating the resistance on a five- or six-point scale respectively. Therefore, it must be remembered that both of these scales are a measure of hypertonia and not a true measure of spasticity.

A comparison of the Ashworth and the Modified Ashworth scales showed that the interrater reliability was better for the Ashworth Scale.[19] Most of the disagreement with the Modified Ashworth scale included the additional rating at the lower end of the scale that may impact the reliability. Several studies investigating only the Modified Ashworth scale found the scale to be more reliable for upper extremity muscle groups,

especially the elbow flexors, than lower extremity muscle groups.[37,38] The studies included adults or adolescents, and it may be more difficult to move the larger and heavier lower extremity consistently through the joint motions compared with the upper extremity. The Ashworth scales are quick and simple to administer, can be utilized with children with cognitive impairments, and do not require specialized equipment.

One of the disadvantages of the Ashworth scales is that they do not truly measure spasticity because they measure only passive movement at a single speed. The modified Tardieu scale assesses the resistance to passive stretch after an initial "catch" or resistance is felt and at varying speeds.[39] The scale also incorporates the joint angle when resistance to passive stretch is encountered (Table 5.2). Both the Ashworth scales and the modified Tardieu scale have been shown to have low interrater reliability and there it is questionable whether they truly measure spasticity when other factors such as contractures may be present.[40,41]

TABLE 5.2.	Tardieu Scale

Velocity of stretch:
V1   As slow as possible (slower than the natural drop of the limb under gravity)
V2   Speed of the limb segment falling under gravity
V3   As fast as possible (faster than the rate of the natural drop of limb under gravity)
V1 measures the PROM; only V2 and V3 are used to rate the spasticity

Quality of the muscle reaction (X):
0   No resistance throughout the course of the passive movement
1   Slight resistance throughout the course of the movement, no clear "catch" at a precise angle
2   Clear catch at a precise angle, interrupting the passive movement, followed by release
3   Fatigable clonus (<10 sec when maintaining the pressure) appearing at a precise angle
4   Infatigable clonus (>10 sec when maintaining the pressure) at a precise angle

Angle of muscle reaction (Y):
Measured relative to the position of minimal stretch of the muscle (corresponding to angle zero) for all joints except hip, where it is relative to the anatomic resting position.

From Boyd R, Graham H. Objective measurement of clinical findings in the use of botulinum toxin type A for the management of children with cerebral palsy. *Eur J Neurol.* 1999;6:S23-S25.

The importance of examining both muscle spasticity and dystonia is to determine their severity and the implications for the development of secondary musculoskeletal deformities such as contracture of soft tissue structures, hip joint subluxation/dislocation, and the risk of developing torsional bony deformities. The information will aid in grading the severity of the movement disorder and will help in determining the deforming or imbalanced forces.

The Fahn–Marsden scale has been used to grade dystonia in adults.[42] The Barry–Albright dystonia scale (BAD scale) is a modification of the Fahn–Marsden scale, which was designed for use with children, including those with cognitive impairments.[43] The BAD scale consists of a five-point ordinal scale that rates the dystonia present in eight areas of the body. The BAD scale has been shown to have very high interrater and intrarater reliability for the total score; the interrater reliability decreases slightly when comparing individual body area scores.[43]

Along with muscle tone, joint ROM is also examined. Although the goniometric techniques used to measure active or passive range of motion (AROM/PROM) in children and adults are similar, age-related differences exist in ROM values between adults and infants and young children. When measuring ROM in children, the most reliable results are obtained when the same examiner evaluates changes in ROM over time. As with adults, variations of 0 to 5 degrees do not necessarily signify change but could be equated to error and variability.

Testing of muscle strength will vary depending on the age and size of the child. Muscle strength testing will help identify muscle activity in specific muscle groups of a child with a spinal cord injury and will assist with developing intervention programs for those children who have undergone soft tissue lengthening procedures. Refer to the outpatient examination section later in this chapter for a more in-depth discussion of muscle strength testing in children.

Testing of cutaneous sensation is especially important for children with a spinal cord injury. Testing techniques do not differ from those with adults; however very young children may have difficulty understanding the directions or expectations. Any identified impairments in cutaneous sensation will assist with determining appropriate transfer techniques to use and what motions to avoid, position changes, and patient education for skin care.

The initial examination after admission to the inpatient rehab unit should include a standardized measure of the child's functional abilities. This standardized measure will help depict how various impairments are impacting the child's activity level and the ability to participate in the community setting on discharge. This functional measure will be monitored periodically throughout the admission and at discharge by the multidisciplinary team involved in the child's care. Standardized functional tests and measures also serve as the outcome data monitoring required by regulatory agencies to monitor patient outcomes and for benchmark data with other facilities nationally.

There are a few nationally recognized outcomes database systems available that will allow a user facility to monitor patient outcome data and benchmark nationally for a pediatric rehabilitation population that encompasses a variety of diagnoses. The most commonly used inpatient rehab database systems are the Pediatric Evaluation of Disability Inventory (PEDI) and Uniform Data System for Medical Rehabilitation (UDS).[12,44] UDS uses the pediatric version of the Functional Independence Measure (WeeFIM II) for the pediatric rehabilitation population.[12]

The PEDI was designed for the functional evaluation of children between 6 months and 7.5 years of age but can be used for older children if their abilities are under those of a 7.5-year-old typically developing child. Function is measured in three content domains: (1) self-care, (2) mobility, and (3) social function. Functional performance also includes the level of caregiver assistance needed to complete a skill such as eating or toilet transfers and records the environmental modifications and equipment required to complete the functional skill. The test can be completed by professionals familiar with the child's functional abilities or through parent interview. The PEDI takes approximately 45 to 60 minutes to complete in its entirety, including the 197 items on the functional scales and the 20 items on the caregiver assistance and modification scales. Intrarater reliability has been shown to be high for both the functional scales and the caregiver assistance scales. Interrater reliability for the functional scales ranges from 0.95 to 0.99, with decreased reliability noted for specific items that are often not observed in the clinic setting such as household chores.[44,45] Interrater reliability has been found to be variable and lower than intrarater reliability, with parent or clinicians who are with the child throughout the day providing higher scores for assistance than clinicians who may see the child only for short time frames.[45] The PEDI has been found to be sensitive to changes in function in an inpatient pediatric population with an acquired brain injury.[46]

The PEDI-CAT (Pediatric Evaluation of Disability Inventory–Computer Adaptive Test) was developed by many of the same authors as the PEDI but is not a replacement for it. The PEDI-CAT serves a broader age range from birth to 20 years of age and includes 276 items across the four domains of daily activities, mobility, social/cognitive domain, and the responsibility domain. The caregiver assistance scale in the PEDI has been replaced by the responsibility domain in the PEDI-CAT. The computer adaptive testing module of the PEDI-CAT also reduces the administration time by individualizing the test to each child on the basis of his or her responses. The PEDI-CAT has been shown to be a reliable and valid assessment tool across a variety of pediatric rehab settings.[47,48] The PEDI-CAT has also been shown to represent a child's activity and participation levels within the World Health Organization's International Classification of Functioning, Disability and Health (ICF) model.[49]

The WeeFIM II is the pediatric version of the Functional Independence Measure (FIM) used in adult rehabilitation and includes a functional assessment, parent satisfaction at discharge, and resource utilization efficiency. The WeeFIM II is a minimum data set and consists of 18 items that measure independence in functional skills across the domains of self-care, mobility, and cognition. The test is designed for use among children and adolescents 6 months through 7 years of age who exhibit a functional or developmental delay. The WeeFIM II may be used with children over the age of 7 years if their skills are at or below those of a typically developing 7-year-old child. There is also a 0 to 3 module that measures the precursors to function in children 0 to 3 years of age. The WeeFIM II test is administered by direct observation or caregiver interview and can be completed in 10 to 15 minutes.[12] Ottenbacher and colleagues found stability in WeeFIM scores across age ranges.[50] This study demonstrated high reliability among raters and over time by the WeeFIM subscale scores with ICC of 0.87 to 0.98. High reliability with an ICC of 0.98 for data collected in-person compared with over the phone was also demonstrated.

All inpatient rehabilitation facilities should be using an outcome measure to monitor change over time with patients. Ideally, the test is one with a national database to allow for benchmarking and improvements in quality of care. The tests discussed previously are all discipline-free assessments, thereby lending themselves for use in an interdisciplinary or transdisciplinary inpatient setting. The WeeFIM is a faster test to administer owing to the limited data set. However, some clinicians may voice concerns that the WeeFIM is not sensitive to small changes in function because of the limited data set.

Functional assessments are not meant to replace other evaluation tools, so other measures such as developmental evaluations, balance tests, timed tests, and other clinical examinations may also be used to complete the evaluation and develop a plan for intervention. Thomas-Stonell and colleagues investigated the responsiveness of nine outcome scales on the World Health Organization's domains of activity and participation.[51] They evaluated 33 children with a mean age of 12.5 years who had sustained traumatic brain injuries and found that the PEDI had a ceiling effect, with 70% of subjects achieving the maximum score by discharge. This study found the WeeFIM and the Child Health Questionnaire (CHQ) to be consistently the most responsive, followed by the Gross Motor Function Measure (GMFM). The combination of the WeeFIM or CHQ, GMFM, and the American Speech-Language Hearing Association National Outcomes Measure System captured all of the improvements cited by parents and clinicians.

Once all of the necessary examination information is obtained, an evaluation and diagnosis are made to facilitate the development of a plan of care.

Evaluation and Plan of Care

Synthesis of the examination findings must also include the parent and/or child's goals and what living situation the child will be returning to on discharge. A return to a home

environment with all rooms on one level and a parent present 24 hours per day will have different functional expectations than a return to a home environment that has a full flight of stairs to enter and no parent or caregiver present during the day. The physical therapist's examination will be incorporated with the evaluations of the other disciplines to provide a unified plan of care that will be presented to the patient and family and carried out in some form by all staff members.

In an inpatient rehabilitation setting, the plan of care is developed through an interdisciplinary team. Often, this will occur at a regularly scheduled care-coordination conference, often called a "staffing" or "rounds," where the child's status is reviewed and progress and impediments toward discharge are discussed. The plan of care, is ideally, an interdisciplinary document that includes the child's functional level based on standardized testing, goals with expected outcomes, length of time to achieve the goals, disciplines involved in the care of the child and their frequency of intervention, and the interventions to be provided to achieve the goals. The plan of care is updated at regular intervals but serves as the template for discharge planning. Ideally, the family and child, if applicable, is involved in the development of the plan of care, which helps serve as an understanding of when to expect the child to be discharged, where the child will be discharged, the child's level of functional independence expected at discharge, and equipment and environmental modifications that may be needed in the home or school environment.

Physical therapists need to understand their role on the interdisciplinary team. Each member should be working toward previously agreed on functional goals and not primarily amelioration of identified impairments. Team members are aware of all of the child's goals and interventions and help to carry over those interventions during their interactions with the child and the family. For example, communication may be a significant activity limitation, and the physical therapist must be able to understand and carry out the communication strategies implemented by the speech pathologist to ensure continuity of care for the child (Display 5.8).

Intervention

The safe return of a child to the home environment at the maximal level of independence should be the driving force behind all interventions. Interventions will be determined by the goals on the plan of care and the expected outcomes

---

DISPLAY
5.8 **Point to Remember—Role of Interdisciplinary Team**

Physical therapists should understand their role on the interdisciplinary team. Each member should be working toward the agreed upon functional goals and not primarily amelioration of identified impairments.

and should focus on improving function. Depending on the extent of injuries sustained by the child and procedures performed, there may be impairments that were identified on the examination that will interfere with accomplishing the functional goals. Remediation of impairments and improving the child's functional status are addressed through interventions described in the Guide to Physical Therapists Practice.[22] A physical therapist would employ these procedures and techniques in the rehabilitation setting just as they would in another setting. A few key elements of interventions that are typically emphasized in the rehabilitation setting are briefly discussed in what follows.

Effective communication with the child, family, and other members of the multidisciplinary team is essential in order to efficiently achieve optimal outcomes for the child and provide high levels of satisfaction for both the child and the family. Communication begins at the time of admission when identifying goals with the family and/or child and extends through to the examination and daily therapy sessions. Time must be taken to explain the interventions, the child's responses and progress, and the adjustments to the child's progress during the delivery of the interventions. Communication extends to all team members and includes formal reporting at care conferences, consults and instruction with other disciplines, outcome reporting, and progress toward discharge. At some point, the physical therapist will need to communicate with professionals in the child's home community such as school personnel, DME vendors, or physical therapists in an outpatient setting closer to the child's home.

During intervention sessions with the child, the physical therapist will often carry over plans implemented by other disciplines to optimize the care provided to the child. Children who are recovering from an acquired brain injury may exhibit confusion or even aggressive behavior, whereas others will have limited methods of communicating their needs. A psychologist or behavior specialist may implement a structured program to be followed by all personnel and family members to provide consistent methods of dealing with inappropriate behavior, whereas the speech pathologist may outline basic methods of communication responses to expect from the child in response to simple questions. To ensure consistency for the child, the physical therapist must understand and seek the communication from other disciplines involved in the care of the child.

In some rehabilitation units, the physical therapist may serve as the case manager for a patient and will need to coordinate care throughout the hospital admission, including follow-up after discharge. Case management or case coordination is a skill that often requires mentoring before a physical therapist is competent to ensure collaboration among team members and an admission with optimal outcomes for the patient.

Instruction to other team members and caregivers is crucial for carryover of goals throughout the day. Areas of patient instruction often include range of motion exercises, donning and doffing of splints or orthotic devices, positioning in bed and/or a wheelchair and transfer techniques. These activities can also be taught to family members to increase their involvement in their child's care and to assist with preparation for discharge.

Therapeutic exercise is a very large category of interventions employed by physical therapists, with many of the techniques utilized in other settings applicable to the rehabilitation setting. Increasing range of motion, improving strength, and increasing endurance for a specific skill or movement is often a focus of intervention for children who have sustained a traumatic injury or undergone a surgical procedure. Children who have sustained a severe brain injury often initially present to the rehabilitation unit with joint contractures that require long-term interventions such as dynamic splinting or serial casting. Serial casts are most commonly applied to the ankle joints to increase dorsiflexion motion and to the elbow or wrist joints to improve extension range of motion. Impairments may need to be addressed, but functional skills should also be addressed simultaneously. Developmental activities for younger children, balance and gait training, and endurance activities are all interventions employed in inpatient rehabilitation.

Functional training is another frequently utilized intervention in the rehabilitation setting. Most current theories of motor development emphasize the multiple subsystems required for movement to occur. These include the musculoskeletal, neuromuscular, sensory, and cognitive subsystems with an emphasis on an opportunity to practice the desired skill. For functional training activities to be effective, the impairments in the subsystems must also be addressed or compensated.

Functional training begins from the time of admission to decrease the activity limitations that may be present at the time of discharge. Early functional training includes bed mobility and transfers and should be carried out by all team members. For functional training to be effective for the patient, communication among staff and with the family is important as well as practice throughout the day for the child. For example, if the child is working on sit-to-stand maneuvers for strengthening or as a component of a transfer, this skill should be practiced not only during the therapy session but also each time the child transfers in and out of bed, from the toilet, or any other surface.

In order to optimize a child's function, or aid in the recovery process, sometimes it is necessary to prescribe or fabricate certain devices or equipment. At the beginning of the inpatient admission, some children will require serial casting and/or orthotic devices to improve and then maintain specific joint range of motion needed for later functional skills. Children who have had a surgical procedure may exhibit ROM that is improved from their preoperative baseline and may require reassessment of the appropriateness of their current orthotic devices. The physical therapist will be asked to provide input on what type of orthotic device is indicated for the child to promote optimal joint alignment, preserve joint motion and integrity and promote function (see Appendix A).

A crucial piece of the ongoing discharge planning is determining what adaptive and assistive devices will be needed in the discharge environment to promote optimal safe function for the child and ease of care for caregivers. Ordering of adaptive and assistive devices, often referred to as DME by third-party payers, involves coordination with multiple team members and the caregivers. Adaptive and assistive devices that may be needed prior to safe discharge ranges from bath and toilet seats to power wheelchairs and lifts for transfers in the home environment.

A home visit by one or two members of the team is an essential piece of prescribing and ordering assistive devices and equipment for the home. The home visit provides crucial information about what type of equipment will work in the home and what devices are necessary for safety. The parents are an integral part of the team because they are the ones who will be using the equipment with the child on a daily basis. The family should be fully trained in the use of the equipment with their child, including direct observation by team members.

Outcomes

Outcomes are based on the goals that were established at admission and reassessed throughout the inpatient episode of care. Goal development can be difficult because there is minimal predictive data for the pediatric rehabilitation population. One study found that length of stay (LOS) varied by diagnosis, in that shorter LOS was seen with children with orthopedic diagnoses as compared with children with spinal cord injuries, who exhibited the longest LOS.[52] Dumas and colleagues investigated the predictive value of several variables in the recovery of ambulation in children who had sustained a traumatic brain injury.[53] For their study, ambulation was defined as "being able to walk indoors without an assistive gait device, support, guarding or supervision for balance on level surfaces." Absence of lower extremity hypertonicity was the strongest predictor of recovery of ambulation by the time of discharge. Severity of injury and lower extremity injury were also factors that helped in predicting the ability of the child to ambulate. This type of information can be very useful to the clinician in developing realistic goals and expected outcomes.

Outcomes are also based on the data from functional assessments such as the WeeFIM and provide the clinician with individual patient outcomes and outcomes by diagnostic groupings for the facility and the nation.

Once the child in an inpatient rehabilitation hospital has reached his potential, demonstrated by meeting all the goals of the program or by a lack of progress toward those goals, the team may consider discharge to home. Some of the factors that may influence this decision are the ability of the child to perform his or her activities of daily living with minimal or moderate assistance from a caregiver, services being required on a less intense basis, and the family being able to manage the child's care and medical needs in the

---

> **DISPLAY 5.9   Point to Remember—Common Discharge Criteria for Inpatient Rehabilitation**
>
> The patient:
> has reached his full potential for independence or can achieve this on an outpatient basis
> no longer requires the comprehensive services of inpatient rehabilitation
> is able to be cared for at home
> can access the level of rehabilitation services on an outpatient basis

---

home environment. Discharge from an inpatient program often involves the transition of rehabilitation services to an outpatient and/or school setting in the child's community (Display 5.9).

In the inpatient rehabilitation setting, the child has been admitted with the focus on therapy goals, recovery or restoration of function, and family caregiver education. From the onset of the admission the focus is on a return to home with the child and family actively participating in several hours of therapy each day, mimicking a more typical daily routine with regularly scheduled meals, dressing and bathing each day, and scheduled times for school or naps as age appropriate. The team is typically a smaller group of professionals who work together regularly and are familiar with carrying over the goals from each discipline during their interactions with the child and family. The physical therapist working in this environment must have strong teamwork and communication skills and have an understanding of a wide range of diagnoses and the DME that may be needed during the admission and for the transition home.

» The outpatient rehabilitation setting

Criteria for admission to an outpatient program will vary among facilities, but most require that, at a minimum, the child is medically stable and has the potential to benefit from outpatient services. Individual facilities may have specific admission criteria related to age or diagnosis, and many will have policies that allow for discharge of the child for attendance failures or a lack of demonstrated progress over a specified period. The ultimate goal of rehabilitation is to have the child reach his or her full potential for independence regardless of the setting. For some individuals, this may occur within a defined period associated with healing and a return to a preinjury physiologic state. For other individuals, this may occur and reoccur over a lifetime because the person with a chronic disability moves through episodes of care associated with the management of a chronic disability.

Outpatient physical therapy services are not a substitute for school-based or early intervention services that address the needs of the child and family in a different context.

School-based physical therapy is mandated by educational law that entitles eligible students to receive services related to their education and that are supportive of the student's individual education plan. Early intervention services are also provided under educational law to eligible families and their children to aid the family in meeting their individual outcomes in accordance with the individual family service plan. Although the interventions provided by the physical therapist may be similar across these settings, the role and intent for the provision of physical therapy services is different.

Outpatient rehabilitation is typically less intensive than an inpatient approach and is directed at a specific activity limitation for a defined episode of care. An outpatient facility may be an outpatient department or satellite center of a pediatric hospital, a freestanding nonprofit organization such as United Cerebral Palsy or Easterseals, or a freestanding private practice. The practice setting will determine the other disciplines that may also provide services and the types of multidisciplinary care that may be available. A private practice may offer only physical therapy services or other rehabilitation services such as occupational therapy. Most of the other types of organizations mentioned will provide multidisciplinary services that are center based. Age ranges and diagnoses served may vary among facilities, and whereas some organizations offer specialty services or expertise in specific diagnostic areas, smaller private practices may limit their patient referrals to those with orthopedic diagnoses only, and yet others may specialize in children with neurologic disorders. Many larger facilities, especially those associated with a hospital, will serve children across a wide age range with varying diagnoses.

Outpatient physical therapy services differ from those provided in an inpatient rehabilitation setting in several key areas. An obvious difference is that the child is now living at home. The home is certainly the ideal environment for the child, but the scheduling of services is different. Physical therapy appointments are dependent on the parent or caregiver's ability to transport the child, parent work schedules, school hours if the child is in school, and the schedules of siblings in the home. In the home, the child is also under the care and decision making of the parent as opposed to the inpatient setting, where a team of professionals is involved in the child's care as well as the parent. The parent often initiates outpatient physical therapy services and is a key factor in the establishment of the frequency of those services and the goals of those services during the child's outpatient episode of care.

The child's initial entry into outpatient services will vary among states depending on direct access regulations and state practice acts. Many states will require a prescription for outpatient physical therapy either at the onset of services or within a defined period after the initiation of services. Even in states with direct access to physical therapy services, a prescription may be required by the payer of those services. As in other settings, the initial visit to an outpatient facility would include an examination and evaluation of the child (Display 5.10).

DISPLAY 5.10   Point to Remember—Outpatient Rehabilitation

Outpatient rehabilitation is typically less intensive than an inpatient approach but is directed at a specific activity limitation for a defined episode of care.

Examination

Much of the same information that is gathered for the inpatient evaluation is part of the outpatient evaluation. Some of the most important initial information to obtain from the parent and/or the child is to determine why they are present for the evaluation. This information can be obtained with questions such as the following: What brings you here? What are your concerns? What would you like to be able to do that is difficult for you right now, or what would you like your child to be able to do that he is having difficulty with right now? Does your child have any pain? These types of questions will help determine the selection of tests and measures and immediately involve the parent or child in the evaluation process and ultimately in the plan of care to be developed.

Answers to the preceding questions will assist with prioritizing and organizing the examination. For example, if the parent states that the child is getting bigger and it is difficult to lift the child, observation of the parent's lifting technique would be appropriate. Observation may lead to education of the parent or show evidence of impairments in the child's joint mobility, weight-bearing ability, or muscle strength. The examination should not be an evaluation of every impairment or body structure and then progress to examining the child's functional skills. Instead, the functional goals should lead the physical therapist to investigate impairments that may be impeding progress toward a specific goal or activity.

A frequent impairment that is often encountered in physical therapy is limitation in joint range of motion. Although the goniometric techniques used to measure active or passive joint ROM in children and adults are similar, several factors must be kept in mind when examining range of motion in children. Age-related differences exist in ROM values between adults and infants and young children. For example, a 6-month-old child will exhibit residual flexion contractures of the hip joints secondary to the remnants of physiologic flexion from intrauterine positioning.

Muscle length tests should also be included in the overall joint motion examination. Specific tests and their procedures do not differ from standard procedures used with the adult population; however, several tests may be used more frequently in pediatrics. Hip flexor muscle length is examined using the Thomas test or the prone hip extension test. Hamstring length is usually examined in adults using the straight leg raise test; however, the passive knee extension test (PKE) is commonly used with pediatrics, as is the measurement of the popliteal angle. The PKE measures the hamstring contracture and not the popliteal angle.[54] The PKE can be used in the presence of a knee flexion contracture and is therefore useful for children who present with involvement of multiple joints.

A variety of methods to examine muscle strength are also available, their use being dependent on the age and ability of the child. For infants and children younger than 3 or 4 years, evaluation of strength is most often accomplished by observing movement and function such as squatting, stair climbing, reaching up on tiptoe, and other biomechanical analyses. A child must be able to follow the directions of the testing procedure to ensure accurate results using either manual muscle testing (MMT) or dynamometry. Handheld dynamometry has been found to be a reliable and sensitive method of examining strength in various populations of children, especially when looking at the same therapist completing the measurements.[55,56] However, the sample sizes for specific populations such as children and youth with cerebral palsy are small and it is therefore difficult to draw strong conclusions about the reliability of the testing.[57] Gajdosik determined that handheld dynamometry could be used reliably with typical developing children between the ages of 2 to 5 years as long as they could follow the directions and understand the command to push as well as agree to participate in the process.[58] Children in the 2-year age range were more likely than the 3- and 4-year-olds to refuse to participate in the testing sessions. Strength may also be reliably tested using isokinetic machines if the child is tall enough to reach the components. The method of strength testing will depend on measurement devices available to the physical therapist, the cognitive status of the child, and the child's ability to adhere to directions.

During the initial examination, a postural screen may be appropriate. The physical therapist examines skeletal alignment in a variety of positions, depending on the age of the child. Skeletal alignment should include spinal and lower extremity alignment and limb length. An example of the basic components of a physical therapy musculoskeletal examination can be found in Appendix B.

A frequent reason for referral to outpatient physical therapy is parental concern about the way their child walks, the presence of an in-toed gait pattern representing the most common complaint. Physical therapists working in a pediatric setting must be aware of the rotational or torsional and skeletal alignment changes of bones and joints that occur with normal growth and development. Often, a parent's concerns can be eased by educating them about the normal development of gait in children. However, these normal developmental processes may be altered secondary to abnormal muscle pull or weight-bearing forces that may be present in a child with a neurologic diagnosis. Therefore, a physical therapist also needs to be able to identify these abnormal deforming forces and potential for development of excessive rotational deformities that may impact function as the child grows.

Staheli has developed a rotational profile to assess lower extremity alignment and assist in determining which component of the lower extremity contributes to the rotational variation.[54,59] The rotational profile consists of six measurements, including (1) foot-progression angle; (2) medial rotation of the hip joint; (3) lateral rotation of the hip joint; (4) thigh–foot angle; (5) angle of the transmalleolar axis; and (6) the configuration of the foot. Normal values have been established for the first five measurements and can be used to determine whether the variation falls within the wide range of normal or whether intervention is indicated (refer to Chapter 15, Orthopedic Conditions).

Lower extremity angular alignment also changes over the course of normal growth and development. An infant who presents with a varus position of the lower extremities will gradually progress to a valgus position by 2.5 to 3 years of age and then to a relatively straight lower extremity position by early school age. Lower extremity angular alignment continues to gradually change over time until skeletal maturity, when girls exhibit a slightly valgus posture and boys a straight or varus position of the lower extremities.

The examination of gait is similar to examining an adult and can be performed through systematic clinical observation or with more objective measures, ranging from video analysis to an instrumented gait laboratory. There are several observational measures such as the Dynamic Gait Index[60,61] or the Observational Gait Scale that was modified from the Physician Rating Scale. These measures can be used clinically to assist with consistency among physical therapists and to document change over time. Many facilities often develop their own check-off gait observation lists that can be easily modified for use with a wide range of children. Whatever the scale or tool that is used for gait examination, the age of the child must be considered and knowledge of the characteristics of early walking incorporated into the exam.

The Berg Balance Scale (BBS) is thought to be the gold standard in functionally measuring balance and was designed to test elderly patients' balance and safety.[62] The Pediatric Balance Scale (PBS) was modified from the BBS and was initially designed for use with school-age children 5 to 15 years of age with mild or moderate balance impairments.[63] Further assessment has found that most children older than 6 years will obtain the maximum score, and, therefore, the PBS is most useful for children under the age of 6 years.[64] The TUG test[15] and the Timed Up and Down the Stairs test[65] may also be useful in the initial evaluation or as a screening tool to guide the examination.

A variety of assessment and evaluation tools are available to determine a child's developmental level or functional abilities. The child's mobility, functional skills, and gross motor abilities can often be obtained through observation and augmented through interview questions. Useful information can often be obtained by asking the parents to report on a typical day for their child. While talking with the parents, the physical therapist should be observing the child's posture, play, spontaneous movements, and activities with relevance to the child's posture, noted asymmetries, and difficulty with age-appropriate skills. The Academy of Pediatric

Physical Therapy of the American Physical Therapy Association (APTA) has developed a resource/fact sheet that lists a multitude of pediatric assessment tools.[66] Although this list is not exhaustive, it does categorize the assessment and evaluation tools reflecting the ICF model, complete with a reference list.

The Bayley Scales of Infant Development, the Bruininks–Oseretsky Test of Motor Proficiency Second Edition (BOTP-2), Canadian Occupational Measure of Performance (COPM), GMFM, Peabody Developmental Motor Scale 2nd Edition (PDMS-2), and PEDI, are all activity or functionally based tests. All have moderate to good reliability ($r \geq 0.50$), and most have established construct or concurrent validity. They can be used as discriminative tools if the focus is directed toward specific items within the test and can also serve the purpose of an initial evaluation or assessment and monitoring progress over time. Caution is warranted, however, because these tests are typically designed for specific age groups and populations and are thus not widely applicable to all children.

The Pediatric Quality of Life Inventory (PedsQLTM) is a quality of life measurement used with children aged 8 to 12 years old. This inventory tool has been shown to have test–retest reliability, sensitivity to changes in quality of life (QOL), and differences between healthy children and children with health concerns.[67] This inventory has been validated with children who have cancer, diabetes, rheumatoid arthritis, and orthopedic conditions.[68] The PedsQLTM has a child's version and a parent's version. The child version asks the child to rate his or her own quality of life in the past month in areas of health and activities, general feelings, getting along with others, and school performance. A five-point scale is utilized, which ranges from 0 = never a problem to 4 = almost always a problem. The items are reverse-scored (0 = 100, 4 = 0) so that the higher the total score, the better the quality of life. The parental version asks questions in the same categories but seeks the parent's perception of how they feel their child does in these same situations. Quality of life is important to consider when examining the effects of rehabilitation services on a child and correlating that change or influence with a meaningful change to the child's participation in meaningful activities.

Once all of the necessary examination information is obtained, an evaluation and diagnosis are made to facilitate the development of a plan of care.

Evaluation and Plan of Care

The physical therapist should review the examination findings with the parent, including any tests scores and their meaning such as age equivalency. A diagnosis is needed to receive payment in the outpatient setting and should be listed on the plan of care. The diagnosis can include the child's medical diagnosis but should definitely include a rehabilitation diagnosis that reflects the examination findings.

Part of any physical therapy examination could include information gained from diagnostic imaging either by report or direct observation of the image. The information gained from this type of test can aid in the selection and prescription of certain interventions and provide information on the patient's response, or lack thereof, to interventions provided. Information gleaned from radiology reports or imaging can also aid with child and family education and provide additional information on the child's condition and prognosis for functional recovery.

In the outpatient setting, the plan of care is developed in coordination with the parent. The parent and the child, if applicable, have identified their goals or concerns that they would like physical therapy to address. The physical therapist may need to guide the parent to goals that can realistically be accomplished within an episode of care. The frequency of services will be determined by goals identified and the effectiveness of the interventions to reach those goals. Parent input and participation is vital in this process. Some children and parents will be able to carry out specific exercises at home on a regular basis and will only need to attend outpatient sessions for updates to this program. Other parents may prefer to attend more frequent physical therapy sessions to ensure consistency of follow-through of work toward the goals.

The duration or episode of care to accomplish the goals and the criteria for discharge should be determined at the onset of physical therapy. If increased ankle joint dorsiflexion ROM to improve gait is a goal, the child may initially only need to attend physical therapy as frequently as the serial casts need to be changed. The frequency may increase as the ROM is obtained and the intervention shifts toward functional training. An increased frequency level may be needed if the child is initially using specialized equipment such as a body weight support device for gait training. Other children may benefit from services once a week with a parent who is able to follow through on a program several times a week at home. The Academy of Pediatric Physical Therapy of the APTA has published a fact sheet that guides the reader through decision making to determine the frequency of outpatient services for children with chronic conditions and any existing evidence to support those decisions.[69]

Some third-party payers will require that the plan of treatment be sent to them or the child's pediatrician/primary care physician for review and authorization for a specified number of physical therapy visits. These reviewers often request that scores from an objective measure or standardized test be included on the plan of treatment for measurement of functional change over time. Scores could include developmental ages or functional scores from standardized assessments or timed scores such as the Timed Up and Go or timed walk tests.

Intervention

Just as in the inpatient setting, the interventions will be determined by the goals on the plan of care, the expected outcomes, and should focus on improving the function of the child in their home and community setting. Intervention may also be focused on training of the parent or caregiver if a change in status such as growth or weight gain has affected how they accomplish daily living skills and transfers in the home. The Guide to Physical Therapist Practice describes the interventions that will be utilized to improve the child's functional status.[22] The key points that have a different emphasis in the outpatient setting are emphasized in what follows.

Coordination and communication differ significantly in an outpatient setting from those in an inpatient facility. The multidisciplinary team that may be involved in the child's care is no longer under one roof, and regular meetings between team members rarely occur in this setting. The physical therapist may need to request information from other medical professionals to learn the child's full medical status and plan. An organized intentional effort will be required to communicate the physical therapy examination findings, plan of treatment, and progress of the child to other medical professionals participating in the care of the child. The physical therapist may need to refer the child for other services or consult with equipment vendors, orthotists, or other providers to further define and augment the plan of care. Coordination of additional services and consultations requires time as well as effective communication skills. It is important to remember in this setting that HIPAA regulations must be adhered to when communicating patient information with other professionals or organizations, including sharing information with the school-based physical therapist.

In the inpatient setting, instruction often occurs initially with other members of the interdisciplinary team to ensure carryover of the treatment plan. In the outpatient setting, instruction is focused on the child and the parent. The physical therapist must communicate with the parents to determine what is their current level of understanding of their child's diagnosis and care, how the parent best learns, and what are the barriers to carrying out a home exercise program. A study by Rone-Adams and colleagues concluded that parental stress is one factor that interferes with compliance of home programs.[70] Client instruction focuses on activities for carryover at home that can be incorporated into the child's day or trials of functional skills practiced during the outpatient visit. Feedback from the parent at subsequent therapy visits will help to determine the compliance and the effectiveness of training and carryover of new skills in the home setting (Display 5.11).

Most interventions that are utilized in other settings can also be incorporated into the outpatient therapy session. Many children attending outpatient physical therapy will at some point require an adaptive or assistive device, a topic that is presented later in this section.

Therapeutic exercise and strengthening have long been used by physical therapists for orthopedic conditions. Strengthening and resistive exercise programs can yield positive improvements in impairments and function for children with neurologic diagnoses. Children with cerebral palsy exhibit significant weakness in their muscles compared to their able-bodied peers while children who have sustained a traumatic brain injury have lost muscle strength owing to inactivity and possible loss of refined movements. Strengthening programs, as well as increased activity levels, will benefit children of all ages with a neurologic diagnosis.

Flexibility exercises and endurance conditioning programs may also be appropriate for many children with a wide range of diagnoses, including neurologic conditions, musculoskeletal injuries, rheumatology conditions, and obesity, as well as those children recovering from a transplant procedure or oncologic medical treatment. The physical therapist will need to design a program based on the child's age, present level of conditioning, and resources available.

Functional training will be determined by the goals developed in the plan of care with the parent or caregiver. Functional training typically involves transfer training, mobility training, or training in the use of a new adaptive or assistive device to promote increased independence for the child. Specific conditioning or training programs such as treadmill training with and without body weight support systems and constraint-induced movement therapy are examples of interventions that have demonstrated positive outcomes for young children and adolescents of varying diagnoses. This evidence of varying interventions for children with cerebral palsy has been synthesized by authors and formulated in a report that highlights effective interventions as well as ineffective interventions that should not be utilized.[71,72]

The physical therapist working in the outpatient setting must be frequently communicating with the parent to determine whether adaptive devices would ease the burden of care in the home or facilitate functional independence in the child. Progress as well as growth may necessitate a change in either an orthotic or assistive device. The physical therapist in the outpatient setting is frequently relied on to provide significant input in determining the type of orthotic device that is most beneficial for the child. Progression in the use of assistive devices is often determined by the physical therapist. Equally important is an understanding of a child's ambulation potential and the ability to identify an alternative method of mobility when appropriate.

For ease in ordering assistive and adaptive devices, an effective working relationship should be established with local vendors for DME. Most third-party payers now require that the child have trialed a device prior to ordering and that several styles of the same device are trialed. For example, if the

---

DISPLAY 5.11 **Point to Remember—Home Exercise Programs**

Home exercise programs should focus on activities that can be incorporated into the child's routines and activities of the day.

physical therapist is helping the family order a bath seat for home, the child should be trialed in several styles of seats prior to submission of the final order. The physical therapist may be requested to write a letter of medical necessity (LMN) to explain the device, how it benefits the child, how it will increase function or ease of burden of care at home, and what other devices were trialed that were not optimal for the child. Information that supports the use of the particular device should be added to the letter and functional levels or safety concerns that would justify the need for the device are always beneficial. (An example of an LMN can be found in Appendix C.)

The vast array of wheelchairs, both power and manual, and especially the options to safely access and drive a power wheelchair, make it almost impossible to remain competent in all of the options available to a child and family. For this reason, not all outpatient centers are able to prescribe sophisticated power wheelchairs, seating systems, and driving array options for children. Specially trained personnel who work in a multidisciplinary team are needed for these unique and expensive equipment options. The team usually consists of a physician, physical therapist, occupational therapist, rehabilitation engineer, and, possibly, a case manager or social worker. The Rehabilitation Engineering and Assistive Technology Society of North America (RESNA) offers credentialing examinations both for providers to evaluate and train a patient in the use of equipment and for vendors who sell and service assistive technology devices.

The outpatient physical therapist plays an important role in instructing both the child and the family members in the safe use of assistive devices. When the family receives the device, the physical therapist needs to ensure that the child and family are able to competently and safely use the device. If the device is delivered to the home and the physical therapist cannot make a home visit, arrangements should be made so a representative from the vendor delivering the equipment or a home health physical therapist can instruct the family in the safe and proper use of the device.

Outcomes

Expected outcomes are based on the successful achievement of the goals established at the outset of the episode of care. Children who have sustained a musculoskeletal injury can often be expected to return to their baseline level of function in a short time. Defining the expected outcomes for children with neurologic diagnoses can be more difficult but can help assist with defining the duration of the episode of care. The Gross Motor Function Classification System provides not only a classification for children with cerebral palsy but also an evidence-based prognosis regarding the child's expected gross motor progress.[73] A prognosis for expected outcomes will assist the physical therapist and family with planning the intervention strategy and monitoring the child's progress over time.

Summary

The physical therapist is an integral part of the rehabilitation team serving a child in either the inpatient or the outpatient setting. Many pediatric rehabilitation hospitals were started more than 100 years ago to care for children with impairments as a result of polio or other congenital orthopedic conditions. Today, facilities provide comprehensive multi- or interdisciplinary services aimed at restoring of function for children and adolescents who have congenital conditions, sustained injuries, have illnesses, or have undergone surgery. In addition, today's inpatient and outpatient facilities are influenced by many federal and state laws and regulations as well as external accrediting agencies such as CARF to protect the patient's rights and to promote quality and patient satisfaction. Major differences between inpatient and outpatient service provision are seen in the frequency and type of services available and the health and availability of the patient.

The role of the physical therapist and the communication needed may change depending on the setting, but the physical therapist is a key member to help identify the activity limitations of the child. The parents also serve as vital members of the team, and the physical therapist must communicate with the parent to develop appropriate goals, establish an appropriate plan of care, and efficiently provide interventions that will optimize the child's functional skills and ease the parent's burden of care. The progress that is often accomplished by a child in the rehabilitation or outpatient setting can be very rewarding for all members involved and reinforces the successful teamwork and communication that fostered the child's progress toward functional independence.

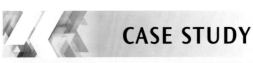

CASE STUDY

JOANN. IN-PATIENT. STATUS POST POSTERIOR SPINAL FUSION

Medical Diagnosis

Scoliosis, s/p Posterior Spinal Fusion (PSF) with bone graft.

Joann is a 14-year-old female who has a medical diagnosis of a 40-degree right thoracic adolescent idiopathic scoliosis (AIS). The scoliosis was corrected surgically through the placement of Herrington rods and spinal fusion using a bone graft from the right iliac crest. Currently, Joann is s/p surgery day 1. She is in pain, which limits her motion, and is lethargic secondary to anesthesia (Impairments). She is unable to perform bed mobility without assistance, transition to sit independently, or ambulate independently secondary to pain and decreased endurance (Functional limitations). Her limitations impair her from exploring her environment and, at present, from going back to school (Disability).

Systems Review

Caridovascular/pulmonary: From medical record: HCT 35%; HgB 15 g per dL. Body temp is 37°C. Patient is on 2 L of oxygen via nasal cannula. From monitor: BP 120/80; RR 12; pulse 84 bpm regular. Pulse Ox. is 97%.

Neuromuscular: Gross sensation to touch intact in the lower extremities. Patient is on IV Morphine, PCA.

Musculoskeletal: Gross ROM of the upper extremities (UEs) is within functional limits (WFL). Gross lower extremity (LE) active movement is limited secondary to pain. Supine posture is unremarkable. Patient is 5 feet 4 inches tall and weighs 135 lb.

Communication: Not impaired.

Integumentary: No prior surgery to low back reported.

Test and Measures

Patient is alert and oriented ×3. Her mother is present. Parent reports that Joann lives at home with both parents and two younger siblings. Parent reports that there are five steps to get into the house and another 12 to go to the second floor, which contains Joann's bedroom and the only bathroom in the house. There is a handrail on the right. The school that Joann attends is a single-story building.

Joann reports no episodes of urination. She has not been out of bed since surgery. She has not taken any food by mouth since before surgery. She complains of feeling light-headed and nauseous but has no episodes of emesis. Joann rates pain 7/10 in her back and right hip, in the area of the iliac crest. Sensation to light touch and sharp/dull discrimination is intact along the dermatomes L3 to S1.

Leg lengths appear equal. In supine, the legs are externally rotated equally.

No edema noted in the lower extremities.

Capillary refill time is less than 3 seconds in both feet.

Bilateral UE strength is 5/5 in upper trapezius, middle deltoids, biceps, triceps muscles. Grip strength is symmetrical bilateral with appropriate co-contraction of the muscles that cross the wrist joint noted. Bilateral LE ankle dorsiflexion and plantar flexion strength are 5/5. Other MMT deferred secondary to the patient's report of pain with hip and knee movements when supine.

Limitations in trunk range of motion secondary to pain and postsurgical precautions. Pain in back increases to 9/10 when transitioning supine to sit. Pain decreases when in stance. Pain is localized to the back and right hip with no radiation reported.

Impairments include:

Pain

Impaired joint mobility

Decreased range of motion

Decreased endurance

Limited independence in ADL

Diagnostic pattern: Impaired Joint Mobility, Motor Function, Muscle Performance, and Range of Motion Associated with Bony and Soft Tissue Surgery.

Goals

1. Patient will transition supine to sit with minimal assistance to allow her to function in her home with the assistance of one parent.

2. Patient will transition to sit to stand independently to allow her to rise from the toilet.

3. Patient will ambulate 200' over level surfaces within 1 day in order to allow her to access rooms in her home.

4. Patient will ascend and descend 15 steps with the assistance of a handrail in order to access the second floor of her house.

5. Caregivers will be able to verbalize precautions to excessive spine movements during the healing phase of surgery in order to decrease the risk of injury to the surgical site.

Physical Therapy Interventions include:

Patient Education

1. Education regarding the effects of morphine on feeling light-headed, dizzy, and nauseous.

2. Deep breathing and pursed lipped breathing exercises will aid in pain management.

3. The importance of deep breathing for pain management and walking to aid in gastrointestinal mobility. When moving do not hold your breath.

4. Reinforced logrolling and use of upper extremities to move from a side-lying position to sit with proper breathing. Movement will initially cause some discomfort, but once up and walking she should feel better, and the pain will subside.

Aerobic capacity/endurance; body mechanics; muscle performance; gait:

Elevate the head of the bed (HOB) to 60 degrees for 10 minutes to allow for her to adjust to the upright position.

Have her move to the edge of the bed (EOB), then placing her feet on the floor.

Assist her to transition sit to stand. Once standing, Joann should keep her eyes open and focus on breathing.

Begin ambulation with moderate assist (2 points of contact on the patient). Measure distance in feet, noting standard tiles on hospital floors are typically one foot long.

Return to the room and sit upright in the chair for at least 1 hour.

Provide additional pillows to the back of the chair to allow for a more upright posture.

Caregiver Education

Instruct family or nurse in proper guarding or assistance of Joann to transition her sit to stand or sit to supine safely.

Treatment

Second visit in the afternoon, repeat morning activities. Increase endurance and add step-ups or stair climbing.

Outcome

Patient has met 4/4 (100%) of the goals stated in her initial evaluation.

Parents (caregivers) were able to verbalize precautions to excessive movement of the spine.

Patient is safe to discharge to home with her parents. The physician will decide when the child can return to school.

Reflective Questions

1. Often, patients who undergo spinal stabilization via autographs have pain at the donor site post surgery. Joann had significant pain at the donor site. How do you think this may affect her rehabilitation?

2. How would the interventions differ if the scoliosis was caused by a nonmalignant tumor or an asymmetry in muscle tone?

3. If Joann remains on IV pain meds, ascending and descending 12 stairs would be limited secondary to the IV pole and pump. What alternate therapeutic exercises can be incorporated into her program to promote stair negotiation?

REFERENCES

1. Sultz H, Young K. *Health Care USA. Understanding Its Organization and Delivery.* 4th ed. Jones and Bartlett; 2004.
2. The US Department of Health and Human Services, Programs and Services. HHS.gov/programs
3. Available at Congress.gov Read H.R. 4449 Self Determination Act of 1990.
4. US Department of Health and Human Services, HIPAA for Professionals. HHS.gov/hipaa for professionals.
5. US Centers for Medicare and Medicaid "Read the Affordable Care Act". Healthcare.gov/glossary/affordable-care-act
6. Available at Congress.gov Read The Assistive Technology Act of 2004.
7. US Department of Labor, Americans with Disabilities Act. dol.gov/general/topic/disability/ada
8. US Department of Health and Human Services and Administration for Children and Families, Child Abuse and Prevention Treatment Act. acf.hhs.gov/cb/focus-areas/child-abuse-neglect
9. Centers for Disease Control and Prevention, Standard Precautions for All Patient Care. Accessed February 11, 2021. https://www.cdc.gov/infectioncontrol/basics/standard-precautions.html
10. The Joint Commission Standards and Performance Improvement. www.jointcommission.org
11. Commission on Accreditation of Rehabilitation Facilities Standards. www.carf.org
12. Uniform Data System for Medical Rehabilitation, WeeFIM II. udsmr.org/products-pediatric-rehab
13. Donahoe B, Turner D, Worrell T. The use of functional reach as a measurement of balance in boys and girls without disabilities ages 5 to 15 years. *Pediatr Phys Ther.* 1994;6:189-193.
14. Volkman KG, Stergiou N, Stuberg W, et al. Factors affecting functional reach scores in youth with typical development. *Pediatr Phys Ther.* 2009;21(1):38-44.
15. Williams E, Carroll S, Reddihough D, et al. Investigation of the timed "Up and Go" test in children. *Dev Med Child Neurol.* 2005;47:518-524.
16. Manworren R, Stinson J. Pediatric pain measurement, assessment and evaluation. *Semin Pediatr Neurol.* 2016;(3):189-200.
17. Michaleff ZA, Kamper SJ, Stinson J, et al. Measuring musculoskeletal pain in infants, children, and adolescents. *J Ortho Sports Phys Ther.* 2017;47(10):712-730.
18. Wong D, Hockenberry-Eaton M, Wilson D, et al. In: Whaley L, Wong DL, eds. *Nursing Care of Infants and Children.* 2nd ed. CV Mosby, Inc.; 1991.
19. Beyer J, Aradine C. Content validity of an instrument to measure young children's perception of the intensity of their pain. *J Pediatr Nurs.* 1986;1(6):386-395.
20. Bieri D, Reeve RA, Champion DG, et al. The faces pain scale for the self-assessment of the severity of pain experienced by children: development, initial validation, and preliminary investigation for ratio scale properties. *Pain.* 1990;41:139-150.
21. McGrath P, Seifert CE, Speechley KN, et al. A new analog scale for assessing children's pain: an initial validation study. *Pain.* 1996;64:435-443.
22. *Guide to Physical Therapist Practice 3.0.* American Physical Therapy Association; 2014. http://guidetoptpractice.apta.org/
23. Puthucheary ZA, Rawal J, McPhail M, et al. Acute skeletal muscle wasting in critical illness. *JAMA.* 2013;310:1591-1600.
24. Pollack MM, Holubkov R, Funai T, et al. Pediatric intensive care outcomes: development of new morbidities during pediatric critical care. *Pediatr Crit Care Med.* 2014;15(9):821-827.
25. Kudchadkar SR, Ajohani OA, Punjabi NM. Sleep of critically ill children in the pediatric intensive care unit: a systematic review. *Sleep Med Rev.* 2014;18:103-110.
26. Manning JC, Pintu NP, Rennick JE, et al. Conceptualizing post intensive care syndrome in children: the PICSp framework. *Pediatr Crit Care Med.* 2018;19:290-300.
27. Cuello-Garcia CA, Mai SHC, Simpson R, et al. Early mobilization in critically ill children: a systematic review. *J Pediatr.* 2018;203:25-33.
28. Wieczorek B, Ascenzi J, Kim Y, et al. PICU Up!: impact of a quality improvement intervention to promote early mobilization in critically ill children. *Pediatr Crit Care Med.* 2016;17:e559-e566.
29. Fink EL, Beers SR, Houtrow AJ, et al. Early protocolization versus usual care rehabilitation for pediatric neurocritical care patients: a randomized controlled trial. *Pediatr Crit Care Med.* 2019;20:540-550.
30. US Department of Health and Human Services. CMS Inpatient Rehabilitation Facility Prospective Payment System; Medicare Learning Network. March 2020. https://www.cms.gov/Outreach-and-Education/Medicare-Learning-Network-MLN/MLNProducts/Downloads/InpatRehabPaymtfctsht09-508.pdf
31. Teasdale G, Bennett B. Assessment of coma and impaired consciousness: a practical scale. *Lancet.* 1974;2:81-84.
32. Simpson D, Cockington R, Hanieh A, et al. Head injuries in infants and young children: the value of the pediatric coma scale. Review of the literature and report on a study. *Childs Nerv Syst.* 1991;7:183-190.
33. Hagen C, Makmus D, Durham P, et al. Levels of cognitive functioning. In: *Rehabilitation of the Head-Injured Adult: Comprehensive Physical Management.* Professional Staff of Rancho Los Amigos Hospital; 1979:87-90.
34. Ewing-Cobbs L, Levin H, Fletcher J, et al. The children's orientation and amnesia test: relationship to severity of acute head injury and to recovery of memory. *Neurosurgery.* 1990;27:683-691.
35. Ashworth B. Preliminary trial of carisoprodol in multiple sclerosis. *Practitioner.* 1964;192:540-542.
36. Bohannon R, Smith M. Interrater reliability of a modified Ashworth scale of muscle spasticity. *Phys Ther.* 1987;67:206-207.
37. Hass B, Bergstrom E, Jamous A, et al. The inter-rater reliability of the original and of the modified Ashworth scale for the assessment of spasticity in patients with spinal cord injury. *Spinal Cord.* 1996;34:560-564.
38. Clopton N, Dutton J, Featherston T, et al. Interrater and intrarater reliability of the modified Ashworth scale in children with hypertonia. *Pediatr Phys Ther.* 2005;17:268-274.
39. Boyd R, Graham H. Objective measurement of clinical findings in the use of botulinum toxin type A for the management of children with cerebral palsy. *Eur J Neurol.* 1999;6:S23-S25.
40. Yam WKL, Leung MSW. Interrater reliability of modified Ashworth scale and modified Tardieu scale in children with cerebral palsy. *J Child Neurol.* 2006;21(12):1031-1035.
41. Alhusaini AA, Dean CM, Crosbie J, et al. Evaluation of spasticity in children with cerebral palsy using Ashworth and Tardieu scales compared with laboratory measures. *J Child Neurol.* 2010;25(10):1242-1247.
42. Burke R, Fahn S, Marsden C, et al. Validity and reliability of a rating scale for the primary torsion dystonias. *Neurology.* 1985;35:73-77.
43. Barry M, VanSwearingen J, Albright A. Reliability and responsiveness of the Barry-Albright dystonia scale. *Dev Med Child Neurol.* 1999;41:404-411.

44. Haley S, Coster W, Ludlow L, et al. *Pediatric Evaluation of Disability Index: Development, Standardization and Administration Manual.* New England Medical Center Hospitals; 1992.

45. Nichols D, Case-Smith J. Reliability and validity of the pediatric evaluation of disability inventory. *Pediatr Phys Ther.* 1996;8:15-24.

46. Tokcan G, Haley S, Gill-Body K, et al. Item-specific functional recovery in children and youth with acquired brain injury. *Pediatr Phys Ther.* 2003;15:16-22.

47. Dumas HM, Fragala-Pinkham MA. Concurrent validity and reliability of the pediatric evaluation of disability inventory-computer adaptive test mobility domain. *Pediatr Phys Ther.* 2012;24(2):171-176.

48. Dumas HM, Fragala-Pinkham MA, Rosen EL, et al. Pediatric evaluation of disability inventory computer adaptive test (PEDI-CAT) and Alberta infant motor scale (AIMS): validity and responsiveness. *Phys Ther.* 2015;95(11):1559-1568.

49. Thompson SV, Cech DJ, Cahill SM, et al. Linking the pediatric evaluation of disability inventory-computer adaptive test (PEDI_CAT) to the international classification of function. *Pediatr Phys Ther.* 2018;30(2):113-118.

50. Ottenbacher K, Msall M, Lyon N, et al. Interrater agreement and stability of the functional independence measure for children (WeeFIM): use in children with developmental disabilities. *Arch Phys Med Rehabil.* 1997;78:1309-1315.

51. Thomas-Stonell N, Johnson P, Rumney P, et al. An evaluation of the responsiveness of a comprehensive set of outcome measures for children and adolescents with traumatic brain injuries. *Pediatr Rehabil.* 2006;9:14-23.

52. Kim CT, Greenberg J, Kim H. Pediatric rehabilitation: trends in length of stay. *J Pediatr Rehabil Med.* 2013;6(1):11-17.

53. Dumas H, Haley S, Ludlow L, et al. Recovery of ambulation during inpatient rehabilitation: physical therapist prognosis for children and adolescents with traumatic brain injury. *Phys Ther.* 2004;84:232-242.

54. Staheli L. *Practice of Pediatric Orthopedics.* Global Health; 2008.

55. Effgen S, Brown D. Long-term stability of hand-held dynamometric measurements in children who have myelomeningocele. *Phys Ther.* 1992;72:458-465.

56. Willemse L, Brehm MA, Scholtes VA, et al. Reliability of isometric lower-extremity strength measurements in children with cerebral palsy: implications for measurement design. *Phys Ther.* 2013;93(70):935-941.

57. Mulder-Brouwer AN, Rameckers EAA, Bastiaenen CH, et al. Lower extremity handheld dynamometry strength measurement in children with cerebral palsy. *Pediatr Phys Ther.* 2016;28(2):136-153.

58. Gajdosik C. Ability of very young children to produce reliable isometric force measurements. *Pediatr Phys Ther.* 2005;17:251-257.

59. Staheli LT, Corbett M, Wyss C, et al. Lower-extremity rotational problems in children. *J Bone Joint Surg.* 1985;67A:39-47.

60. Marchett GF, Whitney SL. Construction and validation of the 4-item dynamic gait index. *Phys Ther.* 2006;86(12):1651-1660.

61. Lubetzky-Vilnai A, Jinikowic T, McCoy SW. Investigation of dynamic gait index in children: a pilot study. *Pediatr Phys Ther.* 2011;23(3):268-273.

62. Kembhavi G, Darrah J, Magill-Evans J, et al. Using the berg balance scale to distinguish balance abilities in children with cerebral palsy. *Pediatr Phys Ther.* 2002;14:92-99.

63. Franjoine MR, Gunther JS, Taylor MJ. Pediatric balance scale: a modified version of the berg balance scale for the school-age child with mild to moderate motor impairment. *Pediatr Phys Ther.* 2003;15(2):114-128.

64. Franjoine MR, Darr N, Held SL, et al. The performance of children typically developing on the pediatric balance Scale. *Pediatr Phys Ther.* 2010;22(4):350-359.

65. Zaino CA, Marchese VG, Westcott SL. Timed up and down the stairs test: preliminary reliability and validity of a new measure of functional mobility. *Pediatr Phys Ther.* 2004;16(2):90-98.

66. American Physical Therapy Association, Academy of Pediatric Physical Therapy. Resource/fact sheet: list of assessment tools categorized by ICF model. 2013. www.pediatricapta.org

67. Varni J, Burwinkle T, Seid M, et al. The Peds-QL as a pediatric population health measure: feasibility, reliability, and validity. *Ambul Pediatr.* 2003;3:329-341.

68. Varni J, Seid M, Kurtin P. PedsQL 4.0: reliability and validity of the pediatric quality of life inventory version 4.0 generic core scales in healthy and patient populations. *Med Care.* 2001;39:800-812.

69. American Physical Therapy Association, Academy of Pediatric Physical Therapy. Resource/fact sheet: intensity of service in an outpatient setting for children with chronic conditions. 2012. www.pediatricapta.org

70. Rone-Adams S, Stern D, Walker V. Stress and compliance with a home exercise program among caregivers of children with disabilities. *Pediatr Phys Ther.* 2004;16:140-148.

71. Novak I, McIntyre S, Morgan C. A systematic review of interventions for children with cerebral palsy: state of the evidence. *Dev Med Child Neurol.* 2013;55:885-910.

72. Novak I, Morgan C, Fahey M, et al. State of the evidence traffic light 2019: systematic review of interventions for preventing and treating children with cerebral palsy. *Curr Neurol Neurosci Rep.* 2020;20(2):1-21.

73. Rosenbaum PL, Walter SD, Hanna SE, et al. Prognosis for gross motor function in cerebral palsy, creation of motor development curves. *JAMA.* 2004;288:1357-1363.

Orthotic Devices

Orthotic devices are listed by body parts. A brief description of the orthotics common application in the pediatric population is provided.

A. Orthotic devices for the neck and trunk:

Cervical Collars: Use to support or immobilize the cervical spine. Often used after trauma, until the cervical spine has been radiographically examined and cleared of any injury or malalignment.

Thoracolumbosacral Orthosis (TLSO): Often used in the management of spinal scoliosis or when immobilization of the spine is warranted. A one-piece or two-piece custom molded TLSO provides support to the trunk. A bi-valved (or two-piece) TLSO is easier to don.

Abdominal Binder: Used to support the abdominal contents. May be used status post kidney transplant, when the new kidney is placed in the lower anterior abdomen for ongoing protection, or with placement of pharmaceutical pumps.

B. Orthotic devices for the lower extremity

Hip Abduction Wedge or Pillow: Maintains the hip joint in abduction.

Standing, Walking, and Sitting Hip Orthosis (SWASH brace): Assist in maintaining the hip joint in alignment during these activities.

Reciprocating Gait Orthosis (RGO): HKAFO with a mechanical assist for reciprocal lower extremity movements. Often used with children who have spina bifida or spinal cord injuries to make ambulation more energy efficient.

Knee–Ankle–Foot Orthosis (KAFO): Use for support of the knee, ankle, and foot during standing or ambulation. Quadricep muscle strength and knee joint stability are major factors in determining the need for a KAFO versus an AFO. Typically include a hinge at the knee joint that may be locked for standing activities and unlocked for sitting.

Knee Immobilizers: Immobilize the knee joint, typically in extension, for medical reasons or if the quadricep muscle is too weak to hold the knee in extension. Act as a temporary device if recovery is expected quickly or while waiting for the permanent orthotic device.

Ankle–Foot Orthoses (AFO): Commonly used to maintain proper alignment of the ankle and foot during weight-bearing activities. The upright aspect can influence knee control or positioning during ambulation. The ankle joint can either be fixed or allow for a certain degree of plantar and/or dorsiflexion of the talocrural joint. AFOs are also used for muscle tone reduction in the lower extremity.

Foot Orthoses (FO): Used to provide support to the subtalar joint, especially with inversion and eversion, in addition to the midfoot articulation, with supination and pronation of the foot. Provides support to the arches of the foot. Can also be used for muscle tone reduction.

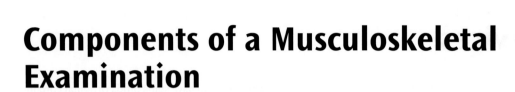

Components of a Musculoskeletal Examination

Joint or Body Segment	Normal Findings	Interventions for Abnormal Findings
Head	- Fontanels—closed by 18 months - Head Circumference—refer to head circumference charts - Symmetry of Cranium	- If closed early, refer to MD - Refer to MD if large head circumference for age compared with weight and height, if cranium asymmetric, child irritable; may indicate early closure of cranial sutures. - Asymmetry or plagiocephaly—could be due to head preference to one side or torticollis. Positioning to encourage head symmetry; may require cranial band for severe cases.
Neck	Symmetrical ROM and position	- If asymmetric in infants look for torticollis, palpate muscle tightness. - If asymmetric in preschool and school-age child, check for other signs of neuro. Involvement such as falling, ataxia, headache—refer immediately to MD; may be early symptoms of posterior fossa tumor. - If asymmetric in an older child or adolescent, is there a mechanism of injury?
Trunk	- Trunk Symmetry (scoliosis screen) - A/P curvature of the spine—not present in infants. Cervical and lumbar lordosis develops as a child gains head control and prone skills. - Symmetrical excursion during breathing with minimal use of accessory muscles	- Asymmetric positioning—check for scoliosis Scoliosis secondary to asymmetric muscle pull with neurologic diagnosis—consider positioning, seating system, etc. Idiopathic scoliosis—refer to MD Kyphosis—positioning to increase trunk extension
Shoulder	Full ROM present at birth except shoulder abduction limited to 130 degrees. Actively moves UE's from birth with movements and reaching becoming more refined during first year. Symmetry of landmarks such as nipple line, scapula, and muscle bulk.	- Full shoulder abduction ROM present by 3 months. - Lack of active movement or symmetrical movement may be early signs of neurologic disorder. - Holds UE in shoulder extension with IR and minimal active movement at shoulder, elbow, and/or wrist. May indicate brachial plexus injury. - Congenital elevation of scapula indicative of Sprengel deformity. Associated with other musculoskeletal anomalies; requires orthopedic workup. - Asymmetric muscle bulk may indicate absence or hypoplasia of muscles such as Poland syndrome or absence of the pectoralis major muscle. - Scapular winging-WB and NWB. Indicative of weakness. If asymmetric and accompanied by shoulder retraction, may be an early sign of neurologic involvement. Intervention focuses on achieving full scapular mobility and increasing stability of surrounding muscles. - Pain or lack of active movement at the shoulder in the school age or adolescent requires full musculoskeletal assessment of the shoulder.

Joint or Body Segment	Normal Findings	Interventions for Abnormal Findings
Elbow and forearm	Newborn: Flexion contracture 25–30 degrees Normal elbow motion and alignment throughout childhood and adolescence.	- Full elbow extension present by 3–6 months. - Limited forearm supination and prominent radial head indicate radial head dislocation. May be congenital or result of trauma.
Wrist and hand	Full ROM present at birth. 2–3 months: reaches and grasps for toys, brings hands to mouth. Raking grasp present 6–8 months Refined pincer grasp present by 12 months. Handedness not apparent until 4–5 years of age.	Child should not show strong preference for one hand before age 4 years.
Hip and femur	Newborn: Hip flexion contracture 30–50 degrees Hip abduction and ER posture Hip IR/ER: 35–90/50–90 degrees* Femoral anteversion 40–60 degrees Femoral antetorsion 35–40 degrees Lateral bowing of femur *Lateral rotation is greater than medial at birth, but exact numbers are variable. Toddler (1–2-year-old): Hip flexion contracture 10–20 degrees at 1 year of age, reduces to <5 degrees by 2 years and resolves by 3 years of age. Hip IR/ER: lateral rotation decreases and internal rotation increases from birth values but slightly greater ratio of ER to IR. By 3 years of age, IR is slightly greater than ER. Femoral anteversion decreases significantly from birth to 2 years. School-age: Hip IR/ER ratio: IR slightly > ER. Femoral antetorsion: Near 20–25 degrees by 4 years and <20 degrees by age 5 years. Adolescent: Hip IR/ER ratio: Ratio near equal in 14-year-olds, then begin trend of ER slightly > IR. Femoral anteversion: Adult values of 5–16 degrees by 16 years of age. Femoral antetorsion: By 16 years approaches adult values of 5–16 degrees.	- Hip flexion contracture decreases to 10–20 degrees by 1 year and 0–5 degrees by 3 years of age. - Asymmetric hip abduction ROM: look for developmental dysplasia of the hip (DDH). Barlow and Ortolani tests used 0–2 months. Asymmetric thigh and gluteal folds, asymmetric hip ROM and positive Galeazzi sign (femoral shortening with hip flexed) in children older than 2 months. Refer to the orthopedist. - Decreased spontaneous or active movement of the hip may be indicative of synovitis or osteomyelitis. - Onset of limp in 4–10-year-olds may indicate Legg–Calve–Perthes disease. PT exam findings include limited hip IR and abduction on the affected side without history of trauma, limp, Trendelenburg sign may be present; refer to orthopedist. - Onset of limp or pain in knee or groin in young adolescent may indicate slipped capital epiphysis (SCFE). PT exam findings of minimal hip IR, leg held in ER and slight abduction may be consistent with SCFE.
Knee and tibia	Newborn: Knee Flexion contracture 20–30 degrees Tibial varum 15 degrees Lateral tibial torsion 0–5 degrees, gradual increase through childhood. Toddler (1–2-year-old): Knee flexion contracture resolved Tibial varum <5 degrees Lateral tibial torsion near 5 degrees Midchildhood to Adult: Tibial varum 0–2 degrees Mean of 22–25 degrees lateral tibial torsion with a range of 0–40 degrees.	- Knee flexion contracture may persist or develop with abnormal muscle pull or development as seen with cerebral palsy or myelomeningocele. - Excessive tibial varum with severe bowing of proximal portion of tibia may indicate Blount disease. Tibial varum of Blount disease progresses with time; physiologic tibiofemoral angle improves with time. - Complaint of in-toeing: Age related, reference rotational profile. Not correctable by type of shoes worn, shoe inserts, or cable twisters. - Medial tibial torsion is indicative of abnormal or imbalanced muscle pull.
Leg (tibiofemoral angle)	Newborn: Genu varum 15–17 degrees 18 months: Nearly straight 2–4 years: gradually progresses to genu valgum with peak of 15 degrees near 3.5 years. 7 years: Adult values of 5–8 degrees genu valgum (females slightly greater valgum than males).	- Natural course of genu varum as an infant, progressing to genu valgum as a preschool-age child with decrease to mild genu valgum by 7 years of age. Natural course includes broad ranges of normal. If excessive or asymmetric may require surgical correction through stapling or osteotomy.

Joint or Body Segment	Normal Findings	Interventions for Abnormal Findings
Foot and ankle	Newborn: Ankle dorsiflexion 40–80 degrees Ankle plantarflexion neutral to 20 degrees Ankle dorsiflexion decreases to 45–50 degrees by 3 months. Non-weight bearing: calcaneal varus of 10 degrees and forefoot varus of 5–10 degrees. In weight-bearing position, calcaneal valgus of 5–10 degrees with no apparent longitudinal arch. Toddler (1–2 years): Ankle dorsiflexion 0–45–50 degrees Ankle plantarflexion 0–20–30 degrees Forefoot varus neutral Stands in calcaneal valgus posture—pronation normal aspect of development. Longitudinal arch may be present in sitting but not in stance. Gait—developing heel strike. 4–7 years of age: Adult gait pattern established. Longitudinal arch present by age 4 years in stance. Stance in 0–2 degrees calcaneal varus.	- Multiple congenital foot anomalies and deformations are possible. May be due to intrauterine positioning or failure of development of the foot. Examples include clubfoot deformity (talipes equinovarus) and metatarsus adductus. Less severe forms respond to serial casting; severe forms of equinovarus will require surgical correction. Positional deformations of the foot often associated with DDH. - Toe walking—may be idiopathic or neurologic in origin. Check for spasticity of plantar flexors or ankle clonus; check ankle dorsiflexion ROM needed for normal gait pattern. Limited ankle dorsiflexion may respond to serial casting and/or use of orthotic devices. - In-toeing may result from multiple causes. Shoe inserts and orthopedic shoes will not correct in-toeing gait.

A/P, anterior/posterior; ER, external rotation; IR, internal rotation; MD, medical doctor; NWB, non-weight bearing; WR, weight bearing.

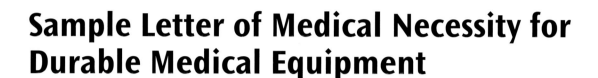

Sample Letter of Medical Necessity for Durable Medical Equipment

Patient's Name: Caleb
Date of Birth:
Date of Assessments:
Diagnosis and ICD 10 Code(s):
Name of Physical Therapist:
Name of Authorizing Physician:
Phone Number:

Equipment Prescribed: Quickie 7r Ultralightweight wheelchair with depth and height adjustable backrest, fold down back, tension adjustable backrest, seat cushion, 4-inch caster aluminum front wheels, marathon plus rear wheels, angle-adjustable flip back footrest with leg straps, padded push away armrests, positioning belt and standard side guards

Medical history

Caleb is an intelligent and active 12-year-old boy with a medical diagnosis of lipomeningocele. He has undergone multiple tethered cord releases, most recently in October 2017. Caleb wears KAFOs and ambulates independently for short distances of 15 to 20 feet with frequent use of furniture or walls to maintain his balance. He currently utilizes a manual wheelchair for all long-distance mobility outside the home. He independently and safely maneuvers his manual wheelchair, including on grades and around corners. He has outgrown his current chair, and it is becoming unsafe because of his height and the short seat depth. He transfers in and out of his wheelchair independently.

Caleb sits independently and exhibits good trunk control.

Caleb requires an ultralightweight manual wheelchair for independent mobility within his community as well as his own home. An ultralightweight wheelchair will allow him to be independently mobile at a level at which he can keep up with his siblings and peers in his home as well as the community setting. Caleb is active in his church youth organization and attends many events necessitating him to interact with his peers. He also participates in adaptive sports such as Miracle League baseball and various other organized activities within his community.

Histories

Additional History: Caleb is followed in the spina bifida clinic at _____. He has had multiple tethered cord releases, with the most recent in October 2017. Caleb has also undergone several orthopedic procedures for correction of his valgus foot deformities; the most recent was a bilateral distal medial tibial stapling and lengthening of his peroneal tendons.

Therapy History: Receives PT once a week at _____ with strong carryover of activities at home by his family. He attends Cyber School.

Primary assessment

Home and School Environment: Caleb lives in a multistory house with a ramp to enter the home. He can manually propel a wheelchair up and down this ramp. The hallways and doorways on the first floor of the house are wide enough to accommodate his wheelchair. His bedroom is on the second floor, and he scoots up and down the stairs to his bedroom. The home has hard wood and laminate flooring on the first floor. The family owns a van and truck and are able to transport the ultralightweight wheelchair in their vehicles. Both mom, dad, and his older siblings are able to independently lift the chair in and out of the vehicles.

Orthotics

Knee–Ankle–Foot Orthoses bilaterally
Adaptive Equipment: Caleb has a standard forward-facing walker that he uses when he is fatigued and must ambulate in areas that are not wheelchair accessible.
Current Functional Status:
Current bed mobility is reported as complete independence.
Current car transfer level is reported as independent for the van, minimal assistance for the truck
Current toilet transfer level is reported as independent.
Current dressing is reported as requiring minimal assistance for shoes only when wearing KAFOs. All other dressing is independent.

Current Toileting: Independent with catheterization program, supervision for bowel program

Current grooming/hygiene is reported as requiring supervision/reminders, which is typical for his age.

Pain Evaluation: No report of pain at rest and throughout the day since his tethered cord release. Caleb does complain of fatigue in his legs after assisted standing activities or periods of ambulation.

Integumentary Assessment: Caleb has not had skin breakdown on his sacral area. He is knowledgeable about skin care and understands the importance of pressure relief and frequent skin checks. He is independent with skin checks related to the fit of his KAFOs and performs these skin checks at least of twice daily. He alerts his parents to any reddened areas.

Posture: Caleb independently sits on the floor or in an armless chair with an erect trunk and excellent head and trunk control. He exhibits good trunk righting skills and accurate protective reactions in sitting.

Cognition/Perception Evaluation

Cognition/Perception Skills are age appropriate.

Assessment of communication reveals that the patient is verbal.

The patient is oriented ×3.

The patient follows multistep directions.

The patient demonstrates age-appropriate problem-solving skills.

The patient is alert, interactive, cooperative, very socially engaged.

Short- and long-term memory is intact.

The patient's attention span is age appropriate.

Muscle Tone Assessment: Flaccid lower extremities except for active hip flexion bilaterally and hip abduction with scores of 3 or less using an MMT.

Range of Motion: Passive range of motion of neck, trunk, and upper extremities within normal limits.

Bilateral lower extremity passive range of motion within functional limits with hip flexion contractures of approximately 25 degrees noted and bilateral contractures of his feet.

» Strength assessment

Neck, trunk, and bilateral upper extremity strength is within normal limits

Left Lower Extremity Strength Assessment:

Hip flexion: 2+/5.

Hip extension: 2−/5.

Hip abduction: 2/5.

Knee flexion: 1/5.

Knee extension: 2−/5.

Ankle plantar flexion: 0/5.

Ankle dorsiflexion and inversion: 0/5.

Toe flexion: 0/5.

Toe extension: 0/5.

Right Lower Extremity Strength Assessment:

Hip flexion: 2+/5.

Hip extension: 2/5.

Hip abduction: 2/5.

Knee flexion: 1/5.

Knee extension: 2/5.

Ankle plantar flexion: 0/5.

Ankle dorsiflexion and inversion: 0/5.

Toe flexion: 0/5.

Toe extension: 0/5.

Sensation: Normal throughout head, trunk, and upper extremities; absent sensation from midthighs to toes bilaterally. Impaired sensation over gluteal and perineal areas.

Upper Extremity Assessment: The patient exhibits: right hand dominance.

Antigravity movement of the Left Upper extremity is intact; Right Upper extremity is intact.

Reaching skills of the Left Upper Extremity are efficient; Right Upper Extremity are efficient.

Grasping skills of the Left Upper Extremity are efficient; Right Upper Extremity are efficient.

Release skills of the Left Upper Extremity are efficient; Right Upper Extremity are efficient.

Bilateral coordination is efficient.

» Mobility

The patient demonstrates the ability to roll to the left and right independently.

The patient demonstrates the ability to transition from supine to sitting independently.

The patient demonstrates the ability to transition from sitting to supine independently.

The patient demonstrates the ability to scoot independently.

The patient demonstrates the ability to crawl on hands and knees independently.

The patient demonstrates the ability to transition from sitting to standing at a support requires use of KAFOs.

The patient demonstrates the ability to transition from standing at a support to sitting requires use of KAFOs

The patient demonstrates the ability to transfer to and from bed/chair independently

The patient demonstrates the ability to transfer to and from toilet independently

The patient demonstrates the ability to ambulate on a level surface requires use of KAFOs and only for distances less than 50 feet.

The patient demonstrates the ability to propel a manual wheelchair independently

Ambulation and Gait Assessment: Caleb walks independently using his KAFOs for short distances, of a maximum of 50 feet but frequently holds on to objects and walls to maintain his balance. Caleb has difficulty standing and uses furniture or a wall to maintain his balance. Caleb does have a walker for use with ambulation in tight spaces but utilizes his wheelchair for any distance mobility needs, especially outside of the home.

» Durable medical equipment recommendations

Quickie 7r Ultralightweight Wheelchair

From Caleb's medical background, functional needs, family needs, and chairs that were trialed, it is recommended that Caleb obtain a Quickie 7r Ultralightweight wheelchair. This ultralightweight chair will provide Caleb with independent mobility so that he is at an activity level where he can interact with his peers and family and keep pace with them, whether indoors or outdoors. Caleb also trialed several other lightweight wheelchairs, but both he and his parents strongly preferred the Quickie 7r Ultralightweight wheelchair. The Quickie 7r chair was much less bulky for Caleb, and he could propel and maneuver the chair easier and faster on both inside and outside surfaces.

The Quickie 7r will also provide Caleb with growth to meet his needs for the next 3 to 5 years. To maximize his functional independence, he requires the following accessories for his chair.

Tension Adjustable Back

Owing to his excellent trunk control and upper extremity strength, Caleb will benefit from a low-profile back for his wheelchair to promote optimal self-propulsion biomechanics and to avoid overuse injuries of his upper extremities. This type of backrest can provide the cueing that Caleb requires to prevent excessive posterior pelvic tilt and kyphotic posture that will affect his ability to self-propel the chair.

Seat Cushion: A 2-inch seat cushion is required for skin protection. Caleb has not had sacral skin breakdown; a cushion is needed to ensure skin integrity.

Aluminum Soft Roll Caster Wheels: These soft roll front caster wheels are necessary for shock absorption over uneven or bumpy surfaces. Caleb is an active boy who uses his wheelchair outside with his family and friends on solid surfaces, but also on uneven surfaces such as grass or gravel/dirt areas.

Schwalbe Marathon Plus Evolution Rear Wheel Tires: The Schwalbe Marathon rear wheel tire is a high-pressure inflation tire that offers low resistance for a smooth ride and easier maneuverability. In addition, these wheels are puncture resistant and offer excellent traction on wet surfaces.

Angle-Adjustable Flip Footrest: Caleb requires angle-adjustable footrests to provide an adequate contact surface for his feet for good sitting support and posture. Caleb currently wears KAFOs, and they do not allow him to alter his ankle position to accommodate a flat footrest. Caleb also requires the footplate to flip back out of the way for standing transfers into and out of his chair. He can transfer in and out of the chair from the floor if the footrest is flipped out of the way; he can flip the footrest away independently. If the footrest does not flip out of the way, Caleb is unable to transfer into and out of the chair independently and safely.

Calf Strap: The leg strap will help keep Caleb's feet securely on the footplate while propelling his chair. This is important from a safety standpoint to prevent his feet from sliding backward off the footplate and underneath the seat of the chair, especially if he is not wearing his KAFOs.

Padded swing-away armrests: Caleb requires armrests to provide upper extremity support while he is at rest seated in his wheelchair. He also uses the armrests during transfers into and out of the chair but will need to swing them out of the way to access lower height tables, desks, and so on.

Side guards: Caleb requires the plastic side guards for safety. The side guard keeps his clothes from getting caught in the spokes of the wheels, which could cause the chair to tip or cause Caleb's clothes to restrict his breathing and overall movement.

Rear Antitips: Antitips are required for safety in the wheelchair because they prevent backward tipping of the chair.

Autobuckle positioning belt: Caleb requires a positioning belt to keep him securely positioned in the chair while he is self-propelling. The belt keeps his hips positioned back in the chair, preventing a posterior pelvic tilt that encourages a rounded back or kyphotic posture. The positioning belt also prevents excessive front-loading of the wheelchair that could cause it to tip forward. Caleb can independently buckle and unbuckle this type of positioning belt.

Summary

Overall, the Quickie 7r manual wheelchair with the listed accessories will provide Caleb with the most efficient independent mobility for the foreseeable future. Caleb is a bright and energetic 12-year-old boy who is currently dependent for mobility outside the home if he does not have a wheelchair. This chair will significantly increase his independence and will facilitate interaction and participation in activities with his peers and family. Caleb enjoys participating in adaptive sports and playing outside, and this wheelchair will allow him full access to those activities. The lightweight qualities of this wheelchair and accessories will also facilitate his endurance for increased independence as he progresses through adolescence.

Thank you for your assistance in obtaining this chair for Caleb. With your approval of this piece of equipment, you will greatly increase the quality of life for Caleb by providing him with a means of independent mobility that he will use in his home and community setting daily. If you have any questions regarding Caleb or the above information, please contact me at _____. Thank you for your time and consideration.

Sincerely,

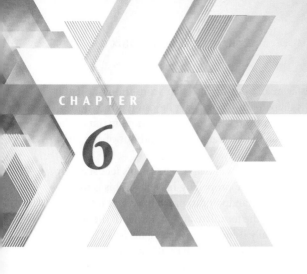

6

Physical Therapy in the Educational Setting: From Early Intervention to School Age

Rita Geddes

>> Introduction

In educational settings, physical therapy services are currently guided in large part by the Individuals with Disabilities Education Improvement Act (IDEA) of 2004 (Public Law [PL] 108-446). IDEA defines physical therapy as an *early intervention service* for infants and toddlers and a *related service* that is provided if it enables a preschool or school-aged child to benefit from special education services.[1] Physical therapy services in the early intervention setting aim to support families in promoting their infant or toddler's development, learning, and participation in family and community life. Physical therapy services in the preschool and school-aged environment aim to promote a student's participation in school-related activities and to prepare the student for further education, independent living, and employment beyond school.

Prior to the 1970s, children with significant physical and/or intellectual disabilities in the United States were typically excluded from public schools. Parents were often encouraged to have their child with a disability live in an institutional setting, and if they declined, parents were forced to pay tuition for their children to attend a segregated school or keep the child at home. In the 1960s, parent advocacy groups joined forces under the "normalization movement." President John F. Kennedy (who had a sister with a developmental disability) and his administration were strong supporters of the normalization movement. In the 1970s, these advocacy groups supported legal cases that resulted in landmark decisions of the Supreme Court, paving the way for the legislation that guides services in educational settings to this day.

The Rehabilitation Act of 1973[2] and the Education for All Handicapped Children's Act of 1975 (PL 94-142)[3] are the key legislative components that guide physical therapy services in educational settings. Section 504 of the Rehabilitation Act states that "no otherwise qualified disabled individual would be excluded from the participation in, be denied the benefits of, or be subjected to discrimination under any program or activity receiving federal financial assistance."[2] The Education for All Handicapped Children's Act, passed in 1975, went on to define the responsibilities of the public schools in providing a "free and appropriate education" (FAPE) for all school-aged children with disabilities[3] (see Table 6.1 for definitions of key terms).

TABLE 6.1.	**Key Definitions from Individuals with Disabilities Education Act (IDEA)[89]**

Child with a disability—A child having an intellectual disability, hearing impairment (including deafness), speech or language impairments, visual impairments (including blindness), serious emotional disturbance, orthopedic impairment, autism, traumatic brain injury, other health impairments, or a specific learning disability; and who, by reason thereof, needs special education and related services

Free Appropriate Public Education (FAPE)—Special education and related services that are provided at public expense, under public supervision and direction, and without charge; meet the standards of the State Education Agency (SEA), including the requirements of this part; include an appropriate preschool, elementary school, or secondary school education in the state involved; and are provided in conformity with an individualized education program (IEP) that meets the requirements of 1414(d)

Individualized Education Program—A written statement for each child with a disability that is developed, reviewed, and revised in a meeting in accordance with Section 1414(d) (ages 3–21 yr)

Individualized Family Service Plan (IFSP)—A written individualized plan developed by a multidisciplinary team, including the parents, as required by Subsection 1436(e), including a description of the appropriate transition services for the infant or toddler (ages birth to 3)

Least Restrictive Environment (LRE)—Each public agency must ensure that to the maximum extent appropriate, children with disabilities, including children in public or private institutions or other care facilities, are educated with children who are nondisabled; and special classes, separate schooling, or other removal of children with disabilities from the regular educational environment occurs only if the nature or severity of the disability is such that education in regular classes with the use of supplementary aids and services cannot be achieved satisfactorily.

Local Educational Agency (LEA)—A public board of education or other public authority legally constituted within a state for either administrative control or direction of, or to perform a service function for, public elementary or secondary schools in a city, county, township, school district, or other political subdivision of a state, or for a combination of school districts or counties as are recognized in a state as an administrative agency for its public elementary schools or secondary schools

Related Services—Transportation and such developmental, corrective, and other supportive services as are required to assist a child with a disability to benefit from special education. The disability may include speech-language pathology and audiology services, interpreting services, psychological services, physical and occupational therapy, recreation, including therapeutic recreation, early identification and assessment of disabilities in children, counseling services, including rehabilitation counseling, orientation and mobility services, and medical services for diagnostic or evaluation purposes. Related services also include school health services and school nurse services, social work services in schools, and parent counseling and training.

Special Education—Specially designed instruction, at no cost to the parents, to meet the unique needs of a child with a disability, including instruction conducted in the classroom, in the home, in hospitals and institutions, and in other settings; and instruction in physical education

Zero Reject—A principle that ensures that all children receive a free and appropriate public education, no matter how severe their disability. A child may not be excluded because a school district feels they are too disabled to learn, has inappropriate behavior caused by their disability, or has a contagious disease unless there is a high risk that the student will infect other students.

Several key concepts from PL 94-142 are still central to current regulations. *Zero reject* was a revolutionary concept at the time, assuring that no child could be excluded from receiving an FAPE regardless of the severity of their disability. For the first time ever in the Unites States, children with a disability such as cerebral palsy (CP), Down syndrome, and muscular dystrophy were eligible to go to school with nondisabled peers! Related services, including physical therapy, were mandated if needed to support a child's ability to benefit from their educational curriculum. PL 94-142 also defined the *least restrictive environment* (LRE), provided rights for *parent participation*, and developed the concept of an *individualized education program* (IEP). All these concepts remain central to current legislation, impacting the provision of educational services to a child with a disability and will be discussed in further detail.

The Education for All Handicapped Children's Act was amended in 1986,[4] again in 1991,[5] and subsequently in 1997 as the IDEA.[6] The most recent reauthorization was the IDEA of 2004.[1] The 2004 reauthorization was founded, in part, on the concept that IDEA's implementation has been impeded by low expectations, and an insufficient focus on applying replicable research on proven methods of teaching and learning for children with disabilities. Almost 30 years of research and experience has demonstrated that the education of children with disabilities can be made more effective by:

- having high expectations for such children and ensuring their access to the general education curriculum in the regular classroom, to the maximum extent possible, in order to:
  - meet developmental goals and, to the maximum extent possible, the challenging expectations that have been established for all children; and
  - be prepared to lead productive and independent adult lives, to the maximum extent possible. (§1400.c.(4)-(5)(A)(ii))[7]

Thus, the changes in the 2004 reauthorization focus heavily on raising expectations for outcomes of children with disabilities. IDEA legislation and elevating expectations for students with a disability were further strengthened by PL 114-95, the Every Student Succeeds Act of 2015.[8]

» Federal regulations

Individuals with Disabilities Education Act

IDEA is the prevailing legislation that guides and defines physical therapy service provision in educational settings. IDEA is divided into four components:

Part A: General Provisions
Part B: Assistance for All Children with Disabilities
Part C: Infants and Toddlers with Disabilities
Part D: National Activities to Improve Education of Children with Disabilities.

According to the General Provisions component,

> Disability is a natural part of the human experience and in no way diminishes the right of individuals to participate in or contribute to society. Improving educational results for children with disabilities is an essential element of our national policy of ensuring equality of opportunity, full participation, independent living, and economic self-sufficiency for individuals with disabilities. (§1400(c)(1))

The General Provisions section indicates that the purpose of IDEA is

> to ensure that all children with disabilities have available to them a free appropriate public education (FAPE) that emphasizes special education and related services designed to meet their unique needs and prepare them for further education, employment, and independent living. (§1400(d)(1)(A)) (see Table 6.1)

Part B outlines assistance for school-age students with disabilities, whereas Part C provides guidelines for infants and toddlers with disabilities. These components will be discussed in greater detail in the next section. Part D pertains to defining the role of the educational system, and it defines grant options to fund technology assistance, parent training centers, and personnel development.

The Rehabilitation Act of 1973

The Rehabilitation Act of 1973 was a groundbreaking legislation that supported the notion that children with disabilities should be provided equal opportunities compared to their nondisabled peers.[2] Today, Section 504 of the Act is used to support services for children who have a disability but are not in need of special education services. For example, a 504 Plan may be developed to address the health needs of a student with diabetes or severe asthma. Section 504 Plans are commonly used by physical therapists (PTs) when a student is able to function independently in academic classes but may need adaptations in an area such as school mobility. For example, a student who walks with a walker may be able to complete all academic work independently and within the same time constraints as their nondisabled peers. They may,

however, need assistance with emergency evacuations, increased time to transition between classes, special transportation, etc. As a result, such adaptations for students who are not in need of special education services typically are defined in a Section 504 Plan and serve as a legal document setting the standard to which the educational agency can be held.

Americans with Disabilities Act

The Americans with Disabilities Act (ADA) (PL 101-336), passed in 1990, provided civil rights protection to individuals with a disability. In the educational settings, this legislation primarily addresses construction standards to reduce mobility barriers and promote accessibility.[9] Although school buildings are not required to be retrofitted across the board, they are required to improve ADA compliance when a facility undergoes renovation. Since the passage of the law, therefore, accessibility in public schools has improved steadily as buildings have been renovated, thus decreasing the need for PTs in educational settings to develop individual plans for student accessibility.

Health Insurance Portability and Accountability Act/Family Educational Rights and Privacy Act

PTs in educational settings are still bound by the Health Insurance Portability and Accountability Act of 1996 (HIPAA).[7] Additionally, therapists must comply with the regulations outlined in Family Educational Rights and Privacy Act (FERPA),[10] a federal law that protects the privacy of student education records. The law applies to all schools that receive funds under an applicable program of the US Department of Education. FERPA permits parents access to student records, provides them with the right to request corrections of records, and requires parent permission to release information beyond demographics from a student record.

In addition to the federal regulations outlined earlier, educationally based PTs must remain current on relevant case law. Concepts in the IDEA and other regulations are continually challenged by parents and school districts. The resulting decisions can result in landmark changes in the provision of services in educational settings.

» Individuals with disabilities education act part C: Infants and toddlers

In 1986, PL 99-457 was enacted and served to expand the services provided under PL 94-142 to infants and toddlers with disabilities.[3] Rationale for the expansion included, reducing educational costs by minimizing the needs of the child by the time he/she reaches school age, minimizing the risk of institutional living, and maximizing a young adult's ability to live independently in society. This policy addresses the statewide development of multidisciplinary agencies to provide services for infants and toddlers with disabilities, coordination for payment of services, and expansion of services. PTs are listed as qualified early intervention service providers under this section (in contrast to related service providers under

Part B). Under current IDEA regulations, Part C indicates that early intervention services are

> designed to meet the developmental needs of an infant or toddler with a disability, as identified by the individualized family service plan team, in any 1 or more of the following areas: physical development; cognitive development; communication development; social or emotional development; or adaptive development. (§1432.(4)(C)(i-v))[1]

Additionally, it indicates that services:

> to the maximum extent appropriate, are provided in natural environments, including the home, and community settings in which children without disabilities participate.((1)§1432.(4)(G))

Services provided under Part B of IDEA already had a network of public school systems to support implementation. With the expansion to infants and toddlers, however, no such system was in existence. As a result, Part C required the development of state interagency coordinating councils to oversee the development and implementation of the early childhood programs. The composition of the council is well defined in the legislation and must include parents, service providers, a state legislator, a foster care representative, a mental health agency representative, and a coordinator of education of homeless children and youth, among others.[1]

Other services, in addition to physical therapy identified for early intervention in the regulations include family training, counseling, and home visits; special instruction, speech-language pathology and audiology services, and sign language and cued language services; occupational therapy, psychological services, service coordination services, and medical services only for diagnostic or evaluation purposes; early identification, screening, and assessment services; health services necessary to enable the infant or toddler to benefit from the other early intervention services; social work services, vision services, assistive technology devices, and assistive technology services; and transportation (§1432.(4)(E)). Part C places heavy emphasis on services being provided in the child's natural environment, which is often the child's home.[11]

Examination/Evaluation under Part C

Parents are essential members of the child's team; so parent permission is required prior to an examination and evaluation. Use of a norm-referenced test is required for infants and toddlers. Criterion-referenced tests can also be used to help guide services but they cannot be used for determining eligibility.[11] Part C provides the states discretion in defining "developmental delay," so it is possible that a child is determined to be in need of services in one state and not in need of services in another state. Definitions of developmental delay currently vary from 25% to 50% or 1.5 to 2 standard deviations below in norm-referenced tests.[12] The PT is typically a member of a team conducting a "multidisciplinary assessment of the unique strengths and needs of the infant or toddler and the identification of services appropriate to meet such needs"[1] (§1436.a.1).

When selecting assessment tools, the evaluation team must choose tools with proven reliability and validity. Cultural sensitivity must also be considered because norm references can be impacted by cultural differences.[13] In selecting a tool, consideration should be given to the potential needs of the child and family. For example, a child who was born prematurely and is considered high risk for CP has different potential needs than one who is being evaluated for autism.

For this younger population, commonly used norm-referenced tests include:

1. *Bayley Scales of Infant and Toddler Development, Fourth Edition (Bayley-4)*—a standardized, norm-referenced test recently revised to measure a child's competency in five major developmental domains that correspond with those stipulated in IDEA: cognitive, language, motor, social–emotional, and adaptive behavior (the latter two assessed by parental response to a questionnaire).[14]
2. *Brigance Inventory of Early Development III (IED III)*—a comprehensive tool containing over 100 assessments that are aligned to state and national standards and IDEA requirements. Used to provide ongoing assessment, monitor progress, and write Individualized Family Service Plans (IFSPs). The IED III contains criterion-referenced and norm-referenced measures, but only norm-referenced measures can be used to determine eligibility.[15,16]
3. *Hawaii Early Learning Profile (HELP-Strands)*—a family-centered, curriculum-based assessment tool[16,17]
4. *Peabody Developmental Motor Scales 2 (PDMS-2)*—a standardized, norm-referenced test of motor skills in children from birth to 5 years. Six subtests assess motor skills in the following areas: reflexes, stationary, locomotion, object manipulation, grasping, and visual motor integration. A motor activities program with instructional objectives, reasons for teaching the skill, examples of related skills as they occur in the natural environment, and suggested instructional strategies supplements the assessment.[18]
5. *Pediatric Evaluation of Disability Inventory—Computer Adaptive Test*—a functional assessment instrument for the evaluation of children with disabilities from 6 months to 7 years. Based on the interview with a primary caregiver, the inventory measures functional status and change in three domains: self-care, mobility, and social function. The standard score, which is norm referenced, can be used to determine eligibility but the scaled score, which is criterion referenced, cannot.[19,20]
6. *Developmental Assessment of Young Children, Second Edition (DAYC-2)*—The DAYC-2 is a norm-referenced measure of early childhood development in the domains of cognition, communication, social–emotional development, physical development, and adaptive behavior of children from birth through 5 years 11 months. The DAYC-2 has proven validity and reliability using a sample of 1,832 children.[21]

An additional tool to assess the infant or toddler's participation in play as well as parental abilities to promote continued development may also be considered, as these tools can be relevant in guiding interventions and determining service levels. For example, the Keys to Interactive Parenting Scale (KIPS) is a valid, reliable, and culturally sensitive test that assesses whether parental behavior positively promotes the child's development. Tools such as this can help identify families that are in greater need of education in strategies to help promote development of their child as well as document outcomes of interventions via retesting.[22,23] Similarly, the Test of Playfulness can be used to gain knowledge of the child's approach to play to develop individualized interventions that promote playfulness.[24-26]

The Gross Motor Function Classification System (GMFCS) provides a way to classify children with CP based on functional abilities and limitations, using a 5-level classification system across four age band groupings. Distinctions between levels of the GMFCS reflect varying levels of severity of motor impairments in sitting, transfers, walking, and wheeled mobility. Level I represents the least impairment (walking without limitations), whereas Level V represents the most severe impairment (dependency of transport in a manual wheelchair). The GMFCS provides a valid and reliable avenue for communication between families and professionals, as well as a grouping variable for program evaluation and clinical research.[27-29] The GMFCS can be used in clinical practice to predict gross motor function, provide a means for collaborative goal setting, predict a need for assistive technology, and guide decisions regarding dosing of interventions.[30]

Individualized Family Service Plan

Under Part C of IDEA, when, as a result of the evaluation, a child is determined to have a development delay by the multidisciplinary team, an IFSP must be developed. The IFSP must be developed by a multidisciplinary team that includes the parents and must include a description of appropriate services to support the child's transition to school-age services. According to IDEA, the IFSP must be evaluated annually but should be reviewed with the family at a minimum of 6-month intervals. State regulations determine timeliness of assessment, IFSP development, and initiation of services.

The IFSP must include at a minimum the following elements[1]:

1. Statement of the infant's or toddler's present levels of physical development (vision, hearing, motor, and health), cognitive development (thinking, reasoning, and learning), communication development (responding, understanding, and using language), social or emotional development (feelings, playing, and interacting), and adaptive development (bathing, feeding, dressing, etc.) based on objective criteria

2. Statement of family's resources, priorities, and concerns related to enhancing the development of the family's infant or toddler with a disability

3. Statement of the measurable results or outcomes expected to be achieved for the infant or toddler and family; the criteria, procedures, and timelines used to determine the degree to which progress toward achieving the results or outcomes is being made; and whether modifications or revisions of the result or outcomes or services are necessary

4. Statement of specific early intervention services based on peer-reviewed research necessary to meet the unique needs of the child and family including frequency, intensity, and method of delivering services

5. Statement of natural environments in which early intervention services will appropriately be provided

6. Projected dates for initiation of services and the anticipated length, duration, and frequency of the services

7. Identification of the service coordinator from the profession most immediately relevant to the needs of the infant or toddler and family

8. Steps to be taken to support the transition of the toddler with a disability to preschool or other appropriate services (which must include a formal plan and team conference 3 to 9 months prior to anticipated transition)

9. Provision for parental consent

Part C: Provision of Physical Therapy Services—Team Models

Unlike services provided under Part B, physical therapy services can be a primary service under Part C. In other words, physical therapy may be the only service a child receives. When a child has needs in other areas as well, a service delivery model must be chosen by the child's team. IDEA defines the "team" as multidisciplinary, and that is often the model for examination and evaluation. For interventions, however, teams may be transdisciplinary.[31] King et al. identified the key components of a transdisciplinary approach as a multidisciplinary assessment using standardized and informal measures, role release of therapists (a provider utilizing strategies and techniques from other disciplines), and intensive and ongoing interaction among team members. Although there are limitations and challenges to this model, there are also many potential benefits such as improving efficiency of service delivery (e.g., in rural areas)[32] and the need for parents to develop a working relationship with one or a few rather than numerous service providers. In the transdisciplinary model, the PT could be a primary coach and be required to supply parent education for other disciplines. Therefore, extensive consultation with other disciplines, experience, and cross-training are integral aspects of the transdisciplinary service delivery model.[31]

Other options for service delivery models include multidisciplinary, where each team member provides services specific to their discipline only, and interdisciplinary, where roles are somewhat more relaxed. In the interdisciplinary model, a PT is responsible for parent training and providing interventions related to the areas assessed by the PT. However, the therapist may incorporate strategies from other service providers to promote global progress, but the PT is not responsible for monitoring and reporting on the progress as in the transdisciplinary model. For example, strategies from a speech and language pathologist to promote improvement in communication skills may be utilized during a gross motor activity. In the interdisciplinary model, communication among members is a key factor of the interdisciplinary team so that each discipline is aware of key components of interventions for the disciplines involved.

Part C: Provision of Physical Therapy Services: Natural Environment and Parental Involvement

Services under Part C are typically provided in a child's natural settings, such as the child's home, daycare, or closest playground that the family routinely accesses with the goal of improving the child's ability to participate in family and play activities. Lestari and Ratnaningsih[33] confirmed that participation in modified games resulted in improvements in physical, cognitive, and social development of kindergarten students. When selecting strategies and equipment, however, the therapist should be aware of what is available to the child and family when the therapist leaves. If the family does not have access to the adapted equipment or modified games, then practice and generalization to daily routines cannot be expected. The PT should be aware of what toys, equipment, etc., are available in the home and develop adaptations to support the child's ability to use the toys safely and effectively when the therapist is not present. The same parameters apply to the daycare or preschool environment for toddlers with disabilities.

Nwokah et al. investigated the dilemma of poverty related to the availability of play materials and determined that PTs and occupational therapists (OTs) providing services to infants and toddlers were likely to take toys into the home but they were less likely than other providers of services to use their own toys during play.[34] The study also found that early childhood professionals across disciplines indicated that they commonly lent or gave toys to families. Toy-lending libraries are another source of material for families to support a child's participation in play activities outside of therapy.

IDEA recognizes the value of minimizing potential developmental delay by promoting intervention during the critical period of brain development from birth to 3 years (IDEA 1431.a.1). Prior to this landmark legislation, infants and toddlers had inconsistent access to interventions, resulting in the development of secondary disabilities. Primary impairments are identified at diagnosis, whereas secondary impairments evolve over time, possibly as a result of the primary impairment.[35] The primary disability is not the reason for the lack of skill development. Rather, it is the lack of opportunity at the critical time in brain development. So, a basic tenet of early childhood services is to

empower parents and families with the skills needed to prevent secondary deformities and delays. Much research has been done to support this concept for a variety of disabilities. Jeffries et al. reported that primary impairments with young children with CP occur in muscle tone and quality of movement and secondary impairments in range of motion, strength, and endurance.[35] Also of note is that the degree of impairment increased as the GMFCS level increased. Similarly, in a report of the results of a scoping review of the best practice principles for management of children with developmental coordination disorder (DCD), Camden et al. identified a key theme:

Professionals and families working together to offer evidence-based services fostering function and participation and preventing secondary consequences. The authors identified the following key supporting principles:

> Principle 2.1 The integration of child and family views in assessment, goal-setting and intervention which recognizes the impact of DCD and the contextual life of the family, and ensures meaningful action.
> Principle 2.2 Interventions should be evidence-based, foster function and participation, and prevent secondary consequences.[36]

This supports the notion that the aim of interventions for this age group should focus on promoting participation in activities that are common to nondisabled peers to promote development of cognitive and motor learning and prevent secondary impairments. By imbedding intervention strategies into daily routines and providing knowledge of interventions to primary caregivers, the opportunity for practice and progress is greatly enhanced.[37,38]

The largest study aimed at OTs and PTs providing services to infants and toddlers at risk of or diagnosed with CP indicated that infants at risk of CP do receive a reasonable amount of therapy that is occurring in their homes. Additionally, most therapists utilize child-initiated, activity-based, and task-oriented motor training strategies, which have proven efficacy. Therapists are not, however, adequately incorporating the use of proven techniques such as constraint-induced movement therapy (CIMT) and parental coaching and education.[39] To maximize the early motor development of children with CP and, thereby, minimize the development of secondary impairments, therapists providing early intervention services should include sensitive, evidence-based assessment tools, promote parent engagement using home programs and formal goal-setting assessment tools, incorporate activities that facilitate activation of lower limb muscles using concentric and eccentric exercises such as sit-to-stand and step up and down activities, use modified CIMT and bimanual training when asymmetric hand movement is present, educate the parents about the appropriate use of toys, advise parents to provide infants with variable practice, provide parents with evidence-based information related to the importance of proper sleeping and feeding, and provide parents with prognostic information to help them develop realistic expectations.[39-44] Recent research has led to a proliferation of knowledge that can improve the efficacy of interventions for infants and toddlers who have primary impairments, thus minimizing secondary impairments.[45-48] Disseminating this information and translating it into everyday practices is a critical challenge for providers of early intervention services.

» Individuals with disabilities education act part B (3 to 21 years)

Examination/Evaluation

In contrast to Part C, physical therapy for school-age children is defined as a related service so it cannot be a child's only special education service. Physical therapy examination/evaluations should be conducted as part of a multidisciplinary team, including the child's parent(s). Depending on the student's disability and needs, some other examples of team members may be, but not limited to, speech and language pathologist, OT, school psychologist, behavioral analyst, teacher of the visually impaired or hearing impaired, orientation and mobility specialist, nurse, or social worker. Before a child can receive special education services, including related services, an individual initial evaluation of the child must be conducted to see if the child has a disability and to determine whether the child is eligible for special education.[1] Informed parent consent must be obtained before this evaluation may be conducted, and once parental consent is received, the local education agency (LEA) has 60 calendar days to complete the assessment.

The evaluation cannot rely on one standardized test to determine eligibility. IDEA dictates that:

In conducting the evaluation, the local educational agency shall—

a. use a variety of assessment tools and strategies to gather relevant functional, developmental, and academic information, including information provided by the parent, …

b. not use any single measure or assessment as the sole criterion for determining whether a child is a child with a disability or determining an appropriate educational program for the child; and

c. use technically sound instruments that may assess the relative contribution of cognitive and behavioral factors, in addition to physical or developmental factors.[1] (§1414.a.1.b.2)

Therefore, PTs cannot rely on one measure for the examination/evaluation process. Rather, a variety of strategies including norm-referenced, criterion-referenced, and/or ecologic assessments should be utilized (Table 6.2). The purpose of the examination is to determine whether

TABLE 6.2. Common Assessment Tools	
Tool	Ages/Grades
School Function Assessment[63]	Grades K–6
Test of Gross Motor Development-3[90,91]	3–12 yr through 10–11 yr
6-Minute Walk Test[92-94]	Ages 4–12
50-Foot Walk Test[95,96]	Grades K–6
30-Second Walk Test	Ages 5–17
Timed up and down stairs	Ages 8–14

a child has a disability and whether the disability results in a need for special education services. A child is determined to be in need of special education services if they have a disability in one of the identified categories (autism, deafness, deaf-blindness, emotional disturbance, hearing impairment, intellectual disability, multiple disabilities, orthopedic impairment, other health impairments, specific learning disability, speech or language impairment, traumatic brain injury, visual impairment, including blindness) and "by *reason thereof*, needs special education and related services."[1] The evaluating team, including the parents, should collectively make that determination. For PTs, use of a strengths-based approach is preferred because, by noting the areas of strength, the therapist can identify the foundation from which to build new skills and foster confidence for the child.

Developing the Individualized Education Program: Goals and Interventions

If the child is found to need special education services, then a meeting to develop goals and other supports detailed in the IEP must be held within 30 calendar days of the completion of the evaluation report. Goals in the educational setting have developed and changed over time and serve multiple purposes. Years ago, educationally based goals were more discipline specific and tended to be written at the impairment level (e.g., student will improve range of motion),[49] but today, participation-based goals are identified as the current standard of "best practice" for goal writing.[11,49] The development of participation-based goals should be a team effort. Wynarczuk et al. conducted small focus groups totaling 20 PTs to understand how PTs are developing goals and to identify factors that facilitate or hinder participation-based goal development. The results indicated that therapists must first have a thorough understanding of the student (i.e., age, intrinsic motivation, health, diagnosis, educational qualification category, and educational program) and then must work cooperatively with other IEP team members to develop shared responsibility for student goals.[49] Such role release and relinquishing of impairment-based focus often proves challenging for PTs. Thus, an awareness of the current standards of best practice, self-reflection on personal practices, and guidance in goal development is needed, especially for therapists who are new to educational settings.[49] A variety of tools, such as the Canadian Occupation Performance Measure (COPM) and the Goal Attainment Scaling (GAS), can aid with the development of collaborative goals.[50,51] Chiarello encourages participation to be a theme embedded across the Doctor of Physical Therapy (DPT) curriculum and recognizes the importance of physical therapy students learning and practicing the art of participation analyses, teaming, and coaching to support the achievement of participation-based goals in the future.[52] Goals not only serve as indicators of student progress but can also be used to identify therapist and program outcomes.[53,54] Therapists and supervisors may use this information to identify needs for professional development and to track the use of best practices.[55]

Although IDEA requires discipline-free "measurable annual goals" as part of the IEP,[1] short-term objectives are not required by current federal legislation, although state and local regulations and practices may vary. Well-developed goals should be functional in nature (part of the student's typical school day), measurable, and generalizable:

Functional: Improvement will increase a student's ability to interact with people and objects within the daily school environment and improve independence of function. The skill would have to be performed by someone else if the student could not.[11]

Measurable (including performance criteria, conditions, and time frame): A skill is measurable if it can be seen and/or heard, can be directly counted (frequency, duration, or distance measures), and lends itself to determination of performance criteria. The baseline and sought-after conditions for performance should be clearly stated, linked to a standard, and, whenever to the extent practicable, linked to an assessment that is valid and reliable.

Generalizable: Goals should be written with the long-term awareness of the importance of the skill. The aim of a goal should not be to accomplish a task in an isolated therapy room but aimed at natural school environments.

Goals should always be stated as behaviors the student will demonstrate and not what will be done with or to the student. In an impairment-based system, improving range of motion to a specific level might be a viable goal. In the school-based setting, however, although improved range of motion may be needed to allow for functional positioning during a desktop activity, the ability to *access and participate* in a desktop activity is the goal rather than the improvement in range of motion (Table 6.3).

Once the goals are developed, the *IEP team* should decide whether or not skilled physical therapy intervention is needed for the child to make progress toward their individual goals. In a study of 22 state and LEA practice guidelines, Vialu and Doyle identified five common questions to help guide the decision for skilled PT intervention[56]:

1. Are the student's disabilities or performance limitations adversely affecting his/her education?
2. Is the student's PT need educational, and not only medical?
3. Is PT necessary for the student to benefit from his/her education?
4. Does the student have the potential to improve access to his/her education and achieve educational outcomes with PT intervention?
5. Does the student require the level of expertise of a PT to achieve educational goals?

If the answer is "yes" to these five questions, then physical therapy services may be needed to help a student make progress toward their individual goals. Wynarczuk et al.

TABLE 6.3.	Integrated Goal Examples			
Time Frame	Condition	Student	Activity	Criteria
Describe when the desired outcome will be achieved	*Describe when and where the activity will take place*	*Name the student*	*Describe the desired activity and the level of prompts or assistance*	*Indicate the performance level for achievement*
In 1 yr	When transitioning between her classroom and lunch	Tiffany	Will walk with adult supervision from a distance of greater than 5 feet, without using an assistive device	Across 3 consecutive weeks of school from a baseline of 0 weeks
In 1 yr	When preparing to leave the classroom	Joey	Will independently participate in at least 50% of physical education activities from a baseline of 20%	Across 3 consecutive weekly physical education classes
In 1 yr	When arriving to school	Rasheen	Will independently exit his bus and report to homeroom within the school-wide time frame	Across 15 consecutive days of school from a baseline of 0 days

found that a goal can have a significant impact on the nature of services, intervention strategies, teaming, and the flexibility of services. Additionally, factors that helped promote participation-based goals included "collaborative school cultures, educational team engagement, a value on participation, and continuing professional education."[49] Support from the educational team helped to foster the development of goals related to participation when integrated service delivery models were frequently utilized. Self-reflection on goal development and how it relates to practice in schools can help advance the use of participation-based goal development.[55,57]

Tremendous variability in practice exists throughout the country in determining whether related services, such as physical therapy, are needed for a child to make progress toward their goals. Kaminker et al. found significant differences in the frequency and context of service delivery recommendations based on the geographic region of practice.[58,59] It is still unclear as to whether the variation comes from staffing availability, employee status (contractor vs. district employee), and/or overuse of a direct service model.[60] As the research into best practices in educational environments progresses and outcomes from specific service delivery models are determined, perhaps such inconsistencies will be mitigated in the future.

To this end, a landmark study for school-based physical therapy, entitled PT Related Child Outcomes in the Schools (PT COUNTS), was conducted. Effgen et al. utilized a practice-based evidence methodology to "investigate changes in students' participation in school activity, self-care, posture/mobility, recreation/fitness, and academic outcomes, and the relationships of these changes to characteristics of school-based therapy."[61] One hundred nine PTs from all geographic regions in the United States participated and collected data for 296 students aged 5 to 12 years across a 6-month time span. To provide uniformity of data collection, the School-Physical Therapy Intervention for Pediatrics (S-PTIP) form was developed as a documentation tool, determined to be valid, and training was provided to all therapists involved.[61] GAS, an individualized, criterion-referenced outcome measure with proven reliability, validity, and responsiveness in children with CP, was utilized as an outcome measure.[62] GAS is a 5-point scale with the baseline defined at −2 and the desired outcome at 0, with −1 indicating progress toward the goal and +1 and +2 exceeding expectations. The School Function Assessment (SFA), a criterion-referenced measure of a student's performance of functional tasks, was also utilized as an outcome measurement tool.[63] This was the first educationally based study in the United States to investigate the links between outcomes and the type, frequency, and method of delivery of services.

The results of this investigation have provided much needed hard evidence to help determine how and what services are being delivered, as well as to help guide physical therapy interventions in schools in the future. The study

determined that PTs were not using interventions that lacked evidence such as neurodevelopmental treatment (NDT) and passive range of motion (PROM), but they also were not using interventions with a more solid research foundation such as CIMT and cardiopulmonary interventions.[64] The study also indicated that, in contrast to best practice, the majority of interventions were provided individually and not integrated into school activities, and this was especially true for students with GMFCS Levels I–III. Also, services levels tended to remain stable over time rather than fluctuate based on students' needs from year to year. The ratio of direct services to services spent on behalf of the student (e.g., staff training, equipment management, and documentation) was roughly 2:1.[36]

When looking at outcomes using the GAS, students who received more mobility-based interventions exceeded academic goal expectations.[65] This supports similar findings that physical activity has a positive influence on cognition, brain structure, and function.[66] Progress toward posture and mobility goals was positively associated with student practice of self-care activities and negatively associated with cognitive–behavioral strategies. For recreation and fitness goals, interventions addressing mobility for playground access, cognitive–behavioral, and functional strengthening activities were positively correlated.[65] When looking at outcomes using the SFA, mobility interventions demonstrated clinically significant correlation with relationship to participation. For mobility, motor learning and cardiopulmonary conditioning interventions and student's engagement in the activity were positive correlates. For recreation, interventions for mobility, playground access, sensory interventions, and students' active participation were positive correlates along with spending less time on sensory integration, orthoses, and equipment training. Passive interventions such as equipment training, orthoses management, and hands-on facilitation techniques were negatively correlated with better outcomes on the SFA. This research supports the concept that the application of motor learning theory (set goals that are meaningful to the child, engage the child actively in the problem-solving/practice process, consider the stage of learning when developing/adjusting interventions, and provide fading assistance/feedback) is beneficial in school-based practices. So, the application of the concepts of motor learning theory is more effective in achieving positive outcomes than passive interventions, and integrating routine practice of motor tasks, such as self-care skills, can lead to improvement in other areas such as postural control.[65,67] By optimizing interventions and service delivery strategies, therapists can maximize their own efficiency by providing sufficient interventions to allow progress toward goals while avoiding excessive interventions that serve to remove a child from his/her academic tasks and add to therapists' workloads.[68] These findings help to justify the need for collaboration and training of support staff, so that practice of the desired skills can occur on a daily basis, rather than just when the PT is present.[36,62,64,67]

Supplementary Aids and Services

The supplementary aids and services (SAS) section of the IEP is the portion of the IEP where any adaptations (accommodations or modifications) that will be carried out when the PT is not present should be clearly defined. An accommodation does not alter the curriculum expectations; so a child with an accommodation would be expected to perform on grade level with support. An example of an accommodation would be the use of a specialized seating system and assistive technology to provide postural support during writing activities. In this case, the student would be able to write on a similar level to his or her same-grade peers with these accommodations in place. A modification, on the other hand, addresses changes to the curriculum when the expected grade-level performance is beyond the ability of the student.[1] An example of a modification would be that the student types one sentence instead of two full paragraphs. PTs commonly make recommendations in this section for adaptations (accommodations or modifications) to functional positioning, school mobility, support for activities of daily living, and participation in gross motor activities (Table 6.4).

Location of Interventions

Physical therapy services provided to school-age children are intended to be provided in their natural school environment. IDEA indicates that "special classes, separate schooling, or other removal of children with disabilities from the regular educational environment occurs only when the nature or severity of the disability of a child is such that education in regular classes with the use of supplementary aids and services cannot be achieved satisfactorily."[1] Additionally, the APTA Academy of Pediatric Physical Therapy defines "best practice" as providing services in the "classroom or other places that support the student's special education program."[11] In 2015, Thomason and Wilmarth found, however, that the majority (69%) of PTs providing services in education settings are still providing services in a private therapy room or isolated area within a school. The three most frequent barriers to inclusive services were identified as teacher attitudes/misinformation, therapist workload/difficulty scheduling, and parent expectations/misinformation. Specific comments were made by respondents that strength, balance, and endurance training activities cannot occur or are not practical when integrated into the classroom.[69]

Such beliefs are flawed in that they do not account for the role of meaningful physical activity in providing opportunities for strengthening and motor skills development. When a child does not participate in key elements of their curriculum such as recess and physical education class, they miss out on the routine practice required to build strength, endurance, and foundational motor skills, and they experience less opportunity to practice motor skills compared to their typically developing peers. So, a child who needs *more* practice to master motor skills is exposed to significantly *less* opportunity for practice. The end result is increased risk of secondary impairments and movement farther away from rather than closer to the curve of typical development. To illustrate this, Mâsse et al. studied participation in activities among children with neurodevelopmental disorders and disabilities utilizing a representative sample of Canadian children and found that children with motor disorders participate in less supervised and unsupervised physical activities both in school and in the community.[70] Fox et al. also demonstrated that children with Down syndrome engage in less physical activity than their nondisabled peers and do not meet the guideline of 60 minutes of moderate to vigorous exercise per day.[71] Similarly, Potvin et al. compared the participation of 30 children diagnosed with high-functioning autism (HFA) to that of 31 typically developing peers in a comparison group.[72] Stanish et al. demonstrated that this trend continues into adolescence as 35 adolescents with autism spectrum disorder participated in approximately 20 minutes per day less of moderate to vigorous physical activity than the 60 typically developing adolescents and fell far short of the recommended 60 minutes per day of moderate to vigorous physical activity.[73] The increasing pool of data that examine the level of participation in physical activities indicate that children with developmental and/or physical disabilities routinely participate in less physical activity than typically developing children[74] and that increased opportunity for practice can have a beneficial impact on participation.[67,75-77]

Palisano et al. proposed a consultative and collaborative model for the implementation of participation-based occupational and physical therapy services.[78] Although the case study of the model applied to community-based services, the implications are the same for school-based therapies: "real-life experiences enable children to learn new activities and develop skills that optimize their participation and self-determination."

TABLE 6.4.	Supplementary Aids and Services (SAS)
Need	**SAS**
Postural Control	Physical therapist (PT) will develop a chart of preferred and nonpreferred positions for use in the classroom. Personal care assistant will use the chart as a visual reference for the student.
Self-Regulation of Mobility	Visual chart of hall-walking rules to be placed at the doorway for review prior to entering the hallway Preinstruction in expectations on a daily basis Fade from use of direct verbal prompts to indirect verbal to gestural prompts Have student rate her performance compared to adult rating at least once a day using the terms not so good, okay, or really good
Participation in Recess Activities	Provide three choices prior to recess PT to provide initial direct instruction and guided practice in playground access Provide weekly opportunities for extra practice for playground access

So, if the focus of school-based physical therapy intervention is on meaningful participation in recess activities, functional school mobility, and physical education class, then the student will be exposed to opportunities to improve strength and endurance on a daily basis with the goal of preventing secondary impairments. Thus, physical therapy services integrated into these key settings, aimed at the promotion of participation in routine motor skill practice, can have a profound impact on a student's function in the long term.

Progress Reporting and IEP Revisions/Updates

According to IDEA, parents should receive periodic reports on the progress the child is making toward their annual goals. The frequency of progress reporting is vague in the IDEA statute and is therefore left to the discretion of the states. Although goals should be integrated and transdisciplinary, the PT will likely provide the written progress report if the goal is within their scope of aimed interventions. The IEP must be updated at least annually, and PTs typically provide input to several sections of the IEP: present levels of functional performance, how the student's disability impacts their participation and progress in the general education curriculum, strengths, needs, SAS, and specially designed instruction (SDI)-related services (including frequency, intervals, and location of interventions), extended school year, goals, and transition services. When updating an IEP, present levels of functional performance should include progress toward previous goals and (if applicable) progress/recommendations for SAS or SDI as well as information about the student's level of independence and physical participation in daily school routines and activities such as school arrival and pack-up, participation in physical education class and recess, level of independence of classroom and hallway mobility, access to transportation, and functional positioning. Any changes over time in the goals and SAS should be clearly identified in the present levels of functional performance as well as in the respective sections of the IEP.

Transition to Adulthood

PTs can play a vital role in preparing a child for transition to adulthood including postsecondary education, vocational training, employment, independent living, and community participation.[1] Application of motor learning theory in early years can help a child master prerequisite motor and self-help skills that are integral to vocational activities and tasks. Addressing community mobility and independent living challenges provides a foundation for accessing vocational and recreational opportunities in the community. Resources for participation in community activities, such as adapted sports and other recreational opportunities, can also be invaluable to support community participation after transition to adulthood. The PTs' role in transition should be a focus of future research so that established standards can be developed to help promulgate the inclusion of PTs in transition teams.

Funding

The mandate of IDEA is to provide FAPE to qualified individuals with disabilities, and IDEA now impacts the education of 7 million American children with disabilities, but the cost can be staggering to states and LEAs.[79] The federal government initially intended to pay the 40% per pupil increase in cost of educating a child with a disability compared to a general education student.[79,80] The actual federal allocation has always been less than half the amount promised (14.3% in 2019), however, resulting in a significant burden for the states and LEAs. In 1988, PL 100-360 was enacted to allow states to utilize Medicaid funds to supplement the cost of providing related services for eligible children.[81] Rules and regulations about Medicaid eligibility and allocation of funds vary from state to state but are frequently restricted to direct service, which can limit the ability of providers to select a delivery mode that is most appropriate and is the most efficient use of resources.[64] Private insurance may also be billed if parents give informed consent to do so, but it is important that they are aware of specifics of their policy so that they do not negatively impact long-term coverage (e.g., a policy that has lifetime caps on therapy services). A large number of professional organizations have formed a funding coalition and developed a proposal for full funding by the federal government that could be phased in over a predetermined time period, thus reducing the burden on local LEAs.

Moving Forward—Knowledge Translation

Historically, research into school-based practices occurred less frequently than research for pediatric inpatient, outpatient, and rehabilitation interventions. This may be due to the fact that the percentage of PTs providing school-based services was relatively low. In recent decades, however, that trend has turned and an increasing volume of literature is being published on the provision of school-based services. This may be due, in part, to the increasing number of PTs working in educational settings. In 1988, the author's first year of working in schools, there were 2,999 PTs working in school settings providing services to children from 3 to 21 years. By 2015, that number nearly tripled to 8,355 therapists, indicating an increase in available data sources and a need for investigations to refine best practices.[60,82]

Despite having an increase in research into the provision of services in educational environments, the knowledge is not consistently translating into practice. In a large online survey study of 561 PTs providing services in educational environments, poor agreement was found between what therapists indicated was ideal practice and what they reported as actual practice in all but seven questions, and 42% of therapists indicated that direct "hands-on" therapy delivery was ideal and 57% reported that they "usually" use this delivery model. Additionally, 51% indicated that therapists should ideally work within natural environments, whereas only

45% "usually" do and 36% do so only occasionally.[83] These statistics are congruent with previous studies, indicating a gap between the desire for best practice and the reality of using outdated models of service delivery.[84] These statistics are in contrast to the team concept of working collaboratively to provide evidence-based services that foster function and participation, thus preventing secondary impairments. Experienced and novice clinicians are encouraged to continually reflect on their knowledge and skills, and the articles "Updated Competencies for Physical Therapists Working in Early Intervention"[85] and "Updated Competencies for Physical Therapists Working in Schools"[86] are a good place to start. The American Physical Therapy Association and the Academy of Pediatric Physical Therapy have a wealth of resources for therapists to utilize for self-reflection, professional development, and parent education (Table 6.5).

When choosing a physician for a serious medical condition such as cancer, one would not choose a provider who bases their intervention solely on what the physician knew to be true when they graduated from medical school. A patient assumes that the physician will stay current with outcome studies and update intervention plans accordingly to provide the best chance for a positive outcome. Children with disabilities deserve no less from their related service providers! A sufficient knowledge base now exists that provides therapists with at least a starting point as to interventions that work and those that are ineffective. When therapists update their practices based on research to the extent practicable, they provide the children they serve the opportunity to reach their maximum potential. The challenge for therapists new to the field of early intervention and educationally based services is to translate this and future knowledge gained from research into actual practice across the country.[87,88] Each and every child that is served deserves no less!

TABLE 6.5.	APTA/APPT Resources
APTA	**Guide to Physical Therapist Practice[97]**
APTA Section on Pediatrics	List of examination/evaluation tools Legislative information about IDEIA Brochure, *Providing Services Under Individuals with Disabilities Education Act (IDEA) 2004* Links to Internet resources Manual, *Providing Physical Therapy Services under Parts B and C of IDEA*
APTA Pediatric Listserv	Ongoing e-mail discussion forum for current issues in pediatric physical therapy. Available to all members of Section on Pediatrics
APTA Section on Pediatrics School-Based Special Interest Group	National organization working to provide opportunities for school-based physical therapists to confer, meet, and promote high standards of practice. Fact sheets, references, and training tools are available.
Pediatric Physical Therapy	Monthly peer-reviewed publication of Section on Pediatrics

APTA, American Physical Therapy Association; APPT, Academy of Pediatric Physical Therapy; IDEIA, Individuals With Disabilities Education Improvement Act.

REFERENCES

1. Individuals with Disabilities Education Improvement Act of 2004. Public Law 108-446; 2004.
2. Section 504 of the Rehabilitation Act. U.S. Congress. Senate. 1973.
3. Education for All Handicapped Children Act. Public Law 94-142. U.S. Congress. Senate, 94th Congress; 1975.
4. Education of the Handicapped Act Amendments of 1986. Public Law 99-457.
5. Individuals with Disabilities Education Act Amendments of 1991. Public Law 102-119; 1991.
6. Individuals with Disabilities Education Act Amendments of Public Law 105-17; 1997.
7. Health Insurance Portability and Accountability Act of Public Law 104-191; 1996.
8. Every Student Succeeds Act of Public Law 114-95; 2015.
9. Americans with Disabilities Act. Public Law 101-336; 1990.
10. The Family Educational Rights and Privacy Act of 20 U.S.C. § 1232g; 34 CFR Part 99; 1974.
11. McEwen I. *Providing Physical Therapy under Parts B and C of the Individuals with Disabilities Education Act (IDEA)*. American Physical Therapy Association; 2009.
12. Shackelford J. *State and Jurisdictional Eligibility Definitions for Infants and Toddlers with Disabilities under IDEA*. Issue No. 20 February 2006. Accessed June 18, 2019, NECTAC Notes.
13. Santamaría-Vázquez M, Maturana AMA, Blanco VG. *Analysis of PEDI Normative Data Between Spain and the United States*. Pediatric Physical Therapy. 2016;28(2):232-237.
14. Bayley N, Aylward GP. *Bayley Scales of Infant and Toddler Development*. 4th ed. NCS Pearson; 2019.
15. Brigance AH, French BF. *Brigance Inventory for Early Development III*. Curriculum Associates; 2013.
16. Toland MD, Gooden C, Li Z. *Reliability Evidence for the Hawaii Early Learning Profile Birth-3 Years: Interrater Agreement with Child Assessment Crediting—Final Report*. University of Kentucky; 2015.
17. Li Z, Gooden C, Toland MD. Reliability and validity evidence for the Hawaii early learning profile, birth-3 years. *J Early Interv*. 2019;41(1):62-83.
18. Folio MR, Fewell RR. *Peabody Developmental Motor Scales, Second Edition (PDMS-2): Examiner's Manual*. Pro-Ed; 2000.
19. Haley SM, Coster WJ, Dumas HM, et al. *The Pediatric Evaluation of Disability Inventory (PEDI)—Computer Adaptive Test*. Center for Rehabilitation Effectiveness-Care, Boston University; 2012.
20. Shore BJ, Allar BG, Miller PE, et al. Evaluating the discriminant validity of the pediatric evaluation of disability inventory: computer adaptive test in children with cerebral palsy. *Phys Ther*. 2017;97(6):669-676.
21. Judith KV, Maddox T. *Developmental Assessment of Young Children—Second Edition (DAYC-2)*. Pro-Ed; 2013.
22. Comfort PR, Gordon M. The keys to interactive parenting scale (KIPS): a practical observational assessment of parenting behavior. *NHSA Dialog*. 2006;9(1):22-48.
23. Comfort M, Gordon PR, Naples D. KIPS: an evidence-based tool for assessing parenting strengths and needs in diverse families. *Infants Young Child*. 2011:56-74.
24. Bundy A. *Test of Playfulness Manual*. Colorado State University; 2010.
25. Okimoto AM, Bundy A, Hanzlik J. Playfulness in children with and without disability: measurement and intervention. *Am J Occup Ther*. 2000;5:73-82.
26. Bundy AC, Waugh K, Brentnall J. Developing assessments that account for the role of the environment: an example using the Test of Playfulness and Test of Environmental Supportiveness. *OTJR*. 2009;29(3):135-143.
27. Morris C, Bartlett D. Gross motor function classification system: impact and utility. *Dev Med Child Neurol*. 2004;46(1):60-65.
28. Morris C. Development of the gross motor function classification system. *Dev Med Child Neurol*. 2008;50(4):249-253.

29. Palisano R, Rosenbaum P, Bartlett D, et al. Content validity of the expanded and revised gross motor function classification system. *Dev Med Child Neurol*. 2008;50(10):744-750.

30. Deville C, McEwen I, Arnold, SH, et al. Knowledge translation of the gross motor function classification system among pediatric physical therapists. *Pediatr Phys Ther*. 2015;27(4):376-384

31. King G, Strachan D, Tucker M, et al. The application of a transdisciplinary model for early intervention services. *Infants Young Child*. 2009;22(3):211-223.

32. Bell A, Corfield M, Davies J, et al. Collaborative transdisciplinary intervention in early years—putting theory into practice. *Child Care Health Dev*. 2010;36(1):142-148.

33. Lestari L, Ratnaningsih T. The effects of modified games on the development of gross motor skill in preschoolers. *Int J Eval Res Educ*. 2016;5(3):216-220.

34. Nwokah E, Hsu HC, Gulker H. The use of play materials in early intervention the dilemma of poverty. *Am J Play*. 2013;5(2):187-218.

35. Jeffries L, Fiss A, McCoy S, et al. Description of primary and secondary impairments in young children with cerebral palsy. *Pediatr Phys Ther*. 2016;28(1):7-14

36. Camden C, Wilson B, Kirby A, et al. Best practice principles for management of children with developmental coordination disorder (DCD): results of a scoping review. *Child Care Health Dev*. 2015;41(1):147-159.

37. Logan SW, Schreiber M, Lobo M, et al. Real-world performance: physical activity, play, and object-related behaviors of toddlers with and without disabilities. *Pediatr Phys Ther*. 2015;27(4):433-441.

38. Zeng N, Ayyub M, Sun H, et al. Effects of physical activity on motor skills and cognitive development in early childhood: a systematic review. *Biomed Res Int*. 2017:1-13.

39. Gmmash AS, Effgen SK. Early intervention therapy services for infants with or at risk for cerebral palsy. *Pediatr Phys Ther*. 2019;31(3):242-249.

40. Morgan C, Darrah J, Gordon AM. Effectiveness of motor interventions in infants with cerebral palsy: a systematic review. *Dev Med Child Neurol*. 2016;58(9):900-909.

41. An M, Palisano RJ, Yi CH, et al. Effects of a collaborative intervention process on parent empowerment and child performance: a randomized controlled trial. *Phys Occup Ther Pediatr*. 2019;39(1):1-15.

42. Morgan C, Novak I, Dale RC, et al. Single blind randomised controlled trial of GAME (Goals—Activity—Motor Enrichment) in infants at high risk of cerebral palsy. *Res Dev Disabil*. 2016;55:256-267.

43. Surkar SM, Edelbrock C, Stergiou N, et al. Sitting postural control affects the development of focused attention in children with cerebral palsy. *Pediatr Phys Ther*. 2015:16-22.

44. Van der Linde BW, van Netten JJ, Otten B, et al. Activities of daily living in children with developmental coordination disorder: performance, learning, and participation. *Phys Ther*. 2015;95(11):1496-1506.

45. Blauw-Hospers CH, Hadders-Algra M. A systematic review of the effects of early intervention on motor development. *Dev Med Child Neurol*. 2005:421-432.

46. Cardoso A, de Campos AC, dos Santos MM, et al. Motor performance of children with Down syndrome and typical development at 2 to 4 and 26 months. *Pediatr Phys Ther*. 2015;27:135-141.

47. Chiarello LA, Palisano RJ, Orlin MN, et al. Understanding participation of preschool-age children with cerebral palsy. *J Early Interv*. 2012;34(1):3-19.

48. Gannotti ME. Coupling timing of interventions with dose to optimize plasticity and participation in pediatric neurologic populations. *Pediatr Phys Ther*. 2017:S37-S47.

49. Wynarczuk KD, Chiarello LA, Fisher K, et al. Development of student goals in school-based practice: physical therapists' experiences and perceptions. *Disabil Rehabil*. 2019;42:3591-3605.

50. Brewer K, Pollock N, Wright V. Addressing the challenges of collaborative goal setting with children and their families. *Phys Occup Ther Pediatr*. 2014;34(2):138-152.

51. Carswell A, McColl MA, Baptiste S, et al. The Canadian occupational performance measure: a research and clinical literature review. *Can J Occup Ther*. 2004:210-222.

52. Chiarello L. Excellence in promoting participation: striving for the 10 Cs—client-centered care, consideration of complexity, collaboration, coaching, capacity building, contextualization, creativity, community, curricular changes, and curiosity. *Pediatr Phys Ther*. 2017:S16-S22.

53. Chiarello LA, Effgen SK, Jeffries L, et al. Student outcomes of school-based physical therapy as measured by goal attainment scaling. *Pediatr Phys Ther*. 2016:277-284.

54. Academy of Pediatric Physical Therapy. Appraisals, task force on school-based physical therapy performance. School-Based Physical Therapy Special Interest Group. www.pediatricapta.org. Accessed December 2, 2019.

55. Wynarczuk KD, Chiarello LA, Gohrband CL. Goal development practices of physical therapists working in educational environments. *Phys Occup Ther Pediatr*. 2017;37(4):425-444.

56. Vialu C, Doyle M. Determining need for school-based physical therapy under IDEA: commonalities across practice guidelines. *Pediatr Phys Ther*. 2017;29(4):350-355.

57. Wynarczuk KD, Chiarello LA, Fisher K, et al. School-based physical therapists' experiences and perceptions of how student goals influence service and outcomes. *Phys Occup Ther Pediatr*. 2019:1-22.

58. Kaminker MK, Chiarello LA, Chiarni-Smith JA. Decision making for physical therapy service delivery in schools: a nationwide analysis by geographic region. *Pediatr Phys Ther*. 2006:204-213.

59. Kaminker MK, Chiarello LA, O'Neil ME, et al. Decision making for physical therapy service delivery in schools: a nationwide survey of pediatric physical therapists. *Phys Ther*. 2004:919-933.

60. Effgen SK, Myers CT, Myers D. National distribution of physical and occupational therapists serving children with disabilities in education environments. *Phys Disabil Educ Relat Serv*. 2007:47-61.

61. Effgen SK, McCoy SW, Chiarello LA, et al. Physical therapy-related child outcomes in school: an example of practice-based evidence methodology. *Pediatr Phys Ther*. 2016;28(1):47-56.

62. Novak I, McIntyre S, Morgan C, et al. A systematic review of interventions for children with cerebral palsy: a state of the evidence. *Dev Med Child Neurol*. 2013;55(10) 885-910.

63. Coster W, Deeney P, Haltiwanger J, et al. *School Function Assessment*. The Psychological Corporation; 1998.

64. Jeffries LM, McCoy SW, Effgen SK, et al. Description of the services, activities, and interventions within school-based physical therapist prctices across the United States. *Phys Ther*. 2019;99(1):98-108.

65. Chiarello LA, Effgen SK, Jeffries LM, et al. Relationship of school-based physcial therapy service to student goal achievement. *Pediatr Phys Ther*. 2020;32(1):26-33.

66. Donnelly JE, Hillman CH, Castelli D, et al. Physical activity, fitness, cognitive function, and academic achievement in children: a systematic review. *Med Sci Sports Exerc*. 2016;48(6):1197-1222.

67. Callanen A. Developmental Coordination Disorder (Physical Therapy)—CE Module. CINAHL Rehabilitation Guide, EBSCO Publishing. http://eds.a.ebscohost.com/eds/pdfviewer/pdfviewer?vid=6&sid=67501176-0302-4fbc-abe8-a90ba96c7a7a%40sessionmgr4007. Accessed November 9, 2018.

68. Effgen SK, McEwen I. Review of selected physical therapy interventions for school-age children with disabilities. *Phys Ther Rev*. 2008;13(5):297-312.

69. Thomason HK, Wilmarth MA. Provision of school-based physical therapy services: a survey of current practice patterns. *Pediatr Phys Ther*. 2015;27(2):161-169.

70. Mâsse LC, Miller AR, Shen J, et al. Patterns of participation across a range of activities among Canadian children with neurodevelopmental disorders and disabilities. *Dev Med Child Neurol*. 2013;55(8):729-736.

71. Fox B, Moffett GE, Kinnison C, et al. Physical activity levels of children with down syndrome. *Pediatr Phys Ther*. 2019;31(1):33-41.

72. Potvin MC, Snider L, Prelock P, et al. Recreational participation of children with high functioning autism. *J Autism Dev Disord.* 2013;43(2):445-457.

73. Stanish H, Curtin C, Must A, et al. Physical activity levels, frequency, and type among adolescents with and without autism spectrum disorder. *J Autism Dev Disord.* 2017:785-794.

74. Schenker R, Coster W, Parush S. Neuroimpairments, activity performance, and participation in children with cerebral palsy mainstreamed in elementary schools. *Dev Med Child Neurol.* 2005:808-814.

75. Srinivasan SM, Pescatello LS, Bhat AN. Current perspectives on physical activity and exercise recommendations for children and adolescents with autism spectrum disorders. *Phys Ther.* 2014;94(6):875-889.

76. Adair B, Ullenhag A, Rosenbaum P, et al. Measures used to quantify participation in childhood disability and their alignment with the family of participation-related constructs: a systematic review. *Dev Med Child Neurol.* 2018;60(11):1101-1116.

77. Kafri M, Osnat AE. From motor learning theory to practice: a scoping review of conceptual frameworks for applying knowledge in motor learning to physical therapist practice. *Phys Ther.* 2019;99(12):1628-1643.

78. Palisano RJ, Chiarello LA, King GA, et al. Participation-based therapy for children with physical disabilities. *Disabil Rehabil.* 2012;34(12):1041-1052.

79. Dragoo KE. *The Individuals with Disabilities Education Act (IDEA) Funding: A Primer.* Congressional Research Service; 2019.

80. National Center for Education Statistics. Children and youth with disabiltiies. https://nces.ed.gov/programs/coe/indicator_cgg.asp. Accessed May 2019.

81. PL 100-360. Medicare Catastrophic Coverage Act of 1988. July 1, 1988.

82. OSERS. *40th Annual Report to Congress on the Implementation of the Individuals with Disabilities Education Act, 2018.* Department of Education; 2018.

83. Effgen SK, Kaminker MK. Nationwide survey of school-based physical therapy practice. *Pediatr Phys Ther.* 2014;26(4):394-403.

84. Schreiber J, Stern P, Marchetti G, et al. School-based pediatric physical therapists' perspectives on evidence-based practice. *Pediatr Phys Ther.* 2008;20(4):292-302.

85. Chiarello LA, Effgen SK. Updated competencies for physical therapists working in early intervention. *Pediatr Phys Ther.* 2006;18(2):148-158.

86. Effgen SK, Chiarello LA, Milbourne SA. Updated competencies for physical therapists working in schools. *Pediatr Phys Ther.* 2007:266-274.

87. Damiano DL, Leonard R. 2014 Section on pediatrics knowledge translation lecture: clinicians and researchers on the same path toward facilitating family goals for mobility and participation. *Pediatr Phys Ther.* 2015;27(2):105-12.

88. Arbesman M, Lieberman D, Berlanstein DR. Method for the systematic reviews on occupational therapy and early intervention and early childhood services. *Am J Occup Ther.* 2013;67(4):389-394.

89. US Department of Education. IDEA. https://sites.ed.gov/idea/statute-chapter-33. Accessed November 7, 2019.

90. Webster EK, Ulrich DA. Evaluation of the psychometric properties of the test of gross motor development—third edition. *J Motor Learn Dev.* 2017:45-58.

91. Ulrich D. *Test of Gross Motor Development: Examiner's Manual.* 2nd ed. Pro-Ed; 2000.

92. Fitzgerald D, Hickey C, Delahunt E, et al. Six-minute walk test in children with spastic cerebral palsy and children developing typically. *Pediatr Phys Ther.* 2016;28(2):192-199.

93. Fiss AL, Jeffries L, Bjornson K, et al. Developmental trajectories and reference percentiles for the 6-minute walk test for children with cerebral palsy. *Pediatr Phys Ther.* 2019;31(1):51-59.

94. Lammers AE, Hislop AA, Flynn Y, et al. The 6-minute walk test: normal values for children 4-11 years of age. *Arch Dis Child.* 2008;93(6):464-468.

95. David KS, Sullivan M. Expectations for walking speeds: standards for students in elementary schools. *Pediatr Phys Ther.* 2005:120-127.

96. Christensen C, Haddad A, Maus E. Reliability and validity of the 50-ft walk test for idiopathic toe walking. *Pediatr Phys Ther.* 2017:238-243.

97. American Physical Therapy Association. *Guide to Physical Therapist Practice.* 3rd ed. APTA; 2014.

7

Adaptive Equipment

Terri Wonsettler

>> Introduction

The ability of a person to function in daily life relies on context. *Functioning*, as defined by the World Health Organization (WHO) in the International Classification of Functioning, Disability, and Health (ICF), refers to all body functions, activities, and participation.[1] *Disability* is a term for impairments, activity limitations, and participation restrictions.[1] ICF also lists environmental factors that interact with these components.[1] Children with disabilities often need help interacting within their environments. This help may come from family members, teachers, peers, and health care professionals such as physical and occupational therapists (OTs). Physical therapists and OTs are able to teach a child to function in a variety of environments and to transfer functional skills to newly encountered environments through direct treatment and consultation, often incorporating adaptive equipment into the plan of care. The use of adaptive equipment is an intervention strategy known to improve function and to mitigate negative environmental or contextual elements that can be barriers to the child's participation.[2]

Physical therapists have many assistive products at their disposal to help children with disabilities with positioning, mobility, activities of daily living (ADLs), and interacting with various environments. *Assistive technology* (AT) is an umbrella term covering the systems and services related to the delivery of assistive products and services.[3] These products or services are generally referred to as *adaptive equipment.*

Most adaptive equipment can be classified as assistive, alternative, or augmentative technology.[4,5] *Assistive technology (AT) devices* include any item, piece of equipment, software program, or product system that is used to increase, maintain, or improve the functional capabilities of persons with disabilities.[4] Devices such as modified eating utensils that are easier to grip with a hand that has limited range of motion (ROM) and orthotic devices that stabilize a particular joint(s) to allow for safe and energy-efficient ambulation are examples of AT. *Alternative technology* provides a substitute means toward the same end function, such as using a wheelchair for mobility in the community instead of walking.

An *augmentative device* supplements an inadequate function, but the child's unaided function remains. This would be the case for a child with dysarthria who can be understood by his family, but needs a speech-generating device (SGD) to be understood by unfamiliar listeners.[4]

Adaptive equipment can also be classified as low-technology (low-tech), mid-tech, or high-tech devices.[2] Examples of low-tech devices are pencil grips or eating utensil grips, using a bench to add foot support in front of a chair or toilet, or using a pointer to indicate choices on a communication board. Mid-tech equipment includes relatively complicated mechanical devices such as powered toys, recording devices, and wheelchairs. High-tech equipment uses complex electronic devices and includes note-taking devices, screen readers, computers with voice recognition or voice output software, electronic communication devices that use eye gaze to elicit digital speech, and powered wheelchairs.[4,6,7] Physical therapists can often assist a family to employ low-tech devices either as a therapeutic tool or as a temporary solution to improve until a high-tech device can be obtained.

Many new commercially available products are being developed continually in an attempt to meet the equipment needs of children with disabilities. Customized equipment can be fabricated to meet individual specifications for a child. The great variety of products and materials available and the constantly changing market present a challenge to the therapist who provides parents with suggestions regarding equipment. How can students, recent graduates, or physical therapists with minimal experience working with children acquaint themselves with these products and feel confident guiding families to make adaptive equipment choices for their children? What conditions should be evaluated before making decisions regarding adaptive equipment? What is the true role of adaptive equipment for children with physical disabilities? Are there particular contraindications for use of adaptive equipment? These questions are addressed in this chapter, the main goal of which is to provide the student and the therapist who is inexperienced in pediatrics with a theoretical construct to facilitate decision making about adaptive equipment, regardless of familiarity with any particular piece of equipment.

The equipment discussed in this chapter provides the child with an adaptive means to participate in activities similar to his/her typically developing peers. The children who benefit from AT can have significant physical limitations affecting their postural control and motor skills, including the ability to sit and engage in floor play with siblings, sit at the dinner table with family, hold his/her head upright to eat, stand, crawl, or walk in their home or environments. These limitations can also affect their ability to sit safely in a car seat, sit independently during toileting or bathing, transfer to different areas, participate in recreational activities, or even maintain a safe position in bed. These children can lack the skills needed to interact with toys, feed themselves, complete schoolwork, or use their speech to communicate with others.

Children who appear to have less severe physical involvement such as poor endurance, hypotonia, and pain can also benefit from AT to keep up with the activity level of their typical peers. For example, a child with hypotonia or a cardiac condition may be able to ambulate on even surfaces throughout the home, but lacks the endurance to ambulate through a long corridor or over uneven terrain independently or safely. He or she would be at risk for falls and would likely benefit from a manual or powered wheelchair to safely and independently maneuver through school hallways between classes, stores in the community, corridors at medical buildings, and outdoors while attending/engaging in sporting events with family or friends. It is important that the physical therapist collaborates with the child, family, and treatment team to consider all areas of the particular child's life and determine whether adaptive equipment can be used to compensate for a physical impairment or remediate skills for function.

» Common types of adaptive equipment

The common types of adaptive equipment that are considered for children with disabilities are as follows, with brief descriptions.

- Seating and positioning components: These include any seat cushions, backrests, headrests, footrests, or other supports that can be added to or configured with an adaptive positioning device. These can also be used to adapt off-the-shelf toys or chairs for the child's use.
- Adaptive positioning chairs: These are chairs adapted to provide additional support that cannot be provided by a standard chair. These often provide options for height adjustment to allow the child to be raised or lowered between table height and floor height (Fig. 7.1).
- Seated wheeled mobility devices: Adaptive strollers and manual and powered wheelchairs make up the three general categories of wheeled mobility devices that can

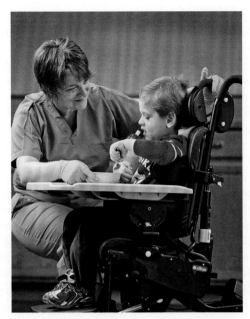

FIGURE 7.1. Rifton Activity Chair on high–low base.

provide the child with mobility and maximal independence during any stage of development. Most of these devices can be configured to offer optimal postural support using adjustable seating and positioning components, as well as providing adjustments within the frames. These are discussed in detail later in this chapter.

- Standers: These support the child in various standing positions, and are typically categorized by supine, prone, multiple-position, sit-to-stand, and dynamic standers. These are discussed in detail later in this chapter.
- Gait trainers, walkers, and crutches: These provide varying degrees of support to the child to work on components of ambulation/mobility.
- Patient lifts/transfer devices: These consist of low-tech devices such as transfer boards/disks used in traditional therapy, or high-tech devices such as manual or power-operated hydraulic lift systems or overhead lifts. The high-tech devices are often necessary for a larger child who is becoming difficult for caregivers to transfer. Consideration for the child being transferred to all pertinent areas is important, including to bed, shower, or toilet. Transferring to the car and in the community is also important, and may entail the use of AT devices. In many instances, once a child reaches 50 lbs, home health agencies require the use of patient lift systems to prevent injury to the caregiver.
- Adaptive floor positioning devices: These include low-tech devices such as wedges or benches, or more complex positioning systems such as side-lyers, corner chairs, and prone positioning equipment. These are often considered for the early intervention population or for children with complex physical impairments who have limited positioning alternatives.
- Adapted car seats: Special needs car seats offer more support or restraint options than do traditional off-the-shelf car seats. There are a number of different options available to accommodate a child with postural limitations and cognitive/behavioral impairments requiring escape-proof vehicle restraints.
- Bathing/showering/toileting equipment: These offer additional support for increased independence and safety with toileting, bathing, or showering. There are a number of options for stand-alone or combination devices. The physical therapist can assist the team by determining safe transfer options and postural supports/control.
- Adapted beds: These encompass beds that provide positioning options and protection from injury as well as beds that are for safety, to prevent a child from climbing or falling out of bed. The physical therapist can use knowledge of appropriate positioning techniques to assist the family and treatment team to determine optimal positioning options in the bed.
- Home and accessibility modifications: Although these modifications do not fall into the durable medical equipment (DME) category, they are a vital consideration when choosing adaptive equipment for a child. Home accessibility modifications include structural modifications such as widening doorways or installing ramps, stair lifts, and grab bars, and can also include electronic adaptations, environmental control systems (ECSs) to control door openers, lights, televisions, and temperature, among other items.
- Vehicle modifications: These can include consideration of ramps, wheelchair, or equipment lifts, or modifications to accommodate various adaptive car seats. The physical therapist can work with the family and team to assist with planning for vehicle modifications depending on the patient's skills and equipment needs.
- Adapted toys: These can range from adapted bicycles or sporting equipment to allow for participation in sports or recreational activities to adapting a battery-operated toy with a single switch to provide a child access to compensate for fine motor impairment.
- Adapted communication/computer technology: Although these devices are typically addressed by other professionals such as OTs, speech language pathologists, or rehabilitation engineers, it is important for the physical therapist to have a general understanding of the benefits of this equipment for the children they serve, and to consult with the treatment team regarding the child's positioning supports and physical access to the devices. Integrating these technologies is important when a child is using any type of positioning device such as a stander, wheelchair, or floor positioner.

Although the specific brands/models of equipment are constantly evolving, common types of equipment are discussed, along with approaches to practical clinical decision making. Although there are some scientific and objective guidelines on which to base a decision about adaptive equipment, a therapist must trial equipment with a child and use clinical reasoning to assist with decisions for the AT.

» Role of adaptive equipment

Adaptive equipment is becoming increasingly necessary as an adjunct to direct treatment. No child can realistically receive the constant handling needed throughout the day to prevent abnormal movement patterns and postures or to support more independent function. Although the physical therapist may teach families, day care providers, and teachers about methods of handling the child to encourage optimal development and function, the child must be allowed time to move, explore, and relax without constant assistance. The increased cost of direct care and the increasing number of children needing therapeutic intervention suggest a need for alternatives to direct patient handling.

One alternative is the use of adaptive equipment to facilitate correct positioning during a child's free independent time. Adaptive equipment can also provide reinforcement and use of positions, movements, and skills introduced to the child during treatment sessions. Similarly, abnormal or undesirable positions or movements can often be prevented or slowed by use of appropriate equipment.

Known benefits of using adaptive equipment include improved function, increased functional independence, increased control over one's environment, improved sense of autonomy and self-determination, increased motivation, enhanced social interactions, enhanced visual attention and perception, improved cognition, and improved ability for parents, other caregivers, and teachers to assist the child with function.[8] Adaptive equipment can facilitate the performance of skills that a child might otherwise be unable to accomplish, thereby promoting motor, sensory, cognitive, perceptual, emotional, and social development.[8,9] Adaptive equipment may help improve a child's performance over capacity. Capacity refers to what physical function a child can do, generally within a specific environment and without using aids.[1] For example, a child who does not have the capability to ambulate independently may use creeping as his primary form of independent locomotion. Although creeping may work in the home, it is not an appropriate form of locomotion in many community environments. Therefore, the child's performance (what he actually does in various places and situations)[1] lags behind his capability. In this case, he can locomote independently in the home, but not in the community. This child's need for a locomotive form in the community could be addressed by providing him with a wheelchair, raising his level of performance. As an alternative, if he learns to walk using an upper extremity gait aid such as a walker or gait trainer, he could improve his capacity for independent ambulation over time.

A child's motor performance may exceed his demonstrated capability, as scored on a standardized test, or his performance may lag behind his capability owing to environmental barriers. Among children with the same diagnosis and similar capability in gross motor skills, there may be different levels of performance, depending on the environment, social expectations, and time constraints.

In addition to having direct therapeutic benefits to improve a child's independence, adaptive equipment can play an important role in decreasing the demands on the caregiver by assisting with daily management of the child at home. An adaptive shower chair can safely position the child so that the caregiver can focus on the specific components of bathing. An adaptive positioning chair can help the child maintain trunk and neck alignment, so the caregiver can provide appropriate tactile or physical cues for safe feeding. A wheelchair or stroller can be used during long shopping trips to increase efficiency, yet promote participation with the parent's activity if ambulation is too inefficient in that situation.

It is important to understand the caregiver's goals and perspective when addressing adaptive and AT needs. For instance, one may think that a patient lift system would be beneficial to a family; however, oftentimes, the caregivers continue to manually lift the child owing to time constraints or because this has become part of their routine. It is often not until the caregiver has an injury or physical limitation that they employ a patient lift.

Although adaptive equipment should be prescribed with the goal of achieving maximum benefits with the least restriction, this ideal approach may occasionally need to be compromised. For example, ideal goals may not be possible because of architectural or financial barriers that prohibit using or obtaining certain adaptive devices. When barriers (behavioral, architectural, or financial) exist, the therapist must analyze the short-term needs of the family and the long-term goals for the child before making a decision or recommendation.

» Professionals involved with choosing adaptive equipment

Decisions to use adaptive equipment should be made in collaboration between the physical therapist, the family, and others who are involved in the child's life. This may include the OT, speech language pathologist, teacher, nurse, aide, and doctor. The child's input is also vital. Involvement of the DME dealer who is providing the equipment is extremely important. A dealer with qualifications to provide complex rehabilitation technology (CRT) with representatives who are credentialed Assistive Technology Professionals (ATP) certified through the National Registry of Rehabilitation Technology Suppliers (NRRTS) is essential for provision of customized and complex AT.[10] Sometimes, it is necessary to have the manufacturer's representative involved when dealing with complex equipment.

Because technology progresses at a rapid pace, expecting all physical therapists or treatment team members to have a thorough knowledge of the specific assistive devices available would be unrealistic. Although AT is a specialty area, it is pertinent for the physical therapist to recognize that there is technology available that may benefit the child and to familiarize yourself with local programs or professionals who can conduct comprehensive evaluations. A referral to a specialized program would be appropriate for a child who has complex needs, and can consist of a team of professionals who may be certified ATP. The ATP certification recognizes demonstrated competence in analyzing the needs of consumers with disabilities, assisting in the selection of appropriate AT for the consumer's needs, and providing training in the use of the selected devices.[11] There are currently postgraduate educational programs dedicated to becoming specialized as an ATP. This entails completion of a combination of continuing education, a specific number of work service hours related to AT, and passing a certification examination. One must continue to meet the qualifications to maintain the certification. This is available for rehabilitation professionals, including, but not limited to, physical therapists and OTs, speech language pathologists, and rehabilitation engineering technologists (RET). A RET is a professional who applies engineering principles to the design, modification, customization, fabrication, and/or integration of AT to persons with disabilities.[11] A Seating and Mobility Specialist (SMS) has a specialty certification that recognizes demonstrated competence in seating and mobility assessment, funding resources, implementation of intervention, and outcome assessment and follow-up.[11] Information regarding obtaining certifications or a list of ATP- or SMS-certified professionals can be found by searching the Rehabilitation Engineering Society of North America (RESNA) website www.RESNA.org.[11]

» Precautions when using adaptive equipment

Adaptive equipment continues to evolve and become common in many environments. It is important to be aware that without proper implementation, training, and monitoring by a qualified professional such as the physical therapist, problems may arise from the way equipment is used by various caregivers. The safe use of the equipment, scheduling use of equipment throughout the child's day, psychosocial indications, and overall plan for equipment provision are all important factors when implementing AT.

Safety Issues

Ensuring the safe and correct use of the equipment is a top priority. The child and caregivers must be taught the correct methods of donning, doffing, and using equipment. Strategies such as color coding and numbering straps to make sure they are fastened to the proper endpoint in the proper sequence help avoid mistakes in donning the device. Specific safety features of the equipment, such as pelvic belts, positioning of shoulder harnesses, and use of wheel locks during transfers should be reviewed. The effects on the child should also be reviewed, such as monitoring for pressure injuries, or signs that the child is not tolerating the position in the equipment. This is particularly helpful when caregivers include a number of people in addition to the parents, such as

grandparents, babysitters, day care staff, teachers, and teachers' aides.

All adaptive equipment used with children should be inspected frequently to ensure the integrity of the equipment for continued safe utilization. Needed repairs should be addressed with preemptive action to avoid the likelihood of equipment breakdown that could cause injury or abrupt loss of function. Liability issues with custom-fabricated equipment must be addressed.

When implementing mobility equipment, the child's cognitive and judgment abilities as well as the safety of the environment should be addressed. Are the areas of the home or school child-proofed? Particularly when introducing power mobility, can the child maneuver within his environment, in terms of both his own safety and the safety of others?

To further avoid unsafe circumstances and injury, equipment should always be used in the intended manner for which it was manufactured. The therapist, along with the equipment provider, is responsible for instructing the child and caregivers in the use of the AT and should not assume that safe use of equipment is common knowledge.

Balance between Equipment Use and Function

A carefully developed plan for therapeutic use of adaptive equipment is important, considering both the benefits and the potential deleterious effects of the equipment. Scheduling use of a particular piece of equipment throughout the day is important to avoid unintentional consequences which can compromise a child's development or safety. Despite the benefits of a particular device, it may not provide a rich environment for exploration or for learning new movements and transitions from one position to another. Gross motor development in typically developing children requires learning through doing, moving, and feeling. Sensory input, particularly vestibular, proprioceptive, and tactile, is required to produce optimal motor output that is both effective and varied. Static positioning, which occurs when some adaptive equipment is used excessively, can inhibit the development of motor skills by modifying sensory input, reducing spontaneous movement activity, and limiting opportunities to move and explore.

Use of equipment that places the child in static postures for frequent prolonged periods can also lead to other complications, such as joint contractures or pressure injuries, either of which may eventually require surgical intervention. Movement, by its very nature, is dynamic and requires the skillful coordination of both agonist and antagonist muscle groups to complete normal patterns of movement. Although equipment can support a child in a therapeutic static position to address some physiologic needs, the opportunity to experience the antagonist movement pattern is denied. For example, a device for side-lying provides an opportunity for the child to play while placed in neutral midline orientation. Although neutral midline orientation may be an appropriate goal, an asymmetric orientation is not inherently undesirable. An asymmetric orientation is a normal precursor to weight shifting, lateral flexion, and intra-axial rotation, and should not be completely excluded from the child's positioning by overreliance on the side-lying device. The therapist is responsible for teaching balanced movement patterns and positions. The person responsible for positioning a child must be aware of the benefits of various positions and must avoid constant and unchanging positioning habits that might interfere with the child's development of balanced movement and postures.

Anyone who has responsibility for the child must understand the therapeutic goals of using equipment and monitoring its use to maximize the benefits and minimize the deleterious effects.

Careful scheduling of equipment positioning is very important. Care must be taken not to continuously "transfer" the child between devices, so that the equipment becomes a substitute for handling or positioning of the child or providing independent movement experiences. This occurrence can be a detriment to parent–child relationships and a barrier to continued skill acquisition. Equipment is not a substitute for treatment or providing times of free movement or having hands-on interaction with the child. Poor balance of equipment use may restrict the learning of active postural transitions and movement for exploration, two major aspects of normal motor development. Just as appropriate equipment can be useful for satisfying the overall needs of a child, overuse or misuse of equipment can be detrimental.

The physical therapist can work with the school team to establish an equipment schedule for the child. For instance, the child can sit in a supportive wheelchair or positioning chair during classroom instruction so he can focus on the cognitive learning task, and then ambulate between classes or "run an errand" using his gait trainer in the hallways. This provides the child with the support needed to focus on academics while also providing a means for working on gait and endurance by ambulating throughout the day. It is important to support the family and to help them understand the positive role of equipment in their lives rather than as a replacement for improving physical skills such as ambulation. Without the collaboration between the physical therapist and the team of professionals who work with the child, a balance of equipment use versus facilitation of skills will not occur.

Planning for the Future

With the increasing difficulty in receiving reimbursement for expensive equipment for the child with a physical disability, the therapist must anticipate and plan carefully for the child's physical growth, developmental changes, and acquisition of new skills, and must understand the progression typical of their diagnosis. The inexperienced therapist may overlook the changing needs of the child. For instance, a child who requires a wheelchair that has a heavy durable seating system to proximally support the head and neck for feeding and swallowing alignment during the early years may need a lighter weight wheelchair and seating system in the near future to facilitate functional self-propulsion. Despite the initial advantages of the wheelchair with a heavy aggressive seating system, meeting the child's needs for a lighter weight wheelchair as he/she gains proximal control may not have been the optimal choice for future mobility and socialization needs. Predicting the child's needs in the areas of growth and development, education, and recreational alternatives (e.g., wheelchair sports) is a monumental task, but one in which physical therapists must often participate at the request of insurers as well as local and state funding agencies. It is important to carefully and thoroughly document the child's body measurements and level of functioning at the time of equipment recommendation so that changes can be clearly and objectively noted when new more appropriate equipment needs to be justified.

Therapists must learn how various agencies and providers prefer to reconcile future needs and reimbursement patterns with the child's current needs. Insurance plans may dictate coverage for a specific DME device, such as a wheelchair, only once every 3 to 5 years. Funding limitations must be considered and contemplated carefully. The consequences of miscalculations in these decisions may be a child poorly accommodated in a device that does not meet the current needs or that will meet the needs for only a short time. In such instances, the therapist may explore difficult alternatives, such as borrowing or adapting existing equipment until the child is eligible for new equipment. Many communities are establishing lending programs for adaptive equipment, which can be found online. This has helped provide options for children as they await funding for the recommended equipment. Clearly, in addition to a child's current age and developmental level, growth and developmental change are critical aspects to consider when selecting adaptive equipment.

Psychosocial Issues

Carefully selected and implemented adaptive equipment can offer many opportunities and increase a child's independence, but equipment can also be psychosocially disadvantageous. Some of the more complex equipment often has a way of drawing attention to a child's disabilities and differences. At times, the extensive equipment can have the appearance of "overtaking" the child. The physical framework of the equipment can actually separate the child from his/her peers, which can be emotionally and socially challenging for the child with a disability. A child strapped into plastic, wood, and metal often seems to be the recipient of fewer hugs and physical affection. This may be simply because of the physical barriers caused by the equipment, but it may also be the result of adults and children who feel intimidated by the equipment and are fearful of disturbing something if they get too close to the child. Equipment manufacturers are continually modifying their designs to address this issue. As the physical therapist who is working with the child, take into account these barriers and provide options and choices that will reduce these barriers and be aesthetically pleasing to the child and family. The therapist may also assist to integrate the child and equipment into the classroom environment and facilitate interaction with other children to increase acceptance and inclusion.

On the positive side, equipment that increases a child's mobility and functional independence such as power mobility and integrated wheelchair standers[12] has been shown to lead to better success with all types of mobility and to enhance a child's cognitive, perceptual motor, and psychosocial development.[9,12]

» Determining a child's equipment needs

The primary therapist or team who provides routine care for a child should have established continually evolving short- and long-term goals for the child. Eventually, it may become clear to the therapist and/or team that adaptive equipment is needed to achieve some functional goals. Sometimes, because of the size or nature of the facility at which the child is treated or because the primary therapist lacks experience working with and recommending equipment, a referral to an outside agency, clinic, or therapist who is certified as an ATP or SMS may be helpful to determine needs and equipment to meet those needs. Whether the child is referred to a program specializing in AT or directly to an equipment vendor's establishment, the provision of appropriate equipment depends mainly on detailed and accurate information about both the child and the child's environment.[13] The primary therapist should either be present during the equipment evaluation or provide a detailed report with a summary of the child's needs and recommendations for equipment to ensure an accurate evaluation of the child's needs.

An initial determination of the child may include a thorough mat examination, a movement examination, an interview of the caregivers and child (when developmentally appropriate), an environmental review, and an evaluation of the child in relation to a specific piece of equipment.[13] Because of time restrictions, the examination may concentrate on one specific type of equipment or functional need (e.g., sitting), and additional examinations may be required for other equipment needs. Once the proper equipment has been ordered and received, the primary therapist should examine the child with the equipment to ensure that it suits the child and meets the identified goals. The child and the caregivers must be instructed in its correct use.

Examination and Evaluation of the Child

The parameters to be considered when evaluating a child's need for adaptive equipment are similar to those of most other examinations. The goal of such an examination, however, is to direct the therapist to the most appropriate equipment options available. A number of AT assessment tools have been developed.[14-16] The child, family, home, school, and other natural environments are evaluated, along with the child's current medical status and medical history. Many of these tools are available on the Internet. A therapist may

want to consult some of the existing tools and use them in part or totality as guidelines. Although every child is unique, using an assessment tool can strengthen the clinical decision-making process.

A vital part of the examination is to conduct a thorough mat observations, both in supine and sitting, particularly for the child with neuromotor deficits. The following specific items summarize what should be considered during the examination and evaluation of the child.

Range of Motion/Orthopedic Issues

Examining both active ROM and passive range of motion (PROM) is extremely important when determining adaptive equipment for an individual. If ROM limitations are not taken into consideration when setting up the equipment, optimal positioning, comfort, pressure relief, and function in the equipment will not be achieved. The critical areas that would affect positioning in adaptive equipment are as follows:

- Pelvic alignment: Examining for pelvic rotation, obliquity, and flexibility in the anterior/posterior planes will have a direct bearing on the way a seating system or piece of equipment is configured. A pelvic deformity will most likely need to be accommodated using a customized seat cushion.
- Hips: ROM of all planes of movement should be observed. The degree of hip flexion that can be obtained without affecting the position of the pelvis, both with the knee extended and with the knee in varying degrees of flexion should be examined. Typically, 90 degrees of hip flexion would be the recommended angle for functional sitting; however, restrictions in hip flexion and the effect on the pelvic position will override this concept. Checking for restrictions in abduction/adduction will affect the alignment of a person's femurs on the seat cushion, or the lower extremity (LE) position when using a stander. The amount of available hip extension and abduction will affect the standing position and equipment choice as well.
- Knees: The amount of knee extension available with and without hip flexion is crucial to setting up the optimal footrest or backrest angles of a seating system and will provide information pertinent to choosing the correct type of stander for the individual. If the child has hamstring tightness affecting the available knee extension, there will be an impact on the pelvic position and the footrest position of a seating system.
- Ankles: The available ankle ROM will affect the position and type of footplates for both sitting and standing.
- Trunk/neck: The trunk should be examined for flexible and fixed ROM. If there is a notable fixed or flexible spinal curvature or rotation, it would be important to know whether there is an orthotic device being recommended while sitting and/or standing, or whether surgical intervention is being planned. This would affect the type of equipment supports that are recommended. The ability to achieve midline and upright alignment of the trunk is

crucial to an individual's positioning in any type of equipment and has a direct effect on neck positioning/alignment for function.

- Upper extremities: Shoulder and elbow ROM restrictions that could have an overall effect on the backrest and upper body supports should be examined.

In some cases, it is recommended that the individual consult with an orthopedic or physical medicine and rehabilitation specialist to help determine whether orthotics, medication, or surgical intervention are necessary before making a final equipment decision. It is extremely important that the primary physical therapist working with the child address these issues before or as part of the equipment evaluation.

Muscle Tone

The therapist must evaluate patterns of movement with regard to decreased or increased muscle tone, tone dominance, and dystonia (uncontrolled, involuntary, extraneous movements). Does the child exhibit hypotonia or hypertonia, and to what degree? Is the dystonia of mild, moderate, or severe magnitude? Does the child have cortical control, manifested by a voluntary ability to initiate a pattern of movement? Does the child compensate, whether volitional or not, for uncomfortable positioning and/or movement? Is the child pursuing medical treatment such as medication or surgery that will have an effect on the tone?

A child's muscle tone and spasticity management need to be considered when in all positions, whether or not they are using adaptive positioning devices. Muscle tone has a significant effect on the child's ability to assume and maintain postural alignment and has an impact on the equipment choices. Positioning devices such as standers, adaptive seats, chairs, and floor positioners often have a modifying effect on muscle tone in these children. For instance, a child who has significant extensor tone or dystonia, as seen with many children with cerebral palsy, may exhibit extensor thrusting patterns, making it difficult to maintain positioning in a seat. This may result in the hips sliding forward on the seat cushion or the LEs pushing into full extension, leading to secondary issues of pressure injuries from the excess pressures placed on the edge of the seating system components, and can lead to equipment frequently breaking, because it will not withstand the heavy extraneous movements. This will have a significant impact on equipment choices and the way in which the equipment is configured. In some cases, a custom-contoured seat and back system or dynamic hardware components may be helpful. Many children have a significant degree of spasticity that results in a tendency for asymmetrical positioning and alignment. This is commonly seen with children who have had an anoxic event or traumatic brain injury. It is important to determine what type of supports and positioning can help the child assume and maintain midline symmetrical alignment.

In contrast, a child who has hypotonia may need to have more supportive equipment that will allow gravity and external supports to assist to maintain postural alignment. Tilt orientation may help the child maintain his head and upper trunk in an upright position. Many children have a number of mixed tonal impairments that will have an effect on their positioning and equipment needs.

Functional Muscle Control/Strength

Once ROM and tone are addressed, a positioning system that will provide adequate proximal support as a basis for maximal motor control and functional strength can be configured. This will allow the child to more effectively operate a powered wheelchair, propel a manual wheelchair or gait trainer, use a walker or access other technology such as communication devices/computers, or to safely participate in care activities such as feeding/swallowing, self-feeding, or play.

Manual muscle testing should be completed if possible, because this is objective information that may help justify a particular type of equipment. The degree of strength and motor control needed for functional use of the device must be determined. For example, use of a manual wheelchair requires adequate trunk control, upper extremity strength, and coordination. If the child does not have adequate skills, a standard manual wheelchair may not be an appropriate choice for independent mobility. A powered wheelchair that requires less strength and motor control may be more functional for the child. A powered wheelchair also has options for control that do not require upper extremity function. A physical therapist or an OT should be aware that there are alternative options for maneuvering a powered wheelchair using a hand-controlled joystick, including repositioning the joystick for easier access, using different joystick tops, reprogramming the joystick parameters, or using an alternative joystick that requires less pressure and movement to operate. There are many other types of powered wheelchair controllers that can be accessed using different body parts and movements, including a head array of switches or sip-and-puff controller. If a child has a consistent body movement and has adequate judgment and cognition, a means of control can be identified with the right equipment. If this is the case, a specific detailed assessment by an experienced ATP can help the therapist identify alternative methods for optimal management of the equipment. In choosing a motorized device, the strength and motor control of the upper extremities or alternative body parts to control the device are only two considerations. One must also evaluate cognitive, sensorimotor, and coping abilities, as discussed later in this chapter.

Strength plays a vital role in choosing standing and gait equipment for a child as well. The type of stander and orientation offered will differ, depending on the child's upper extremity or LE strength and his/her ability to maintain head/trunk control.

The child's needs will change depending on their stage of development, lifestyle, and activity choices. For a child who is able to ambulate, but has hypotonia, pain, or issues with endurance, the type of mobility device can vary. It is pertinent to evaluate their functional mobility for ambulation and endurance for ambulation and then consider the goals for a wheeled mobility device. For example, a child who has se-vere hypotonia such as a child with Ehlers–Danlos syndrome (EDS) may be able to ambulate in the home and classroom, but may need to use a wheelchair when in the community. A child who is elementary school aged and uses a walker to navigate in school may wish to consider a manual or pow-ered wheelchair once entering a larger middle school, for energy conservation purposes. On the same note, a child who uses a manual wheelchair in middle school may want to consider a power assist system or powered wheelchair upon entering high school or college, to contend with the distances and outdoor maneuvering required. These are all factors that must be carefully considered and discussed with the child, caregivers, and treatment team, because each situ-ation is individualized.

In addition to the importance of addressing position-ing for mobility, it is vital to establish appropriate seating/positioning to address the child's access to other technology devices, such as augmentative communication or computer technology, or any environmental controls. The stability provided by the positioning device should be a substantial base of support to access these technologies using any body movement including hand, LE, upper extremity, head/neck, or even eye gaze control. A child's ability to control move-ments to access this equipment should be considered in all pertinent environments/equipment configurations. The physical therapist plays a vital role in providing information regarding the child's optimal movement patterns to the eval-uation team or DME provider.

Reflexes

A change of position with respect to gravity will also affect a child whose motor patterns are influenced by developmen-tal reflexes. The prone or supine position may increase or decrease the impact of the tonic labyrinthine reflex on the child's posture or movement. Because inadvertent facilitation of primitive or pathologic reactions may create a block in the normal developmental pattern, each piece of equipment should be evaluated for its effect on reflexes. For example, some devices for mobility, such as tricycles and bicycles, may facilitate a persistent asymmetric tonic neck reflex (ATNR). As the child pushes the pedal with the right foot, the head is turned toward the right side to enhance the effectiveness of the push. The child reverses this pattern when pushing with the left foot. The ATNR can also have an impact on the setup of a powered wheelchair joystick or communication/com-puter device. A child with ATNR may have optimal control of his hand movements to access this technology when his arm is fully extended. A careful balance of his extended up-per extremity position and head position in relation to keep-ing his visual fields intact must be addressed.

Under some circumstances, the only means for function is to use a primitive reflex. For example, the ATNR can have an impact on the setup of a powered wheelchair joystick or communication/computer device. A child with ATNR may

have optimal control of his hand movements to access this technology when his upper extremity is fully extended. A careful balance of his extended arm position and head po-sition in relation to keeping his visual fields intact and safe must be addressed. The use of devices to restrict or inhibit the influence of primitive reflexes is more common, thus providing an opportunity for the development of more nor-mal and symmetric patterns of movement.

Sensation/Skin Integrity

Children with diagnoses affecting sensation, such as spina bifida or spinal cord injury, offer different challenges when choosing and developing programs with adaptive equip-ment. A priority for a child with impaired or absent sensa-tion is to provide safe seating and upright positioning that is pressure relieving. The therapist should thoroughly examine the child's sensation through testing and consultation with the child and family, because they would likely have a keen awareness of the sensory impairment. Observing all areas of the person's skin is of significant importance. Particular attention must be paid to the skin over the spinal cord le-sion and to bony prominences, including the ischial tuberosi-ties, greater trochanters, sacrum, coccyx, femoral and tibial condyles, tibial tuberosities, fibular heads, and malleoli. The scapular areas and elbows can also be an area of concern. These bony prominences must also be monitored in a child with intact sensation but with limited ability to reposition because of poor motor control, weakness, or severe spas-ticity. As a child grows and gains weight, the pressure over these areas increases; therefore, pressure should continue to be monitored as they develop. It is ideal to evaluate pressure distribution and relief on a sitting surface using a pressure mapping system, which is a computerized system that mea-sures the interface pressure; in this case, between the user and the sitting surface.[17,18]

This is typically used by a qualified therapist or equipment provider who is an ATP.

Cognitive, Sensorimotor, and Social/Emotional Status

Many physical therapists are not trained specifically to evalu-ate cognition, some sensorimotor skills, or social/emotional development; however, it is critical to consider these areas when evaluating for adaptive equipment. The pediatric cli-ent's ability to functionally use adaptive equipment depends on a combination of physical abilities and cognitive, psycho-social, and sensorimotor skills including perception, motor planning, and reaction time. Neurosensory development and stimulation are integral to the development of motor skills as well as cognitive skills in the typically developing in-fant.[19] Although intelligence quotient (IQ) is not considered to be a good determinant of power-mobility potential, for example, other cognitive skills are key, including judgment, problem-solving abilities, and an understanding of cause and effect, direction, and spatial relationships.[9] Motivation, intel-ligence, and normal perception often overcome even severe physical impairments. The opposite is also true. Limitations in cognition, perception, or social/emotional skills may result in function that is lower than would be predicted by physical findings alone.

To develop realistic goals for a child, the physical therapist must take into consideration the whole child, and must integrate information obtained from the caregivers, teacher, social worker, OT, speech language pathologist, psychologist, and any other professionals working with the child to establish a therapeutic plan.[20] The stages in a child's life, environment, and caregiver expectations have a significant effect on the child's equipment needs at a given time. For instance, as an infant, the focus is typically on the child's physical developmental skills. At this point, many parents can have difficulty accepting adaptive equipment, because this may be a sign that there is permanent disability. When a child reaches preschool age, the need for seating and wheeled mobility may increase for participation with peers in the classroom and on the playground/outdoors. As the child moves on to elementary school, it can become even more important to maneuver between classes with peers and have an appropriate place to sit in a variety of classrooms. A stroller base may be inappropriate for a number of children in this situation. As the child approaches middle school or high school, the need for energy conservation and joint protection becomes paramount. Although the preteen may have the ability to propel a manual wheelchair, he/she may be more efficient at using a power wheelchair, power assist, or power add-on system. This will allow the person to expend less energy on mobility and focus on academics and socializing with peers. As the teenager prepares for postsecondary options such as vocational training or college, increased efficiency, energy conservation, and other functions may become priorities. A child who requires much care and is dependent also incurs changes in priorities as he/she moves through life stages. A younger child can be easily transferred to a variety of positioning devices throughout the school day. As the child ages and/or becomes bigger, there is less opportunity to transfer to various devices, and therefore multifunctional positioners can become more important and useful to meet their needs for positioning programs. Children who are graduating from high school and entering adult day programs need to have equipment that can be used throughout the day, with more adjustable positioning options to ensure they are obtaining pressure relief and having toileting, hygiene, and transfer needs met as easily as possible. The therapist plays a significant role in guiding the caregivers and child through this process, educating them to plan for the future.

Functional Skills

Examining functional skills requires integration of all available information, in an attempt to determine why a child behaves in a certain manner. The physical therapist must discover what functions the child is able to perform and how, what functions he or she is unable to perform and

why, and why the child does not do more. For example, if a 2-year-old child is not rolling or exploring the environment, the therapist must first assess why the child does not move and explore. Does he or she have a cognitive disability that limits the natural curiosity to explore the environment? Is the child afraid of moving because of visual, hearing, or other sensory impairments? Does the child exhibit a strong ATNR that acts as a physical limitation to rolling? Is abnormal muscle tone in certain body segments a barrier to movement? Has the child been placed in devices at home that limit the opportunity to develop independent mobility? Once a determination has been made as to why a child has delayed motor skills and decreased mobility, realistic recommendations for a therapy plan and adaptive equipment can be offered. Adaptive equipment can be used to both provide improved positioning and independent mobility and to provide opportunities to facilitate growth in the areas of cognition, initiation for movement, and socialization. It is important to provide opportunities for children to obtain some form of independent mobility at as young an age as possible to provide experiences to facilitate cognitive growth, initiation for movement, and decrease the chance for learned helplessness. The team should continue to monitor mobility with and without adaptive equipment to facilitate physical development of skills as well as to foster the skills obtained through independent mobility.[21,22] When a child has severely limited mobility without reasonable short- or long-term expectations of gaining device-unaided mobility, it would be appropriate to introduce mobility-related adaptive equipment for the purpose of remediation of the problem(s).

The child with profound cognitive deficits may not use equipment that is provided because he or she lacks the motivation to explore his or her environment. For the child with visual or hearing impairments to learn to manipulate the environment, methods for exploration of that environment need to be improved by first addressing the specific sensory impairment. If a child lacks experience in exploring the environment owing to lack of opportunity, the therapist must offer as much freedom of movement and equipment-free mobility as is possible and educate the family about the importance of providing the child with opportunities to move. On the other hand, sometimes equipment can be used therapeutically to provide opportunities for partial participation with mobility. A child may participate in using a powered wheelchair with assistance, for the purpose of moving toward and away from objects, increasing their attendance to visual stimuli and/or their understanding of cause/effect through independent movement. Although equipment may eventually play a role in each of these situations, adaptive equipment should supplement and complement function with the least amount of restriction to the child.

The child who is physically limited may show great improvement in cognitive ability, social interaction, and independence when mobility is improved.[9,21,22] When adaptive equipment or devices are used judiciously, the improvement in mobility should occur without increases in abnormal reflexes or patterns of movement in children with sensorimotor impairments.

Examining a child's ROM, muscle tone, motor control, strength, reflexes, sensation, perception, cognition, social/emotional skills, and functional abilities is an integral component of the examination of the child. When these parameters are considered and the reasons for a child's motor behaviors are understood, goals and appropriate intervention strategies can be planned for the child, including recommending appropriate adaptive equipment.

Standardized or Objective Test Measures

The use of standardized tests or objective measures can be used to support decisions to use adaptive equipment in certain situations. For instance, with a child who has a diagnosis that results in joint pain or low endurance, it may be beneficial to conduct a 6-minute walk test[23] or a Borg Rating of Perceived Exertion Scale[23] to determine whether a wheelchair would benefit them for long-distance mobility. Use of a pulse oximeter to measure blood oxygen levels can be helpful to determine the effects of positioning for a child with significant motor impairment. Observation of the child's posture and gait pattern over the extended time or evaluation of blood pressure and/or oxygen saturation level can be beneficial in both assisting with decision making and in justification to a funding source that a wheelchair is indeed a medically necessary option. The Functional Mobility Assessment is a very useful tool to assist the child, therapist, and family to prioritize needs for AT. This is a simple and validated consumer-centered questionnaire measuring a person's satisfaction in performing common mobility-related activities of daily living (MRADLs). This can be used as an outcome measure to compare scores before and after being provided with a mobility device, such as a wheelchair, walking aid, or prosthetic device.[24]

The Power-mobility Community Driving Assessment (PCDA) and the Power-mobility Indoor Driving Assessment (PIDA) maneuvering of powered wheelchairs can both be used to assist with decision making as well as to validate decisions for power mobility to caregivers and funding sources.[25]

Evaluation of Environmental Accessibility

Evaluating the ability to use the equipment in the home, school, and community environments, as well as the ability to transport the equipment between environments is of great importance. The home environment, opportunities in the home, and parental expectations have been shown to influence the development of a child, including motor development.[26,27] Acquiring, learning to use, and following through with adaptive equipment for a child will be highly influenced by the child's family, home, and other natural environments. Overall, physical therapy goals for the child

using adaptive equipment must be compatible with the goals of all caregivers. This is essential for enabling a child to participate well in both school and home domains.[2,20] Because adaptive equipment is often used across multiple settings, problems sometimes arise from conflicting needs and disparities between caregivers. These conflicts over adaptive aids may arise in particular for the child who lives in a community residential setting owing to the need for collaboration among several different caregivers or rotating staff.

Useful information can be obtained by asking the family members about their expectations for the device being considered. This opportunity for family members to express their opinions promotes a dialogue between family and therapist, allowing the therapist to assist them to establish realistic goals. Collaboration between all people involved is imperative to ensure support and optimal outcome and may require compromise.

Objective data about the family and home include the following categories and questions.

Physical Layout of the Home

Is the residence a house or an apartment, rented or owned? Is there more than one residence?
Is this a multiple-level home, ranch, or split-level residence?
Is there a level entrance into the home, and, if so, are there opportunities for accommodations to be made? (ramp, elevator, porch lift)
Is there a way to get the equipment from a vehicle or bus stop into the home for use or at least into a garage for protection from the elements?
Is there space for equipment use and storage?
Are the structure and size of the home adequate for equipment to be used in the home?
How large are the rooms, and is there an open floor plan?
How many steps are found in the home?
How wide are the doorways and hallways?
Are bathrooms, tubs, and toilets accessible?
What type of floor coverings are in the home?

Often, the therapist can help narrow the equipment choices so that the DME representative can then take the equipment to the home to ensure accessibility with the family.

Community Factors

The community is a very important factor and affects equipment choices. Considerations are as follows:

- Does the family live in a rural, urban, or suburban environment?
- What type of terrain exists just outside the home? Are there paved sidewalks, dirt, or gravel driveways?
- Are there social or sporting activities to attend that entail access to terrain or other accessibility issues?

Transportation Factors

The ability to transport the adaptive equipment using a personal motor vehicle or public transportation must be considered, particularly when choosing a wheeled mobility device. In the case of a very young child who will ride in the vehicle using a car seat, the ability to disassemble the equipment and load in/out of the vehicle is paramount. If a family has a sedan with a trunk, the equipment must be easily folded or disassembled for transport. A sport utility vehicle will typically provide more space with less disassembly necessary; however, the equipment will need to be light enough to lift into the rear of the vehicle. A minivan or an adapted van can provide more space and an easier option for loading the equipment. These factors can have a direct impact on equipment choices and may entail compromises. Ramps or vehicle modifications may be needed to accommodate some equipment, such as a standard powered wheelchair or a heavy wheelchair with a tilt-in-space system. Also consider whether the young child can be safely accommodated in an off-the-shelf car seat versus requiring a special needs car seat. Special needs car seats are discussed later in this chapter.

When a child becomes larger and it is too difficult to transfer into a car seat or there is life-sustaining medical equipment that needs to be transported, it may become necessary to remain seated in the wheelchair during vehicle transport. The wheelchair or stroller would be used as the vehicle seat. This would necessitate a vehicle that has been modified to load the occupied wheelchair into the vehicle and to be secured with an appropriate tie-down system. A separate occupant restraint would be needed to restrain the child. American National Standards Institute (ANSI)/RESNA WC19 is a voluntary standard that specifies design requirements for wheelchairs that are suitable for use as seats in motor vehicles.[28-30] WC20 is a standard related to the wheelchair or stroller seating systems used for vehicle transport.[31] These standards continue to be developed to increase the level of wheelchair occupant safety and crash protection during transit. Many of the wheelchair mobility devices have options to be equipped with WC19 transit options, which can include tie-down hooks on the frame and tether straps that are used to secure the wheelchair/stroller into a motor vehicle. The mobility devices typically need to be specifically configured to qualify as WC19 compliant. To qualify as WC19 compliant, the equipment must be set up with the transit option, including the frame and seating system components that were used during an intense and costly forward-facing crash-testing procedure. Oftentimes, the wheelchair/stroller frame has the option for tie-down hooks that would provide a consistent and safe place to attach the securement straps for vehicle transport; however, the seating system or other wheelchair components that are necessary for the child will negate the WC19 compliance. Although at this time specific laws do not require that a mobility device be WC19 compliant to be transported with an occupied in a motor vehicle, it is highly recommended that as best practice, transit options

be considered for your clients.[28,29] The concept of using transit options continues to evolve.

Public transportation is another factor that needs to be addressed. Whether a child will be transported to/from school by the caregiver/family or in a school bus with wheelchair accommodations versus while seated in a car seat is considered. Some public transportation companies require that the wheelchair or adapted stroller be equipped with tie-down hardware on the frame to transport the device. The availability of privately owned vehicles and/or public transportation is important when the therapist is considering the type of mobility equipment to be purchased.[28,29] The therapist can provide education to the family and assist them in making decisions regarding safety and needs of the child and family.

In contrast to a child who is younger and/or dependent in a motor vehicle, the physical therapist must consider vehicle use for teenagers or young adults who may be considering driving a motor vehicle. Will the person need to drive the wheelchair into the adapted vehicle and drive the vehicle while seated in the wheelchair? Will the person wish to transfer into the vehicle seat and then need to independently load the wheelchair into the vehicle? These options should be factored into the decision-making process. The physical therapist can assist the person to learn the skills needed to manage the transfers and the equipment safely and to use proper body mechanics. Referral to a program specializing in adapted driving can be helpful for the person to determine needs for adapted driving controls and vehicles.

It is essential to educate and assist the family to prepare for the future needs of their child to establish long-term plans for accommodation. Understanding the child's development, diagnosis, and skill progression or regression is important. Providing a family with resources to explore local companies who deal with adapted vehicles can be useful for planning.

Socioeconomic Factors

The cost of equipment and funding resources may have a serious impact on the final decision regarding adaptive equipment for the child with a disability. When making a decision about adaptive equipment, the therapist, often in conjunction with a social worker, must examine insurance coverage, other third-party payment systems, funding agencies within the community, and potential rental options. Before equipment is ordered, it is essential that the availability and source of funding is determined. Size of the family, daily routine, and the time available to spend with the child with special needs, as well as potential options for others to help the family, must be considered. Compliance with the suggested use of adaptive equipment may ultimately be the main consideration in the decision-making process. If there is little realistic expectation that the child will benefit from having the equipment or that the equipment will be used by the family, there may be little justification for its purchase.

Cultural Factors

In addition to socioeconomic factors, other cultural factors must be considered and respected. Increasingly, physical therapists and other health care professionals find themselves working with clients whose culture differs considerably from the dominant culture of the community or from their own culture. It is the therapist's responsibility to learn enough about a child's culture to effectively and competently provide interventions, including recommendations for adaptive equipment. Some cultural issues that need to be addressed include the following:

Who makes the decisions in the family?

Are there cultural sensitivities regarding receiving financial aid to purchase equipment?

Does the equipment being considered violate any religious beliefs of the family?

If there are language barriers, do the family and child understand the need for the equipment and the process for acquiring the equipment?

Will language differences interfere with teaching the family and the child proper use of the equipment, and can these problems be overcome?

Is the home structure amenable to safe and easy use of the equipment being considered?

Are there cultural beliefs that preclude the use of certain equipment? For example, in some cultures, technology such as electricity or computers is not used in the home. These beliefs may affect the use of powered wheelchairs, home-suctioning equipment, and some communications aids.[32]

Educational Setting

The physical therapist must consider the school setting in which the child may spend a large portion of the day. He or she must determine whether the child is enrolled in a specialized school for children with disabilities or mainstreamed into a regular school and/or classroom. In a specialized school, teachers and staff are usually accustomed to implementing AT, and these teachers will initiate the purchase or procurement of the equipment. Whether in a specialized school or regular community school, the therapist can facilitate smooth implementation of the equipment into the classroom. The following factors should be addressed by the team members to ensure successful integration of the technology into the child's school environment[8]:

- Complete a multidisciplinary evaluation in the child's natural environment.
- Include the child, family, and all team members in the decision-making process.
- Plan for the use of specific adaptive equipment in the school environment, by including the equipment in the Individualized Education Plan (IEP) and linking the equipment to the educational goals.
- Educate all staff involved in the operation of the equipment and the goals for equipment use.

- Establish a plan for scheduling use of equipment with the child and sharing equipment among other children. Clearly mark the equipment adjustments or provide simple resources for staff to ensure ease of setup and proper alignment/use of the equipment specific to each child.
- Continually monitor the child and equipment for growth adjustments or adjustments due to progression or regression of skills.
- Assist in solving problems related to care of the equipment, such as portability, storage, and charging.

Common barriers to successful implementation of AT into a school setting are as follows[8]:

- Lack of funding for the high cost of equipment
- Need for repairs that can take a long time, leaving the child without the technology
- Lack of on-site support for repairs, troubleshooting equipment failures
- Insufficient formal training in use of the equipment for the therapists or educational staff
- Resistance of staff to implement equipment

When the child is mainstreamed into a regular school, teachers and staff may be reluctant to accept adaptive equipment because of their limited experience with devices. This reluctance may be related not only to the health and developmental needs of the child but also to concerns about time, space, liability, and education in use of these devices. A thoughtful compromise is often necessary to meet the physical, educational, emotional, and social needs of the child with a disability.

The Individual with Disabilities Education Improvement Act (IDEA, 2004), Part B, provides for AT and AT services deemed necessary for a child to access an education. The IEP should include the specific device and its features, the educational goals for use of the device, and the specific AT services needed for a child to achieve the goals of the IEP, as well as definitive outcome criteria to measure the child's progress. Any equipment that is included in the IEP must be paid for by the school, unless parents choose to purchase the device.[33,34] The IDEA laws are more completely presented in another chapter.

Examples of equipment that might be recommended for use in the classroom to address physical impairments and disabilities include the following:

- Special chairs, seating devices, or adaptations to the regular desk chair
- Wheelchair trays or easels
- Wedges for seating in chairs
- Standers, gait trainers, or walking aids
- Floor positioners for alternative positions or circle time with peers

The physical therapist can be a valuable resource for teachers and other staff by making suggestions and helping procure equipment that can enhance a child's educational experience. Often, a piece of adaptive equipment can make the difference between a child feeling fully included in, rather than excluded from, classroom work and activities.

» Equipment selection

When the child's examination is completed and goals are established, the necessary types of equipment are determined. Equipment can be purchased, rented, borrowed, or, in some cases, where only simple adaptations are needed, fabricated by the child's family or others who have the skill and are familiar with the child.

General Considerations for Equipment

Many companies manufacture devices and equipment that are similar in concept. Criteria that must be considered in choosing a specific device include the following:

- *Dimensions of the apparatus.* The therapist must work with the DME provider to determine which product will best accommodate the child's growth or changes in physical function. Consider the child's diagnoses and typical disease progression. If a child is predicted to have significant physical regression entailing the need for a more support and less streamlined seating system, consider a wheelchair frame that has a built-in system for growth adjustability.
- *Weight, size, and manageability.* Is the device easy to use, and can it be stored? Can it be transported if necessary? Does it fold or disassemble in some way that makes storage and transport easier?
- *Availability of optional adaptations.* Are there parts that help improve the fit and specificity of the device? Are these options cost-effective, easily adjusted, and durable?
- *Reputation of the manufacturer.* Is the product covered by a warranty? Has the company previously provided support when problems with equipment have arisen? Is service readily available, and is equipment for trial use available? Will a company representative instruct the therapist and other appropriate staff in optimal use of the device?
- *Promptness of delivery or repairs:* Is the product kept in stock by most local DME dealers or manufacturer's representatives? Is there a backlog of orders that will delay the equipment's delivery? Is the product customized?
- *Cost.* Is the price reasonable or will less costly alternatives provide the same benefits?
- *Aesthetics.* Is the device aesthetically acceptable to the child and family or might it be rejected on this basis?

Most adaptive equipment manufacturers also have websites, with continually updated descriptions of equipment and information about new equipment and pricing. Many also have printed brochures or catalogs available. Local DME dealers with extensive experience with the equipment can play a vital role in answering many questions. Physical therapists in local hospitals or in the community can recommend dealers who have experience with certain types of equipment or provide the services specific to the client's situation. The therapist should not feel obligated to order from any dealer or person in particular. Although one equipment representative might be knowledgeable about wheelchairs, another person may have more experience with standing devices or ADL equipment. A list of qualified AT providers (dealers and evaluating therapists) can also be located at www.resna.org.[11]

Purchasing/Funding for Equipment

The cost of adaptive equipment and other aids for accomplishing ADLs can be an obstacle to a child's achievement of maximum functional potential. Limited living space and storage in most homes underscores the obvious impracticality of a child obtaining every promising piece of equipment available. Also, some assistive devices may have a limited period of usefulness for a particular child owing to growth or the child's making progress or, in some cases, regressing. Cost can be a primary limitation.

Funds available to pay for health care for children, with or without special needs, as well as eligibility requirements to access those funds, vary greatly among the states or geographical areas. Likewise, the ability of a family to obtain health care or purchase equipment for a child may depend on whether they have private or public insurance.

When one considers lifetime health care costs for families of children with special needs, it is easy to see how adaptive equipment, some very costly, can be difficult to obtain, maintain, and replace as the child grows and changes. Many children with congenital pathologies and impairments require new equipment frequently, over many years in a lifetime, in the presence of other exorbitant and rising medical expenses.

The physical therapist and OT should work in concert with the child and family, caregivers, teacher, physician specialist, primary care physician, ATP, and other health care professionals. The process of equipment procurement must include prioritizing equipment needs, and sometimes opting for a less expensive or complex device, or even sacrificing some adaptations to enable the family to acquire another device to meet a second functional need.

Although renting, borrowing, trading, and fabricating some equipment may be viable options, in some cases, purchasing equipment is the best or only option. How does a family pay for equipment? What resources are available to help parents pay for adaptive equipment?

A number of resources are available to pay for adaptive equipment, but will vary depending on certain conditions and qualifications. The funding options are continually evolving; however, many options have existed for a long time. Briefly, the following resources will purchase or help a family purchase equipment for children, some through the age of 21 years[34-36]:

1. Private medical insurance[37]
   - If the equipment is medically necessary
   - If prescribed by a physician
   - If the family's policy covers adaptive equipment
   - Depends on policy; some limit number of devices in a lifetime or limit frequency of replacement

2. IDEA[37]
   - Under Part B of IDEA, equipment in the child's IEP is paid for by the school district.
   - Under Part C, the district pays for the equipment if it is in the IFSP (Individual Family Service Plan).
   - Part C will not pay if other private or public resources are available.
   - If state or federal laws say parents have to contribute something in the Early Childhood Program, perhaps on a sliding fee basis, parents may pay part; however, the child cannot be denied the equipment or service if parents are unable to pay.
3. Medicaid[37]
   - For families with low income; Medicaid eligibility requirements are determined by each state; age of eligible children varies by state.
   - Jointly funded by Federal-State medical insurance program,[47] coverage varies by state.[37]

Medically necessary AT services are covered under Federal Medicaid law, and AT devices that are considered DME are often offered under a state's Medicaid regulations. Regulations vary between states.

4. Early and Periodic Screening, Diagnosis, and Treatment (EPSDT) program[37]
   - Included in all state Medicaid programs, required by federal government
   - Requires states to provide for children 0 through 21 years of age
   - Physical therapy and DME services not included in the standard state Medicaid plan *may be* reviewed for Medicaid coverage under EPSDT policy.[38]
   - Family must meet state's financial eligibility requirement for Medicaid.
   - Covers AT, but is an often overlooked resource
5. Katie Beckett Waiver/TEFRA (Tax Equity and Fiscal Responsibility Act) state plan option[39]
   - Waiver program for medical assistance for children who do not qualify for Medicaid because of parents' income
   - Waiver was enacted to support home and community care instead of institutionalization for children who need long-term, institutional-level care.
   - For eligibility, only the child's income is considered.
   - Policies vary among states; not available in all states.
6. Children's Health Insurance Program (CHIP)[37]
   - Provides health coverage to children in families with incomes too high to qualify for Medicaid, but cannot afford private coverage
   - Jointly funded by federal and state governments
   - Administered by the states
7. State AT Loan Programs[37]
   - Loan program available in many states, via Assistive Technology Act of 2004
   - Low interest loans and long repayment schedules

Used Equipment-Assistive Technology Reutilization The Pass It On Center: A National Collaboration for the Reutilization and Coordination of Assistive Technology maintains a national database of AT reuse programs in the United States to help people with disabilities acquire reused AT across the country.[40]

8. Community Philanthropic and Service Organizations and Clubs and National Organizations[35,37]
   - Local community service organizations such as the Lions, Masons, Shriners Hospital for Children, Kiwanis Clubs, Civitan, Rotary Clubs, Knights of Columbus, and local churches, synagogues, and mosques[35,37]
   - National organizations such as Easter Seal Society, Muscular Dystrophy Association, United Way, United Cerebral Palsy Association, Juvenile Arthritis Association, and March of Dimes

The Academy of Pediatric Physical Therapy of the American Physical Therapy Association (APTA) publishes a fact sheet that lists numerous sources that can provide a therapist with additional information about funding for adaptive equipment.[35]

Most funding sources, especially private insurance, require a physician's prescription if they pay for AT.[37] Regardless of requirement for prescription, having one at the beginning of the process usually helps ensure a smoother process and improves the likelihood of securing funding. Sometimes in educational settings, a child's care becomes fragmented because of disagreement among health care professionals about the role of the child's physician in recommending or prescribing rehabilitation therapies and DME. However, in the best interests of the child, it is imperative that all who are involved in the child's health care and education work together to optimize the child's potential. Collaboration between the child's therapists and physicians, including having a physician-written prescription for adaptive equipment, can improve coordination of care, avoid duplication of services and conflicting recommendations, and prevent unnecessary expenses.[41]

In addition to a prescription, a letter of medical necessity is often required when ordering adaptive equipment. The letter of medical necessity must be written by the certified or licensed professional who performed the evaluation of the child (a PT, OT, or ATP and physician). When pursuing insurance funding, it is pertinent that all components of the equipment be justified medically.[42] For children and youth younger than age 21, medical necessity is defined in federal law by Medicaid, and refers to the requirement that requested health care, diagnostic services, treatment, or other measures be necessary "to correct and ameliorate defects and physical and mental illnesses and conditions."[43] Many other funding sources abide by these same guidelines. It is important to justify that the AT is needed to correct, compensate for, or improve a condition or prevent it from worsening.[43] If funding for equipment is denied, it is highly recommended that an appeal be filed by the child's caregiver, which may require that an additional appeal letter be written. Many of the equipment manufacturers provide support and sample letters of medical necessity for their products.

As a child ages, there may be increased need for adaptive equipment, yet funding for this equipment may decrease. AT must be available to children younger than age 21 in accordance with the EPSDT requirements of the Medicaid Act; however, states and areas differ in their coverage as children and youth transition into adulthood.[43]

Issues surrounding the funding for adaptive equipment must continue to be a topic of conversation, study, and research for physical therapists and other professionals involved in the care of children with disabilities, particularly in light of changing health care policy.[44]

Some types of equipment for short-term use can be rented. However, if particular customized features are needed in a device, the likelihood of finding the precise, appropriate equipment is decreased. Often, concessions can be made regarding some equipment options if renting the equipment proves to be highly cost-effective. Compromising correct fit and safety for the sake of cost-effectiveness should not be an option.

Renting or Borrowing Equipment

Some communities have what is commonly referred to as an *equipment closet* or *equipment lending library*. These closets, usually run by not-for-profit organizations or agencies, are repositories for used equipment in good repair that are no longer in use. This equipment is made available for other children and parents to borrow for the period needed, often until the child outgrows the equipment.

Also, in today's Internet-connected world, it is not unusual, through social media, personal websites, or support groups, for parents to make contact with other parents who have adaptive equipment that is no longer being used. These parents with unused devices are often willing to sell or give away useful equipment or trade for another piece of equipment. However, the same exceptions and cautions mentioned regarding renting equipment also apply to borrowing or buying used equipment from equipment closets or other individuals.

Fabricating Equipment

An abundance of commercially available equipment today offers therapists, families, and children numerous options. Not only is there a wide variety of equipment types that help a child function in multiple environments but considerable competition also exists among manufacturers and vendors regarding proprietary variations in similar types of equipment. Consequently, the need to fabricate equipment instead of purchasing commercially available equipment has declined considerably. Nonetheless, fabricating instead of purchasing a simple piece of equipment is sometimes a practical choice, especially when there are limited financial resources that may be better spent purchasing highly complex equipment.

The decision to fabricate equipment is based on many variables that must be considered carefully, including who will build the equipment, the cost of building the device, who will pay for the equipment, and liability issues. Asking some carefully framed questions may help the therapist make a decision about whether to advocate homemade adaptive equipment.

- Will the physical therapist be building the equipment, or be serving as a consultant to other builders? Other people who might build equipment for children include commercial woodworkers, woodworking hobbyists, volunteer organizations with appropriately skilled members, and the child's parents.
- Is making the equipment cost-effective? Items that must be accounted for include tools, space needs, building materials, time for planning and designing, and time for measuring and building. In making a decision, the advantages of customized homemade equipment must be weighed against the expense of designing, planning, and building the apparatus. Will adapting a commercially available device be a better compromise?
- Will parents pay out-of-pocket, or will insurance companies pay for the cost of homemade equipment?
- Who will pay for potentially costly errors if the equipment is fitted incorrectly or is inappropriate when completed?
- Who assumes liability for the correct and safe use and performance of equipment made by a therapist, hobbyist, or volunteer? This is an important consideration in today's society wherein manufacturers are liable for the safe use of their products. If a child is injured or otherwise harmed using noncommercial equipment, the person who made the equipment may be legally and financially responsible.

Materials commonly used for homemade equipment include wood, ABS Plastic, Ethafoam, PVC pipe, and tri-wall (triple wall) cardboard. Tri-wall consists of triple-thickness corrugated cardboard that is lightweight, firm, and inexpensive. Tri-wall is fast and easy to use, although its use requires an electric saw, glue gun, and hand tools, such as a hammer, screwdriver, and utility knife. Although it is not waterproof, tri-wall can be treated with tape or fabric for sealing and preservation. Tri-wall is less durable than is wood, which makes it most appropriate for temporary or trial pieces of equipment, or for children who are growing rapidly. As with wood, tri-wall is a firm, solid medium and may require padding for comfort. Many therapists consider tri-wall useful for adding firm support to an off-the-shelf stroller, fabricating a floor-sitting device, or fabricating a tray surface to support upper extremities or place supplies for the child/s access. This can also be used to make supports for a tray, such as elbow or forearm blocks, or for makeshift positioning of switches or communication equipment. Although selection of a design and measuring the child and the tri-wall are time-consuming chores, actual building with tri-wall is a fast process. Working with this material is noisy, messy, and potentially dangerous because of the tools. A separate workplace is recommended. As with wood, family members and volunteers can be recruited to make devices from tri-wall. Special training is usually necessary, and many parents are reluctant to try because

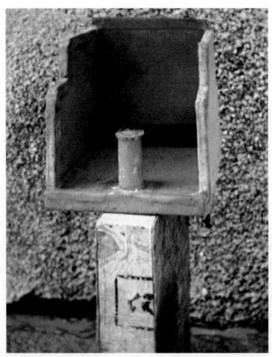

FIGURE 7.2. Seat insert custom fabricated from tri-wall.

of fear of mistakes and failure. Judicious support and praise for the family member can help overcome reluctance, and the parent may become an essential part of the team that is making the adaptive equipment for the child. A seating insert made from tri-wall is shown in Figure 7.2.

In spite of the potential drawbacks, some therapists still choose to fabricate equipment themselves or have a parent do so. This may be particularly useful for the young child who is growing rapidly or for the child whose need is only temporary. In each of these situations, a simply made piece of equipment could satisfy the short-term needs of the patient. The child could use the fabricated equipment until it is outgrown, at which time another piece could be made, or if growth has slowed, a commercially available piece could be substituted. One of the main reasons for building equipment in the past was that commercially available equipment often did not satisfy the needs of a child with unique problems. However, meeting the unique needs of people to enhance function has become the primary emphasis of professionals in the rehabilitation field, including those who design and manufacture adaptive equipment. This recent emphasis has resulted in a wider variety of and improvement in commercially available devices.

» Equipment for positioning

General uses for equipment as an adjunct to treatment have been presented, but benefits can also accrue with proper equipment and frequent changes in position. Among those benefits are temporary inhibition of pathologic tone and movement, temporary reduction of abnormal reflexes,

reduction of asymmetries, improved circulation, improved bone health, improved upper extremity functioning, prevention of soft-tissue contractures and pressure injuries, and improved communication and cognitive and personal–social development. Some of the issues involved in providing children with equipment to support various activities and the sitting, standing, and side-lying positions are now addressed.

Sitting

The sitting position is optimal for upper extremity function, and is therefore important for the child and the adult. Maintained sitting posture is a goal achieved by most typical infants before 1 year of age, and sitting is required for many functions throughout life. By watching children in preschool and kindergarten, it is apparent that a goal of many teachers is sitting for a reasonable amount of time during group activities. Children in the early school years younger than 7 years of age also require frequent changes in position. They prefer to play and work in the prone position, standing by a table, and in other positions that allow for easy transitional movements and change. Sitting, as a position for optimal function, occurs only after the children learn to sit for prolonged periods. When sitting, the weight of the trunk is transferred to the support area mainly through the ischial tuberosities and surrounding tissues. Proper sitting alignment is thought to enhance overall functioning by providing an adequate and secure base of support, inhibiting abnormal tone, providing a stable base from which the upper extremities can function, and improving perception of the environment. There are also significant social benefits to being upright in sitting and being able to move.

The first consideration when selecting a chair or other seating device is the intended purpose of the chair. Chairs can be function-specific. A lounge chair is uncomfortable when a person is eating a meal, yet a straight-back chair with little padding is undesirable for relaxation. Similarly, a therapist must consider function when recommending chairs for children with special needs.

A child's sitting ability without devices helps define the basic purpose of a chair or wheelchair. A child who is a *hands-free sitter* needs a chair to provide a comfortable and stable base of support for functional activities. The purpose of a wheelchair for this child is to provide mobility in addition to the stability. A child who depends on his upper extremities for support to sit independently, a *hands-dependent sitter*, needs seating that effectively stabilizes, centers, and supports his pelvis and trunk so that the child can use the arms and hands for functional skills rather than supporting sitting. A child unable to self-support at all for independent sitting is considered a *propped sitter*, and needs more complex seating that will provide total body support.[6]

Many therapists believe customized seating is preferable, especially a wheelchair. In lieu of a totally customized chair, the following general parameters should be considered, whether choosing a conventional chair, a commercially available adaptive seat, a custom-constructed chair, or a wheelchair.[45]

General Principles for Seat Setup

- Seat height: The height of the chair seat should allow the feet to be placed flat on the floor or on a footrest. Height should be such that with feet flat, the femurs are fully supported. Generally, if ROM permits, hips are flexed to at least 90 degrees. Slightly more hip flexion can be even more desirable to prevent extensor posturing in children with tone issues. Comfortable placement of the feet should prevent pressure from the front edge of the seat on the popliteal fossae.[45]

- Seat depth: The seat should be shallow enough to provide for flexion of the knees without pressure in the popliteal area and without a slouching or kyphotic posture. This posture occurs when the child's pelvis pulls into a posterior tilt and hips slide forward on the seat to allow the knees to flex over the edge of a seat that is too deep. This results in sacral sitting, because the child transfers weight to the chair seat through the sacrum rather than through the ischial tuberosities. Typical sitting posture requires anterior pelvic tilt. The seat should be deep enough to allow maximal distribution of weight.[45] If the seat is too shallow, weight is borne over a smaller area of the body, thereby increasing pressure per square inch on the posterior thighs and increasing the risk of pressure injuries. Many children lack the PROM to achieve anterior pelvic tilt.

A seat that is too shallow decreases the hip flexion to less than 90 degrees because the distal aspects of the thighs are not supported by the seat. This increased extension at the hips may cause the child to slide out of the chair. In a child with extensor hypertonia, increased extension of the hips may also trigger increased extensor tone throughout the body. A good rule of thumb for determining seat depth for children is to have one to two fingers of width between the edge of the seat and the popliteal fossa. Keep in mind that as the child grows, the length of the femur will increase and the space between the edge of the seat and the popliteal fossae will naturally increase.

- Cushions/padding: Cushions or padding can help to limit pressure on the 6-mm^2 surface of each ischial tuberosity that normally bears most of the weight in sitting, which allows for increased sitting tolerance.[46] However, surfaces that are too soft increase the difficulty with which postural changes are made during sitting, and this lack of postural change can lead to back strain and potential skin breakdown. Foam, gel, or air cushions can be used, depending on the properties needed by the child. As far back as the 1940s and 1950s, therapists have valued the constructs set by Bengt Akerblom, who judged movement while sitting to be the most important requirement of a comfortable chair.[47] He designed a chair that allowed for various conditions (i.e., the trunk away from the back support, sitting with lumbar support, or reclining back with both lumbar and thoracic support). These options reduce muscle strain and increase tolerance.[47]

- Backrest: Trunk musculature and spinal ligaments must be considered when sitting to avoid back discomfort. The anterior and posterior longitudinal ligaments of the trunk provide their best support with the back in neutral position. Increasing the normal lordosis may stretch the anterior longitudinal ligament, whereas exaggerated kyphosis will stretch the posterior longitudinal ligament and may cause posterior protrusion of degenerating intervertebral discs. These changes produce low back pain and may cause difficulty in achieving adequate thoracic and lumbar extension needed to rise from sitting. The chair backrest should accommodate adequate movement while in the chair, to help offset muscular fatigue and for pressure relief. However, the backrest should also provide adequate support of the trunk to prevent muscular fatigue. Support for the weight of the trunk reduces the muscular work of sitting. The height of the backrest must be appropriate for the individual child. The child who needs extensive head, neck, and trunk support needs a tall backrest that extends to shoulder height, with a head support that can be adjusted in the anterior/posterior plane. Such a child may also benefit from a reclining backrest, which can provide periodic relief for muscles to combat fatigue.[48] Finally, support for the lumbar curve and allowance for the posterior protruding sacrum and buttocks need to be taken into account in effective seating.

- Seat-to-backrest angle: The angle formed between the seat and the backrest of a chair is arguably most comfortable between 95 and 110 degrees. However, this angle may cause the person to slide forward, particularly those with increased extensor tone in the hips and back musculature. Using a wedged cushion, with the greatest height in the front, may help counteract this problem. Bergan suggests that chairs will provide a child with the best sensory feedback when the child's spatial orientation is that of sitting with a slight inclination backward.[49] The word *dump* in wheelchair seating refers to the number of inches closer to the ground the back of the wheelchair seat is, compared with the front of the wheelchair seat, thereby providing a slightly backward spatial orientation, as described by Bergan. Dump can be accomplished or enhanced in any chair using a wedged cushion, as described earlier, or the dump can be built into the chair[48] by decreasing, to less than 90 degrees, the angle between the seat and the backrest.[45]

Orthopedic and biomechanical needs of all children must be individually considered when establishing a seating system. Although most therapists use an empirical or trial-and-error approach to determine an appropriate seated position for a particular child, most agree that a stable pelvis serves as the keystone for seating, especially for children with neurodevelopmental disorders. Once the pelvis is aligned properly, the trunk, head, and extremities have a more stable base. This often means that fewer assistive devices and wheelchair options are necessary for optimal function.

- Seat orientation: The amount of rearward or forward tilt in the seat can be arranged to accommodate the child's postural needs. Rearward tilt can allow gravity to assist with lack of neck or trunk control. Forward tilt can place the load through the child's feet and LEs and facilitate extension or a more upright posture, in addition to possibly being a more "alerting" position.
- Armrests: Armrests should be positioned to bear approximately 50% of the weight of the child's arms. Armrests are also used to move from a sitting to a standing position and vice versa, to perform transfers and sitting push-ups for regular and frequent pressure relief for the buttocks. Armrests that are too low or too high decrease the mechanical advantage of the flexed elbow when the individual performs sitting push-ups and transfers.

The specific approaches to, options for, and adaptations of seating are too numerous to review here and are constantly evolving. However, providing seated weight bearing on the ischial tuberosities, maintaining a slight lumbar lordosis, positioning the hips and knees in at least 90 degrees of flexion, and maintaining full surface contact with the feet are principles that are fairly consistently applied to seating most children with impairments and disabilities. Variations of these basic concepts may be applied, based on a child's diagnosis and his individual clinical presentation, particularly with children who have sensation impairments.

Seating Considerations for Specific Diagnoses and Impairments

The criteria and limits described for seating are applicable to all types of seating systems and for all diagnoses and impairments. The emphasis may change with the diagnosis and impairments, but the concepts are constant.

Appropriate seating for the child with cerebral palsy and similar neuromuscular disorders must consider the effects of various seating or wheelchair components on muscle tone, abnormal reflex activity, and function. Increase in extensor tone in the LEs, with increased hip adduction and internal rotation, thought to accompany the sling effect of most standard wheelchair seats and backrests is a common problem associated with wheelchair seating of a child with cerebral palsy. A solid seat and solid backrest can reduce this sling effect.

A slightly closed hip angle ends to break up strong extensor patterns due to hypertonia, which can reduce the likelihood of compensatory posterior pelvic tilt that may result in increased kyphosis, scapular protraction, and hyperextension of the cervical spine. Avoiding these postures by establishing proper hip positioning facilitates upper extremity function/control and flexor–extensor balance of the cervical muscles. This change may produce positive consequences for swallowing, breathing, stability, and motor control of the neck and trunk. This position of hip flexion greater than 90 degrees may also decrease the probability of the child's LEs thrusting into an extension pattern and keep the child from sliding out of the chair. As noted previously, careful examination of ROM, muscle tone, and functional control is vital to setting up appropriate seat-to-back angles.

In addition to altering the hip angle, the chair itself may be tilted anteriorly or posteriorly, relative to the floor, as described previously, until the desired results of positioning are achieved. Issues of concern with these adjustments, whether through chair dump or tilt, include pelvic alignment for stability while sitting and the effects on tone of the various angles of the hip and of the seat itself. Perception and hand function will also be altered because differing angles and positions are used. Therefore, an individualized approach examining the effects of each change in position is necessary to determine optimal seating arrangements for children.

Once it appears that the various angles of hips, seat, and chair have been established and pelvic stability has been achieved in the child with cerebral palsy, the therapist must consider the trunk, head/neck, and LEs. The amount of knee flexion needed to provide stability and full contact weight bearing through the feet should be examined. A good starting point is to determine how close to the common position of 90 degrees of knee flexion can be achieved. Some children lack the passive knee flexion ROM to even 90 degrees of knee flexion; therefore, the footrests or footplates of a chair may need to allow the knees to be slightly extended. More commonly, many children with spasticity, hypertonia, or hamstring tightness lack the passive knee extension to achieve 90 degrees of extension. In this case, the footrests may need to be set up so the feet can be "tucked" closer to the frame of the wheelchair. If the lower legs are not provided with the setup to accommodate these limitations, the position of the hips, trunk, and neck will subsequently be affected. Likely this will result in hips sliding forward on the seat. It is also important to address the amount of pressure being placed on any one part of the foot. Too much weight bearing on the anterior plantar surface of the foot can result in a primitive extensor thrust pattern in children with neuromotor impairments that will significantly reduce stability. The flexibility and alignment of the ankles is also important to address. Many chairs have options for adjustable footplates that will accommodate a fixed ankle position due to soft-tissue limitations or for children who are wearing orthotics and have a fixed ankle position.

Alignment of the trunk should encourage maximal symmetry and stability, yet provide for movement and active postural adjustment. A headrest or support should be used only if needed to improve positioning, stabilize the head and neck for functional activities such as feeding/swallowing or engaging in visual activities, or to protect the child when being transported. The ultimate goal of the sitting position should be to align the child without restricting the movements and postural adjustments available to the child. Reevaluation of the seating device is ongoing, and is necessary as the child grows, has physical changes, or acquires new skills.

The seating/positioning concerns are different for children with nonprogressive or progressive weakness, paresis, or paralysis, as seen in muscular dystrophy, spinal muscular atrophy, myelomeningocele, or traumatic spinal cord injury. The height of armrests, type of footrests, dump, tilt, and recline are important factors for successful transfers, mechanically efficient wheelchair push-ups for pressure relief, sit-to-stand, and stand-to-sit. The ability to recline a chair or wheelchair is particularly helpful for children with extreme or progressive weakness because it is easier to achieve periodic rest in a recumbent position. This is true both for the relief of general fatigue and changing, and sometimes limiting, the gravitational influence on various muscles. Also, as strength declines in progressive disorders, muscle imbalance in the trunk may lead to an asymmetric sitting posture, which can be alleviated by strategically placed pads or customized seat cushions and backrests for positioning, appropriate height armrests, and upper extremity support surfaces or trays, which can provide and encourage postural symmetry when seated. A child with myelomeningocele or traumatic spinal cord injury may benefit from seat cushions that have both positioning and pressure-relieving qualities, as well as wheelchair or chair functions that will enable the ability to perform pressure relief measures due to inherent sensory deficits. The child or teenager with the propensity to pressure injuries of the ischial tuberosities may be better served to offload the ischial tuberosities.

The therapist needs to educate the child and caregivers to carefully monitor for reduced joint motion secondary to static positioning, disruption of skin integrity as a result of prolonged use of a seating device without changing positions, limited ability to change position thus risking skin breakdown in a child with impaired sensation, and reduced independent functional mobility resulting from overuse of seating devices. To address these issues, equipment manufacturers continue to research and develop cushions comprising pressure-relieving properties and building dynamic features and adjustable seat adjustment functions into the frames of chairs.

Specialized Sitting Devices

Various specialized chairs are available commercially or can be constructed for particular seating problems. Chairs that incorporate the basic principles of seating, as discussed in this chapter, can have special adaptations that facilitate or accommodate a specific posture. Two examples of specialized chairs that are available are the corner chair and the bolster chair. The corner chair (Fig. 7.3) is a chair that has lateral supports for the upper trunk. These supports position the child in shoulder girdle protraction, a strategy that tends to decrease extensor spasticity in children with tone problems such as cerebral palsy. Bolster chairs are chairs with a bolster-type seat (Fig. 7.4). These

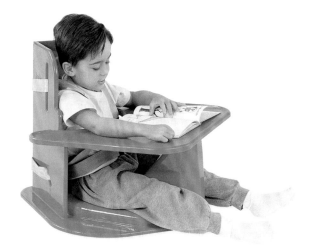

FIGURE 7.3. Tumble Forms corner chair.

chairs also aid in inhibiting excessive extensor tone and hip adduction in children with cerebral palsy by flexing and abducting the hips. An adjustable bench can be very useful, because this can be positioned into an anterior tilt, with blocks placed anterior to the knees to facilitate anterior pelvic positioning and trunk control while supporting the knees to prevent the hips from sliding forward on the bench. Sitting in these types of chairs while engaging in functional activities will help the child work on developing core trunk and neck control, as well as develop upper extremity function. This type of equipment can be used as an adjunct to hands-on therapy.

Many other specialized chairs and seating aids can be found by perusing equipment company catalogs and websites. Products are continually evolving, and often a commercial device is available to meet a child's specific seating needs.

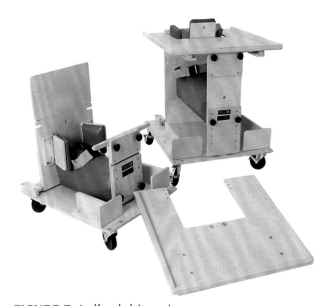

FIGURE 7.4. Kaye bolster seat.

Standing

The upright standing posture is the foundation for many functional activities in addition to bipedal locomotion. Standing and bearing weight through the LEs can also promote circulation, bone mineral density, respiratory endurance, gastrointestinal function, integumentary health, improved/ maintained LE ROM, modulation of spasticity, upper extremity function, vertical access (vertical reach), and social interaction with others.[12,50,51] For a child with limited options and opportunities for moving, appropriate adaptive equipment for standing provides another alternative for positioning throughout the day to help reduce or prevent skeletal deformities.[12]

Equipment for assisted standing is commercially available in a variety of forms, and is categorized according to the function and whether they provide static or dynamic standing opportunities. As the physical therapist, it is essential to choose the appropriate type of stander to support the child's goals. As with all adaptive equipment, it is important to consider the child's needs over the next several years, given the available funding options. Planning for approximately 3 years of growth or physical change is appropriate if it is expected that insurance will fund the equipment.

General Standing Principles

When considering adaptive standing equipment for a child, the therapist must carefully evaluate the child's PROM, muscle control, and orthopedic status to ensure proper LE alignment for weight bearing. Limitations of the child's hip, knee, and ankle PROM or leg-length discrepancies can have an effect on how the child is able to achieve a standing position and how the equipment should be configured. Information about the placement of the hip joint and whether there is a subluxation or dislocation is important. Results of a study conducted by Martinsson and Himmelman "The Effect of Weight Bearing in Abduction and Extension on Hip Stability in Children with Cerebral Palsy" indicate that standing programs for young children should include positioning in hip abduction. This study concluded that 1 year of weight bearing with the maximum achievable abduction (25–30 degrees) and 0 degrees of hip extension for at least 1 hour per day improved hip status both in children following adductor–iliopsoas tenotomy and in children without surgery. It is suggested that children be positioned with 30 degrees of abduction for at least 60 to 90 minutes per day. Several types of positioning standers can be set up to achieve 30 degrees of hip abduction. Correct weight bearing for normal standing requires dynamic pressure through the heels, with the center of gravity passing slightly posterior to the ankle joint.[52]

Muscle tone, stability, and strength of the joints are also important, because the ankle must be aligned and well supported during weight bearing. LE orthotics may be considered to maintain proper ankle alignment during standing. Knee hyperextension must be prevented when standing.

The child's spinal alignment and trunk/head control should also be evaluated to determine how much support might be needed to achieve the standing position. Often, a trunk or neck orthosis is necessary to maintain proper alignment during use of a stander. As the physical therapist, it is important to continually monitor and address these factors.

Standing Devices

There are several types of standing devices that can be set up in various configurations to accommodate the individual child.

STATIC SINGLE AND MULTIPOSITIONAL STANDERS These are standers that position the child in a static position of either prone or supine. The single-positioning standers are usually small in size for fit into a home or crowded school environment, and are helpful for facilitating neck and trunk control, upper extremity and LE strength/function, and gaining endurance. The single-position standers are usually easy to set up and are situated close to the floor to allow the child to be at peer level. Supports can be adjusted or removed as the child gains motor control or works on strengthening goals. Some models will provide the option of positioning the hips into abduction. The limitations for static standers include providing only one positioning option and requiring a dependent transfer into the device. The multipositioning standers have the option of being configured into supine, prone, or upright standing. These are generally a bit larger than are the single-position standers and more complex to reconfigure, but offer many options for physical changes and functions for the child that can be provided with a single piece of equipment.

PRONE STANDERS Prone standers are used frequently for children who require, but cannot achieve, the position of hands-free upright standing or its approximation. The child is placed in the prone position in the device. The trunk, pelvis, and LEs are all supported. The angle can then be adjusted between prone and slightly less than 90 degrees angle to the floor, depending on the child's goal. When the device is positioned closer to horizontal, the demands on the neck and thoracic extensors are greater owing to body weight and gravitational forces. The child is required to stabilize shoulder girdle musculature and weight bear through the upper extremities. There is less benefit of LE weight bearing. As the device is adjusted toward a more upright position, the child benefits from the physiologic changes associated with weight bearing through the LEs, shifting weight through either upper extremity, and increasing freedom to reach and use hands functionally while upright. The child benefits from the social and perceptual opportunities afforded by an upright position. As positioning components are removed, the child can work on head and trunk control in the upright position. Alternative positioning devices can be used in conjunction with the prone stander to accommodate limitations, such as using a trunk or neck orthosis to assist with alignment to benefit from the adjustments of the stander.

Correct weight bearing for normal standing requires dynamic pressure through the heels, with the center of gravity passing slightly posterior to the ankle joint. This is not feasible with the prone positioning stander; therefore, the goals for the prone stander must be carefully evaluated.

Although the child may appear to adapt well to the prone stander for 1 hour each day, the child's positioning and response should be continually monitored. Changes to the position would be needed if abnormal extensor tone, cervical hyperextension, scapular retraction, high guard position of the upper extremities, or postural asymmetry is noted over time.

Providing the opportunity for a child to interact with peers during play or school situations is an important benefit of using a prone stander. Being able to work at a table or play at an elevated sandbox with peers has important social and emotional benefits. Prone standers usually have an option to order casters to enable the child to be moved from place to place while standing. A prone stander may be incorporated into a dynamic stander by providing large wheels for self-propulsion.

SUPINE STANDERS A supine stander is an alternative to the prone stander, and may better meet the needs of children with a goal of achieving a fully upright position. A supine stander allows weight bearing through the trunk and LEs, with the degree of weight bearing proportional to the angle of the supporting surface. The child is secured around the trunk, hips, and knees, with these areas as close to erect standing alignment as possible. With those criteria achieved, the supine stander is angled toward a 90-degree upright position. Unlike the prone stander, the supine stander does not provide for weight bearing for the upper extremities, and LE weight bearing occurs through the heels rather than through the forefeet. This makes the supine stander a better option when working toward weight-bearing alignment for ambulation. The supine stander also affords the child the numerous physiologic benefits of upright weight bearing provided by the prone stander and allows the child to perceive and interact with the environment from an upright posture. Variations of the supine stander are shown in Figures 7.5 and 7.6.

As with all adaptive devices, the supine stander must include a careful examination of the child for compensations, some of which may be pathologic. Commonly noted

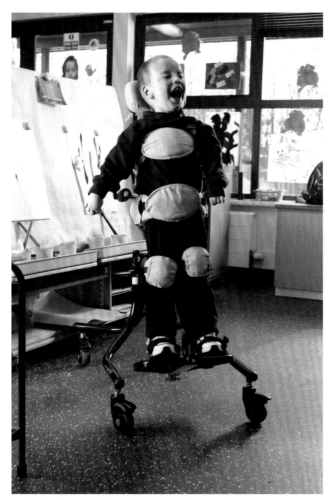

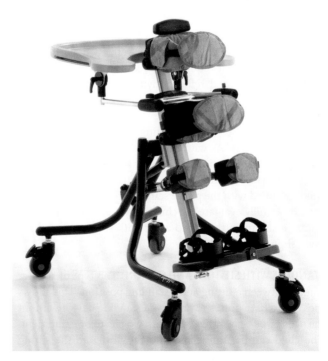

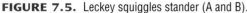
FIGURE 7.5. Leckey squiggles stander (A and B).

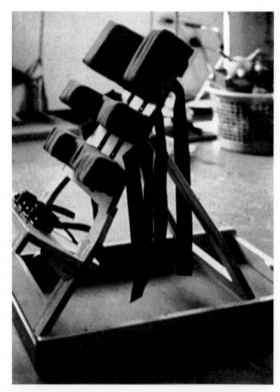

FIGURE 7.6. Supine stander custom fabricated from wood. It is padded for comfort, and was designed and built entirely by parents.

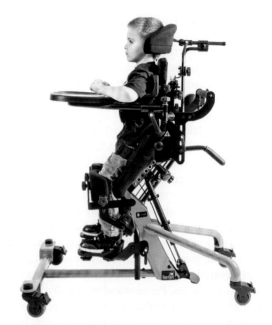

FIGURE 7.7. Easy Stand Bantam sit-to-stand stander.

deviations with use of a supine stander include thoracic kyphosis with forward protrusion of the head, hyperextension of the cervical spine, and asymmetry secondary to imbalanced muscle control. If tolerance for an upright position is limited and the child is reclined, increased evidence of ATNR and the Moro reflex may be seen. These abnormal reflexes may occur in a supine or semi-reclined position for any child with poorly integrated developmental reflex activity. Because normal development requires the acquisition of antigravity control, the increased reflex activity in a supine or semi-supine position may be counterproductive. Upper extremity function for the child in a supine stander usually requires a special table or easel, thus restricting the child's participation in group activities. As with other pieces of adaptive equipment, periodic evaluation is necessary to determine the long-term benefits associated with the supine stander for a given child. As noted with the prone stander, the physical therapist should carefully evaluate the child's physical functioning and the necessity for orthotics to assist with support and alignment should be considered.

STANDERS WITH SIT-TO-STAND OPTION This type of stander adjusts between a sitting and a standing position. This allows the user to have both a sitting and a standing device without the need to be transferred between two pieces of equipment. The child can be transferred into the device in the sitting position, making transfers easier and potentially less dangerous, particularly if the child is large or has behavioral issues

that affect transfer safety. This device increases the ease of a child attaining a standing position with or without assistance. This also provides a gradual transition from sitting toward standing to accommodate a person with hip or knee muscle contractures. The device can be gradually raised toward a standing position and stopped at the position of limitation. These are typically larger in size than are static standers and are situated high off the ground, which can affect a child's interactions at peer level (Fig. 7.7).

INTEGRATED WHEELCHAIR STANDING DEVICES A wheelchair standing device is a standing device integrated into the child's personal wheelchair. It can be controlled either manually or through power, and it can be part of a manual or powered wheelchair base. The advantage of the wheelchair stander is that the child can stand without having to be transferred to another device.[12] The child may stand more frequently and randomly, may be more independent in achieving the standing position, can accomplish functional reach at different heights, and has increased vertical reach, in addition to the other benefits of upright standing. Also, the risks involved with transfers to a standing device are eliminated, and the child and family have one less piece of equipment to accommodate.[12]

Integrated wheelchair standers provide dynamic loading of the LEs and the benefits of dynamic weight bearing during the rise-to-standing and stand-to-sit activities. Dynamic loading also occurs with the child in different standing/semi-standing positions, due to changing skeletal alignment and varying amounts of weight bearing in diverse positions. A child can move in the environment while standing in the wheelchair stander, thereby gaining increased functional opportunities and dynamic loading through the vibration effects by moving across different surfaces and thresholds.[12]

DYNAMIC STANDERS Dynamic standing can be achieved in several ways. Some standers have separate footplates that can shift horizontally and vertically to simulate the weight-bearing changes similar to loading and unloading the extremities during gait. Although appropriate body support is maintained, these standers allow body sway during standing, creating a dynamic weight-bearing environment. Dynamic standing is thought to more effectively increase the loading effects on the long bones for maintaining or increasing bone mineral density.[50,51] Some dynamic standers provide spring actions to allow for lateral weight shifting to simulate a natural gait pattern for the child to promote independent exploration of the environment. Another type of stander is the mobile stander, which is configured with large wheels to allow for upper body rotation over the pelvis, freedom of movement of the upper body, and self-propulsion of the device while in the standing position. Mobile standers create a vibration type of dynamic input as the stander moves over various surfaces and thresholds. They provide significant benefits, because they are low to the ground placing the child at peer level for interaction, increase the child's potential for independent mobility, and increase the means for upper extremity use for propulsion. The dynamic standers do not provide the abducted hip position and still require assistance for transfers (Fig. 7.8).

Positioning on the Floor or Bed

As an alternative to being positioned in a chair or stander, a child is typically positioned on the floor, on the couch, or in bed. It is important to explore ways to support the child appropriately in these positions with the caregiver. Twenty-four-hour postural care is vital, because children with severe neuromotor limitations show prolonged immobilized posture during nighttime sleep. These children have limited movement and are vulnerable to the force of gravity because

their variety of positions is limited. They are a risk particularly during growth spurts. Poor alignment during the day and nighttime can lead to long-term problems such as scoliosis and hip dislocations. Prolonged asymmetrical posture, such as having the head turned to one side or knees falling into opposite direction for prolonged periods, can lead to postural deformities of the spine and pelvis. Children with low muscle tone are also at risk for postural deformities of the hips because they commonly lie in supine with hips abducted. Exploring positioning items designed for children with special needs and using or adapting off-the-shelf items is essential.[53]

Side-lying

Supporting a child side-lying in bed or on the floor is particularly useful for young children or large children with low developmental function who require an alternative to sitting. Side-lyers are commercially available (Fig. 7.9); however, the position can be achieved using pillows, straps, and other commonly available items. This can be achieved on the floor, or in bed, and allow the child to have an alternative position in others' homes or in school. When using a side-lyer, the objective is to place the child in a side-lying position, according to the following criteria:

- The trunk should be as symmetric as possible.
- The head should be supported, in neutral alignment with the trunk.
- Weight-bearing limbs (upper extremity and LE touching the surface) should be slightly flexed.
- Non–weight-bearing extremities should be free to move. This position encourages play in midline, dissociation between the limbs, and symmetric and neutral head and trunk alignment. It is also a position that is neutral regarding most abnormal reflex activity. Straps are commonly used to support the trunk, the pelvis, and, occasionally, the weight-bearing LE. Pillows or pommels usually support the thigh in a neutral position for hip abduction/adduction and internal/external rotation. The device should accommodate the child on either side unless circumstances prevent the child from freely lying on each side. Frequent reassessment is required to prevent compensations while using or after being removed from the side-lyer.
- Areas of potential problems include neck hyperextension from pushing against the head support and flexion/retraction of the shoulder on the non–weight-bearing side. These problems may occur with a child who exhibits

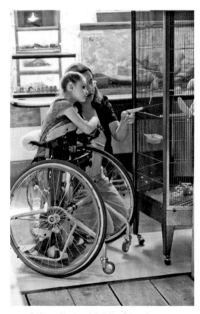

FIGURE 7.8. Rifton Prone Mobile Stander.

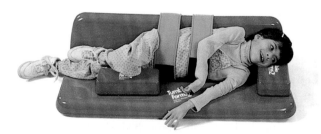

FIGURE 7.9. Tumble Forms Side-Lyer.

extensor hypertonicity. When using a side-lyer, the therapist must be careful when aligning the child with chronic hyperextension of the neck or with a tracheostomy. Improper positioning in either of these cases could cause airway obstruction and compromise the child's ventilation.

- Positioning can be alternated to either side. The side-lyer provides easy manipulation of toys and objects because one hand is stabilized against the surface in midline alignment.

Supine

When lying supine, pillows and soft straps can be used to support the LEs to avoid excessive hip abduction and to compensate for knee and/or hip flexion contractures. Pillows or blankets can be used to "fill in" the spinal concave curvatures for comfort and support. If a child has gastrointestinal issues such as reflux, it is beneficial to use a wedge to incline the trunk.

Prone

Lying prone can be a good alternative for respiration and for prolonged stretching of hip flexors and anterior trunk musculature. This is an excellent position to work on strengthening the neck and the upper thoracic and shoulder girdle musculature. The physical therapist must monitor neck alignment and allow for clearance for breathing.

In any lying position, care should be taken to carefully monitor areas of pressure, particularly the heels or bony prominences. Pressure-relieving mattresses or overlays may be indicated.

There are beds designed for positioning children with special needs; however, the use of positioning supports can be applied, as long as there are considerations for safety.

Overall Considerations for Positioning

Although not a complete list of positioning devices, examples have been provided to illustrate the issues to be considered in choosing and using equipment for positioning, the benefits of various positioning devices, and some of the possible negative consequences. Physical therapists who work with children and adaptive equipment will be required to suggest the frequency and duration of use and endurance, which depends on variables that change daily. Rather than suggesting specific lengths of time for use, the therapist may choose to let the warning signs of fatigue guide the usage. Those warning signs include difficulty maintaining the desired posture, increased asymmetry, complaints of discomfort, facial expressions signifying discomfort or displeasure, and verbal requests to be moved. The therapist can recommend using a device until any one of those warning signs is apparent or a maximum time limit has been reached. Depending on the child and the type of equipment, 60 to 90 minutes is a recommended time frame for a child who can make few, if any, postural adjustments. For a child who is able to make postural adjustments while in the equipment, varying the distribution of weight bearing, for example, 1 hour at a time,

is probably a maximum. It may be worthwhile to encourage attempts to increase endurance gradually over the course of several weeks or months, realizing that minor variations in tolerance will occur daily. Because daily variations in activity level are normal for everyone, we should acknowledge these variations in the child with physical disabilities.

Prolonged positioning in any one posture is contraindicated. In addition to fatigue, negative effects of prolonged positioning include pressure injuries, joint stiffness, and decreased passive and active range caused by hypertonia and/or immobilization.

» Equipment for mobility

In addition to providing assistance with positioning, adaptive equipment can supplement a child's existing manner of independent locomotion or offer mobility to children who otherwise have no means for locomotion. Some devices, such as scooter boards, chairs with floor mobility bases, pre-wheelchair devices, and other devices used on the floor, are appropriate only within the home or classroom. These low-tech premobility devices can be used to provide the child with a play activity that will facilitate the cognitive and perceptual skills needed for mobility if they otherwise have limited floor mobility skills. They can initiate moving from place to place, and they can experience and experiment with figure ground and spatial orientation skills needed for future maneuvering of other wheelchair devices that will make it possible to be mobile within the community. These devices can also be helpful in emotionally preparing parents for the mobility equipment that will be inevitable for their children. When children are very young, parents often need to be focused on the child's medical stability and acceptance of a specific diagnosis. The therapist plays a vital role in supporting the family through this acceptance and showing them ways to prepare the child for function as he/she develops. Oftentimes, it is difficult for parents of infants and young toddlers to accept that a child will need to use adaptive equipment for mobility. The therapist can use these low-tech mobility devices during play to bridge the gap between independent mobility without an assistive device and use of a wheelchair or other higher tech mobility device. Therapists can also assist families to contact parent support groups specific to the child's diagnosis, which can be very helpful in facilitating acceptance and moving forward with adaptive equipment. In addition to providing the child with a play activity that will allow them to work on perceptual, cognitive, mobility, and social skills, use of these low-tech devices can be a means of building core strength and extremity strength necessary for sitting and use of mobility aids.

Scooter Boards

These are flat, padded board with casters. While prone on the board, a child propels using hands to push across the floor. Scooter boards are especially helpful for the toddler or young child who has no prone locomotion and is limited in floor play and exploration.

Crawling Devices

These are set up to support a child in a four-point creeping position to facilitate crawling, and are generally set up with a suspension harness attached to a frame with casters (Fig. 7.10). The device is adjustable to allow for varying degrees of weight bearing through the extremities. This can be useful for the development of head and trunk control, increased tolerance to the prone position, development of co-contraction of muscles, as well as improving initiation for mobility and the visual spatial skills needed in preparation for independent mobility.

Tricycles

Riding a tricycle is a fun and functional way for some small children to locomote, as well as build strength and provide cardiovascular activity. Specially adapted tricycles are available commercially (Fig. 7.11), or a standard tricycle can be modified. Modifications may include vertically turned handgrips (to inhibit flexor hypertonia of the trunk and facilitate antigravity trunk extension in children with tone disorders), abduction pommels, back supports, and foot straps. Foot straps are usually applied at the angle of the foot and lower leg, rather than across the toes, similar to ankle straps on wheelchair footplates. This placement prevents a stimulus to the ball of the foot that might cause uncontrolled plantar

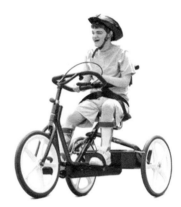

FIGURE 7.11. Rifton Adapted Tricycle.

flexion and increase abnormal extensor tone in the LEs and trunk. Tricycles, although sometimes awkward to transport, are appropriate for use within the community and can be an important adjunct to a child's independence, peer interaction, and integration of play skills.

Bicycles

Bicycles for older children provide functional mobility and recreation. Adapted bicycles are available commercially, and many can be further modified. Typical seating adaptations include seatbelts and backrests, pedal and brake modifications, and wheel modifications that include a third or fourth wheel. Also, the method for propelling the bike can be modified, including hand cycling. For some children, adapted bicycles offer longer distance mobility, energy conservation, and exercise opportunities. Because a bicycle is a mode of transportation and recreation for children without disabilities, using a bike can help a child to fit in with peers more readily.

Chairs with Floor Mobility Bases

These are low-tech lightweight positioning chairs that can support the child in upright sitting and can be attached to a wheeled base that is low to the ground (Fig. 7.12). The child can use his/her feet to move the chair on the floor. This is also helpful for providing the child with a means to initiate self-mobility and begin to develop the figure ground and visual spatial relationships needed for mobility. This also provides a supportive floor position for the child to engage in floor play at the level of peers at home or school, and to allow caregivers to be face to face with the child during interactions, rather than supporting them from behind on the floor. This is pertinent in development of communication and cognitive and visual systems.

Pre-wheelchair Devices

These devices allow very young children to play on the floor at peer level while providing large wheels that they can propel using their hands, similar to propelling a manual wheelchair.

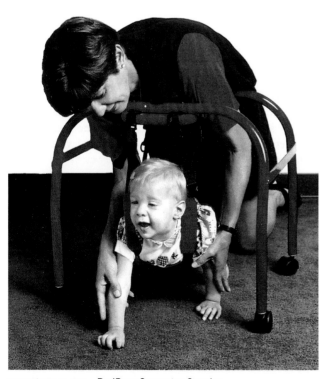

FIGURE 7.10. RedBarn Creepster Crawler.

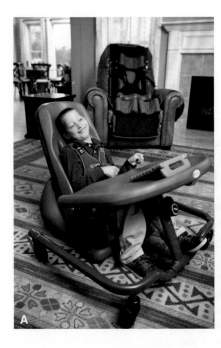

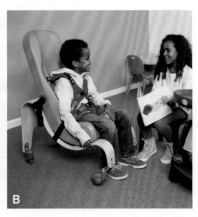

FIGURE 7.12. A: Special Tomato floor sitter chair on stationary base with mobile tray. **B:** Special Tomato floor sitter chair on mobile base.

These typically support the child in a long-sitting position. Several commercial designs are available (Fig. 7.13). Sometimes this type of device is used for a toddler-aged child who will inevitably obtain a manual wheelchair and will learn how to self-propel in a wheeled device using the hands.

Adapted Battery-Operated Ride-On Toys

Many children like to use battery-operated cars for a fun outdoor activity at home. These are typically operated using a foot pedal to "go" and a steering wheel. Many children who have physical impairments are unable to maintain upright sitting posture in the toy vehicle or operate the foot pedal or steering wheel. These toy cars are mid-tech devices that can be adapted by providing simple positioning supports to assist the child to maintain sitting balance. The electronics can be adapted to facilitate the child to use a switch to make the car "go" or "stop." These are referred to as modified ride-on cars (ROCs).[21,22] Go Baby Go Connect[54] is a national program

in the United States that will adapt the vehicle for a specific child. This is a wonderful precursor to prepare a child for power mobility. As the physical therapist working with very young children, it is important to identify that these types of adaptive equipment exist, and to explore means of obtaining the equipment or referring the family to programs that can help them trial or obtain the devices.

Segways

The Segway®, a two-wheeled, dynamically stabilized device that runs on large format batteries, is a personal transporter.[55] Although not originally designed for persons with disabilities, teens and young adults have found the Segway to be a transporter that provides a safe and efficient means to get around campus without automatically being seen as disabled. The original Segway requires being able to stand on the device, but new accessories are being developed, including seats. The scooter or Segway may be preferred for an older marginal ambulator who requires a device for long distances.[56]

Scooters

A three- or four-wheeled scooter is much less expensive than is a standard motorized wheelchair. It can be disassembled into components that are lighter and easier to load into a car or public transport vehicle and is relatively simple to learn to operate and maintain. The scooter is usually equipped with a captain's style seating system. A person can most easily and safely use a scooter if he/she has the sitting balance and upper extremity function to be able to reach the tiller with two hands to operate and steer the device without losing balance. The scooter is not meant to be safely used on uneven terrain.

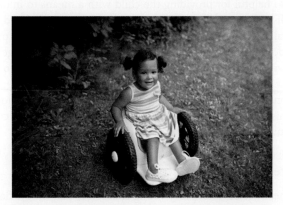

FIGURE 7.13. Bella's Bumbas Pre-wheelchair device.

Scooters are often found in department or grocery stores and some outdoor facilities such as zoos and amusement parks as an option for people who only require limited us of a power wheeled mobility device.

Manual Wheeled Mobility Devices

Recommending a wheelchair for a child requires an understanding and application of all the criteria previously discussed about proper alignment and positioning in sitting. It is also beneficial to know about the options available when recommending a wheelchair and the compromises involved when selecting certain options. This is where involving a DME provider is indicated, because he/she can discuss the comparative adaptability, durability, cost, and features of wheelchairs and other equipment supplied by competing manufacturers, and possibly refer to a specialized AT professional or program for complex cases.

When preliminarily considering a wheelchair for a child, it may be easiest to discuss options by looking at a typical order form for a pediatric wheelchair. These forms are found on the specific manufacturer's website and are traditionally completed by the DME provider in collaboration with the child, family, and therapist.

When matching a child with a wheelchair for mobility, it is important to initially determine the child's potential for dependent versus independent mobility. Exclusively dependent wheelchair mobility should be reserved for children who, for some reason, cannot attain independent mobility with either a manual or powered wheelchair. Dependent mobility may be the goal for children unable to operate a manual or powered wheelchair because of insufficient upper extremity function, limited fine motor control, lack of judgment, insufficient cognitive skills, or profound and multiple physical impairments and disabilities. Unfortunately, some children are dependent for mobility because of environmental or societal barriers such as lack of funds for a powered wheelchair, lack of means to transport a power chair, or inaccessibility of the home. In this case, it is important to collaborate with the team of professionals to refer the family to a case manager or social worker who can assist the family to work toward overcoming these barriers. Wheelchairs for dependent mobility of children include strollers, transport or travel chairs, manual wheelchairs, and reclining and tilt-in-space wheelchairs. Because the goal of enhancing a child's independent function is paramount, feasible options for achieving some degree of independent mobility should be explored before deciding on dependent mobility.

If a child can attain independent wheeled mobility with an appropriate wheelchair, will reaching this goal be most likely attained by a manual or powered wheelchair? Reasons for opting for a powered wheelchair include (1) severe trunk and/or upper extremity weakness, (2) paresis, paralysis, or dyskinesias that preclude manual wheelchair propulsion, (3) inadequate upper body control, (4) poor endurance, (5) respiratory compromise, (6) the need to transport a number of heavy medical equipment devices on the wheelchair, (7) function in more challenging environments such as outdoors or in the community (8), high metabolic costs of propelling a manual wheelchair, (9) and concerns about secondary impairments from overuse injuries acquired from long-term manual propulsion of a wheelchair.[9,45,57] Well-meaning health care professionals may suggest that selecting a powered wheelchair will lead to the child gaining weight or losing muscle strength owing to lack of exercise. This is not a good rationale for choosing a manual wheelchair. As stated earlier, the choice of a primary mobility device should be determined to provide optimal independence. A child who uses power mobility should exercise to prevent disuse weakness and weight gain, but his ability to be mobile in the community should not be connected to his exercise habits.[9]

There are several categories of wheelchairs or seated wheeled mobility devices. It is important explore with the child and the family their potential for independent mobility and have a general understanding of the options available. It can be helpful to provide them with pictures or websites to explore the equipment before the evaluation. Your input and information regarding the child and personal situation is extremely valuable to the dealer you are working with or the specialized team that may be evaluating the child. That way, the equipment type can be narrowed, resulting in a more efficient evaluation. In addition, the family can be "ready" to process and focus on the details of the equipment choices. Sometimes the equipment that may seem best for the child may not work in terms of accessibility to their current home or vehicle. All of this information is important in making final equipment decisions.

The equipment categories and general information are as follows.

Adapted Positioning Strollers

Adapted strollers are primarily used for children who are dependent for mobility. Some strollers have complex positioning systems for the child who needs substantial postural support. These positioning strollers usually have predetermined options for support and offer seat adjustments such as tilt-in-space, recline, and elevating leg rests. These strollers do not typically have the flexibility to accommodate a child who has severe hypertonia or spinal deformities, or the durability of a manual wheelchair in terms of withstanding heavy extraneous movement patterns. With many of these strollers, the seat can be removed to attach to the frame in the forward- or rear-facing positions or offer an additional indoor base that adjusts to various heights including floor level.

Fold-and-Go Strollers

These strollers are similar to umbrella strollers. Some offer soft positioning supports and these can be ordered in larger sizes to accommodate adults.

Jogging Strollers

These have three wheels and resemble the off-the-shelf jogging strollers. Some brands can accommodate positioning cushions for added support.

One is commonly exploring strollers for the child who is very young, possibly the first seated wheeled mobility device being explored for a child. The therapist must make sure that the needs of the child over the net 3 to 5 years are considered, particularly if this is being funded through insurance. In addition, at this stage of equipment provision, the aesthetics of the device is often of high importance. Many families often are seeking a positioning stroller that appears to look similar to other off-the-shelf strollers. It is very important to attend to the emotional aspect of equipment provision.

Manual Wheelchairs

When considering manual wheelchairs, noted that almost any seating system component, meaning seat cushion or backrest, headrest, or additional support, can be interchanged or used with any manual wheelchair frame. Manual wheelchair frames are often considered in the following categories.

ULTRALIGHTWEIGHT RIGID FRAMES These are used for people who can self-propel functionally and need to preserve shoulder integrity. These are the lightest frames and have adjustable wheel axles so the wheelchair can be set up in relation to the user's body shape and size, for a biomechanical advantage when propelling. Typically, the person using this type of wheelchair does not need a heavy aggressive seating system. This frame does not fold from side to side, rather the backrest folds forward into a box-shaped frame (Fig. 7.14). For a smaller child, this does not make a large difference when loading into a vehicle; however, for a teenager or adult-sized child, make sure this will fit into the vehicle, particularly if this is a sedan with a small trunk. Have the user disassemble the wheelchair and place it into the trunk to assure fit, and that they can load it into the vehicle if the person is going to be a driver and will need to complete the process themselves.

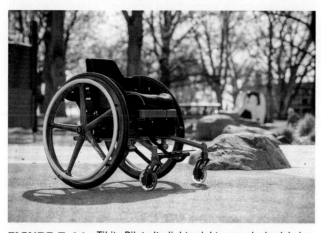

FIGURE 7.14. TiLite Pilot ultralightweight manual wheelchair.

LIGHTWEIGHT FOLDING FRAMES These wheelchairs can be folded side-to-side when disassembled and are not as light as the ultralightweight frames. Although this style of wheelchair is light enough to be self-propelled and can have an adjustable wheel axle, a folding wheelchair frame is typically not as efficient to self-propel, because there is a small amount of "flex" in the frame. This has growth adjustment and can often accommodate a more aggressive seating system.

ADJUSTABLE POSITIONING FRAMES These frames are used for people who are primarily dependent for mobility and need to have some degree of tilt or recline to assist with postural control or pressure relief due to a severe physical limitation. They typically have smaller rear wheels because they do not have to be accessed for self-propulsion. They are usually heavier in overall weight, because there are more parts to the frame. These wheelchairs are offered in both folding and rigid models. The folding models are less likely to withstand heavy extraneous movements, and are typically recommended if the vehicle cannot accommodate a frame without disassembling. The rigid frame is usually very durable and heavy; therefore, consideration of the means for transport and use of ramps, vehicle lifts, is of significant importance.

There are several types of adjustment options, as follows:

- Tilt-in-space: This is used to allow gravity to assist with positioning and for pressure relief. The hip angle remains constant, and the entire seating system tilts rearward. Some wheelchairs can be configured so that the seat will also tilt 5 degrees forward to assist with transfers.
- Recline: Only the backrest opens and the hip angle changes. This allows gravity to assist with positioning and provides a means for pressure relief. Be careful of the shearing of the backrest along the skin of a person's back if they are prone to pressure injuries. This is also not commonly used for people who have extensor tone, because they might push into extension when the backrest is reclined.
- Elevating leg rests: These are usually used in combination with the reclining backrest to prevent the hips from moving forward on the seat because of overstretching of the quadriceps muscles.
- Dynamic components: Many manufacturers have options for wheelchair frame components (or seating system components) that have a dynamic quality to them. As the user pushes against a component, the hardware allows the component to "give" a few degrees with the movement, and then return to the initial position. This is commonly used for the seat-to-back connection, which will allow the backrest to slightly recline as the person pushes into full body extension, and then returns to the upright position when relaxed. This has several functions. If the backrest moves into slight recline as the person applies extension forces to the backrest, the hips are less likely to slide forward on the seat cushion. If this component is used with a properly supportive seating system, the hips are likely to

fall back into place once he/she relaxes; thus, the child's positioning will likely remain intact. This can place less pressure overall on the user's joints and increase the life of the wheelchair components because of less forces being placed on the body and the hardware. Dynamic footrests and headrests are also commonly used. It is crucial that the therapists have a good idea of where the movements are initiated and the strength of the movements to determine the optimal dynamic components.

Powered Wheelchairs

For children who are not independently mobile with a manual wheelchair because of any of the previously described impairments or disabilities, a powered wheelchair may be considered.

These are typically maneuvered using a joystick; however, there are a number of other options for power-mobility access, which are discussed here. Many powered wheelchairs have the capability to accommodate ECSs and augmentative communication technology and can allow for changes in position. The standard powered wheelchair is very heavy, does not disassemble easily into component parts, and generally requires a van for transport and ramps or a level entrance into the home. Therefore, accessibility needs to be thoroughly discussed with the family if power mobility seems to be the direction in which the child is going in terms of independent mobility. Help prepare a family for this, because they are often making decisions about purchasing a new vehicle or moving into a new home. They need guidance about the types of equipment they may need to be accommodating. Many insurance companies will not approve payment for a powered wheelchair if there is not a home assessment completed to ensure accessibility.

Powered wheelchairs can accommodate more aggressive seating systems and can be configured with a number of different manual or electronic seating adjustments. Each seating adjustment needs to be medically justified to a payer. Given here are a few of the common powered wheelchair seat adjustments and typical justifications. Typically, insurance companies are asked to pay for powered wheelchairs; however, in some situations, vocational rehabilitation or other resources can be found to assist with nonmedically justifiable components. The DME representative can assist you with funding questions.

Seat Adjustments and Justifications

- Power tilt-in-space: pressure relief, to allow gravity to assist with positioning, to reduce fatigue, to assist with transfers or repositioning
- Power recline: to provide pressure relief, allows gravity to assist with positioning, to assist with transfers or repositioning, to provide prolonged stretch/change of position to the hips for ROM and pain relief; to allow for diaper changes, hygiene or toileting, use of urinals,

catheterization when in the community (changing tables too small, unsafe, infection/germ avoidance) and access to G-tube
- Power leg rest options: Elevating leg rests provide PROM to LEs, provide hamstring stretch, used in combination with recline to avoid overstretching quadriceps muscles. Also, some powered wheelchairs have articulating leg rests to assist with transfers.
- Power seat height adjustment: To raise or lower the seat for level transfers, reach high or low surfaces, to adjust to peer level, see in crowded environments, improve independence with mobility-related ADLs, such as reaching door openers, elevator buttons, security systems, kitchen or bathroom sinks, and so on; ultimately, this can increase employability and independent living skills. This is difficult to obtain funding through medical insurance at times; however, vocational rehabilitation funding can be an option.
- Active reach: provides varying degrees of anterior seat tilt and/or backrest incline to facilitate forward reach and initiate standing for transfers.[42]
- Power seat to floor: Limited pediatric wheelchairs use this feature to lower to the floor for small clients or children to transfer from floor into the seat of the wheelchair, and then electronically raise to standard seat height.
- Power standing: Provides a standing feature without having to transfer, increase ease for male using a urinal, manage pants when toileting in the community or if more than one caregiver is needed for transfers, clothing management, weight-bearing through LEs for increased bony density/integrity, improved bowel/bladder function, increased ability to reach higher places, completed mobility-related ADLs such as reaching door handles, lights, alarms, sinks, and making light meals can ultimately improve employability in the near future or affect options for living arrangements/day programs for children as they approach young adulthood.

Other Powered Wheelchair Options

In addition to the seating systems and seat adjustments, powered wheelchairs have other variables that must be considered depending on the child's needs, skills, and the environment. For instance, there are varying degrees of suspension offered, which can have a great impact on the child or young adult who needs shock absorption to decrease the chance of sudden movements that will affect positioning, elicit a startle reflex, or affect pain.

There are different drive wheel configurations, including front-wheel drive, mid-wheel drive, rear-wheel drive, and hybrid drive, which can affect turning radius, accessibility, intuitive maneuverability of the wheelchair, and access to varying terrain in the environment. It is extremely important that the user has the opportunity to trial the drive wheel configuration and the specific wheelchair being recommended to assure that all needs are being addressed and met.

Drive Controls

A significant part of an evaluation for power mobility is the user's ability to safely maneuver the wheelchair. Power mobility was formerly considered for adults or for children who were older, under the mistaken impression that a child needed to be older to have the sufficient cognitive development to learn to control a powered wheelchair. The use of power mobility for very young children has evolved significantly over the years.

According to studies cited in the RESNA Position on the Application of Power Wheelchairs for Pediatric Users, early utilization of power mobility for the appropriate child enhances independence, improves psychological development, and enables children to grow to become productive and integrated members of society. Without efficient independent mobility, learned helplessness can develop both from a cognitive and physical standpoint. The ability to safely use a powered wheelchair is directly related to the child's developmental cognitive level. Age, limited vision or cognition, motor impairment, or the ability to use other forms of mobility should not, in and of themselves, be determining factors to rule out power mobility.[9,21] Studies have shown that early access to power mobility improves the child's overall psychosocial and emotional development, in addition to facilitating development of visual spatial skills, and initiation for movement and socialization.

Clinical experience shows that 11- to 12-month-old children have the ability to operate a powered wheelchair.[9] The integrated development of locomotion, cognition, and perceptual-motor abilities in infancy and toddlerhood, and studies of very young children with impairments support the consideration of power mobility for very young children as a means of achieving independent locomotion.[9]

A child who has physical impairments should not be denied the opportunity to move himself from place to place at the same age as a child who has typical physical development. The modified ROCs[54] discussed earlier are an excellent way to introduce a very young child, younger than age 2 years, to wheeled mobility. The ROCs provide that child with the opportunity to learn cause/effect, stop and go, which is the most basic skill necessary for the child to begin power mobility. This can help the child independently gain an understanding of figure ground, and their body position in relation to objects in the environment. After learning these concepts, the ability to learn how to turn in relation to objects or the desired destination is incorporated. As the child gains an understanding of go, stop, and turns, he can begin to refine skill development to maneuver through obstacles, large and small areas, and can begin to learn safety.[21,22] Use of a standard joystick operated with the hand is often the most straightforward means of accessing a powered wheelchair. If this is physically difficult for the child, there are many different ways to configure the joystick, including programming the joystick parameters, using a different joystick top that may be easier to grasp, or moving the joystick to a different location. A physical therapist can assist with

positioning the child in the wheelchair with optimal support and assist with joystick positioning. Some children have an easier time reaching the joystick presented at midline. Children with poor strength and endurance often use both hands to operate the joystick at midline. Use of positioning devices to stabilize the hand or wrist can be explored. It is most important to establish the easiest and safest position for which to place the hand on the joystick, maneuver the wheelchair, independently stop, and remove the hand from the joystick. In some situations, the child has better control of turns when the joystick is configured in the reverse position, where he must pull the joystick to move in the forward direction, and turns are configured appropriately. If a standard joystick does not work for the child, there are many different joystick styles/types that can be trialed, including light touch joysticks, very small joysticks, and trackpad-style joysticks. Some children prefer to use a joystick positioned by their foot, behind the head, or near the chin. If a joystick is not used, there are options for switch-controlled driving, in which any number of single switches can be mounted near any body part to control the wheelchair. A common setup is a head array that contains switches embedded in the headrest pads and requires the child to push back to activate "forward," and turn his head left and right to activate corresponding left and right turns. In other cases, only one movement is consistently available and controlled, allowing the child to use single-switch scanning to choose wheelchair directions. Many other users have good control of "sipping" and "puffing," and will use a sip-and-puff system to maneuver the wheelchair. These are all options that entail access to specialized equipment that can be provided by the DME or manufacturer's representative. It would not be expected for a therapist who does not specialize in AT to have deep knowledge about this equipment, but rather to recognize that there are viable options for the child, and to consult with the appropriate professionals. As the therapist, knowledge of the child's consistent movement patterns and postural needs is vital.

Integration with Function and Other Assistive Technology

Once the details of a child's positioning and mobility needs are established, a comprehensive review of their functional status and all they need to accomplish from the wheelchair level should be done. Some of those issues are as follows:

- Revisit whether the equipment choice/setup will affect other functional skills, such as the ability to perform independent or dependent transfers, the ability to access a toilet or use a urinal from the wheelchair level, the effect of trunk, head/neck positioning for feeding, and the ability to access other technology from the wheelchair in the given position. There may need to be changes or adjustments to the configuration to better accommodate these needs. Collaborating with other team members is vital to ensuring that the configuration is optimal.

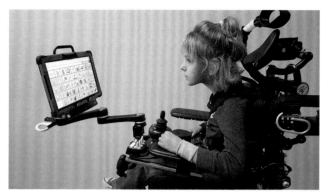

FIGURE 7.15. Augmentative communication device mounted to powered wheelchair using Mount 'n Mover mounting system.

- Integration with other AT: Often, if the child has minimal available controlled movement, it is necessary to use one controller to also operate other assistive devices. For instance, many of the powered wheelchairs offer Bluetooth capability to enable the child to use the joystick to remotely operate a cursor on the computer, a communication device, or an ECS. The therapist involved with choosing a powered wheelchair should find out from other team members if the child needs to have this access to other technology from their wheelchair. The appropriate wheelchair model will be necessary to have this capability, whether it is used now or in the near future.
- Mounting of other equipment to wheelchair: In addition to having access to other technology from the powered wheelchair, mounting and integration of other devices with the wheelchair is pertinent. This would include mounting systems to secure an augmentative communication system to the wheelchair (Fig. 7.15), mounts for switches or control interfaces, additional head supports that may be necessary to use during feeding, visual activities, door opener devices, phone holders, cup holders, intravenous (IV) poles for feedings, ventilator trays, oxygen, or other life-sustaining equipment. Another specialist such as an ATP or a DME provider can assist with the specifics of the actual equipment, the primary physical therapist or OT should provide this information about the additional equipment that needs to be accommodated.

Combination Wheelchairs

In some cases, a person might need a combination of wheelchair components or options to meet their needs. In this case, a combination setup would be beneficial.

Manual Wheelchair with Power Add-On System

This comprises a manual wheelchair base (folding, rigid, or tilt-in-space) with a power add-on system that can be configured by adding wheels that contain motors, a small battery pack, and a joystick to the manual frame. This can be

disassembled fairly easily, and is lighter in weight than is a standard power wheelchair. The power option can be disengaged so that caregiver can still push the wheelchair if the user is unable to maneuver in a given situation. Situations where this might be useful include the following:

- Poor accessibility to transfer a standard powered wheelchair into the home—power option can be stored in garage or vehicle trunk. Lighter weight manual wheels can be used in the home.
- Family or caregiver is not equipped to transport a standard power wheelchair.
- User has fluctuating physical capabilities depending on the environment—the user may be able to self-propel efficiently on level surfaces at school or home; but needs the power add-on system when in the community, crossing outdoor school campuses, or attending sporting or community events, and shopping.
- Child is learning to maneuver a powered wheelchair, but is not yet safe or skilled enough to use a standard powered wheelchair functionally or safely. This is an option where being able to disengage the motor and allow the caregiver to push the wheelchair can be very beneficial when in the community.

Keep in mind that this system is not as durable or rugged to handle heavy outdoor use compared to a standard powered wheelchair. This is for moderate outdoor use, and does not provide the child with the opportunity to change seat adjustments through electronics. This system is not as programmable as a standard powered wheelchair; therefore, it would be most beneficial if the user had the opportunity for a trial before recommendation.

Power Assist Systems

There are several systems that can be attached to a manual wheelchair to provide a "burst" of power to assist when the user pushes on the wheel rim or activates the system. This can be beneficial for someone who has excellent self-propulsion capabilities, but has issues with strength, endurance, shoulder integrity, or has barriers such as hills, grades, or long distances to contend with in the environment. This is commonly used in combination with an ultralight weight manual wheelchair frame. New power assist systems continue to evolve as the effects of prolonged wheelchair propulsion on joints is researched.

When exploring wheeled mobility options with children and their families, provide ongoing support and information about the available options that can meet their immediate needs, as well as their needs over the next 3 to 5 years. Again, consideration of the child's diagnosis, progression or regression of skills, home and vehicle setup, and school/work/community needs is vital. Consider the child and caregivers' emotional acceptance of any adaptive equipment and the changing needs as the child moves through stages of development.

Recreational Wheelchairs

The options for wheelchairs that can be used specifically for recreation are becoming increasingly popular. These devices can be set up specifically to meet the needs indicated for a particular sport. For instance, a wheelchair used for basketball or tennis would require that the wheels be set up with a large degree of camber so that the wheelchair can be maneuverable for quick changes in direction, yet remain stable to prevent falls. These usually require a low center of gravity for stability. These usually have thin high-pressure tires for performance. A wheelchair used for hunting, fishing, camping, farming, or hiking would be set up for all-terrain access, with larger wheels with treads and a high amount of torque. These types of wheelchairs are typically not covered through private insurance. It is helpful to assist the child and family to research local adaptive sports opportunities, so the child is aware and feels comfortable with recreational activities. Many times, the local program will provide equipment for use during the activity.

Wheelchair Fitting/Options

As noted previously, almost any wheelchair frame can accommodate any seating system, including the seat and back cushions and any additional positioning components. Once there is a general understanding of the wheelchair type and configuration and the possible seating system adjustments needed, the details of the seating system should be addressed. The general seating principles discussed previously for chair setup are incorporated when choosing seating system components and integrating a seating system with a wheelchair frame.

The physical therapist should consider the following criteria for wheelchairs, and also the principles of seating discussed earlier in this chapter:

1. Seat width should allow for growth or developmental changes, considering puberty, potential growth spurts, and weight changes. Accommodation to avoid contact of bony prominences with wheelchair seating components is important. The width of the wheelchair should accommodate various clothing thickness, including outerwear for cold winter climates. Most vendors consider 1 inch on each side to be appropriate. For users who are self-propelling, the width should be as narrow as possible to efficiently reach the wheels for propulsion and provide an appropriate shoulder position to prevent injury. With the small child with shorter arms, it is often beneficial to move the armrests out of the way during propulsion to reach the wheels more easily. Be aware of the ability to adjust the wheelchair frames for growth in width over the life of the wheelchair. The DME representative or manufacturer's representative can assist with choosing the optimal wheelchair width with respect to the user's position and integration of the recommended seating system. These professionals can also assist with modifying the wheelchair frame setup should there be a change to the seating system components.

2. Seat depth should permit comfortable knee flexion without popliteal pressure. A sling backrest or an aftermarket backrest that can provide varying degrees of support can be used, depending on the child's needs for positioning. Some wheelchair frames have adjustable depth hardware to allow the back canes to be moved rearward to accommodate growth. To maximize growth potential, mounting an aftermarket backrest in front of the back canes can increase the amount of available growth in seat depth. Of course, this would all have a bearing on the relationship of the child's body and the wheel position for propulsion and the center of gravity of the wheelchair, affecting stability and tipping of the wheelchair. Best practice is to position the rear-wheel axle as far forward as possible without compromising rearward stability of the wheelchair or interfering with the front casters.[11,45] Axle plate adjustments that adjust both horizontally and vertically are available, but the extent of modification depends on many factors, including the frame size of the chair. When establishing seat depth setup of a tilt-in-space wheelchair, consider the weight of the seating system, which may be heavier and deeper in size, as well as any medical equipment that may be mounted to the rear of the wheelchair, which could cause rearward tipping of the wheelchair. All this has a bearing on the overall setup of the wheelchair.

3. Pelvic/LE support: Once the seat depth and width is established, the pelvis is stabilized in the correct position, taking into account the information obtained through the physical examination/mat examination (ROM, tone, strength, etc.). If the pelvis is not in a stable optimal position, the rest of the body will not be aligned or have sufficient stability or mobility. There are many different cushions with varying degrees of support offered. A basic general use cushion is used for comfort and is light in weight, and can be used for someone who has good postural control and is using the wheelchair for endurance reasons rather than for positioning or pressure relief. There are contoured cushions that will provide minimal, moderate to aggressive contouring to provide a more definitive place for the ischial tuberosities and femurs to align symmetrically. Some of these cushions can be modified to accommodate a pelvic obliquity or rotation using inserts or components. They also have other positioning components that can be placed on the cushion to maintain hip adduction or abduction positioning. These are considered positioning cushions. Many cushions have pressure-relieving properties that can be achieved using a variety of mediums, including foams, gels, or air. If the user has issues with pressure injuries, it is highly recommended they be evaluated through a specialized program with a qualified therapist and DME representative. A pressure mapping assessment would be extremely beneficial, particularly when the child lacks sensation or is unable to communicate.

4. Pelvic/seat belt: A pelvic positioning belt is needed to stabilize the pelvis in place on the recommended seat cushion. This can be positioned at different angles, depending on the child's needs, spasticity, and the shape of the cushion. If a child has excessive extensor tone, it can help to use a four-point pelvic positioning belt, which has two points of contact on each side, and prevents the belt from sliding up toward the abdomen.

5. Gravity assistance: There are several ways to use gravity to assist with postural alignment in a wheelchair, depending on the frame of the wheelchair. As stated previously, wheelchair dump can be accomplished by setting up the frame so that the front seat height is higher than is the rear seat height, in relation to the floor. This change allows gravity to assist to maintain the child's trunk in an upright position so that he/she can free the upper extremities to self-propel and to avoid sliding hips forward on the seat. For manual or powered wheelchairs that are not being self-propelled, use of the tilt-in-space option allows the child to have frequent changes in body position, while being provided with gravity-assisted positioning and maintaining the seat-to-back relationship. This can effectively address a variety of issues that can compromise the child's comfort, health, and well-being, including problems associated with physiology, alignment, biomechanics, transfers, and deformity prevention.[48] Another means of using gravity to assist with postural alignment is use of a reclining backrest, where the seat-to-back angle changes, but the seat-to-floor relationship remains the same. A power reclining and/or tilt-in-space chair makes it possible for a child to independently achieve pressure relief and a resting position throughout the day without requiring frequent transfers.

6. Trunk support: The type and size of backrest can vary greatly depending on the child's needs. For instance, if a child has excellent postural control or does not need to use the wheelchair as a primary sitting device throughout the day, an upholstered backrest might suffice, and will make the wheelchair itself lighter in weight and easier to fold/disassemble for transport. Otherwise, a solid backrest that provides postural support can help provide pelvic stability for increased propulsion efficiency and upright trunk alignment. There are many different backrests commercially available that provide varying degrees of lateral trunk support, swing-away lateral support hardware to allow for transfers or accessing G-tubes, and foam inserts to facilitate midline upright trunk alignment or lumbar support. There are also options for custom molding of backrests to accommodate a flexible or fixed spinal curvature (Fig. 7.16). There are different mediums to provide pressure relief and air exchange for users who have difficulty with temperature regulation. For a person who is self-propelling, the preferred backrest height is below the scapulae, for optimum freedom of movement and clearance. This also allows the user to

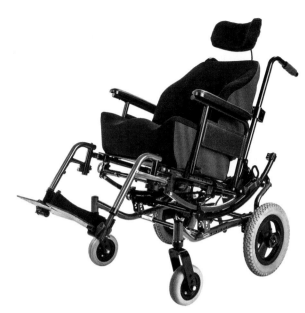

FIGURE 7.16. Precision Rehab Manufacturing Signature Fit custom-molded seating system on manual tilt-in-space wheelchair.

rotate and reach behind the wheelchair or hook an arm over the back cane for pressure releases. Keeping the backrest as light in weight as possible would be optimal. Many children with poor postural control require that the backrest to be higher and more contoured. These backrests can be heavier and more cumbersome, but are necessary to provide adequate support. Attention must be paid to the height of the backrest in relation to adjustment of any other positioning components, including headrests and anterior chest supports. These solid backrests usually offer quick-release hardware that allows the backrest to remove easily for disassembly.

Head/neck supports: Posterior head/neck supports, or headrests, are needed when a wheelchair has a tilt or recline function. Headrests are also needed when a child is being transported in a motor vehicle while seated in the wheelchair (refer to the section Transporting a child in a motor vehicle). These can be mounted with removable quick-release hardware for children who only need the headrest during certain situations. Many headrests that offer support are available, depending on the child's need. It should be considered whether the child needs only slight posterior support as a tactile cue, or a support contoured around the suboccipital area of the head to facilitate improved positioning in the anterior/posterior plane. Some children need lateral head supports to maintain midline alignment. There are some headrests that are open around the upper portion of the head, yet provide substantial support at the neck and shoulder areas. These typically have additional swing-away pad components to provide upper head support, used particularly during transport or when fatigued. Some headrests offer built-in switch mounts to access other technology using a single switch, such as a communication device. Some headrests have an integrated wheelchair controller, which is discussed in a later section. Several headrests offer an anterior component at the neck, chin, or forehead level for added support. A therapist would not be expected to have significant knowledge about the specific headrests that are available, rather the type of support that would benefit the child. When significant support is needed by a child who may be using additional technology, a team approach to choosing a head support and the use of head/neck movements or eye movements to access technology is very important. In addition, the other team members can provide important information regarding the necessary head positioning for safe swallowing, breathing, oral motor control, and use of visual fields.

7. Foot support: There are several factors that can affect the selection and position of wheelchair footrests/footplates, including the child's physical status obtained through the mat examination, method of transfer, and the size of the wheelchair and casters. The position of the footplate will be influenced by the available knee flexion and tonal influences discussed earlier in this chapter. The DME representative can assist to establish a setup that will avoid interference of the footplate with the front caster and footplate to ground clearance. An angle-adjustable footplate would be necessary to provide full foot contact, particularly if a child has PROM limitations or is wearing a foot orthotic with fixed ankle position. The ability of the footrests to swing away for transfers or accessibility is an important consideration. Most rigid wheelchairs have a fixed front end and do not have the option for swing-away removable footrests. They do commonly have the option of a flip-up footplate if needed. If the wheelchair has a reclining backrest, elevating leg rests are useful; however, these are much heavier than are standard leg rests, and can affect the maneuverability of the wheelchair because of the overall dimensions. They can have a negative effect on positioning because when they are elevated, they lengthen the hamstrings and cause the pelvis to posteriorly tilt and slide forward on the seat, subsequently risking pressure injury with prolonged use. If needed, it is necessary to monitor and change positions in the wheelchair to ensure positioning and pressure relief are maintained. A single calf strap with one footplate or heel loops at the back of each footplate can keep the feet from sliding rearward off the footplate. Maintaining stability of the feet on the footplates is another important factor. Simple Velcro straps can be used across the instep of the foot, the ankle, or the toes. There are a variety of different strap closures and foot positioners available. The stability needed and the child's independence with management of the supports must be considered.

8. Arm support: Armrests can improve symmetrical body alignment in midline and help prevent the child from getting his/her hands caught in the wheels of the wheelchair. Armrest height should be comfortable, should allow reduced weight bearing through the shoulders, and should allow easy access to the wheels for propulsion.[45,58] Essentially, the type of armrest should be dictated by ease of management. Removable armrests can provide the benefits of armrests when needed, but can be removed for ease of some types of transfers and for moving the wheelchair into close proximity to a table or desk.

9. Wheels and casters: The size and setup of the wheels and casters have an overall impact on the stability and maneuverability of the wheelchair itself, which affects the user's ability to propel the wheelchair, transfer from an appropriate seat height, and access a variety of terrain in the environment. Stability of a manual wheelchair depends on the height of the person's center of mass (affected by the individual's height and the height of wheelchair seat), placement of the rear-wheel axle relative to the center of gravity, and the width of the base, that is, the distance between the two rear wheels on the floor. Improved lateral stability can be achieved by increasing rear-wheel camber. The vertical angle of the wheels, or camber, dictates the maneuverability of the wheelchair and the overall width of the wheelchair. By angling the wheels inward at the top, the distance between the wheels and the floor becomes greater, thereby enlarging the base of support and increasing lateral stability. A greater degree of wheel camber will make the wheelchair easier to maneuver through quick turns, as is necessary for most wheelchair sports, such as basketball and tennis. For a child who is self-propelling, the size and position of the rear wheel is crucial to having a biomechanical propulsion advantage. Ideally, the elbow should be in 100 to 120 degrees of extension when the child grasps the hand rim at its highest point.[45,58] This optimal elbow angle is a product not only of wheel diameter but also of seat height, including the height of the appropriate wheelchair cushion, armrest position, and placement of the rear axle. When the arm is allowed to hang comfortably down by the side of the wheelchair, the fingertips should fall near the midpoint of the wheel axle. The front caster position can also have an effect on the overall stability of the wheelchair. Some wheelchair frames have options for a flared front caster housing to increase stability. This can be a nice safety feature for the young child who may not have the safety judgment to avoid traversing steeper grades or uneven terrain at high speeds. The child's specific environment and activity level will influence decisions about the wheels and casters. The wheel or caster type can have a significant impact on the performance of the wheelchair on various types of terrain. Pneumatic tires can provide a smoother ride (adding some shock absorbency), but require considerable maintenance for consistent and proper inflation pressure. Underinflated tires increase the effort of manual propulsion. For small children, the child's weight may not justify the need for pneumatic tires considering the extra maintenance

required, but in older, heavier children, riding on rough terrain is easier when using pneumatic tires. Airless inserts in the tires can be used to prevent flat tires or air loss if the child lives in a rural or urban area, where there is a high chance of tire punctures. Large treads will be better for outdoor terrain use, where thin high-pressure tires will perform better indoors and for sports requiring quick turns. The caster size will also have an effect, because the smaller casters are more maneuverable, and the wider larger casters will not be as likely to become caught in terrain/ruts.

10. Wheel locks (brakes): These should be positioned for ease of management and can be operated either by pushing or pulling, with or without extensions, depending on the child's preference and abilities. There are other styles of wheel locks, depending on the manufacturer, some of which are mounted underneath the seat, attendant wheel locks accessed from behind the wheelchair, or hand-operated wheel locks and braking mechanisms attached to the push handles.

11. Anti-tip tubes: These are safety components mounted to the bottom of the rear of the wheelchair, which help prevent the wheelchair from tipping rearward. These must be used during transport in a motor vehicle and are very necessary to use when tilting and reclining a wheelchair, or when heavy medical equipment is mounted to the rear of the wheelchair. If a caregiver moves these out of the way for foot clearance when pushing a wheelchair, they are required to replace them into position for safety.

12. Upper extremity support surfaces: These are trays that are particularly helpful for children, especially the school-aged child. This provides support to the upper extremities, can help relax the upper body by providing a place for support, and is a place on which to mount/position material that must be manipulated or used for ADLs, and school or play tasks. This can be composed of a clear or opaque material. Although a clear tray will allow the user to see more items if self-propelling the wheelchair, it can be distracting for a child with a visual impairment. It is important to discuss the needs with the treatment team.

13. Push handles: Manual wheelchairs or strollers for children who are dependent on or independent with mobility can be outfitted with an extended push handle to assist with maneuvering the wheelchair long distances or up/down curbs or steps. There are a number of options available, depending on the manufacturer. Consider the height of the caregivers and the position of the push handles if the wheelchair device is tilted or reclined.

Once specifications for a wheelchair are finalized and all team members are in agreement with the choices, documentation must be completed by the evaluator to justify payment for the equipment. The type of documentation required differs depending on the funding source. Typically, an extensive evaluation with an accompanying letter of medical necessity is required. Equipment components are itemized, and justification must be medical in nature. It is helpful to state the less costly alternatives that have been ruled out and what medical effects would occur if the equipment is not provided.[41] Therapists should always remember that equipment is expensive and, more importantly, will affect the quality of the child's life for the next 3 to 5 years.

Gait Trainers and Walkers

A gait trainer is a wheeled device that assists the person to learn to ambulate or return to ambulation. A gait trainer may be used on a long-term basis to provide a means of independent ambulation, or may be a step in the continuum of developing independent ambulation with less support such as a wheeled walker or forearm crutches.[59,60] There are many types and styles of gait trainers offering a range of support and options, depending on the child's needs (Fig. 7.17). A gait trainer will not offer the controlled positioning of a stander, but will provide assistance by unweighting the support and providing some postural alignment to work on gait training. Some gait trainers support the child in a more anteriorly tilted or prone position, providing a saddle-type seat, chest support, and hand holds. This position can facilitate the user to initiate stepping. There are leg supports available to keep the hips from excessively adducting and to limit the movement of the LEs. The setup of this type of gait trainer does interfere with the user being able to get up close to tabletops or people, because the support components are in front of the user. There are other gait trainers set up with posterior support, where the user is in a more upright position, and can use the saddle seat, upper body supports, and leg positioners. This type of gait trainer allows the child to be positioned close to tables and people.

For children who need less support, a posterior walker can be used. This facilitates the child to stand upright, and offers an array of components to stabilize the hips as well as various upper extremity supports. These can be provided

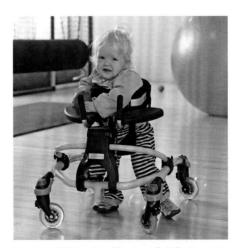

FIGURE 7.17. R82 by Etac Mustang Gait Trainer.

with or without a seat for rest periods. The more traditional forward walkers are used for those who have more postural control and need the support for balance and safety.

Gait trainers and walkers are not only a means of independent ambulation for some children but are also beneficial in other ways: They make possible upright position for social interaction and upper extremity function and offer many benefits of LE weight bearing (discussed earlier in this chapter). The weight-bearing benefits are considered noteworthy because the weight bearing is dynamic and comes from intermittent loading, a strategy that has been found to improve cortical bone mineral density.[51,61] It is extremely important that the intended function of a gait trainer and the progression of the child's skills over the next 3 to 5 years is carefully considered when addressing this type of equipment. It is pertinent that any equipment be trialed by the child before actually prescribing. Funding considerations are important, because in some areas, medical insurance will not fund both a gait trainer and a stander. The DME dealer can be very helpful in determining a plan for the equipment progression and funding options.

Other Mobility Aids

A variety of other mobility aids may be used, depending on the child's impairments and degree of involvement. Mobility aids commonly used with adults can be used with children and include the following:

- Forearm (Lofstrand), platform, or axillary crutches
- Canes (J-cane, T-cane, quad-cane)
- Walkers (wheeled, reverse wheeled, platform, walkers with upturned handgrips)
- General LE orthoses (supramalleolar orthosis [SMO], ankle–foot orthosis [AFO], knee–ankle–foot orthosis [KAFO], and hip–knee–ankle–foot orthosis [HKAFO])
- Specialized orthotic devices (parapodiums, reciprocating gait orthosis)

» Adaptive car seats

Age-appropriate restraints and seating for a child, with or without special needs, in the back seat significantly reduces serious injury in automobile accidents.[62] The American Academy of Pediatrics (AAP) recommends that all children younger than age 13 years ride in the rear seat. As of 2018, the AAP recommended that children be placed in rear-facing car safety seats as long as possible at least until age 2 years or until they reach the maximum height and weight for that particular car seat; and then they graduate to a forward-facing car seat until height and/or weight reach the manufacturer's limit. The AAP further recommended that a belt-positioning booster seat be used when any child has outgrown a forward-facing car seat and should be used at least until the child is 8 years of age, and has reached approximately 4 feet 9 inches in height, according to the

manufacturer's instructions. The child who has not yet reached the suggested height at age 8 should continue to use the booster until reaching the height requirement. The AAP maintains a current list of approved car seats along with recommendations for selecting an appropriate car seat and the correct and safe usage of car seats.[62] Children who need to lie flat during transport because of impairments or disabilities should be in a crash-tested car bed.[62]

In the United States, vehicle safety restraints for the transport of infants and young children are required in all 50 states. In spite of this requirement, nonuse of vehicle restraints for young children with disabilities remains a problem.

Parents may ask a physical therapist or OT familiar with their child's impairments and needs for advice or suggestions regarding appropriate and safe car seats. This includes a standard car safety seat that meets federal motor vehicle safety standards if possible; using rolled towels to give lateral support in the safety seat if needed, without interfering with the seat's harness system; not modifying the car safety seat restraints; turning off airbags if the child must ride in the front seat; moving seat back as far as possible if the child must ride in the front seat; securing all medical equipment under the child's seat or on the floor; and having an adult ride in the back seat with the medically fragile child.[62] Simple modifications, such as adding an abduction pommel, a small seat wedge, or lateral supports to a standard car seat, can be made, as long as the integrity of the seat and safety are not compromised by the adaptation.

Although an appropriately fit standard child car seat should be used if it meets the child's safety needs, for children with complex involvement, a special needs car seat is needed. These seats tend to be more expensive than are standard car seats, but should be used when the standard car seat cannot adequately provide for the child's safety.[62]

A number of vehicle safety restraints for children with special health care needs are currently available. These have different options for positioning, including lateral trunk and hip positioners, footrests, head supports, abductor pommel, seat wedges, and pressure-relieving foam. Some special needs car seats have safety locks to prevent children from unlatching the harness or retainer clip. There are options for seats that turn 90 degrees toward the door to transfer more easily into the seat. The various special needs car seats install into the vehicle in different ways. The physical therapist should consult with the DME provider regarding seats that could meet specific needs for a child with a disability. The National Center for Transportation of Children with Special Health Care Needs provides resources with the most up-to-date guidelines approved by the AAP or safety restraints for children with special health care needs.

The therapist can determine optimal positioning within the car seat using trial equipment and provide information to the family regarding the vehicle setup necessary for safe installation; however, the family is responsible for actually installing the car seat in the vehicle. There are adaptive car seat programs and local Certified Child Passenger Safety Technicians (found on the Internet) to install the car seats and ensure safe setup.[63]

A child being transported in a wheelchair should have head support,[30,31] and the wheelchair should be secured with a four-point tie-down device. Lap trays and other equipment attached to the wheelchair should be removed and secured separately.[31] Another option is to transfer the child from a wheelchair to a certified transit wheelchair.[30] However, these chairs are frequently not available for a given child.

A child's safe transport in a school bus also needs to be addressed. The AAP recommends that a child who weighs under 80 lbs and can be reasonably transferred or can assist with transfers to a Child Safety Restraint System (CSRS),[64] which provides safe support, such as a conventional car seat, special needs car seat, safety vest or harness, or five-point harness integrated into the bus seat, should use this mode of school bus transport. These need to be secured following federally developed safety guidelines for school buses that transport children with special needs, which are available on the National Highway Traffic Safety Administration website.[64,65] If transferring into a CSRS is not safe or possible, transport in a wheelchair or device that meets the voluntary industry standards of the ANSI-RESNA is recommended.

Medical equipment, such as a ventilator or oxygen, is often transported with the child. Any medical equipment, including unoccupied wheelchairs, also needs to be secured within the vehicle for the safety of all occupants, whether in private or public transportation.[64]

» Equipment for infants and toddlers

When considering the needs of the infant and the toddler and the availability of devices, one must remember that these younger children are often undiagnosed or may have a developmental delay that may not result in long-term disability. Children who are developing typically and who require long periods of hospitalization for cardiac, pulmonary, gastrointestinal, and other disorders may benefit from types of apparatus that enhance motor development. Positioning for infants and young toddlers to safely and successfully complete ADLs must be considered.

Feeding/Seated Activities

Standard highchairs and strollers can be used for these children, as long as they are providing appropriate alignment and support for safe feeding and swallowing. Specially designed adaptive highchairs and strollers are also available if their needs cannot be met using standard off-the-shelf equipment or with simple adaptations. Seating equipment for feeding may offer a stable, symmetrical position that allows for optimal oral motor function, head righting and control, and freedom of movement of the upper extremities. A good feeding posture for all infants includes being semi-upright or sitting upright and in slight trunk and neck flexion, to avoid hyperextension of the trunk and neck to aid in swallowing. Establishing foot support for stability is also important as a base of support for safe swallowing and for oral motor skills.

Concepts of seating and positioning already discussed in this chapter should be applied to strollers and highchairs. For example, the toddler who is able to sit in a highchair or stroller should have adequate hip flexion (90 degrees) and support to facilitate trunk symmetry and midline use of the hands. Keep in mind that in addition to eating in the home, these children also need to be appropriately positioned when being fed in the community, usually while seated in their stroller. The original umbrella or sling-style strollers encourage adduction and internal rotation of the hips and posterior tilt of the pelvis, which are not components of good postural alignment for sitting and are not suitable for many infants and toddlers with disabilities. Some contemporary strollers called umbrella strollers have a solid seat and back, which do not create the same kind of postural deviations as the original-style umbrella strollers.

Floor Play

Physical therapy interventions for the infant and toddler who have been hospitalized for long periods should concentrate on encouraging normal development of controlled motor patterns. The therapist should assist the parents to find ways to facilitate movement and provide support as needed to allow for functional movement when the child is seated on the floor. Continue to monitor these children to determine if they progress without the need for adaptive equipment or need the equipment to meet their functional needs.

Bathing/Toilet Training

Infants are typically bathed using an off-the-shelf infant tub until they outgrow the device or become too difficult to manage because of neuromotor impairments. The therapist should continually monitor whether solutions are necessary for providing additional support in the standard bathtub or shower. There are bathtub supports that are designed for the child who can sit in the bottom of the bathtub, but has poor sitting balance and needs additional trunk support. There are also adjustable bath slings available to meet the needs of a child who continues to be dependent and who needs to be in a tilted/reclining position for safety.

» Equipment for hospitalized children

Normal motor development is an integrated process that requires sensory input and freedom to respond to that input through general motor output, exploration, and play. Normal patterns of movement develop when agonist and antagonist muscles learn balanced and synergistic cooperation. Because equipment may disrupt or interfere with this process by limiting or restricting sensory input and movement, using equipment for infants and toddlers is almost always discouraged.

Movement in hospitalized children is often restricted by monitors, telemetry devices, and therapeutic medical equipment. It would be counterproductive to the child's motor development to add apparatus to these medically necessary devices. The objective for the hospitalized child is often to provide optimal freedom of movement within the limits imposed by medical interventions and equipment. Physical therapy for hospitalized children should encourage increased activity, if safe, and should facilitate movement patterns that, because of the external limitations, are difficult for the child to initiate. As the child's medical status improves, or when the child returns home, equipment use should still be limited, except when indicated to promote physical control or safety.

Ventilator-dependent children represent a growing population with major equipment needs. With increasing frequency, the physical therapist is asked to assist in the discharge planning and management of ventilator-dependent children. Technologic advances have prolonged life expectancy for many children with chronic illnesses. Portable ventilators and third-party funding have aided in transforming these once chronically hospitalized children into active members of the community. They often return home, attend local schools, and participate in recreational and social activities in the community. Such participation requires a transport system for essential life-support equipment, which may include a portable ventilator and battery, humidifier, oxygen source, airway suction unit with catheters and hoses, a bag valve mask (manual resuscitator), a bag of medical supplies, and other items.

An innovative approach must be taken with this population to address developmental, orthopedic, and respiratory needs. It is essential to work with a DME dealer who can assist in meeting the unique needs of these children by addressing positioning concerns and the mounting/securement and weight distribution of life-sustaining medical equipment to the mobility device. The system shown in Figure 7.18 is designed to meet the specific needs of both the child and family. The child can recline or sit upright using an age-appropriate and cost-effective mobility device that is aesthetically pleasing and manageable. Figure 7.19 shows a special needs positioning stroller with the medical equipment secured to the stroller. As the child grows and independent mobility becomes likely, manual or motorized wheelchairs can be adapted for the child's use.

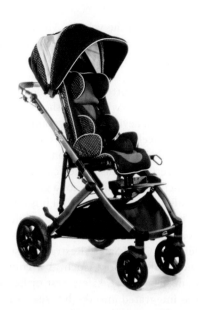

FIGURE 7.18. Sunrise Medical Zippie Voyage positioning stroller.

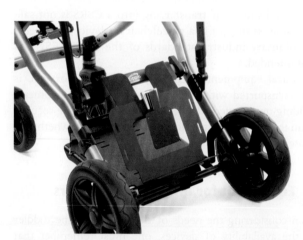

FIGURE 7.19. Sunrise Medical Zippie Voyage Stroller ventilator tray.

» Equipment for activities of daily living

It is crucial that therapists collaborate with all team members regarding goals for participation in ADLs.

Toileting and Bathing

In addition to the simple bath supports mentioned earlier, there are many options for supportive bath seats or slings that can fit into the bathtub or hydraulic bath lifts onto which the child can transfer and then be lowered into the bottom of the bathtub. For the larger child, the transfers into the bathtub become an issue; therefore, tub transfer benches, or sliding bath seat systems may be a consideration.

Providing appropriate positioning and equipment can facilitate healthy bowel and bladder function and toilet training.[66] Although achieving good positioning for toileting may be as simple as using a footstool with some children, others require more support and, therefore, more complex seating arrangements. Toilets may be modified by adding reducer rings with or without abductor pommels, handholds or grab bars, back supports, and footrests. Essential to good positioning on the toilet is for the child's hips and knees to be flexed to 90 degrees or greater with full contact foot support. This position helps limit extensor spasticity in those children affected by hypertonia and also helps children coordinate their muscles to void and to feel secure. Because many children need to sit on the toilet for a prolonged period, it is vital that the pressure of the toilet seat on bony prominences be addressed. Prolonged excess pressure on the hard toilet seat can be a source of pressure injuries to the coccyx and ischial tuberosities if the positioning on the toilet seat is not addressed.

There are a number of different shower/commode chair combinations that offer extensive support and can be used by a child of any size, with a variety of options for bases that can be either propelled by the child or the attendant/caregiver. The child's physical needs and the setup and accessibility of the environment are factors in choosing appropriate bathing/toileting equipment. An OT typically addresses the child's ADL and hygiene needs; however, it is important for the physical therapist to understand the equipment options that are available and to provide input regarding transfers and positioning needs. The DME dealer and/or the manufacturer's representative can assist to determine equipment models that can be trialed by the child (mock usage) and trialed in the home to ensure accessibility.

Feeding

Keeping a growing child nourished in the face of physical impairments can be very challenging for parents and a source of great frustration for the child and parent alike. As with bathing and toileting, good positioning is the first rule of order for feeding a child, whether for independent self-feeding or assisted feeding. Applying basic principles of seating, as discussed earlier, whether in a standard high chair, a regular kitchen or dining chair, or with the help of an adaptive seating device, can (1) improve the child's alignment and stability for safe feeding and swallowing, (2) make it possible for a child to be an independent feeder, (3) improve the caregiver's ability to feed the child, and (4) limit the need for other extensive feeding aids. Feeding aids can be found in rehabilitation catalogs and websites.

Playing

Toys are the tools of children's work, which is to play. Playing with toys enhances a child's sensorimotor, cognitive, psychosocial, and motor development. Often, children with impairments will need help with positioning for play. Play positions should vary and be developmentally appropriate, and the support for positioning can be from an adult or from simple equipment.

Children with certain impairments may be unable to play with many commercially available toys. With a bit of creativity, many toys can be adapted for children, perhaps by changing the switching mechanism on a toy or adapting a toy so that a child can grasp it more easily. In addition to adapting toys, consideration of a child's developmental level and abilities is important when selecting toys. Parents and therapists should not overlook toys made especially for children with special needs; these can be found on the Internet or in special needs catalogs. Also, with the growing emphasis on universal design, more toys found in traditional toy stores, both today and in the future, may be age- and ability-appropriate for children with various impairments. Therapists can help parents find the best toys for their children. After all, providing children with suitable toys and objects for play is an important aspect of nurturing children and helping them learn in all domains of development.

» Access technologies

Access technologies are described as "Technologies that translate the intentions of the user with profound physical impairments into functional interactions such as communication or environmental control."[67] A specific access solution consists of the technology, a user and user interface, a task, and an environment or access site that typically changes throughout the user's day. Access technologies continue to develop to allow a person with severe physical impairments to control items in their environment, operate computers, and use augmentative communication devices. Mechanical methods of access can include directly making selections using a keyboard, remote control, or a set of choices using a voluntary body movement. For people lacking coordinated control, direct selection can be inefficient or result in poor alignment, fatigue, or pain with repeated access. The physical therapist and OT can work with the team to ensure that the child is posturally well supported when using the device and that the access technology is set up for the most efficient use. Many children with severe motor impairments lack the graded control to access technology in this manner, but have consistent movements necessary to access single switches to indirectly access[68,69] and operate a device using a variety of scanning methods. This entails a systematic representation of options appearing in timed intervals from which the user selects by activating a single switch or array of switches. Historically, the user interface for available access technologies has been a mechanical switch activated by changes in displacement, tilt, force, or air pressure, and is controlled by a specific physical movement of the user. These mechanical switches are reliable, available, and relatively simple to operate. However, a user must have a minimum of one consistent movement to control a mechanical switch. This can make it less than ideal for the person who may lack the physical strength and endurance, mental endurance, and/or experience pain when using this movement repeatedly over time.[69] There are many types of switches that require varying amounts of force and provide different feedback to the user, including visual, auditory, tactile, and proprioceptive feedback. The physical therapist and OT can assist to determine consistent movement patterns and feedback necessary for a child to effectively and efficiently activate technology using specific control interfaces. More complex options available for control interfaces include switches that detect respiratory signals that can be translated into messages using Morse code signals,[68] fiberoptic switches that require minimal movement to "break" a beam of light, electromagnetic proximity switches that activate when the user places a body part near the switch, or voice-activated switches that react to sound.[68] These types of switches will open up an array of options for the child with severe physical impairments who may have minimal movements, but have the ability to vocalize, or even control an eye blink.

More complex access technologies include use of head movement detection, eye gaze, or eye tracking. These systems require significant proximal support for the child to stabilize his/her neck for consistent and refined head or eye movements. The setup and positioning of the device or camera detecting the movements is crucial to the success of the system. The physical therapist and OT are vital team members in assisting with this setup, monitoring the child's movements, endurance, and any pain that could occur with the repetitive movements. Education to the teachers, speech language pathologists, family, and child is crucial to meeting physical needs related to use of access technologies.

Voice recognition systems are now mainstreamed with the disabled and nondisabled population, and an excellent method for accessing technologies. These systems have become increasingly easier to use with less training required.

Brain–computer interface (BCI) solutions in which neural signals in a person's brain can be translated by a computer to access technology continue to evolve.[68,69] Options for BCI include either invasive interfaces involving implanted electrodes and interconnections with the user's peripheral nerves or noninvasive interfaces that use external devices to monitor brain activity.[68,69] As wearable technosensor technology develops in the nondisabled community, researchers continue to work on developing options for people with disabilities.[69]

In addition to the electronic access technologies, physical modification to the environments in which a person uses adaptive equipment (e.g., ramps, lifts, grab bars) can optimize a person's interaction with the environment.

Augmentative and Alternative Communication Systems

Communication systems are a subgroup of access technologies. Although most of this chapter has focused on adaptive equipment relative to positioning, mobility, and ADL needs (i.e., the physical needs of the child), it is important that we give brief consideration to communication devices. These devices may be equipment used by a child who is deaf or hearing impaired or has primary speech deficits, partial sight, blindness, or motor impairments.

Physical therapists must be generally familiar with communication equipment for two reasons. First, interactions with children in the therapeutic environment necessarily require the ability to communicate with them. This brief synopsis is intended to broadly familiarize the reader with various types of communication devices that may be encountered. A second reason for physical therapists to have an understanding of adaptive communication systems is that many of these strategies require controlled movement as the user interface. Knowing about these systems can help the physical therapist address movement issues to facilitate the child's successful use of a communication strategy. The physical therapist at times may work closely with a speech and language pathologist in developing appropriate motor control for a communication system.

Children with hearing impairment may need hearing aids, amplified telephones, or classroom amplification systems. They also use some of the gestural communication systems, described in the next section, such as American Sign Language (ASL), which do not require adaptive technology.

Alerting devices that use visual or vibratory cues to alert a hearing-impaired person to a telephone, doorbell, smoke alarm, alarm clock, or automobile horn are important aids for both function and safety. Using the telephone to communicate with persons who are nonhearing or hearing can be accomplished with a telecommunication device for the deaf (TDD) or Telecommunication Relay Service.[70]

People with visual impairments can compensate for or augment their vision using a number of low- or high-tech devices, including magnification devices, screen readers, optical readers,[71,72] or use of Braille technology.[6,33,73] Often, children work with Certified Orientation and Mobility Specialists, who assist the child with basic movement and mobility, perceptual skills, and physical capacity, both indoors and outdoors.[72] The physical therapist can work in collaboration with this specialist to provide cohesive strategies for the child.

Augmentative communication strategies are classified as unaided, nontechnologic devices or SGDs, or neuro-assisted devices. Unaided strategies can be gestures or eye-pointing, and require no instrumentation or adaptive equipment. Movement, generally of the face and upper extremities, is used to transmit messages visually. Smiling, nodding, shaking of the head, and other head and eye movements and hand gestures are typically used gestural communication strategies.

In addition, several gestural communication systems may be used. These include ASL, finger spelling, gestural Morse code,[6,68] and print-on-palm tracing.[74]

Nontechnologic-aided communication uses gesture-assisted strategies that can include low-tech devices such as communication boards or books with a display of a symbol system that is activated by gesture or movement, or simply a display of a few objects requiring the child to gesture by pointing to their choice using a finger or hand to relay a message.[75]

SGDs are accessed in the same way; however, they produce either digitized or text-to-speech output, or a combination of both when activated. High-tech SGDs or gesture-assisted systems require consistent movement of any body part to activate a control interface, infrared sensing device, eye gaze, or head tracking device to access this technology to make choices.[75] Nontechnologic-aided, communication-assisted devices may be composed of simple visual symbol sets such as photographs, drawings, the alphabet, and printed words on a display, or more complex language systems that continue to be developed. A speech language pathologist can explore the most appropriate symbol or system based on the child's language skills. Augmentative and alternative communication (AAC) devices are available commercially; however, they are generally most effective for function when they are customized for a specific child through thorough evaluation and trial.

Neuro-assisted strategies also use a display, but unlike the gesture-assisted strategies that rely on manipulation of a switching mechanism, this display is activated by bioelectric or physiologic signals from the body. BCI technology discussed earlier is an example of this strategy. The same displays are used as in the gesture-assisted systems, but the switches are controlled by surface electrodes on the scalp (electroencephalogram) or a selected muscle (electromyogram).[68,69] The evolving technologies of electrocorticography and intracortical recordings, both with BCIs where electrodes are implanted in the brain, are neural-assisted technologies. This type of access technology is most needed in the child with motor impairments so severe that the child is unable to control body movements adequately for gesturing.[69]

Environmental Control Systems

A person with a disability needs to function in a variety of environments. Therefore, the ability to perform specific functions in everyday life must be considered relative to context. Sometimes, a particular environment renders a person unable to effectively interact with and control the environment, making function more difficult or perhaps impossible. According to the ICF, disability is operationally defined as "capacity limitation which hinders the ability to execute needed activities and thereby participation in a given environment."[76] This could be due to architectural or attitudinal barriers within a society. Environmental contexts in which a child must function vary, depending on the individual child and the age, interests, and family culture. Broadly, children need to function in the home, at play, and at school, and the older teenager and young adult may need to function in a work environment. Changing the environment to optimize a person's functional participation can be accomplished through providing architectural modifications such as building ramps, modifying doorways or installing lift systems, or through implementation of ECSs.

ECSs are another subgroup of access technologies. An ECS is described as a system of technologic devices that has been designed to enable individuals with limited movement to exert some control over their immediate environment.[77] ECSs consist of an interface unit, a processing unit, and an actuating unit. The interface unit is any form of switch or access technology, discussed earlier in this chapter, that establishes a link between the device being accessed and the user. This can be a simple single switch, or can be more complex, such as using the powered wheelchair controller or the AAC device as the access method. The processing unit interprets the input and issues an output signal. The actuating unit receives the command and carries out the desired task. Depending on the age, a child needs a reasonable ability to control the home and play environment. Adapting a battery-operated toy with a single switch can provide the child with severe motor impairments the means to play independently and initiate play. Controlling an electronic device such as a blender, light, or fan will allow the child to participate in activities at home with the family or in school with the classroom. More complex ECSs will enable control of room lighting, television, kitchen appliances, heating and air conditioning, doors, windows, and window shades, which can greatly increase a person's independence and self-confidence. ECS users with severe disabilities have described improvement in their quality of life and reported a greater sense of control.[77]

Although the access technologies described earlier, including the emerging BCIs, have been used mostly as communication access technologies, they have potential as means to control the environment as well.

» Universal design

Universal design is a concept that refers to "the development of products and environments that are universally usable, that is, usable by all people, to the greatest extent possible, without the need for adaptation or specialized design."[78] This idea considers the broadest range of users and goes beyond the prescription approach of legibility legislation,[79] and is based on an understanding that all people can find certain types of equipment and environmental design to be helpful in daily life.[6,33] Ramps, elevators, automatic doors, recorded books, and talking computer software are examples of putting the concept of universal design into practice in today's society. As this concept continues to grow and be embraced by more people, the benefits for persons who have impairments and disabilities will also expand, improving access to better interactions with others and to more environments.

The growing industry of high-technology equipment such as notebook or tablet computers, smart phones, and e-readers exemplifies how universal design has been embraced in today's culture. These devices are developed and produced to increase the ease, speed, and access to communication, knowledge, and entertainment for people of all abilities. Children with impairments and disabilities are using these high-tech devices with increasing frequency, mostly for communication and entertainment. Communication programs that are compatible with these devices have been developed. Some of these devices can be used for environmental control and are extremely helpful in the classroom. These devices are portable, readily available, relatively inexpensive, and adaptable to a child's individual needs and abilities. Use of these ordinary high-tech devices emphasizes the similarities among children with and without disabilities. For a child, using devices that are used by peers rather than using medical devices can be empowering and motivating.

Summary

The purchase, building, and use of adaptive equipment can be complex and time-consuming aspects of pediatric physical therapy. The available options are so numerous and ever changing that even the most experienced physical therapist is unlikely to feel that all equipment has been considered before making a choice. The safest and most realistic approach to the selection of adaptive devices for children lies in a theoretic construct based on (1) careful evaluation of the child, (2) assessment of the environments in which the child functions, and (3) assessment of the family and other caregivers. The goals and abilities of the child must be agreed upon before therapeutic needs can be met with various types of equipment. When this information is known, the therapist can develop a therapeutic program that includes safe and effective use of equipment without unwanted negative effects. When the child's needs and goals are considered, the specific details of the numerous devices available become less intimidating and confusing. Frequent reexamination by the therapist will ensure that the child receives continuing benefits from adaptive equipment. Input from teachers, aides, parents, and the child will provide valuable feedback regarding the child's use of the equipment. The scheme suggested in this chapter provides the therapist with a framework for documenting the needs of the child, selecting or making appropriate equipment, evaluating the effects of the equipment, and reassessing the child's status periodically.

Anyone procuring or fabricating equipment on a regular basis should keep records of the various devices, manufacturers, and vendors used. Records should indicate ease of fit, wear of the device (how well it holds up over time), feedback from children and families, and the efficiency of customer service, including the elapsed time from placement of an order to delivery of equipment. Records are a useful resource for future recommendations and orders. In addition, the records may provide the basis for quantitative data regarding effectiveness of and deficiencies in various adaptive devices.

Keeping abreast of new developments and trends in the field of AT is essential to optimize function in the children whom physical therapists evaluate and treat. The professional literature and the Internet are two of the best resources to help therapists generate ideas for using adaptive aids and equipment and to stay informed.

REFERENCES

1. World Health Organization. *Towards a common language for functioning, disability and health ICF.* Accessed December 16, 2012. http://www.who.int/classifications/icf/training/icfbeginnersguide.pdf
2. Murchland S, Parkyn H. Promoting participation in schoolwork: assistive technology use by children with physical disabilities. *Assist Technol.* 2011;23:93-105. doi:10.1080/10400435.2011.567369
3. World Health Organization. *Assistive technology.* Published May 18, 2018. Accessed July 17, 2020. http://www.who.int/news-room/fact-sheets/detail/assistive-technology
4. Desch LW, Gaebler-Spira D. Prescribing assistive-technology systems: focus on children with impaired communication. *Pediatrics.* 2008;121:1271-1280. doi:10.1542/peds.2008-0695
5. Assistive Technology Industry Association. *What is AT?* Accessed July 17, 2020. https://www.atia.org/home/at-resources/what-is-at
6. Peterson JM, Hittie MM. Inclusive Teaching: The Journey Towards Effective Schools for All Learners. 2nd ed. Pearson Education Inc; 2010.
7. University of Kentucky Assistive Technology (UKAT) Project. *UKAT toolkit.* Accessed August 8, 2020. http://edsrc.coe.uky.edu/www/ukatii/
8. Copley J, Ziviani J. Barriers to the use of assistive technology for children with multiple disabilities. *Occup Ther Int.* 2004;11(4):229-243. doi:10.1002/oti.213
9. Rosen L, Plummer T, Sabet A, et al. RESNA position on the application of power mobility devices for pediatric users. *Assist Technol.* 2017;1-9. doi:10.1080/10400435.2017.1415575
10. National Registry of Rehabilitation Technology Suppliers. Accessed August 15, 2020. https://nrrts.org
11. Rehabilitation Engineering and Assistive Technology Society of North America. Accessed August 16, 2020. https://www.resna.org
12. Dicianno BE, Morgan A, Lieberman J, et al. Rehabilitation Engineering & Assistive Technology Society (RESNA) position on the application of wheelchair standing devices: 2013 current state of the literature. *Assist Technol.* 2016;28(1):57-62. doi:10.1080/10400435.2015.1113837
13. Isaacson M. Best practices by occupational and physical therapists performing seating and mobility evaluations. *Assist Technol.* 2011;23:13-21. doi:10.1080/10400435.2010.541745
14. Numotion. *Functional mobility and wheelchair assessment.* Accessed February 21, 2021. https://www.numotion.com/Numotion/media/NuDigest-Whitepapers/Houston-Methodist-fillable_018-(1).pdf
15. Wisconsin Assistive Technology Initiative. *AT assessment forms.* Accessed February 21, 2021. http://www.wati.org/free-publications/
16. Georgia Project for Assistive Technology. *AT consideration checklist.* Accessed February 21, 2021. https://gpat.gadoe.org/Georgia-Project-for-Assistive-Technology/Pages/default.aspx
17. Park MO, Lee SH. Effects of seating education and cushion management for adaptive sitting posture in spinal cord injury: two case reports. *Medicine (Baltimore).* 2019;98(4):e14231. doi:10.1097/MD.0000000000014231
18. Teleten O, Kirkland-Kyhn H, Paine T, et al. The use of pressure mapping: an educational report. *Wounds.* 2019;31(1):E5-E8.
19. Marshall J. Infant neurosensory development: considerations for infant child care. *Early Childhood Educ J.* 2011;39:175-181. doi:10.1007/s10643-011-0460-2
20. Karlsson P, Johnston C, Barker K. Stakeholders' views of the introduction of assistive technology in the classroom: how family-centered is

Australian practice for students with cerebral palsy? *Child Care Health Dev.* 2017;43(4):598-607. doi:10.1111/cch.12468

21. Huang HH. Perspectives on early power mobility training, motivation, and social participation in young children with motor disabilities. *Front Psychol.* 2018;8:2330. doi:10.3389/fpsyg.2017.02330

22. Feldner H. Impacts of early powered mobility provision on disability identity: a case study. *Rehabil Psychol.* 2019;64(2):130-145. doi:10.1037/rep0000259

23. O'Donnell DE, D'Arsigny C, Fitzpatrick M, et al. Exercise hypercapnia in advanced chronic obstructive pulmonary disease: the role of lung hyperinflation. *Am J Respir Crit Care Med.* 166(1):663–668.

24. Kumar A, Schmeler MR, Karmarkar AM, et al. Test-retest reliability of the functional mobility assessment (FMA): a pilot study. *Disabil Rehabil Assist Technol.* 2013;8(3):213-9. doi: 10.3109/17483107.2012.688240. Epub 2012 May 22. PMID: 22612721.

25. Powermobilityalberta. Accessed August 8, 2020. Powermobilityalberta.wordpress.com

26. Schnackers M, Beckers L, Janssen-Potten Y, et al. Home-based bimanual training based on motor learning principles in children with unilateral cerebral palsy and their parents (the COAD-study): rationale and protocols. *BMC Pediatr.* 2018;18(1):139. doi:10.11886/s12887-018-1110-2

27. Bartlett DJ, Fanning JK, Miller L, et al. Development of the daily activities of infants scale: a measure supporting early motor development. *Dev Med Child Neurol.* 2008;50(8):613-617. doi:10.1111/j.1469-8749.2008.03007.x

28. Manary MA, Ritchie NL, Schneider LW. WC19: a wheelchair transportation safety standard—experience to date and future directions. *Med Eng Phys.* 2010;32(3):263-271. doi:10.1016/j.medengphy.2009.08.012

29. Complexchild. *Car seats for children with special needs.* Updated 2019. Accessed August 16, 2020. https://complexchild.org/articles/2011-articles/october/carseats/

30. Buning ME, Bertocci G, Schneider LW, et al. RESNA's position on wheelchairs used as seats in motor vehicles. *Assist Technol.* 2012;24(2):132-141. doi:10.1080/10400435.2012.659328

31. University of Michigan Wheelchair Transportation Research Institute. *Wheelchair Transportation Safety. WC20: Seating Systems.* Accessed August 6, 2020. Wc-transportation-safety.umtri.umich.edu

32. Ripat J, Woodgate R. The intersection of culture, disability and assistive technology. *Disabil Rehabil Assist Technol.* 2011;6(2):87-96. doi:10.3109/17483107.2010.507859

33. Dell AG, Newton DA, Petroff JG. Assistive Technology in the Classroom: Enhancing the School Experiences of Students with Disabilities. 3rd ed. Pearson Education, Inc.; 2016.

34. American Physical Therapy Association Academy of Pediatric Physical Therapy. *Assistive technology and the individualized education program.* 2007. Accessed August 8, 2020. https://pediatricapta.org/includes/fact-sheets/pdfs/AssistiveTechnology.pdf

35. American Physical Therapy Association Academy of Pediatric Physical Therapy. *Resources on reimbursement for pediatric physical therapy services and durable medical equipment.* 2007. Accessed August 8, 2020. https://pediatricapta.org/includes/fact-sheets/pdfs/ReimbursementBrochure.pdf?v=1

36. Medicaid.gov. *Children's Health Insurance Program (CHIP).* Accessed July 3, 2020. https://www.medicaid.gov/chip/index.html

37. Early Childhood Technical Assistance Center. *Funding sources for assistive technology.* Accessed July 3, 2020. https://ectacenter.org/topics/atech/funding.asp

38. American Physical Therapy Association Academy of Pediatric Physical Therapy. *What providers of pediatric physical therapy services should know about Medicaid.* Reimbursement Committee of the Section on Pediatrics, APTA. Fact sheet. 2009. Accessed August 15, 2020. https://pediatricapta.org/includes/fact-sheets/pdfs/09%20Medicaid.pdf

39. The Catalyst Center. *The TEFRA Medicaid and state plan option and Katie Becket waiver for children: making it possible to care for children with significant disabilities at home.* Accessed July 3, 2020. https://ciswh.org/wp-content/uploads/2016/07/TEFRA.pdf

40. Pass It On Center-The National AT Reuse Center. Accessed August 15, 2020. https://pioc.gatech.edu

41. Long F. *Creating a bulletproof letter of medical necessity.* Rehab Management. Published July 29, 2015. Spinal cord injury, Stroke 6. Accessed February 21, 2021. https://rehabpub.com/conditions/neurological/stroke-neurological/creating-bulletproof-letter-medical-necessity/

42. Permobil. http://www.permobil.com

43. National Academies of Sciences, Engineering, and Medicine Division; Board on Health Care Services; Committee on the Use of Selected Assistive Products and Technologies in Eliminating or Reducing the Effects of Impairments. Coverage or relevant products and technologies. In Flaubert JL, Spicer CM, Jette AM, eds. The Promise of Assistive Technology to Enhance Activity and Work Participation. National Academies Press; 2017. https://www.ncbi.nlm.nih.gov/books/NBK453296/

44. Solanke F, Colver A, McConachie H; Transition collaborative group. Are the health needs of young people with cerebral palsy met during transition from child to adult health care? *Child Care Health Dev.* 2018;44(3):355-363. doi:10.1111/cch.12549.

45. RESNA. *Position on the application of ultralight manual wheelchairs.* Approved by RESNA Board of Directors, March 7, 2012. http://www.rstce.pitt.edu/RSTCE_Resources/RSTCE_Res_Doc/RESNAPosUltralightManWheelchairs.pdf

46. Chen YL, Yang PJ. A preliminary study of the measurement of external ischial tuberosity width and its gender differences. *J Phys Ther Sci.* 2016;28(3):820-823. doi:10.1589/jpts.28.820.

47. Akerblom B. *Chairs and sitting.* Paper presented at: The Symposium on Human Factors in Equipment Design. Proceedings of the Ergonomics Research Society, (pp. 29-35) V. 2. 1954; Sweden.

48. Dicianno BE, Arva J, Lieberman JM, et al. RESNA position on the application of tilt, recline, and elevating legrests for wheelchairs. *Assist Technol.* 2009;21(1):13-24. doi:10.1080/10400430902945769.

49. Bergan A. Positioning the Client with Central Nervous System Deficits: The Wheelchair and Other Adapted Equipment. 2nd ed. Valhalla Press; 1985.

50. Low SA, Westcott McCoy S, Beling J, et al. Pediatric physical therapists' use of support walkers for children with disabilities: a nationwide survey. *Pediatr Phys Ther.* 2011;23:381-389.

51. Paleg GS, Smith BA, Glickman LB. Systematic review and evidence-based clinical recommendations for dosing of pediatric supported standing programs. *Pediatr Phys Ther.* 2013;25(3):232-247. doi:10.1097/PEP.0b013e318299d5e7.

52. Martinsson C, Himmelmann K. Effect of weight-bearing in abduction and extension on hip stability in children with cerebral palsy. *Pediatr Phys Ther.* 2011;23(2):150-157. doi:10.1097/PEP.0b013e318218efc3.

53. Sato H, Iwasaki T, Yokoyama M, et al. Monitoring of body position and motion in children with severe cerebral palsy for 24 hours. *Disabil Rehabil.* 2014;36(14):1156-1160. doi:10.3109/09638288.2013.833308.

54. *Go Baby Go Connect program.* Accessed August 15, 2020. https://www.gbgconnect.com

55. Segway. Accessed August 15, 2020. Segway.com

56. Sawatzky B, Denison I, Langrish S, et al. The Segway personal transporter as an alternative mobility device for people with disabilities: a pilot study. *Arch Phys Med Rehabil.* 2007;88:1423-1428. doi:10.1016/j.apmr.2007.08.005

57. Jones MA, McEwen IR, Neas BR. Effects of power wheelchairs on the development and function of young children with severe motor impairment. *Pediatr Phys Ther.* 2012;24:131-140. doi:10.1097/PEP.0b013e31824c5fdc

58. Boninger ML, Baldwin M, Cooper RA, et al. Manual wheelchair pushrim biomechanics and axle position. *Arch Phys Med Rehabil.* 2000;81(5):608-613. doi:10.1016/S0003-9993(00)90043-1

59. Lovelace-Chandler V, Earl D. Commentary on "Pediatric physical therapists' use of support walkers for children with disabilities: a nationwide survey." *Pediatr Phys Ther.* 2011;23:390. doi:10.1097/PEP.0b013e3182356576

60. *R82 by Etac.* Accessed August 16, 2020. http://www.R82.com

61. Damcott M, Blochlinger S, Foulds R. Effects of passive versus dynamic loading interventions on bone health in children who are non-ambulatory. *Pediatr Phys Ther.* 2013;25:248-255. doi:10.1097/PEP.0b013e318299127d

62. O'Neil J, Hoffman B, AAP Council on Injury, Violence, and Poison Prevention. Transporting children with special heath care needs. *Pediatrics.* 2019;143(5):e20190724. doi:10.1542/peds.2019-0724

63. National Child Passenger Safety Certification. Accessed August 15, 2020. http://cert.safekids.org

64. O'Neil J, Hoffman BD, Council on Injury, Violence, and Poison Prevention. School bus transportation of children with special health care needs. *Pediatrics.* 2018;141(5):e20180513. Erratum in *Pediatrics.* 2018;142(1):e20181221. doi:10.1542/peds.2018-1221

65. National Highway Transportation Safety Administration. https://www.nhtsa.gov

66. Rogers A. *Toileting initiative produces great results.* Published March 20, 2017. https://www.rifton.com/adaptive-mobility-blog/blog-posts/2017/march/toilet-initiative-special-needs-students

67. Tai K, Blain S, Chau T. A review of emerging access technologies for individuals with sever motor impairments. *Assist Technol.* 2008;20(40):204-219. doi:10.1080/10400435.2008.10131947

68. Elsahar Y, Hu S, Bouazza-Marouf K, et al. Augmentative and Alternative Communication (AAC) advances: a review of configurations for individuals with a speech disability. *Sensors (Basel).* 2019;19(8):1911. doi:10.3390/s19081911

69. Koch Fager S, Fried-Oken M, Jakobs T, et al. New and emerging access technologies for adults with complex communication needs and severe motor impairments: state of the science. *Augment Altern Commun.* 2019;35(1):13-25. doi:10.1080/07434618.2018.1556730

70. National Institute on Deafness and Other Communication Disorders. *Assistive devices for people with hearing, voice, speech or language disorders.* Accessed August 14, 2020. https://www.nidcd.nih.gov/health/assistive-devices-people-hearing-voice-speech-or-language-disorders

71. American Foundation for the Blind. *Technology resources for people with vision loss.* Accessed August 14, 2020. https://www.afb.org/blindness-and-low-vision/using-technology

72. Shah P, Schwartz SG, Gartner S, et al. Low vision services: a practical guide for the clinician. *Ther Adv Ophthalmol.* 2018;10:2515841418776264. doi:10.1177/2515841418776264

73. Willings C. *Strategies and tips for selecting the right assistive technology for students who are blind or visually impaired.* Accessed February 21, 2021. https://www.teachingvisuallyimpaired.com/at-instruction.html

74. American Association of the Deaf Blind. Accessed February 21, 2021. http://www.aadb.org/factsheets/db_communications.html

75. Waller A. Telling tales: unlocking the potential of AAC technologies. *Int J Lang Commun Disord.* 2019;54(2):159-169. https://doi.org/10.1111/1460-6984.12449

76. Hirani SA, Richter S. The capability approach: a guiding framework to improve population health and the attainment of the Sustainable Developmental Goals. *East Mediterr Health J.* 2017;23(1):46-50. doi:10.26719/2017.23.1.46

77. Myburg M, Allan E, Nalder E, et al. Environmental control systems—the experiences of people with spinal cord injury and the implications for prescribers. *Disabil Rehabil Assist Technol.* 2017;12(2):128-136. doi:10.3109/17483107.2015.1099748

78. Pennick T, Hessey S, Craigie R. Universal design and the smart home. *Stud Health Technol Inform.* 2016;229:363-365.

79. Mosca EI, Capolongo S. Towards a universal design evaluation for assessing the performance of the built environment. *Stud Health Technol Inform.* 2018;256:771-779.

Orthotics and Prosthetics

Jill Cannoy, Karl Barner, Brian P. Emling, Rebecca Hernandez,
Gerald Stark, and Richard Welling, Jr.

» Overview of pediatric management

Children are not small adults. As simple as this sounds, growing children, who require orthotic and prosthetic devices often present with complex interdependent, multisystem involvement. A multidisciplinary team approach is best suited to provide a comprehensive evaluation and collaborate on interventions that meet the child's and family's needs. A board-certified orthotist or prosthetist should be a part of the rehabilitation team dictated by the child's diagnosis and physical impairments. Other members of the multidisciplinary team may include a referring physician, physical therapist, occupational therapist, social worker, and at the center of the team, the child and family. The purpose of the multidisciplinary team is to work together to better serve the needs of children and their families. The multidisciplinary team must be aware not only of the child's physical needs, but also of the psychological and psychosocial needs of the child and family, as well as the resources available to them.

It is the responsibility of individuals within the multidisciplinary rehabilitation team to be knowledgeable about the most current advances in their focus areas to assist families in making informed decisions for their child. Because no single individual or discipline can have access to all necessary expertise and knowledge needed to optimize patient care, they must all work collaboratively to achieve a successful outcome.[1]

Certified orthotists and prosthetists are health care professionals, who design and fit custom orthoses (braces) and prostheses (artificial limbs) in order to help facilitate age-appropriate development, preserve and restore function, and promote a meaningful quality of life.[1]

The role of the certified orthotist is to evaluate posture, alignment, and function of patients presenting with musculoskeletal or neurologic impairments that contribute to functional limitations and disability, by designing, fabricating, and fitting orthoses, and custom-made braces. In collaboration with the rehabilitation team, the orthotist evaluates the child's function and expectations of the family before designing the orthosis.

Similarly, the role of the certified prosthetist, within the multidisciplinary team, is to evaluate posture, alignment, and function and design and maintain prosthetic devices for children presenting with limb differences, partial, or total absence. The prosthesis should match the child and family's functional and cosmetic expectations. Orthotists and prosthetists provide ongoing care to adjust the devices and education to the child and as the child grows and develops.[1]

The role of the physical therapist (PT) within the multidisciplinary team is to maximize the child's function within their degree of impairment, while also serving as an advocate, teacher, and mentor for the child and family. The PT is often the member of the multidisciplinary team that interacts with the child and family on a regular basis and may serve as a liaison between the family, physician, orthotist, prosthetist, and additional members of the medical team, to ensure that the medical management of the child supports their ability to meet their functional goals.[2]

A physical therapist working with children should be knowledgeable in the areas of gross motor, fine motor, and cognitive development in order to identify primary impairments in each. At examination, the PT must identify the child's primary impairments, activity limitations, and participation restrictions, as well as child and family goals and personal and environmental factors that may impact care. The PT must then assess the knowledge gained at the time of examination and throughout treatment to support age-appropriate function and development. Subsequent treatment interventions targeting range of motion (ROM), strengthening, gait training, and functional activities are dependent on the child's age, underlying medical or neurologic conditions, interests, as well as the family's ability to assist in the child's care. Each child that presents for PT will have unique and variable needs, requiring the therapist to assess the priorities of the child and family frequently to develop treatment strategies that support these needs and to maximize patient function in their environment. PT intervention and treatment should be meaningful and fun, while ultimately meeting the goals of the multidisciplinary team and family.

The utilization goal of any orthotic or prosthetic device should be to improve patient function, support development, and address primary impairments that may be limiting the child's function in their environment. Pediatric sensory, motor, and cognitive development are dependent on the experiences and interactions of the child within their environment. When choosing an appropriate orthotic or prosthetic device, the device and componentry should meet the demands of the child, while complementing age-appropriate function and development to support child and caregiver goals, by matching the child and caregiver's cognitive level for use.

Children are constantly changing in terms of their physical, mental, and personal development. Therefore, orthotists and prosthetists should be aware of the impact physical impairments have on development and work closely with the family and therapists to maximize the child's function. The ever-evolving dynamic nature of a child means that the fitting priorities, expectations, and functional goals are continually shifting not only with the child, but also with the parents and child's therapists. The involvement of the parents and therapists means that constant communication and a personal trust must exist between the orthotics and prosthetics (O&P) clinician, parents, therapist, and child.

Often, difficulties can arise from misunderstandings of the expectations and limitations of the technologies or processes. Therefore, education about the design, fabrication, fit, and function of the orthotic or prosthetic device is imperative throughout the continuum of care. Anticipating changes resulting from a child's growth and functional demands is essential and an important strategy to support future decisions. Constant and empathetic communication is the most effective and critical tool when treating children who present with physical challenges. Open communication also reaffirms the orthotic and prosthetic goals that are prioritized as follows: (1) Optimize function, (2) Correct or prevent further progression of the deformity, (3) Protect the segment, and (4) Pain management. At times, these goals may conflict with one another or may be difficult to achieve all at once. In those cases, the priorities are reinforced, and consensus is found within the multidisciplinary team.

Neurologic Development

A child's neurologic development is dependent on interaction and involvement in his or her environment. This may be more challenging in children presenting with congenital or multisystem impairments, because interaction within their environment is essential for brain development. Previously, it was thought that motor development increased with cognitive capacity; however, it is now understood that motor development increases neurologic development.[3]

Importance of Upright Positioning on Musculoskeletal and Cardiopulmonary Health

The use of orthotic and prosthetic devices is intended to preserve overall mobility and activity expectations of the child as well as aid in normal cardiopulmonary development. Exercising and stretching muscles, even those pathologically involved, helps increase ROM, decreases contractures, and provides better balance and stability. Loading of the appendicular and spinal skeleton also aids in joint function and bone deposition, avoids calcium depletion, and decreases the chance of osteoporosis in the future.[4]

» Orthotic interventions

Initiating Orthotic Treatment

Orthoses are classified as durable medical equipment (DME) requiring a physician's order detailing the devices needed. Although a physician's order is necessary for device provision, identification of the initial need is often discovered by allied health professionals, that is, physical therapists and/or occupational therapists. Children who have musculoskeletal impairments or who are developmentally delayed are likely to enter therapy where a thorough evaluation will isolate the muscle groups that could benefit from additional support. A therapist's understanding of orthotic devices can impact outcomes, even shortening the therapeutic timeline for achieving the determined goals. Referring physicians can provide a detailed order indicating position, range, and restrictions or, alternatively, a general order leaving the decision up to the certified orthotist. Whoever evaluates the deficits, multidisciplinary communication is integral to ensuring the design of a device that supports the patient's development and functional needs.

Orthotic Terminology

Orthotic device nomenclature is largely based on the joint(s) the device is intended to control, resulting in standardized acronyms. Variations from the base acronym are intended to describe a function of the basic device. For example, an ankle foot orthosis (AFO) merely indicates a device for the ankle and foot; however, an articulated ankle foot orthosis (AAFO) describes a function of the base acronym (AFO). Since the 1960s, the O&P field has been working toward standardized nomenclature because of the many devices previously named by the developer or region where the device was made, for example, Boston Thoracic Lumbar Sacral Orthosis (TLSO), developed in Boston, MA, or the Rigo Cheneau Brace, developed by Dr. Manuel Rigo and Dr. Jacques Chêneau.

Despite the field's attempt to standardize nomenclature, some orthoses remain named for the function they serve or are based on device appearance. An example of a functionally named device is the reciprocating gait orthosis (RGO); the RGO is a hip–knee–ankle–foot (HKAFO) harnessing trunk flexion and extension to generate a reciprocal gait. The halo is an example of an appearance-based device that is intended to immobilize the cervical spine by the fixation of a ring to the skull, then secured to a torso section.

Orthotic Function/Goals

With a constantly changing child presentation, the orthotist must treat the immediate needs while anticipating and designing an orthosis for the future. A deep understanding of normal motor development will benefit the treating team in order to identify deficits and determine what support is needed (see Chapter 1, Typical Development for details). A team treating a child with an orthosis should understand and foresee the functional impact of a device in order to set appropriate therapeutic goals.

Benefits of orthoses may include the following:

- Improving, controlling, or limiting joint movements
- Simulating an eccentric or concentric muscle function
- Managing/improving ROM
- Providing kinesthetic feedback

- Pain relief
- Protection against self-injury
- Wound and fracture healing

Indications for orthotic management are muscular deficits, neuromuscular involvement, contractures, joint instability, fractures, pain, joint malalignment, longitudinal asymmetries, or scoliosis. The team approach in addressing all the child's needs should be addressed at the initial evaluation. Goals for orthotic usage and the amount of time the child uses the device should be determined and shared with the parent/caregiver. Improper use of a device could lead to internal or external injury of the child, orthosis failure, and failed outcomes.

When evaluating a child, there are many important factors to consider and balance. The indications for orthotic treatment, home/school environment, ease of use of orthosis for caregivers, goals, and activities should be included in the treatment plan process to ensure optimal outcomes. Discussions with the family about the advantages and disadvantages of an orthosis should be discussed prior to orthotic fabrication.

Most patients should follow up with the orthotist within a couple of weeks of delivery to assess function, skin conditions, and integrity of the orthosis. Regular follow-ups are dependent on the child's needs, but general follow-up should occur every 3 to 4 months. Any safety, skin, or pain concerns should be addressed as they arise.

Orthotic Design

Orthoses utilize leverage from above and below a joint axis or fracture site to stabilize the region. Orthoses utilize three-point pressure systems that apply moments to control or stabilize a body segment. Three-point pressure systems should optimize leverage for control without resisting desired ROM for activities or causing internal complications. Some ROM may be limited by the device in order to control the anatomy being stabilized. Multiple three-point force systems can be used in one device in order to stabilize a body segment or joint in multiple planes.

Children generally require custom devices because of congenital abnormalities that cannot be accommodated by noncustom devices or because they have developed contractures affecting normal anatomic alignment or because their stature lies outside the size ranges available for a noncustom device. Custom devices incorporate bony anatomy reliefs to offload the prominences prone to skin breakdown accompanied by specialty padding. In order to provide a custom device, the process begins by capturing the child's anatomy (Fig. 8.1).

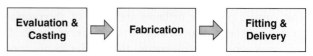

FIGURE 8.1. Custom device workflow.

Noncustom orthoses can be adjusted to fit a child's general needs and are likely to incorporate materials that can be modified, manually bent, or thermoformed in order to improve fit and function. Oftentimes, these devices can be delivered the same day the child was evaluated.

Types of Orthoses

Pediatric orthoses can be split into three categories: positional, contracture management, and functional devices. Each category requires the use of different materials and components to ensure device function meets the needs of the child.

Positional orthoses are used to control a limb, torso, or cranium for a person that is at risk of developing contractures, for stabilizing a surgery or fracture condition, and for protection from pressure sores or getting injured from the environment around them. These orthoses are often padded and designed to reduce contact in the areas that are susceptible to injury.

Contracture management devices can be broken down into the following subcategories: static/passive, static progressive, and dynamic. Static devices are considered a positional orthosis and used to reduce the risk of contractures, stabilize a body segment and/or offload and protect the skin. These orthoses are often well padded and have a broad surface area to minimize pressure on sensitive areas. Children with neuromuscular involvement or paralysis often receive positional devices for long-term use, although these devices are widely used in the acute setting to maintain ROM. Static progressive orthoses incorporate joints with incremental ROM settings that can be easily adjusted on the basis of the patient's needs or therapeutic goals.

Dynamic orthoses are used to provide a constant stretch to contracted musculature in order to improve ROM. These devices most often use an internal joint spring where tension can be increased or decreased to apply a higher or reduced force, respectively. Dynamic orthoses tend to be more complicated to use and more costly, which should be considered in the rehabilitation plan because a simple low-weight device may be more beneficial.

When contracture management devices are used properly, outcomes are positive. However, brace compliance remains challenging in children because a stretch is often perceived as being uncomfortable. As an alternative to orthotic contracture management, therapists often use serial casting or manual joint mobilization. The team should evaluate the child's home situation, expected compliance, cognition/motivation of the child and family, and how long the child has had a contracture before deciding the best course of treatment. A contracture that has been present for an extended period and has a firm end ROM feel is likely to require a surgical release.[5-7]

Materials

Most custom pediatric orthoses are made of thermoplastics that have been vacuum formed to a model of the child's body segment. High-temperature thermoplastics are most commonly used, including polypropylene and copolymer.

Some orthoses are fabricated from carbon and acrylic resins. Padding can be added during the fabrication process or during the fitting/follow-up appointments. Materials have certain indications depending on the individual needs and goals. Straps are an integral part of the orthosis and the three-point pressure systems used to control the foot and ankle. Selection of brace design and appropriate materials are essential for optimizing the child's function while reducing the risk of integumentary or secondary concerns.

Tuning

In addition to design and materials, tuning the orthosis is essential to proper function. Tuning of lower extremity devices was made popular by Elaine Owen, MSc, SRP, MCSP, who has contributed a wealth of research on the use of orthoses. Elaine's work has focused on:

- The sciences of kinematics and kinetics in the normal and abnormal human gait cycle
- Algorithms designed to choose the proper clinical path
- Determining the proper lower extremity orthotic design and shoe modifications needed to optimize gait (Fig. 8.2).[8]

A functional weight-bearing lower extremity orthosis must be tuned to ensure the patient can maintain a stable upright position and to promote smooth gait while accommodating joint contractures or angular deformities. The patient should undergo a thorough examination to determine the functional limitations with strength and ROM, joint alignment, and balance. If a patient's alignment cannot be corrected, the orthosis will need to accommodate the deformity. An orthosis should be designed to provide stability only when needed in the gait cycle.

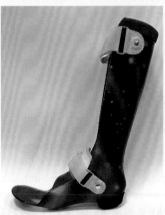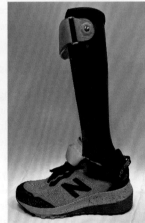

FIGURE 8.2. Left: Solid ankle AFO for patient with a plantar flexion contracture. **Right:** Wedged heel on the AFO, additional external shoe wedging at the heel in addition to the 3/8″ heel incorporated into the shoe's sole. AFO wedging with additional shoe wedging results in a shank to vertical angle (SVA) in 10 degrees inclination.

>> Upper and lower extremity orthoses

Upper extremity functional orthoses are often used to optimize the wearer's independence by holding the hand, wrist, or elbow in position to improve function or aid in the performance of activities of daily living (feeding, hygiene, and dressing).

Every orthosis will have variations based on the child's need, geographic, clinician and/or physician preferences. The following chart is basic information regarding details of indications and goals associated with the devices. Padding, specific materials, trim lines, shoes/modifications, and fasteners should be determined prior to orthosis fabrication (Table 8.1).

TABLE 8.1.	Summary of Lower Extremity Orthoses			
Photo of the Orthosis	Device	Patient Presentation	Materials	Biomechanic Principles
	Foot orthosis (FO)	• Pes planovalgus (mild/moderate) • Accessory navicular • Posterior tibialis dysfunction • Metatarsalgia • Toe walking • Foot pain	Foam top layer (optional) Firm base made of thermoplastic, carbon, crepe, or cork	• Longitudinal and/or transverse arch support • Extrinsic support to improve/accommodate malalignment • Shock absorption
	UCBL, University of California Biomechanics Laboratory	• Pes Planovalgus (moderate/severe) • Plantar fasciitis • Metatarsus adductus	Thermoplastic	Stabilizes foot/ankle complex in coronal and transverse planes Reduces stress on plantar fascia
	Supra Malleolar Orthosis (SMO)	• Moderate to severe pronation or supination • Balance problems in early ambulation • Toe walking	Thermoplastic	Stabilizes foot/ankle complex in sagittal and transverse planes
	Posterior Leaf Spring (PLS) Ankle Foot Orthosis (AFO)	• Drop foot • Charcot Marie Tooth • Peroneal palsy with mild to moderate medial or lateral instability	• Thermoplastic • Carbon graphite options are also available and may be used with an FO, UCBL, or SMO for more foot alignment support.	**Swing** toe clearance (concentric simulation of dorsiflexors) **Stance** loading response (eccentric simulation of dorsiflexors) and slight tibial forward inclination resistance based on design (eccentric simulation of gastrocnemius and soleus) • Stabilizes foot/ankle complex in sagittal and transverse planes

(continued)

TABLE 8.1.	Summary of Lower Extremity Orthoses (*continued*)			
Photo of the Orthosis	**Device**	**Patient Presentation**	**Materials**	**Biomechanic Principles**
	Articulating Ankle Foot Orthosis (AAFO) with dorsiflexion (DF) assist/ plantarflexion resist	Mild drop foot/slap with medial and/or lateral instability	Thermoplastic	**Swing** toe clearance (simulates concentric contraction of pretibial muscles) **Stance** loading response (eccentric simulation of dorsiflexors) Provides transverse and medial and lateral stability of the foot and ankle complex
	Articulating Ankle Foot Orthosis (AAFO) with plantar flexion (PF) stop	Toe walking Mild to moderate genu recurvatum not associated with significant spasticity Moderate to severe M/L instabilities of foot/ankle **Best if patient has strong voluntary controlled gastrocnemius/soleus muscles and quadriceps**	Thermoplastic with plastic/rubber/metal joints	**Swing** toe clearance **Stance** Provides transverse and medial/lateral stability of the foot and ankle complex Encourages knee flexion moment at initial contact through midstance. Provides transverse and M/L stability of the foot and ankle complex. Allows DF and advancement of the contralateral limb
	Articulated AFO with adjustable joints	The sagittal alignment of the ankle joints can allow free motion, stops, or dynamic springs to simulate eccentric/concentric muscle actions.	Thermoplastic, carbon, or metal/ leather with metal joints Occasionally not utilized because of increased weight, bulk, and cost associated with the ankle joints	**Swing** toe clearance **Stance** Provides transverse and medial/lateral stability of the foot and ankle complex. Can be set up in multiple configurations to match the patient's needs
	Solid Ankle Foot Orthosis (SAFO)	Moderate to severe hypertonia/spasticity severe rheumatoid arthritis of foot and ankle	Thermoplastic or carbon	**Swing** Toe clearance Provides transverse and M/L stability of the foot and ankle complex **Stance** Encourages knee flexion moment in initial contact to midstance. Resists excessive knee flexion and ankle DF. Provides M/L stability of the foot and ankle complex
	Floor Reaction Ankle Foot Orthosis (FRAFO) with the foot in neutral slight plantar flexion ankle alignment	Weak quadriceps or Gastrocnemius/Soleus muscle groups	Thermoplastic or carbon	**Swing** toe clearance **Stance** Provides transverse and M/L stability of the foot and ankle complex Encourages knee extension moment or less knee flexion moment to prevent knee forward buckling.

TABLE 8.1.   Summary of Lower Extremity Orthoses (*continued*)

Photo of the Orthosis	Device	Patient Presentation	Materials	Biomechanic Principles
	Floor Reaction Ankle Foot Orthosis (FRAFO) for crouch gait	Lower-level paraplegia (Spina bifida/Spinal Cord Injury [SCI]) associated with hip and/or knee flexion contractures or dorsiflexion contractures Spasticity associated with hamstrings/knee flexion contractures	Thermoplastic or Carbon	**Swing** Toe clearance **Stance** Decreases the crouch gait and keeps torso vertical and center of mass in middle of the foot Provides transverse and M/L stability of the foot and ankle complex
	Knee Ankle Foot Orthosis (KAFO)	Low-thoracic/high lumbar-level paraplegia severe knee hyperextension M/L instability at the knee Blount disease	Thermoplastic, carbon and metal Metal uprights and joints with locking/unlocking options Stance control options that allow free motion knee joints in swing/locked in stance Microprocessor control for larger teenagers	**Swing** toe clearance M/L stability for the knee/ankle in preparation for initial contact **Stance** AFO section provides M/L stability of the ankle, swing phase control, ground reaction forces on the knee Knee joint and thigh extension provide M/L knee support Locked knee joints option provides maximal sagittal plane support but unlock for sitting
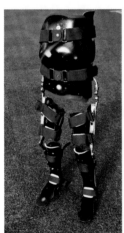	Hip–Knee–Ankle–Foot Orthosis (HKAFO)	Thoracic level Paraplegia associated with spina bifida, SCI, spinal muscular atrophy (SMA), or muscular dystrophies Cerebral palsy (Typically GMFCS [Gross Motor Function Classification System] level III, IV)	Thermoplastic, carbon, and metal Metal uprights and joints with locking/unlocking options	**Swing** phase clearance Prevents scissoring **Stance** Maximum support for lower extremities in all three planes and lower torso
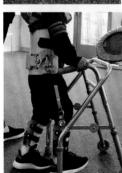	Reciprocating Gait Orthosis (RGO) Hip Knee Ankle Orthosis	Low-thoracic to midlumbar paraplegia Must have good upper extremity and cognitive abilities.	Thermoplastic, carbon and metal Metal uprights and joints with unlocking and locking into reciprocal action	**Swing** phase clearance Assists in advancement of the lower limbs **Stance** Maximum support for lower extremities and lower torso

AFO photo used with permission from Becker Orthopedic. All other table photos used with permission from Children's Healthcare of Atlanta, Orthotics and Prosthetics Department.

» Cranial remolding orthoses

Infants between the ages of 3 and 18 months, presenting with diagnoses of plagiocephaly (diagonal asymmetry of the skull), brachycephaly (a skull presentation with occipital flattening and wider and taller parietal areas), scaphocephaly (a skull presentation with an elongated anterior/posterior dimension and a flatter and taller parietal area), or a combination of the foregoing asymmetries may be candidates for orthotic treatment with cranial remolding orthoses (CRO). Prior to initiation of a CRO an in-depth past medical history should be reviewed for complicating medical conditions such as craniosynostosis or hydrocephalus.

Scaphocephaly and brachycephaly standards are measured by measuring the width of the head and dividing it by the length of the head and then multiplying it by 100 to get a percentage. Two standard deviations above the mean are considered brachycephalic (over age 6 months: boys 91.2%, girls 87.5%). Many sites consider over 90% to be brachycephalic. Two standard deviations below the mean are considered scaphocephalic.[9]

Plagiocephaly is a diagonal asymmetry of the skull that can result in medical concerns regarding ear, eye, and jaw alignment. Plagiocephaly is often associated with torticollis. If the child has torticollis, it is highly recommended to have a physical therapy examination and necessary intervention.[10] Severe or unresolving torticollis may require a surgical release. Different scales consider cranial vault asymmetry (CVA) to be in a normal range if below 3 to 6 mm, and significant asymmetries are considered above 12 to 15 mm of asymmetry.[11] Other scales look more at the percentage of diagonal asymmetry, called the cranial vault asymmetry index (CVAI).[12] It is recommended that physical therapists follow the American Physical Therapy Association's (APTA's) Congenital Muscular Torticollis Clinical Practice Guideline for treatment of torticollis.

CROs are custom-made orthoses that encourage symmetric growth to improve head shape as it grows. Prior to CRO intervention, head control is required, and 2 months of repositioning is recommended. CRO's redirect outward circumferential growth by providing contact with the head where prominent (bossed regions) and relief where desired (flattened regions). In addition to bossed area contact, contact is also required at the base of the occiput and the cheeks. A well-fitting helmet will have minimal rotation or tilt on the child and may lie just superior to the eyebrows. Occasional contact with the ears or depression of an eyebrow while the helmet is in place is not uncommon. The authors' institution has found that most infants wear the helmets for 3 to 5 months, when the helmet is worn for the recommended 23 hours per day. Discontinuation of the helmet occurs when the head shape has improved to parent and clinician satisfaction, the child is repositioning on their own, and torticollis is resolved.

Other Cranial Orthoses

Orthotists may provide protective helmets, off the shelf or custom, which are used to help prevent self-injury, to protect children diagnosed with epilepsy, or protect the brain following craniotomy. Protective helmets are offered in a hard or soft shell and can have various face shield options.

» Spinal orthoses

Spinal orthoses are used to reduce trunk motion or stabilize curve progression by controlling the spine or segments of the spine. Spinal orthoses are available for pain and postoperative management of scoliosis/kyphosis or to provide head and trunk support. The segment of the spine impacted will dictate the size of the orthosis required. Device nomenclature remains consistent with orthotic devices of the extremities, for example, cervical thoracic lumbar sacral orthosis (CTLSO) to lumbar sacral orthosis (LSO). A HALO device does not follow traditional nomenclature and is intended to stabilize the upper thoracic and/or cervical spine. In more recent years, HALOs have been used for HALO-gravity traction on children with severe scoliosis. Thermoplastic materials are most common because they are easily cleaned and durable while allowing for small changes to occur in an office setting. With broad coverage of the torso, thorough skin inspections are vital to prevent skin breakdown.

Fracture Management and Postoperative Orthoses

Spinal orthoses are commonly used for the treatment of acute and chronic low back pain. Spondylolisthesis is a condition where one vertebra slides anteriorly with respect to the adjacent inferior vertebra. This painful condition can be managed with a lumbar sacral orthosis, which induces a posterior pelvic tilt thus improving alignment of the vertebra involved and offloading axial pressure through the vertebral columns. The LSO for spondylolisthesis is traditionally a semirigid thermoformed plastic that is custom made for the patient. Alternatively, off-the-shelf custom-fit LSO devices can incorporate rigid panels into a corset design, which can be helpful in reducing pain by limiting lumbar motion and increasing intra-abdominal pressure.[1]

Fractures occurring in the thoracic and/or thoracolumbar region are typically managed with a TLSO to provide stabilization inferiorly and superiorly to the fracture site. TLSOs should allow hip flexion to 90 degrees for seated comfort and posteriorly should permit toileting without the need to remove the device. Caregivers should carefully perform skin checks, paying close attention to the waist, axilla region, and surgical sites where shear forces or trim edge pressure could cause breakdown. Therapists in the acute care setting will work on transitions to bedside and safe transfers. Fracture management TLSOs are commonly fabricated as bivalve, meaning they have an anterior section and a posterior section, and then closed laterally with velcro straps. The bivalve design makes for easier supine donning by logrolling the child laterally, placing the posterior section, then logrolling to supine, followed by placement of the anterior section. Once donned, with assistance from the therapist, the child can logroll to the side and raise to a seated position at bed. A gait belt over the brace is recommended for safety during ambulation.

Cervical and thoracic injuries are managed with cervical thoracic orthoses (CTOs). In the authors' experiences, CTOs are not well tolerated because movement in the thoracic section causes movement of the cervical section and pressure on the mandible. CTOs often incorporate shoulder straps that can be a source of skin irritation. Therapists should pay special attention to the mandible, base of the occiput, and shoulders for possible skin breakdown.

Finally, as mentioned in the opening section, HALOs are intended to stabilize the cervical spine. The HALO ring is secured to the skull with pins that are torqued to a specific measure of pounds of tightness, that is, approximately half that of adults. The secured HALO ring is then attached to a thoracic section and kept in place until adequate healing has occurred. Because the HALO vest is not removed, sponge baths are necessary for daily hygiene. Pin site cleaning is necessary to prevent infection. Once the HALO is removed, the child may be placed into a cervical collar for a short period to strengthen neck musculature before discontinuation entirely by the physician.

Scoliosis

Orthoses for the treatment of scoliosis are most commonly fabricated from thermoplastic material, integrating various foams to distribute corrective force pressure, protect bony anatomy, or prevent edge pressure at trims. Congenital scoliosis occurs owing to abnormal spine development in utero and may go undetected until outward clinical signs are observed, for example, head tilt, rib prominence, or trunk asymmetries. A TLSO may be used to prevent curve progression or compensatory curve development while the child grows and delay surgery to allow for increased respiratory function.

Idiopathic scoliosis can occur at any age as the child grows and orthotic treatment is intended to prevent progression during periods of growth. Typically, the younger the child, the more likely progression is to occur.[13,14]

Idiopathic scoliosis can be divided into infantile scoliosis (birth to 3 years), juvenile scoliosis (3 to 9 years), and adolescent scoliosis (10 to 18 years). TLSOs for the treatment of scoliosis have regional names, such as Boston TLSO, Providence TLSO, Rigo System Cheneau (RSC), and Boston Bending Brace. The Providence TLSO and the Charleston Bending Brace are two nocturnal devices and are not intended for upright use.[15,16] The Boston TLSO and RSC TLSO are full-time wear devices and have been shown to be effective in preventing curve progression in the treatment of Adolescent Idiopathic Scoliosis.[17] In younger children (3 to 4 years of age), a process called EDF casting (elongation, de-rotation, flexion) may be used to reduce the curve or correct it. Oftentimes, bracing supplements EDF casting as a means of a break from casting or a transition out of the casting process. Initiating bracing in the juvenile or adolescent population generally begins when a curve progresses over 20 degrees.

As the child grows, the corrective forces do not align with the curve or curves, necessitating a change in the design. The use of Schroth Therapy, developed in Europe in the early 1900s, has been increasing in the United States, with physical therapists becoming certified. Schroth Therapy is often used in conjunction with bracing, primarily the Rigo Cheneau Brace. TLSOs for the treatment of scoliosis are discontinued by physicians once the child has reached skeletal maturity when curve progression is unlikely.[18]

Neuromuscular scoliosis is identified at younger ages because of the underlying condition affecting trunk musculature. The goals of orthotic management in the neuromuscular population are to prevent curve progression and improve trunk and head control. Orthotic management can provide support or apply corrective forces intended to reduce the scoliosis present. High-magnitude corrective force may not be well tolerated and could cause enuresis, emesis, or skin breakdown. Common modifications to TLSOs in the neuromuscular population are large belly holes that can provide access to g-tubes or bilateral trochanter extensions that can improve sitting balance. A supportive custom wheelchair with lateral thoracic supports and seating to reduce the risk of pressure ulcers may be more beneficial for a child in a wheelchair. Caution should be exercised, and the child's skin carefully watched if a TLSO is attempted to be incorporated into existing custom seating. Refer to Chapter 15, Orthopedic Conditions for ongoing discussion on PT's involvement in the treatment of adolescent idiopathic scoliosis.

The use of orthotic devices for trunk stability is increasing for children with low tone, delayed milestones, or underlying sensory conditions. Soft elastic fabrics offer increased support while allowing unimpeded trunk motion. These fabric TLSO designs can incorporate removable thermoplastic uprights, malleable uprights, or panels that can be modified or altered for changes to support magnitude.

» Limb deficiency

A child with a limb deficiency requires a family-centered care approach with a team of specialists who have a keen understanding of limb deficiencies with regard to congenital versus acquired limb deficiencies, advantages or disadvantages of the various amputation levels, amputation and revision surgeries, the basic components of a prosthesis, and the need for functional training following prosthetic fitting.

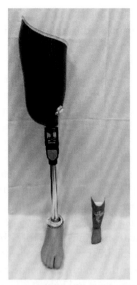

FIGURE 8.3. Limb deficiency is a lifelong condition.

Limb deficiencies in children are the result of either a congenital skeletal anomaly that may or may not require surgical revisions to facilitate prosthetic fitting or an acquired amputation resulting from trauma or disease.

Families of newborns diagnosed with a limb difference often describe their experience as "confusing, isolating, and a period of mourning." It is important that the child and family are followed by the multidisciplinary team so that their questions and concerns may be answered and the family may be able to enjoy their newborn experience with acceptance and relief. Multidisciplinary intervention may occur during the prenatal stage when a limb difference is noted on ultrasound.

The timing of prosthetic fitting in these cases will vary greatly with respect to the etiology of the limb deficiency and their developmental stages. Prosthetic treatment is an ongoing, lifelong commitment to ensure the physical, emotional, and mental well-being of the child with a limb deficiency. Each child undergoing prosthetic treatment presents different challenges at the various stages of development. Peer support for the child and family is exceedingly beneficial throughout the continuum of care (Fig. 8.3).

Congenital Limb Difference and Acquired Difference

Limb difference is a more inclusive term that provides a description for many congenital presentations that include limb absence of fingers, hands, feet, or longitudinal segments as well as additional fingers or toes. Past terms of limb absence were amelia or hemimelia but were regarded as vague and nondescriptive and have since been replaced with International Standards Organization, ISO, and standards for describing limb differences as longitudinal deficiencies and transverse deficiencies.[2]

Longitudinal deficiency refers to the absence of a long bone segment that is absent or partially missing. This usually results in altered positioning of the hands or feet. Surgical intervention may be needed to centralize the affected limb if the segment of the limb distal is determined to be functional. If there is not adequate function, amputation of the distal limb and subsequent fitting of a prosthesis may provide a better functional outcome. The determination of the course of treatment should involve the medical team, the family, and, if age appropriate, the patient.

Transverse deficiency is absence of the entire segment, often secondary to amniotic band syndrome. This description corresponds to the absence of an entire limb segment. The presentation of these deficiencies is described in similar fashion as acquired amputations in adults (i.e., above knee and below knee in lower extremity and above elbow and below elbow in upper extremity).

It is important to note that lower extremity prostheses are often described by their functional level: below knee and above knee. Use of these terms does not provide a full description of the child's limb deficiency. For example, a child with PFFD (proximal femoral focal deficiency) who has had a Syme amputation and anatomic knee arthrodesis, would utilize an above knee prosthesis, or a child with a rotationplasty prosthesis would utilize a below knee prosthesis. These conditions are discussed in more detail within the Orthopedic Chapter. It is important that the team recognize their anatomic deficiencies and how that relates to their outcomes and function with a prosthesis.

The considerations for amputation of a child and for that of an adult are not the same. Often, disarticulation amputations are preferred to maintain the child's ability to distal weight bear through the end of the limb and greatly reduce the risk of bony overgrowth, but it does present challenges with regards to prosthetic components due to space constraints with a long residuum. Growth restriction by disrupting the growth plate allows the length of the limb to slow so there can be end bearing with the prosthetic joint at the correct level such as at the knee or ankle.

» Introduction to prosthetic terminology

A prosthesis can be broken down into its various components, listed from closest to the body to the most distal. The socket of the prosthesis provides the interface between the patient and the prosthesis. Sockets are custom made to the child, via either cast or measurement. The suspension is the manner in which the prosthesis is held on to the residual limb. This may be suction, vacuum, locking liner, a sleeve, anatomic suspension, or a belt for lower extremity or harness for upper extremity. For lower extremity deficiencies, there may be components such as a mechanical hip joint, knee joint, and foot, depending on the level of amputation. In recent years, the development of prosthetic components has allowed for more customization of

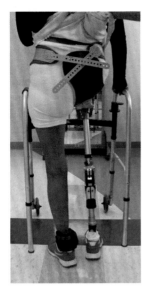

FIGURE 8.4. Hemipelvectomy prosthesis.

a device to enable improved function for children in their environments.

Prostheses can be described as either endoskeletal or exoskeletal. Endoskeletal prostheses consist of modular components that are lightweight and easily adjusted for growth. Exoskeletal prostheses can be more appropriate for young children owing to their increased durability. For upper extremity deficiencies, there may be a shoulder joint, elbow joint, and a terminal device, again depending on the level of amputation. Significant thought and consideration go into the design of a prosthesis so that optimal functional outcomes are achieved. Regardless of the advanced technology available for components, the socket fit is of utmost importance, along with suspension and alignment (Fig. 8.4).

» Prosthetic management of lower extremity limb deficiency

Children present several engineering design paradoxes in that although they are smaller in stature and their limbs proportionally smaller, they often generate force and impulse loads that rival an Olympic athlete. Although the prosthetic componentry on the market is roughly 70% of adult-sized components, the pediatric population often challenges the physical limits of these designs because of their increased physical demands. The small size of pediatric componentry presents material and design challenges for engineers and prosthetists attempting to create systems that are lightweight but that can withstand higher load ratings.

This is compounded by limited surface areas to apply corrective three-vector force loads. One advantage over adult management is that the pediatric skeleton is still developing, so this can be used to hold the proper alignment, while the force of growth can be used to allow migration of the body segments into proper positioning. However, the application

of concentrated and strong forces could iatrogenically produce unexpected and adverse results at the growth plates, if not monitored, such as suspension over distal condyles for lower or upper limb prostheses.

Infants and Toddlers

Children with a lower limb deficiency and with no comorbidities should be evaluated and treated as a typically developing infant, with established goals of sitting, crawling, pulling to stand, acceptance of a prosthesis, and, finally, independent ambulation. If surgical revision is necessary prior to the initial prosthetic fitting, it should be done when the baby is sitting independently and crawling so a prosthesis can aid the infant to pull to stand up. In this author's experience, infants tend not to have complications with edema, phantom pain, delayed wound healing, or the need for desensitization, as normally seen in adults with amputations.

Traditionally, functional prosthetic knees have not been used until 3 to 5 years of age; however, emerging research and anecdotal evidence shows that the use of a prosthetic knee with an extension assist component included and the stance control feature removed allows children to learn improved control of the knee.[19] It has been shown that children will learn to extend and lock the mechanical knee using their own musculature while having a more symmetrical and reciprocal crawling and gait pattern. As children become more confident in independent ambulation, their control of the prosthetic knee improves, and toddlers then continue to reach developmental milestones, consistent with age-appropriate development. A new prosthesis is typically required every 12 months owing to longitudinal and circumferential growth of their residuum, along with outgrown or broken componentry (Fig. 8.5).

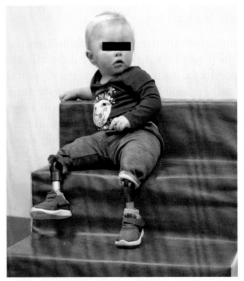

FIGURE 8.5. Toddler with bilateral above knee prostheses.

School-aged Children

For school-aged children with lower extremity limb differences, it is important to maintain a well-fitting prosthesis that allows a child to be independent and keep up with peers. The prosthesis must be able to be worn all day at school without discomfort and to allow for independent donning and doffing and toileting. Physical therapy should focus on function within their school environment and overall endurance. Prosthetic component choice will be determined on the basis of the child's functional needs and their activity level, as well as limitations of clearance and desired cosmesis. All efforts should be made to allow children at this age to maintain the same function and participate in all activities as those of their peers. At all stages of development, the child should be seeing his or her prosthetist on a regular basis to keep up with growth and needed repairs of their prostheses.

During this age, the limb deficiency team begins to see more children with acquired amputations. These amputations are related primarily to trauma, but children at this age also have an increased incidence of amputations related to solid tumor diagnoses. Different from congenital limb differences, those with acquired amputations may have complicating medical, physiological, and psychological factors. Depending on the cause, those with traumatic amputations may present with other injuries, including spinal cord injuries, traumatic brain injuries, fractures, lacerations, and degloving injuries. For those children with solid tumor diagnoses, treated with amputation, their rehabilitation pathway is often complicated and delayed, secondary to chemotherapy side effects and generalized debility. Postoperatively, both acquired and traumatic amputations require edema control and shaping to prepare the residual limb for prosthetic fitting.

The initiation of prosthetic intervention is dependent on the child's wound healing and comorbidities, and the goal of prosthetic and physical therapy treatment is to restore function to the presurgical state.

Adolescents and Teens

Older adolescents and teens with limb deficiencies present unique challenges for their families and the care team. It is very important for the team to listen to and support the teens because they are subject to peer criticism, body image issues, and self-esteem concerns. They have concerns about the future and transitioning into college and the workforce. Social work, psychology, and peer support networks should be offered and encouraged.

Componentry structural failure is a common challenge among adolescents and teens. Some teens may request cosmetic or realistic looking prostheses. Adult componentry is typically used and high-functioning carbon or fiberglass composite feet and hydraulic knees are used, along with microprocessor technology for those with above knee prostheses. Again, physical therapy is crucial in transitioning these young adults into more advanced components. If the teens

are active in competitive sports, activity-specific prostheses may be needed.

» Prosthetic management of upper extremity limb deficiency

Upper extremity limb deficiency in pediatrics presents unique challenges, particularly with regard to function and cosmesis. For congenital amputees, the function of the prosthesis will change throughout their natural development. The design of the prosthesis will need to change accordingly. For traumatic amputations in older children, return of the lost function will drive prosthetic design. In both cases, the need for acceptable cosmesis owing to the visibility of the hands may play a larger role in prosthetic design than would be seen in lower extremity.

Types of Prostheses

There are three types of upper extremity prosthesis, based on their terminal device, that is, hand.

- Nonarticulated upper extremity prostheses are those that have a terminal device that does not move without the use of the opposite hand. The prosthesis provides equal arm length, support for bimanual activities, and cosmesis. These prostheses are not prone to breakage because they have no moving parts and little to no maintenance. They are very lightweight and function to act as an assist for stabilizing objects.
- Body-powered prostheses are those that have a terminal device that is controlled by harness and cable that is secured by the contralateral shoulder. Through the excursion of shoulder flexion and glenohumeral adduction of the involved side, the terminal device can be voluntarily opened or closed. There are several different types of terminal devices, including both hands and functional prehensors or hooks. With training and practice, body-powered prostheses can provide an increased level of proprioception and control of grip strength over other devices.
- Externally controlled prostheses are those that have terminal devices that are driven by electrical motor(s) that receive input signals from either myoelectric surface electrodes or electrical pull/push switches. These devices allow for increased function compared with a passive prosthesis and improved cosmesis, grip strength, and minimal cable excursion needs compared with body-powered prostheses. These devices may require additional training to become proficient as a user because they may use only small contractions of muscle or fine movement to operate. If the patient or family is not willing to devote themselves to mastering the fine control of the device, they may ultimately be disappointed in the function it provides. Current myoelectric devices have limited use in the pediatric setting, secondary to their size, weight, and maintenance needs. Some teens may be able to use adult components, depending on their size, which improves the selection of myoelectric hands available (Fig. 8.6).

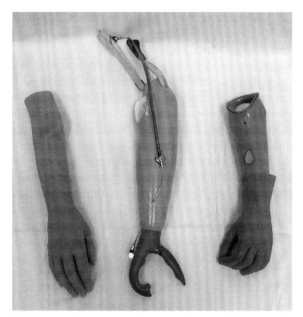

FIGURE 8.6. Three below elbow prostheses: A high-definition nonarticulated, body-powered voluntary closing, and externally powered myoelectric.

Infants

One common heuristic for initiating prosthetic care is "Sit to Fit." As the child is beginning to sit up without support, they will benefit from a prosthesis that supports the trunk during independent sitting, bimanual play, and gross motor exploration and provides equal body symmetry. At this stage, the prosthesis lays a foundation for future prosthetic use (Fig. 8.7).

Infant prostheses use a passive terminal device, which may be shaped with a cupped hand or in a three-jaw chuck position for holding devices, such as a pacifier or food. For the child with an above elbow deficiency, the prosthesis may not include an elbow joint, because the child does not have the ability to control it. The "banana" shape of the prosthesis allows the child to use it for balance.

Toddlers

Between 18 months and 3 years of age, children have a need for greater control of the terminal device. Their fine motor skills are developing, such as grasping, cutting, and use of utensils. As a result, the design of their prosthesis may need to change from a passive device to one with an active terminal device. Children can be fit with either body-powered or external power devices at this point.

Earlier fitting of a body-powered device is possible because of the simplified instructions the child needs to follow to see immediate response from the device. However, as the child progresses from training to playing, he or she may struggle with maintaining the body positions necessary to operate the terminal device. Older toddlers (~3 years of age) may be fit with a myoelectric prosthesis, since they may understand the necessary contraction of the flexor and extensor muscles of the arm to control the device. The first device is often set up as a "cookie crusher" or voluntary opening (Fig. 8.8).

As children advance into school age, they have further need for increased fine motor control. Activities such as cutting paper, writing, and independent dressing and eating require them to manipulate and hold objects with both "hands." Depending on when the child begins using his or her prosthesis, further training may be required within the school or with a therapist who specializes in prosthetic training. Other activities, such as bike riding, sports, or outdoor activities, may require the child to develop other skills with their prosthesis or, if necessary, obtain a prosthesis designed for a specific activity. Myoelectric prostheses, with proper training, provide great function and grip strength, but patient selection is important, because this age is not known to care for devices.

It should be noted that many children at this age may choose to abandon the prosthesis for various reasons. One

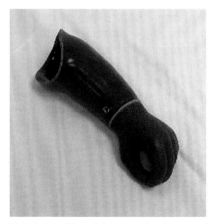

FIGURE 8.7. Below elbow infant prosthesis.

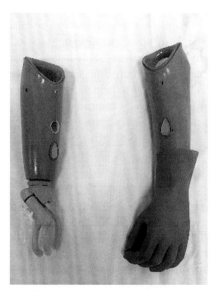

FIGURE 8.8. External powered myoelectric prosthesis, without and with a cosmetic glove.

drawback for prosthetic wear is that it may restrict sensation of the child's residual limb. In certain cases, the child may feel that the prosthesis excessively limits tactile sensation, or it could be that they are not as functional with the terminal device. They may simply feel more functional without the prosthesis and abandon it or return to it later.

This is also the age when an acquired amputation becomes more possible, secondary to trauma. In this event, considerable effort should be made to fit the patient with a device as quickly as possible. The "Golden Period" for fitting is 30 days from amputation; however, delays in healing and contracture management may make this difficult to achieve. The type of prosthesis may be determined by the hand that was lost. The loss of the dominant hand typically precludes the selection of a more functional hand, that is, body powered or myoelectric, while the loss of the nondominant hand may result in the selection of a passive device with improved cosmesis. This factor is not age dependent and plays a role in upper extremity limb loss for adolescents and teens as well.[20]

Adolescents and Teens

For older children and young teens, acceptance of prosthetic use can be attributed to two main factors: activity limitation and cosmesis. For those who are limited in an activity, activity-specific devices (i.e., music and sports) may become a desired option. For those focused on cosmesis, a high-definition custom silicone passive prosthesis can provide a realistic appearing upper extremity, providing increased patient confidence and self-assurance. Body-powered prostheses are seldom used at this age, secondary to diminished cosmesis and limited task-specific function.

Partial Hand Prostheses

Limb difference or acquired amputation, particularly in congenital partial hands, are unique and can be challenging to fit with a "standard" prosthetic design. Many of these children can complete activities of daily living; however, it may take them considerably more time and effort. In these cases, device(s) can be designed to help with each task and reduce patient workload. Increased communication between members of the multidisciplinary team is vital to help optimize function.

Summary

The physical therapist, orthotist, and prosthetist should closely collaborate to determine the prosthetic and orthotic goals of the prescribed device and how it will improve function, while closely monitoring alignment, biomechanic, or integumentary issues that may arise. As children are regularly growing and their level of activity is constantly changing, regular follow-up and assessment within the multidisciplinary team is needed, to ensure their orthotic or prosthetic device is fitting and functioning to meet their current developmental goals and needs.

Regardless of age, the goals of O&P intervention and physical therapy should be to provide individualized care to ensure that children are reaching age-appropriate developmental milestones to reach full functional potential and participate in any activity they choose while encouraging healthy habits. Treating the child as a person and not a diagnosis and involving them in every aspect of their care while ensuring that they are receiving adequate support throughout the continuum of care will yield optimal outcomes.

CASE STUDIES

M.M.

History: Background of Patient

M.M. is a 17-year-old Caucasian woman with a diagnosis of spina bifida. M.M. was diagnosed with a lower lumbar level myelomeningocele at birth, with associated hydrocephalus, shunted shortly after birth.

M.M. is followed by multiple specialists and within the multidisciplinary spina bifida clinic. Her past medical surgical history is significant for the following:

- Right lower extremity: release of peroneus longus and brevis, Achilles tendon release, distal tibial medial malleolar hemiepiphyseal screw tethering, medial displacement osteotomies with calcanei
- Left lower extremity: tenotomies of the Achilles, peroneus longus, and peroneus brevis, distal tibial medial malleolar hemiepiphyseal screw tethering, medial displacement osteotomies with calcanei
- Shunt placement and revisions
- Bladder repair

M.M. is a community ambulator at baseline, has bilateral forearm crutches but prefers not to utilize them in the home or community setting. There is no current or past history of wheelchair use.

M.M. has a history of bilateral lower extremity heel ulcers and blisters and sores on lower extremities from crawling around her home, she presents with bilateral callous formation over her knees and dorsum of her feet. M.M. was noted to have absent sensation below the level of her ankles.

M.M. presents to the multidisciplinary spina bifida clinic and is evaluated by Physical Therapy and O&P.

The following are noted on evaluation:

- Lower Extremity Strength:
  - Hip flexors 4/5
  - Hip extensors 2+/5 right, 3/5 left
  - Quadriceps 4/5
  - Hamstrings 4/5
  - Dorsiflexors 0/5
  - Plantarflexors 0/5

- Lower Extremity Range of Motion
  - 15 degree right knee flexion contracture
  - 5 degree hyperextension at left knee
- Gait: Trendelenburg Gait, left > right
- Postural Assessment:
  - No concerns for scoliosis
  - Lower extremity alignment:
    - Hindfoot valgus
    - Forefoot abduction
    - Left genu valgum

M.M. has had no previous PT intervention. She was previously fit with bilateral lower extremity orthoses, which were noted to be no longer fitting appropriately.

Previous lower extremity orthoses:

- Bilateral floor reaction AFO's (FRAFOs)
- FRAFOs no longer fitting appropriately (fit approximately 23 months ago)
  - Left lower extremity in significant valgus—inadequate bracing support
  - Gapping at bilateral patellae, significant ankle flexibility

Determined to need new bilateral lower extremity orthoses:

- Transitioned to a left knee ankle foot orthosis (KAFO), for improved support and to minimize risk of ongoing development of chronic left knee instability
  - Single upright free motion knee joints with valgus control strap and solid ankle, to support weak gastrocnemii/solei
- Right FRAFO set with a dorsiflexion angle of 5 degree and shank to vertical angle (SVA) at 15 degrees to accommodate knee flexion contracture and weak extensor muscles

Gait assessed while wearing new bilateral lower extremity orthoses, compared with barefoot gait with GAITRite® Mat evaluation. The following were noted:

- Decreased crouch
- Improved balance/self-reports of feeling "more stable"
- Decreased Trendelenburg gait
- Narrow base of support
- Improved foot/ankle alignment—less toe out
- Decreased pelvic rotation
- Slower gait speed

M.M. to continue to be followed by PT for ongoing therapy and will be followed within the O&P department for assessment and maintenance of bilateral lower extremity orthoses.

M.M. reporting that she plans to attend college this fall and reports concerns with the hilly terrain and distance between classes on campus.

Discussion Questions

1. What primary impairments and activity limitations might you want to target during physical therapy treatment?
2. What are some instances in which you would want M.M. to return for ongoing assessment with her primary orthotist? Name some signs/symptoms of adverse orthotic wear.
3. What other members may be a part of M.M's multidisciplinary team?

JENNA

HPI: Jenna is an 8-year-old girl who was diagnosed with an osteosarcoma in her right femur. She underwent chemotherapy and surgical resection. Owing to the size and location of the tumor, the surgeons performed an above knee amputation. Her past medical history is otherwise nonsignificant. She lives at home with her mother and brother in a two-story house. Her father lives nearby in an apartment. She attends third grade in a public school but has been out of school since her surgery. She received Physical Therapy while she was an inpatient after her surgery.

PT Examination: (6 weeks post surgery)

She comes to outpatient PT after being fitted with her prosthesis. Her ROM and upper extremity strength in her bilateral upper extremities are within normal limits. Her left lower extremity ROM and strength are within normal limits. Her right hip flexion is full and right hip extension is −20 degrees. Her right lower extremity hip strength is 3−/5 in all motions.

Residual Limb Edema/Scar: Sutures were removed, incision is healed, small open area noted at the incision site. Patient reports phantom sensations.

Function: She is independent with bed/mat mobility. She ambulates with Lofstrand crutches without her prosthesis on level surfaces and stairs independently. With her prosthesis, she requires contact guard assistance for ambulation with Lofstrand crutches. Her gait is significant for decreased weight bearing over the right lower extremity as well as decreased hip extension on the right. She is unable to maintain standing without upper extremity assistance or her crutches.

Prosthesis: She was fitted with a standard prosthesis with a custom total contact socket, single axis knee joint with knee drop locks that allow the ability to lock the knee or keep it freely moving. She has a standard solid ankle cushioned heel (SACH) foot.

Treatment Plan: Jenna was seen 3 times a week for PT. Her prosthetist worked closely with her PT. Adjustments were made to her prosthesis as needed. Activities included stretching and strengthening of right lower extremity, especially the right hip, gait training, and stair climbing with and eventually without crutches. Sessions also addressed endurance, balance, and coordination activities.

Goals for the outpatient PT episode of care:

1. Independent ambulation on level surfaces without crutches and supervision for safety.
2. Independent ascending and descending stairs with use of railing for safety.
3. Independent transfers without assistive device, including floor to stand.
4. Independent donning and doffing of prosthesis.

Long-term goal:

1. Community ambulation without assistive device and supervision.

Coordination of care: Jenna's outpatient team worked closely with her school PT after Jenna was found eligible for school PT services through a 504 plan. Family training was also done with both her mother and father and other significant caretakers.

Follow-up: Jenna continued to be followed in the amputee clinic at her medical institution. She also followed up with her prosthetist for prosthesis adjustments and modifications as she became stronger and more active. She continued with episodes of PT when she had new goals that she wanted to achieve as she got older. She remained cancer free and went on to graduate high school and college and eventually went on to become an oncology nurse at the same children's hospital where she was treated. Today, she is happily married and expecting a baby.

Discussion Questions

1. What primary impairments and activity limitations early on might you want to target during physical therapy treatment?

2. What are some instances when you would want Jenna to return for ongoing assessment with her primary prosthetist? Name some signs/symptoms of adverse prosthetic fit?

3. What other members may be a part of Jenna's multidisciplinary team?

REFERENCES

1. Lusardi MM, Nielsen CC. *Orthotics and Prosthetics in Rehabilitation*. Butterworth-Heinemann; 2000.

2. Krajbich JI, Pinzur MS, Potter BK, et al. *Atlas of Amputations and Limb Deficiencies*. American Academy of Orthopedic Surgeons; 2016.

3. Diamond A. Close interrelationship of motor development and cognitive development and of cerebellum and prefrontal cortex. *J Child Dev*. 2000;71(1):44-56.

4. Karimi M. Determination of the influence of walking with orthosis on bone osteoporosis in paraplegic subjects based on the loads transmitted through the bones. *Clin Biomech (Bristol, Avon)*. 2013;28:325-329.

5. Morcende J. Radical reduction in the rate of extensive corrective surgery for clubfoot using the Ponseti method. *Pediatrics*. 2004;113(2):376-380.

6. Karol L. Surgical management of the lower extremity in ambulatory children with cerebral palsy. *J Am Acad Orthop Surg*. 2004;12(3):196-203.

7. Garwood C. Soft tissue balancing after partial foot amputations. *Clin Podiatr Med Surg*. 2016;33:99-111.

8. Owen E. The importance of being Ernest about shank and thigh kinematics especially when using ankle-foot orthoses. *Prosthet Orthot Int*. 2010;34(3):254-269.

9. Xia JJ. Nonsurgical treatment of deformational plagiocephaly: a systematic review. *Arch Pediatr Adolesc Med*. 2008;162(8):719-727.

10. Stellwagen L, Hubbard E, Chambers C, et al. Torticollis, facial asymmetry and plagiocephaly in normal newborns. *Arch Dis Child*. 2008;93:827-831.

11. Mortenson PA, Steinbok P. Quantifying positional plagiocephaly: reliability and validity of anthropometric measurements. *J Craniofac Surg*. 2006;17:413-419.

12. Holowka MA, Reisner A, Giavedoni B, et al. Plagiocephaly severity scale to aid in clinical treatment recommendations. *J Craniofac Surg*. 2017;28:717-722.

13. Weinstein S. Adolescent idiopathic scoliosis. *Lancet*. 2008;371 (9623):1527-1537.

14. Asher M. Adolescent idiopathic scoliosis: natural history and long term treatment effects. *Scoliosis*. 2006;1:2.

15. Roland d'Amato C, Griggs S, McCoy B. Nighttime bracing with the providence brace in adolescent girls with idiopathic scoliosis. *Spine*. 2001;26:2006-2012.

16. Davis L, Murphy J, Shaw K, et al. Nighttime bracing with the Providence thoracolumbarsacral orthosis for treatment of adolescent idiopathic scoliosis: a retrospective consecutive clinical series. *Prosthet Orthot Int*. 2019;43:158-162.

17. Weinstein S, Dolan L, Wright J, et al. Effects of bracing in adolescents with idiopathic scoliosis. *N Engl J Med*. 2013;369:1512-1521.

18. Gavin T, Pathwardhan A. Chapter 15: Orthotics in the management of spinal dysfunction and instability. In: Lusardi M, Nielsen C, eds. *Orthotics and Prosthetics in Rehabilitation*. 2nd ed. Saunder: Elsevier; 2007:397-425.

19. Geil M, Coulter C, Schmitz M, et al. Crawling kinematics in an early knee protocol for pediatric prosthetic prescription. *J Prosthet Orthot*. 2013;25(1):22-29.

20. Malone J. Immediate postsurgical management of upper extremity amputation: conventional, electric and myoelectric prostheses. *Orthot Prosthet*. 1981;35:1-9.

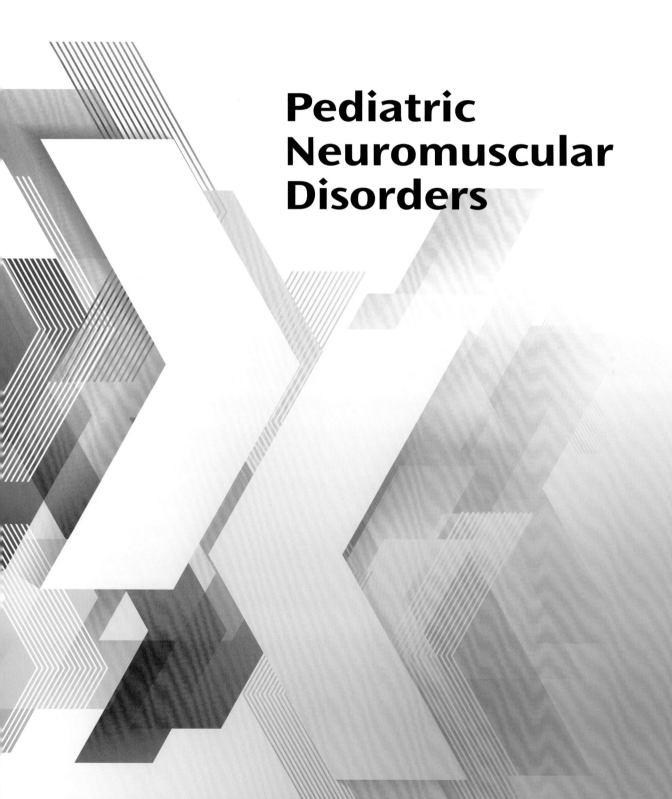

Pediatric Neuromuscular Disorders

III

Pediatric Neuromuscular Disorders

Cerebral Palsy

Jason Beaman, Faithe R. Kalisperis, and Kathleen Miller-Skomorucha

›› Definition

The International Workshop on Definition and Classification of Cerebral Palsy met in 2007 to refine the existing definition and classification of cerebral palsy (CP). They agreed upon the following definition of CP:

Cerebral palsy describes a group of permanent disorders of the development of movement and posture, causing activity limitations that are attributed to non-progressive disturbances that occurred in the developing fetal or infant brain. The motor disorders of CP are often accompanied by disturbances of sensation, perception, cognition, communication and behavior as well as seizures and secondary musculoskeletal problems.[1,2]

Historically, children were diagnosed with CP if the insult occurred prenatally, perinatally, or neonatally. On the basis of the current definition, no upper age limit has been determined for neonatal onset.[1] For this reason, children are being diagnosed with CP throughout infancy and early childhood. Although CP is not considered to be a progressive disorder, its presentation can change over time based on the child's experience, environment, and brain maturation.[3]

›› International classification of functioning and health

In an effort to create a common language around function, disability, and health, the World Health Organization (WHO) created a framework in 2001 to describe the many factors that influence each. In 2007, the WHO built on the original International Classification of Functioning, Disability, and Health (ICF) to create a framework that gives special consideration to the effects of rapid growth and significant change through the first 18 years of life. The International Classification of Functioning, Disability, and Health Children and Youth (ICF-CY) version considers the context of family, development, participation, and environments because each of these factors uniquely impacts the pediatric population.[4] These interactions are multidimensional, not hierarchical in nature. Meaning, the components influence a child's activity performance interchangeably. In this context, successfully performing functional activities is strongly influenced by health conditions, body structures and function, participation, environmental factors, and personal factors. For children and youth with CP who present with multidimensional factors, working within the ICF framework has shifted the focus from just impairment-level concerns. It calls attention to the complex interrelationship of factors the clinician must consider when working with children and youth with CP. Examination, treatment, plans of care, and goals should take into consideration all aspects of the ICF. Given here is an example of how the ICF-CY framework could be applied to a child with the goal of being able to independently walk with his walker for short distances (Fig. 9.1).

» Prevalence

In 2013, Oskoui et al. published a systematic review and meta-analysis on the estimated prevalence of CP, including a total of 49 studies reviewed. The study considered the overall prevalence of CP worldwide, the prevalence of CP in relation to birth weight, and the prevalence of CP in relation to gestational age.[5] The overall prevalence of CP is 2.11 per 1,000 live births.[5] Children born with birth weights between 1,000 and 1,499 g have a significantly higher prevalence of CP than those born with a birth weight ranging between 1,500 and 2,499 g. Children born with birth weights over 2,500 g have the lowest prevalence of CP.[5] It is also necessary to consider the influence of gestational age because it affects the prevalence of CP. The prevalence was higher in children born before 28 weeks' gestation, with those born at 23 weeks' gestation having the highest prevalence of CP. Overall, the estimated prevalence of CP has been relatively stable.[5,6]

» Etiology

There is no single specific cause of the constellation of symptoms known as CP. Rather, risk factors for CP can result from an event that affects the fetal and neonatal developing brain. When considering the underlying mechanisms that can lead to the development of CP, it is important to consider events that occur during three critical periods, which include the prenatal, peripartum, and neonatal periods. Prenatal events are thought to be responsible for about 75% of all CP. Perinatal asphyxia is thought to cause 6% to 8% of CP, with the underlying causes being unpreventable, and 10% to 18% of CP is thought to be caused by events occurring postnatally.[7] See Figure 9.2 for the associated risk factors for examples of associated risk factors in each

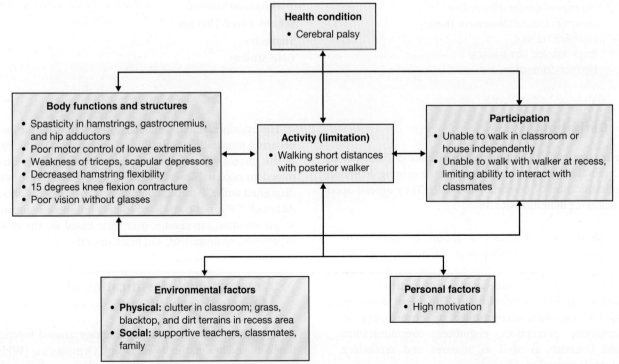

FIGURE 9.1. The International Classification of Functioning, Disability, and Health-Children and Youth (ICF-CY) model demonstrating the Health Disability Continuum. (Reproduced with permission from World Health Organization. *The International Classification of Functioning, Disability and Health: Children & Youth Version (ICF-CY).* 2007. https://apps.who.int/iris/bitstream/handle/10665/43737/9789241547321_eng .pdf)

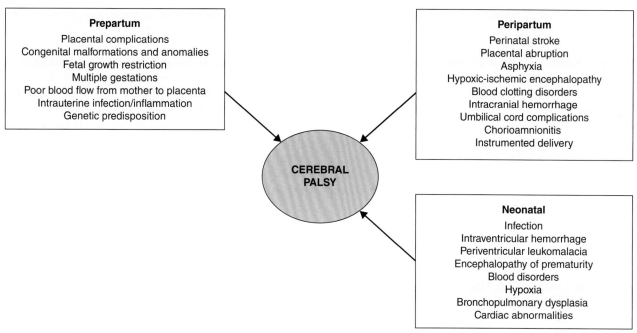

FIGURE 9.2. Associated risk factors in prepartum, peripartum, and neonatal periods. (From Stavsky M, Mor O. Mastrolia SA, Greenbaum S, et al. Cerebral palsy - trends in epidemiology and recent development in prenatal mechanisms of disease, treatment, and prevention. *Front Pediatr.* 2017;5(21):1–10; Papavasileiou A, Petra M. Risk factors for developing cerebral palsy. In: Miller F, Bachrach S, Lennon N, et al., eds. *Cerebral Palsy.* Springer; 2018.)

period.[3] Any one risk factor or interplay of several risk factors could lead to the diagnosis of CP.

Current research is looking into the possibility of variances in genes critical for fetal neurodevelopment. Although one specific gene is not being targeted, researchers are looking into several genes whose variance may be seen more frequently in certain populations of children with CP.[3] Finding a genetic marker will add to the factors associated with the diagnosis of CP.

» Diagnosis and prognosis

CP is one of the most common disabilities diagnosed in childhood. Although the etiology and pathophysiology are complex, achieving an early medical diagnosis of CP in infants and children is possible and beneficial. The path to diagnosis, however, varies depending on whether the infant or child has experienced an event or has a factor associated with CP. If there are no major peripartum risk factors, the diagnosis of CP may be delayed. If risk factors are present, the child and family are often screened earlier and closely followed up as the child grows and develops.[8] For diagnostic purposes, when CP is suspected, the medial team relies on a combination of developmental screening tools and neurologic assessments. The following tools have been highlighted as having good predictive validity for detecting CP in infants before 5 months of age. These include magnetic resonance imaging (MRI), 86% to 89% sensitivity; Prechtl Qualitative General Movement Assessment (GMA), 98% sensitivity; and the Hammersmith Infant Neurological Examination (HINE), 90% sensitivity.[9]

After 5 months' corrected age, the tools that are the most predictive for determining risk for CP are MRI, 86% to 89% sensitivity; HINE, 90% sensitivity, and the Developmental Assessment of Young Children (DAYC), 83% C-index. Other standardized neuromotor assessment tools include Alberta Infant Motor Scale (AIMS), the Motor Assessment of Infants (MAI), the Neuro-Sensory Motor Development Assessment (NSMDA), and the Test of Infant Motor Performance.[8,9] Initiation of therapy during this period of rapid growth and development enables the clinician to take full advantage of the neuroplasticity of the brain.

The signs and symptoms of CP may be apparent in early infancy. Infants presenting with abnormal muscle tone, atypical posture, and movement with persistence of primitive reflexes may be diagnosed earlier than 2 years of age.[10] Milder cases of CP may not be diagnosed until 4 to 5 years of age.[11] Evaluation of the child's motor skills, neuroimaging, and evidence that symptoms are not progressing are key elements of this diagnosis. A correlation between clinical findings and neuroanatomy is possible to a limited degree. Neuroimaging of the brain, such as cranial ultrasound, computed tomography (CT), and MRI, can show the location, type, and extent of brain damage. Cranial ultrasound is often used for the high-risk preterm infant, because it is less invasive than are other imaging techniques. MRI imaging is often preferred, because it provides greater detail of brain tissue and structure.[11] Of the children with CP, 70% to 90% have abnormalities on a brain MRI. The physician should be cautious when interpreting neuroimaging, because the extent of damage to the brain tissue may not correlate directly with physical presentation or functional abilities.[10] When neuroimaging of the brain is unremarkable, other diagnoses that mimic the signs and symptoms of CP may be considered, such as mitochondrial and metabolic disorders and transient dystonia.

Cerebral hemorrhages may be associated with CP. These hemorrhages are labeled as intraventricular hemorrhage (IVH), bleeding into the ventricles; germinal matrix hemorrhage (GMH), bleeding into the tissue around the ventricles; and periventricular intraventricular hemorrhage (PIVH), bleeding into both areas. Periventricular cysts (PVCs) may form in these same areas as the acute hemorrhage resolves.[10] There are known risk factors for hemorrhages including mechanical ventilation and injury during critical periods of brain development. Notably, periventricular white matter is most sensitive to insult and injury between 24 and 34 weeks of gestation.[11,12]

Hemorrhages are graded in increasing severity from I through IV. The grade of bleed alone cannot predict the development or severity of CP.[10] Palmer indicated that cranial ultrasound should be used for low-birth-weight infants to detect grades III and IV hemorrhages, IVH, cystic periventricular leukomalacia (PVL), and ventricular enlargement.[13] After term age, cranial ultrasound and MRI are used to identify cystic PVL and ventriculomegaly, which are associated with subsequent development of CP.[7,13] PVL is the major cause of CP in infants born preterm.[12] The extent and location of white matter damage can lead to different subtypes of CP. Localized damage to the cortical spinal tracts often results in spastic diplegia, and when the lesions extend laterally, quadriplegia is often the result.

Data gathered from multiple countries has shown that the life expectancy for adults with CP is markedly similar to that of the general population. However, individuals with CP who have severe cognitive disability, swallowing impairments leading to aspiration and/or pneumonia, nutritional concerns, or spinal deformities may have a shortened life expectancy.[14] Studies have reported that individuals with CP, who present with a Gross Motor Function Classification System (GMFCS) level V, have a greater risk of dying at a younger age because of medical complexities. This reference also highlights that adults in the United States with CP die from similar age-related causes of death such as cancer, major organ failure, or circulatory problems; however, they tend to die at an earlier age as compared to the general population.[14,15] This may be due to poorer overall health, but the true cause is unknown.

» Clinical classification

The goal of any health care classification system is to help guide clinical decision making with regard to treatment and outcomes. Many methods of classifying children with CP have been used in the past 70 years. Traditionally, classification of CP has focused on pathophysiology or neuroanatomic location of the brain lesion (pyramidal or extrapyramidal), the number and parts of the body involved,

and the type of muscle tone or movement disorder present. Today, CP continues to be defined by the motor type, such as spastic, hypotonic, dyskinetic, or ataxic, by the body parts involved, such as hemiplegic, diplegic, or quadriplegic, and by the functional skills of the child, captured in the assigned GMFCS level.[1,16] In addition, CP classifications used in the United States, Australia, and Europe are slightly different when describing the subtypes of spastic CP, the most common motor type.[17] Australian CP registries use the convention that describes the number of limbs affected, including monoplegia, diplegia, hemiplegia, triplegia, and quadriplegia. European CP registries use either unilateral for one side of the body affected, or bilateral for both sides of the body affected. In North America, both conventions of classifying spastic CP subtypes are used. It is important to have an understanding of the difference in naming conventions for CP around the world to properly understand the types of CP being discussed in clinical conversation and within research from around the world. This section discusses the classification systems, motor types of CP, and distribution based on both topographic categories.[17]

Functional Classification Systems

With the influence of the ICF, the WHO's framework for measuring health and disability, it is important to consider the child's functional mobility and the child's activity and participation within the home and community. In 1997, Palisano and colleagues[18] developed the GMFCS, which is a classification system based on the gross motor function of children with CP. The GMFCS was developed to fill the need to have a standardized system to measure the "severity of movement disability" in children with CP.[18,19] Classifying an infant or child according to functional abilities and limitations improves communication between health care professionals and families in regard to determining the child's current and future needs. In addition, the GMFCS is helpful for stratifying children into more homogeneous groups for research purposes and program evaluation. As a result, recent research has shown that the GMFCS classification is helpful in predicting future motor function.[20] There are five levels of classifications, each level representing a clinically distinct level of function. Distinctions between levels focus on functional limitation, the need for assistive technology for mobility, and, to a lesser extent, quality of movement. Furthermore, the GMFCS describes gross motor abilities at each level across four different age brackets (<2 years, 2 to 4 years, 4 to 6 years, and 6 to 12 years.[21] Level I describes the child with the most independent function. These children can walk without limitation, but have some difficulty with higher level motor skills involving speed, coordination, and balance. Level V describes the child who presents with severe limitations in head and trunk control, who has restrictions in voluntary movement, and who requires assistance for all functional mobility.[18,19] The GMFCS is described in Figure 9.3.

GMFCS E & R between 6th and 12th birthday: Descriptors and illustrations

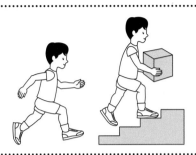

GMFCS Level I

Children walk at home, school, outdoors and in the community. They can climb stairs without the use of a railing. Children perform gross motor skills such as running and jumping, but speed, balance and coordination are limited.

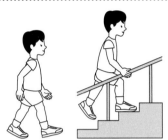

GMFCS Level II

Children walk in most settings and climb stairs holding onto a railing. They may experience, difficulty walking long distances and balancing on uneven terrain, inclines, in crowded areas or confined spaces. Children may walk with physical assistance, a hand-held mobility device or used wheeled mobility over long distances. Children have only minimal ability to perform gross motor skills such as running and jumping.

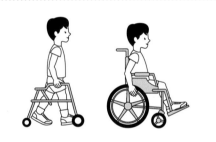

GMFCS Level III

Children walk using a hand-held mobility device in most indoor settings. They may climb stairs holding onto a railing with supervision or assistance. Children use wheeled mobility when traveling long distances and may self-propel for shorter distances.

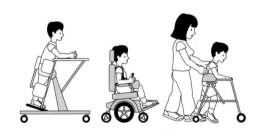

GMFCS Level IV

Children use methods of mobility that require physical assistance or powered mobility in most settings. They may walk for short distances at home with physical assistance or use powered mobility or a body support walker when positioned. At school, outdoors and in the community children are transported in a manual wheelchair or use powered mobility.

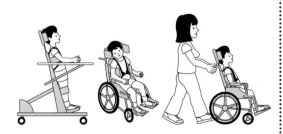

GMFCS Level V

Children are transported in a manual wheelchair in all settings. Children are limited in their ability to maintain antigravity head and trunk postures and control leg and arm movements.

GMFCS descriptors: Palisano et al. (1997) Dev Med Child Neurol 39:214-23
CanChild: www.canchild.ca

Illustrations Version 2 © Bill Reid, Kate Willoughby, Adrienne Harvey and Kerr Graham, The Royal Children's Hospital Melbourne   ERC151050

FIGURE 9.3. Gross Motor Function Classification System (GMFCS—expanded [E] and revised [R]). (Used with permission from illustrations copywrite @Kerr Graham, Bill Reid, Adrienne Harvey. The Royal Children's Hospital Melbourne.)

In addition to the GMFCS, several other similar CP-specific five-level classification systems have been developed. The Manual Ability Classification System (MACS) is a five-level scale used by clinicians to describe levels of fine motor function.[22] The Communication Function Classification System (CFCS) is used to describe expressive and receptive language in children with CP.[23,24] The Eating and Drinking Ability Scale (EDACS) describes five levels of safe and efficient eating for children with CP.[25] The Visual Function Classification System (VFCS) for children with CP was created to classify how children with CP use their vision in everyday life.[26] Classifying children with these five scales creates a comprehensive representation of the functional level of the child with CP and consistent language for communication and collaboration among physicians, clinicians, and researchers who work with children with CP (Fig. 9.4).

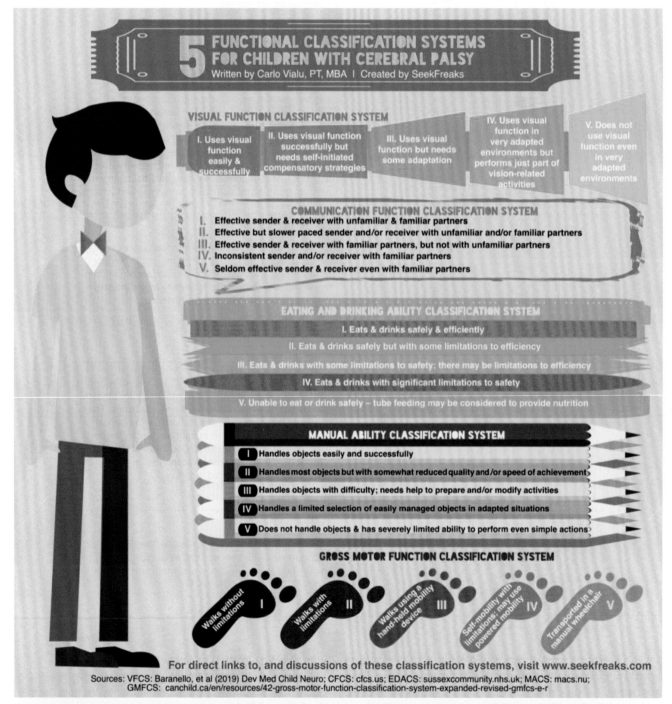

FIGURE 9.4. 5 Functional Classification Systems for children with cerebral palsy. (From Vialu C. 5 Functional classification systems for children with cerebral palsy—2019 update. *SeekFreaks.* October 5, 2019. https://www.seekfreaks.com/index.php/2019/10/05/5-functional-classification-systems-for-children-with-cerebral-palsy-2019-update/)

Motor Type

SPASTIC Spasticity occurs in approximately 75% of all children with CP. It is the most common neurologic abnormality seen in children with CP, including those with diplegia, hemiplegia, and quadriplegia.[10,27] Bevans and Tucker stated that the distribution of spastic CP is monoplegia (<1%), diplegia (29% to 36%), hemiplegia (29% to 39%), triplegia (2%), and quadriplegia (23% to 33%).[17] Spasticity is a complex motor abnormality, often difficult to describe, but a common definition is "hypertonia in which resistance to passive movement increases with increasing velocity of movement."[1] Spasticity causes significant histologic changes, including decreased longitudinal growth of muscle fibers, decreased volume of muscle, change in muscle unit size, and change in muscle fiber type.[10] The muscle changes with spasticity can cause secondary disorders such as hip joint subluxation or dislocation, scoliosis, knee joint contracture, and torsional malalignments of the femur and tibia, among others. These changes often have significant effects on function, including altered gait patterns, difficulty assuming and sustaining developmental positions, and difficulty performing self-care activities such as toileting, bathing, dressing, and self-feeding.

DYSKINETIC Dyskinesia and other movement disorders generally result in uncontrolled and involuntary movements that can include athetosis, rigidity, tremor, dystonia, ballismus, and choreoathetosis.[10,14,27–29] Common abnormalities found in imaging include deep gray matter lesions and, to a lesser extent, periventricular white matter lesions.[30] Athetosis always has involuntary movements that are slow and writhing; abnormal in timing, direction, and spatial characteristics; and are usually large motions of the more proximal joints.[10,27,28] Athetosis is rare as a primary movement disorder and is most often found in combination with chorea.[1] Athetosis is most commonly a secondary movement disorder in conjunction with spasticity. The cortical–basal ganglia–thalamic loop is a sensory and motor feed-forward and feedback circuit, and when impaired, results in athetosis. Older individuals with athetoid CP are at risk for acquiring significant neurologic deficits owing to intervertebral disk degeneration and instability in their cervical spines. After a radiologic study of 180 subjects, Harada and associates found that disk degeneration occurred earlier and progressed more rapidly in subjects with athetoid CP than in those without CP. Advanced disk degeneration was found in 51% of those studied, which is eight times the typical frequency.[31] Individuals with athetosis typically initiate and attempt control of movement with the jaw and head. This eventually causes musculoskeletal changes such as cervical instability, potential high spinal cord injury, temporomandibular joint dysfunction, and or spinal stenosis. Of note, when athetosis is the primary movement disorder, the cognitive ability of these children tends to be underestimated owing to associated dysarthria. In fact, these children tend to have normal to above-normal intelligence. Rigidity is much less common, is felt as resistance to both active and passive movement, and is not velocity dependent.[27] Tremor, a rhythmic movement of small magnitude, usually of the smaller joints, rarely occurs as an isolated disorder in CP, but rather in combination with athetosis or ataxia.[10] Dystonia is a slow motion with a torsional element that may involve one limb or the entire body and in which the pattern itself may change over time.[10] Ballismus is the most rare movement disorder and involves random motion in large, fast patterns, usually of a single limb.[10] Choreoathetosis involves jerky movement, commonly of the digits and varying in the ROM.[10,14]

ATAXIC Ataxic CP is primarily a disorder of balance and control in the timing of coordinated movements along with weakness, incoordination, a wide-based gait, and a noted tremor.[27,28] This type of CP results from deficits in the cerebellum and often occurs in combination with spasticity and athetosis.[27] The cerebellum is a major sensory processing center, and when impaired, ataxia will result. In contrast to other types of CP, a specific lesion is less common with neuroimaging, and one recent study found lesions in only 39% of children with ataxia.[30] Children with ataxia have difficulty with transference of skills, and may benefit from a specific task-oriented approach to treatment. For example, to master stepping onto and off the school bus, it is most effective to practice the skill using bus steps.

HYPOTONIC Hypotonia, or low tone, is a less common and variable muscle tone pattern. Hypotonia differs in pathophysiology from the more common "high tone" or spastic patterns of CP. Unlike spastic CP, hypotonia is often correlated with a congenital abnormality, such as lissencephaly.[10] Children diagnosed with hypotonia also commonly present with poorly defined chromosomal abnormalities.[32] As future research on the influence of genetics and CP emerges, the link between hypotonia and chromosomal disorders may be better understood. Numerous variations of chromosomal disorders that may help explain the wide variety of functional abilities in this subtype of CP exist. Children with hypotonic CP often develop the skills needed for ambulation and typically present as a GMFCS level II or III.[32] Children with hypotonia may also present with a mixed tone pattern, having both hypotonia in the neck and trunk and spasticity in the extremities. Hypotonia in a child with a chromosomal influence and/or congenital brain abnormalities is typically permanent. In some infants, however, hypotonia can be the initial tonal pattern observed with evolution to a movement disorder or spasticity with age. For example, an infant who presents with generalized hypotonia through the trunk and extremities can develop spasticity beginning distally and progressing proximally as toddlers.

Distribution

HEMIPLEGIA/UNILATERAL Hemiplegia is a subtype of spastic CP in which the child's upper extremity (UE) and lower extremity (LE) on the same side of the body are affected. More recently, this subtype of CP is referred to as unilateral CP. Four main types of brain lesions result in unilateral CP. Periventricular white matter abnormalities have been reported as the most common diagnostic finding in children with hemiplegic CP.[33] Cervical–subcortical lesions, brain malformations, and nonprogressive postnatal injuries have also been identified as the main causes of hemiplegia.[34] The UE is typically more affected than is the LE, and both tend to have more distal involvement than proximal involvement. Muscle spasticity on the affected side decreases muscle and bone growth, resulting in decreased ROM. Therefore, children with hemiplegia often present with contractures and limb-length discrepancies (LLDs) on the involved side. The affected side of the child with hemiplegia often presents with scapular protraction, elbow joint flexion, forearm pronation, wrist joint flexion with ulnar deviation, posterior pelvic rotation, hip joint internal rotation and flexion, knee joint flexion, and ankle joint plantar flexion.

Children with hemiplegia tend to achieve all gross and fine motor milestones, but not within the typical time frame. For example, children with hemiplegia tend to walk between 18 and 24 months, but present with gait deficits. In addition, acquisition of bimanual hand skills is delayed because of the neurologic impairment of the affected UE; for example, cutting food using a fork and knife. Two widely known standardized assessments are used to evaluate the quality of UE function in children with hemiplegia: the Shriners Hospital for Children Upper Extremity Evaluation (SHUEE)[35] and the Assisting Hand Assessment.[36] Cognitive function is typically normal in these children, and as adults they are able to work and participate in a variety of professional settings. Similar to children with spastic diplegia, children with spastic hemiplegia have a higher incidence of social and emotional deficits. These include emotional disorders in 25%, conduct disorders in 24%, pervasive hyperactivity in 10%, and situational hyperactivity in 13%.[14] Overall, children with hemiplegia require minimal equipment or self-care/school accommodations. They may benefit from orthotics, assistive devices such as a cane, adaptive self-care equipment, or accommodations because of visual impairments (Fig. 9.5).

DIPLEGIA/BILATERAL Diplegia is one of the most common forms of spastic CP.[30] A white matter infarct in the periventricular areas caused by hypoxia can lead to spastic diplegic CP.[30] It primarily affects bilateral LEs, with mild involvement of the UEs, resulting in issues with gait, balance, and coordination. In standing, children with diplegia often present with an increased lumbar spine lordosis, anterior pelvic tilt, bilateral hip internal rotation, bilateral knee flexion, in-toeing, and equinovalgus foot position. There tends to be a discrepancy between UE and LE function in children

with this form of CP, with the LEs being more affected than are the UEs and the trunk. Overall, there is a large range in the level of motor involvement for children with diplegia. Gait deficits such as equinus and crouched gait posture tend to be the area of greatest concern for these children (refer to the section "Gait" for further details). Owing to bilateral LE spasticity and weakness, energy expenditure is much greater during ambulation, resulting in poor endurance and decreased functional mobility at home and within the community. Children with diplegia generally have normal cognition, but may have some social and/or emotional difficulties. Children with diplegia often require assistive devices such as a posterior walker or forearm crutches. A scooter or wheelchair may be necessary for long-distance mobility.

QUADRIPLEGIA Quadriplegia is a subtype of CP in which volitional muscle control of all four extremities is severely impaired. This subtype is also often accompanied by neck and trunk involvement. As with diplegic CP, periventricular white matter lesions are the most frequently observed neuroimaging findings in children with quadriplegic CP. Extensive lesions affecting the basal ganglia or occipital area often lead to visual impairments and seizures, both commonly seen in children with this subtype of CP.[12] Cognition can vary from normal to severely impaired, and is unique to each child with quadriplegia. It is important to note that children with quadriplegia who are unable to speak are often regarded as being cognitively impaired. However, once they are provided a means of effective communication, some are able to demonstrate age-appropriate levels of understanding and critical thinking.[16] Gross and fine motor abilities vary widely in children with quadriplegia, from being ambulatory for household distances with an assistive device to being dependent for all care. The equipment needs for these children are considerable through the lifespan. Common equipment

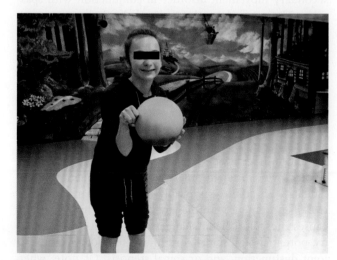

FIGURE 9.5. A child with cerebral palsy (CP) Gross Motor Function Classification System (GMFCS) level II with dystonic unilateral/hemiplegia.

recommendations include mechanical lift systems, wheel-chairs, standers, gait trainers/walkers, feeding systems, bath systems, and toileting systems. Home modifications should be considered for children with severe disabilities to maximize the child's independence with transfers and mobility, to ease caregiver strain, and improve safety for the child and caregiver.

>> Physical therapy management

Physical Therapy Examination

According to the Guide to Physical Therapist Practice 3.0,[37] the management of the infant, child, and adolescent with CP consists of the PT examination, evaluation, diagnosis, prognosis, interventions, and outcomes. The purpose of the PT examination is to discover the functional abilities and strengths of the child, determine the primary and secondary impairments (compensations used because of the primary impairments), and discover the desired functional and participation outcomes of the child and family. The therapist must use an organized approach to information gathering, including a complete and thorough history, systems review, and appropriate tests and measures.

History

HISTORY OF PRESENT ILLNESS The therapist gathers key elements about the child's current needs and why the child was referred to PT services through chart review and or parent interview. The therapist also collects information on child and family concerns, as well as their hopes for the child's short- and long-term abilities. It is important to focus on gathering the information given:

- Recent medical, pharmacologic, or surgical interventions that may have resulted in a need for a PT examination
- Current surgical or other precautions
- Medical complication as a result of recent medical intervention
- Current level of function
- Function before intervention and if there has been a recent decline or improvement in activity and participation at home, at school, or within the community

MEDICAL HISTORY
- Birth history: gestation age, complication during pregnancy and/or delivery, injury/illness after delivery
- Past medical procedures
- Comorbidities
- Full medication list (including over-the-counter [OTC] and home remedies)
- Respiratory issues

DEVELOPMENTAL HISTORY
- Time frame for milestone acquisition
- Functional gains or decline

- Use of or need for assistive devices, braces, assistive technology (adaptive equipment for activities of daily living [ADLs], wheelchairs, positioning devices, speech-generating devices)

SOCIAL HISTORY
- Family support
- Cultural and language consideration
- Barriers to success (transportation, access, family stressors, financial limitations)
- Home setup
- School setup, and academic and therapeutic resources
- Access to community activities and participation: sports, leisure activities

Systems Review

Within a review of systems, the therapist looks at the child as a whole. With information gathered from the parent interview and history, the therapist must determine which body systems require attention, either through PT intervention or referral to another specialist. A general understanding of the key components of these systems and how they affect the child and adolescent with CP is a fundamental aspect of the PT examination.

NEUROMUSCULAR SYSTEM The neuromuscular system is the primary system affected in children and youth with CP. Many of the motor impairments that result in challenges in functional mobility, activity, and participation are secondary to the mechanism of brain injury or encephalopathy.[38] The link between the central nervous system (CNS) impairments and the disability presentation, however, is not well understood. The neuromuscular system integrates the conceptual idea of movement and the plan for movement executed by the musculoskeletal system.[38] Motor control is essential for movement that is accurate, controlled, and well-timed.[38,39] For children and youth with CP, the pathophysiology of abnormal motor control results in imprecise and inefficient movement patterns. As a result of the central pathology, the peripheral information sent to the musculoskeletal system develops abnormally. This results in abnormal muscle tone including hypertonia or hypotonia and/or movement disorders including dystonia, athetosis, chorea, hemiballismus, and tremors.[38]

Neuromuscular problems can be attributed to abnormalities in three subsystems of motor control: muscle tone, motor planning, and balance. Most of the motor impairments in children and youth with CP are due to abnormalities in these areas.[38] Abnormalities in muscle tone often present as spasticity, which is described later. Motor planning abnormalities result in difficulty with constructing and executing a sequence of events to complete a functional activity. These are often described as movement disorders and include dystonia, athetosis, chorea, hemiballismus, and tremors. Generally, the basal ganglia and its connections to the cerebral cortex are involved in these disorders. Balance dysfunction is described as ataxia and is typically due to insults to the cerebellum and its connections to the cerebral cortex.

Miller defines muscle tone as the proper tension a muscle sustains for postural control and the tension needed to prepare for smooth, efficient, and accurate movement. Muscle tone is also often described as the stiffness present in a muscle when it is moved passively. Abnormal muscle tone can be described as high (hypertonicity), low (hypotonicity), or fluctuating.[38] The presence of high or low tone will affect the child's ability to learn and carry out basic functional mobility tasks such as standing and walking. To understand the atypical movement and motor control that occurs in children with CP, there needs to be an understanding of the neural and nonneural components of muscle lengthening. Neural components typically come from the CNS and result in increased muscle activation. It results in spasticity, which is often considered the most common motor impairment in children with CP.[40] Spasticity is the result of an upper motor neuron lesion, and is defined by Lance as "a motor disorder characterized by velocity dependent increase in tonic stretch reflexes (muscle tone) with exaggerated tendon jerks, resulting from hyperexcitability of the stretch reflex as one component of the upper motor neuron syndrome."[41] The nonneural components are described as physiologic changes in muscle tissue, such as contracture, that are examined during passive movement. The current postulation is that changes occur over time at the muscular level because of the abnormal neural input.[42]

Clinically, it may be difficult to tease out the difference between the neural and nonneural components of muscle tone. Often, in the clinic, the therapist will complete a tone examination to help determine the type of tone present and how it affects task performance. As the examining PT, it is important to have an understanding of spasticity, and whether the changes in muscle tone are due to spasticity or the presence of contracture.

MUSCULOSKELETAL SYSTEM Within the systems review, the musculoskeletal system is also a key area of focus for the child and youth with CP. As stated earlier, many secondary impairments of the musculoskeletal system are a result of issues that arise from the neuromuscular input and abnormal communication from the CNS to the peripheral muscles and joints. The following section highlights the common impairments and musculoskeletal deformities that are often seen in children with CP. Attention is given to the examination of the spine, trunk, pelvis, and lower limb.

Examination of the Spine and Trunk Examination of the child's passive and active trunk movement is an essential part of the PT examination. The therapist must document any deviation from normal in the spinal curves, or an asymmetry in the arch of the ribs, noted with forward bending. It is important to note if there is scoliosis, excessive kyphosis and/or lordosis, and whether the curves are structural or functional. The most common spinal deformity for children

with CP is neuromuscular scoliosis. Children at GMFCS levels IV and V are at the greatest risk for developing neuromuscular scoliosis. Neuromuscular scoliosis is thought to be the result of poor motor control, muscle imbalance, muscle weakness, and spasticity. Progression of neuromuscular scoliosis does not respond well to bracing; however, spinal orthoses are sometimes recommended to improve comfort and positioning. The overall incidence of scoliosis for children with CP is 20% to 25%, with a higher risk for the development of scoliosis in those with quadriplegic CP at 64% to 77%.[43] It is important to monitor and watch the progression of spinal curvature because it can directly impact pulmonary function, overall lung volume, and gastrointestinal (GI) function.[44] Children with CP GMFCS levels III to V should be screened yearly for the development of spinal curves starting at age 8.[45]

In addition to examination of the spine, it is also important to complete a thorough examination of the trunk. The therapist should examine the amount of postural control present throughout the trunk. Children and youth with CP tend to have decreased active balance of trunk flexors and extensors when in an upright position, with difficulty sustaining their postural muscles. In addition, respiratory function should be examined with the child in various functional positions. Visual and/or tactile examination of accessory muscle activation and rib movement with breathing, especially in sitting and standing, can reveal important information regarding respiratory function. The presence of flaring of the lower rib cage can be indicative of a lack of trunk and pelvis stabilization using the abdominal oblique muscles, which subsequently can lead to a mechanical impairment of the diaphragm muscle action.

Examination of the Hip Joint and Pelvis The child with CP, most typically with spastic diplegia or quadriplegia, commonly has tightness in the hip flexors, adductors, and internal rotator muscles with resultant limitation in hip extension, abduction, and external rotation. Owing to abnormal muscle pull around the hip joint, hip joint surveillance is a very important aspect in the management of children with CP. This is best managed by a team approach, with consistent screening of the hip joint by clinical examination and periodic radiographic imaging, when appropriate. Neuromuscular hip dysplasia is a common radiographic finding that generally occurs between 2 to 8 years of age, but can occur any time until skeletal maturity.[46] Hip joint subluxation, dislocation, or dysplasia occurs slowly over time due to abnormal muscle forces on the developing hip joint. This may be due to increased spasticity of the hip adductors.[46] Children with CP who are GMFCS levels III to V are at greatest risk for developing hip dysplasia. The examining PT should take consistent ROM measurements of hip abduction, and watch for signs of hip pain. Hip subluxation is difficult to examine via physical examination. Any child younger than 8 years of age with hip abduction of less than 45 degrees on either side should be referred to an orthopedic surgeon for further evaluation.[10] An apparent

LLD may also be noted in a child with suspected unilateral hip subluxation/dislocation. The subluxed or dislocated hip is typically shorter than is the contralateral limb owing to the great majority of subluxations being superior and posterior.[10,47]

Femoral Anteversion Femoral anteversion is a torsion or internal rotation of the femoral shaft on the femoral neck. At birth, an infant has approximately 40 degrees of femoral anteversion, as measured by the angle between the transcondylar axis of the femur and the femoral axis of the neck. The neonate also has 25 degrees of flexion contracture of the hip due to intrauterine positioning and physiologic flexor tone. In the progression of typical development, hip flexors lengthen as the result of gravitational pull while the child is lying in either a prone or a supine position. Active extension and external rotation of the hip tighten the anterior capsule of the hip joint, thus producing a torque or torsional stress that decreases the anteversion that is present from birth.[48] In addition, normal hip extensor and external rotator activation pull on the femur at their attachments on the proximal femoral growth plates, further decreasing the anteversion of the hip. As a result of these forces acting on the femur, 15 degrees of femoral anteversion is typically reached by 16 years of age.[49,50] Femoral anteversion is determined by biplane roentgenograms. Anteversion may be suspected on the basis of a simple clinical test. Internal and external rotation of the hip are tested with the hip in a position of extension (i.e., with the child in a prone position with knee joints flexed). Femoral anteversion may be suspected when external rotation at the hip is substantially less than is the internal rotation.

The infant or child with CP often has overactivity and shortening of the flexors of the hip and poor control of extensors and of external rotators of the hip. Beals,[51] in 1969, studied 40 children with spastic diplegic pattern CP and found that the degree of femoral anteversion was normal at birth. However, this study also revealed that the amount of anteversion did not decrease over the first few years of life, as occurs with typically developing children. After 3 years of age, Beals also reported that no significant change in anteversion occurred regardless of age or ambulation status. At skeletal maturity, the children with CP in this study had a mean of 14 degrees greater anteversion than did the children without CP.[51]

Staheli and associates[52] found greater angles of anteversion of the femur in the involved LE of a group of children with hemiplegic CP than was found in their uninvolved limb. This finding can be easily explained by the consistently poor activation of extensors and external rotators of the hip, preventing the decline in anteversion seen in normal development.

Excessive femoral anteversion is hypothesized to place the hip abductors at a biomechanical disadvantage when walking by decreasing the functional lever arm relative to the hip joint center during the stance phase of gait.[53] Recent studies have also shown that increased femoral anteversion is a cause

of lower limb deformity[54] and gait dysfunction.[55] Femoral derotational osteotomy is the treatment of choice to correct excessive femoral anteversion, typically occurring when the angle is greater than 30 degrees.[56]

Examination of the Knee Joint It is essential to examine sagittal plane knee positioning when examining the child with CP. Oftentimes, these children will present with a crouched gait or knee flexed gait pattern. Less common but still of concern is the child with genu recurvatum. Both issues result in serious gait abnormalities. The child with CP may have limited knee flexion or extension as a result of inadequate length of the quadriceps or hamstrings. The length of the medial and lateral hamstrings and the rectus femoris, all of which cross two joints, should be measured through goniometry. Passive straight leg raise or measurement of the popliteal angle will indicate the degree of hamstring tightness. It is also necessary to examine the positioning of the patella because patella alta is very common in children with CP. Chronic crouched gait causes overstretching of the quadriceps muscles and knee extensor mechanism, which leads to the patella alta. This occurs in 58% to 72% of children with spastic CP.[57] Patella alta decreases the ability of the patella to create optimal knee extension force with functional mobility, and can be painful.

Tibial Torsion Tibial torsion describes a twist of the tibia along its long axis so that the leg is rotated internally or externally. The specific angle of torsion can be determined in two ways: (1) transmalleolar axis (TMA) by the intersection of a line drawn vertically from the tibial tubercle and a line drawn through the malleoli and (2) thigh–foot angle (TFA), which is the angle formed by the TMA and the thigh, measured with the child in prone and the knee joint is flexed to 90 degrees (Fig. 9.6).

Similar to the femur, the tibia undergoes developmental torsional changes. The malleoli are parallel in the frontal plane at birth. During infancy and early childhood, the tibia rotates externally, which places the lateral malleolus in a posterior position relative to the medial malleolus. The progression from relative internal to external tibial torsion is attributable to changes in force on the tibia arising from the decrease in femoral anteversion that occurs as the child grows. As discussed earlier, femoral anteversion does not decrease normally with growth, often resulting in compensatory external tibial torsion to maintain the foot facing forward.

Examination of the Foot Foot deformities are some of the most common musculoskeletal impairments reported in children and youth with CP.[58] In the examination of the foot, special attention should be given to the integrity of the talocrural joint and subtalar joint, alignment of the forefoot and toes, presence of soft-tissue contractures, and the impact of muscle tone on the mobility and stability of the foot.[58] Ankle equinus is a foot deformity that occurs due

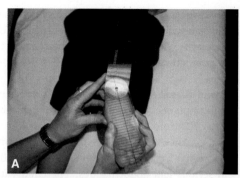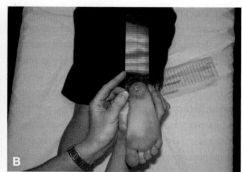

FIGURE 9.6. A: Tibial torsion thigh–foot Angle (TFA): Position the patient prone with knee flexed to 90 degrees and the ankle in neutral DF with subtalar joint (STJ) in neutral position. Place the goniometer along the long axis of the plantar surface of the foot, bisecting the heel. The TFA is formed by the angle between this line and the line bisecting the posterior midline of the femur. Note internal or external rotation. **B:** Transmalleolar axis (TMA): Position the patient prone with knee flexed to 90 degrees and the ankle in neutral DF with STJ in neutral position. Placing the goniometer on the plantar surface of the heel, align one arm parallel to the line intersecting the medial and lateral malleolus. The TMA is formed by the angle between this line and the line bisecting the posterior midline of the femur. Note internal or external rotation.

to overactivity of the plantar flexors. This overactivity due to muscle spasticity generally presents as toe-walking as a child with CP starts to walk. For ambulatory children, the amount of equinus and toe-walking tends to peak between the ages of 5 and 6 years. This spasticity-induced equinus affects muscle growth and ROM of the ankle joint.[58] Ankle equinovarus is another foot deformity that often develops in children with CP, especially unilateral or hemiplegic CP. Owing to the presence of ankle equinus, the forefoot will often fall into adduction resulting in an equinovarus foot position. Another foot deformity is the planovalgus foot. This is the most common collapse type of foot deformity for children with CP. In planovalgus feet, the forefoot falls into abduction, the hindfoot falls into valgus, and the midfoot is in dorsiflexion (DF). This type of foot deformity may also be described as a foot with "midfoot break." This type of deformity should be monitored until the age of 7 years, at which time it either corrects itself or becomes stable. It is often not until the adolescent growth spurt that planovalgus feet progress or become painful when walking.[58] It is also important to take note of the position of the great toe. Often, a bunion with hallux valgus will develop over time because of planovalgus feet. This is often a concern of child and their families because it is a deformity that they often are very aware of when they look down at their feet.[58]

Lower Limb-Length Discrepancy Measurement of the lower limb length should be done with the child in supine, the pelvis level in all planes, the hips in neutral rotation and abduction or adduction, and the knees fully extended. Measurements are taken from the anterior superior iliac spine to the distal aspect of the medial malleolus.

Staheli and associates[52] studied the inequality in lower limb lengths in 50 children with spastic hemiparesis. Of the 16 children who were older than 11 years of age, 70% had a significant discrepancy in limb length. Ten children had a discrepancy of 1 cm or more, and two children had

discrepancies of greater than 2 cm between the involved and uninvolved limbs.

Correction of a discrepancy in the lower limb length using a shoe lift is not advocated by some sources.[48] Children with CP, however, who have asymmetry in muscle tone, muscle activation, posture, and movement are placed at even greater risk for muscle shortening and scoliosis when a discrepancy in lower limb length exists. Such a child will try to equalize the length by ambulating with the shortened limb in plantar flexion with the heel off the floor, thus maintaining a continually shortened position of the ankle plantar flexors. When a full-length shoe lift is used to correct the discrepancy in length, the child should be observed in a standing posture for symmetry of the posterior iliac spines, anterior superior iliac spines, and the iliac crests. When the child wears an orthosis, the shoe lift thickness must take the thickness of the orthosis into account when determining the necessary thickness of the lift. Shoe lifts can be placed inside the shoe or applied to the shoe sole relatively inexpensively.

CARDIOVASCULAR/PULMONARY SYSTEM REVIEW In addition to being the result of direct trauma to the brain in the prenatal, perinatal, or neonatal periods of development, CP can be a secondary injury resulting from serious cardiovascular and/or pulmonary system abnormalities. A 2018 study revealed that 12.6% of children diagnosed with CP and a congenital anomaly have cardiac anomalies.[59] There is also a reported increase in CP diagnosis during the neonatal periods when there is evidence of respiratory distress syndrome. Furthermore, infants born with congenital heart defects who undergo surgical repair anecdotally have shown an increased tendency toward a diagnosis of CP. In 2012, the American Heart Association with the approval of the American Academy of Pediatrics issued a scientific statement acknowledging an increased incidence of developmental disorders, delays, and disabilities among neurodevelopmental outcomes for children with congenital heart defects. The most common congenital heart defects include tetralogy of Fallot, transposition of the great arteries, total anomalous pulmonary venous connections, tricuspid valve abnormalities, and truncus arteriosus. Although the data are not robust, it can be safely stated that children with congenital heart disease are at higher risk for also eventually having a diagnosis of CP.[60]

In addition to the cardiovascular and pulmonary issues related to the diagnosis of CP in some children, the therapist must also consider the overlap of system involvement for all other children and youth with CP. Respiratory involvement such as asthma, sleep apnea, and aspiration pneumonia are all common comorbidities for children and youth with CP.[61] One study of children with CP from the Australian Cerebral Palsy Register reported that 58% had cough and wheezing signs of asthma, 10% reported obstructive sleep apnea, and 40% had dysphagia with fluids that could lead to aspiration pneumonia.[62]

Cardiovascular and pulmonary fitness is another key area to consider when reviewing these systems. Although these systems are not directly affected by the neuromuscular dysfunction, the resulting decrease in functional mobility leads to secondary changes in both the cardiovascular and respiratory systems.[63] In recent years, there has been increased attention and focus on this area of rehabilitation within the CP population, particularly as it related to activity and participation levels of the ICF. By school age, many children with CP are already presenting with decreased levels of both aerobic and anaerobic fitness. These decreased levels can impact their physical activity, participation level, and the overall energy expenditure while walking. Rapid growth in adolescence tends to result in a further decline in physical activity and functional mobility.[64,65] Increased energy demands and the physical strain of activities such as walking result in accelerated fatigue and decline in walking tolerance. As a result, adolescents with CP are predisposed to increased inactivity and a decline in participation.[65] Improved levels of physical fitness can influence activity levels and decrease deconditioning and loss of mobility.[66] Lifelong participation in both aerobic and anaerobic activities is critical to improve and then maintain overall cardiopulmonary health and physical fitness.[67]

INTEGUMENTARY SYSTEM The integumentary system totals approximately 16% of an individual's total body weight, and thus cannot be ignored in the examination of the child with CP.[68] Knowledge of common skin issues in youth with CP is an important role of a physical therapist. Skin checks at the beginning and throughout a physical therapy examination is critical in determining areas of concern. The National Ulcer Advisory Panel defines pressure injuries as

> localized damage to the skin and underlying soft tissue usually over a bony prominence or related to a medical or other device. The injury can present as intact skin or an open ulcer and may be painful. The injury occurs

as a result of intense and/or prolonged pressure or pressure in combination with shear. The tolerance for soft tissue for pressure and shear may also be affected by microclimate, nutrition, perfusion, co-morbidities and condition of the soft tissue.[69]

The skin and soft tissue of the child with CP differs from that of their typically developing peers and can be impacted by the medical complexity of the child. For example, children with CP GMFCS levels III to IV have greater amounts of fat in their tissues as compared to those children with CP who are GMFCS levels I and II.[70] Skin and soft-tissue changes combined with general lack of movement in this group make them the most susceptible for skin breakdown.

There are many reasons that redness, abrasions, surgical wound dehiscence, and pressure sores can occur in children with CP. Any of these problems can result from poorly fitting UE or LE braces, poor positioning in sitting or standing systems, poor skin safety (shear forces) with bed mobility, increased pressure due to a medical device such as facemask or cast, and/or poor skin healing following surgical intervention. It has been reported that children who undergo neuromuscular spinal fusion may end up with a deep wound infection 9.3% of the time due to multiple factors including postoperative skin breakdown.[71] Furthermore, pressure sores are another important concern, especially for children of GMFCS levels IV and V. These children spend the majority of their days in their personal wheelchairs. Long periods of poor positioning in their seating system compounded with limited attention to periodic position changes can result in pressure sores in even young children with CP. It has been suggested that it is helpful to reposition more frequently than every 4 hours for children at increased risk for skin breakdown.[72,73]

Skin breakdown or irritation can happen in any region of the body and at any age. Owing to the negative health implications of an untreated wound, identifying any integumentary abnormality is paramount. All areas of concern found during the PT examination should be clearly documented, including data about color, size, and location of skin breakdown. Taking pictures of any skin issues and including them in the electronic medical record is highly recommended. In addition, it is important to take note of what may have caused the redness and address this, if within the PT scope of practice. Often, referral to other specialty care providers or other members of the child's care team is indicated. Immediately discussing areas of concern, no matter how small they may initially appear, with the child's caregivers is imperative. Caregivers should be instructed to carefully track any potential integumentary issues at least daily and attempt to identify variables at home and/or school that may be contributing factors.

Sensory Functions and Pain The clinicians' understanding of sensory functions and pain, because they influence a child's ability to successfully perform a functional and self-care task, will help shape a holistic therapeutic approach. On the basis of the ICF framework, sensory functions and pain refer to afferent stimuli carried to the brain from the peripheral nervous system.[4] The processing of this information happens cortically. Children with CP will often present either hyporesponsive or hyperresponsive to sensory stimuli. This is often a complex presentation, because it is due to the type(s), intensity, or timing of sensory stimuli. Deciphering whether the child is experiencing difficulty registering peripheral sensory stimuli or processing this information centrally is a challenge. In treatment, working through the peripheral sensory systems to improve the child's level of acceptance of specific sensory information will enhance the processing potential of central sensory systems. The sensory functions that can directly be addressed in therapy include vision, hearing, vestibular, proprioception, and touch. Pain is a prominent sensory function that often impacts children with CP and strongly influences a child's ability to complete functional tasks. This aspect of sensory function must be closely monitored throughout mobility and task performance whether it is through self-report from the child or via nonverbal communication (e.g., grimacing, vocalizations).

Cognition, Learning Style, and Communication Ability According to the ICF framework, mental functions refer to global and specific functions of the brain.[4] This considers more than just a child's level of cognition. When considering functional mobility and ADL training, it is of the utmost importance to have an understanding of the child's mental functions because they relate to the specific functional skill being addressed. The child's orientation to place, to others, and to space aids in the understanding of the environment and the functional performance in that environment. It is important to take note of the child's energy and drive functions, which include energy level, stamina, motivation, as well as impulse control. Attention functions such as sustaining attention, shifting attention, and dividing or sharing attention to a task are a necessary part of the learning process. Furthermore, memory functions including short-term (30-second duration) and long-term memory (consolidated short-term memories), as well as memory retrieval and processing, all need to be considered. Perceptual functions also play an important role in functional task performance, because these are integral to the way the child's body recognizes and perceives sensory stimuli.[4] Functional ADL training requires the child to have basic cognitive functions, which allow the child to have a fundamental understanding of objects and experiences and the ability to apply that knowledge to functional task performance. Depending on the complexity of the functional task or motor skill, higher level cognitive functions including judgment, problem solving, and cognitive flexibility will also need to be considered. If mental functions are diminished, the clinician will need to adjust the environment or treatment techniques and goals to address these deficits.

A comprehensive examination of speech and language is not within the scope of practice of the PT; however, the PT can offer important information to the speech-language pathologist (SLP) regarding the speech and language abilities and quality of respiration of the infant and child on the basis of observations made during physical therapy evaluation and treatment. A comprehensive examination of the mobility and control of the thorax is essential and will assist the SLP in attaining the outcomes established for the child. The mobility of the vertebral column and the rib cage has a great impact on the effectiveness of respiration and breath support for vocalization. It also has an impact on pulmonary hygiene, because improved rib cage mobility and deeper respirations help air to flow in the lungs. Rib cage mobility and abdominal support provide a good basis for speech control and voice quality. In obtaining information about the child's expressive communication, the PT should consider the following questions:

- Did the infant/child hear your voice or other environmental sounds as noted by becoming quiet or looking in the direction of the stimulus?
- Did the child understand questions asked during the evaluation, and did he or she follow step-by-step directional commands?
- Did the infant/child vocalize or verbalize during the assessment? What types of sounds were made? Did the infant/child repeat or stutter speech sounds?
- If the child was verbal, were the words intelligible? Was breath support adequate for speech or was the child able to speak in only one- or two-word utterances owing to poor control of respiration? Are the expressive language skills delayed for the infant/child's chronologic age?
- If the child was nonvocal, was there another means of communication used (i.e., gestures, sign language, manual language board, electronic communication system)? Did the child use eye localization, pointing, or another means within this alternate system?
- Was the infant/child's communication at a functional level?

The therapist should also ask whether the parents/caregivers or teachers have noted any problems with the child's speech or related functional areas, such as difficulty sucking, swallowing, chewing, feeding, or drinking.

These observations and questions can assist in making a referral to an SLP who will perform a more detailed assessment. As appropriate, the SLP can institute a therapeutic program that can be augmented during physical therapy sessions (Fig. 9.7).

Tests and Measures and Outcomes
The Physical Therapist Guide to Practice lists 26 categories of potential impairment, functional limitation, or participation restriction in which the therapist may consider a test or measure to collect objective data (Table 9.1).[38] Discussing potentially useful tests and measures in all these 26 categories is beyond the scope of this chapter. In this section, we focus on the most common tests, measures, and outcomes used in a

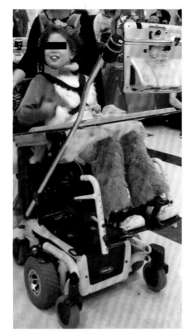

FIGURE 9.7. A 12-year-old young lady participating in her school costume parade using her communication device.

physical therapy examination, during evaluation and at discharge. Data collected with tests and measures are important not just to determine the primary impairments, functional limitation, and participation restrictions of the child but also critical in determining the intervention and progress toward

TABLE 9.1.	List of Tests and Measures (As Written in Guide to Physical Therapist Practice, 3.0)

Aerobic capacity/endurance
Anthropometric characteristics
Assistive technology
Balance
Circulation
Community, social, civic life
Cranial and peripheral nerve integrity
Education life
Environmental factors
Gait
Integumentary
Joint integrity and mobility
Mental functions
Mobility including locomotion
Motor function
Muscle performance
Neuromotor development and sensory processing
Pain
Posture
Range of motion
Reflex integrity
Self-care and domestic life
Sensory integrity
Skeletal integrity
Ventilation and respiration
Work life

goals during therapy. Consistently measuring outcomes in children with CP is a national priority.[74] Outcomes are necessary to identify what interventions, as well as dose of each intervention, are most beneficial to children with each type and severity of CP. When measuring improvements during an episode of physical therapy care, it is important to remember that change may occur in discrete components of the whole goal. Change may also not occur, because of a variety of reasons. When change does occur, it is necessary to be able to show that the change was a product of the intervention and not solely a product of growth and maturation. Adding to the complexity of choosing the most appropriate test or measure is the fact that no two children with CP present the same. Differences in physical function, distribution of involvement, social/family dynamics, comorbidities, cognitive function, surgical history, family/child's goals, age, available equipment, and many other potential variables all factor into selecting tests and measures. Taking a thorough history and having sound knowledge of available tests and measures will help guide therapists to the best tests and measures. The following section describes the clinical utility of several tests and measures/outcome tools commonly recommended when examining a child with CP. The tests and measures are organized by area of concern.

AEROBIC CAPACITY/ENDURANCE Using measurement tools that have been developed, tested, and validated for children with CP is a key component of a PT examination of cardiorespiratory function.[63,64] In the past, information has been gathered on overall physical activity levels through self-reported surveys. However, owing to the inherent limitation of self-reported surveys, the method of choice to measure physical activity is an accelerometer-based motion sensor.[75] The Step Watch, Actigraph, Body Media SenseWear, VitaMove, Uptimer, and Global Positioning System are among several technology options available to monitor and measure walking activity and physical activity in youth with CP. These accelerometers measure motion of a particular body segment or limb as it moves through space. When using a Step Watch, for example, once placed on the ankle and calibrated to the gait cycle of a child, it can be used to accurately count "steps" taken for a specific time frame. This allows the therapist to track walking and physical activity during day-to-day activities at home and school, and in community-based activities[76] (Fig. 9.8).

BALANCE In the world of CP, many terms are commonly used to describe the control of balance and posture including postural control, postural stability, static balance, dynamic balance, and dynamic stability.[77] Unfortunately, these terms often have slightly different meanings depending on the person using each term. A recent Delphi study elaborated on a consensus definition of postural control, created by clinical and research experts in postural control in children with CP, to improve communication among therapists. The group defined postural control as "control of the body's position in

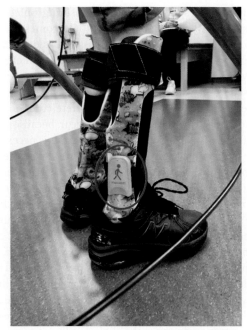

FIGURE 9.8. Step Watch, functional activity monitoring system.

space for postural orientation and postural stability."[77,78] The Delphi group further clarified that the terms *postural stability* and *balance* were "synonymous." *Balance* is also typically defined as the ability to maintain the body's center of mass over its base of support. Although the terms *balance* and *postural control* are still used interchangeably by many clinicians, it is important to understand that balance is considered a subelement of postural control.[77]

Balance has been described as the "foundation for all voluntary motor skills."[79] For humans to be functional, postural orientation and balance must be maintained in a variety of positions and through a variety of activities. Most children and youth with CP experience postural control issues throughout their lives. Even in high-functioning children with CP, falling happens frequently. Boyer and Patterson found that more than half of GMFCS level I children fall at least once per week and more than half of GMFCS level II children fall at least once per day.[80] Owing to this ongoing problem, postural control should be measured and tracked throughout childhood and into adulthood.

Postural control is influenced by complex interactions between our three sensory systems (vision, proprioception, and vestibular) and our motor system (neural control of muscles as well as muscle flexibility and strength).[81] The specific cause of each child's balance and postural orientation issues depends on the region of the brain injured as well as the resulting impairments. Postural control issues in children with CP can be broken down into impairments of one or several separate domains, including the following:

1. Musculoskeletal impairments such as decreased joint ROM and muscle strength required to maintain an upright posture

2. Sensory system impairments such as decreased vestibular, visual, or somatosensory function

3. Anticipatory balance impairments such as poor feed-forward postural adjustments required to transition from sitting to standing

4. Decreased adaptive mechanisms to perturbations resulting in loss of balance when a child's balance is pushed from behind[78]

Despite lifelong issues from one or more postural control–related impairments, postural control often improves throughout early childhood, just at a slower pace than that in typically developing peers.

There are many tools available to test postural control in children and youth with CP. Unfortunately, no test or combination of postural control tests are currently considered the "gold standard" for all children with CP. The great majority of tests that are available only measure one or a few components of postural control. Postural control tests can be very technical such as a computerized posturography or a subtest of a global gross motor evaluation such as the "balance subtest" of the Bruininks–Oseretsky Test of Motor Proficiency, second edition (BOT-2). They can also be a simple functional test such as the Timed Up & Go, or a more comprehensive assessment tool measuring multiple components of postural control such as the Kids-BESTest and the Early Clinical Assessment of Balance (ECAB).

In typically developing individuals, computerized posturography is considered the "gold standard" for balance assessment. Unfortunately, computerized posturography is not typically a good choice for children with CP. The required prolonged standing without movement does not make it feasible for many children with CP. In addition, computerized posturography requires expensive equipment that is not available in most clinics or schools. Lastly, data collected via computerized posturography has a questionable link, at best, to the functional balance of any child with CP. Developmental scale balance subtests such as the BOT-2 subtest are also often an inferior choice because they are not functional and are not responsive to small improvements in functional balance in most children with CP.

Functional postural control tests, on the other hand, appear to have the best potential to measure meaningful improvement (Table 9.2). These balance tests give the indications, pros, and cons of several simple functional tests, as well as more comprehensive postural control tests, with research supporting their use in children with CP. Unfortunately, a recent literature review concluded that there is a general lack of good methodologic studies for all balance tests.[82] One recently developed balance test, the ECAB, has been well researched.[83–85] It is a comprehensive balance test for children 12 years old and younger that addresses several dimensions of balance including head and trunk control, protective responses for sitting balance, maintaining upright posture in both sitting and standing, and making adjustments for voluntary movements in standing.[85] Besides it being valid in children with CP who are 12 and younger and having high

TABLE 9.2. Balance Tests			
Test	Indications	Pros	Cons
Pediatric Balance Scale	• GMFCS I–III • Measures static and dynamic balance in child with mild to moderate balance issues	• Most items functional • Minimal equipment • Inexpensive • Quick to administer • Reliable, valid, and responsive to change[365] • Minimal detectable change = 1.59 points (at 90% confidence interval)[365]	• Ceiling effect in higher functioning children • Requires child to be able to follow directions • No CP norms • Not appropriate for GMFCS IV–V
Early Clinical Assessment of Balance	• GMFCS I–V • Measures global balance issues including: 1. Head and trunk control 2. Protective responses in sitting 3. Maintaining upright posture in sitting and standing 4. Making adjustments for voluntary movements in standing	• Measures multiple pieces of balance • Can be used for all GMFCS levels • Quick to administer • Free form and video training available • Valid for children with CP < 5 y/o • High interrater and test–retest reliability • Standard error of measurement = 3.6 • Minimal detectable change = 10 for 2- to 8-y/o[366] • Developmental trajectories for each GMFCS available to predict changes in balance over time[367]	• Ceiling effect in higher functioning children • Requires direction following • Not researched in children older than 12
Timed Floor to Stand	• GMFCS I–III • Difficulty getting up from floor and walking	• Very quick to administer • Minimal equipment • High intrarater, interrater, and test–retest reliability • Good face validity[368] • Mean and SD determined for 5- to 14-y/o TD children	• Requires child to follow directions • No CP norms • Not appropriate for GMFCS IV–V • Not exclusively a balance test
Timed Up & Go	• GMFCS I–III • Decreased walking speed • Decreased balance with short-distance ambulation	• Very quick to administer • Valid and reliable for GMFCS I–III, 3- to 10-y/o[369] • Median, mean, and standard error of measurement for GMFCS I, II, III[370]	• No validity/reliability for 10+ y/o • Not appropriate for most GMFCS IV and V • Not exclusively a balance test • Requires child to follow directions
Segmental Assessment of Trunk Control	• Test static, active, and reactive control in sitting • Best for GMFCS III–V	• One of few sitting balance tests • Can be used with GFMCS IV–V • Excellent reliability in CP[371] • Good validity[372]	• Responsiveness to change undetermined • Strapping system required • Exclusively a sitting postural control test
Trunk Control Measurement Scale	• Measure static and dynamic trunk control in sitting at edge of mat or table with all orthoses/braces removed	• One of few sitting balance tests • Static and dynamic balance tested • Reliable and valid in children with CP 5 y/o and older[373]	• Requires child to follow directions • GMFCS I–V tested • Only sitting balance tests

CP, cerebral palsy; GMFCS, Gross Motor Function Classification System; SD, standard deviation; TD, typical development.

interrater and test–retest reliability,[83,84] the ECAB is easy to administer and one of the only balance tests that is appropriate for children of all GMFCS levels. What really separates this tool from other pediatric balance tests is its longitudinal trajectories and reference percentiles. The ECAB longitudinal trajectory curves provide valuable information to therapists and families on the balance of a child compared to average values of other children their age and GMFCS level. The published reference percentile curves can also be used to compare progress to peers with CP at the same functional level and age.[85]

MUSCLE PERFORMANCE/STRENGTH Muscle weakness is a common impairment in children and youth with CP, and often plays a major role in limiting independence in functional activities.[86] Determining the location and extent of muscle weakness in the child with CP is important because of known links between strength, walking, and gross motor function.[87–90] Options for measuring muscle strength include isokinetic testing, manual muscle testing (MMT), handheld dynamometry (HHD), and functional strength testing. Isokinetic testing, although advantageous in several ways over isometric testing, is not discussed because it is primarily being used in a research setting. MMT continues to be the most common strength measure used by pediatric therapists treating children with CP. MMT can be useful to examine general strength deficits in extremity muscle groups, but is often less helpful in tracking changes in strength over time. A recent study showed that manual muscle test scores were a very poor predictor of strength when compared to HHD.[86] This study concluded that all major muscle groups with an MMT score of 3 or higher should be tested with an HHD to record maximum voluntary contraction. When using HHD, research supports therapists performing two or more trials with each muscle group to improve reliability.[91,92] Despite low-level evidence supporting HHD use, research has not yet definitively determined its reliability in children with CP.[92]

An argument can be made that measuring strength functionally is more important in most cases when examining a child with CP. The Five-Repetition Sit-to-Stand has been well studied in children with GMFCS levels I to III.[93] Administration is quick, and it has been found to be significantly correlated with isometric LE strength, Gross Motor Function Measure (GMFM) scores, and gait function. Also, because a minimal detectable change has been calculated, therapists can easily determine whether improvement made after therapeutic intervention is significant.[93]

HHD, MMT, and functional strength tests are appropriate only for children who have the cognitive ability and motor control to perform them correctly and with maximum effort. When this is not the case, therapists must carefully observe movement within functional activities to gain basic knowledge of muscle performance (Fig. 9.9).

RANGE OF MOTION Joint ROM measurements are an important part of the physical therapy examination of a child with CP. This is due to frequent limitations found in hip extension, hip abduction, hip rotation, knee extension, ankle DF, elbow extension, and many other joint motions of the child with spastic CP.

Spasticity, muscle weakness, and general lack of movement due to decreased motor control all contribute to decreased limb movement in children and youth with CP. As a result of not being able to consistently move through a joint's full ROM, joint contracture frequently becomes a secondary impairment. With knowledge of these postural and movement consequences, the therapist must be aware of joints at risk for contracture and deformity. Goniometric joint motion and flexibility measurements of areas of high risk should be consistently documented and tracked starting in infancy to determine whether contractures are developing.

The popliteal angle, although not a measure of joint ROM, is also an important measurement, especially when making decisions regarding treatment of the child with crouched gait. The popliteal angle is used as a measure of hamstring contracture in children with CP. A large popliteal angle, measured from the vertical to the lower limb segment, is often an indicator of the need for intervention to minimize crouch gait in the child with spastic diplegic CP.

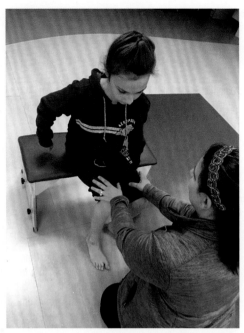

FIGURE 9.9. Five-repetition Sit-to-Stand Test for muscle performance/strength assessment for a young lady with unilateral/hemiplegic cerebral palsy (CP).

Determining the effect of interventions on ROM and hamstring contracture requires taking careful goniometric measurements. Sadly, there are few studies regarding the reliability of goniometry in children with CP,[94,95] with the results varying from poor to good reliability.[94,95] Despite its drawbacks, goniometry is still the method of choice in measuring ROM and hamstring flexibility in children with CP. It is important to note that spasticity can significantly affect the accuracy of ROM measurements. To improve accuracy when taking goniometric measurement, the child's limb should be positioned properly, and then moved slowly to limit the influence of spasticity.

MOTOR FUNCTION

Global Gross and Fine Motor Tests and Measures The GMFM is currently considered the "gold standard" for determining gross motor ability in children with CP.[96] This measure requires a therapist to observe the child with CP attempting to perform various gross motor tasks with the child's best attempt of three recorded. All the test items are scored on a 4-point scale (0–3), where 0 typically indicates not initiating the task, 1 indicates initiating the task, 2 indicates partially completing the task, and 3 indicates completion of the task. The original GMFM consisted of 88 items divided into five dimensions: (1) lying and rolling, (2) sitting, (3) crawling and kneeling, (4) standing, and (5) walking. To improve interpretability and clinical usefulness of the GMFM, the GMFM-66 was developed, consisting of 66 items from the original GMFM-88.[97] Although eliminating 22 items does cut down administration time, a computer and software download (the Gross Motor Ability Estimator-2) is required for data entry. The GMFM-66 gives a total score, standard error of measurement, and 95% confidence interval. The GMFM-66 is highly reliable and sensitive to change. In addition to the GMFM-66, two other more abbreviated versions of the GMFM were created to decrease the burden of time required to complete. The Gross Motor Function Measure—Item Sets (GMFM-IS) and the Gross Motor Function Measure—Basal and Ceiling (GMFM-B&S) typically take approximately 15 to 25 minutes to complete, and have both been found to be valid and reliable tools for children with CP.[98] Regardless of the version chosen, the GMFM is appropriate for children of all GMFCS levels.

For high-functioning children who eventually achieve perfect scores on the GMFM, other global motor function tests such as the Peabody Developmental Motor Scales–second edition (PDMS-2), Pediatric Evaluation of Disability Inventory (PEDI), Pediatric Evaluation of Disability-Computer Adaptive Test (PEDI-CAT), or BOT-2 may be appropriate to track gross motor change. Although not appropriate for all children with CP, the PEDI, PEDI-CAT, PDMS-2, and short versions of the BOT-2 have been found to be valid and reliable tests of motor function in children with CP.[99–102] Regardless of the motor function test and measure used, the therapist should ascertain the following from each motor skill observed:

1. How the particular skills are accomplished
2. The degree of assistance required
3. At what point assistance was necessary
4. Whether the child accomplishes the task using compensatory movement that will lead to structural changes and potential deformity

The Quality of Upper Extremity Skills Test (QUEST) is a widely recognized UE movement assessment for children aged 2 to 12 with CP, because it can be administered with those who have unilateral or bilateral involvement.[103] It is a 34-item criteria-referenced measure that evaluates the quality of UE function in four domains: dissociated movement, grasp, protective extension, and weight bearing.

SPASTICITY SCALES Examining a muscle's neuromotor response to passive stretch is the easiest and classic clinical approach to measuring spasticity. The Modified Ashworth Scale and the Modified Tardieu Scale are the two most common spasticity scales used as part of a physical therapy examination for children and youth with CP.[42] The Modified Ashworth Scale is a subjective ordinal scale that classifies the resistance of muscles felt during a single, quick passive stretch.[104] The Modified Tardieu Scale uses a very similar ordinal scale to measure resistance to passive stretch, but does so with a "slow as possible" passive stretch and then with a "fast as possible" stretch.[105] In addition to recording the angles measured after slow and fast stretches, the goniometric difference between the maximum angle achieved with slow stretch (R2) and the angle of first resistance with the quick stretch (R1) is documented. The clinical significance of the difference between R2 and R1 has been debated, but it is

hypothesized to represent the arc of motion in which spasticity is affected.[105] The larger the arc between R2 and R1, the more severe the spasticity. See Table 9.3 for detailed descriptions of both scales. Although both spasticity scales are frequently used by clinicians, the Modified Tardieu Scale is becoming increasingly popular because of the two different test velocities more clearly defining the velocity-dependent aspect of spasticity. Despite questionable reliability, with formal training, these spasticity measures can provide valuable information regarding the degree of spasticity in all limbs of a child with CP.[42,105] In addition, neither scale can definitely conclude the physiologic cause of an abnormal resistance to stretch. Another issue with both scales is that they only measure "passive" spasticity. Spasticity is most problematic for children with CP when attempting to move functionally. Neither the Modified Ashworth Scale nor the Modified Tardieu Scale scores are able to predict "functional" spasticity often seen during purposeful movement such as walking, reaching, or transitioning from sitting to standing. This "active" spasticity can only be subjectively described for each static and dynamic functional skill observed during the examination.

GAIT TEST AND MEASURES When evaluating the gait mechanics of a child with CP, instrumental gait analysis is the gold standard. The components of a thorough gait analysis include kinematics, kinetics, electromyographic (EMG)

TABLE 9.3. Descriptions of Modified Tardieu Scale and the Modified Ashworth Scales

Modified Tardieu Scale
Spasticity grade
0 No resistance throughout the course of the passive movement
1 Slight resistance throughout the course of the passive movement, with no clear "catch" at precise angle
2 Clear catch at precise angle, interrupting the passive movement, followed by release
3 Fatigable clonus (<10 s when maintaining pressure) occurring at precise angle
4 Infatigable clonus (>10 s when maintaining pressure) occurring at precise angle
5 Joint immovable

Modified Ashworth Scale
Spasticity grade
0 No increase in muscle tone
1 Slight increase in muscle tone, manifested by a catch and release or by minimal resistance at the end of the range of motion when the affected part(s) is moved in flexion or extension, abduction or adduction, etc.
1+ Slight increase in muscle tone, manifested by a catch and release or by minimal resistance throughout the remainder (less than half) of the range of motion when the affected part(s) is moved in flexion or extension, abduction or adduction, etc.
2 Marked increase in muscle tone, manifested by a catch in the middle range and resistance throughout the remainder of the range of motion, but affected part(s) easily moved
3 Considerable increase in muscle tone, passive movement difficult
4 Affected part(s) rigid in flexion or extension

data, measurement of videotape recordings, energy expenditure, and clinical observation.[106] A gait analysis laboratory uses cameras linked to a computer to track reflective markers placed on specific parts of a child's body as the child ambulates down the walkway. The cameras send digitized information to the computer regarding the trajectory of each marker in three dimensions. This data, when analyzed, provides kinematic information such as spatial movement of various joints of the body.[106] Force plates built into the floor of the laboratory record kinetic information such as ground-reaction forces, joint power, and joint moments as the child walks over them. The information collected from all pieces of the gait analysis is presented as graphic and numeric data. Within the gait laboratory, often there is a physical therapist, biomedical engineer, and an orthopedic surgeon who work together as a team to interpret the information generated from the gait analysis. Recommendations for surgical intervention, bracing, physical therapy, and/or referral for other testing are then made depending on the objective data gathered in the gait analysis.

Unfortunately, not every therapist has access to a state-of-the-art gait analysis laboratory, where instrumental gait analysis is performed. Therapists instead can use detailed Observational Gait Analysis (OGA) as an effective way to document many of the gait abnormalities described earlier. When first learning to evaluate gait in the child with CP, a video of the child walking is extremely helpful. The video of the child's gait should be taken from the front, back, and each side. The child should be barefoot, with shorts to allow visualization of the thigh, knee, leg, ankle, and foot. Over the past two decades, a variety of gait examination tools have been created to evaluate the gait of children with CP using video recordings. In these tests, the children walk a predetermined distance and walk at a self-selected speed.[107] The Observational Gait Scale (OGS) is a 24-item scale that assesses gait via video, addressing all three planes of movement.[107,108] The Salford Gait Tool (SF-GT) is an ordinal scale that looks at the gait of children with CP in the sagittal plane.[107,109] OGA is also an ordinal scale, with 10 items, that looks at the hip, knee, ankle, and pelvis in all three planes in both stance and swing phases of gait.[107,110] The Edinburgh Visual Gait Score (EVGS) is a video gait assessment tool that looks at 17 gait parameters of the foot, knee, pelvis, and trunk in the sagittal, frontal, and transverse planes during swing and stance phases of gait.[107,111] The Physician's Rating Scale (PRS) looks at six parameters of hip and knee movement in stance and swing phases of gait. It also scores initial foot contact, stance phase, foot contact, and timing of heel rise.[107,112] In a systematic review of these tools, it is reported that none of the tests are able to reproduce the consistency of evaluation of gait by instrument gait analysis. However, they do report their value in the clinic. The authors concluded that the OGA was a poorly designed outcome tool and is not recommended; the OGS has limited reliability, validity, and clinical use; the PRS has several versions, limited scope of gait parameter assesses, and limited reliability and validity results. The SF-GT shows good concurrent validity and reliability, but only looks

at sagittal plane deviations in gait. Finally, The EVGS looks at gait in all three planes, and also has good reliability and validity. The authors summarize that the EVGS is the most comprehensive OGS, and can be used by clinicians of all levels to evaluate gait in children with CP. They also reinforced, however, that none of the measurements are equal to the data obtained with instrumental gait analysis.[107]

MOBILITY INCLUDING LOCOMOTION Mobility tests and measures for children with CP are numerous in the literature. This makes choosing the best tool for each child challenging. This decision can be made much easier by considering the child and/or family's therapeutic goals. Common walking goals include, but are not limited to, walking faster, walking longer distances, walking with better mechanics, fall less with walking, walking with a less restrictive assistive device, walking without braces, and walking more independently at home, school, or in the community. If the goal is to fall less frequently with community walking, a self-reported outcome tool such as the Gillette Functional Assessment Questionnaire may be the best option to capture improvement in this skill.[113] If the goal is to change gait mechanics, such as improve consistent heel contact in the early stance phase of gait, the OGS or the EVGS (described in the earlier section) may be the best tools. If the child's goal is to walk more independently at home, at school, and within the community, and/or to walk more independently without an assistive device, the Functional Mobility Scale (FMS) is an excellent option to track change. The FMS measures a child's ability to walk over a 5-, 50-, and 500-m distance and the need for an assistive device (Fig. 9.10). These distances represent mobility within the home, school, and community environments. Unlike the GMFCS level that does not change significantly over time, the FMS score can change, particularly following a surgical intervention.[21]

For children with the goal of increasing mobility, speed, and/or endurance, there are several timed ambulation and wheelchair propulsion tests available to the therapist. The 6-minute walk test is the most studied of these tests. This test is a self-paced, submaximal walking test often used to measure functional exercise capacity and walking endurance. The 6-minute walk test is a reliable test for older children and adolescents with CP and GMFCS levels I and II.[114] Additional benefits of the 6-minute walk test are the developmental trajectories and reference percentiles available for children 3 to 12 years of age with GMFCS levels I to III.[115] The longitudinal developmental trajectories give therapists valuable information regarding a child's walking endurance compared to children the same age and GMFCS level. The reference percentiles allow the therapist to track the distance walked in 6 minutes over time and compare that to other peers of the same walking ability and age. Similar to GMFM scores, 6-minute walk test distances increased the most, on average, between 3 and 5 years of age. Children classified at GMFCS level II progress their walking distance over the longest time, and many did not plateau even at 12 years of age.[115] Short-distance ambulation and short-timed tests are more appropriate

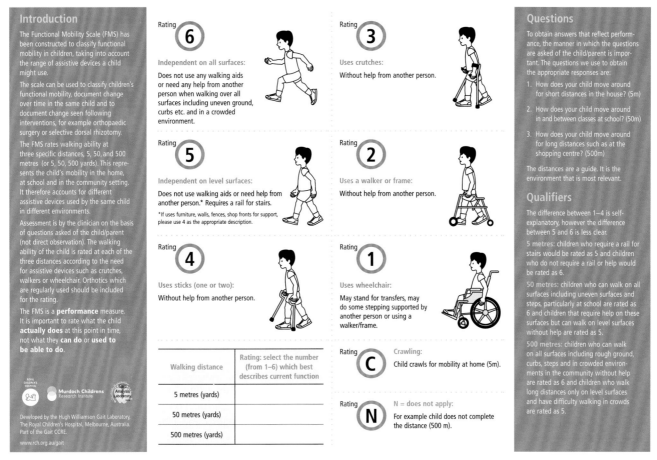

FIGURE 9.10. The Functional Mobility Scale (FMS).

to measure changes in walking speed with therapeutic intervention. The 10-m walk test and 1-minute walk test are both reliable, appropriate options for children with CP.[114,116] For children with CP at GMFCS levels II to IV who use a manual wheelchair as the primary means of mobility, the 6-minute Push Test is a great option to measure submaximal exercise tolerance and functional wheelchair propulsion endurance. In addition to having excellent reliability, the mean distance traveled and standard deviations have been separately calculated for GMFCS levels II, III, and IV.[117]

PAIN An evolving understanding of pediatric pain has focused attention on measurement properties, interpretability, and generalizability of pain intensity measures for children and adolescents.[118] Self-report pain scales include, but are not limited to, the 11-point Numeric Rating Scale (NRS-11), Color Analog Scale (CAS), Faces Pain Scale–revised (FPS-R), and Wong-Baker FACES Pain Rating Scale (FACES). Each relies on the child's expressive communication and cognitive abilities to report pain levels. For those with CP, wide variability of motor and cognitive abilities exist, potentially making self-report challenging. In this case, care providers' ratings are often used in combination with self-report, or specialized pain scales designed for children with cognitive impairments are utilized. Behavioral pain assessment scales including, but not limited to, Face, Legs, Activity, Cry, Consolability Scale

(FLACC), Noncommunicating Children's Pain Checklist–Postoperative Version (NCCPC-PV) and Children's Hospital of Eastern Ontario Pain Scale (CHEOPS) rely on caregiver report to measure intensity of pain.[119,120] The treating therapist must clearly document the child's intensity of pain related to evaluation and intervention and make clear distinctions about onset and resolution of pain.

SELF-CARE AND DOMESTIC LIFE Examination of the self-care skills for the child and youth with CP is traditionally one of the main areas of concern for the occupational therapist (OT). The PT should have the basic knowledge to examine self-care and fine motor and play skills, and make referrals to other specialists as needed. A child following a more typical continuum of self-care skill development will hold a bottle with one or both hands at 4.5 to 6 months of age, finger-feed many soft foods at 9 months, pull off his or her socks while seated at approximately 12 months, will hold out arm and push arm through sleeve at 12 months, will bring filled spoon to mouth (messily) at 12 to 14 months, will attempt to put socks on at 24 to 28 months, and will remove unfastened garment at 24 months. It is not until 3.5 to 4 years of age that a child will begin to button large buttons on a coat, zip a coat, or attempt to tie shoes. Play skill development is important to understand, because this skill set provides the basis on which more refined fine motor and bimanual hand skills are developed. A child following a more typical continuum of fine motor and play skill development will clap at approximately 7 to 9 months, place toy into open container without support of container's surface at 7 to 8 months, poke an object with index finger at 9 to 10 months, point to object at 11 to 12 months, and demonstrate a fine pincer grasp (small object held between tip of thumb and tip of index finger) at 11 to 12 months of age.[121] The developmental continuum is not a rigid process, and is influenced by many factors; therefore, children may master certain skills earlier or later than stated.

Information obtained from parents, caregivers, or teachers may alert the therapist to the need for intervention related to the child's functional abilities during feeding, dressing, toileting, bathing, and prehensile and manipulation skills for play and school function. Direct clinical observation of a child's performance of basic self-care skills, including removing and replacing socks, shoes, and coat, can be very informative of a child's level of independence in these areas. As the child moves to perform these tasks, the therapist can evaluate sitting balance, mobility and control of head and trunk, weight shifting through pelvis, and use and mobility of the arms.

A 2011 study conducted by Chen et al. examined quality of life in ambulatory children with CP. This study determined that fine motor functions, including dexterity and visual motor control, "were the most important motor factors associated with health-related quality-of-life" issues.[122] When gathering information about quality of life for children and youth with CP, it is most often done through self-reported or parent-reported surveys. Health-related quality of life (HRQOL) measures focus on gathering information about physical, mental, emotional, and social well-being. They can be used to measure change over time or determine the effects of specific interventions. One of the primary goals of treatment and management of children and youth with CP should focus on improving HRQOL. Owing to the heterogeneous nature of CP, there is no gold standard tool for measuring HRQOL in children with CP. There are a few HRQOL measures that have been validated for children with CP, including the Cerebral Palsy Quality of Life Questionnaire (CP-QOL-Child and CP-QOL-Teen),[123] Caregivers Priorities and Child Health Index of Life and Disabilities (CPCHILD),[124] Pediatric Quality of Life Inventory 3.0 Cerebral Palsy Module (PedsQL-CP),[125] and the DISABKIDS[126] (Fig. 9.11).

» Physical therapy evaluation, diagnosis, and prognosis

Within the physical therapy evaluation, the therapist synthesizes the information gathered during the examination. The therapist takes into consideration medical history, review of systems, and tests and measures. The primary impairments, functional deficits, and activity and participation goals are then used to create a PT diagnosis and design an appropriate plan of care. Determining a physical therapy "prognosis" can be a challenge owing to the complexity of a child with CP. Reviewing the evidence regarding the typical development

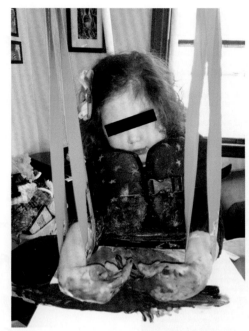

FIGURE 9.11. External upper extremity (UE) support system to paint a picture.

of gross motor function of children with differing severities of CP is often helpful. Following the development of the GMFCS, Rosenbaum and Hanna and colleagues developed predictive gross motor function curves for children at each GMFCS level. A curve showing typical gross motor function progression as children aged was developed for each GMFCS level. These curves aid physicians and therapists in predicting gross motor changes in children with CP as they age.[127] They are also helpful tools to educate parents on the likely gross motor progression their child may make with growth and typical therapeutic/medical interventions. These assist the therapist, child, and parents in establishing realistic and achievable motor goals. The curves show that most children with CP, regardless of their GMFCS level, will near or reach a plateau in gross motor function between 5 and 7 years of age. Higher functioning children (GMFCS I–III), on average, will continue to progress in motor skills longer than do lower functioning (GMFCS IV–V) children. After reaching a plateau, the curves are shown to remain constant up to 12 years of age for all GMFCS levels.[127] More recently, Hanna and colleagues looked more closely at the gross motor function during adolescence and early adulthood to determine whether gross motor function would remain the same or decline.[128] Adolescence is a critical time of transition, because bodies rapidly grow and mature. As a result of rapid growth, children are at a higher risk for developing secondary complications such as joint contractures or muscle stiffness. Hanna's study confirmed what many therapists already knew, that children with lower functional abilities (GMFCS levels III, IV, and V) are at risk for decreased motor capabilities as they progress toward young adulthood (Fig. 9.12)

These levels showed a slight, but consistent, trend toward a decline in gross motor function during adolescence.[128]

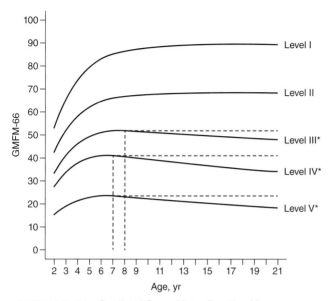

FIGURE 9.12. Predicted Gross Motor Function Measure (GMFM) scores as a function of age by Gross Motor Function Classification System (GMFCS) level. *GMFCS levels with significant average peak and decline. Dashed lines illustrate age and score at peak GMFM66. (Taken from Hanna S, Rosenbaum P, Bartlett D, et al. Stability and decline in gross motor function among children and youth with cerebral palsy aged 2 to 21 years. *Dev Med Child Neurol.* 2009;51(4):Figure 1.)

It should be noted that there was a wide variation in skill achievement and decline recorded among children in these studies. Therefore, absolute statements about gross motor prognosis based on the Rosenbaum and Hanna curves should be made cautiously. Although the curves can provide general prognostic information for gross motor development in children with CP, children may experience positive or negative changes in gross motor function throughout childhood and adolescence. Decreased function may occur due to medical issues such as illness, uncontrolled seizures, obesity, or injury, to name a few. Increased function, slightly above expectations, may be possible with evidence-based therapeutic, neuromedical (such as baclofen pump insertion), and/or surgical intervention. In addition, many children are in the "gray area" between GMFCS levels and may achieve gross motor skills more commonly seen at the next highest level. Rosenbaum and colleagues believed that a leveling off in gross motor function by no means suggests that further therapeutic intervention would be unnecessary or unhelpful. In fact, Hanna's study suggests that continuing to be active and focusing on maintaining function in adolescence is of utmost importance to prevent loss of function in adulthood.[128] From clinical experience, most children at GMFCS levels III, IV, and V are not destined to decline in motor function as they age as long as they receive appropriate care and guidance. Emphasis on function and participation in an environment that is supportive and meaningful to them has been shown to help children and youth with CP maintain functional mobility.[88,128]

» Goal development

When writing specific, measurable, achievable, realistic, relevant, and timed goals (SMART),[129] it is important to consider all factors that shape a child's experience. Therapeutic goals are best defined in collaboration with the family, child, and clinician. The Goal Attainment Scale (GAS) also utilizes these principles, and has recently been used to monitor therapy changes over time and to evaluate the effectiveness of treatment plans and services. Specific information about the child's goals, parents' goals, and vision for the child's functional skill development can be gathered during an initial parent–child interview. When considering a formal goal-setting process, recent studies have shown that there is greater change in self-care and mobility activities when the children and their families are involved in the goal-setting process as compared to therapy carried out without a specific goal.[130] It is not an understatement to suggest a child and family's level of investment in the therapy process starts when a clinician invites them to define what is most important to them at the start of a plan of care.

Gait

One of the questions most frequently asked by parents and caregivers on being told their child has CP is "When will my child walk?" Walking is one of the most complex human functions, making this prediction very difficult in young children with CP. As per Beckung et al.'s[131] review of 10,000 children with CP in Europe, 54% of children with CP walk without an assistive device, 16% walk with an assistive device, and 30% were nonambulatory. The GMFCS is also helpful to estimate future ambulation potential in children with CP. The GMFCS is a reliable and valid system that classifies children with CP by their age-specific gross motor activity.[132] The GMFCS describes the major functional characteristics of children younger than 2 years old, 2 to 4 years old, 4 to 6 years old, and between 6 and 12 years old with CP within each level. Rosenbaum et al.[132] used the GMFCS to assist clinicians and caregivers in looking at the infant/child and make predictions for functional mobility on the basis of the findings of the GMFCS. They plotted the patterns of motor development on the basis of longitudinal observations of 657 children with CP and felt that the findings would help parents understand the outlook for their child's gross motor function based on age and the GMFCS level.[132] This may be a more accurate way of predicting future ambulation skills than were previously used means such as tracking motor skill acquisitions like sitting independently by 2 years of age.[133]

It is extremely helpful to understand typical gait and how the impairments in the child with CP influence his or her ability to ambulate. The prerequisites of normal gait in the order of priority are (1) stable lower limb in stance phase, (2) clearance of ground by foot in swing phase, (3) proper positioning of the foot in DF in terminal swing, (4) adequate step length, and (5) maximal energy conservation.[106,134] Damage to the CNS causes loss of selective motor control, abnormal muscle tone, imbalance between muscle agonist and antagonist, and poor equilibrium reactions. As a consequence, many or all of these prerequisites of normal gait are absent in children with CP[106] (Fig. 9.13).

It is best to observe one region of the body at a time through several gait cycles before moving up to the next region. First, observe the foot position at initial contact. Is there heel strike, flat foot, or forefoot contact? When the foot is in midstance, are the toes pointing out or in (referred to as *internal* or *external foot progression angle*)? Identify foot alignment at push-off (varus or valgus position) when observing from the front and laterally. Consider the knee/thigh region, and observe the child laterally for degree of knee flexion and extension during swing phase and knee angle/stability during stance phase. Does the knee flex excessively or hyperextend during stance phase? Does the knee flex enough during swing to prevent toe drag? Observe from the front for knee position during swing and stance phases. Is the knee in valgus during swing and stance phases? Do the medial aspects of the knees touch? Observe the hips from the side, note the amount of hip flexion during late swing, and hip extension at push-off. Does the child achieve hip extension during late stance or stay in flexion? Does the child hyperflex or abduct at the hip during swing? When observing the pelvis and spine, focus on pelvic tilt, pelvic rotation, lordosis, and trunk alignment during all phases of gait. Is there excessive anterior pelvic tilt with increased lumbar lordosis throughout the gait cycle? Does the child have to excessively rotate his or her pelvis and trunk to assist swing of the lower limb? Does the child elevate the pelvis to prevent the toe from dragging? Lastly, observe the head, arms, and trunk (often referred to as the *HAT segment*). Does the head and trunk laterally flex to one side when swinging with the opposite side? Do the arms swing normally or remain in a fixed posture? Once the observation of each region is completed, watch the body move as a whole without focusing on a particular region to identify other important gait characteristics such as speed, fluidity of movement, stride length, and stride width.

Common Gait Deviations

When discussing gait and gait deviations, it is helpful to understand the link between the primary gait problems and their underlying etiology. Table 9.4 lists the most common gait deviations seen in children with CP and the primary causes of these deviations. Gait deviations in children with CP typically have four main causes: (1) those caused by weakness, (2) those caused by abnormal bony alignment, (3) those caused by muscle contracture, and (4) those caused by muscle spasticity.[55,135] Owing to the overactive stretch response of key walking muscles, spasticity in these muscles can inhibit motion by firing prematurely, resulting in prolonged and inappropriate muscle action.[135] As ambulatory children with CP grow and mature, the abnormal tone and underlying muscle weakness cause skeletal changes that result in abnormal alignment and joint contracture. Because most children with CP have both spasticity and weakness in more than one muscle, they typically have multiple gait abnormalities.

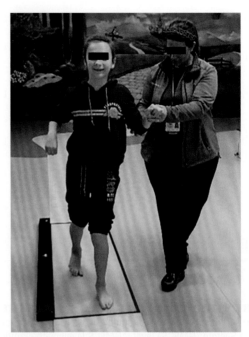

FIGURE 9.13. Foot pressure mapping in the gait analysis laboratory.

There are several classic gait patterns that are characteristic of the different types of CP. These classic gait patterns are described in the following section.

Hemiplegic/Unilateral Gait

Almost all children with hemiplegic-pattern CP will walk, and the great majority of them will be functional ambulators. In fact, most are independent ambulators without an assistive device by 15 to 24 months.[136] Severe cases of hemiplegic-type CP with involved side abnormalities above the knee and mild increased tone and/or muscle weakness of the "uninvolved" side may not ambulate until almost 3 years of age.[10] Beckung et al.[131] found that only 3% of children with hemiplegic CP are not walking by 5 years of age. Severe intellectual impairment was found to be the greatest predictor of not being able to walk by age 5, increasing the risk by 56-fold.[131] Before the age of 2, the majority of children with hemiplegic-pattern CP either toe-walk bilaterally or ambulate with a foot-flat, planovalgus gait pattern.[10] Gastrocnemius spasticity is the primary neuromuscular impairment in both these children, and as contracture develops over time, almost all children with hemiplegic CP will walk on their toes without orthotic intervention.[10] Over time, overactivity of the tibialis anterior and posterior will also often cause the foot to turn inward into equinovarus position. When observing a child with hemiplegic CP walking, asymmetrical weight shift to the involved side is the most obvious feature typically noted. Throughout the gait cycle, the involved UE is often positioned in scapular retraction and the pelvis is rotated posteriorly, when compared with the shoulder and the pelvis on the contralateral side. Arm swing also typically occurs only on the uninvolved side, with the involved UE held in shoulder hyperextension and elbow flexion.

TABLE 9.4.	Gait Deviations and Their Underlying Causes	

Location/Problem	Primary Cause(s)
Pelvis	
Anterior pelvic tilt	Hip flexion contracture/hip extensor weakness
Increased rotation	Decreased push-off from gastrocnemius (gastroc), hip stiffness, hip flexor weakness
Drop of pelvis on swing side	Hip abductor weakness
Hip	
Decreased flexion	Hamstring (HS) or gluteus muscle contractors
	Weak plantar flexors during push-off
	Weak hip flexors
Decreased extension (stance)	Hip flexor contracture; knee flexion contracture
Increased abduction	Weak adductor muscle; abductor contracture
Increased adduction	Adductor contracture/increased tone
Increased internal rotation	Femoral anteversion; increased tone and/or contracture of internal rotators; compensation for external tibial rotation
Increased external rotation	Retroversion of femur; increased tone or contracture of external rotators; compensation for internal tibial torsion
Knee	
Increased flexion at initial contact	Knee flexion contracture; HS tone; toe strike due to plantar flexor tone
Decreased flexion at initial contact	Weak HSs; weak quadriceps
Genu recurvatum in midstance	Increased gastroc tone; weak gastroc; weak HSs
Crouch (stance hip and knee flexion)	Knee joint contracture; HS contracture; hip flexor contracture; poor balance; severe planovalgus feet; ankle equinus
Stiff knee gait	Increased rectus femoris tone; knee stiffness quadriceps contracture; poor push-off from gastroc
Jump knee (knee flex in early stance)	Overactivity of HS
Foot	
Equinus at initial contact	Gastroc/soleus contracture; gastroc overactivity; weak dorsiflexors
Decreased push-off power	Weak gastroc/soleus; severe planovalgus feet
In-toeing (internal foot progression)	Internal tibial torsion; varus feet
Out-toeing (external foot progression)	External tibial torsion; severe muscle weakness; poor balance

Adapted from Miller F. Gait analysis interpretation in cerebral palsy gait: developing a treatment plan. In: Miller F, Bachrach S, Lennon N, O'Neil M, eds. *Cerebral Palsy*. Springer; 2018:1-15. https://doi.org/10.1007/978-3-319-50592-3_96-1

LE gait deviations can vary greatly between those with spastic hemiplegia, but four distinct patterns of gait in children have been described by Winters et al.[137] Type 1, the least involved group, presents with drop foot in swing phase of gait, but has normal DF passive range of motion (PROM). This group also has increased knee flexion at terminal swing, initial contact, and loading response. Hyperflexion of hip during swing and increased lordosis are other compensations commonly seen in this group. Treatment for this group typically includes leaf spring or articulating ankle–foot orthosis (AFO) and tibialis anterior strengthening on the involved side. Type 2, the most common subtype, is significant for plantar flexion throughout the gait cycle, full extension or recurvatum of the knee in stance phase, as well as hyperflexion of the hip and increased lumbar lordosis. Contracture of the triceps surae muscle prevents the tibia from moving forward on the foot during stance phase, resulting in knee extension or hyperextension in middle and terminal stance phase. As a result, advancement of the trunk is limited; therefore, to maintain

the center of gravity (COG) over the foot, the child must hyperflex the hip and extend the lumbar spine. Early treatment for these gait deviations may include gastrocnemius stretching, hinged AFOs with an appropriate plantar flexion stop to prevent genu recurvatum, and botulinum toxin type A (BTX-A) injections into the gastrocnemius.[138] If an Achilles tendon contracture develops preventing proper AFO fit, Achilles tendon lengthening in early grade school, with or without articulating AFO use afterward, is the typical treatment for this situation.[10,138] Types 1 and 2 typically have slight LLDs of 1 to 2 cm. This asymmetry should not be corrected with a shoe lift because this will likely cause problems with toe clearance during involved side swing phase.[10]

In addition to the abovementioned gait deviations, type 3 has decreased knee motion, especially during swing phase, due to quadriceps/hamstring co-contraction. Treatment for type 3 gait dysfunction is similar to that for type 2, with the addition of aggressive hamstring stretching, BTX, or muscle lengthening to overactive/contracted hamstring tendons. Type 4, the most involved group, has additional restricted motion of the hip due to hyperactivity of the iliopsoas and hip adductors. This prevents full hip extension at terminal stance phase.[137] It is not uncommon for children in this group to undergo two to three gastrocnemius and hamstring muscle lengthening procedures owing to more significantly increased muscle tone and contractures. These children often develop significant femoral anteversion, requiring a derotation osteotomy. It should also be noted that type 4 children usually have significant LLDs that may require a shoe lift.[10] In addition to Winter et al.'s[137] findings, a more recent analysis of CP gait determined that the most common gait abnormalities found in children with hemiplegic gait include equinus (64%), stiff knee (56%), in-toeing (54%), excessive hip flexion (48%), and crouch (47%).[139]

Diplegic/Bilateral Gait

Similar to the children with hemiplegic-pattern CP, the gait pattern of a child with diplegia can vary greatly depending on the degree of severity of involvement. Generally, children with spastic diplegic pattern CP ambulate at about half the speed of children without CP.[140] Unlike hemiplegia, there are few children with diplegic CP with only ankle involvement. The great majority of children with diplegic CP have some hip, knee, and ankle involvement. Despite this increased level of involvement, most children with diplegic CP do walk independently, although more severely involved children with diplegic CP require molded ankle–foot orthoses (MAFOs) and an assistive device such as forearm crutches or posterior walker to ambulate.

Bony deformities of the long bones of the lower leg and feet are common in children with diplegic CP.[138] Because LE muscles work best when all the bones are in the line of gait progression, muscle effectiveness is reduced when bony malalignment occurs. This dysfunction is often referred to as *lever arm disease.*[138]

A common combination of bone deformities in children with diplegic CP that results in lever arm disease is internal femoral rotation (anteversion), lateral tibial torsion, and midfoot collapse.[138] Because these bony deformities progress together, the already weak gluteus medius becomes even less effective in controlling hip internal rotation, and the plantar flexors have limited ability to control the progression of the tibia over the foot in stance phase. This causes the hips to internally rotate further and the ankle to drop into excessive DF in the stance phase as well as increased knee and hip flexion. As a result, the foot drops into a more planovalgus position, which is the most common foot deformity seen in children with diplegic CP.

Similar to hemiplegic CP, there are several common gait patterns seen in the child with diplegic CP. The most common gait deviations include stiff knee (88%), crouch (74%), excessive hip flexion (66%), in-toeing (66%), and equinus (58%).[139] A description of several common gait deviations in this group are described in the next section.

EQUINUS When the child with diplegic CP begins to walk, gastrocnemius spasticity commonly causes an equinus gait pattern, with the ankle in plantar flexion throughout the stance phase with hips and knees extended. Sometimes the child may hyperextend his or her knees to get the heels on the ground, which hides the equinus. BTX-A is often used to decrease spasticity in the gastrocnemius muscle in these children to improve stability in stance. Solid or hinged AFOs are the orthotic management of choice for this population.[138]

PLANOVALGUS Planovalgus is characterized as equinus of the hindfoot and pronation of the forefoot and midfoot.[141] Planovalgus is primarily caused by plantar flexor muscle weakness, including the tibialis posterior and exacerbated by the "lever arm disease" described earlier. Planovalgus malalignment maintains the midfoot and forefoot in an "unlocked" position, decreasing stability in midstance. This often results in excessive loading of the plantar, medial portion of the foot. The force-generating capacity of the already weak tibialis anterior and triceps surae is decreased further by the malalignment of the midfoot and forefoot segments. This muscular dysfunction causes the foot to drop into a greater planovalgus position during mid- and late stance and makes effective push-off impossible. Hallux valgus, hindfoot valgus, and external tibial torsion are frequently associated with planovalgus deformity. Planovalgus is also often seen with a crouched gait, which is described here.

CROUCH A crouched gait pattern, with knees and hips flexed throughout the gait pattern, is sometimes seen after growth spurts in the child with diplegic CP.[10] Because the muscles of children with CP are weakest in the shortened range, maintaining normal DF, hip extension, and knee extension in standing and with ambulation becomes increasingly difficult as children gain weight. Generally, this crouched pattern is secondary to overactive hamstrings in stance phase, quadriceps weakness, and triceps surae weakness.[135] In gait, the plantar flexors are of critical importance in maintaining knee extension. During normal gait, the soleus is the only muscle that is active in midstance to control knee extension.[10,134] Because the stance limb is in a closed-kinetic chain, the eccentric activity of the plantar flexors restricts ankle DF, maintaining knee extension through a plantar flexion/ knee extension couple.[134] Plantar flexor weakness limits the effectiveness of this normal mechanism, allowing the limb to sink into crouch. Plantar flexor control of knee extension is further limited by lever arm disease and stance instability created by planovalgus foot deformity. Increased knee flexion throughout stance phase results in excessive demand on an already weak quadriceps muscle. This causes slow progressive stretching of the quadriceps tendon, resulting in patella alta and later patellofemoral syndrome. This progressive quadriceps dysfunction is a vicious cycle, leading to further crouch. Eventually, this will cause hamstring and hip flexor contractures. Decreased knee extension and decreased stride length results in decreased walking velocity.[135] Aggressive hamstring stretching, quadriceps strengthening, and/or modification of bracing (solid AFO or ground-reaction ankle–foot orthosis [GRAFO] to assist the plantar flexors in controlling DF) is indicated with this gait pattern; but often, hamstring lengthening is indicated when contractures develop, to improve knee extension at initial contact. Midstance knee flexion of less than 20 degrees is ideal with increased concern as the angle approaches 30 degrees. After 30 degrees of crouch, a weak, overstretched soleus, tight hamstrings, and quickly fatiguing quadriceps make functional ambulation very difficult. During adolescence, weight gain and rapid increase in height can further contribute to increased crouch. Consistent monitoring of hamstring flexibility, weight, strength, and passive knee extension during this period of growth is necessary to prevent rapid worsening of crouch and subsequent impairments/functional limitations.

JUMP KNEE The jump knee is another gait deviation commonly seen in children with spastic diplegia, with more proximal involvement causing spasticity in the hip flexors, hamstrings, and gastrocnemius.[138] This child presents with anterior pelvic tilt, hip flexion, knee flexion, and ankle equinus.[138] Overactivity of the hamstring muscles produces increased knee flexion in late swing and early stance phases. This child then appears to "jump" owing to a strong quadriceps contraction during late stance phase.[142] The ankle does not progress into greater DF through stance phase as it does in "crouched" gait, also adding to the appearance of a "jump" during the stance phase. Children with this type of gait pattern often require BTX-A injections to the gastrocnemius and hamstring muscles. Orthotic management for children with this gait deviation varies from solid AFOs, hinged AFOs, or GRAFOs, depending on the severity of spasticity/weakness in thigh and ankle muscles.[138]

STIFF KNEE Stiff knee gait is characterized by increased knee extension throughout the swing phase, often owing to overactivity of the rectus femoris.[135] Knee flexion in swing is necessary in normal gait to shorten the swing leg and thus allow the foot to swing through without the toes hitting the floor. Decreased knee flexion thus causes a problem with clearing the swing leg foot. This forces the child to compensate with hip circumduction, vaulting (contralateral plantar flexion and/or abduction in swing phase), posterior pelvic tilt, and/or pelvic external rotation to prevent toe drag.[135] Other causes of decreased knee flexion in swing include slow overall walking speed and lack of swing limb momentum due to hip flexor weakness or poor push-off (Fig. 9.14).

RECURVATUM Recurvatum gait is described as knee extension in early stance progressing to hyperextension in mid- and late stance phases of gait. The most common cause of equinus is overactivity and/or contracture of the gastrocnemius. Increased spasticity of the gastrocnemius causes the ankle to be in equinus at initial contact and remain in plantar flexion throughout the stance phase. This creates an early

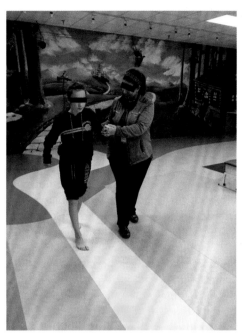

FIGURE 9.14. Gait training with an adolescent with cerebral palsy (CP) Gross Motor Function Classification System (GMFCS) level II with dystonic unilateral/hemiplegia.

knee extension movement, causing the knee to be forced into extension. Gastrocnemius weakness and iliopsoas tightness are also possible causes or contributing factors to knee recurvatum.[10] Repeated stress on the posterior structures of the knee leads to stretching of posterior musculature and, eventually, the posterior capsule of the knee. This can cause chronic, debilitating knee pain in adolescence. Besides the potential for affecting posterior stability of the knee, recurvatum disrupts forward momentum during ambulation, making gait less efficient.[10] Switching to a solid MAFO in children with weak gastrocnemius or increasing the DF angle of a solid or articulating MAFO to 3 to 5 degrees are common changes that often improve back-kneeing.[10]

IDIOPATHIC TOE-WALKING VERSUS MILD DIPLEGIC CEREBRAL PALSY There can be concern and confusion regarding the differentiation between idiopathic toe-walking and spastic diplegic CP. Toe-walking as a toddler is considered a normal variant for new walkers, but is considered abnormal and is classified as idiopathic toe-walking if it persists beyond the first few years of ambulation. Idiopathic toe-walkers typically have normal strength, normal tone, and selective motor control, but still prefer to walk on their toes.[143] Developmental history and physical examination are often helpful in differentiating between idiopathic toe-walking and CP, but are not always sufficient. On physical examination, idiopathic toe-walkers typically have only mild gastrocnemius tightness and no hamstring tightness.[143,144] Hicks et al.[144] found that idiopathic toe-walkers typically have increased knee extension in stance and increased external rotation of the foot with increased plantar flexion. Conversely, they found that children with CP had sustained knee flexion at terminal stance and initial contact.[144] Kelly et al. also showed a difference between the two groups, with idiopathic toe-walkers having initial motion into DF followed by sudden plantar flexion midway through the swing phase, causing the foot to land in equinus. It should also be noted that many idiopathic toe-walkers are able to walk with more "normal" gait mechanics when instructed to do so.[145]

Quadriplegic Gait

Most children with quadriplegic CP are not community ambulators, but many do have some ability to ambulate with an assistive device at home or in a therapeutic setting. Many of these children use a gait trainer in early childhood and then transition to a walker with forearm supports years later. The most common gait deviations seen in this type of CP include stiff knee (93%), crouch (88%), excessive hip flexion (78%), in-toeing (70%), equinus (68%), and excessive hip adduction/scissoring (63%).[10] In adolescence, some of these children lose their ability to ambulate secondary to weight gain and/or growth spurt. Even though functional community ambulation throughout life is not a realistic goal for children with this type of CP, encouraging ambulation is very important. Discussion with the child and family regarding the role of walking is critical early in the therapy process so that the family has time to accept that power mobility will be the best long-term means of mobility from the early school years through the rest of the child's life. Hip subluxation, hip muscle weakness, and osteopenia are all common impairments that can be reduced to some degree with ambulation. Some progress with ambulation can occur up to 12 or 13 years of age in these children.[10] If the child with quadriplegic CP is still using a gait trainer for ambulation at this age, he or she will likely not progress to a posterior walker in adulthood. Discontinuing gait training before adolescence is not recommended, because this training will help children maintain the ability to weight bear with transfers throughout their life. Severe equinovalgus feet, hamstring contractures, hip adductor contractures, hip flexion contractures, and fixed knee flexion contractures are common impairments that limit ambulation in middle childhood and adolescence.[10] Often, these impairments require surgical intervention to prevent the loss of years of ambulation gains. In adulthood, these children should be able to maintain the ambulatory ability they have gained throughout childhood.

Athetotic Gait

The "typical" gait in a child with athetosis is very difficult to describe and even more difficult to address. Athetotic movements are usually first noticed at 2 to 3 years of age. By 3 to 5 years of age, the athetotic pattern is consistent and changes little.[10] Children with milder cases of athetosis have underlying low postural tone that fluctuates to high levels of stiffness. The gait pattern in the LEs is poorly graded and in total patterns of movement. The LE is usually lifted high into flexion and placed down in stance into extension with adduction, internal rotation, and plantar flexion. The hips stay slightly flexed, the lumbar spine is hyperextended, and the thoracic spine is excessively rounded with capital hyperextension, flexion, and rotation of the cervical spine, with the jaw jutting forward and rotated to one side. Orthopedic and physical therapy treatments usually have little effect on athetotic movements. Weighted vests and ankle weights are sometimes helpful in improving balance in this group of children.

Ataxic Gait

The most common features of ataxic gait include general unsteadiness, widened base, irregularity of steps with interjoint incoordination, prolonged stance duration, increased double-limb support duration, slow speed, and large body sways.[146] All gait measurements are highly variable in cerebellar ataxia. Improving gait with physical therapy is not well supported in the literature, but repeated motor training, taping, or light-weighting of the limbs might have some benefit.[146] With this type of gait and owing to profound instability, maintaining balance takes priority over propulsive locomotion that causes several common gait deviations.

» Therapeutic interventions

Multiple factors often come into play when determining the optimal treatment approaches or techniques for working with children with CP. The severity of the child's impairments, the identified functional limitations, and the child and family's goals all influence the design of an effective treatment plan. With the child's goals identified, the PT must analyze the function or task that is desired and carefully choose interventions that will address the impairments that are impeding the child's goal achievement. Answers to the following questions should assist the therapist in selecting and sequencing the appropriate treatment strategies:

- What strengths/competencies does the child possess that will provide a foundation upon which to build toward the functional outcome?
- Which impairments and posture and movement behaviors interfere with the successful completion of the functional outcome?
- How should these impairments be prioritized with regard to the functional outcome?
- What treatment strategies can be utilized to address each of the prioritized impairments?
- In what order must the treatment strategies be sequenced to be most successful?
- What dose of each treatment strategy is best for the child to achieve each functional outcome?

Children with CP face a lifetime of functional challenges that can be ameliorated intermittently with physical therapy. The nervous system of the infant and child with CP is impaired, and the expression of typical motor patterns and skills should not be expected. Therapists should be clear on the purpose and anticipated outcomes of the provision of physical therapy and reinforce that understanding to the parents and caregivers, repeatedly. In general, physical therapy is provided to facilitate the child with CP to become the most independent in performing functional tasks throughout his or her lifetime. The provision of physical therapy should change in frequency and duration as the infant or child grows and develops, with periods of time when the child does not receive formal physical therapy intervention. Therefore, it is paramount that the family and health care providers understand the episodic nature of the provision on physical therapy over the child's lifespan. There will be critical times for formal therapy, times for adjunctive therapies, and times when an independent home or community programs will be adequate to address the current needs of the child.

A question commonly asked by both clinician and parents of children with CP is, "How much therapy is enough?" Recent research highlights the complexity of clinical decision making when determining appropriate and effective plans of care. Studies of clinical effectiveness rely on outcomes that are both quantitative and qualitative. The concept of *dosing* creates a framework in which therapists are challenged to consider the number of sessions, the type of intervention, how strenuous is the activity during each session, and how long the intervention will last when creating a plan of care. A Research Summit was held in 2014 to review the research and discuss dosing options for children with CP. The Research Summit III (Dosing and Motor Learning for Children with an Injured Brain or Cerebral Palsy) was sponsored by the American Physical Therapy Association (APTA) Section on Pediatrics, the National Institutes of Health's Eunice Kennedy Shriver National Institute of Child Health and Human Development (NICHD), and the National Institute of Neurological Disorders and Stroke (NINDS). Participants of the meeting were therapists and academic researchers in the field of pediatrics. The intent of the Summit was to take an interdisciplinary approach to dose-related research for children with CP. The outcome of the Summit was to outline areas of intervention that need further research on clinical effectiveness before dose-related studies can be done. Those involved in the Summit also agreed that the best treatment protocols for children with CP are yet to be determined on the basis of the amount of current research. In summary, dosing decisions are a complex matter and need to involve the family, physician, and therapist.[74]

Currently, there is a national focus on clinical effectiveness for the treatment of children with CP.[74] There is no singular recommended intervention for any specific category of CP because each infant and child presents a unique array of functional competencies, desired goals, functional limitations, and impairments. It is common and necessary to use principles from a variety of treatment approaches for an effective treatment. The therapist must determine the array of methods useful for the child. Displays 9.1 to 9.4 present the typical impairments in four major types of CP. Infants and

---

DISPLAY 9.1   Typical Impairments of the Child with Hypertonia

Neuromotor System
Decreased stiffness in neck and trunk
Increased stiffness in extremities, distal, proximal; varies with type, extent, and location of the lesion
Difficulty grading between CA and reciprocal inhibition (RI), times with excessive amounts of either CA or RI
Difficulty initiating certain muscle groups (i.e., hip extensors and triceps)
Difficulty sustaining certain muscle groups (i.e., thoracic extensors and abdominals)
Difficulty terminating certain muscle groups (i.e., hip flexors, adductors, and internal rotators)
Activation of muscles tends to be in small ranges.
Difficulty with eccentric control (i.e., quadriceps)

Musculoskeletal System
Limited ROM of certain muscles (soft-tissue shortening)
Other muscles are overlengthened (the antagonists)
Decreased ability to generate force in certain muscles, also in spastic muscles
Strength of poor grade
High risk for scoliosis
At risk for hip subluxation and/or dislocation

Sensory/Perceptual System
Decreased tactile and proprioceptive awareness
Difficulty discriminating different kinds of touch
Decreased kinesthesia throughout the body
Decreased vestibular registration
Decreased body awareness
Vision used more in an upward gaze, sometimes asymmetrically

Cardiovascular and Pulmonary Systems
Poor cardiovascular fitness due to decreased mobility
Reduced breath support with flared ribs and tight rectus abdominus

Gross Motor Impairments
Limited independent mobility on the floor or in vertical
May use assistive device for mobility
Poor sitting balance with spastic quadriplegia
Poor higher level balance skills

Fine Motor Impairments
Decreased use of hands owing to use for stability and for assistive device for mobility
Poor grasp and release and decreased in-hand manipulation with spastic quadriplegia

Oral Motor Impairments
Usually noted more with spastic quadriplegia
May have drooling, poor articulation
May have difficulty feeding

Neuromotor System

Decreased stiffness throughout the trunk and extremities

Inability to grade the level of stiffness necessary for functional activities

Extension favored over flexion for function

Difficulty coactivating for stability in trunk and in the extremities in horizontal and vertical positions

Muscle activity is initiated in phasic bursts for functional activity.

Great difficulty sustaining most muscle groups, especially abdominals and gluteals for proximal stability

Muscles tend to terminate passively.

Poor eccentric control of certain muscles (i.e., quadriceps)

Musculoskeletal System

Joints tend to be hypermobile, so the child relies on ligaments for stability.

Stability gained through end-range positioning

Contractures develop secondary to positioning of the arms and legs (i.e., pectorals, tensor fascia latae, flexors of the hips and elbows).

Rib cage at risk for becoming flat/ovoid owing to gravity in supine and prone positions

Difficulty generating force throughout the body

Sensory/Perceptual System

Difficulty with tactile and proprioceptive awareness (requires greater input for the sensory information to register)

Decreased kinesthesia and body awareness

May seek increased sensory input, sometimes in unsafe situations

Decreased ability to use both sides together because a wide base is used for stability

Cardiovascular and Pulmonary Systems

Decreased breath support and shallow breathing with weak abdominals and diaphragm

Poor cough

Decreased cardiovascular fitness

Gross Motor Impairments

Developmental milestones achieved later

May skip creeping on hands and knees

Uses "W" sitting for stability

Lacks higher level balance skills

Uses end-range stability without midrange control

Fine Motor Impairments

Lacks shoulder girdle stability and, therefore, distal strength

Decreased palmar arches

Decreased bimanual skill and in-hand manipulation

Decreased success with independent ADLs

Oral Motor Impairments

Decreased strength of oral motor muscles

Breathy voice and short utterances

Decreased rotary chew ability with inability to handle a variety of textures

Stuffs mouth owing to decreased proprioception

Neuromotor System

Profound global decrease in stiffness, proximal, distal

Poor damping, see high-amplitude and low-frequency oscillations

Difficulty with CA, RI noted much more frequently

Inability to grade initiation or sustaining of muscle activation

Muscle termination tends to be passive.

Difficulty with eccentric control of muscles

Musculoskeletal System

Significant asymmetry of the spine and hips

Joints may be hypermobile owing to excessive RI.

Significant hypermobility at C1 and C6–C7 with increasing age, resulting in possible spinal subluxation

Frequent temporomandibular joint problems

Poor ability to generate force

Sensory/Perceptual System

Vision used in upward gaze

Decreased proprioception, tends to be worse in the UEs than in the LEs

Poor body awareness

Poor kinesthesia

Cardiovascular and Pulmonary Systems

Respiration fluctuates in rate and rhythm

Poor breath support

Gross Motor Impairments

Developmental milestones achieved later

Limited floor mobility with great difficulty sitting on the floor

Delayed acquisition of ambulation skills

Use of "W" sitting for stability

Fine Motor Impairments

Difficulty using hands for tasks because they are used for stability in vertical and on the floor

Decreased bimanual skill and in-hand manipulation

Decreased success with independent ADLs

Oral Motor Impairments

Poor articulation

Breathy voice and short utterances

Prone to temporomandibular joint impairments because of asymmetric use of the facial muscles

Frequent drooling with poor lip closure

Neuromotor System

Tends to have slight decrease in stiffness in trunk, sometimes in the limbs as well

Poor grading of stiffness

Poor damping; oscillations are of high frequency and low amplitude.

Difficulty timing and sequencing initiating, sustaining, and
terminating muscle activation
Decreased ability to grade CA and RI
Poor CA of trunk, hips, and shoulder girdles

Musculoskeletal System
Difficulty generating force
Tends to rest in end range and rely on ligaments for stability

Sensory/Perceptual System (very significant sensory deficits, which are as restricting as the motor deficits)
Relies on vision for balance and postural alignment; therefore,
not free to scan the environment
Visual system with severe nystagmus
Decreased visual perception
Decreased proprioception throughout the body
Increased latency in processing sensory information
Severe postural insecurity; very fearful of movement
Poor vestibular system
Tends to be tactilely defensive with poor discrimination; never
gets sustained input
Difficulty generalizing sensory and motor information to per-
form novel tasks

Cardiovascular and Pulmonary Systems
Often fluctuating with poor proximal stability
Limited mobility impacts rib cage development, especially in
thoracic expansion.
Poor cardiovascular fitness
Shallow and rapid breathing

Gross Motor Impairments
Uses a very wide base to move on the floor independently
Keeps legs flexed in vertical to lower the COG
Pace of development tends to be slower owing to poor bal-
ance in upright.

Fine Motor Impairments
Poor skills due to an inability to grade precise movements
Difficulty with activities requiring dissociation of the arms

Oral Motor Impairments
Wide range of movement
Difficulty with a variety of textures and tastes

children may demonstrate impairments from two or more types of CP. For example, an infant or a child may have spastic quadriplegia with an athetoid component that involves the UEs more than it does the LEs. The information included in these tables is derived from numerous sources.[27,147–150]

Discussions presented in the following section include many of the therapeutic interventions currently utilized or recommended by physical therapists. This list is not intended to be exhaustive, because there are many treatment interventions outside of those listed that are being utilized effectively. The interventions explored in this section include strengthening, flexibility, cycling, neurodevelopmental treatment (NDT), constraint-induced movement therapy (CIMT), treadmill training, robot-assisted gait training, electrical stimulation (ES), aquatics, hippotherapy, virtual reality (VR) training, and community programs.

Strengthening

Strengthening plays an important role in the treatment of the infant or child with CP. Children with CP often present decreased muscle strength and poor selective muscle control.[151] This muscle weakness is due to deficits in motor unit activation, decreased muscle volume, and alterations in muscle length resulting in loss of muscle force, poor coactivation (CA) of antagonist muscle groups, and altered muscle physiology.[152–154] Mobility for children with CP is greatly impacted by both muscle weakness and spasticity. Historically, strengthening was thought to increase spasticity, decrease ROM, and reduce overall function for a child with CP.[155,156] However, these notions have not held up to careful scrutiny.[156–158] In recent systematic reviews of the literature, the authors have found that strength training can increase muscle strength in children with CP, and may improve endurance, cardiovascular health, weight management, maintenance of bone mass, self-perception, and gait function.[155–157,159] One systematic review also determined that there is preliminary evidence to suggest that in addition to strength gains, strength training leads to muscle hypertrophy in children and adolescents with CP.[159]

The question to be determined is, "What is the best strengthening program for children with CP?" The National Strength and Conditioning Association (NSCA) has established strength-training guidelines for children and adolescents.[158,160] Although not based on children with CP, these guidelines are a good framework to use as a starting point in protocol development in CP.[158] In 2016, Verschuren et al. carried out a comprehensive review of randomized controlled trials (RCT) consistent with the training guidelines of the NCSA. He found that the RCT followed all NSCA guidelines except for intensity, mode or exercise, and the duration of the training program. The starting intensity tended to be lower, the types of exercises simpler, and the duration of training longer than were the NCSA guidelines in many of these studies. The general consensus among researchers was that children and adolescents with CP who have never performed resisted strengthening should begin with single-joint activities at a minimal intensity and volume for a few weeks before gradually increasing the dosage and adding multijoint exercises.[161] Table 9.5 describes the recommendations of Verschuren et al. for resistive exercise, cardiovascular exercise, and daily physical activity based on current research.

To have an effective response to strength training, the child must:

1. be at least 7 years old;
2. comprehend the process;
3. consistently produce a maximal or near-maximal effort;
4. be motivated and be able to attend to the task; and
5. have a family that can support the program and the child.[10]

A strengthening program can be especially beneficial following invasive procedures such as dorsal rhizotomy, intrathecal baclofen (ITB) pump insertion, soft-tissue and bony

TABLE 9.5.	Recommendations for Exercise and Physical Activity Prescription among People with Cerebral Palsy

Cardiovascular exercise

Frequency	Start with 1–2 sessions per week and gradually progress to 3 sessions a week
Intensity	>60% of peak heart rate, or >40% of the heart rate reserve, or between 46 and 90% of VO_{2max}
Time	A minimum time of 20 min per session, for at least 8–16 wk
Type	Continuous and rhythmic exercise that involves major muscle groups

Resistance exercise

Frequency	2–4 times a week on nonconsecutive days
Intensity	1–3 sets of 6–15 repetitions of 50–85% of repetition maximum
Time	No specific duration of training has been identified for effectiveness. Training period of 12–16 consecutive weeks
Type	Start with single-joint machine-based resistance exercise, progress to machine/free-weight combination, then multijoint and closed-chain exercises. Be aware that single joint may be optimal for duration of training in children with severe weakness and those that compensate with stronger muscles with multijoint exercises.

Daily physical activity

Moderate to vigorous physical activity

Frequency	at least 5 d per week
Time	60 min
Type	Variety of activities

Sedentary activity

Frequency	7× week
Time	Less than 2 hr per day or break up sitting for 2 min every 30–60 min
Type	Leisure time screen time—television, computer, video games, phone

Source: Verschuren O, Peterson MD, Balemans ACJ, et al. Exercise and physical activity recommendations for people with cerebral palsy. *Dev Med Child Neurol.* 2016;58(8):798-808.

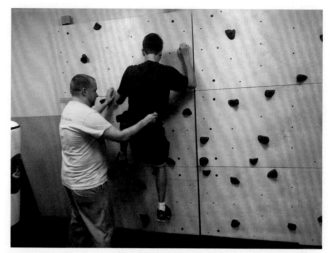

FIGURE 9.15. Functional strengthening while climbing a rock wall.

surgeries, and Botox injections to maximize functional improvement.[10] Further research is needed to determine optimal strength-training protocols for each type/severity of CP (Fig. 9.15).

Strengthening can also be performed without weights by carefully selecting activities that require specific muscle groups and closely resemble the goal activity.[151] For example, if the goal is to transition out of the kitchen chair, practicing sit-to-stand transition from chairs of various heights to strengthen the LE can be done to reach this goal. If the child is too weak or has too little postural control to use external weights or even body weight as resistance, the therapist can position the child to minimize gravity or to provide handling and assistance to complete the motion against gravity. An example of progressing head control against gravity is when the therapist supports the infant in a vertical position with the head aligned over the shoulders so that the infant attempts to balance the head in vertical. The strengthening progression is performed by tilting the infant slightly off vertical alignment, which requires returning the head to vertical and maintaining it there. As strength increases, the ability to return and maintain the head in vertical with eyes parallel to the horizon while the body is taken further toward horizontal should improve. Depending on the severity of the diagnosis, this could happen within a few sessions or over several months or years.

Flexibility

Many factors contribute to limited flexibility in children with CP including spasticity, passive muscle stiffness, and joint contracture.[162] Different factors require different interventions to achieve flexibility goals. Oral and intramuscular medications used to improve flexibility via decreasing spasticity are discussed later in the section "Neuromedical interventions." Here we briefly discuss commonly used techniques available to therapists to improve flexibility.

Passive muscle stretching is one of the most common treatment techniques used by therapists when treating children with CP. Therapists typically prescribe muscle stretching to maintain or increase full joint ROM or muscle flexibility needed for functional activities, to prevent or delay surgery, to minimize contractures, to decrease tone short term, and/or to allow improved active motion with strengthening/functional exercises. Stretching is often considered especially important in children who are not able to move their joints through normal ROMs with functional activities and during periods of rapid growth. Typical stretching protocols include holding stretches of spastic muscles 30 to 60 seconds at a time, for three to five repetitions. Unfortunately, research supporting the use of this type of stretching as the only treatment modality to improve flexibility or contracture is limited.[163–166] A recent systematic review found there were not enough strong studies (levels I and II) to support or disprove using passive stretching as a treatment modality.[164] A recent study did demonstrate that a long-term stretching program (15 minutes of triceps surae stretching 4 days per week for 6 weeks) did increase maximal ankle DF ROM and decreased triceps surae muscle stiffness.[167] Stretching has also been found to reduce severity of tone for several hours in children with CP.[169,168] More research is needed to determine the best parameters for stretching.

Interventions to prevent and treat contractures, especially plantar flexion contractures, are an area of great interest for children with CP. Currently, serial casting is the only nonsurgical intervention that has strong evidence supporting its use in treating plantar flexion contractures.[164,169] It is common for serial casting to be combined with BTX-A injection before casting. A recent systematic review did find that BTX-A injection followed by delayed serial casting was superior to casting alone in PROM improvements.[169] Unfortunately, recent studies have not helped clinicians better understand the impact of serial casting on function or long-term prevention of surgery.[162,169]

Treadmill training is another intervention that has shown the potential to decrease passive stiffness in children with CP. Walking for 30 minutes every day for 4 weeks on an inclined treadmill reduced passive ankle stiffness in children with CP.[170] Other benefits of this training included improved DF during swing phase and heel strike with walking.[170]

Cycling

Cycling is another excellent mode of exercise for children with CP. There are now many models of cycles available that can be adapted to fit children with a wide variety of physical limitations. Besides improving fitness, cycling can also improve social participation, allowing children to cycle with friends and family. A recent systematic review of cycling showed that it can improve muscle strength, balance, and gross motor function in children with CP.[171] Also, a study by Nsenga et al. demonstrated that children with mild CP are capable of achieving fitness levels that are comparable to able-bodied peers, after 8 weeks of cycling for 30 minutes, 3 days per week at a starting intensity of 50% VO_{2max}.[172] Despite these promising studies, an optimal cycling dose and intensity have yet to be determined for children and youth with CP (Fig. 9.16).

Neurodevelopmental Treatment

NDT is a valuable clinical practice model used by clinicians of various disciplines when caring for children with CP. Children with CP show various motor impairments such as muscle weakness, spasticity, limited ROM, and loss of selective motor function. These impairments make the development of gross and fine motor function and mobility difficult. NDT is a multidisciplinary clinical practice model used by OTs and physical and speech therapists when treating individuals with neuromotor disorders such as CP. It is an approach that focuses on an individual's ability to develop or learn a skill,

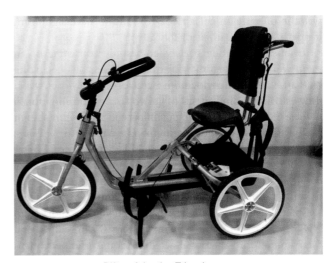

FIGURE 9.16. Rifton Adaptive Tricycle.

taking into account the interaction between intrinsic and extrinsic influences as highlighted by the ICF model.[173] This approach is grounded in improving function and participation by working toward functional goals via problem solving, task analysis, and therapeutic handling.

NDT was founded by Karl and Berta Bobath in 1943. Since that time, advances in the medical field and in the understanding of motor control and motor learning principles have influenced therapeutic approaches across multifaceted domains. In the same way, NDT's theoretic, operational definition and treatment approach has also evolved. The development of movement and skill acquisition, from the hierarchic perspective, is linked primarily to the maturation of the CNS. Within the past 2 decades, the emergence of the Dynamic Systems Theory and Neuronal Group Selection Theory has resulted in a shift in thinking of motor learning principles. Rather than focusing on primitive reflexes, normalizing tone, and facilitating typical movement patterns, the contemporary theoretical framework now focuses on the interplay of all systems, the individuals' abilities, the specific task and its components, as well as the influence of the environment.[130] NDT practice currently draws heavily on elements of Dynamic Systems and Neuronal Group Selection theories conceptualized by Bernstein and Edelman, respectively.[174] These theories have shaped the foundation of the current-day NDT theoretic framework.

The overall body of evidence for NDT clinical research continues to be small and consists of studies with variable study design and strength. On the basis of an evidence report in 2001[175] and a systematic review in 2010,[176] it was stated that there was not enough evidence to determine the efficacy of NDT.[175,176] A more recent systematic review of the effectiveness of multiple modes of therapy used in treating children with CP, including NDT, concluded that level II evidence supported the use of NDT on improving gross motor function. Level IV evidence also indicated that NDT was effective in making improvements on the body structure and function, activity, and participation levels of the ICF.[177] In fact, NDT was the only treatment approach found to have significant impact on all three levels of the ICF.[177,178]

Evans-Rogers et al. performed a study consisting of an intensive NDT program with treatment sessions occurring over a 1- to 2-week period with 5 consecutive days per week, between 2 and 4 hours per day. This study utilized a mixed method design and consisted of 13 parents and their children with a diagnosis of CP ranging in age from 1 to 17 years. Significant quantitative improvements were found using the GAS and Canadian Occupational Performance Measure (COPM) as compared to pre- and postintervention as well as positive qualitative findings identified through a parent questionnaire. This evidence supports the benefits of a short-term NDT intensive program when working with children and their families on functional activities that are important to them.[179] In response to the overwhelming need for further evidence, experts in the field of NDT are in the process of submitting research that further supports the use of NDT as an effective treatment approach for children with CP.[180]

Constraint-Induced Movement Therapy

The foundations for this treatment approach are based on work completed by Edward Taub and his coworkers in the mid-1960s.[17] This research highlighted the importance of cortical reorganization and neuroplasticity, which became the theoretical foundations for CIMT.[181,182] There are three major elements of the CIMT treatment approach: constraint of the less-affected UE with a cast, massed practice of the more affected UE, and intensive shaping techniques used in treatment to train the more affected UE.[182,183] The intensity of treatment is also a hallmark of this technique. Traditional CIMT involved constraint of the less-affected UE 90% of the day over a 2-week period with organized intense intervention for 6 hours per day. Boyd completed a systematic review that looked at several RCTs studying CIMT use for child's with chronic poststroke symptoms that have shown large functional improvements and carryover into daily activities.[183] These studies have also highlighted the fact that the intensity of training and the massed practice elements of this treatment approach are essential components of the effectiveness of this treatment.[183]

CIMT has become widely acknowledged as an effective intervention used with children with unilateral CP.[184–186] This cognitive neurorehabilitation approach centers on the premise that children will experience "learned non-use" if they do not incorporate the use of the more affected UE in activities.[187] Given opportunities to use the more affected UE, the assertion is that the child will begin to use it more spontaneously during bimanual UE tasks. A child-centered CIMT program maintains the foundational tenets of the CIMT approach while incorporating certain changes to the typical adult protocols. Such modifications may include changes to the type of restraint used (cast/sling/glove), intensity of use (number of hours per day), length of program (number of weeks), location of intervention (group/

individual setting), context (community/home/school/camp), and provider (therapist/trained parent).[185,188] Modified constraint-induced movement therapy (mCIMT) may utilize a less intensive means of constraint such as a glove or a mitten rather than a cast for the less-affected UE that is easier to manage and is better tolerated in children. The intensity of treatment may range from less than 3 hours up to 6 hours of intervention a day and from 1- to 2-week intensive periods of treatment.[182,189] A variety of modifications have been detailed in the literature; however, the essential components of intensive practice and constraint of the involved hand remain the same.[190]

When considering this intervention for children with unilateral CP, the focus should be on the importance of helping children learn to incorporate the more affected UE in natural two-handed tasks. There are several massed practice approaches being incorporated with CIMT to help improve spontaneous two-handed use in day-to-day tasks. Some models have integrated CIMT with a "bimanual transfer package" once the restraint period has ended.[191] Others have used a CIMT treatment progression followed by bimanual therapy.[192,193] At this time, limited comparison studies have been published to determine the effectiveness of the hybrid programs as compared to CIMT alone.[187]

There have been several systematic reviews that have evaluated the effectiveness of CIMT in children with hemiplegia due to CP and other causes.[186,194–197] The most recent systematic review by Chiu and Ada only considered randomized trials of reasonable to good quality. They found that CIMT had a beneficial effect compared with no/sham intervention for children with hemiplegic CP. The effect was also found to be beneficial at both the activity and participation levels of the ICF. However, when CIMT was compared with the same dose of upper limb therapy without restraint, CIMT was found to be no more effective.[186]

Coker et al.[182] studied mCIMT treatment on gait characteristics in children with unilateral CP. They theorized that UE and LE benefits could occur simultaneously during mCIMT with cortical reorganization and changes in both UE function and the child's ability to ambulate.[182] Twelve children with unilateral CP participated in five consecutive days of intensive specific treatment for 6 hours a day wearing a resting hand splint covered by a puppet glove on the less-affected hand. The findings did show positive shifts in overall gait performance, including narrowing in heel-to-heel base of support distance, decreased double-limb support time, and increased single-limb support.[182]

Treadmill Training

Treadmill training is a functional treatment in which patients practice walking on a treadmill to improve their ability to walk at home and in the community. On the basis of the task-specific approach to motor learning, if a child with CP is to improve in the skill of walking, intensive training of walking is necessary. Reciprocal treadmill walking may be partially controlled by the spinal cord and can be stimulated in the absence of higher brain center control.[198] Reciprocal stepping is considered to be largely organized by networks of sensory and motor neurons within the spinal cord called *central pattern generators* (CPGs).[199] CPGs are likely activated by the brainstem and basal ganglia, which in turn activate the muscles responsible for cyclic and repetitive walking movements.[200] Treadmill use taps into this automatic reciprocal walking mechanism even when higher brain centers have been damaged.[201]

Partial Body Weight–Supported Treadmill Training (PB-WSTT) is a type of treadmill training in which an overhead harness system is used to support part of the child's body weight. For children and youth with more difficulty performing reciprocal stepping, one or two therapists manually guide the LEs at the foot or lower leg while the child walks to optimize gait mechanics and rhythm of reciprocal movement. By supporting a portion of the child's body weight, those with CP can take reciprocal steps without the fear of falling. The optimal percentage of body weight that should be supported by the harness system is typically individualized for each child to improve gait mechanics and stepping endurance. Recent studies have shown positive impacts of PBWSTT on gross motor function,[201–204] walking speed,[205] and endurance.[206] Owing to common study limitations such as small sample sizes and lack of RCTs, the evidence that PBWSTT results in improvements in gait and gross motor function for children with CP is not conclusive.[207,208] One study suggests that walking with partial body weight support (PBWS) and not progressed by decreasing amounts of support, is no more effective than is traditional overground training without body weight support.[209] Before considering PBWSTT as a treatment modality for a child with CP, it is important to understand its clinical limitations. Maintaining a child's motivation is often challenging owing to the repetitive nature of this type of training. For example, it is not uncommon for the child to hang or lean forward on the harness system because of boredom and fatigue. Combining treadmill training with VR may be one way to improve a child's motivation and maximize its benefits. One recent randomly controlled study found that VR treadmill training with a group of children with GMFCS levels I to III was superior to treadmill training alone in improving gait and balance.[210]

Treadmill training without body weight support has also been studied in children and youth with CP. Basic treadmills are much more readily available in community fitness centers, physical therapy clinics, schools, and homes, making them much more accessible than are PBWSTT systems to children with CP. Simple treadmill training without dynamic body weight support was studied in Greek children with CP and found to have several positive effects.[211] Adolescent children who had treadmill training three times a week for 12 weeks demonstrated significant improvements in walking speed and gross motor function compared with conventional physical therapy.[211] In addition, an RCT of Brazilian children with CP found that treadmill training was superior to overground gait training in improving walking speed, gross motor function, and balance, and in maintaining these gains 4 weeks after the intervention.[212]

Robot-Assisted Gait Training

Robot-assisted gait training (RAGT) is another recently developed therapeutic modality with potential to improve gait. RAGT may be an option for children with some ability to initiate stepping but have limited strength. The robotic walking system typically requires expensive equipment including a robotic exoskeleton, a treadmill, and a harness system for body weight support.[213] In addition, a trained therapy team is required for children to achieve optimal results.[214] Goals of RAGT may include improving weight-bearing tolerance, body alignment, trunk control, ankle control, gait velocity, gait stability, walking endurance, and/or gait symmetry. Although children from GMFCS levels I to V may benefit from RAGT, a trial session is often recommended before deciding to commit to a RAGT program. Femur length, body weight, upright tolerance, and ability to accurately signal pain may restrict a child from participating in a RAGT program. This type of training offers an increase in specificity of gait rehabilitation by allowing a greater amount of stepping practice owing to lower child effort. Gait parameters such as mileage, speed, count steps, guidance forces, and body weight support can be precisely defined for each session, making progression easy to follow.[213] Because RAGT maintains a normal physiologic gait pattern while increasing intensity and frequency, some argue that it offers ideal conditions for gait training. A study by Meyer-Heim et al.[213] in 2009 found that children who participated in RAGT averaged greater than a 15% increase in gait speed. Also, an RCT by in 2017 by Wallard and colleagues reported RAGT improved GMFM scores as well as balance control in 8- to 10-year-olds with CP.[215,216] Despite recent research, there remains limited evidence to the effectiveness of this intervention.[214,217]

Electrical Stimulation

Functional electrical stimulation (FES) is a type of ES that can be used in the treatment of impairments associated with CP. FES is typically used to evoke or assist functional movement that is proposed to improve motor learning.[218] Several types of FES units are available for use, including those that improve hand function, walking mechanics, and cycling ability. Currently, there is a lack of strong evidence supporting or opposing the use of FES in children with CP. Improvements in children with CP have been shown in gait,[219–221] balance,[220] and community participation[221] after FES-assisted ambulation training. Despite its potential benefits, a common concern about trialing FES is that most children with CP may not tolerate the ES. Many clinicians assume that children with CP will respond negatively to the sensation and strong muscle activation. Most research has reported that few children drop out of studies owing to intolerance.[222–224] As with any intervention under consideration, a child's behavioral/ emotional issues, maturity, and cognition need to be considered before choosing FES as a treatment modality.

Aquatics

Aquatic physical therapy is defined by the APTA's Academy of Aquatic Physical Therapy as "the scientific practice of physical therapy in an aquatic environment by physical therapists and physical therapist assistants. Aquatic Physical Therapy includes but is not limited to treatment, rehabilitation, prevention, health, wellness and fitness of patient/ client populations in an aquatic environment."[225] Aquatic therapy is commonly used to treat children with CP. The physical properties of water make an aquatic therapy pool an optimal environment to implement therapeutic exercises. The buoyancy of the water decreases the effect of gravity, allowing for easier movement for children with CP, especially those with limited strength and motor control. As a result, children with a GMFCS level of IV or V can be more physically active when in an aquatic environment. Even despite anecdotal evidence that aquatic therapy may be most beneficial for the most motorically involved children with CP, there is a general lack of research on the effect of aquatic therapy programs on children with a GMFCS level of IV or V. A recent study did show that a 10-week aquatic therapy program, with the majority of the children functioning at GMFCS level IV, made improvement in lying and rolling, crawling, kneeling, and standing dimensions of the GMFM.[226] Several research studies on children with CP with GMFCS levels I to III have found aquatic therapy to be beneficial in improving gross motor function and gait.[227–229]

Hippotherapy

The American Hippotherapy Association (AHA) defines hippotherapy as "how occupational therapy, physical therapy and speech-language pathology professionals use evidence-based practice and clinical reasoning in the purposeful manipulation of equine movement as a therapy tool to engage sensory, neuromotor and cognitive systems to promote functional outcomes."[230] AHA further clarifies that the terms *hippotherapy service* and *hippotherapy programs* are not appropriate. Rather, licensed PTs, OTs, and SLPs incorporate equine movement into their plans of care as a therapeutic tool. The hippotherapy team includes the child, referring physician, therapist specifically trained in hippotherapy, specially trained horse, trained horse handler, and one to two assistants walking next to the horse for safety. Hippotherapy should not be confused with therapeutic riding, which focuses on recreation or riding skills for riders with disabilities.[10,231,232]

Hippotherapy uses the horse's triplanar movement to transmit frequent rhythmical balance challenges to the child when riding the horse.[233] These balance perturbations are postulated to stimulate the child's postural control system

and elicit hundreds or even thousands of righting and equilibrium reactions in a 30- to 45-minute session. Some stables include the care of the horse and the work of the stable in the routine of the therapy, thereby encouraging cognition, following commands, sequencing activities, memory, and psychosocial elements as well as the sensorimotor elements inherent in the activity.

There is a growing body of evidence supporting the use of hippotherapy to improve strength,[218] balance,[234–237] head and trunk control,[238] and motor function[235,239] in children with CP. The triplanar movement of the horse has also been shown to closely resemble the human pelvic motion during gait.[240] As a result, recent research has focused on changes in gait parameters after hippotherapy.[241,242] Studies have shown improved gait speed, step length, horizontal/vertical displacement, and acceleration after children with CP received hippotherapy.[241–244]

Virtual Reality Training

VR is a relatively new treatment approach, with a growing number of studies supporting its use to improve impairments and motor function in children with CP.[245] VR training is suggested to provide a child with real-time sensory feedback of a specific movement or activity. Most VR games are designed to require players to perform repeated body movements at various speeds and in multiple planes of motion in standing or sitting.[246] Other systems are attached to a treadmill or stationary cycle for gait training and/or to improve aerobic fitness. Musculoskeletal, neuromuscular, cardiovascular, and/or pulmonary systems can all be challenged by changing the type, intensity, or duration of game play. There are two basic types of VR systems available for rehabilitation at this time: total three-dimensional immersive using a head-mounted display and projection-based two-dimensional computer games on a flat screen.[246] The majority of the published studies use commercially available, projection-based two-dimensional video game systems as the semi-immersive VR environment.[245] Customizable VR systems are also now available to improve the ability for more children with CP to access this type of intervention. Two systems with this ability are the GestureTek Immersive Rehabilitation Exercise (IREX) and Move it to improve it (Mitii).[246] These systems allow the therapist to achieve an optimal challenge for their patient. Many studies have reported beneficial effects of VR training strategies. A recent meta-analysis by Ghai and Ghai found 88% of VR studies showed significant improvements in gait performance after VR training. In particular, gait velocity, stride length, cadence, and gross motor function improved in children[247] (Fig. 9.17).

Community Programs

In general, children with CP have increased sedentary behaviors compared to their same-aged peers.[248,249] Inactivity puts children at risk for developing medical conditions such

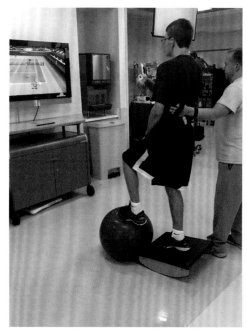

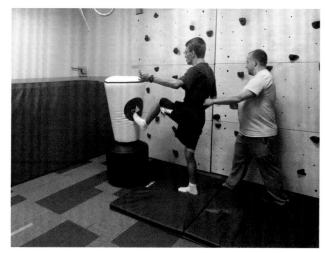

FIGURE 9.18. Balance, strengthening, functional karate kicking. Part of a treatment plan for an adolescent young man with cerebral palsy (CP) Gross Motor Function Classification System (GMFCS) level II with spastic diplegia.

FIGURE 9.17. Virtual reality (VR) and balance training as part of a therapeutic intervention for a young man with cerebral palsy (CP) Gross Motor Function Classification System (GMFCS) level II spastic diplegia, who has a personal goal of playing tennis.

as heart disease, osteoporosis, and diabetes. Outpatient and school-based physical therapy is typically not sufficient to achieve the physical activity needs of children with CP. Formal physical therapy should be supplemented by alternative activities such as community recreational programs.[250,251] With the child's age, functional abilities, level of participation, family support, and contextual factors in mind, alternatives to traditional physical therapy to replace treatment for a specified period of time, or to augment the physical therapy, should be considered. Self-esteem also rises when children with CP can participate in activities with their peers.

Despite all the known benefits of community recreational activities, children with CP participate less in recreational activities than their peers. As physical therapists, we can help decrease or remove some of the barriers that limit participation in these programs. First, therapists can introduce children to activities at a young age that they may not normally be exposed to such as baseball skills, yoga poses, musical instruments, or martial arts techniques during therapy sessions. Once a child identifies an interest in a recreational activity, the therapist should attempt to provide the family with information regarding potential adaptive programs in their area. Most local, regional, and national community programs now have websites that make connecting families much easier than in the past. Frequently found community-based activities include yoga, karate, dance, soccer, baseball, sled hockey, tumbling, swimming, horseback riding, and music lessons. Encouraging early exposure to sports is critical because the skill gap between children with CP and their peers typically widens with age. Trying a new sport later in childhood is

often more intimidating because of the larger skill gap and often results in choosing not to participate. Any of the above-mentioned activities has the potential to enhance the child's current abilities and to build on his or her strengths toward new functional skills. These programs can be very powerful motivators for many children and are physical in nature, which is important for improving overall health and preventing chronic health conditions.

Participation in community programs may need to be supported at times by skilled physical therapy. Targeted functional practice at a particular skill such as catching a ball, balance for yoga, or shooting a basketball may decrease a child's anxiety to try new activity. Once an adequate level of proficiency is achieved in the recreational activity's fundamental skills, a transition to community-based activities will help the child incorporate the skills they have gained in therapy to participate more successfully in their community environment.

There is a growing body of evidence that community recreational activities have numerous physical and quality of life benefits. For example, children with CP who participated in ice skating demonstrated improved gross motor function, walking endurance, and speed.[252] Another study showed increases in HRQOL in youth with CP after 6 months of participation in an active recreation program[253] (Fig. 9.18).

» Adaptive equipment

Adaptive equipment is often a necessary and useful adjunct to treatment of the infant or child with CP. Equipment may offer postural support to the infant or child, or it may aid functional skills and mobility.[10] Any equipment used should be meaningful to the family and easy to incorporate into the family's routines, be comfortable, safe, easy to use, and attractive. Adaptive equipment and its use should coincide with and reinforce functional goals for the child. The equipment should be reexamined frequently and adapted as necessary as the child grows and motor control changes.

Adaptive seating systems and supportive standers are the most common pieces of equipment used by infants and children at home and in the classroom to optimize function; to explore the environment and toys; and to interact with siblings, caregivers, and classmates. The majority of this section focuses on these two specific categories of equipment.

Seating and Positioning Equipment

The wheelchair or stroller system is the most important device for nonambulatory children, because nonambulatory or marginally ambulatory children with CP lack the necessary postural control and coordination to function in a variety of positions. The concept of a specialized stroller or wheelchair for a child with CP is often difficult for families to accept. Caregivers are often hesitant to discuss seating options because it acknowledges the degree of their child's disability. It may take the family some time to accept the need for a supportive seating system for mobility. It is important for the PT to have open discussions with the family regarding seating, but also be sensitive to the psychological process required for the family's acceptance. Caregivers of children who are ambulatory but lack endurance and strength for functional ambulation are often especially resistant to a wheelchair because they believe that their child will stop making progress with walking. This fear should be discussed with such families. Because of functional limitations while in a wheelchair, many children often continue to ambulate at home and school as often as they had before a wheelchair. There is no evidence that the functional ambulation of adults with CP is determined by how much they ambulated as children.[10] In addition to improved efficiency with mobility, an appropriate seating system has been shown to improve UE function,[254,255] enhance respiratory function,[254] improve oral motor function with eating and drinking,[256] and vocalization.[1,257] When caregivers are given a complete picture of all the advantages of an appropriate seating and mobility system, they eventually become more comfortable with utilizing such a device.

When examining a child for adaptive seating, the PT can gain important information from observing the child out of the chair. Questions to consider include the following:

- Can the older infant or child sit independently without external support? If so, what is the child's postural alignment?
- How long can the child sit with optimal alignment of the head and trunk?
- Can the infant or child sit by propping on his or her arms, or is he or she dependent on external support to maintain an upright posture?
- Can the child maintain the pelvis in neutral alignment with the trunk and head held in proper alignment?
- Is the infant or child's posture fixed or flexible?

Seating for a child is a multidisciplinary decision that includes the recommendations of the PT, physician, OT, rehabilitation engineer, and wheelchair vendor. A formal seating clinic allows these individuals to work with the child and family to help make the best decision for seating and mobility. Seating clinics are typically found in pediatric hospitals and some special education schools. The seating team should discuss the goals of the seating system, the child's current and future functional level, the ability of the seating system to function at home and school, available transportation for the wheelchair or stroller, growth needs of the wheelchair, musculoskeletal deformities, and future surgeries/treatments that may affect posture and alignment, the visual and perceptual skills of the child, the behavioral aspect of the child, and any safety issues or concerns should be addressed. At the end of the evaluation, a prescription for a wheelchair/seating system is generated, and the vendor is responsible for obtaining, building, and adjusting the seating system to the needs of the child.

Seating for the Nonambulator

The age and level of function of the child are the most important factors in deciding on a wheelchair or stroller. The child with severe quadriplegic CP who is dependent for all transfers requires supportive seating from an early age, and should be evaluated for his or her first seating system between 1 and 2 years of age. The first chair is often a tilt-in-space seating system combined with a stroller base/frame. The stroller base decreases the total weight of the chair, making it easier for families to transport, and looks similar to typical strollers used for all young children. A tilt-in-space feature in a wheelchair includes a frame that allows the seating system to be tilted backward while keeping the child's hip joints, knees, and ankles at the same angle. Tilt-in-space is necessary to give the head adequate support and thus prevent it from falling forward onto the chest, thereby overlengthening the posterior neck muscles. Typical seating components that aid in positioning are a good pelvic positioner, trunk lateral supports, anterior trunk support, foot positioners, and a head rest. A slide-on lap tray should be included for assisting with UE and trunk support. The tray can also be helpful for feeding, and fine motor and educational activities. Once the child with CP outgrows the stroller-based system, the next seating and mobility system is typically a tilt-in-space wheelchair with more customized seating options to provide postural support for the pelvis and trunk, and for optimal use of the UEs for educational or communication activities.

Power mobility is an option for the school-aged child, but not appropriate for all nonambulatory children with CP. When considering power mobility, practice and careful evaluation of driving controls is necessary to ensure that the child is able to function safely in all environments. Wheelchair transportation and the ability to access the home also need to be considered before committing to power mobility. Children with CP who struggle with increased muscle tone may have success with alternate input controls for driving. This could include a Head Array System, where proximity switches are embedded into the headrest pads. Chin control mini-joysticks and sip-and-puff controls are rarely used for children with CP owing to poor oral motor control in these severely impaired children.

Many children with severe spastic quadriplegic CP will develop significant skeletal deformities and skin issues as they reach adolescence, thus requiring more aggressive support and pressure relief from their seating system. In addition, many of the most severely involved children with CP will develop scoliosis that will require surgical intervention as adolescents. After spinal fusion surgery, significant modifications to the wheelchair are required, including raising the backrest and headrest owing to a total back height increase of 1 to 4 inches in the child. Other common adjustments include removal of custom-molded seat backs/cushions, adjustments to the lateral supports, seat depth, and cutouts on the backrest at the top or bottom of spinal fusion level to prevent excessive pressure[10] (Fig. 9.19).

Seating for the Marginal Ambulator

Children with limited ambulation skills and minimally impaired trunk control are usually prescribed their first seating and mobility system by 3 years of age. The child with strong UEs and sufficient cognitive ability may benefit from a manual wheelchair to allow independent propulsion. If manual propulsion is not feasible because of weakness or decreased motor control, a stroller base may help increase the overall chair height, thereby making dependent pushing of the chair easier for the family. Very early power mobility in this group of children has gained in popularity in recent years. Benefits for children to begin power mobility at a young age include reducing the risk of learned helplessness, promoting self-confidence, increasing learning, and allowing visual development.[258] Many young children with CP with minimal walking

ability fit the profile of "excellent candidate" for early introduction of power mobility, but several factors must be considered before this important decision. Transportation of the wheelchair, safety in all environments, home setup, and cost–benefit analysis are among serious issues to be considered when power mobility is an option. A powered wheelchair is a more appropriate option for these children in later childhood when behavioral maturity, cognitive ability, UE motor control, and caregiver readiness to make the commitment are well determined. The Pediatric Powered Wheelchair Screening Test (PPWST) is a valuable tool designed to assist clinicians in determining whether a child with CP has the cognitive skills to be a successful power mobility user.[259] Most children in this group of CP typically use a joystick with the dominant hand for power mobility, but head and leg switches are also useful for children with more motor involvement. Seating system needs for these children can vary greatly, and may include trunk and thigh lateral supports, chest harness, lap tray, and head support. Swing-away leg rests may be a better choice than are solid leg rests if the child can transfer to standing. These children will spend a majority of their waking hours in their seating system, so consistent evaluation of posture and alignment can minimize secondary impairments associated with prolonged poor positioning (Fig. 9.20).

Seating for the Household and Limited-Community Ambulator

The young household ambulator with minimally impaired trunk control but lacking the endurance to ambulate in the community could consider a special needs stroller that has

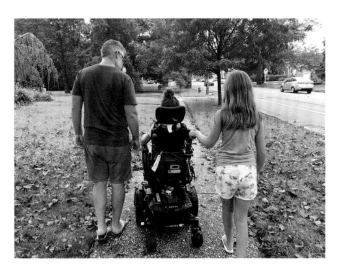

FIGURE 9.19. Power mobility training with family outside in their own own neighborhood.

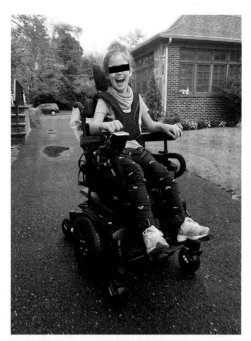

FIGURE 9.20. The joy of independent mobility can truly change a child's ability to interact with their peers, family, and enables greater access to community participation.

the option to be transported on the school bus. Before elementary school, these children work hard to improve their functional ambulation, and families are typically satisfied with a commercially available stroller for longer trips. Once school aged, most of these children are good candidates for either a special needs stroller or a wheelchair with basic seating. Seating system needs for these children are minimal owing to adequate trunk control and decreased overall use. A solid seat and solid back with a seat belt may be all that is required. Older children and adolescents preparing to leave for college often transition to a scooter to allow increased efficiency of movement in the community.

Standers

For older infants or children who are unable to stand independently or for whom sustained standing in proper alignment is indicated, standing systems should be used for external support.[10] A standing program should be initiated by 2 years of age in a child with CP who has not begun standing or ambulating regularly. The potential benefits of a supportive stander include improved weight-bearing tolerance, improved head and trunk control, increased bone density, enhanced hip development and prevention of further LE deformity, sustained muscular stretch of plantar flexors and hip flexors, maintenance of trunk and lower limb PROM, improved coactivation of the LE muscles used for standing, improved respiratory efficiency, improved GI motility, improved circulation/decreased incidence of decubiti, improved renal function, and improved social interaction with peers. A systematic review of standing programs for children and adults, including children with CP, concluded that there was moderate evidence supporting the use of a standing device with children who were not physically active.[260] Regrettably, there are a scarce number of studies that address the optimal dose of a standing program. In a review of the few pediatric studies available, standing was recommended at least 5 days a week to improve bone mineral density (60 to 90 minutes per day), hip biomechanics/stability (60 minutes per day with stander was positioned in 30 to 60 degrees of hip abduction); hip extension, knee extension, and ankle DF ROM (45 to 60 minutes per day; and spasticity 30 to 45 minutes per day).[261] The effect of standing doses above and below the systematic review's recommendations have yet to be determined. The standing program time doses listed earlier should be used only as a general guide. Children with CP often need to be slowly progressed to these doses because of discomfort, anxiety, and potential skin issues.

Once a decision is made to use a stander, a detailed examination should be performed and many factors considered before selecting the most appropriate stander for the child. Information about previous standing equipment, other equipment purchased recently, overall functional level of the child, and expected goals of the stander is extremely important to collect before making the choice of a specific item. This information may move the conversation about equipment in a completely different direction. For example, a common dilemma confronts the child who could benefit from a gait trainer and a stander but owns neither. Usually, third-party payers will only cover the purchase of one of these two types of therapeutic equipment during a specific time frame. If ambulation potential is noted during the evaluation, this must be considered when reviewing standers. A thorough objective examination with attention to head/trunk control in sitting and standing, posture in sitting and standing, and ROM limitations is the next step in the evaluation process. Overall child height, floor-to-chest height, floor-to-elbow height, leg length, lower-leg length, trunk width, hip width, inseam, and weight must be measured precisely. As with a seating system, the child's age and future growth potential are also important considerations. Because of the many pros and cons to each type of stander, several standers may have to be tested before deciding. Besides the obvious benefit of being able to evaluate the posture and alignment of the child during a trial, it is important to determine whether the caregivers can easily and efficiently transfer the child in and out of the stander. Ease of transfer is often the most important factor in compliance with using a stander. After trialing each stander for at least 15 minutes, carefully inspect the skin for pressure areas. Any redness should disappear within 20 minutes of removal from the stander. Once a stander has been chosen, carefully select the accessories required to provide optimal function and that can be removed or adjusted as the child's strength improves.

There are currently four basic stander designs on the market: supine, prone, upright, and sit-to-stand. This section details the basic differences between these stander types. Refer to Table 9.6 for more detailed descriptions of each stander's indications and contraindications. Supine standers start in a horizontal or reclined position with the child lying supine. The child can be easily secured in the device while supine and slowly transitioned to a more vertical position (45–80 degrees of inclination). A tilt table is the most basic type of supine stander, but is rarely the best option for children with CP. More sophisticated models of supine standers are available to meet the complex needs of a child with CP. Supine standers can be ordered with components such as trunk and hip lateral supports, knee pads, hip adduction/abduction support, and head supports. A supine stander is a good option for the younger child with moderate to severe extensor spasticity and poor head control who can be easily transferred via a scoop-dependent lift. Children who would benefit from supine standers have poor head control; therefore, optimal tilt should be just short of full vertical (80 degrees) to prevent the head from dropping into flexion. Children with extreme extensor spasticity are often not good candidates for this type of stander because the posterior pressure often stimulates their extensor muscle tone. Prone standers provide anterior support to the child and, similar to the supine stander, is positioned horizontally for ease of transfer. The available components are similar to those of a supine stander, with the addition of a chin support to aid in head control and positioning when

TABLE 9.6. Guide to Stander Selection

Stander Selection for Children with CP

Type	Indications	Contraindications
Supine 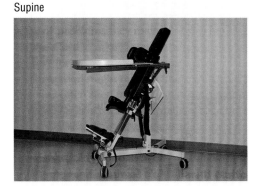	2-yr-old to adult Poor head/trunk control requiring head support or reclined position Flexor tone Tracheostomy Unable to tolerate full upright position	Strong extensor tone Good head and trunk control Significant knee and hip flexion contractures Larger children making transfer difficult for caregiver
Prone 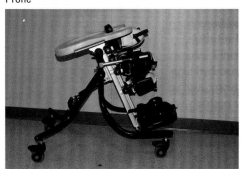	Younger child (often early school aged) Fair or good head control Fair trunk control Goal is to use upper extremities in standing. Goal is to participate in classroom activities while standing. Able to tolerate full upright position Dynamic options available, allowing mobility for children with good UE control	Strong extensor tone Uses extensor tone as main means to extend head and trunk to vertical position Poor head control—only phasic activation of cervical extension Larger children making transfer difficult for caregiver
Upright 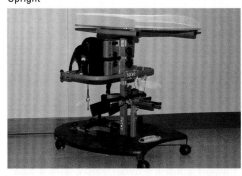	Younger/lighter child Tolerates full upright position for long periods Good head control and endurance Economical choice is important.	Poor head control Excessive flexor or extensor tone Hip or knee flexion contractures Large child
Sit-to-stand 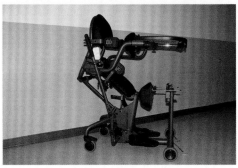	School-aged child or adolescent Good head and fair trunk control Mild hip/knee flexion contractures Child has cognitive and physical ability to transition stander between positions independently.	Poor head control Poor posture when stander in sitting

CP, cerebral palsy; UE, upper extremity

the child is vertical. Prone standers are not recommended for children with poor head control because they do not provide enough support for the child's head and neck. Traditionally, children in prone standers were placed in a slightly forward flexed position (10 to 20 degrees) to encourage activation of their extensor muscles and improve head control. Because maximum weight bearing and most upright functions occur in the fully vertical position, the forward tilted position is not typically recommended for most children. For the child with fair head and trunk control with the goal of improving head control endurance, either a prone or supine stander may be used to achieve optimal weight bearing as well as cervical and trunk alignment. Simple upright standers, or parapodia, are standers into which the child is placed in a standing position. They often do not have support above the pelvis, thus requiring increased trunk and head control. Because most children with CP with minimally impaired head and trunk control have some ambulatory ability, this type of stander is rarely recommended for children with CP. More supportive upright standers are commercially available and can be a good, economical choice for some children with CP. An upright stander is an acceptable choice for a younger child with good head control, some level of trunk control, and impaired LE alignment without external support. In the past decade, the sit-to-stand-style stander has become a very popular model for children with CP. Because of its versatility, a variety of nonambulatory or marginally ambulatory children with CP benefit from this type of stander. The child is usually transferred into this stander via stand- or sit-pivot transfer. Once properly supported at the knees and trunk in sitting, the child is slowly transitioned to a standing position using a manual hydraulic pump or a power-lift mechanism. This type of stander is an excellent choice for a larger child or an adolescent, and for the child with mild hip and knee flexion contractures who cannot stand fully upright. For these children, a sit-to-stand stander can provide a low-load, long-duration stretch to the hip flexors, hamstrings, and posterior knee capsule in addition to the other benefits of standing. Some children stay in this style of stander for several hours at a time, alternating between standing and sitting positions. Although this is a great feature of the sit-to-stand models, it is often difficult to adjust the stander to provide the optimal posture in both standing and sitting. The caregiver or school aide must therefore be trained in making proper adjustments to the stander after each transition in position. Another option in upright and sit-to-stand standers is the "mobile stander." These standers have wheels that the child can access to maneuver in their home and school (Fig. 9.21). These "mobile standers" can be excellent motivators for a child to stand, but they are frequently not appropriate or practical for children with CP to use at home.

Ambulation Aids

Numerous ambulation devices are available to make walking as functional, energy efficient, and safe as possible for

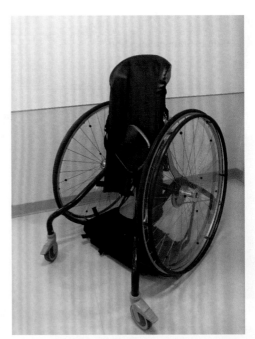

FIGURE 9.21. Mobile stander.

children with CP. Assistive devices improve ambulation independence and endurance for many children at GMFCS levels II to IV by decreasing the body load through the LEs via partial weight bearing through the UEs and improving balance by increasing the base of support via additional points of ground contact. A thorough examination of the child's functional capabilities must be completed before deciding on the best ambulation aid. Communication with the child's team regarding the child's routines, necessary transitions through the day, and distances to be traveled is important before deciding on an ambulation device.

Gait Trainers

A gait trainer is a walking device that provides more trunk and pelvic support than does an anterior or posterior walker. Gait trainers were developed to improve ambulation skills in children who can take independent or assisted steps but lack the balance and motor control to walk safely with a traditional walker. Gait trainers are often used in young children with emerging trunk control and active stepping to assist in progressing toward more independent walking with a posterior walker. In more severely involved children, gait trainers are more often used as a therapeutic tool to enhance physical activity and participation.[262] Common gait trainers include the Rifton Pacer, Mulholland Walkabout, Prime Engineering KidWalk, and the R82 Mustang. The use of gait trainers for children with CP is an area of debate among physical therapists. Those who support gait trainers argue that walking practice will allow children to strengthen muscles used in ambulation, and eventually the child may progress to a less restrictive mobility device. Others support their use to improve bone mineral density, GI function, respiratory efficiency, and social interaction with peers. Opponents argue that gait trainers are expensive, not time efficient to use, difficult to adjust, and rarely lead to improved functional gait. Research supporting gait trainer use is weak and thus not sufficient to determine their clinical effectiveness.[262]

The features of gait trainers vary greatly between models. A four-wheel base and a solid or sling seat that supports the child who cannot maintain standing or who loses balance while walking are common to almost all gait trainers. Some gait trainers, such as the Rifton Pacer by Rifton Equipment, Inc., have many accessories to improve trunk and LE alignment such as trunk supports, forearm prompts, hip guides, and ankle straps to limit LE adduction (Fig. 9.22). Other gait trainers are more similar to a partial weight-bearing gait training system and use battery power, pneumatic power, or springs to partially unweight the child during ambulation. These devices typically do not have as many accessories to improve LE alignment with ambulation, making it a poor choice for children with alignment issues that cannot be easily corrected with orthoses, such as excessive adduction, or scissoring, of the LEs due to adductor muscle spasticity (Fig. 9.23).

Walkers

Historically, owing to the lack of other options, children with CP had to use the forward walkers commonly prescribed to older adults. Posterior walkers were developed to address many of the postural issues caused by children using anterior walkers and are now considered the walker design of choice for most children with CP. Posterior walkers are more energy efficient for children with CP, and improve upright posture[263,264] because the shoulders are held in greater depression with humeral extension, and the scapulae tend to be more adducted, leading to greater thoracic extension. The posterior walker may have either two or four wheels. Logan and associates[263] found that the posterior walker with two wheels increased stride length by 41% and decreased double-limb support by 39% over anterior walkers. However, Levangie and colleagues,[254] in their comparison of posterior walkers with four wheels, posterior walkers with two wheels, and anterior walkers, found that the four-wheel posterior walker was more efficient and allowed more significant increases in

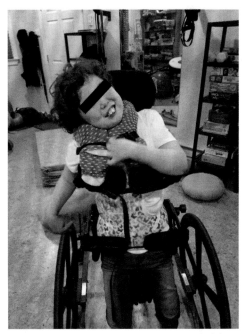

FIGURE 9.23. An adolescent young lady with cerebral palsy (CP) Gross Motor Function Classification System (GMFCS) level V, using head and trunk support to walk with her gait trainer.

the child's velocity, right and left stride length, and left step length. The results of the same study found that children walked similarly with anterior walkers and posterior walkers with two wheels.[264] Although this study is important, each child's ambulation abilities and deficits are unique. An evaluation with multiple types of walkers is necessary to determine which walker affords stability and safety while providing for an energy-efficient gait pattern. Several optional accessories are available for posterior walkers such as forearm supports, locking wheels to prevent motion in reverse, swivel wheels, hip guides, and flip-down seats. Forearm supports are common for children with quadriplegic CP because they typically do not have hand, triceps, trunk, and scapular depressor strength to maintain an upright position without forearm supports. Wheels that lock in reverse are often used with children beginning to use a posterior walker who have limited dynamic balance control and trunk stability to prevent the walker from rolling backward with any posterior loss of balance. Swivel wheels should be considered when the child has mastered forward ambulation and would benefit from the increased freedom and speed of turning. Hip guides should be considered when hip abductor strength is insufficient to keep the pelvis in midline as the child walks in the walker. A classic example of a child who would benefit from hip guides is the child whose pelvis is consistently deviated to one side of the walker, causing the walker to veer to that side with ambulation. A flip-down seat is an option for the child who is able to exceed household distances, but requires rest breaks for longer walks. For the flip-down seat to be functional, the child must be able to balance briefly with one hand on the walker while rotating the trunk to pull the

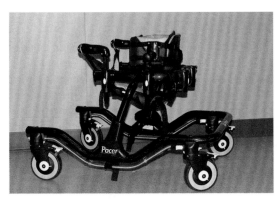

FIGURE 9.22. Rifton Pacer.

seat down with the other hand. Consistent reexamination of a child's ambulation ability is important throughout childhood to determine whether changing these accessories will improve overall function (Fig. 9.24).

Crutches and Canes

Young children with diplegic CP often use upper-body strength to substitute for lack of weight-bearing strength of the legs when using a mobility aide. When taught to ambulate with a posterior walker, children will frequently rely on the arms for much of the weight bearing and simply "toe-touch" in stance phase. Although functionally mobile with a posterior walker, the walking mechanics are not ideal to promote LE strength, balance, and trunk control for ambulation. In addition, relying solely on a posterior walker results in limitations in walking in tighter spaces and uneven terrains. Walkers also cannot be used on the stairs, limiting their usefulness in the community. Children using a posterior walker independently by school age may be evaluated for the use of forearm crutches (also known as Lofstrand or Canadian crutches). Forearm crutches are a better ambulatory aide to improve LE strength because forearm crutches are used primarily to improve balance rather than unweight the lower extremities. Initially, the child will need assistance to learn to rely on the legs for weight bearing and balance while moving the crutches forward. A four-point gait is

initially taught for maximal stability because three points are always in contact with the floor. As the child's coordination and strength improves, a two-point gait pattern and, lastly, a three-point gait pattern can be recommended to keep up with peers. Attempting to progress children with spastic diplegia from a walker to forearm crutches during the early school years is critical because the window for making functional ambulation improvements often closes for children with spastic diplegia as they approach adolescence.

Some children with mild diplegia or moderate hemiplegia who were independent ambulators in middle childhood may choose one or two forearm crutches in adolescence to minimize falls and increase walking endurance. Axillary crutches are not recommended for children with CP. Children who use axillary crutches typically lean forward at the hips and bear most of their weight on the crutches with the axillary pad pressed deep into the axilla. The older child with mild diplegia and normal UE strength may choose a single-point cane as the best long-term device for community-distance ambulation.

» Neurologic interventions to treat muscle spasticity

The treatment of spasticity requires a comprehensive evaluation and monitoring to determine the intervention's effects on function, comfort, and ease of care of the child. In addition, treatments for spasticity may prevent secondary problems such as pain, joint subluxation, and contracture. Functionally, the child may incorporate muscle spasticity to assist with standing, transfers, and stepping. In these cases, interventions to address the spasticity should take into consideration the impact on function versus the management of muscle tone and the long-term orthopedic implications. Conversely, treatment for spasticity can have a very positive effect on overall function and care of the child when combined with physical therapy, proper orthoses, and, when appropriate, serial casting.[168] Spasticity management is a comprehensive approach, and should include appropriate muscle stretching or strengthening, or functional exercises to optimize the benefits of the intervention.

Neuromedical Interventions

Oral Medications

Oral medications are typically used to manage muscle spasticity in children with spastic CP. Although easy to use, oral medications have side effects such as sedation and may lose their effectiveness within weeks.[10] Tilton,[168] however, showed that those sedating effects may improve over several weeks of use. The most commonly used oral spasticity medications for children include diazepam and baclofen. These drugs work by blocking gamma-aminobutyric acid (GABA) in the brain and spinal cord and thereby reduce muscle spasm. Oral baclofen and diazepam both are very sedating, which may impair cognitive functioning in children who use these medications.

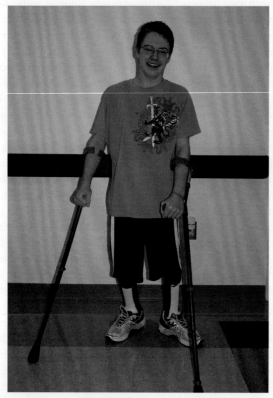

FIGURE 9.24. Adolescent young man with cerebral palsy (CP) Gross Motor Function Classification System (GMFCS) level III with spastic diplegia who ambulates with bilateral forearm crutches.

Conversely, diazepam taken at night may aid sleep and decrease nightly spasm without daytime carryover of drowsiness.[265] Tizanidine and dantrolene sodium are other oral medications reported to decrease spasticity in children with CP, but are not commonly used owing to several negative side effects. There has been limited research on the functional effects of these drugs in children. Therefore, it is important that the physical therapist collaborates with the prescribing physician to ensure that the optimum dosage, which balances spasticity reduction and function in the child, is achieved; and little is known about optimal dosing, safety, and side effects.

Neuromuscular Blocks

Neuromuscular blocks (also called chemodenervation) are chemicals injected near a peripheral nerve or intramuscularly to prevent nerve–muscle transmission.[168] Phenol and ethyl alcohol were the neuromuscular blocks commonly used to treat spasticity in the 1970s. These chemicals are injected perineurally, causing temporary axonal degeneration, although reinnervation occurred over months to years.[168] Studies have shown diminished spasticity with injection of both alcohol[266] and phenol,[267,268] but these chemicals may produce significant pain and dysesthesias after injection, leading to more recent use of BTX neuromuscular blocks.[269]

BTX-A is a neurotoxin produced by *Clostridium botulinum*, an anaerobic bacteria that typically causes food poisoning and tetanus.[10,168] The BTX causes temporary muscle paralysis by binding to synaptic proteins at the neuromuscular junctions, thus preventing the junctions from releasing acetylcholine.[10] The binding is irreversible, and the peripheral nerve must sprout a new fiber to form a new neuromuscular junction.[270,271] This process takes approximately 3 to 4 months.[10] Since 1993, BTX-A injections have been used to treat spasticity in individuals with CP. In 2005, Gough and colleagues called into question the long-term benefit of repeated BTX-A use to treat children with spastic diplegia.[272] At that time, this group suggested a cautious approach to the use of BTX-A because of the lack of evidence about the long-term effects. Recent studies have called into question the effects of BTX-A on PROM, gait kinematic, and overall carryover to functional abilities. Currently, clinical protocols using BTX-A are being scrutinized to determine the true effects on injected muscle for both short-term and long-term benefits, and harm to the muscle. Preliminary evidence shows that muscles injected with BTX-A lose contractile elements that are replaced with fat and connective tissues.[273] As a result, the muscles are weaker and stiffer. Given the current understanding of the effects of BTX-A on muscle physiology, and overall muscle health, BTX-A should be used with caution because more research and studies need to be conducted.

Neurosurgical Interventions

Selective Dorsal Rhizotomy

Selective dorsal rhizotomy (SDR), otherwise known as selective posterior rhizotomy (SPR), is a surgical procedure aimed at reducing muscle spasticity in children with spastic CP. It has been a poorly understood procedure with a low level of evidence supporting its long-term effects on function.[274–279] Child selection is critical to a good outcome because only two types of children are appropriate candidates. The first group includes children who are functionally limited by spasticity but have sufficient underlying voluntary power to maintain and eventually improve their functional abilities. These children typically present with a GMFCS level I, II, or III and have a preoperative GMFM score of 60 or greater.[280] The second group includes nonambulatory children whose spasticity interferes with sitting, bathing, positioning, perineal care, and classroom activities.[277–278] The surgery is typically completed across segments L2–S2,[275,277] or L2–S1,[278] and only a selected number of dorsal rootlets are sacrificed—those that appear to have the greatest influence on the spasticity and produce abnormal movement patterns. Studies have shown the need for subsequent additional treatment of muscle spasticity, such as physical therapy, post SDR.[279]

Intrathecal Baclofen Pump

In addition to being taken orally, baclofen can be delivered to children via a pump surgically implanted subcutaneously or subfascially into the abdomen. A catheter delivers the baclofen from the hockey puck–sized pump to the intrathecal space in the high thoracic region.[281] Many studies have shown the effectiveness of ITB in reducing spasticity in children with CP.[282–284] Traditionally, ITB pumps were selected for children with moderately severe spasticity (GMFCS level IV or V) with the primary goals of decreasing pain/improving comfort, preventing worsening of deformity or function, and improving ease of care.[10,285] In 2011, the results of the largest controlled study of ITB in nonambulatory children with CP determined that ITB decreased muscle tone and spasms, improved comfort and care, but had little impact on function and participation in society 18 months after surgery.[286] Children with minimal or moderate functional limitations were historically not considered candidates for insertion of an ITB pump. A few recent studies, however, have demonstrated improvements in the quality of gait[287–289] and improvements of ambulatory status[290–294] in less severely involved children with CP. On the other hand, nonambulatory children are not likely to become ambulatory as a result of ITB pump implantation.[286,295] This has not been proved to be an absolute rule, but realistic goals need to be discussed with the caregivers of nonambulatory children before surgery to prevent new ambulation skills from becoming an expectation after surgery. In addition to possible ambulation gains, other studies have shown improvements in overall function as measured by the GMFM in mildly, moderately, and severely involved children with spastic and dystonic CP.[296,297] It should be noted that some children (~12% in two studies)[290,293] showed deterioration of ambulation and transfer skills after ITB pump implantation, presumably because of decreased ability to use their muscle stiffness and spasticity, functionally.[290,293]

The PT has several critical roles before and after ITB pump insertion. The therapist can help identify children appropriate for the baclofen pump, assist in the evaluation process to distinguish between spasticity that interferes with function and that which the child is using to function, and assist in setting realistic outcomes before surgery. After pump implantation, PTs can measure extremity and trunk tone to assist in the decision-making process regarding dosage, help the family and child to become acquainted with bodies that feel and move differently, evaluate seating for required modifications (such as moving the position of seat belts and trunk supports away from abdominal surgical site), evaluate new equipment needs, determine rehabilitation service needs, monitor skin integrity, and educate caregivers in postoperative precautions.[285] Postoperative precautions vary among surgeons, but commonly include no hip flexion past 90 degrees, no forced trunk rotation, and lying flat for at least 48 hours after surgery to decrease the incidence of severe headaches secondary to cerebrospinal fluid leaks. Children with the desired outcomes of increased ease of care and decreased pain will not likely require increased frequency of physical therapy, but those with the goal of functional changes may benefit from a "burst" of therapy starting approximately 1 month after surgery.[285]

» Orthopedic interventions

The goal of orthopedic management is to help each child reach optimal functional ability and prevent deformity through detection at an early stage when simple and conservative treatment options may be instituted.[10,298,299] Physical therapy is frequently prescribed by orthopedic surgeons to minimize secondary impairments, such as contracture and muscle weakness, with the goal of delaying orthopedic surgery. The objective is to reduce the number of orthopedic surgeries a child may need before skeletal maturity. When surgical intervention occurs, the goals of surgery should be to improve function, decrease discomfort, and prevent structural changes that may become disabling.[298]

Owing to the fact that children with CP often present with orthopedic impairments at multiple joints, surgical intervention at only one level often does not result in an acceptable improvement in overall alignment and function, and may lead to negative consequences at adjacent joints. Therefore, it has become common practice for orthopedic surgeons to perform multiple orthopedic procedures at the same time, with the goal of improving overall function with fewer total surgeries. This approach, commonly known as single-event multilevel surgery (SEMLS), has become the standard of care in the orthopedic management of children with CP. This technique is especially successful when comprehensive gait analysis is used to help guide surgical decision making.[300–302] The most common orthopedic problems and surgical procedures involving the spine and LEs are addressed in the following sections. Refer to Table 9.7 for definitions of surgical terms commonly used, and Table 9.8 for common

TABLE 9.7.	Orthopedic Surgery Terms
Term	**Definition**
Tendon release/ tenotomy	Complete cut of a tendon
Tendon lengthening	Myofascial lengthening of tendon, often via Z-plasty
Percutaneous lengthening	Tendon lengthening involving small cuts into tendon without opening the area for visualization
Recession	Another term used for myofascial lengthening; usually used to differentiate gastrocnemius lengthening only versus entire Achilles tendon lengthening
Osteotomy	Surgical cutting of a bone with the goal of changing the orientation of the bone
Shelf procedure	Refers to a number of pelvic osteotomies that build a shelf superior to the acetabulum to reduce a dislocated hip
Tendon transfer	Involves cutting one end of a tendon and attaching it to another muscle to change or eliminate the presurgical function of that muscle
Arthrodesis	Fusion of at least two bones

orthopedic surgeries, indications, and typical postoperative recommendations. Postoperative protocols can vary greatly depending on the hospital, surgeon, and the child; therefore, the information presented here should be used only as a guide in planning and implementing a therapeutic program. An understanding of gross motor development and movement compensations in children with different patterns and classifications of CP is necessary to better predict how surgery will likely impact the child's future function. This knowledge is critical to making realistic short- and long-term goals.

Spinal/Neuromuscular Scoliosis

Spinal deformities are very common in children with CP, with neuromuscular scoliosis being the most common pattern of deformity. Neuromuscular scoliosis is primarily caused by an imbalance between agonist and antagonist muscles in the spine. This imbalance often leads to the development of S-shaped or C-shaped curves in the spine that continue to progress throughout childhood. In contrast to the S-shape typical in idiopathic scoliosis, neuromuscular scoliosis in children with CP more frequently has a broad C-shape, typically with left convexity.[303] The incidence of scoliosis is between 20% and 25% in children with CP,[281,304] with the most severe scoliosis typically present in nonambulatory children functioning at levels IV and V on the GMFCS.[305] Most cases of scoliosis present before the age of 10 years,[306] but begin to progress quickly during puberty with curve progression up to 2 to 4 degrees per month.[304] Pelvic obliquity eventually develops owing to the scoliosis extending all the way to the lower lumbar region, which affects sitting posture and balance. As

TABLE 9.8.	Common Orthopedic Surgeries for Children with CP		
Surgical Procedure	**Indications**	**Complications**	**Postoperative Care**
Posterior spinal fusion	Neuromuscular scoliosis	Pancreatitis Wound infection	Log rolling only No hip flexion past 90 degrees No forced trunk rotation
Adductor lengthening	Hip subluxation Adductor contracture Scissoring gait Difficulty with perineal hygiene	Reoccurring contracture Heterotopic ossification Overlengthening (rare)	No precautions WBAT
Pelvic osteotomy	Hip subluxation/dislocation	Internal infection Repeat dislocation Loss of fixation	No hip flexion past 90 degrees No forced hip rotation No adduction past midline WBAT
Femoral varus derotation osteotomy	Increased femoral anteversion Hip subluxation/dislocation	Wound infection Femur fracture	No hip flexion past 90 degrees No forced hip rotation WBAT
Iliopsoas release/tenotomy	Hip flexion contracture in nonambulators	Reoccurring contracture Overlengthening	WBAT No precautions
Psoas lengthening	Hip flexion contracture in ambulatory children	Reoccurring contracture Overlengthening	No precautions WBAT
Hamstring lengthening	Hamstring contracture Mild knee flexion contracture	Reoccurring contracture Overlengthening	Knee immobilizer wear 8–12 hr/d
Posterior knee capsulotomy	Moderate knee flexion contracture	Reoccurring contracture Overlengthening	Strict knee immobilizer use
Rectus femoris transfer	Stiff knee gait	Reattachment of some fibers to quadriceps (rare)	No prone flexion past 90 degrees
Tibial osteotomy	Internal or external tibial torsion	Ankle varus or valgus Compartment syndrome	Short leg cast 6–8 wk WBAT
Tendon Achilles lengthening	Equinus deformity Planovalgus foot	Overlengthening Reoccurring contracture	Short leg casts for 4–6 wk WBAT
Gastrocnemius recession	Gastrocnemius contracture without soleus contracture	Overlengthening Reoccurring contracture	Short leg casts for 4–6 wk WBAT
Subtalar fusion	Severe planovalgus foot	Nonunion Ankle valgus	Short leg casts for 12 wk WBAT
Triple arthrodesis	Severe planovalgus and painful foot	Nonunion Ankle valgus	Short leg casts for 12 wk WBAT
Lateral column lengthening	Planovalgus foot	Reoccurrence of planovalgus	Short leg casts for 12 wk WBAT
Posterior tibialis transfer	Varus foot with tibialis anterior firing throughout swing or stance phase of gait	Over- or undercorrection of varus foot	Casted for 4 wk after surgery WBAT
Anterior tibialis split tendon transfer	Varus foot with tibialis posterior firing throughout stance phase of gait	Over- or undercorrection of varus foot	Casted for 4 wk after surgery WBAT

CP, cerebral palsy; WBAT, weight bearing as tolerated.

the curve increases, the adolescent's scoliosis may cause respiratory restriction, pain, pressure sores, and increased difficulty with hygiene management.[305] Unfortunately, neuromuscular scoliosis is not responsive to orthotic management,[304] and there is no evidence supporting the use of stretching, strengthening, joint mobilization, or ES for treatment. The treatment of choice in children older than 10 years with curves greater than 50 degrees and deterioration of functional skills is posterior spinal fusion.[304] This procedure uses a unit rod, a U-shaped rod with a prebent pelvic section, that is fixed to the ilium, thereby correcting the pelvic obliquity and scoliosis (Fig. 9.25).[306] It is preferable to delay spinal fusion until the

child reaches puberty or has achieved most of the expected growth. The trunk will not be able to grow once the fusion is completed. The complication rate with neuromuscular scoliosis surgery is high, with one study reporting a 68% rate. Common complications include pulmonary issues, wounds, hardware failure, curve progression, pancreatitis, and pseudo-arthrosis.[307] Despite the high complication rate, caregiver and child satisfaction rate is high, and the surgery has been shown to significantly improve the quality of life of the child.[305] After surgery, the therapist should evaluate all seating and standing devices because the alteration in alignment can result in improper support, and skin breakdown or sores, if adjustments

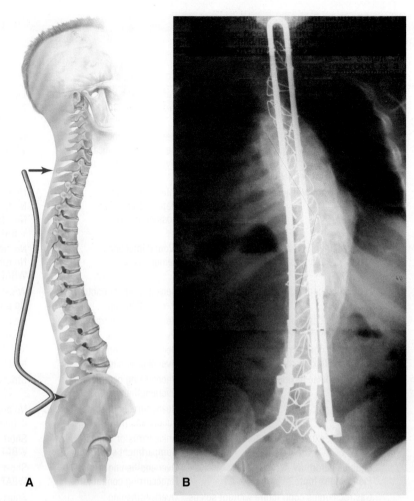

FIGURE 9.25. Posterior spinal fusion: **(A)** Illustration of typical unit pod placement. **(B)** Radiograph showing correction of curve with unit rod.

are not completed in a timely manner. There is also increased potential for improvements in respiratory function after surgery because the lungs will generally have more volume for gas exchange and thoracic expansion improves. This should be addressed during postoperative rehabilitation in addition to functional training.

Hip Joint

A child with CP may require hip surgery for a number of reasons, including to prevent or reduce hip subluxation or dislocation, correct in-toeing with ambulation, eliminate scissoring gait, or improve perineal care in a severely impaired child. Hip abnormalities are common in children with CP, with the reported incidence ranging from 2% to 75%.[47]

Femoral Anteversion

Increased femoral anteversion exaggerates hip internal rotation and can severely affect walking by tripping the child when the toe of one shoe catches the opposite shoe during the swing phase of gait. A femoral derotation osteotomy with blade plate fixation (Fig. 9.26), sometimes with medial

hamstring release, is the standard surgery for this deformity.[10,308,309] Postsurgical management does not include cast or immobilization, and physical therapy begins with PROM on postoperative day 1 or 2. The child is typically transferred out of bed into a wheelchair by day 2. Full weight bearing and assisted ambulation is expected by discharge, which occurs between postoperative days 4 and 7.[10] Physical therapy is directed toward increasing ROM and strengthening the hip muscles for improvement in muscle balance. Functional training is important for the child to learn new ways of moving with the new hip alignment and possible need for better motor control. Improvement to and beyond presurgical status is expected for up to 1 year.[10] Unilateral hip surgery may result in LLD, which must be considered during treatment and in consultation with the surgeon.

Hip Joint Subluxation/Dislocation

The more severe the neurologic involvement of the child with CP, the greater the chance of hip dislocation or subluxation.[310,311] One study by Soo et al.[311] found that the incidence of hip displacement was 0% for children classified as level I on the GMFCS and 90% for children classified as level V.

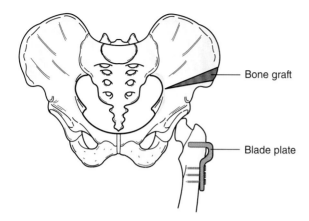

FIGURE 9.26. Pelvic osteotomy with varus derotation osteotomy (VDRO) blade plate fixation.

To understand the progression of hip abnormalities in children with CP, one must first understand normal hip development. Children with and without CP are born with normal hip joints that are in an anteverted position. In the development of the hip joint, balanced muscle use during standing and with ambulation promotes development of the acetabulum, femoral head, and remodeling of anteversion. In children with CP, ambulation is key to preventing hip subluxation. Children who walk independently by age 5 develop the muscle balance necessary to prevent dislocation. Children using an ambulation aid may develop painless subluxation, but seldom require surgical intervention in childhood. The hips of children who do not ambulate may begin to dislocate before age 7.[47] Superior and posterior direction subluxation is the most common pattern of hip subluxation, with adductor muscle spasticity being the primary cause of hip subluxation. Passive hip abduction of less than 40 degrees with hips flexed[47] or 45 degrees with hips extended[10] may be indicative of subluxation requiring further evaluation from an orthopedic surgeon. Although the adductor longus is the primary contributor to adduction of the hip joint, the gracilis and adductor brevis spasticity also contribute to the abnormal forces, resulting in subluxation. The constant co-contraction of the adductors, hamstrings, and hip flexors causes the hips to be held in flexion and adduction and generates excessive forces on the hip. These abnormal and powerful forces usually redirect the femoral head to the superior and posterior aspect of the acetabulum.[47] As subluxation progresses, the femoral head presses up on the lateral edge of the acetabulum, resulting in acetabular flattening and articular cartilage degeneration.[40] In addition to the femoral head changes, the angle of femoral neck inclination remains high and anteversion persists. EMG studies have implicated spasticity of the medial hamstrings and gluteus medius weakness as the muscle imbalance that leads to the internally rotated position of the hips and persistent femoral anteversion.[47] Left untreated, the femoral head may continue to migrate until it is dislocated. Gamble and coworkers[312] maintain that this process occurs over a 6-year period.

Conservative treatment options to prevent or retard progression of the subluxed hip include neurochemical spasticity interventions and passive muscle stretching of the adductors and hip flexors. ITB can help decrease hip joint muscle spasticity in moderately to severely involved children, but BTX is not commonly used owing to the technical difficulty with injections. Proper positioning in a correctly adjusted seating system and routine standing may slow progression. If progression continues, surgery may become necessary. Surgical management is divided into three basic categories: (1) soft-tissue releases to halt early subluxation, (2) soft-tissue and bony osteotomies to slow advancing subluxation due to femoral and acetabular dysplasia, and (3) palliative surgery for the painful, arthritic hip joint.

Postoperative precautions are limited after soft-tissue releases around the joint, which allow for early weight bearing, stretching, and functional strengthening. It is important to train caregivers to appropriately stretch the adductors after surgery to improve the flexibility of the developing scar tissue. Nonadherence to the postoperative stretching protocol may reverse hip abduction ROM gains achieved by surgery and further progress the subluxation. Physical therapy must also include muscle strengthening around the hips to improve muscular balance between the hip abductors and adductors. Standing activities and gait training with manual and visual cuing should be used to improve muscle CA patterns. For children with progressing subluxation or complete dislocation, femoral anteversion, and acetabular dysplasia, combined muscle and bony surgeries are often necessary to realign and stabilize the hip joint.

Chronic, progressive subluxation leads to acetabular dysplasia. The acetabulum has little potential to remodel, even with soft-tissue releases and varus derotation osteotomies (VDROs) to reset the femoral head appropriately in its center.[47] Complete hip joint reconstruction is indicated in these cases, and refers to a combination of muscle releases, reduction of the femoral head into the acetabulum via VDRO, and, lastly, reconstruction of the acetabulum to correct its deformity.[313–316] Acetabular reconstructions, also known as pelvic osteotomies, involve cutting the pelvis and adding bone grafts to create a shelf superior to the acetabulum. These shelf procedures change the orientation of the acetabulum to better hold the reduction of the femoral head after the VDRO (Fig. 9.27). The goal for hip reconstruction is a near-normal joint and normal hip ROM. Postoperative therapy after VDRO and/or pelvic osteotomies varies depending on the surgeon's postoperative precautions and protocol. Common postoperative precautions after bony osteotomies include no hip flexion past 90 degrees, limited hip rotation ROM, and no hip adduction past neutral. Early mobilization and weight bearing after surgery can help prevent skin breakdown, osteopenia, and weakness that occur with immobilization. Typically, the rehabilitation process after hip reconstruction lasts between 6 and 12 months, with return to presurgical function usually occurring between 12 and 24 months. The focus of postoperative therapy should be on

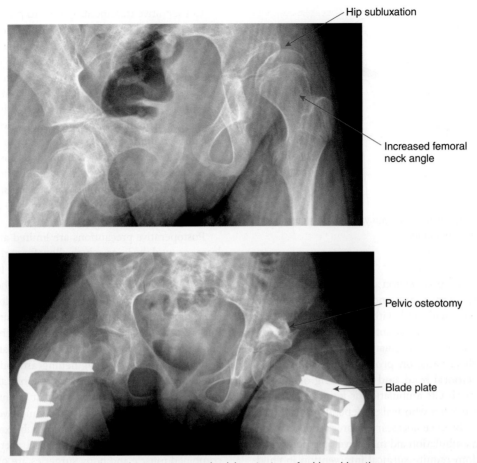

Hip subluxation

Increased femoral neck angle

Pelvic osteotomy

Blade plate

FIGURE 9.27. Pre- and post-varus derotation osteotomy and pelvic osteotomy for hip subluxation.

stretching to maintain improved hip abduction ROM, functional strengthening in standing when possible to achieve improved muscle balance around the hips, and proper positioning when seated.

In the left radiograph, note the superior hip subluxation of the left hip and increased angle of the femoral neck. The right radiograph shows the femoral neck angle decreased to reduce the femoral head into the acetabulum using blade plate for fixation. Also note the bone graft wedge placed to create a superior border of acetabulum.

Palliative surgeries for dislocated hips are reserved for children who have failed reconstruction and continue to be painful. Total hip arthroplasty, with a shoulder prosthesis, or resections of the proximal femur are palliative options. The goal of these surgeries is to remove the source of pain and improve function.[10,312,316]

Hip Adductor Contracture without Subluxation

Indications for management of the hip adductor contracture include the following:

- Improvement in a scissoring gait
- Improvement of femoral head alignment in acetabulum (typically combined with VDRO)
- Improved care of the perineum

Conservative management includes stretching, positioning, and strengthening of the hip abductors to promote muscle balance across the hip joint. The hip adductors can be lengthened in isolation or the iliopsoas can be lengthened as well, depending on the presentation of the child. Typically, there is no period of immobilization postoperatively and ROM/functional strengthening can be started immediately.[10] Hip adductor lengthening is commonly combined with femoral osteotomies and pelvic osteotomies to improve hip alignment.

Hip Flexor Contracture

Hip flexion contractures interfere with balance, posture, and function with standing and ambulation. Compensation occurs typically with excessive extension at the thoracolumbar junction, and the knees remain flexed so that body orientation remains vertical. It is difficult to stretch contracted hip flexor muscles because the pelvis rocks forward into an anterior tilt while extension occurs at the thoracolumbar junction. Surgical intervention involves complete cut/resection of the iliopsoas tendon or tendon transfer to the pelvis or hip joint.[10,16,317,318] This procedure is rarely done in isolation, but rather as one of multiple surgical sites in a child with greater functional limitations. Iliopsoas tendon lengthening recommendations should be made carefully because children often present with increased hip weakness, making function activities such as stair climbing difficult. Physical therapy after surgery should include a daily program of prone-lying to maximize the lengthening into hip extension and strengthening of the hip extensors and abductors. Facilitation of functional skills should continue, with care taken to prevent a return to the child's previous compensatory patterns of movement (Fig. 9.28).

Knee Joint and Lower Leg

Knee Flexion Contracture

Decreased knee extension ROM is a common finding in children with CP. Despite consistent hamstring stretching, knee flexion contractures often develop. Hamstring contracture may or may not affect function in children with CP and may not require aggressive intervention in all cases.[10] In children with spastic diplegic CP, increased knee flexion in stance phase is often at least partially due to hamstring spasticity and contracture. This flexed knee or "crouched" gait usually includes decreased step length, increased knee flexion in stance, decreased knee extension at terminal swing, increased hip flexion, and increased ankle DF in stance. This crouched posture also causes energy inefficiency during gait, partially because of continuous quadriceps firing, which prevents the knee from collapsing into further flexion (see the section "Gait" for a more detailed review of crouched gait).[319–321] Persistent knee flexion eventually leads to contracture of the hamstrings and, in more severe cases, knee joint capsule contracture and shortening of the sciatic nerve.[10]

Lengthening tight posterior structures of the knee to prevent further deformity is the goal of treatment for knee flexion contracture. Consistent hamstring stretching is often the first line of defense against contracture. Therapists should teach caregivers hamstring stretching before hamstring tightness begins to have an adverse effect on function. Knee immobilizer use is another conservative approach being used with some success to reduce hamstring stiffness. Knee immobilizers can be used at various times during the day or while the child is sleeping. Providing the child with a standing regimen can also help prevent knee flexion contracture and may help gain length when tightness is not excessive. When conservative management fails, there are three surgical interventions typically available to improve knee extension, depending on the severity of contracture: (1) hamstring lengthening, (2) posterior knee capsulotomy with hamstring lengthening, and (3) femoral extension osteotomy with hamstring lengthening.

Hamstring lengthening is widely considered to be the surgical procedure of choice for the correction of increased knee flexion.[10,322,323] The hamstrings are usually lengthened distally, and the most common procedures include a combination of Z-plasty/tenotomy of semitendinosus, tenotomy of gracilis, semimembranosus recession/myofascial lengthening, and, sometimes, biceps femoris recession.[10,321,324] Indications for surgical lengthening of the hamstrings include the following:

- Severe kyphotic posture in sitting due to shortened hamstrings
- Fixed knee flexion contracture greater than 10 degrees
- Popliteal angle of greater than 40 to 50 degrees
- Knee flexion of 20 to 30 degrees at foot contact during gait
- Constant EMG activity of hamstrings during stance and/or initial swing
- Knee flexion during midstance greater than 20 degrees[10,324–326]

Several studies have demonstrated improvements in knee extension during stance phase after hamstring release, thus decreasing crouch.[327,328] Quadriceps strength at 30 degrees of knee flexion also increases after hamstring lengthening, which is important to prevent progression back into a more crouched posture.[229] Physical therapy begins postoperative day 1 with knee PROM, bed mobility, weight bearing as tolerated (WBAT), and family education of knee immobilizer use and stretching. Initially, knee immobilizer use is recommended 2 hours on, 2 hours off during the day and on for the entire night. This wear schedule is eventually weaned down to nighttime only.[10] The importance in teaching the caregivers proper intensity and frequency of hamstring stretching cannot be understated. Following hamstring lengthening, it is recommended that the hamstrings are stretched for 30 seconds three times a day starting postoperative day 2 and continuing for at least 3 to 4 months after surgery. Careful monitoring of popliteal angle during rehabilitation is used to determine when the frequency can be slowly decreased. Noncompliance with stretching will result in disorganized scar formation, with the knee in a flexed position causing

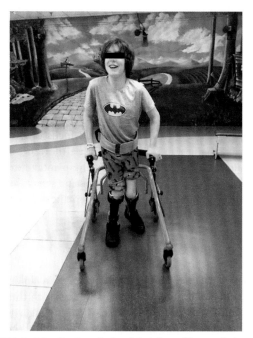

FIGURE 9.28. Postsurgical gait training with a posterior walker.

a reoccurrence of the original contracture. The outpatient PT should initially focus on improving hamstring flexibility, knee extension AROM/PROM, assisted standing with knees extended (using knee immobilizers and/or AFOs), and strengthening of both knee extensors and flexors for improved balance across the joint.[10] Despite surgical lengthening, the hamstring muscles have the potential to strengthen to preoperative levels by approximately 9 months after surgery.[323,329] Once lengthened, the hamstring muscle belly recoils, and sarcomeres are placed on slack. Over time, the number of sarcomeres in the muscle fibers is reduced to restore optimal filament overlap. This process takes several months and explains the extended time required to increase hamstring strength to the presurgical level. Because the hamstrings cross the knee and hip joints, the therapist must also emphasize ROM and strengthening exercises for the hip musculature. AFOs are often required to control DF and crouch in standing and with ambulation. Gait training and balance training are often the emphasis of therapy in later phases of rehabilitation, teaching the child to ambulate and move efficiently in a more upright posture. Functional improvements are not likely to be seen until strength around the knee approximates or exceeds preoperative levels.[323,329]

Although hamstring releases are a relatively simple surgical procedure, there are several noteworthy complications. The most common complication of hamstring lengthening is recurrence of hamstring contracture.[10] This will inevitably lead to return of the crouched/flexed knee gait pattern. In addition to the recurrence of hamstring contracture, crouched gait may return owing to external tibial torsion deformity, quadriceps weakness, or growth spurt.[10,319] Repeat hamstring lengthenings are common due to this functional deterioration, especially if the first surgery occurred in early childhood.[10] Sciatic nerve palsy is also a common complication after hamstring lengthening.[10,321] Hamstring tendon release improves knee extension, but causes the nerves in the popliteal fossa to become taut. These nerves can limit knee extension and can be damaged with aggressive stretching. The PT should examine the child for dysesthesias and ability to wiggle the toes immediately after surgery and for the first several weeks after surgery.[321] Foot swelling can also occur in some cases owing to the sympathetic response to the sciatic nerve stretch.[10] Children with postoperative pain managed with an epidural injection are at increased risk for sciatic nerve pain due to the pain medication masking nerve pain and numbness, which allows the child to tolerate extreme nerve stretches that may lead to prolonged nerve palsy.[321] Genu recurvatum is another complication with hamstring lengthening. Overlengthening results in the hamstring losing the ability to control knee extension in swing phase, thus leading to recurvatum in stance phase.[10,327,328] Knee recurvatum often improves over time, but should be controlled in the short term with a solid or articulating AFO set in slight DF.[10]

For more moderate knee flexion contractures (10 to 30 degrees), posterior knee capsulotomy in addition to hamstring release is indicated.[10] Postoperative management is more involved after capsulotomy, with the knees splinted in extension for 12 to 18 hours per day for 6 weeks and nighttime splinting in extension for up to 6 months.[10] Early knee PROM exercise can prevent knee stiffness, but is much more painful. In addition, the risk of sciatic nerve palsy is greater after posterior knee capsulotomy, requiring careful grading of hamstring stretching. Severe knee flexion contractures (>30 degrees) are corrected with distal femoral extension osteotomy. Rehabilitation after extension osteotomy is extensive, often requiring therapy for greater than 1 year. Postoperative precautions include knee flexion PROM limited to 90 degrees and knee immobilizer use when not in therapy. Weight bearing may or may not be limited depending on intraoperative fixation.[10]

Stiff Knee Gait due to Rectus Femoris Dysfunction

A stiff knee gait pattern can be caused by several impairments, including decreased hip flexor strength, poor ankle strength, femoral anteversion, tibial torsion, and rectus femoris muscle dysfunction.[10] Rectus femoris transfer or release is the treatment of choice for decreased knee flexion during the swing phase of gait due to rectus femoris spasticity or inappropriate activation in early to middle swing phase. When a transfer is performed, typically the gracilis tendon is connected to the distal end of the rectus femoris tendon. In the rectus release, either the origin or insertion of the rectus femoris is detached, but taking care to preserve the remaining quadriceps. BTX injection before surgery can help determine the effect a future rectus transfer may have on the child's gait pattern.

Tibial Torsion

In-toeing or out-toeing due to internal or external tibial torsion are both relatively common in children with CP and typically do not improve with maturity, as seen in children with normal motor control.[16] As with femoral anteversion, internal tibial torsion can cause inefficient gait and tripping. Tibial osteotomy is the only effective surgery to correct internal and external tibial torsion. After surgery, there are usually no precautions or weight-bearing limitations. The lower leg is often casted for 6 to 8 weeks. Rehabilitation is unrestricted after cast removal and should focus on improving walking mechanics and balance. With a more normal foot progression angle, the demands on the plantar flexors and dorsiflexors are changed, requiring specific strengthening to help these muscles handle their new demands.

Ankle Joint and Foot
Equinus Deformity

Equinus, the most prevalent foot deformity in children with CP, results from a muscular imbalance in which the plantar flexors of the ankle are five to six times stronger than are the dorsiflexors[10] when there is spasticity around the ankle. In ambulatory children, the hyperactive stretch reflex of the plantar flexors is stimulated during each stance phase, which contributes to the equinus. Spasticity here is manifested as toe-walking, premature heel rise, or premature ankle plantar flexion moment during gait.[10] Children with more severe involvement may have difficulty with foot placement on the pedals of the wheelchair, assisted stand-pivot transfers, and donning of shoes causing a stretch to the triceps surae triggering spastic equinus. Conservative management should include passive stretching, with care taken to lock the subtalar joint by slightly supinating the foot before stretching into DF, nighttime splinting, and strengthening of the dorsiflexors. A MAFO can help maintain a neutral ankle position, but will neither increase the length of the triceps surae nor allow for any strengthening of the dorsiflexors. If the ankle and foot cannot be brought into a neutral position with the knee in extension, the child will not be able to stand with heels on the ground and will need to compensate in some manner. When an equinus ankle is forced into an orthosis set at 90 degrees, there will be skin breakdown on the heel, or the foot will become hypermobile in the joints distal to the calcaneus. Serial casting offers a conservative method to manage a shortened Achilles tendon, with or without BTX-A injections.[270,330,331] There are a variety of protocols to complete a regimen of serial casting across a joint. The number of casts utilized will vary, but the casting trial will typically continue for 2 to 4 weeks. Care must be exercised to lock the subtalar joint while applying the cast to gain DF of the ankle, to ensure stretching of the gastrocnemius/soleus group, and to prevent hypermobility of the subtalar joint.

Tendo Achilles lengthening (TAL) and gastrocnemius recession are the two most common surgical procedures to treat equinus. TAL is most common, and is indicated for contracture of both the gastrocnemius and soleus muscle.[10,308,332] For children with normal soleus length and contracture of the gastrocnemius, the surgical procedure of choice is a gastrocnemius recession.[9] The Silfverskiöld test is often used to determine the difference between soleus and gastrocnemius flexibility (Fig. 9.29A and B), and is used in conjunction with gait analysis to assist with surgical decision making. The gastrocnemius and soleus are two of the most important muscles in ambulation, making the correct amount of lengthening crucial to improving gait mechanics. The goals of lengthening are to decrease triceps surae spasticity, improve heel contact at initial contact, reduce the midstance plantar flexion moment to near normal, and increase power at push-off.[10,333] Reoccurrence or nonimprovement of equinus gait is the most common complication of TAL and gastrocnemius recession, with a reported rate of 5% to 40%.[10,333–337] Typically, no more than two total lengthenings are required to treat equinus during childhood. Overlengthening is a less common but much more serious surgical complication, resulting in excessive DF in midstance. This gait abnormality is often referred to as *calcaneal gait*[338] and causes an increased crouched position, which further stretches the plantar flexors and shortens the hip flexors and hamstrings.[10] There is no therapeutic or surgical treatment that can correct overlengthening. Long term and, in many cases, permanent use of solid AFOs or GRAFOs is often necessary to prevent further progression of crouched gait.

Postoperative care following lengthening or recession requires that a short leg walking cast be worn for 4 to 6 weeks, set in neutral or slight DF. Ambulatory children typically are able to tolerate full weight bearing in the walking casts within the first few days of surgery. After removal of the cast, the child's ankle muscle will be weak owing to the surgery and weeks of immobilization. It may take several weeks for the child to tolerate standing long periods without the casts. Intermittent solid or articulating AFO use for 3 to 6 months after surgery is recommended to help maintain postsurgical DF gains and assist weight bearing with optimal posture. Each child should have an individualized schedule for AFO wear and use the ankle actively when out of the orthosis to facilitate functional strengthening and skill development. It is important to strengthen the entire ankle, especially the dorsiflexors and plantar flexors after surgery. Some clinicians use neuromuscular electrical stimulation (NMES) or FES to activate the dorsiflexors at the appropriate time. The long-term goal of rehabilitation should be optimal gait mechanics and return to presurgical function approximately 6 to 12 months after surgery.

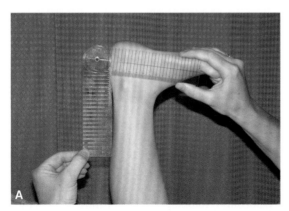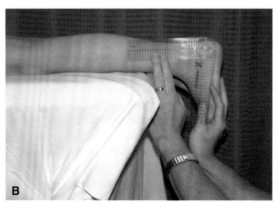

FIGURE 9.29. Silfverskiöld test. Measures the difference in flexibility of the gastrocnemius and the soleus muscles. Soleus length is assessed by recording passive range of motion with knee flexed **(A)**, and gastrocnemius length is measured by recording passive range of motion with knee extended **(B)**.

Planovalgus

A planovalgus foot, commonly known as a *flat foot*, is a deformity caused by multiple factors including spasticity (especially of the peroneals or plantar flexors), LE weakness, ligamentous laxity, genetics, and altered biomechanics during standing and walking.[10] This foot position causes increased pressure on the inside of the foot and great toe during ambulation. This deformity is usually flexible at first, and can be corrected by reducing the subtalar joint and forefoot to a neutral position with the ankle plantar flexed. In severe cases, the foot eventually turns out so significantly that there is virtually no pressure through the plantar surface of the foot. In most children with CP, however, the planovalgus foot never progresses beyond moderate severity and can be managed with correct triceps surae stretching, ankle strengthening, and orthotic shoe inserts. Three situations contribute to more severe planovalgus deformity: (1) spastic peroneal muscles that change the axis of rotation of the subtalar joint to a more horizontal alignment and abduct the midfoot and forefoot; (2) gastrocnemius/soleus contracture causing plantar flexion of the calcaneus; and (3) persistent fetal medial deviation of the neck of the talus.[48] Most children with CP never require surgical intervention for flat feet,[16] but if the planovalgus deformity causes pain or other functional issues with ambulation, there are several surgical corrections commonly used: (1) lateral column lengthening, (2) subtalar arthrodesis,[308] and (3) triple arthrodesis.[10,308]

Lateral column lengthening (also known as calcaneal lengthening) is usually indicated for the milder, more flexible flat foot. This surgical procedure involves an osteotomy of the calcaneus with a bone graft used to maintain the osteotomy open after distraction. This osteotomy lengthens the calcaneus with the goal of pushing the foot into a more supinated position.[10] Subtalar motion is moderately restricted after this surgery, but allows greater three-dimensional motion than does a subtalar fusion and triple arthrodesis. Postoperatively, the child is placed in short leg walking casts until the osteotomy is healed, which takes approximately 10 to 12 weeks.[16] Subtalar arthrodesis is reserved for more severely planovalgus feet in ambulatory children. Surgery involves inserting a bone graft between the talus and calcaneus and then inserting a screw to fuse the bones together in subtalar neutral. Triple arthrodesis is a palliative treatment most often indicated for older children who are nonambulatory or marginal ambulators. The surgical procedure involves subtalar fusion surgery as well as fusion of the cuboid to the calcaneus, navicular to the talus, and first cuneiform to the navicular. Postoperative immobilization with a short leg cast after both fusions is also approximately 12 weeks with WBAT. An orthosis will sometimes be used, depending on the results of the surgery and whether the joint(s) require further stability.[10] Owing to joint fusion, the therapist may note joint hypermobility in joints distal to the fusion. This hypermobility should be monitored and may eventually require orthoses to control instability and prevent pain (Fig. 9.30).

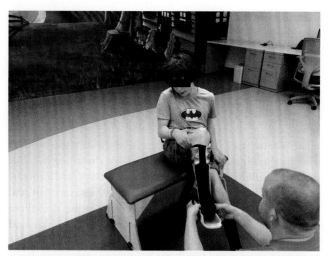

FIGURE 9.30. Donning ground-reaction ankle–foot orthosis (AFO) post orthopedic surgical intervention in preparation for walking.

Varus Deformity

Varus deformity in the ankle is less common in children with CP, and is seen mostly in children with hemiplegia or diplegia. It results from an imbalance between weak peroneal muscles and spastic posterior or anterior tibialis muscles.[308] The varus foot is very unstable and at risk for inversion ankle sprain. Surgery is often delayed until about 8 years of age. The foot is best managed with splinting, stretching, and strengthening until that time. The indication for surgery is a varus foot in stance or swing phase of gait. Surgical procedures performed for this deformity include lengthening or splitting and transferring of either the posterior or anterior tibialis muscle.[10,308,339–341] Postoperatively, the foot is often casted in a neutral or slightly dorsiflexed position for 4 weeks in a short leg walking cast.[10] After the cast is removed, rehabilitation can be performed without restriction or with an orthosis. Therapeutic intervention should emphasize muscle reeducation, particularly when a muscle has been transferred.

>> Lower extremity orthoses

The decision to use an orthosis and the choice of which orthosis to use should be a collaborative decision between the family, orthopedic surgeon, physiatrist, child, orthotist, and PT. In ambulatory children, the selection should also be based on the understanding of the primary gait deviations.[342] Besides gait observations, the PT's contribution to the team includes examination of available ROM, both PROM and AROM; foot alignment and flexibility during weight-bearing and non–weight-bearing situations (structural vs. functional deformity); voluntary control of movement in the leg, ankle, and foot; current functional abilities; and the desired functional and participatory outcomes from the device. Because the foot is used for both stability and mobility, the effects of an orthosis on both functions must be considered carefully. It is important to remember that an orthosis will provide stability, but will also limit the available movement and any opportunity to strengthen the muscles across the joint being stabilized. Because of this restriction of motion, an orthosis should allow as much motion as possible and only control the undesired movement. There are a variety of options available to allow the health care team to choose the least restrictive and most functional orthoses.

When a child is provided an orthosis, the family should be given a specific wearing schedule to prevent skin breakdown, promote improved function during wearing times, and avoid the atrophy that occurs when a joint or limb is immobilized for an extended period. An orthosis for an infant is rare unless there is a structural deformity that can be influenced by immobilization. It is usually when an infant begins consistent weight bearing in standing that an LE orthosis may be considered to manage how the foot contacts the floor.

A common question after fitting a child with a new LE orthoses is "What type of shoes should we buy?" When answering this question, the therapist must consider the family's resources, the width and intended function of the orthoses and shoes, age of the child, the appearance of the shoe, and the environment in which the orthoses will be used. A larger shoe is often required to accommodate the orthosis, but too large a shoe often has a negative impact on gait mechanics. A typical recommendation is not to exceed 1 to 1.5 sizes larger than the shoe size typically worn without the orthosis. Therapist knowledge of shoe brands that are typically wider is helpful in these cases. If the orthoses fit easily into the new shoe when donned for the first time, it is recommended to try at least a 0.5 size smaller. An exception to this rule is the nonambulatory child, in which case comfort and ease of donning is of much greater importance than a snug fit. Many LE orthoses today are molded to stabilize the midfoot and forefoot, which reduces the need for a motion-control shoe with a good arch support. In general, a low-top, wide shoe with a straight last and an insole that is easily removed may be the best choice for most children. Shoes that are manufactured specifically for children with LE orthosis are available today, but many common brands of shoes work as well.

The following section describes the most common orthoses prescribed for children with CP. Table 9.9 details common indications, contraindications, and special considerations for each type of orthoses, which may also be helpful to therapists in their clinical decision-making process.

Ankle–Foot Orthoses

Ankle equinus is the most common joint malalignment in children with CP.[10] For decades, custom-molded AFOs have been the most common method of blocking equinus in children with CP.[343] The modern high-temperature thermoplastics used today for AFOs are able to withstand significant plantar flexion force. Although many variations of AFOs have been studied, there is limited data supporting

one type of AFO over another. Figueiredo et al. reviewed the efficacy of AFOs on the gait of children with CP. The authors concluded that AFOs have a positive effect on ankle ROM, gait kinematics and kinetics, and functional activities related to mobility.[344] Unfortunately, because studies with high-quality methods are lacking, it is difficult to conclude which group of children would benefit from which type of AFO.[344] Given here is the most current evidence supporting the use of the most commonly prescribed AFOs: traditional solid AFOs, articulating ankle AFOs, posterior leaf spring (PLS) AFOs, and GRAFOs. It should also be noted that there are many styles and designs of each type of AFO including the tone-reducing, thin-plastic, wrap-around design commonly used for many children with CP. This design of AFO, commonly referred to as a *dynamic ankle–foot orthosis* (DAFO), was created and popularized by Cascade DAFO, Inc. Although DAFOs are not a different type of AFO, this section also discusses how this design differs from traditional AFO designs.

Solid Molded Ankle–Foot Orthoses

A solid MAFO with anterior tibial strap and anterior ankle strap is a common orthotic design to provide ankle and foot stability, giving a stable base for children to stand. The thick, high-temperature thermoplastic, absence of ankle joint motion, and high calf design of this traditional orthosis allows maximum medial-lateral ankle stability and maximum knee stability in standing, and can resist strong plantar flexor spasticity. The solid AFO has also been shown to increase the plantar flexor moment in terminal stance,[345] normalize ankle kinematics in stance,[346] increase stride length,[346,347] and improve the performance of walking/running/jumping skills as measured by the GMFM.[346] A study conducted by Buckton et al.[346] concluded that most children with spastic diplegia would benefit functionally from a solid AFO or PLS-AFO. The solid AFO is also a good choice for the child with severe equinovarus or equinovalgus deformity. Articulating MAFOs, PLS-AFOs, and DAFOs do not control midfoot and forefoot deformity well and eventually could lead to greater foot deformity. Solid AFOs are also commonly prescribed for children who are short-distance ambulators or nonambulatory. The short-distance ambulator with significant crouch often requires a more traditional, thicker plastic, solid AFO to minimize excessive DF and knee flexion. The main purpose of an AFO for a nonambulating child with CP is to improve ankle position and prevent contracture. Comfort and prevention of skin breakdown is important, and a simple, well-padded solid AFO is an appropriate choice to improve ankle position, minimize skin issues, and allow for an easy application for the caregiver. The drawbacks of this orthosis include overall bulkiness of the plastic, making it difficult for caregivers to find shoes that fit this type of brace, decreased distal muscle activation when balancing in standing,[348] and a negative effect on dynamic balance with functional activities such as transitions to standing and negotiating stairs. An elastic proximal tibial strap is sometimes used to allow a small

TABLE 9.9. **Guide to Orthoses Selection for Children with CP**

Orthoses	Solid Molded Ankle–Foot Orthoses (MAFO)	Dynamic Ankle–Foot Orthoses (DAFO)	Articulated MAFO
	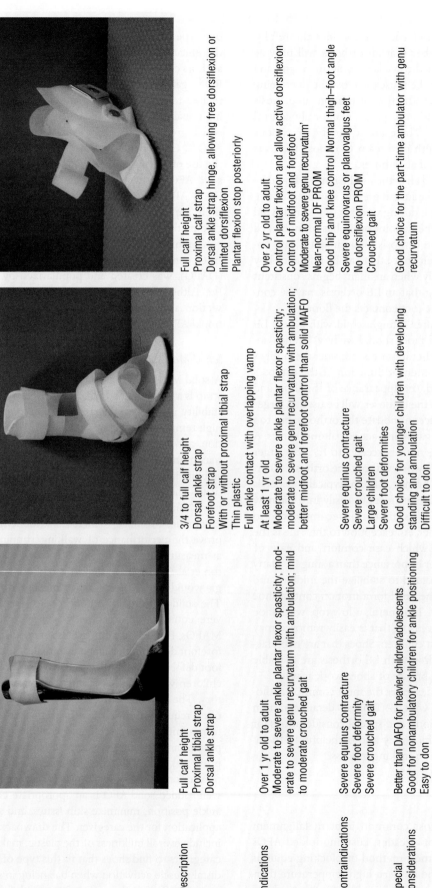		
Description	Full calf height Proximal tibial strap Dorsal ankle strap	3/4 to full calf height Dorsal ankle strap Forefoot strap With or without proximal tibial strap Thin plastic Full ankle contact with overlapping vamp	Full calf height Proximal calf strap Dorsal ankle strap hinge, allowing free dorsiflexion or limited dorsiflexion Plantar flexion stop posteriorly
Indications	Over 1 yr old to adult Moderate to severe ankle plantar flexor spasticity; moderate to severe genu recurvatum with ambulation; mild to moderate crouched gait	At least 1 yr old Moderate to severe ankle plantar flexor spasticity; moderate to severe genu recurvatum with ambulation; better midfoot and forefoot control than solid MAFO	Over 2 yr old to adult Control plantar flexion and allow active dorsiflexion Control of midfoot and forefoot Moderate to severe genu recurvatum' Near-normal DF PROM Good hip and knee control Normal thigh–foot angle
Contraindications	Severe equinus contracture Severe foot deformity Severe crouched gait	Severe equinus contracture Severe crouched gait Large children Severe foot deformities	Severe equinovarus or planovalgus feet No dorsiflexion PROM Crouched gait
Special considerations	Better than DAFO for heavier children/adolescents Good for nonambulatory children for ankle positioning Easy to don	Good choice for younger children with developing standing and ambulation Difficult to don	Good choice for the part-time ambulator with genu recurvatum

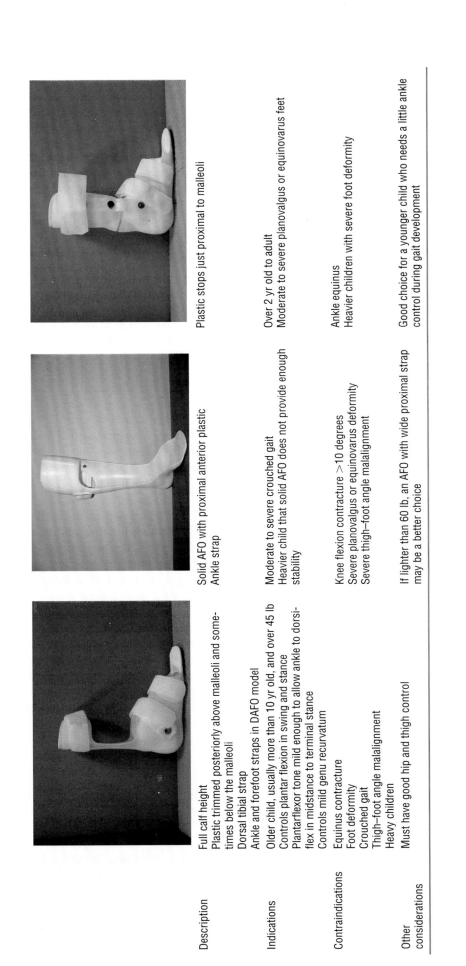

Description	Full calf height Plastic trimmed posteriorly above malleoli and some- times below the malleoli Dorsal tibial strap Ankle and forefoot straps in DAFO model	Solid AFO with proximal anterior plastic Ankle strap	Plastic stops just proximal to malleoli
Indications	Older child, usually more than 10 yr old, and over 45 lb Controls plantar flexion in swing and stance Plantarflexor tone mild enough to allow ankle to dorsi- flex in midstance to terminal stance Controls mild genu recurvatum	Moderate to severe crouched gait Heavier child that solid AFO does not provide enough stability	Over 2 yr old to adult Moderate to severe planovalgus or equinovarus feet
Contraindications	Equinus contracture Foot deformity Crouched gait Thigh–foot angle malalignment Heavy children	Knee flexion contracture >10 degrees Severe planovalgus or equinovarus deformity Severe thigh–foot angle malalignment	Ankle equinus Heavier children with severe foot deformity
Other considerations	Must have good hip and thigh control	If lighter than 60 lb, an AFO with wide proximal strap may be a better choice	Good choice for a younger child who needs a little ankle control during gait development

349

amount of passive DF, thus making it slightly more dynamic in standing.

Articulating Ankle–Foot Orthoses

An articulating AFO includes ankle articulation, allowing free DF and plantar flexion or free DF with a plantar flexion stop. The most frequently prescribed articulating AFO used for children with CP allows for free DF with a plantar flexion stop. These orthoses inhibit plantar flexion hypertonus while permitting free DF, thus giving the child increased ease in rising to stand, negotiating stairs, and ambulating. By allowing free ankle DF and some plantar flexion, they also encourage ankle activation, which may help strengthen the muscles crossing the ankle joint. Significant biomechanical changes were found when the ankle was given freedom to move with an articulating AFO. The benefits included more natural ankle motion during stance, increased stride length, and greater symmetry of segmental LE motion.[345,349–351] Buckton et al.[346] noted that an articulating AFO has a detrimental effect on the gait in some children with diplegic CP, including increased peak knee extensor moment in early stance (leading to recurvatum), excessive ankle DF (which would contribute to crouch), and decreased walking velocity. Night splinting with an articulating AFO combined with an adjustable strap attached at the footplate by the toes can be used in some children to increase the length of the gastrocnemius/soleus group by maintaining a prolonged stretch into DF. Low-load prolonged stretch of the gastrocnemius is an ideal way to slowly improve DF in some children. Lack of comfort and disturbed sleep are common concerns for therapists and families with this type of orthoses. A recent study by Mol et al.[352] refutes that claim and found no statistical significance in sleep disturbances between children using and not using night orthoses.

Posterior Leaf Spring Orthoses

A PLS orthosis is an AFO primarily used for children with foot drop, but with some stability in stance phase.[353] The PLS-AFO design, with the thermoplastic trimmed posteriorly to the malleoli, is strong enough to prevent plantar flexion during swing and stance phases of gait but flexible enough to allow some anterior tibial translation and DF from midstance to the beginning of terminal stance. The PLS-AFO is also proposed to have a "spring effect" at push-off. When the posterior plastic is put on tension as the ankle dorsiflexes, energy is theoretically stored in the plastic and then released to assist plantar flexion during terminal stance. This may decrease fatigue with ambulation in some children with CP.[354] There are multiple strut thicknesses and carbon fiber options available to grade the amount of tibial translation and "spring effect" during ambulation. Thicker plastic posteriorly and/or posterior reinforcement with carbon fiber may be necessary to control more severe crouch in larger children. Ounuu et al.[353] found that the PLS-AFO design improves DF during swing and initial contact and allowed normal DF in midstance, but

does not improve the power-generating capabilities of the ankle in children with CP as its name suggests. Careful consideration should be made before choosing this AFO design for a child with CP owing to its decreased overall stability and decreased subtalar, midtarsal, and forefoot control. For children with foot deformities, PLS-AFOs can be combined with a supramalleolar orthosis (SMO) insert to provide the necessary foot stability.

Ground-Reaction Orthoses

The GRAFO (also known as floor-reaction AFO) is commonly prescribed for ambulatory children who walk with excessive DF and knee flexion (crouched gait) during the stance phase of gait.[342] A floor-reaction brace is both a stance- and swing-control orthosis designed to provide increased resistance to both ankle DF and plantar flexion.[342] A DAFO or traditional AFO also helps control crouch in younger children with CP, but as a child's crouched gait approaches 55 degrees of knee flexion at midstance, a more supportive floor-reaction orthosis is often required. The floor-reaction AFO is more rigid because of increased plastic thickness, a broad anterior wall (supporting either proximal tibial only or whole length of lower leg), and, in some cases, carbon fiber reinforcement.[342] This rigidity provides superior resistance to the strong knee flexion and DF moment in the second rocker of the stance phase. To benefit from this type of orthosis, the child must have at least DF to neutral with the knee extended and less than 20 degrees of internal or external tibial torsion.[10] This orthosis has traditionally not been ideal for children with severe foot malalignments, but newer designs (such as one utilizing an SMO placed within the outer AFO shell) make it an option for some children with mild foot deformities. Rogozinski et al. concluded that the best outcomes with floor-reaction orthosis, as determined by peak knee flexion in midstance, occurred when children had knee and hip flexion contractures less than or equal to 10 degrees. The efficacy of the orthosis in controlling peak knee flexion in midstance was poor in children with knee and hip contractures greater than or equal to 15 degrees, thus making the floor-reaction orthosis a poor choice in these children.[342]

Dynamic Ankle–Foot Orthoses

In the past 20 years, inhibitive AFOs or DAFOs have become very popular as an alternative to conventional AFOs. DAFOs evolved from inhibitive casts used during the 1970s.[355] Inhibitive casts were purported to decrease spasticity by providing a prolonged stretch and pressure on the tendons of the triceps surae muscle and toe flexors and to inhibit or decrease abnormal reflexes in the LE by protecting the foot from tactile-induced reflexes.[356] The footplate in a DAFO is a custom-contoured plate similar to that used with inhibitive casting. It has built-up areas under the toes, lateral and medial longitudinal arches, and a transverse metatarsal arch with recessed areas under the metatarsal and calcaneal pad areas. These features provide support and stabilization to the arches of the foot and position the midtarsal and subtalar joints in a neutral position.[356] "The footplate is designed to reduce abnormal muscle activity and to effect biomechanical changes, including decreased excessive ankle plantar flexion and improved motions of the lower extremity, pelvis, and trunk during standing and gait."[356] Evidence supporting molding the DAFO footplate with pressure points to inhibit tone is very limited, although this is still commonly used in DAFO designs.[10,357] The DAFO also differs from a traditional AFO in that it provides total contact to the ankle with its wrap-around design. The circumferential design with overlapping vamp may improve proprioception, distribute forces over a larger area of skin, and improve overall alignment, but often makes it more difficult for the child or parent to don the orthosis. Because it requires two hands and considerable strength to open the DAFO, many children may not become independent donning this orthosis. Strapping options on a DAFO include a toe loop to stabilize the first digit, a forefoot strap to control forefoot position, and an ankle strap over the talus that holds the heel down into the heel cup. The DAFO is also made of a thinner, more flexible plastic that allows graded motion, unlike the rigid 3/16 inch plastic used in most traditional solid AFOs. This thinner plastic cannot withstand high-stress environments, thus making it ineffective for many children. The thin, total-contact design also cannot be easily modified if skin problems arise or the child has a growth spurt, limiting the overall life of the orthoses.

The effect of DAFOs on gait mechanics and function has not been extensively studied. Currently, there is conflicting evidence that DAFOs significantly change gait parameters or walking kinematics.[347,351,356,358] Radtka[356] found that both DAFOs with a plantar flexion stop and traditional AFOs increased stride length, decreased cadence, and reduced excessive ankle plantar flexion when compared with no orthoses. Lam et al. demonstrated additional biomechanical gait benefits with the DAFO use compared with the traditional AFO. Specifically, study subjects wearing DAFOs demonstrated increased knee flexion at initial contact compared with traditional AFOs.[347] Carlson et al.,[358] on the other hand, found that neither AFOs nor DAFOs significantly influenced stride length or walking speed. The DAFO also was not found to have much effect on walking kinematics.[358] Romkes and Brunner[351] also concluded in their 2002 study that DAFOs did not improve gait significantly, but hinged AFOs did improve gait.

Recent evidence suggests that DAFOs have a positive effect on gross motor function and balance in children with CP. Bjornson et al.[359] reported significant improvements in crawling/kneeling, standing, and walking/running and jumping skills as measured by the GMFM 88 and 66 with short-term DAFO use. Burtner et al.[348] investigated balance differences between children wearing solid AFOs and DAFOs. Their study showed that children wearing the more rigid AFO had a decreased ability to respond to balance threats and substitute with an alternate balance strategy. These issues did not occur in the children wearing DAFOs, suggesting that DAFOs are more advantageous for children with spastic CP when balance is perturbed unexpectedly, such as being bumped into by a classmate or standing on a moving object such as a bus that slows down or speeds up suddenly.[348]

Supramalleolar Orthoses

The SMO is typically indicated for the child with good ankle plantar flexion and DF control but who needs control of planovarus or planovalgus foot position. The SMO typically has trim lines anterior and superior to the malleoli and a molded footplate providing control at the subtalar joint, midfoot, and forefoot. An anterior ankle strap is occasionally necessary to improve the effectiveness of the SMO.[10] The wrap-around thin-plastic design found in the Cascade DAFO, Inc.–style SMO is often a good option for younger children, but may not be strong enough to control the foot in larger or adolescents.[10] SMOs have been shown to improve balance in children with Down syndrome[360] and those with hemiplegia,[361] but studies on the efficacy of SMO use in children with CP are limited.[362–364]

Foot Orthoses

When the child with CP has control of the ankle joint but requires external support when the foot contacts the floor, a foot orthosis is desirable. For children with CP with good ankle and knee control, but poor midfoot and forefoot alignment, a foot orthosis may be beneficial. Foot orthoses include the University of California Berkley Laboratory (UCBL) orthoses and arch supports. UCBL trim lines are inferior to the medial or lateral malleoli, but proximal enough to support the navicular and thus control excessive pronation. The footplate can be proximal or distal to the metatarsal heads, dependent on each child's unique needs. Foot orthoses can be custom molded or purchased OTC from a variety of resources.

Use of a shoe insert is indicated for the following:

- Control of the calcaneus, subtalar, and midtarsal joints
- Improved alignment and stability of the LEs and pelvis
- Management of the forefoot for neutral positioning
- Knee pain secondary to foot pathology

Combining Orthoses

A recent trend in orthotics is to order a brace with multiple parts to provide multiple brace options for the child. One such product is the DAFO TURBO (Cascade DAFO, Inc., Bellingham, WA), which is a combination of an SMO and AFO. This may be appropriate for the young child with spastic- or hemiplegic-type CP. The SMO piece can be used for functional activities that require free DF/plantar flexion, and the combined orthoses can be used when more ankle stability is required. This combination orthoses is also commonly prescribed for the child with such severe plantar flexor spasticity that donning a traditional DAFO is extremely difficult for the caregiver. This design allows the caregiver to more easily don the SMO piece first while maintaining ankle DF. Once the SMO piece is donned, the AFO portion can be attached by keeping the child's heel seated appropriately in the SMO portion.

» School-based therapy

Communication between the school therapist and the child's teacher is essential for appropriate and effective management and education of the child in the classroom. The therapist should obtain information from the teacher regarding the child's daily routine at school. With that information, joint planning for the child can result in an effective and efficient educational program. Major areas of emphasis in school-based therapy services include evaluating any barriers to independence in the classroom or school, evaluating alignment at different times during the day while the child is sitting in their personal wheelchair or classroom seat, and evaluating the opportunities available to stand, and, when applicable, ambulate safely. Consistent movement throughout the day, such as standing, walking between activity centers in the classroom, or participating in physical education class, will provide relief from the sitting position. There should be a sharing of the responsibility, assistance, and supervision required between the classroom staff and the child for quantity and quality of position changes and movement. The physical education teacher should be informed of joint movement goals and specific types or patterns of movement that may either be deleterious or beneficial for the child. There should also be a review conducted with teachers for the purpose of and proper use of splints, orthotics, and other assistive or adaptive devices.

The OT will share information about the child's fine motor, visual motor, visual perception, visual discrimination, and manipulation skills; attention span; cognition; sensory system modulation; emotional level; and adaptive self-help skills. The speech pathologist will inform the team about the child's speech and language capabilities. This information, along with specific suggestions, should facilitate learning for the child.

Therapists should work with the classroom staff to ensure that the personnel work appropriately with the child in the maintenance of correct alignment, relief from prolonged sitting, use of adaptive or assistive devices, and attention to issues regarding safety. Remember, the role of physical therapy in the educational setting is to optimize the child's ability to learn in that environment. This will involve good communication and collaboration with all the members of the child's Individualized Education Plan (IEP) team (Fig. 9.31).

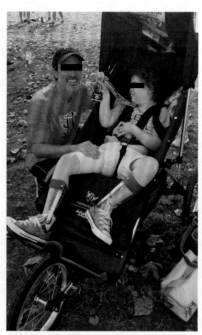

FIGURE 9.31. Family 5K win! The ultimate way to participate in life!

Summary

This chapter explores the distinct challenges facing children and youth with CP, because each child presents with a unique constellation of neuromuscular, musculoskeletal, sensory/perceptual, and cognitive concerns. To be effective in the examination, evaluation, and treatment of children and youth with CP, the physical therapist must consider the complex needs of the child and his or her family. The framework provided by the ICF model allows the physical therapist to categorize the child's strengths and areas of concern while keeping in focus the child and family's activity and participation goals. It is imperative that the physical therapist maintain open communication with the child, the family/caregiver, and the rest of the interdisciplinary team. The ultimate outcome of treatment is to help children maximize their functional independence and help them participate within their home and community to their greatest potential.

Acknowledgments

We thank Jane Styer-Acevedo, PT, for her ongoing mentorship, knowledge, inspiration, and contributions to this chapter. We extend our heartfelt gratitude to Dr. Freeman Miller, Dr. Wade Shrader, and Dr. Jason Howard whose willingness to share their expertise of CP has been critical to our ability to treat our patients effectively and write this chapter. We thank Nancy Lennon, PT, who has been an integral mentor to us as the CP program coordinator at Nemours/Alfred I. duPont Hospital for Children. We also thank Chris Church, PT, for his assistance with the "Gait" section; Gary Mickalowski, CPO, and Heather Mickalowski, CPO, for assisting with the "Orthoses" section; Denise Peischl for her help with the adaptive equipment section; Jeanne-Marie Shanline, MPT, for her contribution to the NDT section; Caitlin Grimes, MS OTR/L for her contribution to the CIMT section, as well as our supervisors and colleagues at Nemours/AI duPont Hospital for Children who have mentored and supported us. Last but certainly not least, we thank our families for supporting our efforts this past year. Their understanding of our motivation to write this chapter has made it possible for us to focus our time and attention to it. This chapter would NEVER have been completed without you.

CASE STUDIES

CASE STUDY 1

Ella is a 5-year-old girl with a diagnosis of left hemiplegic/unilateral-pattern CP referred to outpatient physical therapy owing to decreased left LE flexibility, increased gait dysfunction, and poor overall balance. Ella's parents express concern about Ella's safety at school and on the school playground, because she will enter kindergarten in the fall.

Past Medical History

Ella is a bright and happy 5-year-old girl who was diagnosed with left hemiplegia around 1 year. She was born full term at 38 weeks' gestation. During the birthing process, a fetal monitor showed frequent fluctuations in Ella's heart rate, indicating distress. For this reason, immediately following her birth, she underwent an MRI to determine whether any cerebral insult occurred. This neuroimaging showed a grade IV IVH, enlarged lateral ventricles with the right ventricle larger than the left, increased head circumference, and bulging fontanels. At this time, she also presented with nystagmus. She underwent a shunt placement at 3 months of age owing to congenital hydrocephalus. She was evaluated at 6 months of age by an ophthalmologist who diagnosed her with cortical visual impairment, optic atrophy, and severe visual impairment. An orthopedic surgeon, who gave Ella the diagnosis of left hemiplegia after her first birthday, has also followed her up from infancy.

Developmental History

Ella participated in occupational therapy, physical therapy, and speech and language therapy from birth owing to concerns related to overall developmental delay. She was provided all of these services in her home through an early intervention program to address functional concerns that arose from her left hemiplegia, decreased mobility, and decreased vocalizations. At 5 months, Ella was able to roll from supine to prone and vice versa, initiating both transitions by arching through her back and neck. She was able to sit independently at 11 months, but preferred a "W" position. At 18 months, she began creeping with an asymmetrical "bunny hop" pattern. At 21 months, Ella was able to stand independently with right UE support at the family couch and cruise in both directions; however, she preferred to cruise to the right. At 24 months, Ella took her first independent steps, and was walking consistently without an assistive device at 30 months.

Physical Therapy Examination

Precautions:

Ventriculoperitoneal shunt

Pain:

According to the Wong-Baker Faces Pain Scale, Ella reported a 0/10 pain level related to activities of tasks.

ROM:

Right hip, knee, and ankle: within normal limits (WNL); left hip flexion: 100 degrees, left hip extension: 10 degrees, left knee extension: WNL, left popliteal angle: 35 degrees, left ankle DF with knee extension: −2 degrees, left ankle DF with knee flexed: 5 degrees; right shoulder, elbow, and wrist: WNL; left shoulder flexion: 100 degrees, left elbow flexion: WNL, left elbow extension: 10 degrees, left wrist flexion: WNL, left wrist extension: 15 degrees.

Strength:

MMT bilaterally: right hip, knee, and ankle: 5/5; left hip flexion: 3/5; left hip abduction: 2/5; left hip adduction: 2/5; left knee extension: 3/5; left prone knee flexion: 21/5; left ankle DF: trace.

Muscle tone:

Modified ashworth scale (MAS): left quadriceps: 1/5; left hamstrings: 2/5; three-beat clonus in left ankle.

Sensation:

Intact to light touch, hot and cold, sharp and dull.

Functional Mobility:

Ella is able to transition from sit-to-stand with increased weight shift to the left. She is able to transition from floor to standing through half-kneel, leading with the right LE and pulling up on an object using the right UE. She is unable to hop on the left foot, but can hop three times in a row on the right. She fatigues quickly, and is not able to keep up with her peers on the playground.

Gait/Steps:

Ella is able to ambulate independently with an asymmetrical gait pattern. She presents with decreased stance time and weight shift on the left in stance phase, has a shortened step length on the left, a retracted pelvis on the left, stiff knee on the left during swing, and initial contact with her forefoot on the left. She is noted to have inconsistent mild knee recurvatum during midstance on the left as well. She is able to ascend standard steps with a step-two pattern, holding a railing with her right hand and leading with her right foot. When descending steps, she leads with her left foot while holding the railing with her right hand.

Balance:

Single-limb stance on the right for 5 to 8 seconds; left less than 1 second.

Equipment:

Ella has a solid AFO for her left LE, but parents report that she has not worn them in the past 9 months owing to skin irritation and complaints of pain whenever she wore it.

Physical Therapy Evaluation/Prognosis

Ella is a 5-year-old girl with a diagnosis of left hemiplegia. She presented with left LE weakness, decreased ROM, decreased endurance, gait deficits, and difficulty keeping up with her peers. Overall, her prognosis was favorable. She would be able to safely attend her local public elementary school with some necessary accommodations. She would benefit from continued school-based services and medical-model therapies to support her following a change in status or other medical interventions. She is also involved in a community dance class, which allows her to interact with her peers and work on balance and strengthening in a fun and social setting.

Intervention
Physical therapy intervention one to two times a week, including the following:

Stretching:
Stretching left hip extensors, left hamstring, left gastrocnemius, and soleus, three repetitions with a 30-second hold for each stretch.

Strength Training:
Strengthening of left and right LEs was addressed through play skills, because a formal strengthening program was not appropriate owing to Ella's age. Activities included sidestepping, transitions on and off the floor and from sit-to-stand, and forward and lateral step-ups.

Therapeutic Handling:
Therapeutic ball work to address core strengthening, postural control, and left LE strengthening and stretching; facilitation of agonist/antagonist muscle groups during transitions to promote postural alignment and equal weight shifting.

Bracing:
After Ella achieved 2 degrees of knee-extended DF PROM with regular stretching, an articulating, thin-plastic, total-contact design AFO (Cascade DAFO 2) was recommended for use 6 to 8 hours per day. With her new AFO, Ella almost immediately demonstrated consistent left heel strike, no genu recurvatum, and improved weight shift to the left during stance phase.

Gait Training:
Gait training focused on improving heel strike at initial contact on the left, weight shifting to the left during stance phase, stride length on the left, and pelvic–femoral mobility due to pelvic retraction on the left.

Child/Parent Education:
Home program consisted of stretching and strengthening activities associated with the goals that were being addressed during treatment.

Discharge/Continuum of Care:
Ella's parents have been intimately involved in all intervention decisions and have been excellent advocates for all her needs. She has benefited from a variety of interventions at home, in the medical model, and now in school, and within the community. Ella will most likely continue to make progress toward a productive, full life with her family and friends, given the therapeutic and external support necessary.

CASE STUDY 2
Thomas is a 12-year-old boy with a diagnosis of spastic quadriplegic CP referred to outpatient physical therapy 1 week after extensive surgical interventions including bilateral VDROs, a right Dega procedure, bilateral adductor and hamstring lengthenings, and bilateral lateral column lengthenings.

Past Medical History
Thomas has an extensive medical history. He was born at 29 weeks of gestation and spent 6 weeks in the neonatal intensive care unit (NICU), during which time he was orally intubated for 2 days, then placed on supplemental oxygen via nasal cannula. He had a feeding tube and several other intravenous lines placed during his NICU stay. He underwent cranial ultrasound to determine the extent of his neurologic insult; however, this assessment did not reveal neuroanatomic changes. Thomas had an echocardiogram to rule out cardiac involvement without significant findings. He was discharged from the NICU with an apnea monitor because of respiratory concerns.

Thomas progressed slowly with his gross and fine motor milestones, and often used atypical movement patterns to move. At 6 months, he was able to roll from supine to and from prone, but initiated movement with neck and back extension while rolling his body as a complete unit. Thomas was not able to activate his trunk flexors to allow dissociated movement of his UEs from his LEs while rolling. He first attained stability in sitting using a "W" sit pattern, with an anterior pelvic tilt, bilateral hip internal rotation and adduction, knee flexion, and ankle DF. Thomas' truncal hypotonicity made sitting without assistance or external support difficult and inefficient. He was able to ring-sit and side-sit with minimal to moderate physical assistance.

By 18 months of age, he was able to maintain ring-sitting with bilateral UE support and close supervision. He attempted to creep; however, owing to poor lower limb dissociation was unable to coordinate the sequence needed to reciprocally creep. He moved around his environment by advancing both arms alternately, then both legs simultaneously using extensor tone to initiate the movement, with poor ability to sustain LE hip flexion.

At 18 months, Thomas underwent his first eye surgery due to retinopathy of prematurity (ROP). This was followed by a second eye corrective surgery when he was 2.5 years old. Following his second eye surgery, his visual perception notably improved during ambulation. Gait training was initiated using a gait trainer with a trunk support, hip guides, bilateral ankle prompts, bilateral forearm prompts, and tilted hand grips to accommodate hand placement. By the time Thomas was 2.5 years old, he had progressed from a gait trainer to a posterior walker with hip guides. He ambulated with limited trunk rotation, increased adduction bilaterally during swing phase causing the forefoot to hit the heel of the stance-phase leg ("scissoring"), decreased terminal knee extension in stance phase due to tight hamstrings (crouched posture), and initial contact at his forefoot/toes due to increased plantar flexor tone and decreased ankle ROM. Owing to his inefficient and effortful gait pattern, Thomas used a manual wheelchair for long distances.

To address the spasticity of his LEs, he received BTX-A injections to his bilateral hamstrings, gastrocnemius, and adductors when he was 3 and again when he was 5 years old. He underwent bilateral hamstring lengthenings at age 6 years. At that time, he also had an adenoidectomy to resolve persistent snoring and difficulty sleeping.

Thomas was involved in therapy from a young age. He participated in home-based early intervention services for the first

3 years of his life, received physical and occupational therapies at a children's hospital on an outpatient basis, then moved into weekly school-based services at the age of 5. He had both medically based physical therapy and occupational therapy at a frequency of one to three times a week until the age of 9. His family was very involved in his care and was consistent in helping Thomas carry over a home exercise program, which changed as his functional abilities improved. Thomas was very involved in school activities, and with his improved functional mobility, he did not receive medically based physical therapy after the age of 9.

Prior Level of Function

Thomas underwent extensive surgical intervention at the age of 12 owing to continued growth, weight gain, increased LE spasticity and contractures, increased crouch gait pattern, pain, poor bony alignment, and decreased ability to move around within his home and classroom.

Functional Mobility:

Before surgery, Thomas was able to transition from sit-to-stand and transition into his walker with close supervision. He was able to transition onto and off the floor by pulling up on a stationary object with minimal physical assistance. He required moderate physical assistance to do so using a half-kneel-to-stand pattern.

Gait/Steps:

Before surgery, Thomas independently ambulated with a posterior walker and bilateral Cascade Turbo braces, using a crouched gait pattern with increased adduction across midline during the swing phase of gait. He was able to ambulate household distances and move through his classroom with his walker. He used a manual wheelchair for long distances to minimize fatigue. He was able to manage a curb step given moderate physical assistance.

Bracing:

At the age of 12, Thomas was wearing AFOs with SMO inserts, commonly known as TURBO braces made by Cascade. Before surgery, he presented with an increased crouched gait pattern.

Physical Therapy Examination

Following surgery, Thomas had an acute inpatient stay at a children's hospital where he received physical therapy for bed mobility and transfer training, along with parent education on precautions following surgery. Once he was discharged from the hospital, he returned to undergo an outpatient physical therapy initial examination to determine his postoperative plan of care. The results of this evaluation were as follows.

Precautions:

No hip flexion greater than 90 degrees, no forceful hip internal or external rotation, no adduction across midline; knee immobilizers to be worn 2 hours on, 2 hours off and throughout the night; WBAT in short leg casts.

Pain:

According to the Numeric Pain Scale (0 to 10), Thomas reported a 5/10 pain overall, but reports that his left foot is most painful.

ROM:

Bilateral hip flexion to 90 degrees, hip abduction to 35 degrees, hip adduction to neutral, popliteal angles: 25 degrees, ankle motion not tested secondary to short leg casts.

Strength:

MMT bilaterally: hip flexion: 21/5; hip abduction: 1/5; hip adduction: 2/5; knee extension: 3/5; prone knee flexion: 2/5; ankle testing not possible secondary to short leg casts.

Tone:

MAS: 2/5 in bilateral adductors and hamstrings.

Sensation:

Bilateral LE sensation was intact to light touch, hot and cold, sharp and dull.

Functional Mobility:

Required moderate physical assistance to perform sit-to-stand transfer; floor-to-stand transfer deferred at this time.

Gait/Steps:

Ambulates using a posterior walker for 10 feet and moderate physical assistance, wearing bilateral knee immobilizers and short leg casts.

Balance:

Thomas is able to maintain static standing with both knee immobilizers donned for 5 to 10 seconds without bilateral UE support on his walker; able to stand 30 seconds with UE support on his walker.

Equipment:

Thomas is currently using a manual wheelchair at school, but family notes that his propulsion was slow and inefficient, causing difficulty keeping up with peers. The therapists discussed the advantage of using a powered wheelchair with Thomas and his family, and explained that a powered wheelchair would provide Thomas energy-efficient mobility for long distances in all environments. Thomas and his family are considering power mobility now that he is older, owing to decreased endurance and his inefficient gait pattern. Thomas repeatedly states that he enjoys school and would like to reserve some energy for academics rather than using it all to get from one class to another. His family is in the process of getting a van modified with a wheelchair lift to accommodate the increased weight and size of a powered chair.

Physical Therapy Evaluation/Prognosis

Thomas is a 12-year-old young man with a diagnosis of spastic quadriplegic CP. He recently underwent extensive LE surgery to improve hip joint orientation, increase muscle length, and improve foot alignment. He presents with impairments, including pain, increased LE tone, decreased LE strength, decreased balance, and poor endurance. As a result, he presents with inefficient gait patterns, decreased independence with functional mobility and transfers. The outlook for treatment is good because of his motivation to walk. Thomas, along with his family and therapists, determined that his long-term goal is to walk 25 feet across a stage at school, then stand for about 5 to 10 minutes using his walker alongside his classmates at the end-of-year celebration.

Interventions for first 6 months post the surgery (frequency: three, 60-minute sessions per week postoperatively)

Stretching:

Bilateral hip adduction and hamstring stretching, ankle DF when casts were removed 8 weeks postoperatively, five repetitions with a 30-second hold for each stretch.

Strength Training:

Functional strength training to start, including sit-to-stand repetitions from various seat heights and surfaces, progressing from higher to lower seats with lowest placing hips at a 90-degree angle (using benches, balls, bolsters). Leg strengthening with manual resistance and machines, attention to hip abductors, adductors, extensors and hamstrings, and DF strengthening; use of strength-training machine with resistance high enough to result in fatigue after one to three sets of 6 to 10 repetitions (following NSCA strengthening guidelines); core strengthening using medium therapy ball in supine, prone, and sitting.

Therapeutic Handling:

Functional movement sequences practiced with facilitation to improve CA of LE musculature to promote an active base of support while addressing posture and alignment. Such movement sequences include facilitated weight shifting in standing using parallel bars, progressing to walker with facilitation to gluteals and abdominals given visual cues from a mirror; facilitated step-up with input to gluteus medius/maximus and internal/external obliques.

Bracing:

Following cast removal, he was fitted for molded solid AFOs to limit crouch and promote good foot alignment.

Aquatic Therapy:

Casts were removed 12 weeks postoperatively, thereby allowing Thomas to participate in aquatic therapy. Aquatic activities included standing balance and gait training in shoulder-deep water progressing down to waist-deep water, closed-chain functional strengthening, and kicking with a kickboard for hip strengthening.

Gait Training:

Began with stride stance and pregait activities in standing to increase tolerance for weight bearing and preparation for ambulation; progressed to gait training on even surface using personal posterior walker.

Parent/Child Education:

Review of precautions, transfer training, and home stretching program for hip adductors, hamstrings, and triceps surae (after casts were removed).

Interventions 7 to 18 months postoperatively (physical therapy: two 60-minute sessions per week, no postoperative precautions)

Stretching:

Continue adductor, hamstring, ankle DF stretching, three repetitions with 30-second hold each to maintain gains achieved.

Strengthening:

Progressed resistance with functional closed-chain strengthening and focused single-joint strengthening of muscles, such as the triceps surae, quadriceps, gluteus medius, and maximus, which are important in maintaining optimal upright posture NDT/therapeutic handling:

Incorporated primarily into functional activities to address child/family and therapist-determined goals. Including core strengthening with pelvic weight shifting, flexion with rotation and extension with rotation activities on a therapy ball, foot preparation before standing activities, and facilitated weight shifting and balance training with and without UE support on walker.

Gait Training:

Emphasis on increased walking distance using walker while maintaining optimal posture and alignment to minimize crouch; PBWSTT initiated to increase endurance.

Child/Parent Education:

Emphasis on ambulation and functional strengthening. The family is able to decrease the frequency of stretching to once a day owing to stability of ROM measurements over 8 consecutive weeks.

Discharge/Continuum of Care:

Eighteen months postoperatively, Thomas reached his personal goal of standing for 5 minutes with his walker and walking across the stage at school to stand alongside his classmates during the end-of-the-school-year celebration. At this time, he was discharged from a medically based physical therapy program with a home program. The therapists explained that Thomas' therapeutic needs would be best met using an episodic plan of care, and recommended a physical therapy reevaluation in 6 months' time to determine whether further intervention was needed. Before discharge, Thomas' interests were discussed and options for community activities were provided. In view of the time spent in the pool during aquatic therapy, Thomas will attend an adapted swim program at the local YMCA.

REFERENCES

1. Rethlefsen S, Ryan D, Kay R. Classification systems in cerebral palsy. *Orthop Clin North Am.* 2010;41:457–467.
2. Rosenbaum P, Paneth N, Leviton A, et al. A report: the definition and classification of cerebral palsy April 2006. *Dev Med Child Neurol Suppl.* 2007;109:8.
3. Stavsky M, Mor O. Mastrolia SA, Greenbaum S, et al. Cerebral palsy—trends in epidemiology and recent development in prenatal mechanisms of disease, treatment, and prevention. *Front Pediatr.* 2017;5(21):1–10.
4. World Health Organization, Elibrary, I. 2007. *International Classification of functioning, disability, and health: children and youth version: ICF-CY.* World Health Organization Geneva. Accessed February 20, 2021. https://apps.who.int/iris/handle/10665/43737
5. Oskoui M, Coutinho F, Dykeman J, et al. An update on the prevalence of cerebral palsy: a systematic review and meta-analysis. *Dev Med Child Neurol.* 2013;55:509–515.
6. Van Naarden Braun K, Doernberg N, Schieve L, et al. Birth prevalence of cerebral palsy: a population-based study. *Pediatrics.* 2016;137(1):e20152872.
7. Reddihough DS, Collins KJ. The epidemiology and causes of cerebral palsy. *Aust J Physiother.* 2003;49(1):7–12.
8. Michael-Asalu A, Taylor G, Campbell H, et al. Cerebral palsy: diagnosis, epidemiology, genetics, and clinical update. *Adv Pediatr.* 2019;66:189–208.
9. Novak I, Morgan C, Adde L, et al. Early, accurate diagnosis and early intervention in cerebral palsy: advances in diagnosis and treatment. *JAMA Pediatr.* 2017;171(9):897–907.
10. Miller F. *Cerebral Palsy.* Springer-Verlag, Inc; 2005.

11. National Institute of Neurological Disorders and Stroke. Reducing the burden of neurological disease. *Cerebral Palsy: Hope Through Research*. Accessed February 21, 2021. https://www.ninds.nih.gov/Disorders/Patient-Caregiver-Education/Hope-Through-Research/Cerebral-Palsy-Hope-Through-Research

12. van Haastert LC, de Vries LS, Eijsermans MJC, et al. Gross motor functional abilities in preterm-born children with cerebral palsy due to periventricular leukomalacia. *Dev Med Child Neurol*. 2008;50:684–689.

13. Ferrari F, Cioni G, Einspieler C, et al. Cramped synchronized general movements in preterm infants as an early marker for cerebral palsy. *Arch Pediatr Adolesc Med*. 2002;156(5):460–467.

14. Colver A. Outcomes for people with cerebral palsy: life expectancy and quality of life. *Paediatr Child Health*. 2016;26(9):383–386.

15. Maudsley G, Pharoah PO. Causes of excess mortality in cerebral palsy. *Dev Med Child Neurol*. 2000;42(4):287–288.

16. Miller F, Bachrach S. *Cerebral Palsy: A Complete Guide for Caregiving*. 2nd ed. Johns Hopkins University Press; 2006.

17. Bevans KB, Tucker CA. Classification terminology in cerebral palsy. In: Miller F, Bachrach S, Lennon N, O'Neil M, eds. *Cerebral Palsy*. Springer; 2019.

18. Palisano R, Rosenbaum P, Walter S, et al. Development and reliability of a system to classify gross motor function in children with cerebral palsy. *Dev Med Child Neurol*. 1997;39:214–223.

19. Morris C, Bartlett D. Gross motor function classification system: impact and utility. *Dev Med Child Neurol*. 2004;46(1):60–65.

20. Palisano R, Hanna S, Rosenbaum P, et al. Probability of walking, wheeled mobility, and assisted mobility in children and adolescents with cerebral palsy. *Dev Med Child Neurol*. 2010;52:66–71.

21. Rosenbaum P, Paneth N, Leviton A, et al. The definition and classification of cerebral palsy. *Dev Med Child Neurol*. 2007;49:1–44.

22. Eliasson AC, Krumlinde-Sundholm L, Rösblad B, et al. The manual ability classification system (MACS) for children with cerebral palsy: scale development and evidence of validity and reliability. *Dev Med Child Neurol*. 2006;48(7):549–554.

23. Hidecker MJ, Paneth N, Rosenbaum PL, et al. Developing and validating communication function classification system for individuals with cerebral palsy. *Dev Med Child Neurol*. 2011;53(8):704–710.

24. Compagnoe E, Maniglio J, Camposeo S, et al. Functional classifications for cerebral palsy; correlations between the gross motor function classification system (GMFCS), the manual ability classification system (MACS) and the communication function classification system (CFCS). *Res Dev Disabil*. 2014;35(11):2651–2657.

25. Sellers D, Mandy A, Pennington L, et al. Development and reliability of a system to classify the eating and drinking ability of people with cerebral palsy. *Dev Med Child Neurol*. 2014;56:245–251.

26. Baranello G, Signorini S, Tinelli F, et al. Visual function classification system for children and cerebral palsy: development and validation. *Dev Med Child Neurol*. 2019;62(1) (epub ahead of print).

27. Howle JM. *Neuro-Developmental Treatment Approach Theoretical Foundations and Principles of Clinical Practice*. The North American Neuro-Developmental Treatment Association; 2002.

28. Katz RT. Life expectancy for children with cerebral palsy and mental retardation: implications for life care planning. *NeuroRehabilitation*. 2003;18:261–270.

29. Accardo J, Kammann H, Hoon AH Jr. Neuroimaging in cerebral palsy. *J Pediatr*. 2004;145(2 suppl):S19–S27.

30. Krageloh-Mann I, Cans C. Cerebral palsy update. *Brain Dev*. 2009;31:537–544.

31. Harada T, Erada S, Anwar MM, et al. The cervical spine in athetoid cerebral palsy. A radiological study of 180 patients. *J Bone Joint Surg Br*. 1996;78(4):613–619.

32. Miller F. Hypotonic and special hip problems in cerebral palsy. In: Miller F, Bachrach S, Lennon N, O'Neil M, eds. *Cerebral Palsy*. Springer; 2018.

33. Wiklund L, Uvebrant P. Hemiplegic cerebral palsy: correlation between CT morphology and clinical findings. *Dev Med Child Neurol*. 1991;33(6):512–523.

34. Cioni G, Sale B, Paolicelli PB, et al. MRI and clinical characteristics of children with hemiplegic cerebral palsy. *Neuropediatrics*. 1999;30(5):249–255.

35. Davids J, Peace L, Wagner L, et al. Validation of the Shriners hospital for children upper extremity evaluation (SHUEE) for children with hemiplegic cerebral palsy. *J Bone Joint Surg Am*. 2006;88:326–333.

36. Holmefur M, Krumlinde-Sundholm L, Ellasson AC. Interrater and intrarater reliability of the assisting hand assessment. *Am J Occup Ther*. 2007;61:79–84.

37. Guide to Physical Therapist Practice 3.0. American Physical Therapy Association; 2014. Accessed September 8, 2019. http://guidetoptpractice.apta.org/

38. Miller F. Motor control and muscle tone problems in cerebral palsy. In: Miller F, Bachrach S, Lennon N, O'Neil M, eds. *Cerebral Palsy*. Springer; 2018.

39. Cahill-Rowley K, Rose J. Etiology of impaired selective motor control: emerging evidence and its implications for research and treatment in cerebral palsy. *Dev Med Child Neurol*. 2014;56(6):522–528.

40. Bar-On L, Molenaers G, Aertbeliën E, et al. Spasticity and its contribution to hypertonia in cerebral palsy. *BioMed Res Int*. 2015.

41. Lance J. Symposium synopsis. In: Feldman RG, Young RR, Koella WPE, eds. *Spasticity: Disordered Motor Control*. Yearbook Medical; 1980:485–494.

42. Bar-On L, Harlaar J, Desloovere K. Spasticity assessment in cerebral palsy. In: Miller F, Bachrach S, Lennon N, et al, eds. *Cerebral Palsy*. Springer; 2018.

43. Dabney K, Shrader W. Surgical treatment of scoliosis due to cerebral palsy. In: Miller F, Bachrach S, Lennon N, et al, eds. *Cerebral Palsy*. Springer; 2019.

44. Miller F. Early-onset scoliosis in cerebral palsy. In: Miller F, Bachrach S, Lennon N, et al, eds. *Cerebral Palsy*. Springer; 2018.

45. Miller F. Spinal deformity in children with cerebral palsy: an overview. In: Miller F, Bachrach S, Lennon N, et al, eds. *Cerebral Palsy*. Springer; 2019.

46. Miller F. Hip problems in children with cerebral palsy: an overview. In: Miller F, Bachrach S, Lennon N, et al, eds. *Cerebral Palsy*. Springer; 2019.

47. Valencia F. Management of hip deformities in cerebral palsy. *Orthop Clin North Am*. 2010;41:549–559.

48. Bleck EE. *Orthopedic Management of Cerebral Palsy*. WB Saunders; 1979.

49. Shands AR, Steele MK. Torsion of the femur. *J Bone Joint Surg*. 1958;40A:803–816.

50. Michele AA. *Iliopsoas*. Charles C Thomas; 1962.

51. Beals RK. Developmental changes in the femur and acetabulum in spastic paraplegia and diplegia. *Dev Med Child Neurol*. 1969;11:303–313.

52. Staheli LT, Duncan WR, Schaefer E. Growth alterations in the hemiplegic child. A study of femoral anteversion, neck-shaft angle, hip rotation, C.E. angle, limb length and circumference in 50 hemiplegic children. *Clin Orthop Relat Res*. 1968;60:205–212.

53. Riccio AI, Carney CD, Hammel LC, et al. Three-dimensional computed tomography for determination of femoral anteversion in a cerebral palsy model. *J Pediatr Orthop*. 2015;35:167–171.

54. Lee KM, Chung CY, Sung KH, et al. Femoral anteversion and tibial torsion only explain 25% of variance in regression analysis of foot progression angle in children with diplegic cerebral palsy. *J Neuroeng Rehabil*. 2013;56.

55. Akalan NE, Temelli Y, Kuchimov S. Discrimination of abnormal gait parameters due to increased femoral anteversion from other effects in cerebral palsy. *Hip Int*. 2013;23:492–499.

56. Karabicak GO, Balci NC, Gulfsen M, et al. The effect of postural control and balance on femoral anteversion in children with spastic cerebral palsy. *J Phys Ther Sci*. 2016;28(6):1696–1700.

57. Morrell DS, Pearson JM, Sauser DD. Progressive bone and joint abnormalities of the spine and lower extremities in cerebral palsy. *Radiographics*. 2002;22:257–268.

58. Miller F. Foot deformities in children with cerebral palsy: an overview. In: Miller F, Bachrach S, Lennon N, et al, eds. *Cerebral Palsy*. Cham: Springer; 2018.

59. Papavasileiou A, Petra M. Risk factors for developing cerebral palsy. In: Miller F, Bachrach S, Lennon N, et al, eds. *Cerebral Palsy*. Springer; 2018.

60. Owens L, Shieh E, Case A. Postnatal causes of cerebral palsy. In: Miller F, Bachrach S, Lennon N, et al, eds. *Cerebral Palsy*. Springer; 2019.

61. King KA, Selhorst D. Asthma in a child with cerebral palsy. In: Miller F, Bachrach S, Lennon N, et al, eds. *Cerebral Palsy*. Springer; 2019.

62. Proesmans M. Respiratory illness in children with disability: as serious problem. *Breath*. 2016;12(4):97–103.

63. Lennon N, Miller F. Aerobic conditioning and walking activity assessment in cerebral palsy. In: Miller F, Bachrach S, Lennon N, et al, eds. *Cerebral Palsy*. Springer; 2018.

64. Balemans AC, Fragala-Pinkham MA, Lennon N, et al. Systemic review of the clinimetric properties of laboratory—and field-based aerobic and anaerobic fitness measures in children with cerebral palsy. *Arch Phys Med Rehabil*. 2013;94(2):287–301

65. Balemans AC, Bolster EA. Aerobic and anaerobic fitness in children and youth with cerebral palsy. In: Miller F, Bachrach S, Lennon N, et al, eds. *Cerebral Palsy*. Springer; 2019.

66. Fowler EG, Kolobe THA, Damiano D, et al. Promotion of physical fitness and prevention of secondary conditions for children with cerebral palsy: section on pediatrics research summit proceedings. *Phys Ther*. 2007;87(11):1495–1510.

67. Zwinkles M, Takken T, Ruyten T, et al. Body mass Index and fitness in high-functioning children and adolescents with cerebral palsy: what happened over a decades? *Res Dev Disabil*. 2017;71:70–76.

68. McLafferty E, Hendry C, Farley A. The integumentary system: anatomy, physiology and function of skin. *Nurs Stand*. 2012;27(3):35–42.

69. Freundlich K. Pressure injuries in medically complex children: a review. *Children (Basel)*. 2017;4(4):25.

70. Finbraten A, Martins C, Andersen GL, et al. Assessment of body composition in children with cerebral palsy: a cross-sectional study in Norway. *Dev Med Child Neurol*. 2015;57:858–864.

71. Mohamed AMH, Koutharawu DN, Miller F, et al. Operative and clinical markers of deep wound infection after spine fusion in children with cerebral palsy. *J Pediatr Orthop*. 2010;30(8):851–857.

72. Stansby G, Avital L, Jones K, et al. Prevention and management of pressure ulcers in primary and secondary care: summary of NICE guidance. *BMJ*. 2014;348:1–5.

73. Visscher M, King A, Nie AM, et al. A quality-improvement collaborative project to reduce pressure ulcers in PICUs. *Pediatrics*. 2013;131:e1950-e1960.

74. Kolobe TH, Christy JB, Gannotti ME, et al. Research summit III proceedings on dosing in children with an injured brain or cerebral palsy: executive summary. *Phys Ther*. 2014;94(7):907–920.

75. Ahmadi M, O'Neil M, Fragala-Pinkham M, et al. Machine Machine learning algorithms for activity recognition in ambulant children and adolescents with cerebral palsy. *J Neuroeng Rehabil*. 2018;15:105

76. Bjornson KF, Lennon N. Walking and physical activity monitoring in children with cerebral palsy. In: Muller B, Wolf SI, eds. *Handbook of Human Motion*. 2018;2:1005–1036.

77. Dewar R, Claus AP, Tucker K, et al. Perspectives on postural control dysfunction to inform future research: a Delphi study for children with cerebral palsy. *Arch Phys Med Rehabil*. 2017;98:463–479.

78. Dewar R, Claus AP, Tucker K, et al. Reproducibility of the Kids-BESTest and the Kids-Mini-BESTest for children with cerebral palsy. *Arch Phys Med Rehabil*. 2019;100:695–702.

79. Huxham FE, Goldie PA, Patla AE. Theoretical considerations in balance assessment. *Aust J Physio ther*. 2001;472:89–100.

80. Boyer ER, Patterson A. Gait pathology subtypes are not associated with self-reported fall frequency in children with cerebral palsy. *Gait Posture*. 2018;63:189–194.

81. Niiler TA. Assessing dynamic balance in children with cerebral palsy. In: Miller F, Bachrach S, Lennon N, et al, eds. *Cerebral Palsy*. Springer; 2019.

82. Verbecque E, Lobo Da Costa PH, et al. Psychometric properties of functional balance tests in children: a literature review. *Dev Med Child Neurol*. 2015;57:521–529.

83. Randall KE, Bartlett DJ, McCoy S. Head-to-head comparison of the early clinical assessment of balance test in young children with cerebral palsy. *Pediatr Phys Ther*. 2014;26:332–337.

84. McCoy SW, Bartlett D, Yocum A, et al. Development and validity of the early clinical assessment of balance for children with cerebral palsy. *Dev Neurorehabil*. 2014;17:375–383.

85. Fiss AF, Jefferies L, Bjornson K, et al. Developmental trajectories and reference percentiles for the 6-minute walk test for children with cerebral palsy. *Pediatr Phys Ther*. 2019;31:51–59.

86. Manikowska F, Chen BP, Jóźwiak M, et al. Validation of manual muscle testing (MMT) in children and adolescents with cerebral palsy. *NeuroRehabil*. 2018;42(1):1–7.

87. Damiano DL, Vaughan CL, Abel MF. Muscle response to heavy resistance exercise in children with spastic cerebral palsy. *Dev Med Child Neurol*. 1995;37:731–739.

88. Damiano DL, Abel MF. Functional outcomes of strength training in spastic cerebral palsy. *Arch Phys Med Rehabil*. 1998;79:119–125.

89. Eek MN, Tranberg R, Zugner R, et al. Muscle strength training to improve gait function in children with cerebral palsy. *Dev Med Child Neurol*. 2008;50:759–764.

90. Goh HT, Thompson M, Huang WB, et al. Relationships among measures of knee musculoskeletal impairments, gross motor function, and walking efficiency in children with cerebral palsy. *Pediatr Phys Ther*. 2006;18:253–261.

91. Willemse L, Brehm MA, Scholtes VA, et al. Reliability of isometric lower-extremity muscle strength measurements in children with cerebral palsy: implications for measurement design. *Phys Ther*. 2013;93:935–941.

92. Mulder-Brouwer AN, Rameckers EA, Bastianen CH. Lower extremity handheld dynamometry in children with cerebral palsy. *Pediatr Phys Ther*. 2016;28:136–153.

93. Wang T, Liao H, Peng Y. Reliability and validity of the five-repetition sit-to stand test for children with cerebral palsy. *Clin Rehabil*. 2012;26(7):664–671.

94. Mutlu A, Livanellioglu A, Gunel MK. Reliability of goniometric measurements in children with spastic cerebral palsy. *Med Sci Monit*. 2007;13(7):CR323–CR329.

95. Ten Berge SR, Halbertsma JPK, Maathuis PGM, et al. Reliability of popliteal angle measurements, a study in cerebral palsy patients and healthy controls. *J Pediatr Orthop*. 2007;27:648–652.

96. Russell DJ, Avery LM, Rosenbaum PL, et al. Improved scaling of the gross motor function measure with children with cerebral palsy: evidence of reliability and validity. *Phys Ther*. 2000;80:873–885.

97. Harvey AR. The gross motor function measure. *J Physiother*. 2017;63:187.

98. Brunton LK, Bartlett DJ. Validity and reliability of two abbreviated versions of the gross motor function measure. *Phys Ther*. 2011;91:577–588.

99. Besios T, Aggeloussis N, Gourgoulis V, et al. Comparative reliability of the PEDI, GMFM and TUG tests for children with cerebral palsy. *J Phys Ther Sci*. 2013;25(1):73–76.

100. Shore BJ, Allar BG, Miller PE, et al. Measuring the reliability and construct validity of the pediatric evaluation of disability inventory—computer adaptive test (PEDI-CAT) in children with cerebral palsy. *Arch Phys Med Rehabil*. 2019;100:45–51.

101. Wang HH, Liao HF, Hsieh CL. Reliability, sensitivity to change, and responsiveness of the peabody developmental motor scales—second edition for children with cerebral palsy. *Phys Ther*. 2006;86(10):1351–1359.

102. Selves C, Stoquart G, Render A, et al. Reliability and concurrent validity of the Bruininks-Oseretsky test in children with cerebral palsy. *Biomed J Sci Tech Res*. 2019;18(5):13961–13967.

103. Thorley M, Lannin N, Cusick A, et al. Reliability of the quality of upper extremity skills test for children with cerebral palsy aged 2 to 12 years. *Phy Occup Ther Pediatr*. 2012;32(1):4–21.

104. Bohannon RW, Smith MB. Interrater reliability of a modified Ashworth scale of muscle spasticity. *Phys Ther*. 1987;67:206–207.

105. Gracies JM, Burke BS, Clegg NJ, et al. Reliability of the Tardieu scale for assessing spasticity in children with cerebral palsy. *Arch Phys Med Rehabil*. 2010;91:421–428.

106. Gage JR, DeLuca PA, Renshaw TS. Gait analysis: principles and applications. Emphasis on its use in cerebral palsy. *J Bone Joint Surg Am.* 1995;77(10):1607–1623.

107. Rathinam C, Bateman A, Peirson J, et al. Observational gait assessment tools in paediatrics -a systematic review. *Gait Posture.* 2014;40(2):279–285.

108. Araújo PA, Kirkwood RN, Figueiredo FM. Validity and intra- and inter-rater reliability of the observational gait scale for children with spastic cerebral palsy. *Rev Bras Fisioter.* 2009;13:267–273.

109. Toro B, Nester CJ, Farren PC. The development and validity of the Salford gait tool: an observation-based clinical gait assessment tool. *Arch Phys Med Rehabil.* 2007;88:321–327.

110. Kawamura CM, de Morais Filho MC, Barreto MM, et al. Comparison between visual and three-dimensional gait analysis in patients with spastic diplegic cerebral palsy. *Gait Posture.* 2007;25:18–24.

111. Read HS, Hazlewood ME, Hillman SJ, et al. Edinburgh visual gait score for use in cerebral palsy. *J Pediatr Orthop.* 2003;23:296–301.

112. Koman LA, Mooney JF, Smith BP, et al. Management of spasticity in cerebral palsy with botulinum-A toxin: report of a preliminary, randomized, double-blind trial. *J Pediatr Orthop.* 1994;14:299–303.

113. Novacheck TF, Stout JL, Tervo R. Reliability and validity of the Gillette functional assessment questionnaire as an outcome measure in children with walking disabilities. *J Pediatr Orthop.* 2000;20:75.

114. Thompson P, Beath T, Bell J, et al. Test-retest reliability of the 10-metre fast walk test and 6-minute walk test in ambulatory school-aged children with cerebral palsy. *Dev Med Child Neurol.* 2008;50(5):370–376.

115. Fiss AF, McCoy SW, Bartlett D, et al. On track study team. Developmental trajectories for the early clinical assessment of balance by gross motor function classification system level for children with cerebral palsy. *Phys Ther.* 2019;99(2):217–228.

116. McDowell BC, Humphreys L, Kerr C, et al. Test-retest reliability of a 1-min walk test in children with bilateral spastic cerebral palsy. *Gait Posture.* 2009;29:267–269.

117. Verschuren O, Ketelaar M, De Groot J, et al. Reproducibility of two functional field tests for children with cerebral palsy who self-propel a manual wheelchair. *Dev Med Child Neurol.* 2013;55:185–190.

118. Birnie KA, Hundert AS, Lalloo C, et al. Recommendations for selection of self-reported pain intensity measures in children and adolescents: a systemic review and quality assessment of measurement properties. *Pain.* 2019;160(1):5–18.

119. Merkel SI, Voepel-Lewis T, Shayevitz JR, et al. The FLACC: a behavioral scale for scoring postoperative pain in young children. *Pediatr Nurs.* 1997;23(3):293–297.

120. Hadden KL, LeFort S, O'Brein M, et al. A comparison of observers' and self-reported pain ratings for children with cerebral palsy. *J Dev Behav Pediatr.* 2015;36(1):14–23.

121. Alexander R, Boehme R, Cupps B. *Normal Development of Functional Motor Skills: The First Year of Life.* Therapy Skill Builders; 1993.

122. Chen CM, Chen CY, Wu KP, et al. Motor factors associated with health-related quality-of-life in ambulatory children with cerebral palsy. *Am J Phys Med Rehabil.* 2011;90:940–947.

123. Waters E, Davis E, Mackinnon A, et al. Psychometric properties of the quality of life questionnaire for children with CP. *Dev Med Child Neurol.* 2007;49(1):49–55.

124. Narayanan UG, Fehlings D, Weir S, et al. Initial development and validation of the caregiver priorities and child health index of life with disabilities (CPCHILD). *Dev Med Child Neurol.* 2006;48(10):804–812.

125. Varni JW, Burwinkle TM, Berrin SJ, et al. The PedsQL in pediatric cerebral palsy: reliability, validity, and sensitivity of the generic core scales and cerebral palsy module. *Dev Med Child Neurol.* 2006;48(6):442–449.

126. Mueller-Godeffroy E, Thyen U, Bullinger M. Health-related quality of life in children and adolescents with cerebral palsy: a secondary analysis of the DISABKIDS questionnaire in the field-study cerebral palsy subgroup. *Neuropediatrics.* 2016;47(2):97–106.

127. Rosenbaum P, Walter S, Hanna S, et al. Prognosis for gross motor function in cerebral palsy creation of motor development curves. *JAMA.* 2002;288(11);1357–1362.

128. Hanna S, Rosenbaum P, Bartlett D, et al. Stability and decline in gross motor function among children and youth with cerebral palsy aged 2 to 21 years. *Dev Med Child Neurol.* 2009;51(4):295–302.

129. Bovend'Eerdt TJ, Botell RE, Wade DT. Writing SMART rehabilitation goals and achieving goal attainment scaling: a practical guide. *Clin Rehabil.* 2009;23:352–361.

130. Law M, Darrah J. Emerging therapy approaches: an emphasis on function. *J Child Neurol.* 2014;29:1101–1107.

131. Beckung E, Hagberg G, Uldall P, et al. Probability of walking in children with cerebral palsy in Europe. *Pediatrics.* 2008;121:e187–e192.

132. Rosenbaum PL, Walter SD, Hanna SE, et al. Development and reliability of a system to classify gross motor function in children with cerebral palsy. *JAMA.* 2002;288(11):1357–1363.

133. Watt J, Robertson CM, Grace MG. Early prognosis for ambulation of neonatal intensive care survivors with cerebral palsy. *Dev Med Child Neurol.* 1989;31:766–773.

134. Perry J, Burnfield J. *Gait Analysis: Normal and Pathological Function.* 2nd ed. Slack Inc; 2010.

135. Sutherland DH, Davids JR. Common gait abnormalities of the knee in cerebral palsy. *Clin Orthop Relat Res.* 1993;288:139–147.

136. Beckung E, Hagberg G. Neuroimpairments, activity limitations and participation restrictions in children with cerebral palsy. *Dev Med Child Neurol.* 2002;44(5):309–316.

137. Winters TF, Gage JR, Hicks R. Gait patterns in spastic hemiplegia in children and young adults. *J Bone Joint Surg Am.* 1987;69:437–441.

138. Rodda J, Graham H. Classification of gait patterns in spastic hemiplegia and spastic diplegia: a basis for a management algorithm. *Eur J Neurol.* 2001;8(suppl 5):98–108.

139. Wren TA, Rethlefsen S, Kay RM. Prevalence of specific gait abnormalities in children with cerebral palsy: influence of cerebral palsy subtype, age, and previous surgery. *J Pediatr Orthop.* 2005;25(1):79–83.

140. Mossberg KA, Linton KA, Fricke K. Ankle-foot orthoses: effect on energy expenditure of gait in spastic diplegic children. *Arch Phys Med Rehabil.* 1990;71:490–494.

141. Davids J. The foot and ankle in cerebral palsy. *Orthop Clin North Am.* 2010;41:579–593.

142. Rodda JM, Graham HK, Carson L, et al. Sagittal gait patterns in spastic diplegia. *J Bone Joint Surg Br.* 2004;86(2):251–258.

143. Westberry D, Davids JR, Davis RB, et al. Idiopathic toe walking: a kinematic and kinetic profile. *J Pediatr Orthop.* 2008;28(3):352–358.

144. Hicks R, Durinick N, Gage JR. Differentiation of idiopathic toe-walking and cerebral palsy. *J Pediatr Orthop.* 1988;8:160–163.

145. Kelly IP, Jenkinson A, Stephens M, et al. The kinematic patterns of toe-walkers. *J Pediatr Orthop.* 1997;17(4):478–480.

146. Mochizuki H, Ugawa Y. Cerebellar ataxic gait [in Japanese]. *Brain Nerve.* 2010;62(11):1203–1210.

147. Bly L. Abnormal motor development. In: Slaton DS, ed. *Proceedings of a Conference on Development of Movement in Infancy Offered by the Division of Physical Therapy.* University North Carolina; May 18-22, 1980.

148. Bobath B, Bobath K. *Motor Development in the Different Types of Cerebral Palsy.* William Heineman Medical Books; 1982.

149. Finnie NR. *Handling the Young Cerebral Palsied Child at Home.* 2nd ed. Dalton Publications; 1975.

150. Novak I, Mcintyre S, Morgan C, et al. A systematic review of interventions for children with cerebral palsy: state of the evidence. *Dev Med Child Neurol.* 2013;55: 885-910. https://doi.org/10.1111/dmcn.12246

151. Scholtes V, Becher J, Comuth A, et al. Effectiveness of functional progressive resistance exercise strength training on muscle strength and mobility in children with cerebral palsy: a randomized controlled trail. *Dev Med Child Neurol.* 2010;52:107–113.

152. McNee A, Gough M, Morrissey M, et al. Increases in muscle volume after plantarflexor strength training in children with spastic cerebral palsy. *Dev Med Child Neurol.* 2009;51:429–435.

153. Scianni A, Butler JM, Ada L, et al. Muscle strengthening not effective in children and adolescents with cerebral palsy: a systemic review. *Aust J Physiother.* 2009;55:81–87.

154. Reid S, Hamer P, Alderson J, et al. Neuromuscular adaptations to eccentric strength training in children and adolescents with cerebral palsy. *Dev Med Child Neurol.* 2010;52:358–363.

155. Lee JH, Sung IY, Yoo JY. Therapeutic effects of strengthening exercise on gait function of cerebral palsy. *Disabil Rehabil.* 2008;30(19):1439–1444.

156. Rogers A, Brinks S, Darrah J. A systemic review of the effectiveness of aerobic exercise interventions for children with cerebral palsy: an AACPDM evidence report. *Dev Med Child Neurol.* 2008;50:808–814.

157. Verschuren O, Ketekaar M, Takken T, et al. Exercise programs for children with cerebral palsy: a systemic review of the literature. *Am J Phys Med Rehabil.* 2008;87(5):404–417.

158. Verschuren O, Ada L, Maltais D, et al. Muscle strengthening in children and adolescents with spastic cerebral palsy: considerations for future resistance training protocols. *Phys Ther.* 2011;91:1130–1139.

159. Gillett JG, Boyda RN, Carty CP, et al. The impact of strength training on skeletal muscle morphology and architecture in children and adolescents with spastic cerebral palsy: a systematic review. *Res Dev Disabil.* 2016;56:183–196.

160. Faigenbaum AD, Kraemer WJ, Blimkie CJR, et al. Youth resistance training: updated position statement paper from the national strength and conditioning association. *J Strength Cond Res.* 2009;23(5):S60–S79.

161. Verschuren O, Peterson MD, Balemans ACJ, et al. Exercise and physical activity recommendations for people with cerebral palsy. *Dev Med Child Neurol.* 2016;58(8):798–808.

162. Christensen C. Flexibility in children and youth with cerebral palsy. In: Miller F, Bachrach S, Lennon N., et al, eds. *Cerebral Palsy.* Springer; 2019.

163. Pin T, Dyke P, Chan M. The effectiveness of passive stretching in children with cerebral palsy. *Dev Med Child Neurol.* 2006;48(10):855–862.

164. Craig J, Hilderman C, Wilson G, et al. Effectiveness of stretch interventions for children with neuromuscular disabilities: evidence based recommendations. *Pediatr Phys Ther.* 2016;28(3):262–275.

165. Wiart L, Darrah J, Kembhavi G. Stretching with children with cerebral palsy: what do we know and where are we going? *Pediatr Phys Ther.* 2008;20(2):173–178.

166. Harvey LA, Katalinic OM, Herbert RD, et al. Stretch for the treatment and prevention of contractures. *Cochrane Database Syst Rev.* 2017;1:CD007455.

167. Theis N, Korff T, Mohagheghi A. Does long-term passive stretching alter muscle–tendon unit mechanics in children with spastic cerebral palsy? *Clin Biomechan.* 2015;30(10):1071–1076.

168. Tilton A. Management of spasticity in children with cerebral palsy. *Semin Pediatr Neurol.* 2009;16:82–89.

169. Tustin K, Patel A. A critical evaluation of the updated evidence for casting for equinus deformity in children with cerebral palsy. *Physiother Res Int.* 2017;22(1):e1646.

170. Willerslev-Olsen M, Lorentzen J, Nielson JB. Gait training reduces ankle joint stiffness and facilitates heel strike in children with cerebral palsy. *NeuroRehabilitation.* 2014;35(4):643–655.

171. Armstrong EL, Spencer S, Kentish MJ, et al. Efficacy of cycling interventions to improve function in children and adolescents with cerebral palsy: a systematic review and meta-analysis. *Clin Rehabil.* 2019;33(7):1113–1129.

172. Nsenga AL, Shephard RJ, Ahmaidi S. Aerobic training in children with cerebral palsy. *Int J Sports Med.* 2013;34(6):533–537.

173. Boenig, B. NDT in a Nutshell. NDTA Network; 2005:12.

174. Howle J. Motor control. In: Bierman JC, Franjoine MR, eds. *Neuro-Developmental Treatment A Guide to NDT. Clinical Practice.* Stuttgart, Germany. Thieme. 2016:248.

175. Butler C, Darrah J. Effects of neurodevelopmental treatment (NDT) for cerebral palsy: an AACPDM evidence report. *Dev Med Child Neurol.* 2001;43:778–790.

176. Martin L, Baker R, Harvey A. A systematic review of common physiotherapy interventions in school-aged children with cerebral palsy. *Phys Occup Ther Pediatr.* 2010;30:294–312.

177. Franki I, Desloovere K, Cat J, et al. The evidence-base for conceptual approached and additional therapies targeting lower limb function in children with cerebral palsy: a systemic review using the ICF as a framework. *J Rehabil Med.* 2012;44:396–405.

178. Ganley K. Review of neurodevelopmental treatment. *Dev Med Child Neurol.* 2014;56:1026–1027.

179. Evans-Rogers DL, Sweeney JK, Holden-Huchton P, et al. Short-term, intensive neurodevelopmental treatment program experiences of parents and their children with disabilities. *Pediatr Phys Ther.* 2015;27:61–71.

180. Neurodevelopmental Treatment Association. Accessed September 13, 2020. https://www.ndta.org/Research.

181. Taub E, Uswatte G, Pidikiti R. Constraint-induced movement therapy: a new family of techniques with broad application to physical rehabilitation—a clinical review. *J Rehabil Res Dev.* 1999;36(3):237–251.

182. Coker P, Karakostas T, Dodds C, et al. Gait characteristics of children with hemiplegic cerebral palsy before and after modified constraint-induced movement therapy. *Disabil Rehabil.* 2012;32(5):402–408.

183. Boyd RN, Morris ME, Graham HK. Management of upper limb dysfunction in children with cerebral palsy: a systemic review. *Eur J Neurol.* 2001;8(5):150–166.

184. Novak I, Mcintyre S, Morgan C, et al. A systematic review of interventions for children with cerebral palsy: state of the evidence. *Dev Med Child Neurol.* 2013;55:885–910.

185. Sakzewski L, Gordon A, Eliasson AC. The state of the evidence for intensive upper limb therapy approaches for children with unilateral cerebral palsy. *J Child Neurol.* 2014;29:1077–1090.

186. Chiu HC, Ada L. Constraint-induced movement therapy improves upper limb activity and participation in hemiplegic cerebral palsy: a systematic review. *J Physiother.* 2016;62:130–137.

187. Eliasson AC, Gordon AM. Constraint-induced movement therapy for children and youth with hemiplegic/unilateral cerebral palsy. In: Miller F, Bachrach S, Lennon N, et al, eds. *Cerebral Palsy.* Springer; 2019.

188. Tervahauta MH, Girolami GL, Oberg GK. Efficacy of constraint-induced movement therapy compared with bimanual intensive training in children with unilateral cerebral palsy: a systematic review. *Clin Rehabil.* 2017;31:1445–1456.

189. Facchin P, Rosa-Rizzotto M, Visona Dalla Pozza L, et al. Multisite trial comparing the efficacy of constraint-induced movement therapy with that of bimanual intensive training in children with hemiplegic cerebral palsy: post intervention results. *Am J Phys Med Rehabil.* 2011;90(7):539–553.

190. Eliasson AC, Holmefur M. The influence of early modified constraint-induced movement therapy training on the longitudinal development of hand function in children with unilateral cerebral palsy. *Dev Med Child Neurol.* 2014;57:89–94.

191. Deluca SC, Trucks MR, Wallace DA, et al. Practice-based evidence from a clinical cohort that received pediatric constraint-induced movement therapy. *J Pediatr Rehabil Med.* 2017;10:37–46.

192. Aarts PB, Jongerius PH, Geerdink YA, et al. Effectiveness of modified constraint induced movement therapy in children with unilateral spastic cerebral palsy: a randomized controlled trial. *Neurorehabil Neural Repair.* 2010;24:509–518.

193. Kuhnke N, Juenger H, Walther M, et al. Do patients with congenital hemiparesis and ipsilateral corticospinal projections respond differently to constraint-induced movement therapy? *Dev Med Child Neurol.* 2008;50:898–903.

194. Charles J, Gordon AM. A critical review of constraint-induced movement therapy and forced use in children with hemiplegia. *Neural Plast.* 2005;12:245–261.

195. Chen YP, Pope S, Tyler D, et al. Effectiveness of constraint-induced movement therapy on upper-extremity function in children with cerebral palsy: a systematic review and meta-analysis of randomized controlled trials. *Clin Rehabil.* 2014;28:939–953.

196. Hoare B, Imms C, Carey L, et al. Constraint-induced movement therapy in the treatment of the upper limb in children with

hemiplegic cerebral palsy: a Cochrane systematic review. *Clin Rehabil.* 2007;21:675–685.

197. Huang HH, Fetters L, Hale J, et al. Bound for success: a systematic review of constraint-induced movement therapy in children with cerebral palsy supports improved arm and hand use. *Phys Ther.* 2009;89:1126–1141.

198. Dimitrijevic MR, Gerasimenko Y, Pinter MM. Evidence for a spinal central pattern generator in humans. *Ann N Y Acad Sci.* 1998;16:360–376.

199. Cohen A, Ermentrout G, Kiemel T, et al. Modeling of intersegmental coordination in the lamprey central pattern generator for locomotion. *Trends Neurosci.* 1992;15:434–438.

200. MacKay-Lyons M. Central pattern generators of locomotion: a review of the evidence. *Phys Ther.* 2002;82:69–83.

201. Mattern-Baxter K, Bellamy S, Mansoor J. Effects of intensive locomotor treadmill training on young children with cerebral palsy. *Pediatr Phys Ther.* 2009;21:308–319.

202. Cherng R, Liu C, Lau T, et al. Effect of treadmill training with body weight support on gait and gross motor function in children with spastic cerebral palsy. *Am J Phys Med Rehabil.* 2007;86:548–555.

203. Day J, Fox EJ, Lowe J, et al. Locomotion training with partial body weight support on a treadmill in a nonambulatory child with spastic tetraplegic CP: a case report. *Pediatr Phys Ther.* 2004;16:106–113.

204. Schindl MR, Forstner C, Kern H, et al. Treadmill training with partial body weight support in non-ambulatory children with CP. *Arch Phys Med Rehabil.* 2000;81:301–306.

205. Dodd KJ, Foley S. Partial body-weight supported treadmill training can improve walking in children with cerebral palsy: a clinical controlled trial. *Dev Med Child Neurol.* 2007;49:101–105.

206. Provost B, Dieruf K, Burtner P, et al. Endurance and gait in children with cerebral palsy after intensive body weight-supported treadmill training. *Pediatr Phys Ther.* 2007;19:2–10.

207. Mutlu A, Krosschell K, Spira DG. Treadmill training with partial body-weight support in children with cerebral palsy: a systematic review. *Dev Med Child Neurol.* 2009;51:268–275.

208. Damiano D, DeJong S. A systematic review of the effectiveness of treadmill training and body weight support in pediatric rehabilitation. *J Neurol Phys Ther.* 2009;33:27–44.

209. Willoughby KL, Dodd KJ, Shields N, et al. Efficacy of partial body weight-supported treadmill training compared with overground walking practice for children with cerebral palsy: a randomized controlled trial. *Arch Phys Med Rehabil.* 2010;91:33–39.

210. Cho C, Hwang W, Hwang S, et al. Treadmill training with virtual reality improves gait, balance, and muscle strength in children with cerebral palsy. *Tohoku J Exp Med.* 2016;238(3):213–218.

211. Chrysagis N, Skordilis EK, Stavrou N, et al. The effect of treadmill training on gross motor function and walking speed in ambulatory adolescents with cerebral palsy: a random controlled trial. *Am J Phys Med Rehabil.* 2012;91:747–760.

212. Grecco LA, Zanon N, Sampaio LM, et al. A comparison of treadmill training and overground walking in ambulant children with cerebral palsy: randomizes controlled clinical trial. *Clin Rehabil.* 2013;27(8):686–696.

213. Meyer-Heim A, Ammann-Reiffer C, Schmartz A, et al. Improvement of walking abilities after robotic-assisted locomotion training in children with cerebral palsy. *Arch Dis Child.* 2009;94:615–620.

214. Van Hedel HJ, Meyer-Heim A, Rüsch-Bohtz C. Robot-assisted gait training for children and youth with cerebral palsy. In: Miller F, Bachrach S, Lennon N, et al, eds. *Cerebral Palsy.* Springer; 2019.

215. Wallard L, Dietrich G, Kerlirzin Y, et al. Effect of robotic-assisted gait rehabilitation on dynamic equilibrium control in the gait of children with cerebral palsy. *Gait Posture.* 2017a;60:55-60.

216. Wallard L, Dietrich G, Kerlirzin Y, et al. Robotic-assisted gait training improves walking ability in diplegic children with cerebral palsy. *Eur J Paediatr Neurol.* 2017;21(3):557–564.

217. Lefmann S, Russo R, Hillier S. The effectiveness of robotic-assisted gait training for paediatric gait disorders: systematic review. *J Neuroeng Rehabil.* 2017;14:1.

218. Lee I, Kim J, Lee S. The effects of hippotherapy on spasticity and muscular activity of children with cerebral palsy. *J Korean Soc Occup Ther.* 2019;19:117–124.

219. Ho CL, Holt KG, Saltzman E, et al. Functional electrical stimulation changes dynamic resources in children with spastic cerebral palsy. *Phys Ther.* 2006;86:987–1000.

220. Pool D, Valentine J, Bear N, et al. The orthotic and therapeutic effects following daily community applied functional electrical stimulation in children with unilateral spastic cerebral palsy: a randomized controlled trial. *BMC Pediatr.* 2015;15:154.

221. Khamis S, Martikaro R, Wientroub S, et al. A functional electrical stimulation system improves knee control in crouch gait. *J Child Orthop.* 2015;9:137–143.

222. Prosser LA, Curatalo LA, Alter KE, et al. Acceptability and potential effectiveness of a foot drop stimulator in children and adolescents with cerebral palsy. *Dev Med Child Neurol.* 2012;54:1044–1049.

223. Danino B, Khamis S, Hemo Y, et al. The efficacy of neuroprosthesis in young hemiplegic patients, measured by three different gait indices: early results. *J Child Orthop.* 2013;7:537–542.

224. Seifert A, Unger M, Burger M. Functional electrical stimulation to the lower limb muscles after botox in children with cerebral palsy. *Pediatr Phys Ther.* 2010;22:199–206.

225. Academy of Aquatic Physical Therapy. Original Definition. Accessed February 21, 2021. https://aquaticpt.org/Files/Our%20History%20-%20Original%20Definition.pdf

226. Akinola BI, Gbiri CA, Odebiyi DO. Effect of a 10-week aquatic exercise training program on gross motor function in children with spastic cerebral palsy. *Global Pediatr Health.* 2019;6:1–7.

227. Lai CJ, Liu WY, Yang TF, et al. Pediatric aquatic therapy on motor function and enjoyment in children diagnosed with cerebral palsy of various motor severities. *J Child Neurol.* 2015;30(2):200–208.

228. Gorter JW, Currie SJ. Aquatic exercise programs for children and adolescents with cerebral palsy: what do we know and where do we go? *Int J Pediatr.* 2011;2011:712165.

229. Kelly M, Darrah J. Aquatic exercise for children with cerebral palsy. *Dev Med Child Neurol.* 2005;47:838–884.

230. American Hippotherapy Association. Accessed February 21, 2021. https://www.americanhippotherapyassociation.org/

231. McCloskey S. Notes from Lecture on Hippotherapy at Arcadia University; April 28, 2004.

232. Casady RL, Nichols-Larsen DS. The effect of hippotherapy on ten children with cerebral palsy. *Pediatr Phys Ther.* 2004;16(3):165–172.

233. Willgens A, Erdman E. Using hippotherapy strategies for children and youth with cerebral palsy: an overview. In: Miller F, Bachrach S, Lennon N, et al, eds. *Cerebral Palsy.* Springer; 2019.

234. Silkwood-Sherer DJ, Killian CB, Long TM, et al. Hippotherapy—an intervention to habilitate balance deficits in children with movement disorders: a clinical trial. *Phys Ther.* 2012;92:707–717.

235. Kwon JY, Chang HJ, Yi SH, et al. Effect of hippotherapy on gross motor function in children with cerebral palsy: a randomized controlled trial. *J Altern Complement Med.* 2015;21:15–21.

236. Moreas AG. The effects of hippotherapy on postural balance and functional ability in children with cerebral palsy. *J Phys Ther Sci.* 2016;28(8):2220–2226.

237. Zadnikar M, Kastrin A. Effects of hippotherapy and therapeutic horseback riding on postural control or balance in children with cerebral palsy: a meta-analysis. *Dev Med Child Neurol.* 2011;53(8)684–691.

238. Shurtleff TL, Engsberg JR. Changes in trunk and head stability in children with cerebral palsy after hippotherapy: a pilot study. *Phys Occup Ther Pediatr.* 2010;30:150–163.

239. Park ES, Rha DW, Shin JS, et al. Effects of hippotherapy on gross motor function and functional performance of children with cerebral palsy. *Yonsei Med J.* 2014;55(6):1736–1742.

240. Garner BA, Rigby BR. Human pelvis motions when walking and when riding a therapeutic horse. *Hum Mov Sci.* 2015;39:121–137.

241. Manikowski F, Jozwiak M, Idzio M, et al. The effect of a hippotherapy session on spatiotemporal parameters of gait in children with cerebral palsy—pilot study. *Orthop Traumatol Rehabil.* 2013;15(3):253–257.

242. Mutoh T. Application of a tri-axial accelerometry-based portable motion recorder for the qualitative assessment of hippotherapy in children and adolescents with cerebral palsy. *J Phy Ther Sci.* 2016;28(10):2970–2974.

243. Martín-Valero R, Vega-Ballón J, Perez-Cabezas V. Benefits of hippotherapy in children with cerebral palsy: a narrative review. *Eur J Paediatr Neurol.* 2018;22(6):1150–1160.

244. Mutoh T, Mutoh T, Tsubone H, et al. Impact of serial gait analyses on long-term outcome of hippotherapy in children and adolescents with cerebral palsy. *Compl Ther Clin Pract.* 2018;30:19–23.

245. Ravi DK, Kumar N, Singhi P. Effectiveness of virtual reality rehabilitation for children and adolescents with cerebral palsy: an updated evidence-based systematic review. *Physiotherapy.* 2017;103(3):245–258.

246. Gilbertson T, Hsu LY, McCoy SW, et al. Gaming technologies for children and youth with cerebral palsy. In: Miller F, Bachrach S, Lennon N, et al, eds. *Cerebral Palsy.* Springer; 2019.

247. Ghai S, Ghai I. Virtual reality enhances gait in cerebral palsy: a training dose-response meta-analysis. *Front Neurol.* 2019;10:236.

248. Keawutan P, Bell K, Davies P, et al. Systematic review of the relationship between habitual physical activity and motor capacity in children with cerebral palsy. *Res Dev Disabil.* 2014;35:1301–1309.

249. Carlton S, Taylor N, Dodd K, et al. Differences in habitual physical activity levels of young people with cerebral palsy and their typically developing peers: a systematic review. *Disabil Rehabil.* 2013;35:647–655.

250. Binder H, Eng GD. Rehabilitation management of children with spastic diplegic cerebral palsy. *Arch Phys Med Rehabil.* 1989;70:482–489.

251. Molnar GE. Rehabilitation in cerebral palsy. *West J Med.* 1991;154:569–572.

252. Walsh S, Scharf M. The effect of a recreational ice skating program on the gross motor function of a child with cerebral palsy. *Physiother Theory Pract.* 2014;30:189–195.

253. Slaman J, van den Berg-Emons H, van Meeteren J, et al. A lifestyle intervention improves fatigue, mental health, and social support among adolescents and young adults with cerebral palsy: focus on mediating effects. *Clin Rehabil.* 2015;29:717–727.

254. Nwaobi OM, Smith PD. Effect of adaptive seating on pulmonary function of children with cerebral palsy. *Dev Med Child Neurol.* 1986;28:351–354.

255. Reid DT. The effects of the saddle seat on seated postural control and upper extremity movement in children with cerebral palsy. *Dev Med Child Neurol.* 1996;38:805–815.

256. Hulme JB, Shaver J, Archer S, et al. Effects of adaptive seating devices on the eating and drinking of children with multiple handicaps. *Am J Occup Ther.* 1987;41:81–89.

257. Harris SR. Movement analysis—an aid to diagnosis of cerebral palsy. *Phys Ther.* 1991;71:215–221.

258. Rosen L, Arva J, Furumasu J, et al. RESNA position on the application of power wheelchairs for pediatric users. *Assist Technol.* 2009;21(4):218–226.

259. Furumasu J, Guerette P, Tefft D. Relevance of the pediatric powered wheelchair screening test for children with cerebral palsy. *Dev Med Child Neurol.* 2004;46:468–474.

260. Glickman LB, Geigle PR, Paleg GS. A systematic review of supported standing programs. *Pediatr Rehabil Med.* 2010;3(3):197–213.

261. Paleg GS, Smith BA, Glickman LB. Systematic review and evidence-based clinical recommendations for dosing of pediatric supported standing programs. *Pediatr Phys Ther.* 2013;25(3):232–247.

262. Paleg GS, Livingstone R. Outcomes of gait trainer use in home and school settings for children with motor impairments: a systematic review. *Clin Rehab.* 2015;29(11):1077–1091.

263. Logan L, Byers-Hinkley K, Ciccone CD. Anterior versus posterior walkers: a gait analysis study. *Dev Med Child Neurol.* 1990;32:1044–1048.

264. Levangie PK, Chimera M, Johnston M, et al. The effects of posterior rolling walkers on gait characteristics of children with spastic cerebral palsy. *Phys Occup Ther Pediatr.* 1989;9:1–17.

265. Verotti A, Greco R, Spalice A, et al. Pharmacotherapy of spasticity in children with cerebral palsy. *Pediatr Neurol.* 2006;34:1–6.

266. Tardieu G, Tardieu C, Hariga J, et al. Treatment of spasticity in injection of dilute alcohol at the motor point or by epidural route. Clinical extension of an experiment on the decerebrate cat. *Dev Med Child Neurol.* 1968;10:555–568.

267. Spira R. Management of spasticity in cerebral palsied children by peripheral nerve block with phenol. *Dev Med Child Neurol.* 1971;13:164–173.

268. Yadav SL, Singh U, Dureja GP, et al. Phenol block in the management of spastic cerebral palsy. *Indian J Pediatr.* 1994;61:249–255.

269. Wong AMK, Chen CL, Chen CPC, et al. Clinical effects of botulinum toxin A and phenol block on gait in children with cerebral palsy. *Am J Phys Med Rehabil.* 2004;83(4):284–291.

270. Sutherland DH, Kaufman KR, Wyatt MP, et al. Injection of botulinum A toxin into the gastrocnemius muscle of patients with cerebral palsy: a 3-dimensional motion analysis study. *Gait Posture.* 1996;4:269–279.

271. Fragala MA, O'Neil ME, Russo KJ, et al. Impairment, disability, and satisfaction outcomes after lower extremity botulinum toxin A injections for children with cerebral palsy. *Pediatr Phys Ther.* 2002;14(3):132–144.

272. Gough M, Fairhurst C, Shortland AP. Botulinum toxin and cerebral palsy: time for reflection? *Dev Med Child Neurol.* 2005;47(10):709–712.

273. Multani I, Manji J, Hastings-Ison T, et al. Botulinum toxin in the management of children with cerebral palsy. *Paediatr Drug.* 2019;21(4):261–281.

274. Echols K, DeLuca S, Ramey S, et al. Constraint induced movement therapy in children with cerebral palsy. In: *Proceedings of the American Academy of Cerebral Palsy and Developmental Medicine. Dev Med Child Neurol.* 2001;43.

275. Peacock WJ, Stoudt LA. Functional outcomes following selective posterior rhizotomy in children with cerebral palsy. *J Neurosurg.* 1991;74:380–385.

276. Guiliani CA. Dorsal rhizotomy for children with cerebral palsy: support for concept of motor control. *Phys Ther.* 1991;71:248–259.

277. Abbott R, Forem SL, Johann M. Selective posterior rhizotomy for the treatment of spasticity: a review. *Childs Nerv Syst.* 1989;5:337–346.

278. Oppenheim W. Selective posterior rhizotomy for spastic cerebral palsy. A review. *Clin Orthop Relat Res.* 1990;253:20–29.

279. Tedroff K, Hagglund G, Miller F. Long-term effects of selective dorsal rhizotomy in children with cerebral palsy: a systematic review. *Dev Med Child Neurol.* 2020;62(5):554–562.

280. Dudley RW, Parolin M, Gagnon B, et al. Long-term functional benefits of selective dorsal rhizotomy for spastic cerebral palsy. *J Neurosurg Pediatr.* 2013;12(2):142–150.

281. Lonstein JE. Cerebral palsy. In: Weinstein SL, ed. *The Pediatric Spine: Principles and Practice.* Ravens Press Ltd; 1994.

282. Albright AL, Cervi A, Singletary J. Intrathecal baclofen for spasticity in cerebral palsy. *JAMA.* 1991;265:1418–1422.

283. Gilmartin R, Bruce D, Storrs BB, et al. Intrathecal baclofen for management of spastic cerebral palsy: multicenter trial. *J Child Neurol.* 2000;15:71–77.

284. Hoving MA, van Raak EP, Spincermaille GH, et al. Efficacy of intrathecal baclofen therapy in children with intractable spastic cerebral palsy: a randomized control trial. *Eur J Paediatr Neurol.* 2009;13:240–246.

285. Barry MJ, Albright AL, Shultz BL. Intrathecal baclofen therapy and the role of the physical therapist. *Pediatr Phys Ther.* 2000;12:77–86.

286. Morton R, Gray N, Vloeberghs M. Controlled study of the effects of continuous intrathecal baclofen infusion in non-ambulant children with cerebral palsy. *Dev Med Child Neurol.* 2011;53:736–741.

287. Brochard S, Lempereur M, Filipetti P, et al. Changes in gait following continuous intrathecal baclofen infusion in ambulant children and young adults with cerebral palsy. *Dev Neurorehabil.* 2009;12(6):397–405.

288. Bleyenheuft C, Filipetti P, Caldas C, et al. Experience with external pump trial prior to implantation for intrathecal baclofen in ambulatory patients with spastic cerebral palsy. *Neurophysiol Clin.* 2007;37:23–28.

289. Shilt J, Reeves S, Lai L, et al. The outcome of intrathecal baclofen treatment on spastic diplegia: preliminary results with minimum of two-year follow-up. *J Pediatr Rehabil Med.* 2008;1:255–261.

290. Gerszen P, Albright A, Barry M. Effect on ambulation of continuous intrathecal baclofen infusion. *Pediatr Neurosurg.* 1997;27:40–44.

291. Conclaves J, Garcia-March G, Sanchez-Ledesma M, et al. Management of intractable spasticity of supraspinal origin by chronic cervical intrathecal infusion of baclofen. *Stereotact Funct Neurosurg.* 1994;62:108–112.

292. Fitzgerald JJ, Tsegaye M, Vloeberghs MH. Treatment of childhood spasticity of cerebral origin with intrathecal baclofen: a series of 52 cases. *Br J Neurosurg.* 2004;18:240–245.

293. Gooch JL, Oberg WA, Grams B, et al. Care provider assessment of intrathecal baclofen in children. *Dev Med Child Neurol.* 2004;46:548–552.

294. Brochard S, Remy-Neris O, Filipetti P, et al. Intrathecal baclofen infusion for ambulant children with cerebral palsy. *Pediatr Neurol.* 2009;40:265–270.

295. Pin TW, McCartney L, Lewis J, et al. Use of intrathecal baclofen therapy in ambulant children and adolescents with spasticity and dystonia of cerebral origin: a systematic review. *Dev Med Child Neurol.* 2011;53(10):885–895.

296. Krach L, Kriel R, Gilmartin R, et al. GMFM 1 year after continuous intrathecal baclofen infusion. *Pediatr Rehabil.* 2005;8:207–213.

297. Motta F, Antonello C, Stignani C. Intrathecal baclofen and motor function in cerebral palsy. *Dev Med Child Neurol.* 2011;53:443–448.

298. Sprague JB. Surgical management of cerebral palsy. *Orthop Nurs.* 1992;11(4):11–19.

299. Dormans JP. Orthopedic management of children with cerebral palsy. *Pediatr Clin North Am.* 1993;40(3):645–657.

300. Thomason P, Baker R, Dodd K, et al. Single-event multi-level surgery in children with spastic diplegia. *J Bone Joint Surg Am.* 2011;93:451–460.

301. McGinley JL, Dobson F, Ganeshalingam R, et al. Single-event multilevel surgery for children with cerebral palsy: a systematic review. *Dev Med Child Neurol.* 2012;54:117–128.

302. Godwin EM, Spero CR, Nof L, et al. The gross motor function classification system for cerebral palsy and single-event multilevel surgery: is there a relationship between level of function and intervention over time? *J Pediatr Orthop.* 2009;29:910–915.

303. McCarthy JJ, D'Andrea LP, Betz RR, et al. Scoliosis in the child with cerebral palsy. *J Am Acad Orthop Surg.* 2006;14:367–375.

304. Tsirkos A, Lipton G, Chang W-N, et al. Surgical correction of scoliosis in pediatric patients with cerebral palsy using the unit rod instrumentation. *Spine.* 2008;33:1133–1140.

305. Bohtz C, Meyer-Heim A, Min K. Changes in health related quality of life after spinal fusion and scoliosis correction in patients with cerebral palsy. *J Pediatr Orthop.* 2011;31:668–673.

306. Sarwark J, Sarwahi V. New strategies and decision making in the management of neuromuscular scoliosis. *Orthop Clin North Am.* 2007;38:485–496.

307. Comstock CP, Leach J, Wenger DR. Scoliosis in total-body involvement cerebral palsy: analysis of surgical treatment and patient and caregiver satisfaction. *Spine.* 1998;23:1412–1425.

308. Green NE. The orthopedic management of the ankle, foot, and knee in patients with cerebral palsy. Neuromuscular disease and deformities. *Instr Course Lect.* 1987;36:253–256.

309. Moens P, Lammens J, Molenaers G, et al. Femoral derotation for increased hip anteversion. A new surgical technique with a modified Ilizarov frame. *J Bone Joint Surg Br.* 1995;77(1):107–109.

310. Lonstein JE, Beck RP. Hip dislocation and subluxation in cerebral palsy. *J Pediatr Orthop.* 1986;6:521–526.

311. Soo B, Howard JJ, Boyd RN, et al. Hip displacement in cerebral palsy. *J Bone Jont Surg Am.* 2006;88:121–129.

312. Gamble JG, Rinsky LA, Bleck EE. Established hip dislocations in children with cerebral palsy. *Clin Orthop Relat Res.* 1990;253:90–99.

313. Root L, Laplasa FJ, Brourman SN, et al. The severely unstable hip in cerebral palsy. Treatment with open reduction, pelvic osteotomy, and femoral osteotomy with shortening. *J Bone Joint Surg Am.* 1995;77(5):703–712.

314. Brunner R, Baumann JU. Clinical benefit of reconstruction of dislocated or subluxated hip joints in patients with spastic cerebral palsy. *J Pediatr Orthop.* 1994;14(3):290–294.

315. Atar D, Grant AD, Bash J, et al. Combined hip surgery in cerebral palsy patients. *Am J Orthop.* 1995;24(1):52–55.

316. Barrie JL, Galasko CS. Surgery for unstable hips in cerebral palsy. *J Pediatr Orthop B.* 1996;5(4):225–231.

317. Patrick JH. Techniques of psoas tenotomy and rectus femoris transfer: "new" operations for cerebral palsy diplegia—a description. *J Pediatr Orthop B.* 1996;5(4):242–246.

318. Moreau M, Cook PC, Ashton B. Adductor and psoas release for subluxation of the hip in children with spastic cerebral palsy. *J Pediatr Orthop.* 1995;15(5):672–676.

319. Dreher T, Vegvari D, Wolf SI, et al. Development of knee function after hamstring lengthening as a part of multilevel surgery in children with spastic diplegia. *J Bone Joint Surg Am.* 2012;94:121–130.

320. Gage JR. Surgical treatment of knee dysfunction in cerebral palsy. *Clin Orthop Relat Res.* 1990;253:45–54.

321. Karol LA, Chambers C, Popejoy D, et al. Nerve palsy after hamstring lengthening in patients with cerebral palsy. *J Pediatr Orthop.* 2008;28:773–776.

322. Kay RM, Rethlefsen SA, Skaggs D, et al. Outcome of medial versus combined medial and lateral hamstring lengthening surgery in cerebral palsy. *J Pediatr Orthop.* 2002;22:169–172.

323. Abel MF, Damiano DL, Pannunzio M, et al. Muscle tendon surgery in diplegic cerebral palsy: functional and mechanical changes. *J Pediatr Orthop.* 1999;19:366–375.

324. Jones S, Haydar AJ, Hussainy A, et al. Distal hamstring lengthening in cerebral palsy: the influence of the proximal aponeurotic band of the semimembranosus. *J Pediatr Orthop.* 2006;15:104–108.

325. Root L. Distal hamstring surgery in cerebral palsy. In: Sussman MD, ed. *The Diplegic Child Evaluation and Management.* American Academy of Orthopaedic Surgeons; 1992.

326. Gage JR. Distal hamstring lengthening/release and rectus femoris transfer. In: Sussman MD, ed. *The Diplegic Child Evaluation and Management.* American Academy of Orthopaedic Surgeons; 1992.

327. Chang WN, Tsirkos AI, Miller F, et al. Distal hamstring lengthening in ambulatory children with cerebral palsy: primary versus revision procedures. *Gait Posture.* 2004;19:298–304.

328. Gordon AB, Baird GO, McMulkin ML, et al. Gait analysis outcomes of percutaneous medial hamstring tenotomies in children with cerebral palsy. *J Pediatr Orthop.* 2008;28:324–329.

329. Damiano DL, Abel MF, Pannunzio M, et al. Interrelationships of strength and gait before and after hamstring lengthening. *J Pediatr Orthop.* 1999;19:352–358.

330. Booth MY, Yates CC, Edgar TS, et al. Serial casting vs combined intervention with botulinum toxin A and serial casting in the treatment of spastic equinus in children. *Pediatr Phys Ther.* 2003;15(4):216–220.

331. Mazur JM, Shanks DE. Nonsurgical treatment of tight Achilles tendon. In: Sussman MD, ed. *The Diplegic Child: Evaluation and Management.* American Academy of Orthopaedic Surgeons; 1992.

332. Yngve DA, Chambers C. Vulpius and Z-lengthening. *J Pediatr Orthop.* 1996;16(6):759–764.

333. Kay RM, Rethlefsen SA, Ryan JA, et al. Outcome of gastrocnemius recession and tendo-achilles lengthening in ambulatory children with cerebral palsy. *J Pediatr Orthop B.* 2004;13:92–98.

334. Borton DC, Walker K, Pipiris M, et al. Isolated calf lengthening in cerebral palsy. Outcome analysis of risk factors. *J Bone Joint Surg Br.* 2001;83(3):364–370.

335. Etnyre B, Chambers CS, Scarborough NH, et al. Preoperative and postoperative assessment of surgical intervention for equinus gait in children with cerebral palsy. *J Pediatr Orthop.* 1993;13:24–31.

336. Gaines RW, Ford TB. A systematic approach to the amount of Achilles tendon lengthening in cerebral palsy. *J Pediatr Orthop.* 1987;7:253–255.

337. Rosenthal RK, Simon SR. The Vulpius gastrocnemius-soleus lengthening. In: Sussman MD, ed. *The Diplegic Child Evaluation and Management.* American Academy of Orthopaedic Surgeons; 1992.

338. Segal LS, Thomas SE, Mazur JM, et al. Calcaneal gait in spastic diplegia after heel cord lengthening: a study with gait analysis. *J Pediatr Orthop.* 1989;9:697–701.

339. Kagaya H, Yamada S, Nagasawa T, et al. Split posterior tibial tendon transfer for varus deformity of hindfoot. *Clin Orthop Relat Res.* 1996;323:254–260.

340. Roehr B, Lyne ED. Split anterior tibial tendon transfer. In: Sussman MD, ed. *The Diplegic Child: Evaluation and Management.* American Academy of Orthopaedic Surgeons; 1992.

341. Green NE. Split posterior tibial tendon transfer: the universal procedure. In: Sussman MD, ed. *The Diplegic Child: Evaluation and Management.* American Academy of Orthopaedic Surgeons; 1992.

342. Rogozinski BM, Davids JR, Davis RB III, et al. The efficacy of the floor-reaction ankle-foot orthosis in children with cerebral palsy. *J Bone Joint Surg Am.* 2009;91(10):2440–2447.

343. Rosenthal R. The use of orthotics in foot and ankle problems in cerebral palsy. *Foot Ankle.* 1984;4:195–200.

344. Figueiredo EM, Ferreira GB, Moreira RC, et al. Efficacy of ankle-foot orthoses on gait of children with cerebral palsy: systematic review of literature. *Pediatr Phys Ther.* 2008;20:207–223.

345. Radtka S, Skinner S, Johanson M. A comparison of gait with solid and hinged ankle-foot orthoses in children with spastic diplegic cerebral palsy. *Gait Posture.* 2005;21:303–310.

346. Buckton CE, Thomas S, Huston S, et al. Comparison of three ankle-foot orthoses configurations for children with spastic hemiplegia. *Dev Med Child Neurol.* 2004;46:590–598.

347. Lam WK, Leong JC, Li YH, et al. Biomechanical and electromyographic evaluation of ankle foot orthosis and dynamic ankle foot orthosis in spastic cerebral palsy. *Gait Posture.* 2005;2:189–197.

348. Burtner PA, Woollacott MH, Qualls C. Stance balance control with orthoses in a group of children with spastic cerebral palsy. *Dev Med Child Neurol.* 1999;41:748–757.

349. Middleton EA, Hurley GR, McIlwain JS. The role of rigid and hinged polypropylene ankle-foot orthoses in the management of cerebral palsy: a case study. *Prosthet Orthot Int.* 1988;12:129–135.

350. Carmick J. Managing equinus in a child with cerebral palsy: merits of hinged ankle-foot orthoses. *Dev Med Child Neurol.* 1995;37(11):1006–1010.

351. Romkes J, Brunner R. Comparison of dynamic and a hinged ankle foot orthoses by gait analysis in patients with hemiplegic cerebral palsy. *Gait Posture.* 2002;15:18–24.

352. Mol EM, Monbaliu E, Ven M, et al. The use of night orthoses in cerebral palsy treatment: sleep disturbance in children and parental burden or not? *Res Dev Disabil.* 2012;33:341–349.

353. Ounuu S, Bell K, Davis R, et al. An evaluation of the posterior leaf spring orthosis using joint kinematic and kinetics. *J Pediatr Orthop.* 1996;16(3):378–384.

354. Aboutorabi A, Arazpour M, Ahmadi Bani M, Saeedi H, Head JS. Efficacy of ankle foot orthoses types on walking in children with cerebral palsy: a systematic review. *Ann Phys Rehabil Med.* 2017;60(6):393–402.

355. Hylton N. Dynamic casting and orthotics. In: *The Practical Management of Spasticity of Spasticity in Children and Adults.* Lea & Febiger; 1990.

356. Radtka SA. A comparison of gait with solid, dynamic, and no ankle-foot orthoses in children with spastic cerebral palsy. *Phys Ther.* 1997;77(4):395–409.

357. Kobayashi T, Leung A, Hutchins, S. Design and effect of ankle-foot orthoses proposed to influence muscle tone: a review. *J Prosthet Orthot.* 2011;23(2):52–57.

358. Carlson WE, Vaughan CL, Damiano DL, et al. Orthotic management of gait in spastic diplegia. *Am J Phys Med Rehabil.* 1997;76:291–225.

359. Bjornson K, Schmale G, Adamczyk-Foster A, et al. The effect of dynamic ankle foot orthoses on function in children with cerebral palsy. *J Pediatr Orthop.* 2006;26(6):773–776.

360. Martin K. Supramelleolar orthoses and postural stability in children with down syndrome-Martin replies. *Dev Med Child Neurol.* 2005;47:71.

361. Pohl M, Mehrholz J. Immediate effects of an individually designed functional ankle-foot orthosis on stance and gait in hemiparetic patients. *Clin Rehabil.* 2006;20:324–330.

362. Harris SR, Riffle K. Effects of inhibitive ankle-foot orthoses on standing balance in a child with cerebral palsy. A single-subject design. *Phys Ther.* 1986;66:663–667.

363. Ramstrand N, Ramstrand S. AAOP state-of-the-science evidence report: the effect of ankle-foot orthoses on balance—a systematic review. *J Prosthet Orthot.* 2010;22(10):4–23.

364. Kornhaber L, Majsak M, Robinson A. Advantages of supramalleolar orthotics over articulating ankle-foot orthotics in the gait and gross motor function of children with spastic diplegic cerebral palsy. *Pediatr Phys Ther.* 2006;18(1):95–96.

365. Chen C, Shen I, Chen C, et al. Validity, responsiveness, minimal detectable change, and minimal clinically important change of Pediatric Balance Scale in children with cerebral palsy. *Res Dev Disabil.* 2013;34:916–922.

366. Randall KE, Bartlett DJ, McCoy S. Head-to-head comparison of the early clinical assessment of balance test in young children with cerebral palsy. *Pediatr Phys Ther.* 2014;26:332–337.

367. Fiss AF, Jefferies L, Bjornson K, et al. Developmental trajectories and reference percentiles for the 6-minute walk test for children with cerebral palsy. *Pediatr Phys Ther.* 2019;31:51–59.

368. Weingarten G, Lieberstein M, Itkowitz A, Vialu C, Doyle M, Kaplan S. Timed floor to stand-natural: reference data for school age children. *Pediatr Phys Ther.* 2016;28(1):71–76.

369. Carey H, Martin K, Combs-Miller S, Heathcock JC. Reliability and responsiveness of the timed up and go test in children with cerebral palsy. *Pediatr Phys Ther.* 2016;28:401–408.

370. Zaino C, Marchese VG, & Westcott SL. Timed up and down stairs test: preliminary reliability and validity of a new measure of functional mobility. *Pediatr Phys Ther.* 2004;16:90–98.

371. Hansen L, Erhardsen KT, Bencke J, et al. The reliability of the timed up and go (SATC o) in children with cerebral palsy. *Phys Occup Ther Pediart.* 2018;38(3):291–304.

372. Butler P, Saavedra S, Sofranac M, et al. Refinement, reliability and validity of the segmental assessment of trunk control (SATC o). *Pediatr Phys Ther.* 2010;22(3):246–257.

373. Heyrman L, Molenaers G, Desloovere K, et al. A clinical tool to measure trunk control in children with cerebral palsy: the trunk control measurement scale. *Res Dev Disabil.* 2011;32(6):2624–2635.

Spina Bifida

Elena Tappit-Emas

» Incidence and etiology

Spina bifida is a type of neural tube birth defect causing neuromuscular dysfunction. Until recently, the occurrence of spina bifida approached 1 in every 1,000 pregnancies, making it the second most common birth defect after Down syndrome. The increased availability of maternal vitamin supplements, more accurate prenatal testing, and pregnancy termination options have greatly reduced the incidence of babies born with this diagnosis in much of the world. In the United States, that number has now stabilized at 3.4 per 10,000 live births. Studies examining the possible causes of spina bifida have evaluated genetic, environmental, and dietary factors that might affect its occurrence. However, no single definitive cause, including chromosomal abnormalities, has yet been identified.[1-3]

Many factors may contribute to a baby being born with spina bifida. The presence of a genetic predisposition may be enhanced by numerous environmental influences. Low levels of maternal folic acid prior to conception have been implicated in several studies. Duff and Cooper found a significant, though temporary, increase in the number of children born with all types of neural tube defects (NTDs) on the island of Jamaica who were conceived during the months immediately following Hurricane Gilbert in September of 1988. The typical diet of the island is rich in naturally occurring folic acid or vitamin B-9 from fresh fruit and vegetables. The hurricane destroyed many of the island's crops, and for a temporary period, fresh produce was scarce.[4] This study as well as an annotation by Seller proposed the need to fortify with folic acid commonly eaten foods such as orange juice, cereals, flour, rice, and salt.[5]

In 1992, the U.S. Public Health Service recommended that all women receive a daily dose of 400 μg of folic acid during the months prior to conception and 600 μg through the first trimester of pregnancy. With improved education and the support of the medical community, this level of folic acid can be reached through improved diet, dietary supplements, and fortified foods. Folic acid is abundant in dark green leafy vegetables, beans, nuts and seeds, citrus fruits, enriched grains, pasta, bread, and rice.[6] A diet consistently rich in folic acid can be difficult to maintain. In 1996, the health departments of both the United States and Canada recommended that all cereal grains be fortified with folic acid to enable women to more easily reach this daily requirement. Two years later, fortification was mandated. The U.S. Department of Health and Human Services also set a national objective to reduce by 50% the number of children born with spina bifida.[6-9] The reduction is currently closer to between 26% and 36%, but this improvement is encouraging.[10-12] It appears that the ability of folic acid to significantly reduce the incidence of spina bifida has now directed researchers' attention to the genes involved with folic acid metabolism and transport as the target of further investigation.[13,14] Costa Rica, Chile, and South Africa have joined the United States and Canada, seeing a decline in the incidence of babies born with NTD after folic acid was added to grains.[15]

Maternal use of valproic acid, an anticonvulsant, is also known to increase the potential for spina bifida. It appears that the developing nervous system is especially sensitive to disruption after exposure to this drug.[14] Maternal use of antidepressants has also been examined and is considered another possible risk factor.[16] Maternal hyperthermia caused by saunas, hot tubs and electric blanket use, and maternal fevers during the first trimester of pregnancy were studied, and only the use of hot tubs showed any tendency to increase the risk of spina bifida.[17] It appears in more recent investigations that this has not attracted wide concern.

In the United States, in past decades, the highest occurrence of spina bifida was seen in families of Irish and Celtic heritage, with as many as 4.5 per 1,000 pregnancies. This was thought to be the result of lingering nutritional deficits from the Irish Potato Famine more than 100 years ago, but the true etiology might be the link between a limited diet and an inherent genetic predisposition. Japanese families, with 0.3 per 1,000 pregnancies, historically had the lowest occurrence rate.[18] More recently, as the overall number of affected births has decreased for Caucasian women in the United States, there has not been the same level of decrease seen in babies born to African-American women.[19] Also, the number of affected babies born to Latina mothers has not decreased as much as in the Caucasian and African-American populations.[19] One suspected factor is a change in diet for Latino families. As this group, in the United States, has shifted from rural farms and small towns to large American cities, access to natural folic acid is more difficult. There may also be a genetic resistance to the absorption of folic acid from vitamin supplements, by Latina women, compared with the vitamin in its naturally occurring state. There is added concern about socioeconomic factors that might negatively influence this group. The effects of a language barrier, limited access to prenatal care, and financial challenges adhering to a vitamin and dietary regimen are just a few.

Among all populations, one cannot disregard the influence of religious practice or personal philosophy on a woman's decision to terminate a pregnancy after a birth defect is identified in the fetus. In a recent multinational study, 63% of women opted to end their pregnancy when spina bifida was diagnosed before 24 weeks of gestation.[20-23]

Lastly, for families in which spina bifida is already present, there is a 2% to 5% greater chance than in the general population of having a second child born with the defect. This introductory section includes a great deal of data primarily to illustrate that the number of babies born with spina bifida has been decreasing in this country and around the world. For some groups of women, there remain various confounding factors preventing them from experiencing this decrease.

» Prognosis

In previous generations, long-term survival of children with spina bifida was reported to range from as low as 1% without treatment to 50% with treatment. A survival rate of more than 90% is now expected when aggressive treatment is provided to the spinal defect and its associated problems. This chapter presents the primary problems affecting this population of children, which include hydrocephalus, motor and sensory deficits in the lower extremities, and urologic impairment, as well as the secondary issues such as orthopedic and cognitive/perceptual deficits, which are of clinical significance for the physical therapist (PT).

The use of antibiotics to limit infection in the open spine, starting in 1947, and the surgical insertion of ventricular shunts in 1960 to manage hydrocephalus were two major advances in the treatment of spina bifida. Early and consistent use of clean, intermittent catheterization to completely empty the neurogenic bladder has also dramatically improved the survival rate by controlling urinary tract infection and renal deterioration, both of which have been cited as major causes of mortality. These measures, along with the practice of early back closure, continue to improve the chances of survival of children with spina bifida. As the survival rate improved, an increased awareness evolved for the associated problems that were neither immediately evident nor a priority for treatment in the past. The number of severely affected children who have survived has increased. Additionally, there is an increased number of less severely involved individuals who would not have lived without aggressive treatment protocols. Therefore, the full spectrum and complexity of this

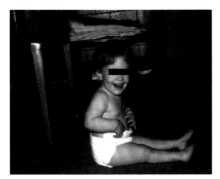

FIGURE 10.1. A young child with spina bifida.

disability can now be appreciated. PTs have the opportunity, not available in previous eras, to work with and learn a great deal from this heterogeneous group (Fig. 10.1).[24,25]

» Definitions

The terms myelomeningocele, meningomyelocele, spina bifida, spina bifida aperta, spina bifida cystica, spinal dysraphism, and myelodysplasia are all synonymous. They are used interchangeably by various medical communities throughout the world. Spina bifida is used in this chapter for consistency. Spina bifida is a spinal defect usually diagnosed at birth by the presence of an external sac on the infant's back (Fig. 10.2). The sac contains meninges and spinal cord tissue protruding through a dorsal bony defect in the vertebrae. This defect may occur at any point along the spine but is most commonly located in the lumbar region. The sac may be covered by a transparent membrane with neural tissue attached to its inner surface, or may be open with the neural tissue exposed. The lateral borders of the sac have bony protrusions formed by the unfused neural arches of the vertebrae. The defect may be large, with many vertebrae involved, or small, involving only one or two segments. The size of the lesion is not by itself predictive of the child's functional deficit or ultimate outcome.[18,25,26]

Several other congenital spinal defects should be mentioned here. *Spina bifida occulta, myelocele,* and *lipomeningocele* are less severe anomalies associated with spina bifida. *Spina bifida occulta* is a condition involving nonfusion of the halves of the vertebral arches but without disturbance of the underlying neural tissue. This lesion is most commonly located in the lumbar or sacral spine and is often an incidental finding when imaging is done for unrelated reasons. Spina bifida occulta may be distinguished externally by a midline tuft of hair, with or without an area of pigmentation on the overlying skin. Between 21% and 26% of parents who have children with spina bifida cystica have been found to have an occulta defect. Otherwise, spina bifida occulta has only a 4.5% to 8% incidence in the general population.[18,25] Neurologic and muscular dysfunction were previously thought to be absent in individuals with spina bifida occulta; however, a high rate of

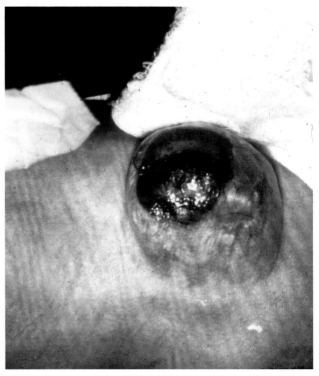

FIGURE 10.2. Spina bifida defect on a newborn before surgical back closure. The term "closure" is used rather than back repair because the damage to the spinal nerves is permanent and cannot be repaired. Incorrect terminology can be misleading to families.

tethered cord, its associated neurologic problems, and, especially, urinary tract disorders in these individuals have been found.[27-29] Refer to additional information regarding tethered cord later in this chapter.

A *myelocele* is a protruding sac containing meninges and cerebrospinal fluid (CSF), but the spinal cord and nerve roots remain intact and in their normal positions. There are typically no motor or sensory deficits, hydrocephalus, or other central nervous system (CNS) problems associated with a myelocele.[26]

Lipomeningocele is a superficial fatty mass in the low lumbar or sacral region of the spinal cord and is usually included with this group of diagnoses. Significant neurologic deficits and hydrocephalus are not expected in children with a lipomeningocele; however, a high incidence of bowel and bladder dysfunction resulting from a tethered spinal cord has been noted in this population as well as subtle changes in distal leg strength and foot function. These findings are usually seen in later childhood or early adolescence, especially after a growth spurt.[30]

» Embryology

Spina bifida cystica, one of several NTDs, occurs early in the embryologic development of the CNS. Cells of the neural plate, which forms by day 18 of gestation, differentiate to create the neural tube and neural crest. The neural crest becomes the peripheral nervous system, including the cranial nerves, spinal nerves, autonomic nerves, and ganglia. The neural tube, which becomes the CNS; the brain, and the spinal cord, is open at both the cranial and caudal ends. Over a period of 2 to 4 days, the cranial end begins to close, and this process is completed on approximately the 24th day of gestation.[14] Failure to close at the cranial end results in anencephaly, a fatal condition. The caudal end of the neural tube closes on approximately day 26 of gestation. Failure of the neural tube to close at any point along the caudal border initiates the defect of spina bifida cystica or myelomeningocele. Common clinical signs of spina bifida include an absence of motor and sensory function (usually bilateral) below the level of the spinal defect and loss of neural control of bowel and bladder function. Unilateral motor and sensory loss has been seen, and the pattern of loss may also be asymmetric, with a higher motor or sensory level on one side than on the other. The functional deficits may be partial or complete, but they are almost always permanent.[25,31,32]

» Hydrocephalus and the Chiari II malformation

Hydrocephalus and the *Arnold–Chiari malformation* are CNS abnormalities that are closely associated with spina bifida. *Hydrocephalus* is an abnormal accumulation of CSF in the cranial vault. In individuals without spina bifida, hydrocephalus may be caused by overproduction of CSF, a failure in absorption of CSF fluid, or an obstruction in the normal flow of CSF through the brain structures and spinal cord. Obstruction by the *Arnold–Chiari malformation* is considered to be the primary cause of hydrocephalus in most children with spina bifida. This malformation, also known as the *Chiari II malformation*, is a deformity of the cerebellum, medulla, and cervical spinal cord. The posterior cerebellum is herniated downward through the foramen magnum, with brain stem structures also displaced in a caudal direction. The CSF released from the fourth ventricle is obstructed by these abnormally situated structures, and the flow through the foramen magnum is disrupted. Traction on the lower cranial nerves also occurs and is associated with the malformation. Studies using magnetic resonance imaging (MRI) have shown that most children with spina bifida have the Chiari II malformation. Among those with this malformation, the likelihood of hydrocephalus developing is greater than 90%.[33-36]

Theories related to the etiology of the Chiari II malformation are of interest. At one time, the primary spinal defect was thought to act as an anchor on the spinal cord, preventing it from sliding proximally within the spinal canal as the fetus grew. Traction on the cord was thought to pull down the attached brainstem structures into an abnormally low position. Hydrocephalus was believed to result solely from the hydrodynamic consequence of this blockage.[37] In 1989, McLone and Knepper more closely linked the occurrence of spina bifida, the Chiari II malformation, and hydrocephalus

at the cellular level.[38] They theorized that a series of interrelated, time-dependent defects occur during the embryonic development of the primitive ventricular system, causing, first, the Chiari II malformation and then the resulting hydrocephalus.[39] Their findings indicate that most affected children have a small posterior fossa that is unable to accommodate the hindbrain and brain stem structures, which may contribute to the abnormal positioning. Significantly, McLone and Knepper found that more than 25% of neonates with spina bifida whom they examined had head circumferences measuring below the fifth percentile. Therefore, neither downward traction from the spinal defect nor pressure from hydrocephalus caused the malformation. They postulated that spina bifida and the accompanying hydrocephalus result from mistimed steps in the development of the ventricular system that is initiated by the failure of the neural tube to close. This explanation has received widespread acceptance among both neuroanatomists and neurosurgeons and should be of interest to PTs who may have wondered about the CNS dysfunction that has been observed in many children with spina bifida. Individuals with spina bifida differ greatly from those who have only hydrocephalus without spina bifida, and they do not resemble those with acquired spinal paralysis either, two groups with whom they have incorrectly been compared. The McLone and Knepper theory begins to offer an anatomic rationale for the CNS abnormalities seen in many of these children and offers a viable basis for continued investigation.[38]

Approximately 2% to 3% of children with spina bifida show significant impairment from the Chiari II malformation[39] (Display 10.1). Tracheostomy and gastrostomy may be life-saving measures for the symptoms, which are reported to resolve in many cases as the child grows and the brain matures. In severe cases, vocal cord paralysis, upper extremity weakness, or opisthotonic postures may be seen. Posterior fossa decompression and cervical laminectomy to relieve

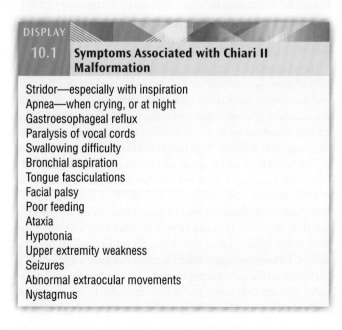

DISPLAY 10.1 **Symptoms Associated with Chiari II Malformation**

Stridor—especially with inspiration
Apnea—when crying, or at night
Gastroesophageal reflux
Paralysis of vocal cords
Swallowing difficulty
Bronchial aspiration
Tongue fasciculations
Facial palsy
Poor feeding
Ataxia
Hypotonia
Upper extremity weakness
Seizures
Abnormal extraocular movements
Nystagmus

pressure on the brain stem and cervical spinal structures are accepted courses of treatment but are associated with varying degrees of success. It is interesting that no correlation has been found between the severity of the Chiari II symptoms and the degree of hydrocephalus seen in the infant or between the child's spinal defect level and these CNS findings. Therefore, attempts to predict which children will experience significant CNS difficulties resulting from the Chiari II malformation have had limited success. Examination by MRI has revealed abnormalities in some children who appear asymptomatic. There is speculation that brain stem auditory-evoked potentials may provide diagnostic assistance. Physicians also believe that there is much to learn at the microscopic level about this abnormality, which may be helpful for further understanding.[18,25,40-43]

» Prenatal testing and diagnosis

Increasingly sophisticated and more widely available prenatal testing has allowed for the early diagnosis of spina bifida. Testing provides information that allows a family to make informed decisions about the pregnancy. As prenatal testing is now more routine than exceptional, a significant number of pregnancies are terminated each year when the results have indicated a high likelihood that the fetus has an NTD.[7,44,45] This is a major factor in the decrease in the number of babies being born with spina bifida. For the family that chooses to bring their baby to term, appropriate and coordinated medical care can be arranged in anticipation of the birth.

Alpha-fetoprotein (AFP) is normally present in the developing fetus and is found in the amniotic fluid. AFP levels reach their peak in the fetal blood and in the amniotic fluid from the 6th to the 14th week of gestation. In the presence of spina bifida, after the 14th week, AFP continues to leak into the amniotic fluid through the exposed vascularity of the open spine. Abnormally high levels of AFP in the amniotic fluid provide strong diagnostic evidence for the presence of an NTD. Testing for AFP by amniocentesis and in maternal blood samples has been responsible for the detection of approximately 89% of NTDs. The tests have the potential for both false-positive and false-negative results. Therefore, AFP results are routinely compared clinically with the results of ultrasound imaging before a definitive diagnosis is made.[25,33]

Improved ultrasound equipment and experienced technicians have enabled obstetricians to observe and document several cranial abnormalities that have a high correlation with the presence of spina bifida in the developing fetus. Because a small back lesion may be difficult to detect, clinicians use the presence of the cranial signs as an indication that the fetus may have spina bifida. One example is in the shape of the frontal bones of the fetal skull. They lose their normal convex shape and appear flattened when spina bifida is present, similarly to the shape of a lemon. The "lemon sign" can be detected before 24 weeks of gestation. It disappears as the fetus matures and the skull becomes stronger or

as hydrocephalus develops and pushes on the flattened skull, reversing its shape into the more typical configuration.[46] Detection of the lemon sign can then be followed by additional ultrasound studies specifically for the purpose of visualizing the back, looking for a lesion.[47-49]

There has been discussion regarding the best method of obstetric delivery when spina bifida is detected prenatally. A Cesarean section is considered to have a protective effect on the sensitive neural tissue of the neonatal back, thus possibly improving the child's ultimate functional status. Cesarean section reduces the trauma to the exposed nerves of the back that may occur during a vaginal delivery. Moreover, a Cesarean delivery avoids the bacterial contamination of the neonate's open spine during passage through the vaginal canal, reducing the risk of the baby contracting meningitis. A Cesarean section also avoids trauma to the back in the case of a difficult or breech presentation, which could also affect the infant's neurologic function. Finally, with early prenatal detection, it is believed that arrangements for the timely back closure surgery at an appropriate hospital can be planned and accomplished more successfully following a scheduled Cesarean section than with an unscheduled birth.[50-53]

» Fetal surgery

Since 1997, several institutions have made efforts to perform fetal surgery to repair the spinal defect prior to birth. This has not replaced the typical neonatal management for most babies born with spina bifida, but is one methodology that obstetricians and neurosurgeons are actively exploring to address the problem, with a highly selective population of mothers and fetuses. Johnson et al. performed prenatal surgery between 20 and 25 weeks' gestation and saw a survival rate of 94% with significant reversals in hindbrain herniation, a significant decrease in the need for shunting secondary to hydrocephalus, and improvement in lower extremity function.[54] Two other studies also demonstrated a lessening of hindbrain herniation, a decrease in the need for shunting, and an older median age for the insertion of the first shunt for those infants who did develop hydrocephalus. In these studies, there was no indication that lower extremity motor function improved with fetal surgery.[55,56] In a 2011 study assessing fetal correction of spina bifida performed at three US surgical centers, Vanderbilt University, Children's Hospital of Philadelphia, and the University of California, San Francisco, the outcome for babies who received this surgery between 19 and 25.9 weeks' gestation was generally positive. Known as MOMS (Management of Myelomeningocele Study), the results indicated that by 12 months of age, 30% fewer babies required shunting for hydrocephalus, and the occurrence and severity of hindbrain herniation was reduced by more than 30%. Additionally, at 30 months of age, babies demonstrated better leg movement by as much as two segmental levels as compared with the predicted movement based on the anatomic location of their lesion. The theory that is propelling this area of fetal intervention is that the amniotic environment is harmful to the exposed neural tissue and actually has a deteriorating effect on the spinal cord if left unprotected through the remaining months of gestation. When fetal repair is performed, the nervous system has additional time to develop in a more normal environment and manner.[3] Follow-up of the original cohort of babies from 1995 until 2019, reported by Houtrow et al. found that many of the benefits of fetal surgery seen early in the child's life continued through school age in both neurologic and motor areas.[57]

All of the prenatal studies identified several and significant risk factors for fetal back repair, which include an increase in infant mortality, premature births and its associated complications, lowered birth weights, and increased infant morbidity. Maternal complications included preterm labor and placental abruption (premature separation) and thinning of the uterine wall that would impact the success of future pregnancies. But, overall, the authors are optimistic that there are significant benefits to be gained by performing fetal surgery and that over time, concentrating on improving the surgical procedure and the maternal/fetal selection will reduce the risk factors and diminish many of the negative results.[3,55,56] Dr. David Shurtleff of the Seattle Children's Hospital and other well-respected researchers who have long been involved with the treatment of children with spina bifida have voiced their concern that larger and more long-range studies are needed before fetal spinal repair can be accepted as the standard of care. At stake is whether the initial improvement in motor and neurologic findings will translate into better functional abilities for the older child in the areas of gait, cognitive ability, sexual function, and bowel and bladder control and whether these functional gains will outweigh the risk factors to both mother and child.[3,58-60]

>> Management of the neonate

General Philosophy of Treatment

Philosophies of treatment for the neonate with spina bifida vary throughout the world and within the United States as well. Because the back lesion was not universally thought to be life threatening, hospitals developed their own protocols for the timing and intensity of treatment for infants. However, comparing the results of studies in which various initial treatment regimens were used supports the efficacy of early medical intervention. Immediate sterile care of the open spine to prevent infection is essential, and surgical closure of the back within 72 hours of birth is now an accepted goal in most institutions.[18,25,61]

The objective of back surgery is to place the neural tissue into the vertebral canal, cover the spinal defect with surrounding skin and fascia, and achieve a flat, watertight closure of the sac (Fig. 10.3). The open spine provides direct access for infection to the spinal cord and brain. Preventing infection and its potential for brain damage can preserve, the child's level of function, both physically and cognitively.

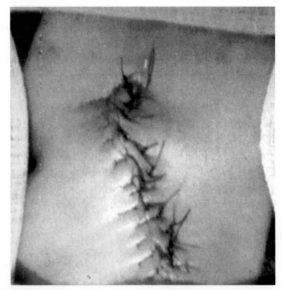

FIGURE 10.3. The same defect shown in Figure 10.2, after surgical closure.

McLone and associates have shown that babies who suffered gram-negative ventriculitis were less adept intellectually than those who had experienced no infection. This study is significant in that intellectual function was otherwise not negatively affected by either the presence of hydrocephalus or the level of lower limb paralysis.[17,61-63]

Many institutions treat children with spina bifida aggressively with immediate back closure and rapid management of hydrocephalus. Others practice selective treatment. That is, more aggressive management is offered to those children who appear to be less physically involved. In these institutions, the care of the neonate with spina bifida will vary depending on the level of lower extremity paralysis and the presence of other complicating factors. Some of the factors that influence treatment decisions include accompanying abnormalities, such as severe hydrocephalus, kyphoscoliosis, and renal problems. Still other institutions work to educate parents regarding their baby's status and the long-term implications that spina bifida will have on all of their lives. The parents may then, with support from the medical staff, thoughtfully decide on a mutually acceptable course of action. During this period of education and planning, which may last several hours or weeks, the infant is usually treated to maintain a stable condition and prevent infection.

Regardless of the treatment protocols, this early period provides time for the medical staff to gather information about the baby. Discussions can begin about the management of hydrocephalus if it is present or orthopedic deformities that are noted and that may need to be addressed in the coming months. It is important to note that an accurate prediction of the infant's functional potential by the medical staff is difficult in these early days even when the baby's problems seem minimal. Many variables will influence the child's medical condition and cognitive and motor abilities in the coming years. Clinicians must be wary about presenting long-term prognostic information about the child's future. The exception to this may be in the case of a child who presents with multiple and significant congenital anomalies as well as spina bifida whose outcome is apparently bleak and for whom aggressive management may not be recommended.[64,65]

Preoperative Examination

In many centers, the preoperative examination is done by one physician experienced in the overall care of children with spina bifida. Consults are then requested as needed for specific services. In other centers, a team of specialists will each evaluate the baby and monitor him or her throughout the course of the hospitalization within their individual area of expertise. These professionals may also comprise the team that will be involved in providing the long-term care of the child after initial treatment, discharge, and into the outpatient clinic setting.

The neurosurgeon is concerned initially with the location and extent of the infant's back lesion. Skin grafting may be necessary to gain adequate coverage over a large area. The presence of congenital kyphoscoliosis presents a complication that may lead to impaired wound healing because of excessive pressure at the suture site. This spinal deformity may have to be addressed and surgically reduced early in the baby's hospital experience. Congenital scoliosis with accompanying fused ribs at the level of the back lesion may be present and usually predicts a rapid progression of the scoliosis during the growth periods of childhood (Fig. 10.4). The

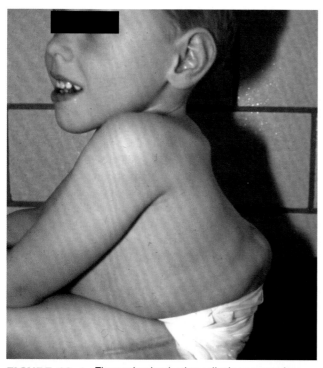

FIGURE 10.4. Thoracolumbar kyphoscoliosis compromises lung function, sitting alignment, balance, and free use of upper extremities.

effect of progressive scoliosis on cardiopulmonary function may ultimately be life threatening, even with spinal bracing and surgical intervention. It will also impact sitting alignment, weight distribution in sitting, and acquisition of upright balance. It is important to note this anomaly as a plan of treatment begins to evolve.

A pediatrician or neonatologist may be consulted to assess the general health of the baby and to identify other congenital defects or cardiopulmonary dysfunction that may be present. The urologist can request urodynamic testing during the early neonatal period. Goals of the urologist include minimizing the effects of a neurogenic bladder on the upper urinary tract and producing urinary continence without compromising the health of the system. The bladder may not relax and empty as it should, and residual urine can become a source of chronic infection. Clean intermittent catheterization is widely accepted as the protocol to follow to accomplish the foregoing goals, and although attention to bladder function may not be indicated until after back closure, it is understood that families will better accept intermittent catheterization as a management strategy if it is discussed and taught to them early rather than later in the infant's life. Intermittent catheterization is recognized as one of the most successful methods to preserve kidney function and prevent deterioration, which can be seen as early as 3 years of age in this population.[66,67]

A comprehensive orthopedic evaluation may not be imperative at this time, but an examination can offer insight into the severity of any orthopedic problems that are present at birth. The need for early corrective surgery, taping, splinting, or casting and its timing can be discussed and will provide additional information and education to the family and the rest of the medical team. Following the evaluation of the lower extremities and spinal alignment, a plan of orthopedic care can be established for the baby's first months of life.[18,25,65,68]

Management of Hydrocephalus

After surgery for back closure, 10% of the infants recover, have their sutures removed, and leave the hospital without further complication. The remaining 90% will begin to develop hydrocephalus. Preoperatively, the open back lesion may have acted as a natural drain for CSF, and when it is closed, the CSF pressure begins to rise in the cranium. Of the 90% of the infants who develop hydrocephalus, approximately 25% are born with evidence of hydrocephalus and need immediate shunt insertion. Studies show that an additional 55% will develop hydrocephalus within several days. The remaining babies will need shunting within 6 months. The neurosurgeon carefully monitors changes in the baby's head circumference, and studies such as ultrasound, computed tomography (CT), or MRI provide baseline information about the size of the lateral ventricles. Later comparisons assist in determining the appropriate time for insertion of a shunt.

Changes in the baby's state can indicate increasing intracranial pressure and the need for shunt insertion.

The enlarged ventricles cause the brain to expand within the flexible cranial vault, and symptoms of hydrocephalus may be seen singularly or in combination. The most common symptoms are "sunsetting," a downward deviation of the eyes, separation of the cranial sutures, noted on palpation, and/or a bulging anterior fontanel.

The increasing fluid pressure may stabilize without surgery in some individuals, but it is impossible to predict when or whether this will occur, how great the pressure will become, or how large the head will expand. Vital signs become depressed and respiratory arrest can occur when pressure, from excess CSF on the brain stem structures, becomes too great. Some individuals may survive without treatment for hydrocephalus, but they can be severely impaired as a result.[18,24,65]

Surgical insertion of a shunt will relieve the signs and symptoms associated with increased intracranial pressure. The shunt is a thin, flexible tube that diverts CSF away from the lateral ventricles. It is secured at the proximal and distal ends and is radiopaque for easy location. The ventriculoatrial (VA) shunt moves excess CSF from one lateral ventricle to the right atrium of the heart. Because infections of the VA system can lead to septicemia, ventriculitis, superior vena cava occlusion, and pulmonary emboli, this location is not commonly used. The ventriculoperitoneal (VP) shunt is currently the preferred treatment for hydrocephalus. Although occlusion of this type of shunt may occur more easily than with the VA shunt, complications associated with the VP shunt are far less severe. As it exits the lateral ventricle, the shunt can be palpated running distally down the side of the neck, under the clavicle, and down the anterior chest wall, just below the superficial fascia. The shunt inserts into the peritoneum, where CSF is reabsorbed and the excess excreted (Fig. 10.5).[67-69] An Ommaya reservoir is used in some institutions to siphon excess CSF for some time into a superficial well that can be emptied by needle aspiration. It would allow observation for cases in which hydrocephalus might resolve and a shunt would not be indicated and will postpone the need for initial shunt insertion until the child is older and more medically stable.

Although shunt insertion is a common procedure performed by the neurosurgical team, it is yet another invasive event for the infant who has already had back surgery. In order to spare the infant a second anesthesia, several centers perform simultaneous back closure and shunt insertion. Advocates of this approach believe that healing of the back wound from the inside is compromised when the CSF pressure is permitted to build. Therefore, more rapid healing of the back wound is expected, and neither negative sequelae nor increased postoperative complications have been reported by performing the double procedure.[70,71]

After surgery, a plan for physical therapy, based on the infant's condition, can be developed. The priority is for rapid healing, an uneventful recovery, and a speedy discharge to home. Individual surgeons have specific protocols, but at minimum it is appropriate to wait at least 24 to 48 hours postoperatively before initiating physical therapy. In many cases, the extent of hydrocephalus prior to surgery will affect the timing of when the baby may receive oral feedings, position changes, range-of-motion exercises, and normal handling in the upright position. Premature aggressive handling after surgery is not appropriate, particularly for the baby who had significant hydrocephalus. Intracranial pressure can drop dramatically after shunt insertion, and vascular insult can occur if the baby is also held upright, too soon after surgery.[65]

» Physical therapy for the infant with spina bifida

Overview

The role of the PT can begin in the early preoperative period before back closure with an examination of the neonate's active lower extremity movement. Ideally, the therapist who provides this preoperative evaluation is able to continue treating the baby throughout the hospitalization. It is also helpful if the same therapist can provide the long-term monitoring and parent education as the baby graduates to the outpatient department or specialty clinic. This staffing approach provides consistent support for parents during a stressful period. Also, the importance of staff continuity becomes increasingly evident as the child grows. When changes in function are suspected, the therapist who is familiar with the infant and has a good baseline of observations and documentation can be a valuable resource for the medical team. When a therapist has monitored the baby through the early period of care, the ability to detect even subtle changes is greatly enhanced.[65]

Manual Muscle Testing

A manual muscle test performed by the PT can provide objective information about the presence of active movement and the quantity of muscle power present in the baby's lower

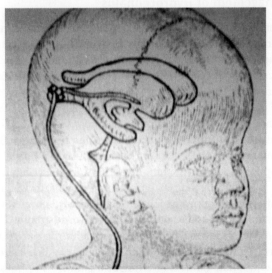

FIGURE 10.5. Location of the lateral ventricles and placement of ventriculoperitoneal shunt.

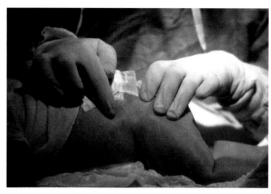

FIGURE 10.7. Tactile stimulation of the infant above the lesion level to elicit movement and palpation during manual muscle testing. Palpation and observation for the presence of the left gluteus medius and maximus muscles.

extremities (Display 10.2). Manual muscle testing should be performed before back surgery whenever possible. Testing may be repeated approximately 10 days after surgery, then at 6 months, and yearly thereafter unless a problem arises, requiring a more frequent schedule. The goal of these early testing sessions is to assist the medical staff to identify the level of the back lesion by assessing the lower extremity movement or lack thereof.[65]

Consideration must be given when positioning the baby for this first muscle test. Depending on the status of the back lesion or surgical site, the infant may be limited to only prone or side-lying. But careful observation and palpation should still allow for identification of most major muscle groups (Figs. 10.6 and 10.7).

A motor level can be assigned according to the last intact nerve root found. Lindseth has defined the motor level as the lowest segmental level at which the child is able to perform antigravity movement through the available range.[72] Although this degree of certainty may not be possible when testing an infant, preliminary identification of the motor level encourages consistency of communication among professionals involved with the baby. Keep in mind that children assigned the same motor level may still vary widely in their muscle strengths, so it is wise to locate and grade the individual muscle groups as soon as it becomes feasible.

It is because of that variability that some clinics prefer not to use the lesion level as a descriptor for the active movement in the baby's legs. Instead, they note the major muscle groups that are present and strong. Still other clinics refer to the area of the spine in which innervation is present based, again, on the results of a manual muscle test. This chapter has referred to the lesion level in all three ways.[73]

Several factors may influence movement during the infant's first hours of life. The effects of maternal anesthesia, increased cerebral pressure from hydrocephalus, and general lethargy and fatigue from a difficult or long labor may depress spontaneous movements. Conversely, these same factors may render the baby hyperirritable to stimulation. The therapist should tickle or stroke the baby above the level of the lesion or around the neck, face, or shoulder as a stimulus to keep the baby awake and moving. Movement of the legs can be observed and contractions palpated by stabilizing the limb proximally in order to avoid misinterpreting the origin of a movement. The principles for muscle testing in the infant population are much the same as those for older children, with the exception, of course, that the baby cannot follow directions. Gentle resistance to movement at one part of the leg may help increase the strength of a movement at a distal part of the limb. Allowing movement to occur at only one joint at a time will also assist in a more accurate interpretation. For example, holding firmly onto the hip and knee in either partial flexion or extension to prevent movement at those joints will enable the therapist to observe and detect weak ankle motion that might otherwise go unnoticed. After locating each movement, the therapist can then examine the general strength of the responsible muscle group. Above all, practice, experience, patience, and ingenuity will improve the accuracy of this early measure of the baby's motor ability.[65,74] This author has stood at the bedside of a newborn with spina bifida and watched an inexperienced clinician stroke the baby's foot and wonder why it was not eliciting any movement; the same clinician, with gentle guidance from PT, tickled the baby's face and thought the kicking movement elicited was an indication that the legs were intact.

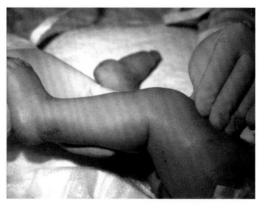

FIGURE 10.6. Palpation and observation of the quadriceps muscle during a preoperative manual muscle test to locate and chart the active muscles in the lower extremities.

The therapist should note whether or not muscles are functioning, which muscles are strong and can move a joint through its entire range, and which are weak and can move the joint only partially. This distinction will help in determining the motor level more precisely. The ability to distinguish between active and reflexive movement, although sometimes difficult during this early period, will also help to more accurately identify the lesion level.[74]

Reflex movement is common in infants with thoracic paralysis. There is usually no active movement at the hip joint, but movement may be noted distally at the knee or ankle. The movement, which may look like fasciculation of the muscle belly or simply a weak, continuous jerking movement of the joint, may be seen when the baby is sleeping or at rest and the other joints of the limb are not moving. Reflex movement is most often observed as flexion of the knee or may be seen at the ankle as either dorsiflexion or plantarflexion. Reflex movement represents sparing of the local reflex arc although cortical control of the movement has been interrupted by the spinal defect. This reflex movement is of concern because of its involuntary nature and because it is usually unopposed by an active antagonist at the same joint. Therefore, this unchecked reflex activity can be a deforming force that often requires intervention. The movement can also be misleading to both staff and family who may interpret the movement as functional motion and think the child's motor level is lower than it is. However, because the movement is not cortically initiated, it seldom has any functional value.[65]

Recording manual muscle testing grades can be modified until the child can be positioned appropriately for gravity and gravity-eliminated responses. Modification is also suggested until the child is older and can be tested with resistance to increase the consistency and reliability of the results. One successful method developed by the physical therapy department at Lurie Children's Hospital of Chicago uses an "X" to indicate the presence of a strong movement, an "O" for an absent response, a "T" for trace movement when a contraction is palpated but movement cannot be seen, and an "R" to indicate reflex movement. This scheme of grading, when combined with the existing scale of "0" through "5," or "absent" through "normal" classification, provides significant information about the lower extremities even in these very young children.

Early manual muscle testing can also deduce muscle imbalance around a joint and its potential for deformity. If a deformity is already present, muscle testing can help ascertain whether the cause of the limitation is passive, as a result of in utero positioning, or active, from movement in one direction with no opposing muscle movement. Distinguishing the etiology of joint deformity is helpful for the orthopedic surgeon who may want to consider early surgery to the lower extremities. The surgeon will want to spare potentially useful muscle function while weakening or eliminating movement that will continue to be deforming in nature. Conversely, if the origin of the movement is uncertain, the surgeon may wisely choose to wait until the child is older

and a more accurate examination is possible before deciding on the type of surgery to perform. Some centers have attempted to use electromyography (EMG) to evaluate lower extremity innervation. EMG studies are interesting from an academic standpoint but have offered little functional information that manual muscle testing does not, and these tests have not been widely used.

There has been poor correlation between early manual muscle testing and the child's ultimate level of gross motor function, so predictions about ambulation potential based on these early examinations must be made carefully. Acquisition of functional skills depends on the innervation and strength of the lower extremity musculature, the child's CNS status, motivation, intellectual capacity, and the family's commitment to long-term compliance, support, and interest. These variables are only a few of the many factors that can influence the functional outcome of the child with spina bifida. Some of these influences are addressed in greater detail in subsequent sections of this chapter.[75,76]

Results of early manual muscle tests (Table 10.1) should be compared with later tests in order to monitor the child's neuromuscular stability. It is a pleasant surprise to find increased movement and/or strength after back closure, but if a decrease in movement is noted, the neurosurgeon should be alerted. Deterioration of lower extremity motor function may indicate a serious problem and should be brought to the physician's attention.[77]

Range-of-motion Examination

Preliminary examination of range of motion (ROM) of the lower extremities can also be performed prior to back closure. Typical, full-term neonates may have flexion contractures of up to 30 degrees at the hips and 10 to 20 degrees at the knees and ankle dorsiflexion of up to 40 or 50 degrees.[78-80] ROM limitations in the baby with spina bifida should not be considered an indication for immediate and aggressive stretching. Early limitations in passive flexibility require a safe plan of management executed over several weeks or months. When it becomes apparent that contractures will be both severe and long lasting, a long-term plan with the orthopedic surgeon can be developed that will likely include a combination of positioning, taping, splinting, and/or surgical correction.

Several common patterns of early joint contractures may be seen in the neonate with spina bifida. One example is the baby with extreme tightness of the hip flexors and adductors with or without the legs held in knee hyperextension (Fig. 10.8). This may be present in the child with a motor level of L-2/L-3 or L-3/L-4 and is caused by the presence of a strong iliopsoas with no opposing force offered from absent hip extensors. There is also no opposing hip abduction at this innervation level. Medial hamstrings, which are primary knee flexors, can exert a secondary hip extension force, but they are absent or weak. If the baby does not have sufficient range of hip extension to safely tolerate prone positioning, the nursing staff and neurosurgeon must be informed in order to prevent fractures of the femur when the baby is

TABLE 10.1. Modified Guide for Manual Muscle Testing of Babies and Young Children			
Lower Extremity Movement	**Active Muscles**	**Contributing Nerve Roots**	
Hip Flexion	Iliopsoas & Sartorius	Lumbar 1,2,3	
	Pectineus & Gracilis	Lumbar 2,3	
Hip Adduction	Adductor Brevis, Longus, Magnus	Lumbar 2,3,4	
Knee Extension	Quadriceps	Lumbar 2,3,4	
Hip Adduction & Ext rotation	External Obturator	Lumbar 3,4	
Ankle Dorsiflexion & Inversion	Tibialis Anterior	Lumbar 4,5	
Ankle Plantarflexion & Inversion	Tibialis Posterior	Lumbar 4,5	
Hip Flexion, Medial Rotation, Abduction	Tensor Fascia Lata	Lumbar 4,5	Sacral 1
Hip Abduction	Gluteus Medius & Minimus	Lumbar 5	Sacral 1
Knee Flexion (Medial)	Semimembranosus & Semitendinosus	Lumbar 4,5	Sacral 1
Large Toe extension, Ankle Dorsiflexion	Extensor Hallucis Longus	Lumbar 4,5	Sacral 1
Extends Toes 2-5, Foot Eversion	Extensor Digitorum Longus & Brevis	Lumbar 5	Sacral 1
Ankle Plantarflexion & Dorsiflexion	Peroneus Tertius	Lumbar 5	Sacral 1
Ankle Plantarflexion & Eversion	Peroneus Brevis	Lumbar 5	Sacral 1
Ankle Plantarflexion & Eversion	Peroneus Longus	Lumbar 5	Sacral 1,2
Ankle Plantarflexion	Gastrocnemius	Lumbar 5	Sacral 1
	Soleus	Lumbar 5	Sacral 1,2,3
	Plantaris	Lumbar 5	Sacral 1,2,3
Knee flexion (Lateral)	Biceps femoris	Lumbar 5	Sacral 1,2,3
Hip Extension	Gluteus Maximus	Lumbar 5	Sacral 1,2
Flexes Large Toe	Flexor Hallucis Longus & Brevis		Sacral 1,2
Flexes Toes 2-5	Flexor digitorum Longus & Brevis		Sacral 1,2,3

Adapted from Hislop HJ, Montgomery J. *Daniels and Worthingham's Muscle Testing: Techniques of Manual Examination.* 8th ed. Saunders; 2007; Sharrard WJW. *The Segmental Innervation of the Lower Limb Muscles in Man.* Arris and Gale lecture given January 1964; Phillips LH, Park TS. Electro physiologic mapping of the segmental anatomy of the muscles of the lower extremity. *Muscle Nerve.* 1991;12(12):1213-1218.

positioned for surgery. Adapted prone positioning in the operating room may be necessary during back closure. A strategy that has been successfully used is to elevate the baby on a small, raised, and padded platform or firm stack of towels with both hips safely flexed over one end while keeping the body supported. Postoperatively, this modified prone position or side-lying will be the safest postures for the baby with these contractures.[63]

Extreme dorsiflexion at the ankle is another contracture seen at birth. The child with an L-5 innervation has strong ankle dorsiflexion, provided by the anterior tibialis and toe extensors, but weak or absent toe flexors and plantarflexion from the gastrocnemius/soleus. This may indicate the need for serial taping or splinting of the ankle to bring it down to 90 degrees, and, in addition, gentle passive exercise can reduce this deformity in a short time.

Provided that the baby is medically stable and the physician agrees, daily ROM exercise for the lower extremities can begin at bedside as early as a day or two after back closure. Although positioning options are limited after surgery, the prone and side-lying positions are adequate to perform all lower extremity motions needed at this time.[18,65]

Postoperative Physical Therapy

In order for the PT to develop a comprehensive and appropriate program for the infant who has undergone back closure and shunt insertion, consideration must be given to both the neurologic and orthopedic findings, and to be most effective, the therapist should also be sensitive to the state of family members, who will become more available as they begin to visit their baby regularly.

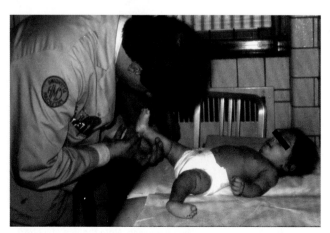

FIGURE 10.8. Orthopedic check in clinic of baby born with extreme hip flexion and knee hyperextension.

Communication with Team Members and Parents

In most cases, the family of an infant born with spina bifida will experience a very different and more stressful postpartum period than they had anticipated. Their baby was probably transferred to another facility shortly after birth to receive specialty care. Often, the needs of the recovering mother are superseded by those of the baby, so it might be difficult for family members to be as attentive to him or her as they focus on the infant. Inaccurate information about spina bifida, in general, and their child, in particular, may further compromise the family's coping skills during this physically and emotionally difficult time. It has been reported that parents were told by staff that their child would be mentally disabled, would never walk, and would require around-the-clock care and, ultimately, institutionalization. These professionals, although well intentioned, are usually not experienced in current methods of evaluation and treatment of children with spina bifida and may only recall information from a previous era in which a bleak outlook for the babies was the norm rather than the exception. This misinformation confuses and frustrates many parents, especially if the specialty team, after assessing the infant, presents what seems to be conflicting information albeit a more optimistic outlook. Therefore, it is important to ensure close communication between the therapist and other team members. All persons working with the infant should know and understand each other's findings so as to avoid contradiction. Information should be provided to the family by the appropriate personnel openly and honestly, but also sensitively.

One objective for the PT should be to reflect a positive and caring attitude during treatment sessions rather than a stiff, impersonal demeanor. This approach can help to normalize the involvement of family members with their infant. Portions of a home program can begin to be taught to the family immediately as a constructive way for the therapist to begin building a relationship with them and as a means of facilitating their interaction with the infant. The therapist and nursing staff can encourage family members to participate in the infant's care as soon as feasible during the hospitalization, to prepare them for providing care at home. Waiting until discharge for home instruction will place unnecessary stress on the family members, who have much to learn from many people, in a short time. Also, an unexpectedly quick discharge may leave little time for family education, which could have been spread over the entire period of hospitalization. After discharge, follow-up sessions can be scheduled during outpatient or clinic visits to help reinforce what has already been taught and to progress the program. Frequent follow-up appointments solely with physical therapy may greatly inconvenience a family and may not be as valuable as periodic sessions, stretched out over a longer period.

Range-of-motion Exercises

Daily sessions for lower extremity ROM exercises can begin after back closure, demonstrated and then taught to parents as soon as feasible. Passive ROM exercises should be brief

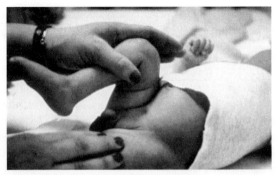

FIGURE 10.9. Range of motion exercises for the lower extremities. Gently combining full flexion of one hip and knee with full extension of the opposite extremity limits the number of movements a parent must learn.

and performed only two or three times each day. It is suggested that parents embed the exercises into a daily routine with their infant, such as during washing and diaper changes, when the baby's legs are normally exposed. The therapist can combine individual leg movements into patterns of movement so the family only needs to learn three or four patterns for their home program. An example that this author found easy for families to learn is to position the baby in supine and flex the hip and knee of one leg up almost to the chest, while simultaneously stretching the opposite leg into full extension. After this pattern has been reversed and repeated several times, both hips and knees can then be held flexed at approximately 90 degrees. The hips can then be abducted at the same time, leaving only the foot and ankle movements to be done individually (Figs. 10.9 and 10.10).[65]

ROM exercises are performed gently with the therapist's hands placed close to the joint being moved, to use a short lever arm, that prevents stress to soft tissue and joints. Several repetitions of each pattern, holding the joint briefly at the end of the range, can maintain and even increase ROM, when there is a mild or moderate limitation. If severe limitations

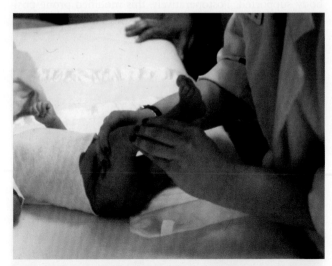

FIGURE 10.10. Placement of the hands as close to the joint as possible for range-of-motion exercises. Note the use of a short lever arm to avoid injury to the joint and surrounding soft tissue.

exist, exercise at that joint may require additional time and repetition. But aggressive stretching should be avoided, regardless of the severity of the contracture.

By participating in the ROM exercises during these early days, parents are encouraged to touch and move their baby's legs while being observed by the therapist. Opportunities to handle their baby with supervision can help alleviate anxiety that many families express about further injuring their infant's back and legs. With the therapist's comforting and supportive words and demonstrations, the exercise program offers a valuable opportunity for the start of positive parent–child interactions.

Passive ROM exercises must continue throughout the child's life. The goal is that the child will eventually learn to perform the exercises independently. Passive exercise is often forgotten by therapists and parents alike as the child becomes more active and therapy begins to concentrate on gross motor activities and gait training. Although one may think these later motor activities are adequate for maintaining joint flexibility, they are not. Regardless of how active the child is, only the innervated portions of the limb are being moved, in only some planes of motion, and often through only part of the full range of the joint. Therefore, if ROM exercises are discontinued, contractures will develop. For some children, it may take years before tightness is noted, whereas for others range is lost very soon. Loss of flexibility invariably leads to compromised function.[18,25,33,65]

Positioning and Handling

Because it is known that babies with spina bifida often do not develop and move in the same way or at the same pace as their peers typically do, the PT should assume responsibility for developing a program of positioning and handling for the hospitalized baby that may be taught to the parents prior to discharge for continuation at home. Although more positioning options are available as discharge nears, during the first few postoperative days the baby may still be limited to prone or side-lying. As the child's medical status stabilizes and tolerance to movement improves, it is advisable that if parents are visiting, they are encouraged to avoid leaving the child in bed, immobile for long periods of time, when he or she is awake. Handling and carrying strategies can be practiced by the therapist and then recommended to the parents. Finding a comfortable chair is most important, and, once seated, the therapist or family member can hold the child prone over their lap, rocking or swaying slowly side to side. This position is restful for the parent and provides novel movement for the infant. The baby may also enjoy a slow walk around the hospital floor while being held up and slightly over the parent's shoulder. This position gives the infant an opportunity to attempt to raise and turn their head. If the supine and sitting positions are contraindicated, parents may gently cradle the infant prone across one forearm. These few position options will provide a small repertoire of acceptable handling strategies when families visit their baby. These positions are also safe for the infant, who needs time to recover and who may not respond well to more aggressive movement and handling. Remember that the primary postoperative goals for the infant are an uncomplicated healing of the back wound, speedy recovery from shunt insertion, and discharge from the hospital.[65]

In many cases, with medical clearance after a few days, short periods of supine and supported sitting in the therapist's arms will not affect the course of healing and may be added to the handling repertoire. This approach will help normalize the baby's experiences during waking hours while being fed or quietly observing the surroundings. It is also useful for the therapist who can note the baby's responses to gravity in each position, feel for changes in muscle tone, particularly through the shoulders and neck, and observe any significant asymmetries. Documenting this information will provide a useful baseline against which to compare later developmental findings.[33,65]

Families should first watch, then work to duplicate, the activities recommended for their baby. Be aware that most parents show some hesitation or anxiety on first handling their baby. Lack of hesitation may indicate a poor understanding of the infant's medical condition and may contribute to poor judgment later in other areas of care. Even for families with experience of raising older children, some initial level of anxiety can be a healthy sign.

As these teaching sessions proceed, the therapist can begin to "role release" some of the ROM and handling activities, delegating them to the parent. As this transition occurs, the therapist can refocus on other areas of the child's plan of care. The therapist may be asked to repeat the lower extremity manual muscle test prior to discharge. He or she can also observe the baby's state, noting changes secondary to hydrocephalus and shunt insertion. Gathering this information may help to identify a later shunt malfunction. If one begins to occur, in addition to the signs and symptoms presented in Table 10.2, a change in the baby's tone, a negative reaction to movement, or increased irritability during movement might be noted.

Family members should be encouraged to actively gather information about their infant as well, mainly by playing with and observing their baby, not only to foster positive interaction but also to aid the medical staff in assessing the infant's function. Over time, interaction with the medical team becomes less frequent as the child becomes more medically stable, and parents' observations can help identify problems, such as a shunt malfunction, early so that appropriate medical care can be sought.

Sensory Examination

The PT can perform a sensory examination on the neonate to determine areas of the infant's lower body and legs that react to or are insensitive to touch. Mapping this sensory information, along with the results of muscle testing, helps to establish the level of the spinal lesion more accurately. This examination will also identify the areas of intact sensation on the baby's trunk and legs so stimulation at those spots will make the baby move. It is the beginning clinician who

TABLE 10.2.	Signs and Symptoms of Shunt Malfunction

Infants
Bulging fontanel
Vomiting
Change in appetite
"Sunset" sign of eyes
Edema, redness along shunt tract

Toddlers
Vomiting
Irritability
Headaches
Edema, redness along shunt tract

School-aged Children
Headaches
Lethargy
Irritability
Edema, redness along shunt tract
Handwriting changes
High-pitched cry
Seizures
Rapid growth of head circumference
Thinning of skin over scalp
Newly noted nystagmus
Newly noted eye squint
Vomiting
Decreased school performance
Personality changes
Memory changes

when performing a manual muscle test strokes the plantar surface of the baby's foot, expecting a reaction. This technique is successful only when the infant has intact sensation at the sacral nerve roots. Most infants with spina bifida have a higher level of sensory deficit and need to be stimulated on the thigh or somewhere on the trunk. The therapist may find that the level of motor function and sensation is not similar in both legs. Be aware that early results of sensory testing can be inaccurate and incomplete and that it is difficult to assess all sensory modalities at this time: light touch, deep pressure, and temperature. A more comprehensive assessment may be indicated when the baby is older.

The sensory information should be shared with the family members, who must learn about their child's skin anesthesia. Educating parents about skin care for the baby is often the shared responsibility of the nursing and therapy staffs. It is sometimes difficult for parents to understand the concept that their baby has areas of the lower body and legs that are insensitive to touch. They may see the lack of movement in the legs but not appreciate the limitations in sensation. The therapist can help the family discover this information on their own. Using a gentle touch, caress, or tickle, a family member can map out areas of responsiveness when the infant is awake and alert. The therapist should never use a pin or other sharp object during testing or when demonstrating to parents. The baby's response to a pinprick is no more valid than its response to a gentle touch, and, furthermore,

seeing staff using a sharp object on their baby may add to the parents' anxieties and concern. This author always demonstrated this concept to new residents and staff so they would not pull out a pen top or paper clip from their pockets.

Insensitive areas of the lower extremities will require protection because the child will be unaware of injury at these areas of denervation. For example, families must always test the temperature of bath water before immersing the child. They cannot rely on the child's reaction to judge whether the temperature is correct. They must be cautious and not allow their child to play with the faucets and inadvertently add hot water that they will not feel. Open space heaters and radiators need covering or relocation to keep a baby from moving on the floor and resting too close, suffering serious burns. Before placing the infant down to play, a search for hidden objects on the floor or in the carpet may prevent an accidental injury from loose tacks or a small sharp toy. When the infant is playing and crawling on the floor, his or her legs and feet should always be covered with tights or socks and pants to avoid rug burns and abrasions. Wearing socks or booties will also help prevent problems when children begin to pull their legs up, reach for, mouth, and even bite at their toes, typically at the age of 6 to 8 months (Fig. 10.11).

Skin insensitivity will remain a concern throughout the child's life. Wearing new shoes or braces, for example, requires vigilance to avoid pressure areas, sores, and abrasions. Normal sensation keeps the typical person from sitting immobile for long periods. Sensory feedback causes weight shift to change weight distribution, relieving pressure and discomfort. People typically move and shift their weight many times during a movie or a dull class. People with areas of insensitivity develop skin problems secondary to prolonged sitting because they do not feel the discomfort and therefore do not shift their weight, change their position, and relieve the pressure. Similarly, discomfort from an ill-fitting shoe makes one quickly become aware of the problem and readjust his/her gait to avoid continued abrasion until

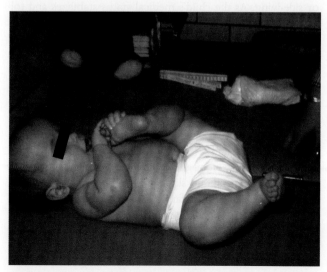

FIGURE 10.11. Socks or booties should be worn to protect insensate toes from inadvertent injury.

one can get off his/her feet or change shoes. For the child without full sensation, such readjustments will not occur, as areas of pressure are not perceived. It is therefore important to gradually introduce the use of a new orthotic. The brace should be worn for only a few hours at a stretch, and the skin should be inspected carefully to determine whether there are any pressure areas. When redness is seen that lasts for longer than 30 minutes, an adjustment to the orthosis is indicated. The child should not be permitted to keep wearing the brace in the hopes that the skin will toughen. Rubbing tea bags or alcohol on the site, as suggested in some home remedies, does not help to toughen the skin. The accommodation to a new brace is best implemented at home, over a weekend or in the evenings, when regular and frequent skin checks can be made. Unless it is clear that this is more successfully implemented at day care or school, it is unwise to have the child wear a new device for a full day until proper fit and good skin tolerance are ensured. If these issues are not initially addressed and the child experiences skin breakdown, it can lead to extended periods of time out of the device, infection, a possible need for hospitalization, and most likely a delay in the progression of the orthotics and gait program. Avoiding many of these scenarios begins with good, precise, and repetitive parent teaching during the early PT sessions in the hospital.[25,33,65]

» Care of the young child

Ongoing Concerns and Issues

As the initial phase of intervention for the baby with spina bifida comes to an end, a plan for long-term follow-up care should be developed. Various approaches to the delivery of medical care are seen, but in the best of cases the ongoing care is delivered by specialists located within one institution. When care is divided among several locations, a new role must emerge for parents, and they become their child's case manager, facilitating continuity of care and communication among the professionals. This added responsibility can be a huge burden for some parents and may result in less-than-optimal care for the child. It appears that, because of the multiple specialty areas needed by the child with spina bifida, care is best delivered by experienced professionals who work together as a coordinated team. That is why many pediatric hospitals have organized a multidisciplinary clinic for children with spina bifida and other similar neuromuscular diagnoses, where several specialists working under the same roof can see the child, preferably on the same day. Families are encouraged to continue their child's care at one of these spina bifida clinics. A team of specialists working together to complement one another benefits everyone. Communication is facilitated and expedited among professionals, and medical information can be more easily shared to increase learning, maintain a current outlook on interventions, and, ultimately, provide the best care. Although these clinic appointments can be very long,

---

DISPLAY 10.3

Goals of Neurosurgical Care for Children with Spina Bifida

Coordinate early care prior to back closure
Assess location and size of the back defect
Perform closure of the back defect
Assess extent of lower extremity paralysis
Assess and treat hydrocephalus
Monitor function of ventricular shunt
Monitor for acute and chronic CNS abnormalities
Monitor for CNS deterioration, tethered cord, and hydromyelia
Provide support/collaboration to clinical team

---

when problems arise, the necessary personnel are often at hand to address the concern and often without the need for scheduling a return visit. With consistency and coordination by the medical staff, parents can start to develop a sense of trust in their team, which will, hopefully, decrease their stress, enable them to cope better with their new responsibilities, and remain focused on addressing the needs of their child.[25,33,65]

The child may have to return frequently to the clinic during the initial years of life for ongoing follow-up by the various specialists. The neurosurgeon will monitor the status of the back closure, look for the presence of hydrocephalus, determine whether shunt placement is necessary, and check that once a shunt is in place, it is functioning well (Display 10.3).[18,68] The orthopedic surgeon will evaluate spinal alignment and limb flexibility, strength, and joint integrity. Plans are made for lower extremity splints and surgery to prepare the child for standing at the optimal chronologic age (Display 10.4).[25,65] The urologist will monitor bowel and bladder function, assess renal status at regular intervals, and plan a course of care that includes intermittent catheterization and possibly pharmacologic management (Display 10.5). At the appropriate time, a bowel program to attain fecal continence will be implemented that may involve scheduled toileting, diet recommendations, medication, biofeedback, and behavior modification approaches (Display 10.6).[65-67,81-83]

As the child's status stabilizes in each of the specialty areas, visits to the clinic will become less frequent. It is not unusual

---

DISPLAY 10.4

Goals of Orthopedic Care for Children with Spina Bifida

Provide pertinent information to family: current and projected issues
Prevent fixed joint contractures
Correct musculoskeletal deformities
Prevent skin breakdown from structural malalignment
Provide resources to achieve best mobility
Monitor for scoliosis
Monitor for CNS deterioration, tethered cord, and hydromyelia
Provide support/collaboration to clinical team

DISPLAY
10.5

Goals of Urologic Care for Children with Spina Bifida

Assess and preserve renal function
Provide for adequate bladder emptying
Provide for urinary continence
Provide resources for bowel management
Monitor for CNS deterioration, tethered cord, and hydromyelia
Provide support/collaboration to clinical team

for a child to be seen every 6 months over several years and then yearly if there are no ongoing problems or major concerns. However, more frequent visits may be necessary if a chronic problem requires close monitoring and intervention.

Developmental Issues

As stated earlier in this chapter, the survival of a greater number of infants born with spina bifida has afforded clinicians working with these children valuable experience and insight into the full scope of the disability and all of its primary and

DISPLAY
10.6

Nutrition and Spina Bifida in Pediatrics

Rebecca Thomas, RD, LDN
Clinical Dietitian, Children's Hospital of Philadelphia

Nutrition-Related Problems	Considerations/Interventions
Obesity	
After 6 years of age, 50% of children with spina bifida are overweight	Consistent eating pattern/meal schedule
Children with spina bifida have a higher percentage of body fat, lower total energy expenditure, and reduced physical activity	Decrease high fat/calorie foods
• Increased risk of decubitus ulcers	Limit juice/soda
• Increased difficulty with mobility	Increase intake of fruits/vegetables
• Decreased social acceptance	Encourage lean meats, low-fat dairy products
	Increase physical activity/physical therapy program
	Decubitus ulcers/wound healing
	High-protein diet
	Additional ascorbic acid and zinc
	Monitor visceral protein stores
	Increase physical activity
	Bone health
	Encourage weight-bearing activity
	Ensure adequacy of calcium, vitamin D intake
Malnutrition	
Caused by limited variability in intake: limited fruits and vegetables, inconsistent eating patterns, overconsumption of foods/beverages with low nutritional value	Encourage varied, balanced diet
	Encourage calorie-dense foods, nutritional supplements if underweight
Abnormal or stunted growth	Daily multivitamin
Owing to poor vertebral growth, atrophy of the muscles in the lower extremities; deformities of the spine, hips, and knees; hydrocephalus; renal disease; prolonged hospitalizations	
• Decreased weight-bearing activity	
• Decreased bone mineralization	
Bowel Continence/Incontinence	
Owing to inadequate fiber and fluid in diet and decreased physical activity	Consistent eating pattern/meal schedule
	Ensure adequate fiber intake via fruits, vegetables, whole grains, nuts/seeds
	Ensure adequate fluid intake
	Encourage physical activity

Suggested Readings

Leibold S, Ekmark E, Adams RC. Decision-making for a successful bowel continence program. *Eur J Pediatr Surg.* 2000;10(suppl 1):26-30.

Littlewood RA, Trocki O, Shephard RW, et al. Resting energy expenditure and body composition in children with myelomeningocele. *Pediatr Rehabil.* 2003;6(1):31-37.

Nevin-Folino NL, ed. *Pediatric Manual of Clinical Dietetics.* 2nd ed. Pediatric Nutrition Practice Group, American Dietetic Association; 2003.

secondary issues. It is apparent that a significant number of children with spina bifida exhibit CNS deficits, which for some can be more detrimental to their function than their lower extremity paralysis. The CNS deficits can have a major impact on the child's acquisition of gross motor, fine motor, perceptual motor, and cognitive skills, and it is critical that the PT understand these problems. The knowledgeable PT can be a resource to other service providers in regard to the array of problems they may be observing.

The Chiari II anatomic malformation was identified and studied for years before discussions began about how this malformation might relate to the developmental dysfunction that was often seen in children with spina bifida. Using MRI studies, the structural abnormalities have been identified and can be visualized.[30] However, as previously noted, MRI studies are inconsistent in predicting the clinical presentation of a particular child. Up to 85% of children with spina bifida have low tone, with minimal to moderate developmental delay. The most common difficulties are delayed and/or abnormal development of head and trunk control and delayed and/or abnormal acquisition of righting and equilibrium responses, which are the necessary foundation skills for higher levels of movement against gravity and complex functional skills. Interestingly, children who have simple hydrocephalus without spina bifida do not exhibit the same movement problems with the frequency or severity shown by children with both spina bifida and hydrocephalus. So when one works with these children, regardless of their age, it is necessary to integrate our knowledge of early motor development with orthopedics, orthotics management, and kinesiology. Although one can only postulate that the Chiari II malformation is a contributor to the movement difficulties one may be seeing, he or she is still compelled to address all of the child's needs to develop a comprehensive plan for successful remediation.[25,33,65,67-70]

The earliest motor problems noted in many infants with spina bifida include prolonged instability of the head and upper body with delayed or weak acquisition of antigravity movement in all positions and weak or delayed righting and equilibrium responses of the head and upper body. The following is a brief description of the development of stability of the head and upper trunk as well as some of the more atypical patterns seen in babies with spina bifida. It is not intended to be a complete analysis of typical motor development. Please refer to the bibliography as well as other sources for more complete information.

The typical baby spends time in all positions right from the beginning of life and experiences the effects of gravity on the head and body in all of these positions. Typical infants will begin to stabilize their head over their shoulders in the supported upright position in their parent's arms. This early stability occurs well before the baby can lift its head up from a prone or supine position. As the baby's head becomes progressively more stable, parents find new and more convenient ways to carry and handle their baby and in less protective ways. This parent–child feedback is most apparent when the baby is held upright in the parent's arms. At first, in the early weeks, the parent's hand is placed behind the baby's head to prevent it from falling backward or to the side. A few months later, this support is withdrawn. Only when the baby is raised or lowered from a crib or changing table or when a sleeping baby is lifted will the head require support. So in just a few months, almost no guarding of the head is required when the baby is awake and carried in an upright position. The parent has responded to the baby's new skills and has, accordingly, changed their style of lifting, holding, and carrying, usually without the need for any therapeutic instruction or expert interventions. For the infant with typical tone, there is a degree of physiologic stability of the head and neck from the tension provided by muscle, tendon, and ligamentous structures. Typical joint proprioception through the cervical spine and the sensitive stretch reflexes of the soft tissue structures of the neck permit the baby's head to fall slowly into gravity with movement or a position change, but only to a limited degree. The head is held reasonably steady without much active or intentional participation by the infant. If the baby is lifted or moved too quickly or the head falls too far, the startle response is elicited, the baby cries, and the parent makes sure not to do that again.

The child with spina bifida who demonstrates poor neck stability secondary to low tone may retain a startle response longer than a typically developing infant. The baby also requires support at the head and neck beyond the time frame that is considered typical. Parents will respond by continuing to provide the needed head support well past the time the baby should maintain his or her head up independently. This begins an abnormal cycle in which the support provided by the parent's hands, while appropriately reacting to the baby's need, actually limits the experiences and opportunities the baby may get to practice and develop better head control, and so the delay can be further prolonged. The infant who has low tone lacks the joint integrity and proprioceptive responses to changes in gravity, or the responses may be slow and weak, permitting the head to fall forward or to the side much farther before the stabilizing responses occur. A mechanical disadvantage compounds the problem as the baby grows. The head becomes larger and heavier, so the task of stabilizing the head using appropriate head righting is made ever more difficult by this additional weight and the relatively weak musculature. When an infant with spina bifida is placed in various positions and makes attempts to stabilize his or her head, compensatory patterns of movement can often be seen. Elevation of the shoulders to "fix" the head in one place is one pattern. This is a developmentally immature alignment for the infant who should have head stability in supported upright by 4 months of age. Stabilizing the head with this shoulder pattern will inhibit the further development of typical head righting skills. The infant should be experiencing and practicing increased freedom of movement and control of the head and neck, separate from the upper extremities.

Compensatory patterns of overusing the arms are seen when the baby attempts to lift his or her head, look around, reach, and play while in the prone position. Side-to-side weight shifting over the hands and arms does not occur easily.

When the child lifts an arm to reach for a toy, the prop is removed, stability is lost, and the head and upper chest fall. The child may figure out how to tilt his or her head to one side for a weight shift and let it hang there to unload one arm and reach for a desired object. Once this compensatory pattern is successful, it may not improve without appropriate intervention. As this scenario plays out, months later, the child who did not develop sufficient head and neck strengths and balance reactions will not develop adequate trunk strength and stability to maintain the body in upright positions and may continue to need help for their upper extremities to prop when placed in sitting. There the child remains stuck, unable to move into or out of the position except in limited, stereotyped ways. To change positions, the child may eventually develop strategies to move, which, however, are usually passive, allowing the body to fall into gravity, involving little muscle activity or control from the neck and trunk. The child may lower his or her head to one side and slowly collapse to the floor or may lean forward and crawl out of the sitting position. Getting into and out of sitting from one side or the other requires balance, control, and strength of the head and trunk in multiple planes of movement, which this child lacks. So getting into and out of the sitting position using only straight plane movements is usually the easiest and most efficient. When the child is in prone or four-point, the child merely pushes his or her body straight backward with their arms, until the buttocks reach the surface, in between the knees. This is one reason children with low tone are seen, with or without spina bifida, successfully get into a "W" sitting posture and remain there. Permitting the baby to use these more passive patterns of movement does not help to further improve strength and coordination of the neck and trunk.

When a typical baby lifts an arm to reach for an object while in prone, a weight shift to one side occurs that activates the neck, trunk, hip, and leg musculature to counterbalance and stabilize the baby's position as they reach. The baby does not depend on upper extremity support to lift the head and can therefore reach without the head and chest dropping. When the forearms are stabilized on the floor, during typical weight shifting and movement in prone, the arms become more externally rotated while the forearms rotate from pronation into supination, with pressure shifting across from the radial to the ulnar surface of the hands. Increased and varied weight bearing and tactile stimulation across the hands help to reduce the sensitivity of the grasp response. This typical upper extremity weight-bearing progression aids in opening the baby's flexed fingers and hands to permit more and varied manipulation of objects and getting objects to the mouth. Experiences in the prone position also provide considerable proprioception through the joints of the upper extremities as well as opportunities to increase control and strength.

The child with spina bifida needs coordination and strength of the upper extremities to use assistive devices for ambulation, to perform activities of daily living, and to manipulate paper and pencil for tasks in school. But using the upper extremities in lieu of head and trunk support will limit

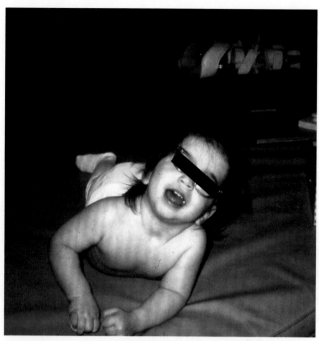

FIGURE 10.12. Leaning the head side to side unweights an arm to creep forward. This is a compensation for the lack of a strong neck and trunk.

the baby's motor experiences of the arms and hands. The shoulders remain elevated to continue providing stability for the head. Arms tend to be held in more internal rotation with scapular protraction. The forearms are pronated with wrist and hand flexion. Weight bearing on the hands may remain limited to the radial aspect (Fig. 10.12).

Paralysis of the lower extremities decreases the total amount of tactile, proprioceptive, and vestibular input that the child is receiving from the body. The degree to which this loss affects the individual depends on the remaining movement and sensation available in the legs, the function of the upper body, and the child's CNS status for processing this tactile input. If a child is able to explore the environment actively and independently, knowledge is gained about the body in relation to the environment. A typical baby has a vast number of movement experiences occurring at the same time, and learning is acquired through many sensory modalities. When movement and exploration are limited, learning is ultimately affected. Lower extremity paralysis, in combination with low tone and poor head control, makes gross motor movement, especially against gravity, more difficult for many children with spina bifida, and this can also affect the child's motivation, confidence, and willingness to move. When movement is more difficult, it can become a negative experience, and learning more sophisticated skills will be impacted.

It is important for PTs to appreciate these impediments on motor learning for the child with spina bifida and use this information to facilitate and encourage early handling strategies for parents that will enhance their baby's development and encourage the acquisition of more typical movement patterns (Figs. 10.13 and 10.14).[84-92]

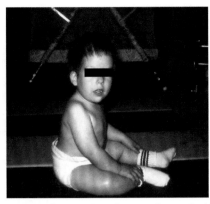

FIGURE 10.13. Good sitting alignment is noted with upper extremities resting on lower extremities to support the upright position.

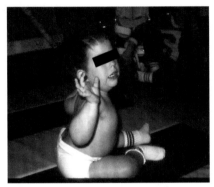

FIGURE 10.14. With upper extremities free in play neck and trunk weakness is revealed which requires addition of strengthening and balance work.

>> Handling strategies for parents

As mentioned earlier, instruction sessions with parents should begin, when possible, before the child is discharged from the hospital and should continue until the parents are comfortable with their handling and acceptable movement and function of the child is observed. Parents should be aggressive in their involvement but tempered by the medical status and age of their baby. Teaching sessions should, ideally, include opportunities for the parents to observe the therapist handling their baby and time to practice with this expert assistance.

Parents often focus on the most conspicuous deficit, their baby's lower extremity paralysis. But the PT has the responsibility of incorporating into the instructional program additional information that will promote the family's understanding of gross, fine, and perceptual motor abilities above the waist. The pace of instruction should be based on the status of the infant and the capacity of the family. Families can be gently alerted, during early treatment sessions, about the developmental delays that may be seen in some children, especially the possible difficulty in developing control of the head and upper body. Parents should not

permit the baby to be held or positioned with the head at severe angles. The presence of hypotonus will influence the acquisition of antigravity head control in all directions, and one must alert caregivers to avoid allowing the overstretching of neck muscles and other soft tissue structures. Adapting the car seat with a soft towel roll to maintain erect head alignment is one useful suggestion. Leaning the seat back will also decrease the effect of gravity on the baby's head and neck.

In supine, the infant will be the most asymmetric until active neck flexion is present to maintain the head in midline, and the baby may have difficulty turning his or her head from side to side because of gravity acting on the head. Abnormal compensatory patterns of movement may be seen when the baby tries to turn, or the baby may be content with keeping the head to one side. The prone position promotes greater symmetry but may be frustrating if neck and upper trunk extensor strength is poor and the baby cannot easily lift and turn the head. Keeping the head to one side in either prone or supine may tire the infant, who may begin to cry. In response, a parent will lift the baby or roll it into a different position. By responding in this manner, the parent unknowingly assumed responsibility for a motor skill that the child should be mastering. Parents should be educated about how their good intentions may actually interfere with appropriate muscle development needed for their baby to move in a more acceptable manner, and they can be instructed in the use of alternative approaches.

Extensive literature is available that describes early motor development of the typical child. From this information, as mentioned earlier, one learns that an infant acquires head and neck stability in upright postures before he or she can lift their head from prone or maintain midline control in supine. Being better able to stabilize the head while upright helps strengthen the musculature needed to lift and control the head in the other positions (Figs. 10.15 and 10.16). Guided by these thoughts, the therapist can recommend that parents offer their baby with spina bifida experiences in all positions with a strong emphasis on upright postures. The push to give the baby "tummy time" is not recommended in these early weeks because it can be frustrating for both child and parent.[33,85-90]

Parents can be taught to carry their awake, alert child in ways that will not require supporting the baby's head and that will facilitate the development of antigravity head control without allowing the head to fall suddenly in an uncontrolled manner, eliciting a startle response. Holding the baby high up on the parent's shoulder rather than at the chest level is one position that can be tried (Fig. 10.17). Another useful strategy is for the parent to sit near a table holding their baby in sitting, facing them, and at eye level. The parent, while engaged in visual and verbal play with their child, is providing experiences for practicing independent head control. The infant can be held around the shoulders at first and then lower, at chest

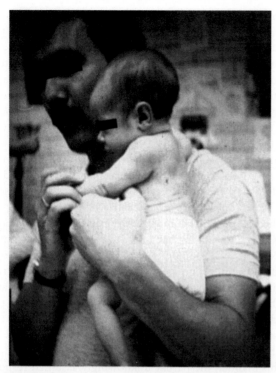

FIGURE 10.15. Typical infant at 4 weeks of age. The infant is stabilizing his head over his shoulders while held in an upright position. Note the erect alignment of the thoracic spine in the infant with typical muscle tone.

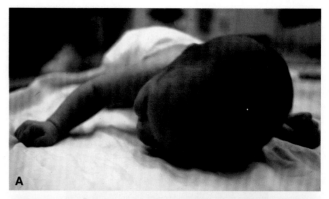

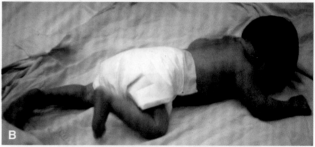

FIGURE 10.16. **A** and **B:** The same infant at 4 weeks of age as shown in Figure 10.15 barely able to lift his head against gravity while prone. He can clear his face and turn his head from side to side.

level, as head stability and control develops. Providing upright experiences, however, does not mean that the child is placed in an infant seat or other sitting devices. More about that shortly.

Parents can be alerted to observe their infant for evidence of prolonged asymmetries. But the therapist should not wait

for asymmetries to be seen. The PT can demonstrate appropriate, symmetric alignment of the baby in various positions that the parent can practice during their normal routines of the day: diaper changes, dressing, meal time, rest, and play (Fig. 10.18). Another position that encourages a more symmetric alignment is with the parent sitting comfortably on a

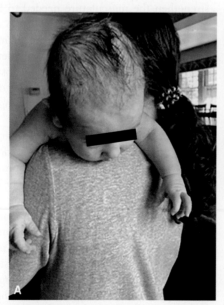

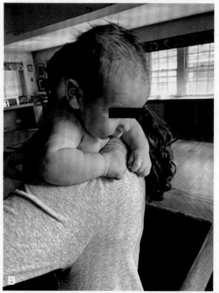

FIGURE 10.17. **A** and **B:** Infant is being carried high on the adult's shoulder to allow independent movement of the head and an improved position of the upper extremities.

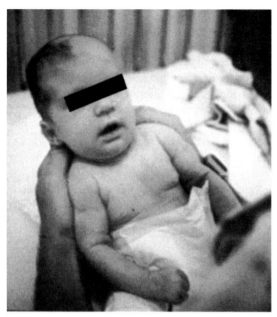

FIGURE 10.18. A suggested position for handling an infant in supine. Note the hand placement of the parent to provide a symmetric midline posture while stimulating the baby in face-to-face play.

soft chair or sofa, legs elevated with hips and knees partially flexed. The baby can be nestled supine, on the parent's legs, face-to-face, with head and body in good midline alignment. From there, head righting activities can be practiced and strengthened.

Children with spina bifida often require long-term therapeutic intervention that may be unavailable or inconvenient in the hospital setting. This is especially true for those babies in whom CNS deficits are seen. Early intervention programs, either home- or community based, are recommended if the program is able to provide the needed therapy services. Ideally, the program should provide support for the family as well. Ongoing assistance is vital once the family leaves the secure environment of the hospital and takes their baby home. The services of a 0- to 3 early intervention program should be provided to families whether they are experienced with older children or are first-time parents. It is interesting that some parents, who have other children, may be accustomed to the range of motor development seen in typically developing infants. They may deny or minimize the developmental delays of their child with spina bifida, regardless of the information they are receiving to the contrary. So the therapist should provide early and consistent input to help parents develop a critical eye and an effective approach that addresses the needs of their child. It is inappropriate to wait until significant delays or abnormalities are seen before referring a child to an intervention program. Communication between the therapists is also of vital importance. Early intervention staff should not be expected to effectively plan a program and work with a child and family without support from the hospital team. Conversely, the early intervention staff can

also provide important insight for the hospital staff. Having worked for many years in both of these venues, the author has found that intra-agency conversations are often not as collegial as they should be.

>> Physical therapy for the growing child

Developmental Concerns

A long-range plan of care should be developed by the PT that is acceptable to the neurosurgeon, orthopedic surgeon, and family. The therapy plan for the young child with spina bifida is based largely on the objective findings by the PT integrated with the concerns of the other specialists. Repeated manual muscle tests and careful observation of the child's development enable the therapist to identify the child's strengths and weaknesses. Intervention can then be directed at both the specific issues related to the lower extremities and the child's overall gross motor development (Display 10.7).

Children with spina bifida need to practice activities to improve righting and equilibrium responses of the head and trunk. When the therapist addresses these needs and sees improvement, there is an important secondary benefit. While the child's automatic balance responses against gravity are being stimulated in all positions, active movement in the trunk and lower extremities can be seen. So these balance responses should become an important part of the child's daily home exercise program because of this two-fold gain.[65]

Sitting, with movement, stimulates the child's balance, improves head and trunk control, increases the child's visual field, and provides an opportunity for many eye–hand experiences. Head righting and equilibrium responses in sitting can be tested and improved by holding the child at the shoulders and slowly tilting him or her backward. Beginning

---

DISPLAY 10.7   Goals of Physical Therapy for Children with Spina Bifida

Establish preliminary motor level by manual muscle test
Provide medical team with accurate information regarding lower limb movement
Perform periodic manual muscle testing for comparison purposes
Provide instruction to family for a long-term home program to prevent lower extremity deformity
Provide home program instruction to facilitate motor development as close to chronologic age as is possible
Assist in determining appropriate orthosis
Facilitate mobility program for ambulation and wheelchair use, where indicated
Provide information about neurologic function to treating physicians
Monitor for CNS deterioration, tethered cord, and hydromyelia
Provide support/collaboration to clinical team

conservatively at 20 to 30 degrees, the infant should respond by holding the head steady and then pulling the head forward, depending on the baby's age and skill level. Next, the therapist brings the infant's body back to midline and repeats the activity to one side, the other side, forward, and to the diagonal directions. If no response occurs in any direction and the child's head hangs, or if the child becomes upset with the activity, the movement may have been too rapid, or the baby was tilted too far. A slower and less challenging movement is used until a response is noted, and one can build from there. Changing the position of the supporting hands may also enable a child to react in the direction that was weaker. With the baby positioned on the lap of the handler, gentle downward pressure through the shoulders and thorax or mild bouncing to stimulate and approximate the joint surfaces of the cervical and thoracic spines may also help. As the child's responses to the tilting become more brisk and strong, the angle of the tilting can be increased. Over time, as the child improves, support can be moved distally to the chest and then to the waist, but the activity continues. During this balance and equilibrium routine, especially when the baby is tilted to the diagonal directions, the oblique abdominals as well as lower extremity musculature will contract in response to shifts in the center of gravity and in an attempt to maintain an upright posture. As equilibrium responses strengthen, active hip flexion, hip adduction and abduction, knee extension, and ankle and foot movements can be seen. In many instances children with limited head and upper body control have started working on righting and equilibrium reactions, and over time a significant improvement was seen not only in these automatic responses at the neck and trunk, but also in the movement and strength of the legs. Working on developmentally appropriate positions and movement patterns is especially helpful to address the lower extremity needs of young children who cannot follow verbal directions and are unable to intentionally participate in strengthening activities.

When asymmetries in the baby's balance reactions are noted to one or more directions, repetitions can be added in those directions or can be performed more frequently, but the stronger responses should still be included and not forgotten. For the young child, it is recommended that these sessions of tilting last only about 2 to 5 minutes and stop if the baby becomes tired or upset. It is advisable to help families identify a few opportunities during the child's daily routine, during which they can practice this activity. For a parent who watches a lot of television, suggest that they work with their baby on these exercises during part of each commercial break. Parents always ask how long they should practice an activity. They can work on this after each diaper change for as long as it takes to slowly sing the ABC song, trying to keep the baby engaged all through the song. The song is used as a timing device. A parent who, while practicing balance, has only got to the letter "G" one day can aim for more of the song the next time. Identifying specific times when the exercises can be practiced and for specific durations may encourage compliance and enable the responses to strengthen more quickly (Fig. 10.19).

In the prone position, neck and thoracic extensor strengthening is achieved as the child attempts and becomes successful at maintaining the head and upper body elevated against gravity without the use of his or her upper extremities. Low back extensors, gluteals, quadriceps, and plantarflexors can be activated during prone extension patterns of movement, provided, of course, that the muscles are innervated. Routine carrying of the infant in the prone position or playing face-to-face with a family member while both are lying on the floor or on a bed will stimulate the baby to hold his or her head erect (Fig. 10.20). As this becomes stronger, the baby can be further challenged with side-to-side weight shifting, which will strengthen the responses and continue to stimulate the muscles of the trunk and lower extremities.

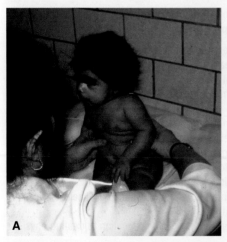 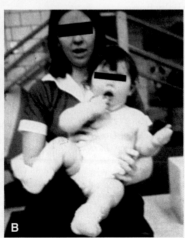 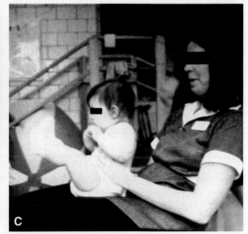

FIGURE 10.19. A–C: Beginning to teach parents in the clinic how to elicit sitting head righting and balance reactions in their baby so they can practice it through their daily routine with their child. They must see it first before they can practice it at home. Challenging the child's balance responses to elicit more sophisticated and stronger upper body reactions and strengthening of the lower extremities as they respond.

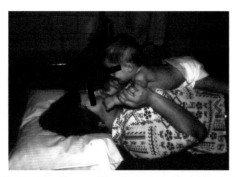

FIGURE 10.20. One position for a parent to interact with her baby to increase the baby's time in prone and facilitate strong neck and back muscles.

As mentioned earlier, in supine the effects of gravity may cause the child to look the most asymmetric. Strengthening of active neck flexion during sitting and tilting activities will carry over and improve the child's active head control in midline when supine, thus decreasing much of the asymmetry. Spending time in supine facilitates beginning eye–hand coordination and bilateral upper extremity play for the typical child. If the child with spina bifida remains asymmetric with the head turned to a preferred side, development of these skills will be hampered. Supine also facilitates disassociation of body parts as the child moves into and out of the position while at play. Through rotation of the thorax on the lumbar spine, the lumbar spine on the pelvis, and the lower extremities on the pelvis, a great deal of strengthening and control of these body parts is gained. When the child holds his or her legs up in supine, extending them to kick and play against gravity, neck flexors and abdominal musculature are strengthened as well as the muscles of the lower extremities. Neck and trunk flexors combine with the extensors to provide for good spinal alignment in sitting, which is another goal for the baby as he or she progresses.

A typical infant, held up in their parent's hands, as early as 2 months of age can bear weight on their lower extremities as a result of the positive support reaction (Fig. 10.21). When

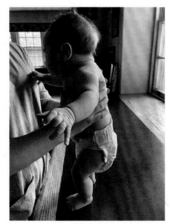

FIGURE 10.21. Supported weight bearing of baby 4 weeks of age.

this novel response is discovered by parents, it is quickly included into the repertoire of positions that parents use to play with their child.

Proprioceptive input through the legs and spine is provided by this weight bearing. Joint compression adds to the sensory input that is important for body awareness and perception of body in space. Standing also provides the baby with a new visual perspective of his or her surroundings. During this early weight bearing, contact between the femoral head and acetabulum, together with muscle contractions around the hip joint, help to stimulate acetabular development, stabilizing the hip. As the child grows, practice in supported standing evolves from being reflexive to being volitional. Upright weight bearing continues to challenge and improve trunk and leg extension, control, and balance against gravity and stimulates available muscles in the trunk and lower extremities that will assist with independent sitting and standing.

Family members should be taught to assist their young child to perform brief periods of supported standing several times each day until the child can stand with less assistance or until a first standing device or bracing is provided for longer periods in upright. Placing the child on a solid table surface, the baby can be supported against the parent's body, and one leg at a time can be stabilized and the body weight lowered onto the leg. The activity does not have to be performed with both legs simultaneously, if this is too difficult (Fig. 10.22). Rolling the baby over a small ball or lowering the child from the parent's shoulder to stand on their lap are two other methods. Many ways can be tried until one is found that is easy and convenient for the parent and success is seen. The important factor here is to get the baby weight bearing as easily as possible for the parent and to continue this briefly but often.[33,65]

Returning to general motor development, as the child with spina bifida becomes more mobile but learns to use his or her arms to compensate for weakness in the trunk and neck, the child may be able to roll over, attain the four-point position, and perhaps pull to stand, if lower extremity innervation is adequate. But this progression, with increased reliance on the arms, and poor trunk strength will ultimately lead to the child requiring a higher level of bracing than the level of the back lesion might indicate, and the child will also require a more supportive assistive device during gait than would otherwise have been predicted. Therefore, during assessment and treatment, it is not sufficient merely to identify that a developmental milestone has occurred. Rather, it is important to assess the quality of the movement, including such considerations as the child's ability to perform the movement against gravity, whether the movement is typical and symmetric in appearance or whether compensatory or abnormal patterns have developed. One can then identify the patterns of movement that need to be enhanced and strengthened as foundations for future skills, as well as the movements that should be avoided or changed.[65] Intervention for the areas of concern can be addressed in a safe and appropriate exercise regimen. The physical therapy plan can include activities

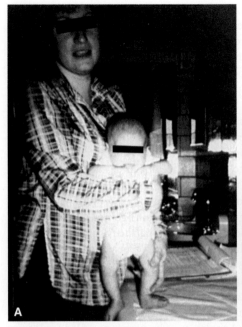
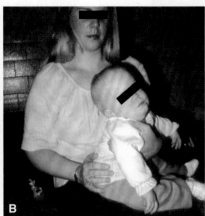
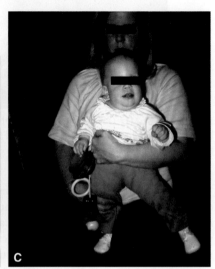

FIGURE 10.22. A: Brief periods of standing throughout the day will help provide for well-aligned weight bearing in the child without fully innervated musculature of the lower extremities. **B:** Baby with low tone sitting and leaning on mom during a clinic visit. Mom is used to this, so her child is given all the support she needs. **C:** Standing with support helps strengthen extensor tone through the neck and body and assists in better alignment.

performed in all positions, the use of gravity to challenge the child, and with varied and changing movement experiences to facilitate motor development. Providing these opportunities increases the likelihood that the child's gross, fine, and perceptual motor abilities will be less negatively affected and that the child's motor skills will be commensurate with the motor level of the lower extremities.[84-92]

Infant Devices

The issue of infant seats and various baby positioning devices always arises during conversations with parents and should be addressed by the therapist as soon as possible. The available literature consistently emphasizes that all infants need to be active to acquire the strength and motor control necessary to move against gravity, attain erect sitting and standing postures, and walk. The infant must receive and integrate vast amounts of sensory and motor information to build a foundation of knowledge about his or her body and to develop the ability to function effectively within the environment. Infant walkers, jumper seats, swings, bouncer chairs, exer-saucer seats, and the excessive use of infant seats can have a negative impact on motor development and sensorimotor learning. So the use of these devices can further delay the development of the baby with spina bifida who is already at risk for motor disturbances.

All infants must experience the upright sitting position because of its influence for mastering many skills. Upright sitting gives the child a new visual perspective of the surroundings and provides the first sensation of the effects of gravity, the weight of the head, and the opportunity to stabilize the head over the shoulders. However, to practice and gain confidence in these early skills, the infant must be stimulated by movement, for example, while being carried in a parent's arms. The experiences of random and varied weight shifting and tilting as the parent moves and walks are physiologically important. Mild bobbing and jerking movements of the head stimulate the stretch reflexes in the joint receptors of the neck, producing muscle contractions that mark the infant's beginning attempts at head control. This stimulation is essential, yet most infant seating devices offer total support, which is unwise for the infant with spina bifida who may be slow to develop head control. Infants with spina bifida need frequent opportunities to participate in activities that challenge the head, neck, and trunk. The infant should be actively moving and turning to see his or her surroundings and to feel and respond to gravity acting on their body parts in different planes. To be seated in a device allows little or no active participation in movement or in the learning process. The device allows the infant to be passive and visually entertained without offering any motor benefits. When the infant tries to move in a seated device, it is common to see an arching or hyperextending of the neck against the back of the device, a pattern that is not conducive to further acquisition of functional skills.

Now consider the child who has sufficient lower extremity function to successfully move around the room in an infant walker. The pelvis and upper body are supported, and the child is often seen with poor alignment or tilted to one side in the walker. Coordinated reciprocal movements of the legs are not necessary to gain momentum in this device, and weight bearing through the legs is often random, momentary, and sporadic. Only a quick, thrusting pattern is necessary to propel the device. It is inappropriate to facilitate and strengthen this pattern because it has no carryover for developing coordinated movements or providing stability to the lower extremities and trunk, both of which are vital components for independent standing and ambulation. Rather, infants should bear weight on their lower extremities while maintaining erect alignment of the trunk and upper body over their legs. Parents who are concerned about the "weak" legs of their infant with spina bifida can be guided and encouraged to provide prone, supine, and standing experiences that require more active participation from the child's whole body, as was mentioned in the previous section, rather than using these devices. Typically, when moving and playing, children use many parts of their body at once. A child who is excited by a bright object or favorite toy will be seen moving his or her arms while also lifting and kicking his or her legs. These movements help strengthen the musculature of the legs and trunk while offering unique sensory stimulation, and parents can be encouraged to play and excite their baby in this manner rather than thinking a device will be helpful.

Parents may initially plan to use these positioning devices for only short periods. But, because most parents strive to keep their children happy and content, the time in these devices often increases insidiously. This further reduces the time the baby spends playing and moving around on the floor in more appropriate activities. In assessing the use of such devices and the type of instruction a therapist may give a parent, one must consider the lifestyle of the family. Many parents spend long periods of time out of the house, in a car, traveling to appointments, going to the supermarket, malls, or other destinations. The infant may go from a car seat into a stroller or shopping cart and back to the car seat. Add to this the time the infant spends sleeping and eating, and it becomes apparent that little time is left for beneficial motor activities. However radical the approach may seem, the therapist may find it best to totally discourage the use of all infant devices. Then, if parents must use an infant seat for a brief period, for example, during mealtime or to keep the baby nearby while cooking, that parent might be more conscientious and remove the baby as soon as possible. Of course, the exception is in the case of a car safety seat, which must always be used when traveling and whose use should be strongly reinforced. This therapist encourages the use of a playpen or pack-n-play at home to keep the baby safe and still allow movement and exploration while a parent must cook, use the bathroom, or otherwise not be able to hold or supervise their baby for certain periods. The pack-n-play can also be moved from room to room so parent and child can see each other.[33,65,85,87-89,93]

>> Orthotics

Introduction to Bracing

A discussion of orthotics for the young child with spina bifida is most logically approached by grouping the children together who share motor levels that will require similar orthopedic and orthotic management. This chapter has considered children with thoracic-level lesions in one group, those with high lumbar L-1 to L-3 lesions in a second group, children with low lumbar L-4 to L-5 lesions in a third group, and those with sacral lesions in a fourth, final group. Early lower extremity management, splinting, standing devices, and bracing for initial standing and ambulation will be discussed for each of the groups and a rough plan of progression suggested. One should be aware that within each group the children may have very different patterns of active movement, strengths, and upright function. Thus, the clinician should remember that each child must be evaluated individually, and, depending on the results, a management plan specific to that child can be developed, with the information in this section serving as a guide.

Philosophies of Bracing

Some clinics follow a bracing philosophy that pre-establishes a plateau of expected maximum function for children on the basis of their lesion level and general gross motor development. Several publications have supported the concept that an ultimate and predictable level of mobility exists for children at each motor level. These approaches advocate establishing reasonable but not unrealistic expectations for each child because much time, effort, and money can be spent on orthotics and physical therapy services to teach gait training and maintain upright skills that, for some children, will be feasible only for a short time in their lives. This philosophy is thought to be an efficient, cost-effective method that supports the concept that later functional outcome can be predicted primarily by the child's lesion level at an early age. Institutions that follow this model are often reluctant to brace a child with a thoracic or high lumbar lesion after the early childhood years, because some literature indicates that most adolescents with high-level lesions are mobile only from their wheelchair and have discarded functional ambulation. There is, however, opposing research that acknowledges a significant number of variables that affect the level of upright performance of a child, among which lower extremity innervation is only one factor. Interest, commitment, and participation by the family and the child's CNS function, motivation, learning capacity, and the desire for movement are just a few of the factors that should be considered when deciding whether to begin, proceed with, or discontinue an ambulation program. An article from a major clinic in Australia identified that the later the child began to ambulate, the earlier he or she was to abandon it. The article also pointed to rapid growth and weight gain, the need for frequent brace adjustments, and other medical problems as factors that stop a child from ambulation even earlier than might have been expected.[94] An editorial by Dr. Malcolm Menelaus stated that early ambulation is important for many physiologic and psychological reasons even if it is abandoned later in the individual's life.[95] Finally, from an ethical standpoint, one might question whether proceeding with or terminating a gait program should be determined by anyone other than the child, as evidenced by his or her abilities, in combination with the family, who is ultimately responsible for their child's program continuity and follow-up care.

The Lurie Children's Hospital in Chicago follows a course of action in which all children who were seen through the myelomeningocele clinic begin a program of early standing and gait training and as the child grows, the clinic staff, parents, school personnel, and the child communicate and share their impressions and experiences, so bracing and ambulation would continue for as long as it seemed reasonable. When a child is considered a household or exercise ambulator and uses a wheelchair for primary mobility, this level of gait is still supported and encouraged by the clinic staff.

Adopting this approach means that more time is required to communicate between various institutions and individuals so that everyone is aware of the ambulation goals and is working toward the same end. Because the child's needs and abilities may be constantly changing, the goals established for mobility also have to be flexible. Changes in medical care for children with spina bifida, as well as advances in orthotics technology and materials, warrant an active and creative approach toward bracing and gait. The end goal is to help each child attain his or her optimal level of performance, regardless of motor level, and to assist the child to maintain this level for as long as it is feasible. Consider just one issue: the physical environment of the child and its impact. In this country, in large and small cities, rural and suburban areas, there can be tremendous variations in the style of architecture and the size of homes or apartments. The condition of sidewalks, yards, or driveways, stairs, accessibility of schools, access to parks and expanses of space to walk and play in, and many other assets or obstacles will influence the child's ability to acquire and maintain gait skills. All factors should be considered when helping to develop a gait program, rather than using the child's lesion level as the determining factor.[33,65,96]

General Principles of Orthotics

Any discussion of bracing raises the fundamental question of whether the child should be braced high and levels of bracing removed as motor control is mastered or whether the child should be braced low, with sections added as the need dictates. Unfortunately, initial orthotic decisions can be imprecise and become more refined only with clinical experience. A brace that is prescribed for a moving, growing, changing child can be correct only for the brief period that the child remains exactly as he or she was when evaluated. That period

may be very short for the 1- to 3-year-old child, longer for the 3- to 5-year old, and longer still for the 14- to 16-year-old teenager. This means that the younger child who is growing rapidly and is very active may require more frequent brace reevaluations, revisions, and repairs. This is not an indication to become frustrated and give up on the ambulation plan but rather to be even more diligent and committed to supporting the ambulation process with the child and family.

Also, in order to make an appropriate brace selection, the effects of CNS dysfunction on the child's ability to move must be considered as well as the motor level of the lower extremities. The orthopedic surgeon, PT, and family should try to gather as much objective information about the child as possible before beginning an orthotics program. The PT, having spent time with the child, should have a good impression of the child's motor capabilities. Also, asking parents to share their perceptions of their child's motor function can identify any differences between home and clinic performance. For example, parents can be asked to describe the ways in which their child likes to play, their child's favorite positions, responses to the upright position, degree of assistance needed to change positions, and the method the child uses to move and explore on the floor. The answers to these questions can give the therapist valuable information about how active the child is, even though the child may be sitting quietly in a stroller in the clinic, throughout this conversation. Sharing of short iPhone video clips, taken while the child is at home playing, has been very valuable for therapists. There have been families who, although excited about the prospects of beginning a bracing and gait program with their child, were able to verbalize that he or she did not seem ready to be upright, follow directions, and walk with braces and an assistive device. Hence, the plan was postponed for a few months to enable the child to begin practicing small parts of the gait program, for short periods each day, until the child seemed more ready and the parents were agreeable. In specific situations, a walker may be introduced in the house so the child begins to see it as a routine piece of furniture and is no longer afraid to hold it. Another child may be placed in their braces and allowed to go through their typical day, but nothing more. Or a child may be braced and propped at the sofa to play, without being asked to move. The ability to break down the process or an activity and introduce it in small portions to the timid or fearful child may make the difference between success or failure, ease or frustration.

Once a brace is fabricated for a child, the family should be shown proper donning and doffing. Appropriate leg coverings should be suggested to protect the child's skin. This therapist recommends a long, boy's tube sock for protection or thin, non-textured tights for both girls and boys. Parents should be alerted as to where and how to look for improper fit of a brace and when a brace modification would be indicated owing to poor fit. Pressure along the medial or lateral borders of the feet, ankles, and knees and the bony prominences of hips and legs should be examined. Parents should be included in the discussion when a change in orthotics is being considered, adding or subtracting a section of the brace on the basis of their child's progression or if problems are encountered. Regardless of the brace, families must know whom to call and what action to take if the brace does not produce the desired result. They should understand that the problems with the brace do not mean that they or their child are failures or are somehow inadequate. Selecting and fitting the appropriate brace for a child is an ongoing process that may take time to perfect. The need for change to an already existing brace program is often based on sound observations and recommendations from parents, who are living and working with their child each day. Families should not have braces sitting in a closet for several months, unused, while awaiting a routine clinic appointment to discuss a problem with the therapist or orthopedic surgeon. Likewise, a poorly fitting brace that might cause serious skin damage should not be worn because the parents want to comply with their home program instructions. Brace changes that require adding a level of support should not be construed as the child's failure, regression, or lack of progress. Rather, it should be handled as a matter of course for a decision that is often difficult and based on both objective and subjective findings.

Decisions to change the bracing level, unlock joints, or change an assistive device should be made after due consideration. The child's attitude toward and readiness for gait training strongly influences the timeliness of these decisions. Generally, the goal is safe and functional ambulation by 5 or 6 years of age in preparation for mobility in school. But, given the numerous tasks and skills to be mastered, this is not a great deal of time in which to prepare. Parents and therapists may feel rushed when the child is nearing school age, but sufficient time must be allowed for mastery of skills at one stage before progressing to the next. Some families are assertive when expressing their desire to have their child standing and ambulating with as little assistance as possible, as soon as possible. This should not rush the clinician into a premature decision that might have a negative effect on the child's outcome. The responsible method of practice is to pace the progression of skills slowly to achieve the safest, most secure, and least stressful result for the child and family, while still moving forward. In keeping with this measured approach, only one change at a time should be made to an orthosis or an assistive device. Unlock the proximal joint of the brace or remove a trunk strap, see the outcome, and allow some time for the child to adapt before making the next alteration. Note that the child has progressed nicely with a walker before trying to transition to crutches. Otherwise, diagnosing the etiology of a problem that may arise becomes more difficult if multiple modifications were made at the same time or over too short a period.

A well-defined orthotics program should begin as early as the child's first days of life after the initial evaluations are concluded. The PT and orthopedic surgeon can discuss the deformities that are present and those that may likely occur secondary to muscle imbalance or bony deformity around a joint. They can then develop a plan of care, including necessary taping, splinting, and bracing, to address the current and/or anticipated problems. Orthopedic surgery and an early orthotics program can then be coordinated to prepare the child for upright positioning close to the typical developmental age of 12 to 15 months, if possible.[25,65,80]

Children with Thoracic-level Paralysis

The child with no motor control below the thorax has flaccid lower extremities and is at risk for developing a "frog-legged" deformity. This posture is also commonly seen in the immobile infant with hypotonia who remains in supine for long periods. The legs are abducted, externally rotated, and flexed at the hips and knees with the feet in plantarflexion. There is no active leg motion to counteract the effects of gravity and reverse this position. Muscle and other soft tissue structures become increasingly tight over a short period without proper attention, and the presence of reflex activity at the knee or ankle can make the posture more resistant. Prone positioning and frequent, daily ROM exercises are advised. Also, gentle nighttime wrapping of the legs in extension and adduction with an elastic bandage can help prevent or minimize the deformity. Flexibility can be gained using these intervention strategies when minimal to moderate tightness already exists, but trying to avoid the problem before it occurs is a primary goal. As the baby grows, a "total-contact" orthosis may be used during nap times and through the night to prevent loss of joint range. Proper fit of the brace will prevent limb movement within the device that can lead to abrasions, and the child should always wear protective tights or long socks. To enable the child to work further on control and strength of the head and trunk, this first orthosis can be adapted with wedged rubber soles so it can be used for brief periods of standing and tilting exercises through the day. During these sessions of standing, the child can practice and become proficient in balance and equilibrium reactions of increasing difficulty (Fig. 10.23). Prone-lying in the splint, while the child is asleep, is recommended to help avoid pressure over bony prominences, such as the ischial tuberosity, sacrum, and calcaneus. Skin breakdown at these sites is common with persistent supine positioning. Inspection of the skin is also essential after each session with the orthosis, and any red marks that do not fade should be brought to the attention of the orthotist for adjustment.

If the child has moderate to severe limitations in hip ROM, it is inappropriate to use an orthosis to force the limbs into better alignment. This is dangerous and can result in skin breakdown and/or a fracture, especially at the proximal femoral neck. Significant limitations in flexibility are managed best by conservative methods of wrapping and gentle stretching with eventual surgical release of the tight soft tissue structures, including the iliotibial band, hip external rotators, and knee flexors. The total-contact orthosis can then be used following surgery to maintain the newly acquired position.

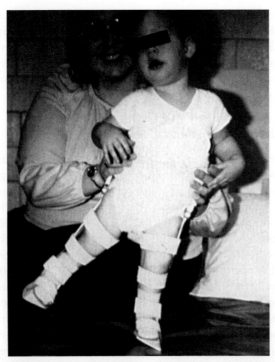

FIGURE 10.23. A total-contact orthosis to be worn at night fitted with wedged soles for periods of standing and weight-shifting activities.

The total-contact orthosis should always include a thoracolumbar section to stabilize the pelvis and lumbar spine. Without this section, the child can wiggle and move and laterally flex the trunk, causing malalignment of the lower extremities, with adduction of one hip and abduction of the other hip, relative to the pelvis. Contractures at the foot will make later brace and shoe fit difficult, so the total-contact orthosis should also include the lower legs and feet to hold the knees extended and the ankles in a neutral/plantigrade position.

For the older child or adolescent with a high thoracic lesion who may no longer be ambulatory, the total-contact orthosis may be appropriate to use at night, to prevent or minimize contractures that can easily develop in individuals who are sitting all day. Also, a lightweight, foot splint or ankle–foot orthosis (AFO) can be fabricated for use during the day to maintain the ankle at 90 degrees and good shoe fit.[25,65]

Children with High Lumbar-level Paralysis

Children with a motor level from L-1 to L-3 will usually exhibit some active hip flexion and adduction, but no other strong movements at the hips or knees are present. Weak quadriceps and medial hamstrings may be noted in some children with an L-3 motor level. To prevent flexion/adduction contractures at the hips, the child with a high lumbar lesion can also benefit from the use of the total-contact orthosis. The splint can maintain hip and knee extension with moderate abduction (approximately 30 degrees) and be

worn during sleep. It can also serve as the child's first standing device.

Children with this degree of lumbar paralysis will usually require an initial level of bracing that supports the hips and lower legs to stand and walk. Bracing at that level is necessary to stabilize extension at the knees and a 90-degree angle at the ankles and to provide medial–lateral control at the hips. Many children with this level of paralysis who have strong trunk musculature, good sitting balance, and intact CNS function may be able to control the rotation and adduction components of hip movement and ambulate without orthotic control at the hips later in childhood, but they will still require bracing above the knees, as well as some type of assistive device such as a walker or crutches.

Hip subluxations and dislocations are common in children with a high lumbar paralysis owing to the significant muscle imbalance around the hip. It can be either unilateral or bilateral. When hip dislocation is detected, therapists and parents should continue passive ROM exercises, with care, to ensure no additional loss of joint flexibility or related muscle shortening occurs. There is often fear that more damage to the joint will occur from ROM exercises, but this is not the case. Rather, more harm is done by discontinuing the exercises and allowing additional adductor and flexor tightness to develop. Much discussion and debate has taken place within the orthopedic community in regard to the optimal surgical approach to the dislocated hip in those with this level of paralysis. The consensus is that surgery to relocate either one or both hips is not indicated. There are many postoperative complications that may be more problematic than the original dislocation. Fractures, pain, and infection can occur as well as a stiff, frozen hip as a result of an open reduction procedure. An immobile hip joint will compromise sitting and standing alignment and often requires additional surgery, if it can be corrected at all. Subsequent dislocation as high as 30% to 45% of the hips is also common, owing to the lack of dynamic forces around the hip to provide joint stability. The hip dislocation does not affect the child's functional abilities in upright. Simple surgical release of soft tissue structures may be decided if the active and unopposed hip flexors and adductors have tightened to the point of restricting range. In the case of a unilateral dislocation, an asymmetric pelvis can result if the involved hip becomes tight. This asymmetric posture creates an uneven foundation for sitting and standing and interferes with proper fit and alignment of braces. Again, addressing the limitation of ROM and achieving a level pelvis without joint surgery is more important than achieving a good looking X-ray. Evaluation for a shoe lift may be necessary for the child with a unilateral hip dislocation in order to equalize leg lengths when the child is upright. Even a small leg-length difference may affect standing alignment and stability of the younger, smaller children and should be addressed.

When hip surgery is performed and the child is immobilized, it is appropriate for the PT to be involved with the child and family for home program instruction. After the hip has healed, intervention with the child and family can help ensure that the hip will remain flexible and the child can return to the standing or gait program.[25,65,97-101]

Orthotics for Children with Thoracic and High Lumbar-level Paralysis

When children with T-12 to L-3 motor levels are almost 12 months old and exhibit adequate head control to be positioned upright, they should be considered for the "A frame," also known as the Toronto standing frame. This device can be used for multiple, short standing sessions during the day in an attempt to duplicate the activities of typical children who pull to stand for short periods but are still predominantly mobile on the floor, on their hands and knees (Fig. 10.24). The device is easy to don and doff, and a schedule of upright positioning for up to 30 minutes, three to five times each day seems manageable for many parents. The device is freestanding and represents the child's first opportunity to be upright without having hands-on assistance from a parent or using their own upper extremities for support. Engaging the child

in finger feeding, block play, and other fine motor activities is ideal during this standing time. Additionally, parents should be instructed to challenge their child while in the device by working on head righting and balance skills. A recommended activity is to slowly tilt the frame in one direction, watching for the child's righting response of the head and trunk. The frame is returned to midline and then tilted in another direction, waiting again for the child's balance response. The frame should be tilted slowly and to a small angle, and all directions should be performed: forward, back, right and left sides, and to the diagonals. This routine is recommended for the first 3 to 5 minutes of each standing session. On the basis of the child's success, increasing the angle of each tilt will further strengthen not only the responses but also the neck and trunk musculature. Again, as mentioned earlier, if asymmetry is seen in the quality of the child's responses, then tilting can be performed more frequently to specific directions to strengthen these weaker reactions. Positioning the child to passively stand in front of the television is not recommended, and unsupervised standing is not advisable because the child's wiggling body can easily topple the device,

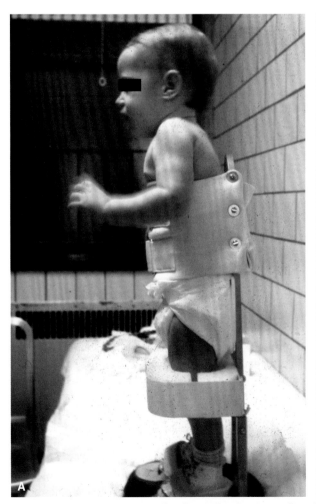 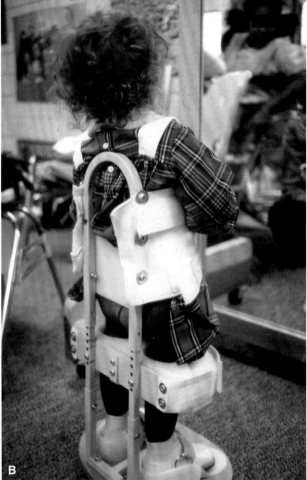

FIGURE 10.24. A: Toronto standing frame showing proper fit and good trunk and leg alignment. Caution not to allow hips to be in flexion or knees in either hyperextension or flexion past neutral. The foam knee pad is truly at the patella and not below. **B:** Rear view showing the location of the upright bar low enough that the child cannot lean her head back and rest on it.

causing injury.[33,65] Several companies offer their version of a standing frame, but the bases are larger, making them stable enough to leave the baby unattended. Unfortunately, this defeats several of the objectives of using the frame: having the parent interact with the child doing fun and beneficial activities and practicing righting and equilibrium reactions with their child.

As the child progresses in developmental activities, such as rolling, getting into and out of sitting, and creeping or crawling, the child may no longer tolerate the immobility of the standing frame. This may indicate a readiness to begin bracing and ambulation training.

Children with moderate to severe CNS deficits and delayed acquisition of head control and upper extremity function may continue to use the standing frame until they are too tall to properly fit into the frame (at about 6 years of age, depending on the child's height and weight). As the child outgrows the frame, either the parapodium or the Orlau swivel walker may be considered. These are two orthotic options that will provide continued and valuable time in an upright posture while providing good trunk and leg alignment and adequate support to meet the needs of the child with significant limitations. Both devices are easy to don and doff, they are simple to size and fit well and are also freestanding. So they require supervision. Regardless of the device chosen, the child should continue an exercise program that includes developmental and preambulation skills to further improve function in the neck, arms, and upper body. While in either device, the child can practice weight-shift activities, as described earlier. For the child in a parapodium, a walker or forearm crutches can be introduced at some point to teach forward mobility using a hop-to gait, if the child has sufficient upper extremity strength and coordination. The Orlau swivel walker has a ball-bearing plate at its base that causes a forward progression on smooth level surfaces without the use of an assistive device. Movement of the Orlau walker requires the child to move their head and shoulders in a side-to-side motion, and that causes the device to unweight on one side and swivel forward. As skills improve, children can progress to different, less supportive and restrictive orthotics, but the child can remain with either of these two devices as long as it will accommodate their growth.[65,102]

For many years, the standard hip–knee–ankle–foot orthosis (HKAFO) was the only option for the child with a high level of paralysis who had graduated from the standing devices and was ready to ambulate. A thoracic extension could be added to the HKAFO for the child with limited trunk control, but this was very confining and limited the child's potential to walk only as a household or exercise ambulator. Another option, the Louisiana State University Reciprocating Gait Orthosis (RGO), originally developed for the adult with traumatic paraplegia, easily transitioned as a viable option for the child with spina bifida. The RGO uses a system of cables with a dual-action hip joint that flexes one hip while maintaining the opposite hip in locked extension for a stable one-legged stance and a reciprocating pattern of gait.

A properly fitted RGO maintains the ankles at 90 degrees, extension at the knee and hip joints and aligns and supports the trunk and pelvis over the legs with lateral thoracic uprights and a strap. Many children who have used the RGO and an assistive device have been able to progress to a more energy-efficient and safer gait pattern than was possible with the HKAFO. As a child's trunk stability improves, the RGO can be modified without decreasing the child's ability. By retaining the cables and dual-action hip joints but removing the chest strap and thoracic uprights, the child can still use the brace mechanism for an assisted reciprocating gait but with less restriction of the upper body.[103-107]

The isocentric RGO is another ambulation option for the child with a high level of paralysis and trunk instability. It eliminates the posterior cable system but maintains the same functional properties as the original RGO. Children accustomed to using the original RGO can easily switch to the isocentric model when they require a new brace owing to growth, or it can be prescribed as the child's first brace.[104]

With hip and knee joints locked, the child ambulating with either of these reciprocating braces and an assistive device performs a lateral weight shift onto one leg and leans slightly back at the shoulders to facilitate the forward flexion of the unweighted leg. Repeating the weight shift to the other side and posterior lean produces forward flexion of the opposite leg. This gait pattern requires no active motor function in the lower extremities, but if active hip flexion is present, it can be utilized to move one leg forward while the weighted leg is still kept stabilized in extension (Figs. 10.25 and 10.26).[104-108]

When using the standard HKAFO with a pelvic band, locked hip and knee joints, and solid ankle joints, the child can learn either a hop-to or swivel pattern of gait using a walker and later master the swing-to or swing-through patterns with forearm crutches as arm strength and control increase. The child with active hip flexors can attempt to walk with one or both hip joints unlocked, using a reciprocating gait pattern. In the absence of innervated gluteals, however, when both hips are unlocked, the child will jackknife forward. To maintain an erect posture, the child must be able to hyperextend the lumbar spine to shift the center of gravity posterior. The child must also use both arms to remain erect by pushing on their assistive device (Fig. 10.27). When unlocking the hip joints of the HKAFO, the lateral metal uprights and pelvic band control for hip adduction/abduction and medial/lateral rotation, motions the child is unable to actively control. For some children with a high lumbar lesion and an intact CNS, the pelvic band may be removed at some point to allow further freedom for transfers and to permit a faster swing-through gait pattern, when the child progresses to crutches. Arm strength, trunk stability, and the ability to hyperextend the lumbar spine are essential for a stable stance without the pelvic band. When these factors are present, the gait of the child will more closely resemble those with acquired, traumatic paraplegia.[104,105]

Regardless of the orthosis, most therapists find that the rollator walker is the most effective assistive device when

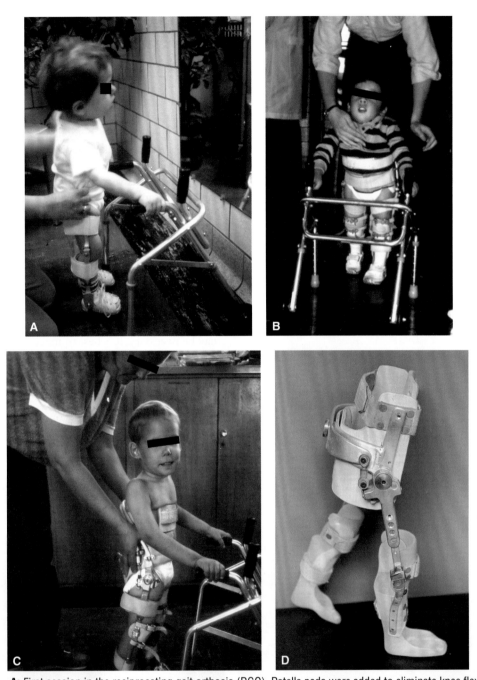

FIGURE 10.25. A: First session in the reciprocating gait orthosis (RGO). Patella pads were added to eliminate knee flexion. Standing at a mirror, mom begins with teaching her son to hold on and not wiggle too much. **B:** In the RGO, a lateral weight shift with a slight tilt backward causes the unweighted leg to swing forward. **C:** Another example of erect alignment in the RGO and an easy, low stress gait training session. **D:** One style of the isocentric RGO. The same principle to elicit a reciprocating gait pattern and without the rear cable mechanism.

gait training is initiated. Configured with two rear legs for stability and two front wheels, the walker is stable and easy to maneuver, and the child does not have to lift the walker to advance it. An anterior-facing walker provides support for the child who needs to lean heavily on the device to keep their trunk erect. Some children may do well with a posterior walker. Beware that initially having all four legs with wheels may be too much movement for the young child to control. Both anterior and posterior facing walkers should

be tried and the correct device chosen, based on the child's performance.

Young children can begin their gait program by first learning to hold their walker for short periods, repeated several times daily. The young child often requires hand-over-hand assistance from an adult. While standing at a low window or mirror, the child is reminded not to let go or move. If they do, allowing them and their walker to tilt and even fall over, in a controlled, protected manner, often reinforces the point.

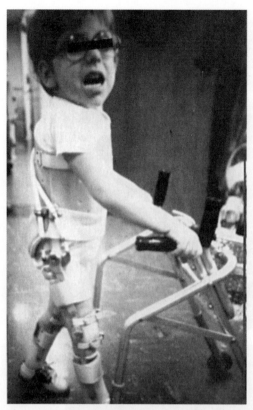

FIGURE 10.26. Several weeks after the first gait training session, the child is independent on level surfaces.

Placing the walker against the wall or mirror stabilizes it in the sagittal plane while the child learns to control the other directions. After a few practice sessions, the child may be moved away from the mirror and shown how to move forward. If possible, the use of parallel bars should be avoided during initial gait training because they provide too much stability, and the young child may develop patterns of leaning and pulling on the bars that will be dangerous when making the transition to a walker that is less stable. Exceptions to this may be made in cases where a child has difficulty learning to use a walker or is very fearful. But before assuming parallel bars are the answer, one should first check that the level of bracing is appropriate. If the child is braced too low, they will feel the need for more support (Table 10.3).

The decision to progress the child from a walker to either axillary or forearm crutches will depend on the child's ability. The child should have a reasonable period of time to walk successfully with the first device before transitioning to another. A typical timeline for progression cannot be easily recommended or predicted, and a degree of experimentation may be necessary. It is best to make the transition by 6 to 8 years of age, when upper extremity strength is sufficient, the child can follow simple cues and verbal directions, and before a child becomes too dependent on the walker or becomes anxious about falling.

A child wearing a body jacket to control scoliosis may find axillary crutches difficult to use. The crutches may be

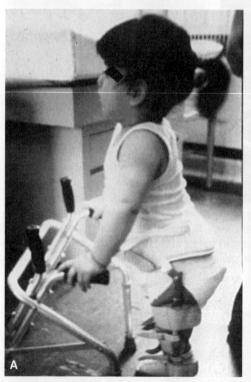

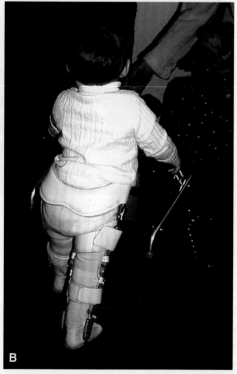

FIGURE 10.27. A: Hip–knee–ankle–foot orthosis (HKAFO) with hip joints unlocked. The child with an L-4 or L-5 motor level maintains balance with a hyperextended lumbar spine and upper extremity support on the walker. The HKAFO is needed to control medial–lateral instability at the hips due to muscle imbalance. **B:** Photo illustrates proper positioning and configuration of the Butterfly pelvic band to assist with passive hip extension when active hip extension is absent.

TABLE 10.3.	Ambulation Sequence: T-12 to L-3 Motor Level		
	CNS Status		
	Typical → Mild Deficit	Mild → Moderate	Moderate → Severe
Preambulation orthosis	Toronto A Frame	Toronto A Frame	Toronto A Frame
Assess	Ambulation bracing at 15–24 mo	Ambulation bracing at 15–24 mo	Continue with A Frame
Ambulation orthosis	HKAFO; locked hips; rollator walker	RGO; thoracic uprights; rollator walker	Orlau swivel walker; no assistive device
Progress	As above, hips unlocked	RGO; remove uprights; rollator walker	RGO; thoracic uprights; rollator walker
Progress	As above, crutches	As above, crutches	
Progress	KAFO, pelvic band removed; crutches	Assess for further changes; consider standard HKAFO or KAFO	Assess for further changes

CNS, central nervous system; HKAFO, hip–knee–ankle–foot orthosis; KAFO, knee–ankle–foot orthosis; RGO, reciprocating gait orthosis.

hard to stabilize and may move against the slippery spinal brace. With HKAFO bracing and a trunk extension, axillary crutches can get caught on the lateral uprights. But axillary crutches encourage a more upright posture, and they may work well for the child who does not have sufficient strength or control of the shoulders and needs this added support for a reciprocating gait or hop-to pattern.

The swing-to and swing-through patterns are best accomplished with forearm crutches, and it has been this author's experience that the vast majority of children with spina bifida who make the transition go from a walker to forearm crutches rather easily. However, the child who is using forearm crutches over several years, leaning forward onto the crutches, can develop an upper thoracic kyphosis and tight pectoral muscles that cause elevation and protraction of the shoulders and scapulae. If these postural malalignments begin to develop, the therapist and family should work together with the child to maintain a flexible, erect thoracic spine and well-aligned shoulders. Prone extension and exercises for shoulder external rotation and depression, in sitting, prone, and/or supine, will help strengthen the rhomboids and lower trapezius muscles and stretch the tightening pectorals, which may help to minimize any permanent structural changes.

By the time the child, with a thoracic or high-level lumbar paralysis, approaches adolescence, he or she may have already chosen to use a wheelchair as their primary form of mobility to be faster and more competitive with their peers. It has been found that girls prefer wheelchair mobility earlier than boys as a result of their earlier puberty and the weight gain and body development that accompany adolescence. As transitioning to wheelchair use occurs, children and families may discard the idea of bracing, standing, and walking. The growth spurts and weight gain that are typical of all adolescents make brace management a serious problem for the child with spina bifida. Braces may require more frequent adjustment, repair, and/or replacement. The child might be spending little or no time standing and walking during the typical school day, so the value of the braces is greatly reduced in their eyes. But spending a full day in a wheelchair increases the likelihood of developing hip and knee flexion contractures and foot deformities. These are common in the nonambulatory adolescent and can impact the child's wheelchair and transfer skills, bed mobility, and skin integrity. Therefore, when wheelchair mobility is chosen, if possible, children should also maintain a program of positioning and physical activity aimed at avoiding joint contractures and musculoskeletal deterioration. Prone positioning in combination with a standing device, parapodium, or braces can be used during prescribed therapy sessions and for certain periods throughout the week, both at home and at school. Embedded into the routines of the home, standing in some manner, for homework, meals, relaxation time, TV watching, and so on will help to maintain the musculoskeletal and physiologic benefits of upright that were discussed earlier in this chapter. Swimming, wheelchair sports and games, wheelchair aerobics, and other activities that help with weight control and improve cardiovascular function can be a part of the child's activity regimen as well. Maintaining and increasing trunk and arm strength and coordination also remain important for the older child/adolescent so that during these times of growth and weight gain, there is no loss of function.[25,94,95,98,109]

Children with Low Lumbar-level Paralysis

Children with L-4 or L-5 motor function usually have strong hip flexors and adductors. Gluteus medius and tensor fascia lata may be present to contribute to active hip abduction, although the strength of these muscles can vary from a "poor" to a "good" grade depending on the contribution from the innervated nerve roots. But hip extension power from the gluteus maximus is absent. Children at this level are at risk for flexion contractures as well as early hip dislocation or later progressive subluxation, depending on the imbalance of strengths of the muscles surrounding the hip joint. Inherent ligamentous laxity in the child with low tone also contributes to hip joint instability.

Manual muscle testing around the knee usually shows strong quadriceps and medial hamstrings (semitendinosus and semimembranosus) but absent lateral hamstring function. Kicking and crawling during the early childhood years can produce an internal tibial torsion deformity from the unopposed stimulation by the medial hamstrings on the tibia. This imbalance of muscle forces contributes to a toeing-in posture during both standing and gait, which may first be observed when the child pulls to stand and begins to cruise.

Careful manual muscle testing is crucial in children with this lower-level lesion because there is considerable variation in active motion seen at the ankle and foot within this population (Display 10.8). Active anterior and posterior tibialis muscles, long and short toe extensors, peroneus longus and brevis muscles, and toe flexors may be noted. If significant imbalance is found, there may be a need for splints for night wear to prevent a progressive loss of flexibility, until corrective surgery is indicated.

With strong dorsiflexors and absent plantarflexors, a calcaneus deformity may have been present at birth, or it may develop through early childhood. An exceptionally high arch, a pes cavus deformity, is caused by the unopposed action of the anterior tibialis and results in a foot with a dangerously reduced weight-bearing surface. The distribution of body weight is limited to the heel and ball of the foot, and pressure problems can quickly develop when the child is standing and walking. Bracing and shoe fit can be difficult, and surgery is often indicated to weaken or eliminate the deforming forces, realign the bones, and provide a greater weight-bearing surface over the entire sole of the foot.[110]

When there is an absence of the plantarflexor (gastrocnemius/soleus) muscles, the various combinations of strengths and weaknesses of the intrinsic foot musculature can produce additional abnormal ankle, foot, and toe alignment and deviations in the weight-bearing surfaces. The orthopedic surgeon may consider muscle-lengthening procedures and tendon transfers in an attempt to balance the dynamic forces around the joints or excise the tendons if active muscle balance cannot be reached. The goal is to attain a flat foot that is easy to fit with bracing and shoes.[110,111] Torosian and Dias stated that deformities of the foot are the most common lower limb problem in the spina bifida population. Foot deformities cause pain, interfere with shoe and brace fit, and negatively affect the child's ability to walk.[112] They specifically addressed the management of severe hindfoot valgus, but the principles are universal to all foot malalignment. A mild deformity may be accommodated by a brace, but if it is severe, the insensate foot requires surgical correction because it is highly vulnerable to pressure sores and ulceration.

The clubfoot deformity, talipes equinovarus, is the most common foot deformity requiring surgical correction for children with an L-4 or L-5 motor level (Fig. 10.28). The diagnosis and management of clubfoot has prompted extensive discussion, but most surgeons now follow a multipronged protocol that includes gentle manipulation and taping as early as the baby's first weeks of life, followed by application of a well-padded splint. Serial casting may be used, but problems can develop from pressure over bony prominences, associated skin irritation, and breakdown. Also, casting may not be precise in applying the appropriate pressures to a small foot with this multiplanar deformity. The clubfoot is often very resistant to conservative treatment, and surgical correction may be inevitable. Recurrence of a clubfoot deformity, secondary to conservative treatment or incomplete surgical correction, can be as high as 68% and may lead to skin problems from a brace and shoe that is difficult to fit.[110] Postoperative gentle passive stretching exercises to maintain flexibility of the foot and a well-padded, properly fitting brace are important, although additional surgery to fully correct the deformity will be necessary in the future. It is reported that when tendon lengthening is used instead of excision of the tendons, the deformity is more likely to recur. Since children with this level of motor paralysis will always need bracing to stabilize the ankle and foot for gait, tendon excision should have no functional impact on the child's level of bracing or ambulation ability. Initially, the midfoot has a prominent medial crease from forefoot adduction. Postoperatively, the foot lengthens as it becomes properly aligned. Prior to surgery, parents can be instructed to perform frequent but

---

DISPLAY

10.8   **Common Foot Deformities in Children with Spina Bifida**

Pes calcaneus, calcaneovarus, calcaneovalgus
Talipes equinovarus or clubfoot
Pes equines or flatfoot
Convex pes valgus or rocker-bottom foot with vertical talus
Pes cavus, high arch with toe-clawing
Ankle valgus, at the mid- or hindfoot

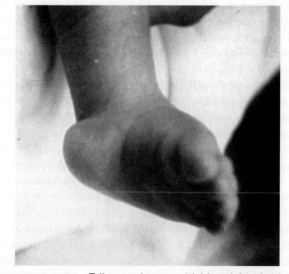

FIGURE 10.28. Talipes equinovarus (clubfoot deformity) in a neonate. She will be treated with serial taping to gently stretch soft tissue structures into a more neutral position followed by surgery.

gentle stretching of the skin and soft tissue structures, especially at the medial aspect of the foot as well as posterior, at the tight heelcord. This has been found to help prevent wound dehiscence, a complication following surgery, when the skin is stretched thin and taut to cover the longer, corrected foot. The more flexible the soft tissue, prior to surgery, the less likely this will occur. The Ponseti method of clubfoot management is popular in many clinics for children with and without spina bifida. This regimen includes serial splinting or casting, surgery to release the tight Achilles tendon, and postoperative stretching and positioning with shoes or splints. The rates of full correction and later recurrence vary with the institution, but it is apparent that attention to the details of skin care and proper alignment in whatever immobilization device is used is paramount.[25,65,113-116]

Regarding hip reduction surgery for the child with an L4 or L5 motor level, the debate continues. When deciding on a course of management, the discussion should focus on the child's motor function, including lower extremity strength and developmental skills and the child's potential to walk with an assistive device versus independently. Surgical correction is considered contraindicated if bracing to the hips and/or assistive devices might always be needed for mobility, because the hip status will not affect these parameters. On the other hand, surgical correction might be considered for the child with good motor control of the trunk and strong quadriceps and gluteus medius musculature. If this child is able to walk with some configuration of AFO or KAFO bracing and no assistive device, a surgeon may choose to address the child's hip(s) to prevent or correct gait deviations that might hamper the child's future unassisted walking. Surgery might also be considered to prevent degenerative changes in the unstable hip. Many surgeons contend that bilateral hip dislocations should never be surgically repaired for fear that postoperative complications could ultimately be more harmful, with minimal functional gains and the greater potential for diminished gait later in life. A unilateral dislocation is usually corrected only in the child with a low level of innervation and intact CNS function who has the potential for ambulation with short bracing and no assistive device.[25,65,117]

It is apparent from this section of the chapter and from the literature that the management of hip dislocations is often a confusing and controversial subject in regard to the child with a low lumbar lesion. The therapist can play an important role in assisting the physician to identify the child's muscle strengths and weaknesses, skills in the upright position, trunk and pelvic alignment, and overall gross motor ability. This information may then enable the physician to better evaluate the treatment options and decide accordingly. It is widely accepted that function, not X-ray findings, should guide this important decision.

Children with L-4 to L-5 paralysis who have significant CNS deficits may be unable to control their trunk in upright positions or move their legs well. This lack of movement often conveys the impression that a higher level of paralysis exists. The therapist and the family should continue their attempts to remediate the effects of any CNS deficit: by improving balance and antigravity strength of the head, shoulders, and trunk. An upright program can begin with a Toronto standing frame and progress to a parapodium and then to the RGO for gait training as feasible. These upright devices can offer a psychological and motivational boost for the family and the child who has been slow to acquire gross motor skills. If gait training is performed patiently and thoughtfully, some measure of success can be realized. In error, a child with poor trunk stability but a low lumbar paralysis might be fitted for bracing that is too low, based solely on the lower extremity muscle testing. The inappropriate orthotics and the resulting tedious and ineffective attempts at gait training can cause great frustration for everyone involved. To avoid these situations, use of the RGO seems to provide significant benefits for this group of children who can then be progressed to a lower brace level at some point in the future, as their strengths and coordination skills improve. This author was recently involved with exactly that scenario, and after many weeks of unsuccessful and frustrating failure to have the child standing and walking, in bilateral AFOs, a higher brace was obtained, and the 2-year-old walked out of the session pushing her walker.[103-105]

Children who have a lesion level at L-4 to L-5 and without any apparent CNS deficit can be provided with bracing according to their need (Table 10.4). Many children at this level are attempting to stand or can already pull to stand by 10 to 12 months of age and will not require a standing frame. If the child can control his or her knees while upright, they can go directly into an AFO (Fig. 10.29). Although some children at this motor level may be able to stand and begin to cruise along furniture and even walk short distances without foot support, the AFO will provide ankle stability for stance and gait, assist in normalizing gait parameters, increase ambulation speed, increase stride length, decrease double support time, and decrease oxygen consumption. The orthosis will also help to control the subtalar joint, preventing heel valgus, and control forefoot adduction/abduction. Care should always be taken that the AFO is set at 90 degrees to give the child a solid foundation for standing and does not permit flexion at the ankle that would translate into compensatory flexion at the knees and hips.[25,65,118] Some clinicians believe that setting an AFO into some dorsiflexion will improve the gait for children with cerebral palsy. This practice does not apply to the child with spina bifida who has paralysis of the plantarflexion musculature that would maintain the ankle at 90 degrees for erect standing. "Twister cables" may be added if tibial or femoral rotation is seen when the child is upright. This is a simple mechanism of a waist band and either plastic or wire cables running laterally down each side, attaching to the proximal lateral aspect of each AFO. They are adjusted to provide the correct amount of rotatory force to better align the foot progression angles of each leg. Internal rotation, emanating from unequal forces at the hip or behind the knee, is very common at this lesion

TABLE 10.4.	Orthotic Management for L-4 to L-5 and Sacral Motor Lesions	
	L-4 to L-5	**Sacral**
Muscles present	Hip flexors and adductors	All, with possible exception of gluteus maximus, gastrocnemius/soleus group, and foot intrinsics
	Quadriceps	
	Medial hamstrings	
	Anterior tibialis	
	Some gluteus medius	
	Some foot intrinsics	
Preambulation orthotics	Toronto standing frame (some children may pull to stand, bypassing the frame, and begin with bracing*)	Usually none needed*
Ambulation bracing	RGO if CNS deficits present	AFO with weak gastrocnemius/soleus or crouched gait. Some need no bracing, but shoe insert may help maintain proper foot alignment
	KAFO with weak quadriceps	
	AFO with good truncal balance, with or without "twisters" if torsion is present*	
Assistive devices	Start with rollator walker and progress to crutches. An independent gait is possible for some, usually with a gluteus medius lurch and lumbar lordosis	Possibly a walker early on; most progress to an independent gait*
Expected functional level	Ambulatory in life unless increased body weight; flexion contractures; poor CNS status; further complications may reduce ambulatory status	Independent gait with moderate to minimal deviations based on patterns of weakness

*Control of upper body and CNS status may modify these levels.
AFO, ankle–foot orthosis; CNS, central nervous system; KAFO, knee–ankle–foot orthosis; RGO, reciprocating gait orthosis.

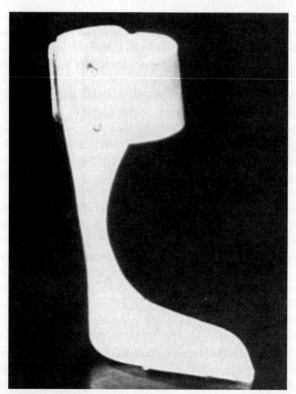

FIGURE 10.29. A plastic ankle–foot orthosis is aligned at 90 degrees or at a neutral position.

level (Fig. 10.30). However, external rotation of both legs or a combination of internal rotation of one leg and external rotation of the other leg have also been seen. Twister cables can be adjusted to control any of these combinations and are valuable in aligning the lower leg for a safer and more cosmetic gait. Twister cables should always be attached to both AFOs. They cannot be used unilaterally. If one leg does not require correction, then the cable on that side can be set at neutral. Twisters can also reduce some of the stance-phase varus or valgus deviations at the knee that are seen during gait, in a limb with excessive torsion. Twisters may also prevent overstretching of the loose ligamentous structures at the knee if the child were to continue walking with the legs malaligned. Over time, with the help of the twister cables, the child may learn to control minimal rotational deviations independently and avoid surgical correction, but, ultimately, surgery to properly align the legs will be indicated for most children. Surgery is usually recommended at around 6 years of age. The procedure should correct the bony rotation at its source, either the femur or the tibia. If the rotation is in the lower leg, tendon transfer of the active and unopposed medial hamstrings to a more midline orientation behind the knee has been performed so that recurrence of the deformity of the tibia is minimized.[65]

A KAFO may be used for the child with weak quadriceps who has difficulty maintaining either unilateral or bilateral

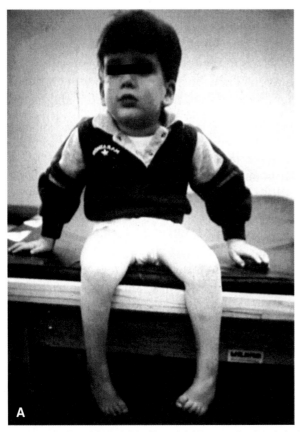 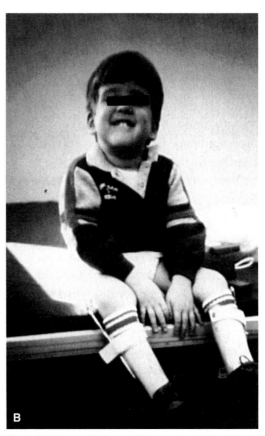

FIGURE 10.30. A and **B:** A child with an L4-L5 motor level and significant in-toeing is seen. Twister cables are attached to his ankle–foot orthosis and set at neutral to control tibial torsion until surgery is indicated.

knee extension when upright. Many braces that cross the knee joint are fabricated with straps across the thigh and lower leg. This author has found that adding a true knee/patellar pad will help maintain better knee extension while reducing the pressure exerted into the other straps. This reduction in pressure decreases the probability of skin breakdown at those sites. Although a pad at the knee adds briefly to the time spent donning and doffing the brace, it is a valuable component that ensures true knee extension that the more proximal and distal straps alone do not offer. Some children who have been ambulatory in bracing with only the thigh and tibial straps have developed a posterior displacement of the tibia relative to the femur from excessive force exerted into the tibial strap during standing and gait. The patellar pad prevents this from occurring. Note, however, that if knee flexion is seen on one side when the child stands and walks, prior to considering the KAFO, a possible leg-length discrepancy should first be ruled out, which would cause the longer leg to flex in compensation.[25,65]

Some clinics have tried a "floor-reaction" or "anticrouch" orthosis for children who have difficulty attaining knee extension. This orthosis is a standard AFO with an anterior shell that should facilitate knee extension at heel strike. The orthosis is theoretically sound and has been used with other motor disabilities. But problems with excessive pressure across

the bony anterior tibia and subsequent skin breakdown have caused some centers to avoid using this brace with the spina bifida population.

A study presented by Hunt et al. explored the use of a hinged AFO that limited mobility at the ankle from 5 degrees of dorsiflexion to 10 degrees of plantarflexion rather than the typical solid ankle. It demonstrated a positive influence on walking velocity; therefore, this brace may warrant further investigation.[119] Allowing dorsiflexion at the ankle that produces consistent knee flexion may have to be monitored by the family and reevaluated at more frequent intervals by the clinician to avoid developing knee or hip flexion contractures that will limit a child's ambulation skills.

Regardless of the orthosis chosen, a careful assessment of the resulting gait pattern should determine the success or failure of a particular device and the need for revision or replacement.

The child with an L-4 or L-5 motor level is often able to begin ambulation with a rollator walker after only a brief demonstration in the clinic. Crutch training for the young child, before the age of 6 years, is often more involved and lengthy, and many clinicians believe that crutches are ill-advised until the child has reached a reasonable level of skill and self-confidence with a walker. The child must have a sufficient attention span to benefit from short training sessions with crutches without excessive frustration. The only experience this author has had with crutch training earlier than 5 years of age was with a young boy whose mother was a PT. She was committed and diligent to have her son enter kindergarten fully ambulatory, safe and independent, using forearm crutches. She was successful in having her son achieve this goal.

Some children with L-4 to L-5 paralysis will attempt independent, unassisted ambulation. Their gait pattern usually includes a hyperlordotic lumbar spine and a side-to-side gluteus medius lurch that can be minimal at first but quite severe as the child grows. The degree of these deviations depends on the strength of the hip extensors and abductors relative to the hip flexors and adductors as well as the stability and control of the trunk and height of the child. Gait will improve when good back and abdominal strength can assist with holding better alignment of the lumbar spine and pelvis, but some degree of deviation will always be seen when there is weakness and/or muscle imbalance around the hip joints. Secondary external rotation and valgus deformities at the knees and ankles can also occur with unsupported gait in children with this level of lesion. For this reason, therapists should vigorously support the continued use of an assistive device through childhood and adolescence, especially for gait outside the home, to prevent overstretching of soft tissue structures and arthritic changes to the joints with accompanying pain. Prevention or minimization of these problems is imperative because they can lead to decreased or total loss of gait skills later in the child's life.

Moderate to severe hip flexion contractures are the single most influential factor leading to the deterioration of ambulation skills. Hip flexion contractures of 20 degrees or more for the child using AFOs and crutches can diminish gait velocity by as much as 65%. For this reason, despite the high degree of activity demonstrated by many children with a low lumbar lesion, ROM exercises remain important. A prone positioning program is helpful to counteract the hyperlordotic posture of the spine and flexion at the hips that is seen during gait. Prone positioning for prescribed periods during the day, as well as through the night, can minimize the development of hip flexion contractures. Activities to maintain spinal mobility and to prevent a fixed lordotic spine should be included. Prone, supine, and sitting activities to address abdominal and back muscle strengths, which will influence balance and spinal alignment, are also recommended for a comprehensive long-term program at school and in the home.[65,76,99,111,114]

Children with Sacral-level Paralysis

The child with a sacral-level lesion will have a higher degree of muscle function throughout the lower extremities than one with any other motor level. But, as with other levels, there remains a great deal of variation among the children in this group as well. Muscle forces around the hips and knees are in better balance, with full or partial innervation of the major muscle groups. At the S-1 and S-2 motor levels, strong knee flexors and gluteus medius are expected, while gluteus maximus and gastrocnemius/soleus are present, but may be weak. Children with S-2 to S-3 motor levels have innervation of all musculature of the hips, knees, and ankles, and "fair" to "good" strengths can be expected. The incidence of hip subluxation and dislocation is lower in this population than at the higher motor levels. If dislocation does occur, surgical intervention is usually recommended primarily to avoid later joint pain, reduce lateral trunk flexing, and improve the biomechanics of the child's gait.[103] Significant hip flexion contractures should not develop, and abnormal torsions of the femur and tibia are not as prevalent as with higher level lesions. Because of the additional musculature available at the proximal joints, through the trunk, hips, and knees, the gait pattern of the child with sacral innervation will more closely resemble a typical gait, although mild to moderate deviations will still be seen.

Manual muscle testing demonstrates that variations in this population are greatest at the foot and ankle with weakness seen in the gastrocnemius/soleus muscle group. Toe flexors may be present and may provide some secondary ankle plantarflexion, but they are usually not strong enough to compensate for a weak gastrocnemius/soleus and stabilize the ankle during stance and through the entire gait cycle. As a result, AFOs would be indicated for these children. If strong plantarflexors are present, external support may not be necessary while the child is young, but close monitoring is necessary, especially during periods of rapid growth and weight gain. The gastrocnemius/soleus may be strong enough to adequately stabilize the tibia of a small child for standing and walking short distances but may not be strong enough for the active older, taller, and heavier child. Gait deviations may begin to emerge as the child grows. As the lever arm of the muscle lengthens, a decrease in muscle efficiency may result. The loss of mechanical advantage at the ankle means that additional strength is needed for stabilization, not available from a partially innervated muscle. The gastrocnemius/soleus helps control the forward movement of the tibia over the foot through the components of the stance phase. When strength is inadequate, a crouched gait may develop, because the tibia is permitted to roll too far forward and too rapidly, forcing the foot into dorsiflexion with compensatory hip and knee flexion. Therefore, the child should always be observed both in static standing and in dynamic gait during each physical therapy or clinic appointment. Flexion contractures, though not expected in children with sacral-level lesions, can develop if this flexed posture is not remediated. The added energy expense of walking with a flexion deformity will also reduce ambulation capacity. Surgical lengthening of tight hamstrings is unusual but might be necessary as a result of these changes in gait, and a previously independent ambulator may need an assistive device for support. The crouched gait and its associated problems can be prevented simply by using a fixed ankle AFO as soon as the child demonstrates a need. The child whose posture is maintained by an orthosis can then go for short periods without bracing, to attend a party or special event, without compromising future potential.[65] The child with a sacral motor level is not intact, as was once thought before more precise testing and close monitoring by physical therapy was feasible. Although the issues that can develop are not as severe as in the children with higher level paralysis, even these problems are not benign.

As PTs becomes more experienced in addressing foot and ankle problems, the child with a sacral-level lesion may benefit from having molded shoe orthotics placed within the shell of their AFO. This may more precisely address any of the hindfoot and midfoot malalignments that can arise as the child grows and imbalances of the intrinsic muscles of the foot become more pronounced. AFOs with articulating ankle joints or an AFO fabricated from a more flexible material that permits limited and controlled dorsiflexion with assisted plantarflexion may be indicated for a specific child who will benefit from the opportunity to have a more dynamic gait, thus allowing them to better utilize the active musculature that is present at their ankle and foot.[119,120]

Compared with the child with a higher motor paralysis, the child with a sacral lesion may not appear to need therapeutic intervention. But they may still exhibit some mild to moderate gait deviations that can be minimized as they mature and are able to participate in their therapy program. Benefits can be gained from therapy to "fine-tune" the child's gait. This program can be delivered during occasional sessions over a long period, with shorter periods of more intense intervention, if deterioration is seen, especially after a growth spurt that may negatively affect the child's alignment. Abdominal strengthening, especially the oblique abdominals as well as the rectus abdominis, and strengthening to the extensors of the trunk and legs, is recommended. The child should also practice correct alignment of the shoulders, trunk, pelvis, and limbs during standing and ambulation.

Tactile, verbal, and visual reinforcement can all be used to help the child learn and maintain proper posture for progressively longer periods. Children involved in a program like this may still exhibit their abnormal gait pattern most of the time, when they are not thinking about how they look. But as the child becomes more skilled, he or she may desire to walk with a corrected pattern, if even for a short period. The child will then have the knowledge and muscle strength to do so. One child, with whom this author worked, ran around the playground at school with moderate lateral trunk flexion to each side, severe lumbar lordosis, and bilateral internal rotation of his legs at every step. When entering the clinic area, however, he was able to align his trunk and maintain an erect, symmetric posture with both feet pointing forward, to walk past the team and show off. His mother always commented that she hoped he could walk down the aisle at his wedding looking like that.

It is a pleasure to work with a child who can reach a high level of motor function. The process of working with a child like this is also an educational opportunity for the clinician. The therapist can learn to more closely observe the child, analyze subtle gait deviations, and determine the source. If trunk and limb weakness contributes to the deviations, an appropriate intervention plan can be developed. Is the deviation from muscle paralysis, low tone or habitual poor posture? Will addition or modification to bracing or an assistive device solve the problem, and what role will exercise play? The development of careful and critical observational skills ultimately benefits all clients, not only those with spina bifida (Fig. 10.31).

Many of the CNS, biomechanical, and neuromuscular factors that negatively influence the acquisition of mobility skills are not as prevalent in children with sacral-level paralysis compared with children with higher levels of paralysis. Fewer children with sacral lesions have hydrocephalus and require a shunt, and fewer exhibit significant hypotonicity

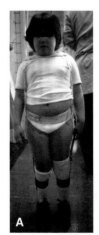 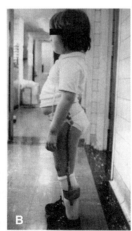 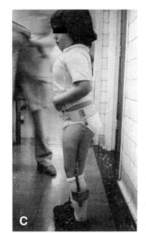 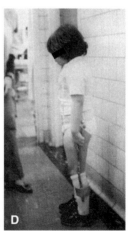

FIGURE 10.31. A: Nine-year-old girl with an S-1 motor level. **B:** An independent gait has been achieved with ankle–foot orthoses and twisters. Note the poor alignment and low tone of the trunk, as well as the anterior pelvic tilt with hip flexion. **C:** Following a long-term program of active exercises for problem areas, she works hard to align the thorax and lumbar spine cortically and improve pelvic alignment. **D:** Increasing success with correct posture, holding during gait, is next.

that is pathologic and affects their gross motor development and function. As a result, children with sacral paralysis who present with hip instability or other joint deviations are usually treated aggressively to preserve their potential for life-long community ambulation.[25,65]

The use of a preambulation or standing device may not be necessary for the child at the sacral level if he or she is developing strong balance responses in the trunk and exhibits a good quality of movement. The child may already be pulling up to stand by 10 to 12 months of age, as expected of a typical child. A foot splint, commonly fabricated to be worn at night to maintain alignment, may also be used during the day to stabilize a weak ankle, enabling the child to stand while awaiting definitive bracing if the need is seen. With the higher level of functional activity of this group of children, care must still be exercised to monitor the fit of all braces and shoes because sensory deficits, especially in the foot, remain a concern.

For the child who does experience CNS difficulties, one can follow the same course of intervention that would be prescribed for a child with a higher level lesion. The program should include activities that address flexion and extension strength against gravity through the head and trunk, as well as balance and equilibrium reactions in all positions. The program should also include passive and active exercises for the lower extremities to prevent joint contractures, and a standing and orthotics program based on the muscle strengths of the legs and the skill level of the child.[65,86-90]

Three-dimensional Gait Analysis

The development of increasingly more sophisticated and more readily available gait analysis technology is providing objective information that enables therapists, orthotists, and orthopedic surgeons to visualize and more accurately understand the gait parameters and deviations of the child with spina bifida. Widely held beliefs and treatment protocols that were developed solely on the basis of observation and anecdotal evidence may now be validated, modified, or discarded by utilizing the three-dimensional information provided by gait analysis. Orthotic prescriptions can be better tailored to the specific needs of the child when the effects of the orthosis can be understood, especially in the sagittal plane kinematics, walking speed, and progression of ground-reaction forces across the foot, and on the three planes of motion of the pelvis, hips, and knees. Vankoski et al. from the gait lab at Lurie Children's Hospital in Chicago found that comparing the gait studies of children with spina bifida with the gait parameters of typical individuals did not provide the most meaningful information to guide and evaluate treatment plans.[121,122] Rather, it was found that children with spina bifida at a given lesion level demonstrate characteristic gait patterns that are reasonably homogeneous. These identifiable patterns have become the baseline from which comparisons can be drawn, enabling the clinician to focus on realistic goals on the basis of motor level and to evaluate more fairly the

result of interventions, either conservative or surgical. Ounpuu et al. found that in the absence of the gluteus medius, gluteus maximus, and ankle plantarflexors, certain compensatory movements at the pelvis and hip were consistently noted to enable children to maintain ambulation without an assistive device. This gait pattern of the child with a lumbosacral-level lesion is characterized by exaggerated movement at the pelvis and pelvic obliquity, increased stance-phase hip abduction, increased stance-phase knee flexion, knee valgus, and increased ankle dorsiflexion.[123,124] In another study, Williams et al. reported a 24% incidence of late knee pain in ambulatory subjects with a lumbosacral-level lesion. Knee valgus, causing the discomfort, was found to result from a combination of internal pelvic and hip rotation and stance-phase knee flexion.[125] The use of gait analysis for early detection of these abnormal knee movements can direct the clinician toward the most appropriate treatment—either surgical intervention such as a tibial derotation osteotomy or the use of KAFOs, to support the knee in extension and avoid pain and joint deterioration. The continued use of crutches was also found to be an important deterrent to arthritic joint changes and pain in this population. Even though the children were able to walk unaided at an early age, continued use of crutches reduced the exaggerated range of movements and joint stress through the lumbar spine, pelvis, hips, and knees, helping to reduce gait deviations and decrease pain in those areas.[120-122] Analysis of the effects of an AFO on gait found that in many of the children examined, less stress was placed on the knee without the brace than was noted with it. This was especially true for children with L-4 to sacral-level lesions.[126] This study is certainly not an indication to stop using a brace for a child with a lumbar or sacral-level paralysis, because the gait deviations that would arise unbraced could be far more disastrous. Rather, this type of analysis may hopefully lead to the development of new orthotics that will provide the needed control at the ankle while avoiding negative influences on the more proximal joints. Three-dimensional gait analysis is also moving the focus away from static X-ray findings toward the child's functional abilities as a parameter to measure the success of conservative and surgical interventions.[100]

Finally, it is interesting to note that even with the high technology of the gait labs in many institutions, the manual muscle test and gross motor assessment provided by the PT remain important components of the child's evaluation for successful development of an orthopedic treatment plan.

» Casting/immobilization following orthopedic surgery

Earlier in this chapter, various deformities commonly associated with different motor levels were mentioned, as were some of the surgical procedures to correct them. After most of these procedures, the child must be immobilized in a cast for a certain period to allow the surgical site to heal undisturbed. The period can vary from 2 to 3 weeks following soft tissue surgery, 6 to 8 weeks for a bony procedure such as a pelvic osteotomy, or sometimes even longer. Casts and their associated immobilization should never be considered a benign treatment modality for the child with spina bifida. Pressure and irritation to insensitive skin are always a risk. Fractures, loss of joint flexibility, and loss of gross motor skills are also complications. Even children with minimal or no CNS deficits can exhibit a loss of postural security and antigravity muscle strength following a period of immobilization. Children with significant CNS problems may regress even further. It is troublesome to see children lose skills that they have acquired after a long struggle.

Most surgeons agree that children with spina bifida should be casted for the shortest possible time needed for adequate healing.[127] Because of problems related to immobility and in order to minimize the number of hospitalizations and anesthesia, some surgeons will try to perform several procedures at the same time so the child is casted only once. The therapist can assist the child and family to make this period less problematic while supporting that surgery and the subsequent casting period are important parts of the child's program to reduce deformity and ultimately maintain or gain function.[65] Returning the child as quickly and as safely as possible to his or her preoperative status, or to an improved status, should be the objective. Recommendations to manage the child in a cast can be discussed with the family prior to surgery whenever possible so the child's needs are understood and adequate preparation can be made at home for the postoperative period. A child undergoing surgery introduces additional stress into the normal routine of family life. Important questions are often forgotten when a family learns that their child will be facing surgery. So the therapist may have to anticipate many issues that families will have to address while their child remains immobile.

A child might be in a hip spica cast following pelvic or hip surgery. If unilateral surgery is performed, the full hip spica may still be used to stabilize the pelvis and opposite limb, thereby ensuring that no movement will occur at the surgical site. With the surgeon's approval, prone positioning will help prevent skin breakdown at bony sites such as the calcaneus and sacrum, and prone positioning will challenge the child to lift and extend his or her head to watch television, read, or play. Prone positioning in a reclining wheelchair or on a scooter board can provide some mobility if the child can manage self-propulsion. This mobility will also reduce the amount of carrying by family members. Similarly, prone positioning on a padded wagon for trips outdoors may help the family survive this period with less anxiety and frustration because the child is occupied and happy. After several days, the physician may permit the child to stand in the cast, a position that can be easily maintained during mealtime and play. To ensure the child's safety, it will be necessary to lean the child forward onto a heavy chair, table, or sofa that will not move. Depending on the child's age and reliability, it may be necessary for a family member to always remain with the child to prevent falling and not merely supervise from a distance. One clever family adapted a hand truck to safely stand and move their taller, heavier preadolescent while she was in a hip spica cast (Fig. 10.32). If the cast is asymmetric, towels can be propped under one foot to level the child, and cast boots will help provide a nonskid surface. Families living in multilevel homes may have to prepare a temporary bedroom on the first floor for an older, heavier child. An old crib mattress or a few thick blankets on the floor can be a comfortable short-term bed. Care should be taken to avoid abrasion to the toes when the child is prone by allowing the feet to hang over the end of the mattress or by placing some small towel rolls under the ankles to lift the toes away from the surface. A foot plate on the cast that extends past the toes is helpful to prevent increasing toe out while wearing the cast. There should always be a sock or other covering to protect toes that are exposed. Instruction should be given to family members for safe lifting and turning the child, using good body mechanics, while also considering the alignment of the child. Getting the child home from the hospital and through the front door of the house may be a challenge and could be addressed.

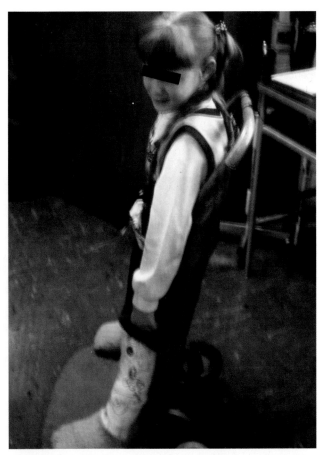

FIGURE 10.32. A parent devises an imaginative and safe way to stand and move their older and heavier child while in a hip spica cast by adapting a commercially available hand truck.

Regardless of the age of the child, daily exercise periods are important to prevent loss of neck and trunk strength and to maintain the automatic balance responses that will be important when the cast is removed and the child resumes his or her daily activities. Several times each day and depending on the age and abilities of the child, he or she should perform a routine of exercises with a family member for 10 to 15 minutes that includes prone lifts for neck and back extensors, shoulders, and arms. Supine head lifting and partial sit-ups for neck and trunk flexors and standing with tilting in all directions completes the home program. As the child attempts these activities, muscles are contracting within the cast as well as those muscles that are visible. The muscle activity places stress on the bones of the lower extremities, thereby reducing bone demineralization and the risk of a fracture when the cast is removed. Postural insecurity is diminished as vestibular and proprioceptive stimulation are provided by these challenging antigravity exercises (Fig. 10.33). Families should be warned to avoid propping their child in a half-sitting position for long periods that will cause pressure at bony prominences, as mentioned earlier, and can contribute to a rounded upper back. Long periods of time in supine should also be avoided.

The child may be readmitted for a brief course of intensive therapy once the cast is removed. Whether therapy is provided to the child as an inpatient or outpatient, the goal should be to ensure his or her rapid and safe return to function following cast removal. Lower extremity ROM and strength, especially at the surgical site, are the immediate concerns, along with improvement in balance and equilibrium responses of the neck and upper body. A return to former function can be achieved soon if the therapist targets all of the child's needs and not the lower extremity ROM alone.

For the child with a high-level lesion, surgery might have been performed to gain passive flexibility for better limb alignment and brace fit. For this child, a review of ROM exercises with parents, an orthotic evaluation, and a review of activities to further improve upper body control may be all that is needed after cast removal. The child may then be monitored, until adequate function is achieved, through an outpatient clinic, community facility, or school-based physical therapy program.

The child with a thoracic or high lumbar-level lesion who demonstrates a significant loss of motion at the hip or knee is at risk for fracture. A brief hospitalization may be indicated to regain lost mobility. The child may also be sent home in a bivalved cast or splint to be worn most of the time and removed only for frequent ROM exercises and sedentary activities until range is regained, if the family is able to comply. Some children are immobilized in their HKAFOs instead of a cast following soft tissue lengthening or tendon excision to allow parents to gently perform ROM exercises and stand their child during the healing process.

Procedures to relocate or stabilize the hip joint(s) in children with L-4, L-5, or sacral lesions can be simple tendon lengthening or more complex femoral or pelvic osteotomy. Admission to the hospital after cast removal following these procedures may be necessary to ensure that joint mobility and balance skills are again safe and acceptable and that the child can resume ambulation.

Reduced mobility in the lumbar spine and the lower extremities is common after a long casting period. After cast removal, it is often difficult for the child to achieve 90 degrees of hip flexion for good sitting alignment because of adapted shortening of the hamstrings and hip extensors. Hamstring, hip and low back tightness cause the pelvis to

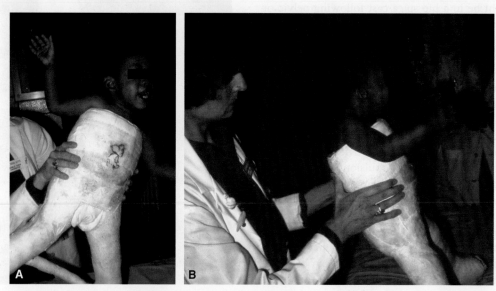

FIGURE 10.33. A and **B:** Child in a hip spica cast following surgery. Standing, when the surgeon approves, approximately 10 days after surgery, is an important aspect of the home program. A short but valuable exercise regime of standing and tilting in all directions for the weeks of immobilization can be shown to the parents.

rock posteriorly, with a secondary thoracic rounding. This posture requires attention. Gentle activities are indicated to increase pelvic and hip mobility and strength. Working with the child to gradually sit up and maintain active thoracic extension along with active hip flexion will help the child return to and hold a 90-degree alignment. It is safer to help the child work on actively holding a more erect sitting position to gain flexibility than to only move the limbs passively and possibly push too hard on a fragile bone. Care should also be taken to avoid allowing the child to sit with a rounded back for extended periods so this poor alignment does not become habitual and compensate for limited range.

Parents should be warned not to initially allow their child to crawl after a spica cast is removed. Crawling requires hip and knee flexion exceeding 90 degrees. Hip rotation is also required as the child moves into and out of sitting and the four-point position. If the necessary flexibility is not present for all of these motions when the cast is removed, fractures can occur.[100,101]

Following surgery at the knee or ankle, children may have either one or two long or short leg casts. The family will require instruction to help their child avoid excessive time in supine or sitting. Besides contributing to skin breakdown, development of flexion contractures is always a major concern. Excessive sitting, crawling, and knee walking with short leg casts will increase tightness of the hip and knee flexors. Information regarding alternative positions should be offered to avoid positions that encourage flexion. Prone-lying is the preferred position, with standing and ambulation the preferred activities, when feasible. When ambulation in the cast(s) is permitted, it is achieved quickly when a walker rather than crutches is used as an assistive device for this temporary period. Crutch training is difficult for an inexperienced child because of the additional weight of the cast, potential lack of adequate balance, poor proprioception, and a possibly malaligned cast. By comparison, instruction with a walker is usually a faster and safer choice. Brief strengthening exercises can be taught for back, hip, and knee extensors, along with exercises for the trunk to help keep the child mobile during the cast period. With such a multifaceted program, the child will be more likely to rapidly return to his or her previous or improved level of function once the cast is removed.[25,33,127-131]

» CNS deterioration

Throughout life, individuals with spina bifida, their family members, and the professionals involved in their care should be vigilant for any deterioration in function that could indicate hydromyelia or a tethered spinal cord. These neurologic conditions can affect the child's mobility, gross motor function, urologic function, fine motor skills, and activities of daily living (ADLs). If diagnosed and treated in time, the effects can be temporary. If left untreated, the symptoms can worsen, and their effects will be permanent. Therapists must be knowledgeable about these problems because they are often discovered by the PT during routine appointments, examinations, manual muscle testing, or in conversation with parents.[25,33,65]

Hydromyelia

Hall et al.[132] conducted a study of children with spina bifida who exhibited rapidly progressive scoliosis and found that CSF had migrated into the spinal cord. Excess CSF was seen collecting in pockets along the spinal cord, creating areas of pressure and, ultimately, necrosis of the surrounding peripheral nerves, causing the scoliosis. Other symptoms found to be associated with hydromyelia include progressive upper extremity weakness and hypertonus. It may be noted that initial examination of the lateral ventricles showed no enlargement and did not indicate that the shunt was malfunctioning. However, revision of the VP shunt produced symptomatic improvement for those children whose diagnosis was made early. Some children required an additional shunt placed at the level of the fluid pockets in the spine to ensure that the excess CSF and its accompanying pressure would be eliminated. Although Lindseth was an orthopedic surgeon, he was a strong advocate of closer investigation in all cases of rapidly progressive scoliosis, regardless of one's clinical specialty. He stated that it is important to always consider the possibility of CNS complications and not treat scoliosis as an isolated musculoskeletal phenomenon. Left untreated, the fluid continues to collect along the spinal cord, causing continued deterioration in both upper and lower extremity function.[25,33,65,132,133]

Tethered Spinal Cord

At approximately 10 weeks of gestation, the vertebral column and spinal cord of the fetus are the same length, and the spinal nerves exit horizontally at their corresponding vertebrae. By 5 months of gestation, the vertebral column has grown more rapidly than the spinal cord, which now ends at S-1. At birth, the cord is at L-3, and by adulthood, the cord is at the L-1 to L-2 vertebral level.

A tethered spinal cord occurs when adhesions anchor the spinal cord at the site of the original back lesion. The child is growing rapidly, but the cord is not free to slide upward and reposition as it should. Instead, it remains bound at the level of the defect. Excessive stretch to the spinal cord causes metabolic changes and ischemia of the neural tissue, with associated degeneration in muscle function. Rapidly progressive scoliosis, hypertonus at one or several sites in the lower extremities, changes in gait pattern, and changes in urologic function may be attributed to this tethering of the spinal cord. Occurrences of increased tone on passive ROM, asymmetric changes in manual muscle testing results, areas of decreasing strength, or complaints of discomfort in the back or buttocks should alert the examiner to consider the presence of a tethered cord.[134,135] Periodic examination by professionals and an alert parent can identify early functional changes associated with this complication so appropriate medical management can be considered (Display 10.9). Petersen suggests, on the basis of his study population, that those children with repaired lesions at levels above L-3 will begin to exhibit symptoms of a tethered cord before age 6 and that those with lesion levels below L-4 tend to become symptomatic after age 6. He also found that children with an unrepaired back defect exhibit symptoms much earlier, regardless of the location of their lesion.[136] When tethering is suspected, imaging may be utilized to confirm the diagnosis, and subsequent neurosurgical release can free the cord. After release, the cord may not migrate to its appropriate position, but further growth of the child may proceed without recurrence of the symptoms, and further degeneration in function may be avoided. If the release is performed in a timely manner, permanent neurologic damage can usually be prevented. However, it is becoming clear that total correction of all the symptoms following surgery cannot be assumed.[65] McLone et al. conducted a study of 30 children who exhibited scoliosis as a symptom of cord tethering and who received surgical intervention to release the spinal cord. The children whose scoliosis showed the greatest improvement were those who had spinal curves of less than 50 degrees. During a 2- to 7-year follow-up, 38% of the children's curves showed progression owing to retethering of the spine, but the remaining children showed a stabilized or improved spinal alignment.[137]

The child who has a thoracic-level paralysis does not have the full complement of active trunk musculature to provide adequate antigravity strength to maintain an erect posture and is always at risk for scoliosis. However, a child with a lumbar or sacral lesion with full innervation of trunk musculature should be evaluated when any curvature develops, especially when it develops over a short time. It is recommended that hydromyelia and tethered cord should always be suspected if scoliosis occurs in a child with a motor level below T-12. Clinics that aggressively treat hydromyelia and tethered cord by surgical correction report a reduction in the overall occurrence of scoliosis that will require spinal fusion in their spina bifida population, compared with data from other sites.[133,138-141]

Scoliosis

The development of a spinal deformity is serious for the child with spina bifida. When scoliosis occurs and trunk alignment is compromised, the child will require additional support to remain erect. If the child must lean on his or her upper extremities to stay up, this compensation directly impacts the child's freedom of movement and increases the energy expenditure for all activities. Propelling a wheelchair becomes more strenuous, because the child must work both to maintain the upright sitting position and to move the chair. In sitting, a moderate to severe scoliosis creates pelvic obliquity that changes the surface area for weight bearing, causing areas of increased pressure that can quickly lead to skin breakdown. The posterior aspects of the thighs and bony prominences of the ischial tuberosity, greater trochanter, sacrum, and coccyx are especially vulnerable. Gait can become more unstable as truncal alignment and balance are affected. Pelvic and trunk asymmetry will affect the fit of the HKAFO and RGO bracing. When braces do not fit and gait is less efficient, the orthotics may not be worn as frequently as they should. This can lead to further deterioration of the child's mobility skills.

The use of a spinal brace or body jacket can be useful for the child without trunk stability or to assist in slowing the progression of the curve, but surgical fusion is inevitable for many children. There are numerous methods for and preferred approaches to spinal fusion, and the periods of immobilization and restrictions on daily activity vary with each. The type of instrumentation employed and the area and extent of the fusion will also influence the child's functional parameters. If the fusion extends to the sacrum, pelvic mobility is diminished and ambulatory ability will be affected. As previously mentioned, gait analysis has shown greater excursion of movement at the pelvis in ambulatory children with spina bifida than in the typical child. Given this information, surgeons avoid fusing down to the sacrum of an ambulatory child as much as possible. For successful and efficient wheelchair propulsion, upper extremity and trunk movement are both necessary. If flexibility of the distal spine is diminished or absent secondary to fusion, an individual can lose independent wheelchair mobility.

Maintaining flexibility and strength in all extremities and preventing skin problems during the postoperative period of immobility, following spinal fusion, should be addressed immediately after surgery, if possible. When a return to full activity is permitted, it is important to reassess the child to determine whether functional skills have been impacted. The PT should be concerned with the child's postoperative activity level and assist with resumption of mobility. Spinal fusion can influence the performance of many ADLs in which the child might have been independent, so adaptive strategies need to be developed in the functional areas that were affected. It is also feasible that once the spine is stabilized, the child may have greater freedom of arm use and might gain skills that were not possible prior to surgery. A comprehensive pre- and postoperative physical therapy assessment and intervention plan is indicated to assist this child and their family.[25,33,65]

» Latex allergy

Allergic reaction to latex by individuals with spina bifida is a serious concern. Latex is a natural rubber used in a wide variety of products that come into contact with human skin and other body surfaces. In the health field, a vast number of commonly used items contain or are made exclusively from latex, which has been depended on for its impermeable qualities and strength while still providing sensitivity to touch. This makes it an excellent material for use in sterile gloves, where it provides protection and prevents the spread of illness. It is durable as well as elastic, which accounts for its popularity and wide usage for various types of flexible tubing and in the toy industry (Display 10.10).

Although it is believed that only 1% of the general population is allergic to latex, various studies have found that 18% to 37% of those with spina bifida exhibit a significant sensitivity to latex. It has also been found that 7% to 10% of health care workers exhibit a latex sensitivity. Allergic reactions may appear as watery and itchy eyes, sneezing, coughing,

---

DISPLAY 10.10 Partial List of Commonly Used Products Containing Latex

Balloons
Pacifiers
Chewing gum
Dental dam
Rubber bands
Elastic in clothing
Beach toys
Koosh balls
Some types of disposable diapers
Glue
Paints
Erasers
Some brands of adhesive bandages
Bulb syringes
Ready-to-use enemas
Ostomy pouches
Oxygen masks
Pulse oximeters
Reflex hammers
Stethoscope tubing
Suction tubing
Vascular stockings
Crutch axillary pads, tips, and hand grips
Kitchen cleaning gloves
Swim goggles
Wheelchair tires
Some wheelchair cushions
Zippered food storage bags

---

hives, and a rash in the area of contact. More severe reactions may produce swelling of the trachea, and changes in blood pressure and circulation, resulting in anaphylactic shock. Diagnosis of latex sensitivity is based on a clinical history, observation of a reaction, and immunologic findings following a skin prick allergy test. The cause, to date, is unknown, but it is theorized that early, intense, or consistent exposure to latex products results in the development of the sensitivity in many individuals. Some of the more dramatic symptoms were believed to be a result of inhalation of the powder contained in many sterile latex gloves. The powder makes the gloves easy to don and doff, but it can become airborne when the gloves are removed. Further investigation found that this was not a consistent irritant.

The U.S. Food and Drug Administration (FDA) and the Centers for Disease Control and Prevention (CDC) continue to investigate the problem and support efforts to find the components of latex that are responsible for the allergy; develop methods of producing safe, nonallergenic rubber; and conspicuously label products containing latex. There has been evidence that the latex allergy is also related to a sensitivity to some foods such as bananas, chestnuts, avocados, and kiwi fruit in some children and adults, and this relationship is also being investigated. A blood test has been developed that is being used during pre-employment testing for health care workers and for those with spina bifida to assist them in avoiding the allergen if the test results are positive.

Some researchers theorize that children with spina bifida develop a latex allergy because of their high level of exposure to materials containing latex, right from birth. One study points out that the presence of spina bifida should be considered a risk factor for a latex allergy. One method employed to prevent latex sensitivity is to practice primary prevention from the first day of life by creating a latex-free environment for the children. In one study employing this strategy for 6 years, the percentage of children sensitive to latex dropped from 26.7% to 4.5%.[142,143]

Advocacy groups are encouraging hospitals to become latex free and have been asking the FDA to ban latex products in all hospitals. It is recommended that parents, older children, and other caregivers carry an autoinjectable type of epinephrine pen that is easy to use in case of a serious allergic reaction. All sensitive individuals should wear a Medic Alert bracelet, necklace, or dog tags. Neighborhood paramedic teams, the fire department, and local Emergency Medical Services who might respond to an emergency call should be alerted that the child has this sensitivity. Keeping a set of nonlatex gloves near the front door for emergency personnel to use, as they enter, is also recommended. Children and families are encouraged to become familiar with products that must be avoided, and a list of commonly used latex products and alternative latex-free items is available from the Spina Bifida Association of America. The Internet can provide many sources of latex information, latex-free products, and resources that can be shared with parents.[144-149]

» Perceptual motor and cognitive performance

Children with spina bifida are a diverse group traversing many domains. Their strengths and challenges are varied, and besides the motor and CNS issues that have already been discussed throughout this chapter, therapists should be aware of possible difficulties that may affect the learning styles and cognitive processing of their patients. This section provides only a brief overview of the vast amount of information that is available regarding perceptual and cognitive performance. Although intervention for these issues may typically fall to the expertise of the occupational therapist or educator, one is encouraged to explore this area because it will directly affect the selection of therapy strategies, teaching methods, and, ultimately, the level of success with the child. A PT can also be a valuable resource for both professionals and families who may be unaware of the link between spina bifida and the difficulties the child may be experiencing.

Great interest and concern has been expressed regarding the intellectual, sensory, and perceptual motor function of children with spina bifida. Studies have shown that the overall intelligence of the children in this population is unrelated to their anatomic motor level, severity of hydrocephalus prior to shunt insertion, or the number of shunt revisions performed. However, several factors that are considered as influencing cognition include delayed treatment of hydrocephalus, episodes of cerebral infection, and the presence of other CNS abnormalities.[41-63]

Intelligence testing for many children with spina bifida places them within the normal range but below the population mean. Willis and associates found that test scores of their subjects were particularly low in performance IQ, arithmetic achievement, and visual motor integration.[151] When the same children were retested at an older age, their arithmetic achievement and visual motor integration scores declined even further, but reading and spelling abilities did not decline. One conclusion of this study was that a visual–perceptual–organizational deficit was present that influenced the child's ability to solve mathematical and visual–spatial problems.[151] These deficits then become relatively more severe as the child ages, when greater accomplishment in math is expected. Standardized assessments reflect the expectation that acquisition of skills will increase with age and educational experience, and therefore the scores declined, over time, in the group that was studied. If early foundation skills are not strong, the development of more advanced, intuitive math processing will be limited.

Other research has noted a high degree of attention deficit or distractibility in some children with spina bifida. These problems were especially profound in children who showed poor language development. These same children had poor development of auditory figure-ground, which allows a child to recognize and attend to relevant features in the auditory environment. A child with difficulty in this area may not be able to identify the primary auditory input such as a teacher speaking and giving directions or dismiss the irrelevant input such as noise from a truck passing by an open window or another child seated nearby. In a rich auditory environment, extraneous sounds easily distract the child from his or her assigned task. These children may perform better in a quiet, secluded site, whereas performance in a typical, busy classroom, for similar tasks, can be poor.

Horn et al. found limited development of language comprehension in many of the children tested.[151] Individual vocabulary comprehension was normal, but comprehension of a story was poor. The children had difficulty identifying and retaining the relevant features of a story while ignoring the unimportant facts. Difficulty learning and memorizing lists of unrelated words has also been noted. However, memory for related facts was better, such as when answering questions about a short story that was read aloud.[151-153]

In all of the studies cited, little information was available regarding the early medical treatment of the subjects, methods, and timeliness of interventions or other complications that may have influenced the child. It is therefore difficult to hypothesize which factors may have been responsible for the problems. Decreased opportunity to develop and practice fine motor and manipulation skills was thought to be a factor.[152] Other negative influences might be the limitations of early mobility that affect the child's experiences: exploring the environment, moving his or her body relative to stationary objects, and manipulating and moving those objects. Theoretical rationales for cognitive dysfunction include potential cerebellar abnormalities associated with the Chiari II malformation that would influence the range, direction, force, and rate of voluntary movements of the body and the manner in which movement is interpreted. Regardless of the cause, however, the learning difficulties that result are notable because they will affect many aspects of the child's ability to function and may limit the child's ultimate successes in school and throughout life.

Finally, an interesting study that examined the deficits in conceptual reasoning abilities found many children with spina bifida to be chatty, friendly, and talkative but with repetitive and nonspecific content in their conversations. Many decades before this study was conducted, the term coined for this language style was "Cocktail Party Chatter" for its old school but obvious reasons. There is quantity but little quality to the child's verbalizations, similar to walking through a crowded party and asking how everyone is doing and other niceties but not processing the answer or going into depth to further a conversation. For the child with spina bifida, it is an organic, processing issue rather than an active behavior or choice that the child is making.[154]

Any discussion of perceptual problems in this population should also address the issue of ocular function. When compared with the typical population, strabismus occurs six to eight times more frequently in children with spina bifida. The lack of conjugate gaze influences spatial relationships

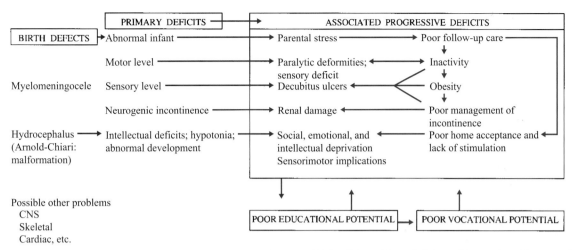

FIGURE 10.34. Primary and progressive deficits in children with spina bifida. (Adapted from Syllabus of Instructional Courses. American Academy for Cerebral Palsy; 1974.)

and constancy of size, and development of normal visual perception and visual–spatial problems during manipulation activities have been noted in some children with spina bifida. Other, more frequent ocular problems include nystagmus, poor ocular motility, and other convergence defects. These abnormalities have been attributed to brain stem dysfunction, although no correlation was made between the severity of the Chiari II malformation and these clinical observations.[155,156]

The consensus seems to be that children with spina bifida need a broad range of movement and learning experiences during their early years. Increased experiences in many sensory modalities may help to decrease the negative impact of any one specific area of limitation. Testing with age-appropriate materials and in an environment where the child can focus on the task is critical. Also, eliminating test items that include a motor component will afford a more accurate and valid result (Fig. 10.34).[150-157]

» Wheelchair mobility

This chapter has devoted much attention to bracing and preparing the child for ambulation, but seated mobility must also be considered for the children for whom it is necessary. Any decision to use one of the many devices available should include input from the child when appropriate, family members, and other professional staff involved with the child. A discussion might first determine the need for and proposed uses of seated mobility. Questions to consider might be whether the device will be primarily for recreation and peer group interaction, indoor or outdoor use, at school, long family outings, or primarily for family convenience and transport.

A first device for the young child might be a hand-propelled "Caster Cart," "Ready Racer," or "The Wheel,"

which are all available through medical supply companies or secondhand via the Internet. Commercially available electric cars and motorcycles can be modified with a hand switch rather than the usual foot pedal configuration, and imaginative parents have been able to adapt leg positioning and trunk support on these items. The devices are relatively inexpensive and low to the ground, facilitating easy transition to the floor or to a standing position. They are cosmetically appealing and are acceptable to those with physical challenges and typical children alike. They can be fast and safe when used in the proper environment, and they provide beneficial stimulation and opportunities for exercise, recreation, and socialization. The child's perceptual skills, upper extremity abilities, and presence of abnormal tone should guide the therapist in selecting whether a manual or battery-operated device is more appropriate. Excessive upper extremity exertion to propel and maneuver a device may frustrate the child and produce an unacceptable change in tone if CNS dysfunction is present. One study of interest examined young children with otherwise poor independent mobility skills who received instruction in using a motorized wheelchair. Most of the children did very well, and the benefits that were noted included increased curiosity, initiative, motivation, communication, exploration, and interaction with objects and people in the environment. There were also significant decreases in dependency behaviors. So rather than limit the child to struggling with a slow ambulation method in environments and situations that might become frustrating, this study supports the idea that, when used appropriately, a self-propelled wheeled or powered device can be an important addition to the child's mobility program and not impact adversely on motivation for ambulation training.[158]

Strollers are available in progressively larger sizes, which can accommodate bracing, and can be used in combination

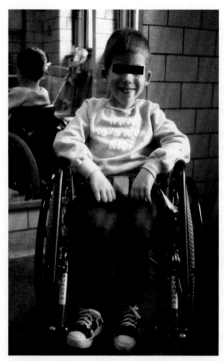

FIGURE 10.35. A lightweight wheelchair is selected for long-distance use in the school and community. This child also uses a reciprocating gait orthosis for shorter distances in the home and school.

with ambulation. To include their child in family events, a stroller can be used until the child is 5 or 6 years old. For a typical child of that age, it is not unusual to alternate walking and riding in a stroller during a long family outing. But care must be taken not to increase the child's dependence on others for mobility as he or she gets older. It is helpful to know which strollers, travel chairs, or wheelchairs can be safely secured on a school bus and what the local regulations are for acceptable school transport. Seated mobility is helpful for the child who is not ready to ambulate all day in school because of limitations in balance or endurance (Fig. 10.35). A wheelchair can be obtained before the child starts school if boarding, exiting, and safe transportation on the school bus will be an issue for the child not yet fully ambulatory. Long distances from the bus loading area into class and to other destinations within the school should be considered because they can be prohibitive for a young child. Other indications for a wheelchair might include the child's lack of efficient mobility, marginally functional or unsafe ambulation, speed of ambulation that is necessary to travel along with peers and/or family, and need for increased recreational activities that would be unavailable with ambulation alone. The child who is ambulatory can be assisted on and off the bus and secured in a car seat or a regular bus seat with a safety belt and/or harness. The child would then be required to ambulate on arrival at school and for the remainder of the day. So obtaining a wheelchair is only the first part in a series of decisions to determine

how, when, where, and in which situations the child will use the chair.

Remember the increased risks for the child in a wheelchair. Abandoning the gait program by the family, even though the child may have the potential to reach a high level of efficient ambulation, is always a risk when introducing wheelchair use. Flexion contractures of the hips and knees, skin and pressure problems, and spinal deformity are other issues affecting the seated child.[131] Therefore, the child should spend time both out of the wheelchair and out of the seated, flexed position every day. Consider a routine that allots time for prone positioning, standing erect in a standing table or in any of a variety of standers while wearing braces, and building in opportunities for ambulation to counteract the effects of sitting.

As the child matures and mobility needs change, a power wheelchair or electric scooter can provide added speed and efficiency. A motorized device, which will conserve energy, may be very important for the individual facing a long and hectic day at school or work. In the area of wheeled mobility, as in many other aspects of care, the skills, imagination, and problem-solving ability of the therapist can be extremely helpful. Developing trusting relationships with dependable vendors and equipment representatives will enable the therapist to remain current in the latest devices that are available and thereby enhance the child's life. In some instances, accessibility limitations at home may prevent a powered device from leaving school with the child each day. Therapists may find themselves in the position of advocating for this part-time device when insurance companies are also paying for bracing and ambulation equipment. They may also find themselves on opposite sides of the discussion with other professionals who want to see their children remain solely ambulatory. Developing a clear and realistic goal, in partnership with the child and family, with a reasonable expectation of the situations in which the child will use wheeled mobility, either manual or powered, will strengthen the discussions with those having opposing views.

A wheelchair cushion should always be included for the individual with spina bifida. Various types of cushions may reduce the development of pressure sores. Several materials are available, including high-density foams and inflatable types, which can be modified for more even distribution of weight when the child exhibits asymmetry. But, regardless of the cushion chosen, activities for pressure relief are still the best means of preventing skin breakdown on the posterior thighs and buttocks and should be performed diligently throughout the day. Frequent wheelchair push-ups, side-to-side weight shifting, and out-of-chair time should be incorporated into the child's daily schedule to provide for regular pressure relief. Also, many methods should be explored that will assist even the young child to become independent in performing these activities, including reminders from a wristwatch alarm, talking clock, or beeper.[65,159]

>> Recreation and leisure activities

As the child reaches elementary school age, he or she will have much less time available for play and movement on the floor. Generally speaking, a full-time school curriculum in an integrated or mainstreamed educational setting provides little chance for consistent recreation. Gym class, with an instructor who is imaginative, motivated, and willing to collaborate with a PT, is ideal. Strategies can be developed to include the student with spina bifida in the regular array of activities the rest of the class is performing. Giving the child the opportunity to participate in the regular physical education curriculum, with adaptations or accommodations, may assist the child to find activities in which he or she is able to participate and those that he or she might also enjoy after school hours. It should never be assumed that the child with spina bifida, enrolled in a regular educational program, will automatically be excused from physical education or not be expected to participate in some aspect of an activity that their peer group is performing. The PT can also collaborate with a willing physical education teacher in developing a modified grading system that will assess what the child is successfully doing in class as opposed to what he or she is unable to perform. This author has assisted all teachers to become more flexible and inclusive of their students with spina bifida.

The child enrolled in a special education curriculum may have periods of physical education as well as scheduled sessions for the development of recreation and leisure skills. Once again, having an innovative and motivated school staff will help to provide the child with experiences that he or she might otherwise have lacked and that may become a lifelong interest or hobby helping to keep them physically active.

But, as is true with the population of typical children, the child with spina bifida is most often dependent on the interest, knowledge, and resources of family and friends to provide them with experiences in new, novel, and consistent recreational pursuits. Identifying activities that can be learned and pursued throughout one's life should be considered an important part of the total care plan for the individual with spina bifida. The PT has a valuable role in assisting the child and his or her family to find appropriate programs that offer wheelchair games and sports or modified programs for the child who is ambulatory with bracing, such as adapted/accessible playgrounds, bumper bowling, or T-ball instead of traditional Little League baseball. Also, increasing numbers of teams are being formed that pair children with special needs with typical teens or young adult volunteers who can assist the child to participate. The child with spina bifida should be encouraged to participate regularly in activities that stimulate cardiovascular health, strengthen muscles, improve eye–hand coordination, maneuver their wheelchairs, and learn sportsmanship, from which all children can benefit. The therapist is commonly asked by families for an opinion or a recommendation regarding adapted bicycles and other home exercise or recreation equipment. Helping to keep the child active, by providing this professional advice to parents, can be a valuable contribution. Often, one may have to go beyond recommendation to provide specific resources, brand names, and contact numbers of reliable vendors, as well as letters to justify the need for the device to insurers. Teaming with children and families for these tasks is time consuming but ultimately invaluable and highly worthwhile for all.

The inclusion and expansion of aquatics within the physical therapy profession has significantly increased the body of research and information available for the therapist who has the opportunity to add aquatics to his or her clinical repertoire. The interest in health and fitness within the general population has resulted in the building of many more pools accessible to the handicapped and available for both recreation and therapeutic purposes. Providing opportunities to explore and enjoy the benefits of moving in water may assist the child with spina bifida to participate in a recreational activity that is also physically beneficial. Learning water safety and basic swimming skills can be taught to the young child and utilized throughout his or her lifetime. Water competency with or without the use of flotation devices can enable the person with spina bifida to experience a level of independent freedom of movement otherwise unavailable on land. More advanced aquatic skills can also be incorporated into a multifaceted therapeutic program that can be designed for an individual and taught and monitored by the PT who has access to a pool facility. Utilizing the natural properties of resistance and buoyancy of the water will strengthen the body and increase cardiovascular efficiency. And, it is fun.

This therapist has found that providing therapy sessions in a pool can be an especially useful tool in the rehabilitation program of the child following orthopedic surgery. Children who are already comfortable in the water are easily motivated to work hard on an exercise program with the excitement and novelty of this environment. Mobilizing a child who has been in a cast or in bed recovering from surgery can be achieved more rapidly in the water than on a mat. Brief, free swim periods can serve as a rest break between the therapeutic activities or as the reward, at the end of a session, for a child who did a good job. When working on a mat program, taking a rest break usually means the child is not moving, but he or she will continue to move when in the water. Lap swims, races, and in-pool team games such as underwater search and retrieve, basketball, volleyball, or tag are just a few of the many possibilities that will have the child moving significantly more than he or she would in a traditional therapy session. But, as in all merging of recreation and therapy, the therapist must not compromise the objectives that must be addressed just to have the child happy and playing. Specific exercise routines must be developed, as they would be for any program, so intervention is truly targeting the appropriate areas of need (Display 10.11).

Provides strengthening to innervated lower extremity musculature, upper extremities, and trunk:

1. Movement of legs in all directions, all planes, with combination patterns of movement not feasible on a two-dimensional gym mat. Can be passive, active, active assistive, and resistive, depending on need
2. Use of flotation device for trunk in deep water with legs in the water, kicking in place against water's resistance
3. Pushing off from side of pool or therapist's hands while prone or supine on water surface to strengthen extension musculature and enjoy the sudden propulsion through the water
4. Swimming laps with only leg motions while holding kickboard or in an inner tube if necessary
5. Lap swims using webbed gloves for added propulsion and resistance and a variety of strokes to address all muscles of shoulders (flotation cuffs can be used around ankles if necessary to prevent legs from dragging on pool floor and provide extension if active gluteal musculature is not present)
6. Resistive swimming with therapist holding legs and preventing forward movement prone or supine
7. Supine, within flotation ring, lifting legs out of water and twisting them side to side for work on all abdominals with assistance as needed to hold legs up
8. Ball toss and catch, basketball, Newcomb or standard volleyball in various water depths, depending on child's age and abilities

» The young adult with spina bifida

The interest in the population with spina bifida should not end when he or she moves on to an adolescent or adult facility for medical care. Although one may not be directly involved with young adults, knowledge about the challenges this age group faces can be helpful for the clinician. Knowing the effects of the aging process on those with spina bifida, the therapist can gain a perspective that is beneficial for those of any age. It is also helpful to have an understanding of the long-range effects of various medical, surgical, therapeutic, and intervention decisions. By knowing how they have evolved and how they have influenced the functioning of the older adult, the approach with children can be improved. One can modify the existing protocols that were not successful and even discard them while developing new and, hopefully, better strategies that will eventually enhance the lives of those of all ages.[160]

Selber and Dias looked at a population of young adults in Chicago with sacral-level spina bifida who had been followed at the same medical clinic and by the same staff who employed many of the same protocols since the subjects were young children. They were treated aggressively for any symptoms of tethered cord and lower limb deformity.

But many of these individuals still shared several complications, including episodes of osteomyelitis, scoliosis, and a decrease in ambulation function. The participants and their families had many opportunities over the years to receive education for skin care and had long-standing relationships with the clinic staff. The bouts of osteomyelitis may have resulted from many factors besides insensate skin or poorly fitting orthotics and shoes. What is most disturbing is that the problems might have been caused by procrastination in seeking treatment when early skin breakdown was noted, especially in the vulnerable foot and ankle areas. The more severe cases resulted in amputation. Another issue found in the study group was that many individuals maintained their community ambulation status but experienced significant knee pain and had to return to using orthotics, crutches, or canes that had been discontinued, to support and stabilize their gait and reduce joint stress. Recall, from earlier in this chapter, that the group of children with sacral-level lesions was thought to be the least affected. These complications should prompt practitioners, clients, and their families to remain knowledgeable about the complicating factors that can impact function at any point along the life cycle, even in the child with minimal muscle deficits.

One can never allow the intensity of therapeutic efforts and interventions to slacken over time, especially when it can potentially have such disastrous results. One may feel this is unnecessarily repetitive, as in several sections of this chapter, but, hopefully, the consistent reinforcement of important information may result in a better outcome for the PT student as well as the child.[161]

Another report that did not specify the lesion levels of the young adults in the study noted a general disinterest in personal care and poor follow-through on hobbies or areas of stated interest and commitments. There was also an inability to organize and complete long-range projects specifically related to school activities, assignments, and term papers. And many of the children appeared stubborn and argumentative. Memory problems, poor comprehension of material, deficits in conceptual reasoning, problem solving, and mental flexibility were all identified as weaknesses in the study population.

With typical adolescents and young adults, there is an evolution of maturity and greater acceptance of responsibility, with increasing ease and compliance in personal care, success at school and in their social lives. But this study demonstrates that the child with spina bifida may inherently be unable to adapt successfully to these mounting expectations unless provided with intervention and supports that focus on remediation of their specific areas of need. It concludes that they should have opportunities to participate in the planning and execution of their own intervention plan to achieve early independence. If the child is actively engaged along with the family, before they have habituated to an excessive level of need and assistance, this action plan has a higher potential for success in the areas in which they may be specifically limited.[154]

In a study conducted through Riley Children's Hospital in Indiana, the parents of adolescents with spina bifida voiced concerns that centered on lifelong issues affecting their children, such as environmental accessibility, transportation in the community, and independence. The teens, however, were more concerned with the immediate issues of finances, medical care, communication and socialization with friends, and peer acceptance. With the exception of medical care, their issues were, again, not too different from what would be expected of their typical peers. The study concluded that attention should be given to assisting this population with social integration, vocational training, and sexual counseling.[162]

The health risks of poor diet, obesity, reduced physical activity, increased TV/computer time and other sedentary activities, and substance abuse have been documented as beginning in childhood in a population of typical young adults.[163] In a study of adults with spina bifida, Dias et al. found that while 50% of the study population was over 30, 80% were living with their parents or other relatives.[164] Although 82% had achieved some level of independence, only 17 got married and were living away from family members. Interestingly, the individual's degree of independence was unrelated to their lesion level or the level of ambulation they had achieved. It may hence be inferred that motivational factors may be absent in the cognitive makeup of some individuals with spina bifida that would compel one person to seek increased autonomy versus the other who will live at home with all of the potential isolation and dependency behaviors that it entails.[164]

Dunne and Shurtleff[165] identified some common complaints from adults with spina bifida that included obesity, incontinence, recurrent urinary tract infections, chronic decubiti, joint pain, hypertension, neurologic deterioration, and depression. Urinary incontinence was also a central issue in a self-rating survey completed by a group of adolescent boys and girls with spina bifida. In general, the girls rated themselves lower in physical appearance, athleticism, and global self-worth than the boys. But both the girls and the boys who were continent rated themselves higher than the children who were incontinent. It appeared from this study that urinary continence was more important than the ability to walk for many young adults.[166]

Urinary tract infection is the most frequently reported cause of morbidity in the adult population. Adults are very concerned about urinary incontinence and its social implications, and a variety of methods are employed to enable them to remain dry and infection free. Urinary diversion is a surgical procedure that allows urine to be accessed by catheter from a stoma in the abdomen or collected in an absorbent pad. It was a preferred solution for many who did not want to depend on performing intermittent catheterization. When residual urine is permitted to remain in the bladder, it becomes a reservoir for bacteria, resulting in a high rate of infection and potential renal damage. An indwelling Foley catheter was used for some, but resulted in a high rate of infection. Other external collecting devices, Valsalva voiding, and diapers were commonly tried with varying results and rates of success. It appears that intermittent catheterization performed diligently and on the recommended daily schedule remains the most successful method for adult management of urinary incontinence and was also associated with the lowest risk of infection or renal damage. But, knowing that organization, compliance, and long-term follow-through may be limited when parents are no longer providing or supervising care, one can see how self-catheterization may be less successful than predicted for the young adult with spina bifida.[167,168]

McLone[169] cited still other problems that were identified by the adult with spina bifida that included a lack of opportunity for job training, lack of viable employment, and decreased ability to achieve psychological and physical independence from family. In two studies, when multifaceted neuropsychological testing was performed on young adults with spina bifida, with and without hydrocephalus, the subjects scored low in areas of verbal learning, verbal recall, and sequencing of complex tasks and exhibited a high rate of attention deficit. They were performing in the average range for delayed memory, spatial memory, and visual recognition memory. In one of the studies, almost 50% of the subjects with spina bifida and hydrocephalus exhibited some type of cognitive impairment even though their full IQ fell within the normal range.[170,171] Thus, one can see how weak verbal recall and sequencing, as well as other areas of challenge mentioned earlier, would significantly impact a person's ability to experience success in school and learn to take control of and manage the complex responsibilities of their day-to-day lives. Working with a variety of people who have different learning styles, one can, hopefully, maximize an individual's learning strengths to help compensate for his or her areas of challenge. There is also improvement in incorporating both high- and low-tech adaptations to assist. So the use of an activity sequencing chart to learn self-catheterization or any multistep procedure seems reasonable. Using photos or pictures for a home exercise program is another adaptation that will avoid having one recall lengthy verbal instructions or read and process descriptions on a handout sheet. Making a video of the client performing their exercise program that can be watched and followed has also been used. Calendars, checklists, or day planners and certainly the use of tablets, iPads, and other electronic devices may help motivate the patient and keep them on track. Although many of these strategies are used with younger children, the need to continue them with older individuals may mean the difference between success and failure, dependence or independence. Family members may also benefit from some of these strategies to aid with their compliance because they are expected to remember many different protocols, exercises, and schedules and may need help with being more organized.

In some school districts, a special education transition plan is included in the student's annual educational program when the child is 14 years old. As a team, the therapist, social worker or counselor, teachers, family, and often the child discuss ideas about what type of educational program might be appropriate for high school and even post-high school study, where the child might be able to receive his or her future education, what type of setting would be best, what type of housing might be required when the child no longer lives at home, and what types of job options could be considered. Sometimes this may seem very premature, but actually for the population with spina bifida, even the child who is younger than 14 years would benefit from a flexible plan that stimulates communication between the medical providers, school staff, and family to minimize or prevent some of the long-term problems that have been listed in the foregoing paragraphs. It appears clear that the adult population has multiple and varied needs and that these needs should be addressed as early and consistently as possible by a comprehensive, multidisciplinary team approach that will efficiently identify and address the issues and make referrals to specialists for interventions to help transition the young patient into a more independent adult.

Summary

There are many aspects of care for the PT to consider when treating children with spina bifida. The information presented in this chapter provides both an historic and contemporary foundation for building an understanding of this complex birth defect. It also poses issues that new approaches, technologies, and research may make clearer in the near future. Most often, the role of the PT is defined by the venue in which one practices and the age of the children in that setting. Therefore, certain sections of the chapter may be more or less relevant than others. Spina bifida is a disability that requires an understanding of the many systems that are affected and how they interact and influence the child's abilities to function through their entire life. Concerns and strategies for intervention suggested throughout this chapter reflect the author's humble philosophy that PTs must be knowledgeable about all of the affected body systems that are common to spina bifida and the trends and protocols being applied to optimize their care. The therapist should be aware of the priorities of the families and the focus of other professionals assisting the child. The true challenge to the PT is to integrate these various perspectives into a creative treatment plan that produces the best result for each child. Beginning with a strong basis in anatomy, neurology, and kinesiology combined with imagination, experimentation, and exploration, the PT will discover new and novel ideas for treatment that will not only advance his/her own clinical abilities to a more sophisticated and successful intervention but, most importantly, will help the child progress to his or her most functional and productive level.

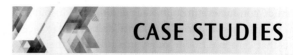

CASE STUDIES

CRYSTAL, 7 YEARS OLD

Significant History
Crystal's back was closed when she was 3 days old, and at 12 days, a VP shunt was inserted to control hydrocephalus. She was discharged to home and had no further complications or shunt revisions. She lives with her grandparents and a younger brother. She attended an early intervention program from 3 to 5 years of age where she received occupational therapy, physical therapy, and speech services. She did not receive early intervention services until age 3 because of multiple moves and poor follow-up with the EI referral. Crystal entered school 2.5 years ago and travels in her personal manual wheelchair, with no bracing. She is followed by a spina bifida clinic at a local pediatric hospital.

Present Findings
Crystal has moderate limitations in expressive and receptive language and cognition. She is in a special education classroom for children with similar learning challenges. Crystal is able to follow simple verbal directions. She is the only student in class with a physical disability. Her gross and fine motor skills are her strength, and she enjoys leaving class to push her wheelchair in the hallways, schoolyard, and gym. Her classroom is on the first floor, in a school with an elevator that is used to transition her to specialty classes and the library. She is catheterized at school 2 times a day, in the nursing suite, which is also on the first floor.

Gross Motor Skills
Crystal is able to perform a sliding transfer with close supervision; from her wheelchair to her classroom chair and back and to the couch in the nursing suite. She is impulsive and may forget to lock her chair, or she might be careless moving her legs. At times, she also forgets to position her chair properly and may require verbal and physical cues. She prefers throwing herself forward onto the couch rather than taking the time for setup and safety. Crystal is able to propel her chair very well and steers it herself in multiple environments. She easily keeps up with her classmates as they transition from the bus, into and out of the building, to lunch, and outdoor recess.

Passive Range of Motion
Last year, Crystal had bilateral hamstring releases and was in long leg casts for 6 weeks. When the casts were removed, she remained with a 15-degree knee flexion contracture on the right and the left knee extended to neutral. When she returned to school after the summer vacation, she had full passive ROM in both hips, but her knees lacked 30 degrees of extension (R) and 15 degrees (L).

Manual Muscle Testing
She has strong arms and trunk and the following bilateral lower extremity active muscle function: "Fair" hip flexion and adduction; "Poor +" knee extension; "Poor +" knee flexion; and "Trace" ankle dorsiflexion. No other active movements are noted.

Upright Mobility

After her casts were removed, she was fitted with an HKAFO with a butterfly pelvic band and drop locks at the hip and knee joints to maintain her in extension. The ankles are solid and set at 90 degrees. The knee pads can be loosened to accommodate her knee flexion. She was taught to perform a hop-to pattern with all joints locked, using a posterior walker. Her grandparents were instructed in brace donning and doffing at the spina bifida clinic. She has been coming to school with her walker and her braces and sneakers in a bag to be donned in school for ambulation training. Multiple calls to her family have produced no change in this routine. She and her family report that she is not wearing her braces at home in the evenings or on weekends. Crystal's grandmother explained that donning the brace in the morning is difficult for her owing to lack of time. It is also not possible to have the classroom staff place her in her brace each day. If the family sent Crystal to school wearing her braces, the school nurse is willing to remove them to perform her late morning catheterizing and put the braces back on her following the afternoon catheterization, but she is resentful that the family will not share this responsibility. It is also difficult to get a commitment from Crystal's grandparents that they will help her stand and practice walking after school and/or on weekends.

Crystal receives a weekly physical therapy session in school, and her program consists of transfer training, gait training/ practice walking, and a strengthening program for her trunk and upper extremities. Active and active assistive ROM is also performed, with an emphasis on knee extension. She is consistently able to ambulate with close guarding for approximately 500 yards before becoming tired. She likes to walk to the school nurse for a visit before returning to her class. Crystal's greatest challenge in upright appears to be her excessive right knee flexion contracture, which causes that leg to be relatively shorter than the left and creates an uneven base of support. When she is upright, her weight bearing is predominantly on the left leg. She must overuse her arms for additional support. She also appears fearful when standing with her posterior walker unless she receives contact guarding and much verbal reassurance.

Action Taken

An anterior-facing rollator walker was tried and she immediately exhibited more confidence, with no decrease in her walking ability. She was also able to keep her upper body erect over the walker. The walkers were switched.

A conference call was held between the school-based PT, the PT who staffs the spina bifida clinic she attends, and Crystal's orthopedic surgeon. We were all in agreement to experiment, and the pelvic band of the brace was removed. The orthotist also added a 2-inch wedged shoe lift under the right shoe to compensate for her right knee flexion, and that gave her a flat surface for standing. Crystal's grandmother was called and attended a clinic appointment to again receive instruction on donning and doffing Crystal's newly modified braces, and the suggestion was repeated by the clinic therapist and physician to have Crystal wear them daily. Her grandmother explained that the long leg braces (KAFO) seem much easier for her to manage. She was

also advised that in a few years Crystal would be nearing adolescence, when she would be less likely to gain new upright skills unless her functional walking significantly improved. Crystal's grandmother left the appointment with a renewed commitment to participate in the gait program.

Results

Crystal is now coming to school wearing her braces each day. Thanks to the assistance of the classroom staff, she sits in class with both knees locked to stretch her knee flexors on the right and to prevent further tightening on the left. Her legs are propped up on a small box because her wheelchair does not have elevating leg rests. She continues to walk with the therapist each week and her distance is charted. Crystal is positioned upright by the classroom staff in a standing box for up to 1 hour each day. It is much easier and quicker for them to lock her knees, and she only requires setup and supervision to pull up to stand. The staff also walks with her from her seat to the standing table and back. It is a short walk, but it gives the staff experience that may be helpful in encouraging them to walk her longer distances in the near future. The standing box has a tray to enable Crystal to participate in her class activities and perform desktop work while standing in it. Because she has active hip flexors, it might be possible to use a reciprocating pattern of leg movement, but a hop-to pattern increases her speed, and she does not have to control for the active adduction of her legs, which would slow her down. She holds her legs together and takes off.

The goal is for her to walk twice a day to the nurse for her catheterizations rather than use her wheelchair. The school nurse is now able to perform the catheterization without removing Crystal's braces, so it is more efficient. Finally, a small picture card has been developed and is attached to her chair for easy access, to remind her of the correct sequencing of steps to set up and safely transfer out of her wheelchair. It also serves as a prompt to the staff, who help her. This adaptation has greatly improved her level of safe and independent transfers. She has begun to practice a standing pivot transfer with her school PT, which will allow her to transfer to many other types of surfaces and heights.

Conclusion

Although the pelvic band was initially appropriate for her lesion level and lower extremity strengths and weaknesses, it appeared that its removal was a key to moving her forward in the standing and gait components of her therapy program. The removal of the pelvic band has not impacted her speed, endurance, or alignment in a negative way. The classroom staff is more energized to be involved, and it is easier for them to assist. Her family has also increased their participation and compliance by sending her to school wearing her braces. Crystal is an exercise ambulatory, and her wheelchair is her dominant mode of mobility. But one of her goals is to maintain her present level of upright skills primarily for weight control; maintaining and increasing strength of her legs, trunk, and arms; and improving cardiovascular function. If she had begun an ambulation program with appropriate bracing earlier in life, it might have resulted in a higher level of upright function. If the family was able to offer more assistance, the clinic might have considered an RGO that would allow Crystal to stand and walk with less effort. It is not a consideration at this time because the RGO is a larger and more complicated device. With continued effort in the gait program by the classroom staff, school nurse, school PT, and the clinic staff, the long-range plan is to increase involvement at home so Crystal will wear her braces and walk on weekends and during extended holiday and summer vacations, at the minimum. If her walking skills improve, additional opportunities to walk longer distances and increased upright time can be added to her daily routine.

ANDREA, 4 YEARS OLD

History

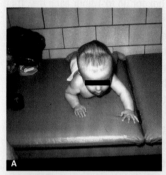
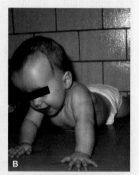
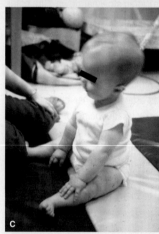
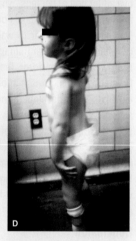

Andrea was seen for the first time in the myelomeningocele clinic at Children's Memorial Hospital in Chicago, now Lurie Children's Hospital, when she was 4 months old. She was born at her regional hospital, where her back was closed but her hydrocephalus went untreated for many months. As her head grew and signs of hydrocephalus were noted, her family looked for another hospital that would treat her more aggressively.

Andrea was seen by the neurosurgeon, urologist, orthopedic surgeon, and PT at that clinic visit, and they agreed on a course of action for her. She was admitted that afternoon and received a VP shunt two days later to relieve her hydrocephalus. After several days of flat bed rest to enable her to recover from surgery and the excess CFS to drain slowly, she was permitted to slowly be held upright and begin her PT program.

Andrea's manual muscle test indicated an L5-S1 motor level with active and strong hip flexors, adductors, quadriceps, and medial hamstrings. She also had a "Poor+" gluteus medius. She had active anterior and posterior tibialis muscles as well. However, her head control and trunk balance were delayed and weak, and although she could push up on her hands to elevate her head, she did not lift her head well or stabilize it when held in supported sitting. She was also rolling by using her arms without lifting her head. The therapist believed this was largely a mechanical issue because of her large head and that although she exhibited hypotonia throughout her neck and body, no other neurologic pathology was noted.

Andrea was referred to Early Intervention, and a phone call to the receiving PT from the clinic therapist was made to share information and begin a relationship that would follow Andrea until school age.

The clinic PT began to teach Andrea's parents a series of exercises for her home program and shared it with the EI therapist:

1. Range of motion was demonstrated with special emphasis on keeping her hips and ankles flexible. She was given night splints for both feet to keep her ankles from tightening into dorsiflexion.
2. Prone play over her mother's lap was successful, and she began lifting her head and reaching for toys without leaning on her arms.
3. Supine pull to sit was shown, and getting Andrea to lift her legs in the air to kick a toy tambourine and bells worked to strengthen her neck and trunk flexors as well as her legs.
4. Sitting and tilting slowly in all directions to stimulate head and trunk righting and strengthen the muscles of those areas was taught.
5. Standing in her mother's arms with weight on both legs and her trunk aligned well was easy because of her active lower extremity musculature, although she had not been weight bearing before.
6. Lastly, in accordance with the clinic's philosophy, the family was asked to avoid using all walkers, jolly jumpers, and other positioning devices that might further delay Andrea's acquisition of motor skills.

She was followed in the clinic, and her development improved quickly. At 8 months, with a stronger neck and trunk, secondary to all of the work she was doing with PT and her family, she was crawling on hands and knees. As she neared her first birthday, she was beginning to pull up in her crib wearing her night splints. Definitive AFOs were fabricated for her, and she began to cruise and let go of support at approximately the same time expected of a typical child. Her gait showed only a moderate lumbar lordosis due to absent gluteus maximus muscles, but all of the work on strengthening had improved her gluteus medius enough to ensure that her pelvis was more stable and that she was able to walk without an assistive device.

Her rapid achievement in gross motor skills and her level of ability in gait could not have been predicted on the basis of the initial impression she presented in clinic. But a sustained and coordinated plan involving family, clinic staff, and community resources enabled Andrea to reach a high level of motor function.

REFERENCES

1. Morrisey RT. Spina bifida: a new rehabilitation problem. *Orthop Clin North Am.* 1978;9:379-389.
2. Myers GJ. Myelomeningocele: the medical aspects. *Pediatr Clin North Am.* 1984;31:165-175.
3. Adzick NS, Thom EA, Spong CY, et al. A randomized trial of prenatal versus postnatal repair of myelomeningocele. *N Engl J Med.* 2011;364:993-1004.
4. Duff EM, Cooper ES. Neural tube defects in Jamaica following Hurricane Gilbert. *Am J Public Health.* 1994;84(3):473-476.
5. Seller M. Risks in spina bifida: annotation. *Dev Med Child Neurol.* 1994;36:1021-1025.
6. Share with women: folic acid—what's it all about. *J Midwifery Womens Health.* 2003;48(5):365-366.
7. MMWR Editorial Note. Center for disease control and prevention. *MMWR Editorial Note.* 2004;53(17):362-365.
8. Ray JG, Meier C, Vermeulen MJ, et al. Association of neural tube defects and folic acid food fortification in Canada. *Lancet.* 2002;360(9350):2047-2048.
9. Frey L, Hauser WA. Epidemiology of neural tube defects. *Epilepsia.* 2003;44(suppl 3):4-13.
10. Centers for Disease Control and Prevention. Trends in wheat-flour fortification with folic acid and iron—worldwide, 2004 and 2007. *MMWR Morb Mortal Wkly Rep.* 2008;57:8-10. Accessed November 2012. http://www.cdc.gov/mmwr/preview/mmwrhtml/mm5701a4.htm
11. Centers for Disease Control and Prevention. Periconceptual use of multivitamins and the occurrence of anencephaly and spina bifida. *MMWR Morb Mortal Wkly Rep.* 1988;37(47):727-730. Accessed November 2012. http://www.cdc.gov/mmwr/preview/mmwrhtml/00001309.htm
12. Mathews TJ, Honein MA, Ericckson JD. Spina bifida and anencephaly prevalence—United States, 1991-2001. *MMWR Recomm Rep.* 2002;51(RR-13):9-11. Accessed February 11, 2021. https://www.cdc.gov/Mmwr/preview/mmwrhtml/rr5113a3.htm
13. Finnell RH, Gould A, Spiegelstein O. Pathobiology and genetics of neural tube defects. *Epilepsia.* 2003;44(suppl 3):14-23.
14. Dias MS, Partington M. Embryology of myelomeningocele and anencephaly. *Neurosurg Focus.* 2004;16(2):E1.
15. Searby L. *Folic acid fortification: the current global state of play.* Nutraingredients.com. News and Supplements. April 2016. Accessed February 11, 2021. https://www.nutraingredients.com/Article/2016/04/22/Folic-acid-fortification-The-current-global-state-of-play
16. Alwan S, Reefhuis J, Rasmussen A, et al. Use of selective serotonin reuptake inhibitors in pregnancy and the risk of birth defects. *N Engl J Med.* 2007;356:2684-2692.
17. Lunsky AM, Ulcicus M, Rothman KJ, et al. Maternal heat exposure and neural tube defects. *JAMA.* 1992;268:882-885.
18. Bowman RM, McLone DG. Neurosurgical management of spina bifida: research issues. *Dev Disabil Res Rev.* 2010;16(1):82-87.
19. Centers for Disease Control and Prevention. *Estimating the prevalence of spina bifida.* Accessed September 2012. http://www.cdc.gov/ncbddd/spinabifida/research.html
20. Smith K, Freeman KA, Neville-Jan A, et al. Cultural considerations in the care of children with spina bifida. *Pediatr Clin North Am.* 2010;57(4):1027-1040.
21. Canfield MA, Ramadhani TA, Shaw GM, et al. Anencephaly and spina bifida among Hispanics: maternal, sociodemographic and acculturation factors in the national birth defects prevention study, birth defects research (Part A). *Clin Mol Teretol.* 2009;85(7):637-646.
22. Arizona Department of Health Services. *Facts about Spina bifida, 1995-2009.* Accessed February 11, 2021. https://www.azdhs.gov/documents/preparedness/public-health-statistics/birth-defects-monitoring/fact-sheets/SpinaBifida.pdf
23. Johnson CY, Honein MA, Flanders DW, et al. Pregnancy termination following prenatal diagnosis of anencephaly or spina bifida: a systematic review of the literature. *Birth Defects Res A Clin Mol Teratol.* 2012;44(1):857-863.
24. Scarff TB, Fronczak S. Myelomeningocele: a review and update. *Rehab Lit.* 1981;42:143-147.
25. Tachdjian MO. Pediatric Orthopedics. Vol 3. 2nd ed. WB Saunders; 1990:1773-1880.
26. Behrman RC, Vaughn VC, eds. *Nelson's Textbook of Pediatrics.* 11th ed. WB Saunders; 1979.
27. Fidas A, MacDonald HL, Elton RA, et al. Prevalence of spina bifida occulta in patients with functional disorders of the lower urinary tract and its relation to urodynamics and neurophysiological measurements. *BMJ.* 1989;298:357-359.
28. Warder DE. Tethered cord syndrome and occult spinal dysraphism. American Association of Neurological Surgeons. *Neurosurg Focus.* 2001;10(1):e1.
29. Tubbs RS, Wellons III JC, Grabb PA, et al. Chiari II malformation and occult spinal dysraphism. Case reports and a review of the literature. *Pediatr Neurosurg.* 2003;39(2):104-107.
30. Kanev PM, Lemire RJ, Loeser JD, et al. Management and long-term follow-up review of children with lipomyelomeningocele. *J Neurosurg.* 1990;73:48-52.
31. Moore KL. *The Developing Human: Clinically Oriented Embryology.* WB Saunders; 1974.
32. Robbins SL. Pathologic Basis of Disease. WB Saunders; 1974.
33. Umphred DA. Neurological Rehabilitation. CV Mosby; 1985.
34. Sharrard WJ. *Neuromotor evaluation of the newborn.* In: Symposium on Myelomeningocele. CV Mosby; 1972.
35. Peach B. The Arnold-Chiari malformation. *Arch Neurol.* 1965;12:165.
36. Peach B. The Arnold-Chiari malformation. *Arch Neurol.* 1965;12:109.
37. McCullough DC. *Arnold-Chiari malformation—theories of development.* Paper presented at: The 2nd Symposium on Myelomeningocele; 1984; Cincinnati, OH.
38. McLone DG, Knepper PA. The cause of Chiari II malformation: a unified theory. *Pediatr Neurosci.* 1989;15:1-12.
39. McLone DG, Dias MS. The Chiari II malformation: cause and impact. *Childs Nerv Syst.* 2003;19(7-8):540-550.
40. Lutschg J, Meyer E, Jeanneret-Iseli C, et al. Brainstem auditory evoked potential in myelomeningocele. *Neuropediatrics.* 1985;16:202-204.
41. Hesz N, Wolraich M. Vocal cord paralysis and brainstem dysfunction in children with spina bifida. *Dev Med Child Neurol.* 1985;27:528-531.
42. Hoffman HJ, Hendrick EB, Humphreys RP, et al. Manifestations and management of Arnold-Chiari malformation in patients with myelomeningocele. *Childs Brain.* 1975;1:255-259.
43. Staal MJ, Melhuizen-de Regt MJ, Hess J. Sudden death in hydrocephalic spina bifida aperta patients. *Pediatr Neurosci.* 1987;13:13-18.
44. Biggio JR, Wenstrom KD, Owen J. Fetal open spina bifida: a natural history of disease progression in utero. *Prenat Diagn.* 2004;24(4):287-289.
45. Palomaki GE, Williams JR, Haddow JE. Prenatal screening for open neural-tube defects in Maine. *N Engl J Med.* 1999;340(13):1049-1050.
46. Thomas M. The lemon sign. *Radiology.* 2003;228(1):206-207.
47. Pilu G, Romero R, Reece A, et al. Subnormal cerebellum in fetuses with spina bifida. *Am J Obstet Gynecol.* 1988;158:1052-1056.
48. Benacerraf BR, Stryker J, Frigotto FD. Abnormal ultrasound appearance of the cerebellum (banana sign): indirect sign of spina bifida. *Pediatr Radiol.* 1989;171:151-153.
49. Nyberg DA, Mack LA, Hirsch J, et al. Abnormalities of cranial contour in sonographic detection of spina bifida: evaluation of the "lemon" sign. *Radiology.* 1988;167(2):387-392.
50. Thiagarajah S, Henke J, Hogge WA, et al. Early diagnosis of spina bifida: the value of cranial ultrasound markers. *Obstet Gynecol.* 1990;76:54-57.
51. Bensen J, Dillard RG, Burton BK. Open spina bifida: does cesarean section delivery improve prognosis? *Obstet Gynecol.* 1988;71:532-534.

52. Luthy DA, Wardinsky T, Shurtleff DB, et al. Cesarean section before the onset of labor and subsequent motor function in infants with myelomeningocele diagnosed antenatally. *N Engl J Med.* 1991;324:662-666.

53. Hogge WA, Dungan JS, Brooks MP, et al. Diagnosis and management of prenatally detected myelomeningocele: a preliminary report. *Am J Obstet Gynecol.* 1990;163:1061-1064.

54. Johnson MP, Sutton LN, Rintol N, et al. Fetal myelomeningocele repair: short term clinical outcomes. *Am J Obstet Gynecol.* 2003;189(2):482-487.

55. Sutton LN, Adzick NS, Bilaniuk LT, et al. Improvement in hindbrain herniation demonstrated by serial fetal magnetic resonance imaging following fetal surgery for myelomeningocele. *JAMA.* 1999;282(19):1826-1831.

56. Buner JP, Tulipan N, Paschall RL, et al. Fetal surgery for myelomeningocele and the incidence of shunt-dependent hydrocephalus. *JAMA.* 1999;282(19):1819-1825.

57. Houtrow AJ, Thom EA, Fletcher JM, et al. Prenatal repair of myelomeningocele and school-age functional outcomes. *Pediatrics.* 2020;145:2.

58. Danzer E, Johnson MP, Adzick NS, et al. Fetal surgery for myelomeningocele: progress and perspectives. *Dev Med Child Neurol.* 2012;54(1):8-14.

59. Verbeek RJ, Heep A, Maurits NM, et al. Fetal endoscopic myelomeningocele closure preserves segmental neurologic function. *Dev Med Child Neurol.* 2012;54(1):15-22.

60. Shurtleff D. Fetal endoscopic myelomeningocele repair. *Dev Med Child Neurol.* 2012;54(1):4-5.

61. Raimondi AJ, Soare P. Intellectual development in shunted hydrocephalic children. *Am J Dis Child.* 1974;127:664-671.

62. McLone DG, Czyzewski D, Raimondi AJ, et al. Central nervous system infections as a limiting factor in the intelligence of children with myelomeningocele. *Pediatrics.* 1982;70:338-342.

63. Ellenbogen RG, Goldmann DA, Winston KW. Group B streptococcal infections of the central nervous system in infants with myelomeningocele. *Surg Neurol.* 1988;29:237-242.

64. Murdoch A. How valuable is muscle charting? *Physiotherapy.* 1980;66:221-223.

65. Schafer M, Dias L. *Myelomeningocele: Orthopedic Treatment.* Williams & Wilkins; 1983.

66. Kaplan G. Editorial: with apologies to Shakespeare. *J Urol.* 1999;161:933.

67. Tanaka H, Katizaki H, Kobayashi S, et al. The relevance of urethral resistance in children with myelodysplasia: its impact on upper urinary tract deterioration and the outcome of conservative management. *J Urol.* 1999;161:929-932.

68. McLone DG. *An Introduction to Hydrocephalus.* Children's Memorial Hospital; 1982.

69. Raimondi AJ. Complications of ventriculoperitoneal shunting and a critical comparison of the 3-piece and 1-piece systems. *Childs Brain.* 1977;3:321-342.

70. Bell WO, Sumner TE, Volberg FM. The significance of ventriculomegaly in the newborn with myelodysplasia. *Childs Nerv Syst.* 1987;3:239-241.

71. Bell WO, Arbit E, Fraser R. One-stage myelomeningocele closure and ventriculo-peritoneal shunt placement. *Surg Neurol.* 1987;27:233-236.

72. Lindseth RE. Treatment of the lower extremities in children paralyzed by myelomeningocele (birth to 18 months). *Am Acad Orthop Surg Inst Course Lec.* 1976;25:76-82.

73. McDonald CM, Jaffe KM, Shurtleff DB, et al. Modifications to the traditional description of neurosegmental innervation in myelomeningocele. *Dev Med Child Neurol.* 1991;33(6):473-481.

74. Daniels L, Williams M, Worthingham C. *Muscle Testing: Techniques of Manual Examination.* WB Saunders; 1956.

75. Strach EH. Orthopedic care of children with myelomeningocele: a modern program of rehabilitation. *BMJ.* 1967;3:791-794.

76. Asher M, Olson J. Factors affecting the ambulatory status of patients with spina bifida cystica. *J Bone Joint Surg Am.* 1983;65(3):350-356.

77. Bunch W. *Progressive neurological loss in myelomeningocele patients.* Paper presented at: The American Academy of Cerebral Palsy and Developmental Medicine Conference; 1982; San Diego, CA.

78. Coon V, Donato G, Houser C, et al. Normal ranges of hip motion in infants. *Clin Orthop.* 1975;110:256-260.

79. Haas S. Normal ranges of hip motion in the newborn. *Clin Orthop Relat Res.* 1973;91:114-118.

80. Banta JV, Lin R, Peterson M, et al. The team approach in the care of the child with myelomeningocele. *J Prosthet Orthot.* 1989;2:263-273.

81. Lie HR, Lagergren J, Rasmussen F, et al. Bowel and bladder control of children with myelomeningocele: a Nordic study. *Dev Med Child Neurol.* 1991;33:1053-1061.

82. Brem AS, Martin D, Callaghan J, et al. Long-term renal risk factors in children with myelomeningocele. *J Pediatr.* 1987;110:51-55.

83. Anagnostopoulos D, Joannides E, Kotsianos K. The urological management of patients with myelodysplasia. *Pediatr Surg Int.* 1988;3:347-350.

84. Mazur JM. Hand function in patients with spina bifida cystica. *J Pediatr Orthop.* 1986;6:442-447.

85. Anderson P. Impairment of a motor skill in children with spina bifida cystica and hydrocephalus: an exploratory study. *Br J Psychol.* 1977;68:61-70.

86. Dahl M, Ahlsten G, Carlson H, et al. Neurological dysfunction above cele level in children with spina bifida cystica: a prospective study to three years. *Dev Med Child Neurol.* 1995;37:30-40.

87. Bobath B. Motor development, its effect on general development and application to the treatment of cerebral palsy. *Physiotherapy.* 1971;57:526-532.

88. Bobath B. The treatment of neuromuscular disorders by improving patterns of coordination. *Physiotherapy.* 1969;55:18-22.

89. Bobath B. The very early treatment of cerebral palsy. *Dev Med Child Neurol.* 1967;9:373-390.

90. Caplan F. The First Twelve Months of Life. Grosset and Dunlap; 1973.

91. Turner A. Upper-limb function in children with myelomeningocele. *Dev Med Child Neurol.* 1986;28:790-798.

92. Turner A. Hand function in children with myelomeningocele. *J Bone Joint Surg Br.* 1985;67:268-272.

93. Cronchman M. The effects of babywalkers on early locomotor development. *Dev Med Child Neurol.* 1986;28:757-761.

94. Williams EN, Broughton NS, Menelaus MB. Age-related walking in children with spina bifida. *Dev Med Child Neurol.* 1999;41(7):446-449.

95. Menelaus M. The evolution of orthopedic management of myelomeningocele. *J Pediatr Orthop.* 1999;18:421-422.

96. Beaty JH, Canale ST. Current concepts review. Orthopedic aspects of myelomeningocele. *J Bone Joint Surg Am.* 1990;72:626-630.

97. Dias L. Orthopedic care in spina bifida: past, present, and future. *Dev Med Child Neurol.* 2004;46(9):579.

98. Stauffer ES, Hoffer M. Ambulation in thoracic paraplegia [Abstract]. *J Bone Joint Surg.* 1972;54A:1336.

99. Hoffer MM, Feiwell EE, Perry R, et al. Functional ambulation in patients with myelomeningocele. *J Bone Joint Surg.* 1973;55(1):137-148.

100. Swaroop VT, Dias L. Orthopedic management of spina bifida. Part I: hip, knee and rotational deformities. *J Child Orthop.* 2009;3(6):441-449.

101. Swaroop VT, Dias L. Orthopedic management of spina bifida. Part II: foot and ankle deformities. *J Child Orthop.* 2011;5(6):403-414.

102. Stallard J, Lomas B, Woollam P, et al. New technical advances in swivel walkers. *Prosthet Orthop Int.* 2003;27(2):132-138.

103. Yngve D, Douglas R, Roberts JM. The reciprocating gait orthosis in myelomeningocele. *J Pediatr Orthop.* 1984;4:304-310.

104. Dias L, Tappit-Emas E, Boot E. *The reciprocating gait orthosis: the Children's Memorial experience.* Paper presented at: The American Academy of Developmental Medicine and Child Neurology; 1984; Washington, DC.

105. Douglas R, Larson PF, D'Ambrosia R, et al. The LSU reciprocating gait orthosis. *Orthopedics*. 1983;6:834-839.

106. Stallard J, Henshaw LH, Lomas B, et al. The Orlau VCG (variable centre of gravity) swivel walker for muscular dystrophy patients. *Prosthet Orthop Int*. 1992;16(1):46-48.

107. Fillauer. Reciprocating Gait Orthosis: Patient Component Selection Guide. Accessed February 14, 2021. https://fillauer.com/wp-content/uploads/2020/03/m009b-rgo-selection-1.pdf

108. Katz DE, Haideri N, Song K, et al. Comparative study of conventional hip-knee-ankle-foot orthoses versus reciprocating-gait orthoses for children with high level paraparesis. *J Pediatr Orthop*. 1997;17(3):377-86.

109. Williams L. Energy cost of walking and of wheelchair propulsion by children with myelodysplasia. *Dev Med Child Neurol*. 1983;25:617-624.

110. Wright JG. Hip and spine surgery is of questionable value in spina bifida: an evidence based review. *Clin Orthop Relat Res*. 2011;465(5):1258-1264.

111. McDonald CM, Jaffe KM, Mosca VS, et al. Ambulatory outcome of children with myelomeningocele: effect of lower extremity muscle strength. *Dev Med Child Neurol*. 1991;33:482-490.

112. Torosian CM, Dias LS. Surgical treatment of severe hindfoot valgus by medial displacement osteotomy of the os calcis in children with myelomeningocele. *J Pediatr Orthop*. 2000;20(2):226-229.

113. Neto J, Dias L, Gabriel A. Congenital talipes equinovarus in spina bifida: treatment and results. *J Pediatr Orthop*. 1996;16:782-785.

114. Schopler SA, Menelaus MB. Significance of the strength of the quadriceps muscles in children with myelomeningocele. *J Pediatr Orthop*. 1987;7:507-512.

115. Arkin C, Ihnow S, Dias L, et al. Midterm results of the Ponseti method for treatment of clubfoot in patients with spina bifida. *J Pediatr Orthop*. 2018;8(10):e588-e592.

116. Gerlach DJ, Gurnett CA, Limpaphayon N, et al. Early results of the Ponseti method for the treatment of clubfoot associated with myelomeningocele. *J Bone Joint Surg Am*. 2009;91(6):1350-1359.

117. Sherk HH, Uppal GS, Lane G, et al. Treatment versus nontreatment of hip dislocations in ambulatory patients with myelomeningocele. *Dev Med Child Neurol*. 1991;33:491-494.

118. Duffy CM, Graham HK, Cosgrove AP. The influence of ankle-foot orthosis on gait and energy expenditure in spina bifida. *J Pediatr Orthop*. 2000;20(3):356-361.

119. Hunt KG. The effects of fixed and hinged ankle-foot orthoses on gait myoelectric activity in children with myelomeningocele. Meeting Highlights of AACPDM. *J Pediatr Orthop*. 1994;14(2):269.

120. Knutson LM, Clark DE. Orthotic devices for ambulation in children with cerebral palsy and myelomeningocele. *Phys Ther*. 1991; 71:947-960.

121. Vankoski S, Dias L. Children with spina bifida benefit from gait analysis. *Standard*. 1997;1:4-5.

122. Vankoski S, Sarwark J, Moore C, et al. Characteristic pelvis, hip and knee kinematic patterns in children with lumbosacral myelomeningocele. *Gait Posture*. 1995;3(1):51-57.

123. Ounpuu S, Davis R, Bell K, et al. *Gait analysis in the treatment decision making process in patients with myelomeningocele*. In: 8th Annual East Coast Gait Laboratories Conference; May 5-8, 1993; Rochester, MN.

124. Duffy CM, Hill A, Cosgrove A, et al. Three-dimensional gait analysis in spina bifida. *J Pediatr Orthop*. 1996;16:786-791.

125. Williams J, Graham G, Dunne K, et al. Late knee problems in myelomeningocele. *J Pediatr Orthop*. 1993;13:701-703.

126. Thompson JD, Ounpuu S, Davis RB, et al. The effects of ankle-foot orthosis on the ankle and knee in persons with myelomeningocele: an evaluation using three dimensional gait analysis. *J Pediatr Orthop*. 1999;19(1):27-33.

127. Porsch K. Origin and treatment of fractures in spina bifida. *Eur J Pediatr Surg*. 1991;1(5):298-305.

128. Drummond D. Post-operative fractures in patients with myelomeningocele. *Dev Med Child Neurol*. 1981;23:147-150.

129. Rosenstein BD, Greene WB, Herrington RT, et al. Bone density in myelomeningocele: the effects of ambulatory status and other factors. *Dev Med Child Neurol*. 1987;29:486-494.

130. Lock TR, Aronson DD. Fractures in patients who have myelomeningocele. *J Bone Joint Surg Am*. 1989;71:1153-1157.

131. Bartonek A, Saraste H, Samuelson L, et al. Ambulation in patients with myelomeningocele: a 12 year follow-up. *J Pediatr Orthop*. 1999;19(2):202-206.

132. Hall P, Lindseth R, Campbell R, et al. Scoliosis and hydrocephalus in myelomeningocele patients: the effect of ventricular shunting. *J Neurosurg*. 1979;50:174-178.

133. Mazur JM, Stillwell A, Menelaus M. The significance of spasticity on the upper and lower limbs in myelomeningocele. *J Bone Joint Surg Br*. 1986;68:213-217.

134. Mazur JM, Menelaus MB. Neurologic status of spina bifida patients and the orthopedic surgeon. *Clin Orthop Relat Res*. 1991; 264:54-64.

135. Jeelani NO, Jaspan T, Punt J. Tethered cord syndrome after myelomeningocele repair. *BMJ*. 1999;318:516-517.

136. Petersen M. Tethered cord syndrome in myelodysplasia: correlation between level of lesion and height at time of presentation. *Dev Med Child Neurol*. 1992;34:604-610.

137. McLone DG, Herman J, Gabriele A, et al. Tethered cord as a cause of scoliosis in children with a myelomeningocele. *Pediatr Neurosurg*. 1990;91(16):8-13.

138. Banta JV. The tethered cord in myelomeningocele: should it be untethered? *Dev Med Child Neurol*. 1991;33:167-176.

139. Flanagan RC, Russell DP, Walsh JW. Urologic aspects of tethered cord. *Urology*. 1989;33:80-82.

140. Kaplan WE, McLone DG, Richards I. The urological manifestation of the tethered spinal cord. *J Urol*. 1988;140:1285-1288.

141. Grief L, Stalmasek V. Tethered cord syndrome: a pediatric case study. *J Neurosci Nurs*. 1989;21:86-91.

142. Hochleiter BW, Menardi G, Haussler B, et al. Spina bifida as an independent risk factor for sensitization to latex. *J Urol*. 2001;166(6):2370-2373.

143. Nieto A, Mazon A, Pamies R, et al. Efficacy of latex avoidance for primary prevention of latex sensitization in children with spina bifida. *J Pediatr*. 2002;140(3):370-372.

144. Centers for Disease Control. Anaphylactic reaction during general anesthesia among pediatric patients, United States. Jan 1990-Jan 1991. *MMWR Morb Mortal Wkly Rep*. 1991;40:437-443.

145. U.S. Food and Drug Administration. *Recommendations for Labeling Medical Products to Inform Users that the Product or Product Container is not Made with Natural Rubber Latex: Guidance for Industry and Food and Drug Administration Staff*; December 2014. Accessed February 14, 2021. https://www.fda.gov/regulatory-information/search-fda-guidance-documents/recommendations-labeling-medical-products-inform-users-product-or-product-container-not-made-natural

146. Meeropol E, Frost J, Pugh L, et al. Latex allergy in children with myelomeningocele. *J Pediatr Orthop*. 1993;13:1-4.

147. D'Astous J, Drouin M, Rhine E. Intraoperative anaphylaxis secondary to allergy to latex in children who have spina bifida. *J Bone Joint Surg*. 1992;74(7):1084-1086.

148. Meehan P, Galina M, Daftari T. Intraoperative anaphylaxis due to allergy to latex. *J Bone Joint Surg*. 1992;74-A:1103-1109.

149. Lu L, Kurup V, Hoffman D, et al. Characterization of a major latex allergen associated with hypersensitivity in spina bifida patients. *J Immunol*. 1995;155:2721-2728.

150. Willis KE, Holmbeck GN, Dillon K, et al. Intelligence and achievement in children with myelomeningocele. *J Pediatr Psychol*. 1990; 15(2):161-176.

151. Horn DG, Pugzles Lorch E, Lorch RF, et al. Distractibility and vocabulary deficits in children with spina bifida and hydrocephalus. *Dev Med Child Neurol*. 1985;27:713-720.

152. Wolfe GA, Kennedy D, Brewer K, et al. *Visual perception and upper extremity function in children with spina bifida*. Paper presented at: The

American Academy of Cerebral Palsy and Developmental Medicine; 1989; San Francisco, CA.

153. Cull C, Wyke MA. Memory function of children with spina bifida and shunted hydrocephalus. *Dev Med Child Neurol*. 1984;26:177-183.

154. Dise JE, Lohr ME. Examination of deficits in conceptual reasoning abilities associated with spina bifida. *Am J Phys Med Rehab*. 1998;77(3):247-250.

155. Lennerstrand G, Gallo JE. Neuro-ophthalmological evaluation of patients with myelomeningocele and Chiari malformations. *Dev Med Child Neurol*. 1990;32:415-422.

156. Rothstein TB, Romano PE, Shoch D. Meningomyelocele. *Am J Ophthalmol*. 1974;77:690-693.

157. Ruff HA. The development of perception and recognition of objects. *Child Dev*. 1980;51:981-992.

158. Butler C. Effects of powered mobility on self-initiated behaviors of very young children with locomotor disability. *Dev Med Child Neurol*. 1986;28:325-332.

159. DeLateur B, Berni R, Hangladarom T, et al. Wheelchair cushions designed to prevent pressure sores. *Arch Phys Med Rehabil*. 1976;57:129-135.

160. Borjeson MC, Lagergren JL. Life conditions of adolescents with myelomeningocele. *Dev Med Child Neurol*. 1990;32:698-706.

161. Selber P, Dias L. Sacral level myelomeningocele: long term outcome in adults. *J Pediatr Orthop*. 1998;18:423-427.

162. Buran CF, McDaniel AM, Brej TJ. Needs assessment in a spina bifida program: a comparison of the perceptions of adolescents with spina bifida and their parents. *Clin Nurse Spec*. 2002;16(5):256-262.

163. Sawin KJ, Brei TJ. Health risk behaviors in spina bifida: the need for clinical and policy action. *Dev Med Child Neurol*. 2012;54(11):974-975.

164. Dias LS, Fernandez AC, Swank M. *Adults with spina bifida: a review of seventy-one patients*. Paper presented at: The American Academy of Cerebral Palsy and Developmental Medicine; 1987; Boston, MA.

165. Dunne KB, Shurtleff DB. *The medical status of adults with spina bifida*. Paper presented at: The American Academy of Cerebral Palsy and Developmental Medicine; 1987; Washington, DC.

166. Moore C, Kogan BA, Parekh A. Impact of urinary incontinence on self-concept in children with spina bifida. *J Urol*. 2004;171(4):1659-1662.

167. Lobby NJ, Ginsburg C, Harkaway RC, et al. Urinary tract infections in adult spina bifida. *Infect Urol*. 1999;12(2):51-55.

168. Campbell JB, Moore KN, Voaklander DC, et al. Complications associated with clean intermittent catheterization in children with spina bifida. *J Urol*. 2004;171(6, pt 1):2420-2422.

169. McLone DG. Spina bifida today: problems adult face. *Semin Neurol*. 1989;9:169-175.

170. Iddon JL, Morgan DJR, Loveday C, et al. Neuropsychological profile of young adults with spina bifida with or without hydrocephalus. *J Neurol Neursurg Psychiatry*. 2004;75:112-118.

171. Barf HA, Verhoef M, Jennekens-Schinkel A, et al. Cognitive status of young adults with spina bifida. *Dev Med Child Neurol*. 2003;45(12):813-820.

ADDITIONAL RESOURCES

Developing child. Harvard.Edu/topics/understanding intervention (research and topics of interest about the benefits of early intervention).

- Scherzer A, Tscharnuter I. *Early Diagnosis and Therapy in Cerebral Palsy*. Marcel Dekker; 1982 (handling strategies for young children).
- Williamson GG. *Children with Spina Bifida: Early Intervention and Pre-School Programming*. Brooks Publishers; 1987 (family concerns and PT/OT interventional strategies).
- Zabel TA, Linroth R, Fairman AD. The Life Course Model Website: an online transition-focused resource for the Spina Bifida community. *Pediatr Clin North Am*. 2010;57(4):911-917.

SOURCES FOR LATEX INFORMATION

American Latex Allergy Association. https://www.allergyhome.org/blogger/the-american-latex-allergy-association-and-latex-allergy/
Food and Drug Administration. www.fda.gov
Spina Bifida Association of America. www.spinabifidaassociation.org

Traumatic Brain Injury

Alison Kreger

» Definition

Traumatic brain injury (TBI) occurs when an external, mechanical force either accidentally or intentionally impacts the head.[1–4] It is not associated with congenital injury or degenerative insult. TBI is characterized by a period of diminished or altered consciousness that ranges from brief lethargy to prolonged unconsciousness to brain death.[1,2,4] Symptoms vary greatly depending on the location of the lesion and the extent of the underlying brain injury. Although approximately 97% of the children who sustain a TBI experience only a mild injury and recover uneventfully, others are left with partial or total functional disability and/or psychosocial impairment.[5] TBI is also referred to as acquired brain injury, head injury, or closed head injury.

» Incidence

In recent years, the number of visits to the emergency room (ER) by children with a suspected head injury has increased to approximately 2.87 billion each year.[4] Overall, brain injury is the leading cause of death and permanent disability in children between 1 and 19 years old.[6] It is also the third leading cause of death in children younger than 1 year of age. In spite of this, the survival rate in children with TBI is better than that in similarly injured adults.[7,8]

Currently, there are two peak periods of incidence of TBI in children that should be monitored. The first occurs in early childhood (younger than 4 years of age) and the second occurs during mid to late adolescence (15 to 19 years of age).[7,9] In every age group, the incidence of TBI is two times greater in boys than in girls, with boys between 0 and 4 years of age having the highest number of hospitalizations and TBI-related deaths.[1,7,10,11–13] Premorbid personality and behavior have been found to predispose children to brain injury.[14] Children who are impulsive and hyperactive, and who have difficulty with attention, are at an increased risk for injury.[14,15] In addition, there is evidence that once a child sustains a TBI, even a mild TBI, the likelihood of reinjury and a lower threshold for damage to the brain increases.[16,17]

Brain injury and death rates vary considerably by race and socioeconomic status. TBI-associated mortality rates are higher in African Americans, followed by Caucasians and then other races.[5,18] For all races, death rates are inversely related to socioeconomic status.[18] Thus, children of families with low incomes have higher death rates than do children of families with upper and middle incomes.

» Causes of injury

Falls

Falls are the leading cause of hospitalization in all pediatric TBIs that require hospitalization or result in death.[1,4,7,18–20] Children younger than 12 months were at the greatest risk of injury from a fall, with 0- to 6-month-olds sustaining the highest rate of moderate injury from falls, including falls from a caregiver's arms.[21] Among preschoolers, 51% of the trauma injuries from falls occur while playing on playground equipment.[18] Older children usually escape severe injury in falls from heights of less than 10 feet.[18,22] Although many falls occur accidentally, falls of less than 10 feet bear investigation for potential child abuse.[18,22]

Motor Vehicle Accidents

Motor vehicle accidents (MVAs) are the leading cause of hospitalization in adolescents and those aged 14 to 44 years old.[4] Between 4 and 14 years of age, the majority of injuries involving a motor vehicle occur when the child is a bicyclist or pedestrian.[9] In contrast, the majority of motor vehicle injuries sustained during adolescence occur when the adolescent is an unprotected occupant in the automobile.[9] MVAs cause the vast majority of serious injuries and multiple trauma in children, with approximately 70% of the children demonstrating various degrees of coma for some time.[18]

Gunshot Wounds

Firearm injuries occur from accidental gun discharges, homicides, and suicides, and they rank second only to MVAs as the leading cause of trauma death in school-age children and adolescents.[23] The incidence of gunshot wounds among male inner-city youth is extremely alarming, because the children are often both the victims and the perpetrators.[24] More than twice as many children survive their injuries as die, with approximately 25% having permanent sequelae.[25]

Abuse/Assault

Physical abuse in infants and young children is prevalent in children 0 to 4 years old.[7–9,19] Approximately 28% of ER visits due to TBI in children younger than 17 years old are due to the child being struck by or against an object.[4] Abuse frequently results in a head injury owing to the vulnerability of the immature brain and the weak supporting neck musculature, such as shaken baby syndrome. Abuse resulting in TBI is characterized by a marked discrepancy between the explanation of how the injury occurred and the nature and severity of the injury. Early identification of abuse is critical to prevent repeated or progressive injury.

Sports/Recreational Activities

Sports and recreational causes account for approximately 29% of the brain injuries to school-age children and adolescents.[18,20] High-risk contact sports, such as hockey, rugby, wrestling, football, boxing, and taekwondo, result in up to half of the injuries.[18,20,26,27] TBI is also seen in other recreational activities when head protection is either not used or forgotten, including in diving, baseball, cycling, horseback riding, and rugby.[13]

» Mechanisms of injury

Acceleration–Deceleration Injuries

Acceleration–deceleration injuries are caused when a moving head hits a relatively fixed object, such as the ground or a windshield, or sustains a high-speed change from acceleration to deceleration. This can lead to coup or contrecoup brain contusions against the skull. The young infant is particularly susceptible to acceleration–deceleration injuries, because there is less restraint of motion in the neck owing to musculoskeletal development.[28,29] Therefore, acceleration–deceleration injury in infancy may result in greater differential displacement of the skull and cranial contents potentially causing shearing injury.[28] The direction of acceleration injuries may be translational (linear) or rotational (angular). Most TBIs are a result of a combination of both translational and rotational injuries.

Translational Injury

In translational injury, the head in motion strikes a stationary object and responds with lateral displacement of both the skull and the brain. The injury that results from the initial impact of the skull on the brain is known as *coup*. The lesion that occurs in the direction opposite to the initial force is termed *contrecoup*. Contrecoup occurs because the brain decelerates against the bony structures of the skull.

Rotational Injury

Rotational injury occurs when the skull rotates as the brain remains stationary. The effect is angular forces on the brain, surface contusions, lacerations, and shearing trauma. Rotational injury can result in either focal or diffuse brain damage. These injuries can occur with MVA involving whiplash with rotation.

Impression Injuries

Impression injuries occur when a solid object, such as a rock or a blunt object, impacts a stationary head. Impression injuries produce skull fracture and a focal lesion at the site of the impact. The presence of a skull fracture is associated with an increased risk of intracranial injury; however, the absence of a skull fracture does not reliably exclude a significant intracranial injury.[30,31]

>> Primary brain damage from trauma

Primary brain damage from trauma is a direct result of the forces that occur to the head at the time of initial impact.[28,30–32]

Concussion

Concussion is a complex pathophysiologic process affecting the brain, and is characterized by headache, altered awareness and cognitive function, and impaired balance immediately following trauma.[33] Impaired consciousness typically lasts a few seconds to several hours, and is related to the transmission of stretching forces to the brainstem as the brain is thrown back and forth in the cranial vault.[34] Concussion can be seen without obvious pathologic changes to the brain; however, it may also be seen with mild diffuse white matter lesions or neurochemical injury.[34] Following concussion, a child may exhibit clinging behavior, disturbances in sleep, irritability, delayed response to others or in understanding, sensitivity to light, nausea, or more distractibility than usual. These behavior changes can last a few days to a few months.[33–35] Children and adolescents may take longer than adults do to recover after a concussion.[17]

Contusion

A contusion is a bruising or hemorrhage of the crests or gyri in the cerebral hemispheres. Contusion can be seen following a crush injury or blunt trauma, or during an inertial load injury, such as acceleration–deceleration of the brain within the skull.[36] Contusions occur most commonly in the frontal and temporal lobes of the brain because of bony irregularities in the cranial vault.[34]

Skull Fractures

Skull fractures are seen in both closed and open head injuries and compound head injuries. Linear comminuted fractures result from an impact with low-velocity objects, and depressed fractures generally result from an impact with higher velocity objects. Linear fractures can produce contusions, hemorrhage, and cranial nerve damage.[28,37] Depressed skull fractures of greater than 5 mm are considered significant.[28] Depressed fractures can produce herniation syndromes, contusions, lacerations, and cranial nerve damage.[28]

Intracranial Hemorrhages

Intracranial injury can occur with or without immediate loss of consciousness or skull fracture.[30,31] Two types of intracranial hemorrhage frequently seen following pediatric TBI are extradural and intradural hematomas. Signs of an intracranial hemorrhage may not appear initially on clinical examination.[31] The rate of blood collection and the location of the hematoma are related to severity and outcome.[38] Intracranial hemorrhage is a common cause of clinical deterioration and death in those who experience a lucid interval immediately after injury.

Extradural Hematomas

Extradural or epidural hematomas develop because of the tearing of an artery in the brain, primarily the middle meningeal artery and its branches. In children, epidural hematomas usually follow skull fracture or bending of the skull into the brain.[29,38] With unilateral epidural hematoma, there is often herniation of the temporal lobe.[39] Coma may ensue and cardiorespiratory arrest is possible. Other signs and symptoms include confusion, headache, nausea, vomiting, and confusion.

Intradural Hematomas

Intradural hematomas include subdural and intracerebral hematomas. Acute subdural hematomas occur secondary to injury of veins in the subdural space causing blood to accumulate as a space-occupying lesion. Subsequent recovery depends on both the time before hemorrhage evacuation and the extent of damage to underlying brain tissue.[29,38] Subdural hematomas are frequently seen with inertial injuries, and occur commonly in the temporal and frontal lobes.[34] Subdural hematomas are associated with higher mortality rates and poorer functional outcomes. Intracranial hematomas can result from trauma or rupture of a congenital vascular abnormality.[40] Very severe injuries may cause large intracerebral hematomas that can rupture into the ventricles, causing intraventricular hemorrhage.[29,34]

Diffuse Axonal Injury

Diffuse axonal injury (DAI) is a microscopic phenomenon, not commonly visible on computed tomography (CT) scan, due to acceleration–deceleration motion that causes shearing damage to white brain matter.[41] DAI is seen following rotational injury within the cranial vault.[28] The shearing trauma results in diffuse disturbance of cellular structures following TBI. DAI is associated with much of the significant brain damage seen in TBI, including sudden loss of consciousness, extensor rigidity of bilateral extremities, decorticate or decerebrate posturing, and autonomic dysfunction.[34]

» Secondary brain damage from trauma

Secondary brain damage from trauma evolves as a result of the pathophysiologic changes initiated by the primary trauma.[28,32] Research suggests that secondary brain damage from trauma develops over a period of several hours or days.[34] Secondary injuries account for a significant amount of the overall damage that occurs in TBI, and prevention of secondary brain damage is a major goal of the acute management of the child with TBI.[38]

Cerebral Edema

Perhaps the most frequently occurring cause of secondary injuries is cerebral edema. Unchecked cerebral edema accompanied by an increase in intracranial pressure (ICP) can lead to multiple cerebral infarctions, brain herniation, brainstem necrosis, and irreversible coma.[29,39] Controlling brain swelling is often difficult, and may require the use of a combination of the following techniques: narcotic sedation, diuretics, barbiturates, systemic neuromuscular paralysis, or hyperventilation.[38,39]

Intracranial Pressure

When a mass, such as a hematoma or cerebral edema, is present following TBI, ICP increases in response to the pressure exerted on the brain. Initial increases in ICP are accommodated by the mechanisms of the ventricular system.[39,42] However, when the compensatory mechanisms are no longer effective, ICP rises.

In infancy, increases in ICP will cause bulging of the fontanels and separation of the sutures. In children older than 5 years of age, as ICP rises, the contents of the cranial vault are forced downward through the foramen magnum.

This causes brainstem compression and may lead to drowsiness, difficulty breathing, and even cardiorespiratory arrest.[28] Prolonged increased ICP may lead to the development of posttraumatic hydrocephalus presenting with incontinence, spasticity, poor appetite, and seizure activity.[28,43,44]

Herniation Syndromes

Herniation syndromes result from displacement of the brain by an expanding lesion and cerebral edema. Depending on the location of the lesion, herniation can cause obstructive hydrocephalus, brain shift past midline, or brainstem compression.[34,45] Herniation can lead to neurologic deterioration of a grave nature, with resultant decreasing levels of consciousness, altered respiration, hypertonicity, hemiparesis, and decorticate posturing.[34]

Hypoxic–Ischemic Injury

The supply of oxygen and nutrients to the brain is dependent on adequate cerebral perfusion. Alterations in cerebral perfusion, raised ICP, or lack of oxygen to the brain may result in hypoxic–ischemic brain damage.[34] Ischemia frequently occurs in the tissue surrounding cerebral contusions or hematomas and ultimately leads to further brain damage. Severe hypoxic injury and diffuse axonal injuries are most likely to cause severe disabilities, including prolonged postcoma unawareness.[29,34,46]

Neurochemical Events

When trauma occurs to the brain, there is a disruption of the blood–brain barrier and a release of excitatory neurotransmitters and oxygen-free radicals into the blood system.[34] Oxygen-free radicals have an extremely toxic effect on the brain and are damaging to cell membranes and vessel walls.[47] The damage from oxygen-free radicals causes internal disruption of neuronal functioning and further brain damage.[47]

» Other consequences from brain damage

Hydrocephalus

Hydrocephalus can be differentiated as either communicating or noncommunicating type. In communicating hydrocephalus, all components of the ventricular system are enlarged, and ICP may only be intermittently elevated. Communicating hydrocephalus is seen in the vast majority of posttraumatic cases.[48,49] Noncommunicating hydrocephalus refers to enlargement of the ventricles of the brain owing to an obstruction of the flow and impaired absorption of cerebrospinal fluid.[49] Children with hydrocephalus may present with changes in mental status, lethargy, nausea/vomiting, headache, gait ataxia, and urinary incontinence.[48] Neurosurgical ventriculoperitoneal shunting procedures are performed in children with hydrocephalus to improve the flow and absorption of cerebrospinal fluid.[48,49]

Seizures

The occurrence of early posttraumatic seizures is more common in children than in adults, with an incidence of approximately 25% in children with a severe TBI.[50] Early posttraumatic seizures in children are frequently of a generalized onset type, such as grand mal and tonic–clonic seizures.[51] Partial or focal seizures and seizures of late onset are uncommon in children.[51] The frequency of seizure activity within the first year of TBI may be predictive of further recurrence.[51] Thus, children who do not experience a seizure within the first 2 years of injury are less likely to develop seizures at a later time.

Infections

Penetrating injuries, such as gunshot wounds and depressed skull fractures, carry an inherent risk of brain infection due to exposure of the neural tissue to the exterior environment. In addition, neurosurgical procedures to insert ICP monitors and shunts for increased cerebrospinal fluid also carry risk of brain infection. Two common infections following penetrating wounds are meningitis and brain abscess.[48] Meningitis may cause symptoms such as fever, headache, seizures, and confusion. Brain abscess may cause bulging fontanels, increased irritability, seizures, and projectile vomiting. The physical therapist (PT) can assist the medical team by monitoring for signs of infection such as fever, headache, confusion, neck stiffness, and signs or symptoms of increased ICP.

Dysautonomia

Dysautonomia, a malfunction of the autonomic system, occurs after brain injury in 13% of children.[52] A combination of fever, tachypnea, hypertension, tachycardia, diaphoresis, or dystonia are indicators of dysautonomia.[52] PTs should be diligent in monitoring the child for signs of dysautonomia to alert the medical team and best manage the symptoms noted. Dysautonomia is associated with poorer outcomes and the need for prolonged rehabilitation.[52]

Endocrine Disorders

Although rare, hypopituitarism and precocious puberty are both reported in children following TBI.[51] Hypopituitarism may present with delays for failed growth and delayed or arrested pubescent development, including amenorrhea, muscle fatigue, decreased energy, and decreased bone density.[53] Linear growth and weight are closely followed up so that the need for medical intervention may be determined. The PT should report any concerns of increased weight gain or the development of secondary sexual characteristics to the child's physician.

>> Predictors of injury severity and outcome

Clinical rating scales are used to standardize the description of patients with TBI, monitor progress, determine a general plan for appropriate medical intervention, predict outcome, and assist with clinical outcomes research.

Predicting recovery and outcome in children with TBI is complex. The rate of recovery following TBI often appears rapid in the first few months, but can continue throughout the 2 years after the injury. After the first year, the incidence of children continuing to demonstrate gains is greater in children with mild TBI; however, in children with severe injury, some improvement is also noted in the second and third years following injury.[54]

Outcomes are affected by a number of factors, including location and morphologic characteristics of the injury, complications that occur during the medical stabilization following the injury, the age of the child at the time of the injury, the length of coma, the duration of posttraumatic amnesia (PTA), the severity of the injury, premorbid psychological and cognitive adjustment, and the family response to the injury. Pupillary response at admission and occurrence of hypothermia were also found to be important factors in determining outcomes post TBI.[29]

Coma Scales

Coma is defined as a complete state of unconsciousness in which the child does not open his or her eyes, follow commands, speak, or react to painful stimuli.[55] To assist with determining the level of unconsciousness, Glasgow neurosurgeons Teasdale and Jennett developed a coma assessment scale (Table 11.1), known as the Glasgow Coma Scale (GCS).[55,56] It is a standardized tool for assessing the neurologic status of a trauma victim and is based on the patient's best response to three categories: motor activity, verbal responses, and eye-opening. For children younger than 2 years old, the Pediatric Glasgow Coma Scale (PGCS) has been developed.[57]

The Pediatric Coma Scale (PCS)[58] has also been found useful in the assessment of outcome in children (Table 11.1) and is used in children 9 to 72 months of age.[58] In addition, the Adelaide Pediatric Coma Scale developed interpretive norms for several age groups between birth and 5 years old (Table 11.2).[28] Children whose coma scores were below the norm for age tended to have poorer outcomes.

Duration of Coma

The duration of coma is directly related to outcome, with outcomes worsening as coma duration increases.[59–61] For the majority of children with mild TBI and loss of consciousness lasting 1 night or less, the results on the long-term outcome measures of cognition, achievement, and behavior are indistinguishable from those of uninjured children.[62,63] In contrast, children with coma lasting more than a few days and moderate

TABLE 11.1.	Comparison of Glasgow Coma Scale and Adelaide Pediatric Coma Scale	
	Glasgow Coma Scale (Adults)	Adelaide Pediatric Coma Scale
Eyes open	Spontaneously 4	
	To speech 3	As in adults
	To pain 2	
	None 1	
Best motor response	Obeys commands 6	
	Localizes pain 5	Obeys commands 5
	Withdraws 4	Localizes to pain 4
	Flexion to pain 3	Flexion to pain 3
	Extension to pain 2	Extension to pain 2
	None 1	None 1
Best verbal response	Oriented 5	Oriented 5
	Confused 4	Words 4
	Words 3	Vocal sounds 3
	Sounds 2	Cries 2
	None 1	None 1

From Teasdale G, Jennett B. Assessment of coma and impaired consciousness. A practical scale. *Lancet*. 1974;2(7872):81–84 and Reilly PL, Simpson DA, Sprod R, et al. Assessing the conscious level in infants and young children: a paediatric version of the Glasgow Coma Scale. *Childs Nerv Syst*. 1988;4(1):30–33.

TABLE 11.2.	Age Norms	
0–6 mo		= 9
6–12 mo		= 11
12–24 mo		= 12
2–5 yr		= 13
>5 yr		= 14

For the Adelaide Pediatric Coma Scale Score.
Source: Kaufman BA, Dacey RG. Acute care management of closed head injury in childhood. *Pediatr Ann*. 1994;23:18-28.

to severe TBI experience a variety of physical, cognitive, language, and psychological sequelae that may improve following the injury or result in permanent impairment.

For children with TBI who had a coma with a duration of 1 week or more and survived, it should be noted that a return to regular education is usually not possible. Rarely do young children stay in a persistent state of coma. Ninety percent have been shown to recover to be moderately disabled or better over a 3-year period.[51]

Depth of Coma

In addition to the duration of coma, the depth of coma, as measured by the PGCS and GCS, is easy to assess and correlates well with prognosis and functional outcome.[61] Using the PGCS, a coma score of 3 or 4 is predictive of a poor outcome, whereas a score of 7 or greater is predictive of a good outcome.[31,64]

Most children who sustain mild brain injury, as determined by the coma scales, are expected to experience a full recovery within several weeks. However, new evidence suggests that following even a mild TBI some children experience problems with balance, response speed, and running agility that persist at discharge.[65] For children who are moderately and severely injured, the degree of initial impairment on a coma scale is related to both the degree of recovery and residual deficit.[66] Strong correlations of depth of coma and outcome severity have been noted, especially in the areas of intelligence, academic performance, and motor performance.[63]

Orientation and Amnesia Assessment

PTA is defined as the interval between injury and the moment at which an individual can recall a continuous memory of what is happening in the immediate environment.[67] Evaluation of PTA in children is challenging, because traditional assessment methods rely on the subject's verbal response. Because standard orientation questions are inappropriate for children owing to their limited cognitive and language skills, the Children's Orientation and Amnesia Test (COAT)[66] was developed. The COAT is reliable for children between the ages of 4 and 15 years.[66] Although the COAT is useful in the age range established, a reliable method of assessing PTA in children younger than 4 years of age has not been established.[68] The Sydney PTA scale has been developed for assessment of children aged 4 to 7 years old, and has been found valuable in indicating TBI severity and aiding in rehabilitation planning.[69]

Duration of Posttraumatic Amnesia

In children, the duration of PTA has been found to be more predictive of future memory function than of coma scales.[66,70] The length of PTA has also been used to classify the severity of TBI. In children with PTA of more than 3 weeks' duration, verbal and nonverbal memory was found to be significantly impaired at both 6 months and 12 months post injury.[66]

Rancho Los Amigos Levels of Cognitive Functioning

The Rancho Los Amigos Levels of Cognitive Function Scale (Rancho Scale)[71] is a descriptive scale of cognitive and behavioral functioning. It is used primarily during inpatient rehabilitation. The Rancho Scale summarizes neurobehavioral function and serves to enhance communication between staff. The Rancho Scale is also useful as a framework for the PT to identify probable treatment issues and to develop treatment strategies on the basis of the current level of cognitive function. The main limitation of the Rancho Scale is that the phases of recovery and prediction of discharge functional ratings are often poorly related. In addition, cognitive function and behavior may fluctuate depending on the environment as well as on fatigue or stress on any given day (see Display 11.1). Predicted outcome is difficult to determine because of the fact that patients may plateau at any point in time at any stage.

DISPLAY
11.1   Rancho Los Amigos Levels of Cognitive Functioning

I. *No response:* Patient appears to be in a deep sleep and is completely unresponsive to any stimuli.

II. *Generalized response:* Patient reacts inconsistently and nonpurposefully to stimuli in a nonspecific manner regardless of stimulus presented. Responses may be physiologic changes, gross body movements, and/or vocalization, and these are often limited and delayed. Often, the earliest response is to deep pain.

III. *Localized response:* Patient reacts specifically but inconsistently to stimuli. Responses are directly related to the type of stimulus presented. May withdraw an extremity and/or vocalize when presented with a painful stimulus. May follow simple commands such as closing eyes or squeezing hand in an inconsistent, delayed manner. May also show vague awareness of self-discomfort by pulling at nasogastric tube, catheter, or resisting restraints. May show a bias responding to familiar persons. Once external stimuli are removed, may lie quietly.

IV. *Confused-agitated:* Patient is in a heightened state of activity, and agitation is generally in response to own internal confusion. Behavior is bizarre and nonpurposeful relative to the immediate environment. Verbalizations frequently are incoherent and/or inappropriate to the environment. May cry or scream out of proportion to stimuli; and, even after removal, show aggressive behavior, attempt to remove restraints or tubes, or crawl out of bed. Gross attention to the environment is very brief; selective attention is often nonexistent. Patient lacks any recall. Has severely decreased ability to process information and does not discriminate among persons or objects; is unable to cooperate directly with treatment efforts. Unable to perform self-care without maximal assistance. May have difficulty performing motor activities such as sitting, reaching, and ambulating on request.

V. *Confused-inappropriate:* Patient is able to respond to simple commands fairly consistently. However, with increased complexity of commands or lack of any external structure, responses are nonpurposeful, random, or fragmented. Demonstrates gross attention to the environment, but is highly distractible and lacks ability to focus attention on a specific task. With structure, may be able to converse on an automatic level for short periods of time. Verbalization is often inappropriate and confabulatory. Memory is severely impaired; often shows inappropriate use of objects; and may perform previously learned tasks with structure but is unable to learn new information. Responds best to self, body, comfort, and family members. May show agitated behavior in response to discomfort or unpleasant stimuli. Can usually perform self-care activities with assistance. May wander off, either randomly or with vague intentions of "going home."

VI. *Confused-appropriate:* Patient shows goal-directed behavior, but is dependent on external input or direction. Response to discomfort is appropriate and is able to tolerate unpleasant stimuli when need is explained. Follows simple directions consistently and shows carryover for relearned/newly learned tasks such as self-care. Responses may be incorrect owing to memory problems, but they are appropriate to the situation. Past memories show more depth and detail than recent memory does. No longer wanders and is inconsistently oriented to time and place. Selective attention to tasks may be impaired. May have vague recognition of staff; has increased awareness of self, family, and basic needs.

VII. *Automatic-appropriate:* Patient appears appropriate and oriented within the hospital and home settings; goes through daily routine automatically but frequently robot-like. Patient shows minimal to no confusion and has shallow recall of activities. Shows increased awareness of self, body, family, food, people, and interaction in the environment. Has superficial awareness of, but lacks insight into, condition; decreased judgment and problem solving. Lacks realistic ideas/plans for the future. Shows carryover for new learning but at a decreased rate. Requires supervision for learning and safety purposes. With structure, patient is able to initiate social or recreational activities.

VIII. *Purposeful-appropriate:* Patient is able to recall and integrate past and recent events and is aware of and responsive to the environment. Shows carryover for new learning and needs no supervision once activities are learned. May continue to show a decreased ability relative to premorbid activities, abstract reasoning, tolerance for stress, and judgment in emergencies or unusual circumstances. Social, emotional, and intellectual capacities may continue to be at a decreased level but functional in society.

From Malkmus D, Booth B, Kodimer C. *Rehabilitation of Head Injured Adult: Comprehensive Cognitive Management.* Downey, CA: Los Amigos Research and Education Institute, Inc; 1980:2.

Pediatric Rancho Scale

The Pediatric Rancho Scale[72] is an adapted version of the Rancho Los Amigos Scale that can be used to evaluate young children between the ages of infancy and 7 years. Similar to the Rancho Scale, the Pediatric Rancho Scale serves to enhance communication of recovery among staff and to assist with developing a framework for treatment management on the basis of the child's cognitive level (see Display 11.2).

Age

The capacity of the brain to guard against and respond to trauma changes with age.[29,58] Although at one time, young children were thought to be spared greater dysfunction following TBI, newer research has demonstrated an increased vulnerability in the young child to the effects of TBI.[29,73–75]

The age of the child at the time of injury also appears to correlate with increased risk for specific impairments.[76] Young children are more vulnerable to the effects of diffuse injury on memory than are older children. Although the plasticity of the developing brain can allow for dramatic recovery of motor function, the effects of a diffuse insult produced by TBI may ultimately result in greater cognitive impairment in the developing brain than in the mature brain.[73,76] Children who experience TBI before the age of 5 years exhibit more profound cognitive deficits than those injured later in

DISPLAY
11.2   **Pediatric Rancho Scale**

V. *No response to stimuli:* Complete absence or observable change in behavior to visual, auditory, or painful stimuli.

IV. *Generalized response to sensory stimulation:* Reacts to stimuli in a nonspecific manner; reactions are inconsistent, limited in nature, and often the same regardless of stimulus present. Responses may be delayed. Responses noted include physiologic changes, gross body movement, or vocalizations. First responses are often to pain. Gives generalized startle to loud sounds. Responds to repeated auditory stimulation with increased or decreased activity. Gives generalized reflex response to painful stimuli.

III. *Localized response to sensory stimuli:* Reacts specifically to stimulus. Responses are directly related to the type of stimuli presented. Responses include blinking when strong light crosses the field of vision, following a moving object passed within the visual field, and turning toward or away from loud sound or withdrawing from painful stimuli. Reactions can be inconsistent and delayed. May inconsistently follow simple commands such as "close eyes" or "move an arm." May show vague awareness of self by pulling at tubes or restraints. May show a bias by responding to family and not others.

II. *Responsive to environment:* Appears alert and responds to name. Recognizes parents or other family members. Imitates examiner's gestures or facial expressions. Participates in simple age-appropriate vocal play/vocalizations. Gross attention but highly distractible. Needs frequent redirection to focus on tasks. Follows commands in an age-appropriate manner and is able to perform previously learned tasks with structure. Without external structure, responses may be random or nonpurposeful. May be agitated by external stimuli. Increased awareness of self, family, and basic needs.

I. *Patient is oriented to self and surroundings:* Shows active interest in environment and initiates social contact. Can provide accurate information about self, surroundings, orientation, and present situation as appropriate to age.

From Professional Staff Association of Rancho Los Amigos Hospital I. *Rehabilitation of the Head Injured Child and Adult: Pediatric Levels of Consciousness, Selected Problems.* Downey, CA: Rancho Los Amigos Medical Center, Pediatric Brain Injury Service and Los Amigos Research and Education Institute, Inc; 1982:5–7.

childhood.[21,76] Moreover, deficits may remain hidden until a time in which the child needs to participate in higher level academic activities.

Function

In spite of improvement in function over time, children with TBI persist in exhibiting lasting differences in balance, gait velocity, stride length, and cadence when compared with healthy peers.[75,77] Even children with a mild TBI have shown problems with balance on the Bruininks Pediatric Clinical Test of Sensory Integration for Balance and the Postural Stress Test at 12 weeks post injury.[78] Such information should be taken into consideration when predicting a return to sports and physical activities that require refined balance skills.

Functional limitations and impairments may also be used to predict discharge status for children with TBI.[79,80] The Pediatric Evaluation of Disability Inventory (PEDI) is used for classification of recovery of function following TBI, and may assist in facilitating optimal service delivery. During admission to a rehabilitation unit, the recovery of walking is a primary goal for children with TBI.[81] Knowing whether the child can ambulate by discharge impacts decisions regarding the discharge environment and the equipment needs at discharge. Four factors associated with a nonambulatory status at discharge include prolonged loss of consciousness, lower extremity (LE) injury, impaired responsiveness, and presence of LE spasticity.[81] In addition, low scores on the PEDI Mobility Functional Skills Scale and a long length of stay were also associated with being nonambulatory at discharge.[81]

Environmental Influences

Children with TBI may be particularly vulnerable to the influence of family dynamics. In families of children between the ages of 6 and 12 years, it has been shown that greater parental distress and burden was associated with poorer fine motor dexterity, behavioral control, and academic performance.[77,82] The negative consequences of the TBI combined with high levels of family dysfunction make it more difficult for the family to support the child's recovery. PTs should consider the influence of the home environment in the prognosis for improvement in the child with TBI, and could include using the Family Assessment Device General Functioning (FAD-GF) Scale to aid in the process.[77]

» Physical therapy examination of the child with traumatic brain injury

When a child with TBI is referred for treatment, a thorough physical therapy examination is necessary to ensure appropriate physical therapy management. The examination (Display 11.3) should contain, but may not be limited to, information on past medical history, etiology of injury, social history and living environment, cognitive/behavioral status, basic sensorimotor status, sensory tolerance, and functional status. While performing the examination, consideration should be given to the child's tolerance level to physical and

DISPLAY
11.3   **Physical Therapy Examination Format**

Medical History

Onset and mechanism of injury (including time frames)

Diagnostic test results (CT scan, MRI, radiographs)

Medical precautions (weight bearing or ROM precautions)

Vital signs

Autonomic nervous system function (history of orthostatic hypertension or dysautonomia)

Social History and Living Environment

Family and support system

Educational/prevocational status

Cognitive/Behavioral Status

Level of arousal

Orientation

Attention

Behavior/affect

Basic Sensorimotor Status

Hearing/auditory processing

Vision, perception, and visuospatial ability

Sensation (light touch, vibration, pain, temperature)

Range of motion

Strength

Muscle tone

Abnormal movement patterns, posture, and reflexes (pathologic reflexes, deep tendon reflexes)

Balance and balance strategies (sitting and standing)

Praxis and coordination

Speed of movement

Endurance

Functional Status

Bed/floor mobility

Transfers/transitions

Sitting and standing skills (static and dynamic)

Ambulation on level surfaces (supports needed)

Stair ascension/descension (supports needed)

Ambulation outside/rough terrain (supports needed)

Advanced gross motor skills/sports

Generalization of functional abilities

Skin integrity

Respiratory status

Bowel and bladder status

Dysphagia status

Medications

Cultural issues

Discharge environment

Memory

Language/communication (productive and receptive)

Executive functions

Neuropsychological or psychological assessments

cognitive input and attention span, because deficits may limit the PT's ability to complete the examination in one session. The PT may also need to incorporate play into the assessment in an effort to enhance cooperation and obtain a more accurate picture of the child with TBI.

Subjective Examination: Patient History

Medical History

The PT should thoroughly review the child's past medical/surgical and current condition before initiating the physical examination. Information should be gathered regarding the mechanism of the injury, severity of damage, and significant changes in the clinical picture over time. The child's history of prior concussions or other cognitive issues should be noted. Particular attention should be given to reports from CT scans, magnetic resonance imaging (MRI) scans, radiographs, and other diagnostic tests.

Social History and Living Environment

Interviewing the parents, siblings, and/or caregivers of the child with TBI is important, because successful therapeutic intervention should be family- and child-centered.[83] The family members are the experts in knowing their child and often can give helpful advice to the therapist regarding the best way to motivate the child in therapy. In addition, information can be gained regarding the conditions and limitations of the home environment, including supports available at home and the physical accessibility of the home. Families should be encouraged to collaborate with the rehabilitation team in the development of an appropriate plan of care and the identification of equipment needs upon discharge. Family or psychosocial information may also be gained by talking to the social worker.

Systems Review

A thorough review of all body systems helps the PT decide which systems will require further testing and often directs the selection of subsequent tests (see Display 11.4). During this review, information that was not noted in the initial history may be obtained and used to inform further examination of concerns.

Objective Examination: Tests and Measures

Children who sustain TBI may experience a complex array of deficits in body structures and functions in physical abilities, emotional development, and cognitive/behavioral functioning (Display 11.5).[77,82]

Cognitive/Behavioral Status

A comprehensive cognitive examination is beyond the scope of practice of the PT. However, cognition should be grossly examined by the PT to assist in determining realistic

Is the patient experiencing any of the following?
  General: Fatigue, sleep disturbance, appetite change, personality change
  Cardiopulmonary: Irregular heart rate or rhythm, blood pressure fluctuations, edema, dyspnea, ventilator use, sputum production, orthostatic hypotension
  Integumentary: Color changes, abrasion, bruising, decubitus ulcer, infection
  Musculoskeletal: Pain, stiffness, swelling, joint limitation
  Neuromuscular: Headache, seizures, spasticity, hypertonicity, hypotonicity, flaccidity, weakness, tremor, gait disturbance, balance loss
  Communication, language, affect, and cognition: Inability to make needs known, altered consciousness, disorientation, memory loss, affect changes, behavioral changes, inability to understand what is said or instructions

treatment goals and appropriate interventions. Physical therapy examination of cognition may include the following areas: arousal/orientation, attention span and focus, behavior/affect, short- and long-term memory, communication, mental flexibility, problem solving, judgment, and insight.

LEVEL OF AROUSAL/ORIENTATION Trauma that damages the frontal lobe and brainstem may result in impairment of arousal and orientation in the child with TBI. In addition, medications used to diminish muscle spasticity, seizures, or pain may decrease arousal.[39] This arousal impairment may be expressed as lethargy, drowsiness, or even coma. Decreased levels of arousal will interfere with the child's ability to attend to pertinent stimuli, follow commands, and benefit from feedback in therapy. The Pediatric Ranchos

Scale can be used to assess arousal and track changes through rehabilitation. Recognizing that children may plateau at any phase of the Scale is important.

ATTENTION Trauma to the frontal lobe may impair attention in the child with TBI. Impairment of attention may affect both the ability to attend to a specific stimulus and to sustain attention over time. Children with TBI who have problems with attention often have difficulty following commands and relearning motor tasks; thus, the impairment may be expressed as distractibility or inattention. This is especially noted when therapy is conducted in busy environments with many distractions. Care must be taken to structure the environment and remove extraneous stimuli as appropriate. Breaking activities down into parts before joining skills together into a full functional task, at times, can help prevent the child from becoming fatigued or frustrated. Working within the child's endurance and tolerance will help facilitate learning and participation.

BEHAVIOR/AFFECT After a TBI, children may display a wide array of problems in behavior and affect (see Display 11.5). Two common changes in behavior noted during the time of rehabilitation are agitation and confusion. Agitation is characterized by a heightened state of activity and a severely decreased ability to process stimuli from the environment in a useful manner. The child who is agitated may be restless, irritable, and combative. Impulsivity and unsafe behavior may be observed because the child acts before thinking and is not paying attention to his or her surroundings. Fortunately, agitation in children with TBI does not last as long as the agitated phase of recovery in adults with TBI.[84]

Behavior Management Confusion is characterized by general disorientation and inability to make sense out

Physical	Emotional	Cognitive/behavioral	Functional
Headaches	Mood swings	Decreased arousal	Limited bed mobility
Dizziness	Denial	Disorientation	Limited transfers
Visual disturbance	Anxiety	Distractibility	Poor sitting control
Visuospatial impairment	Depression	Inattention	Poor standing control
Hearing loss	Irritability	Impaired concentration	Gait impairment
Sensory loss	Guilt/self-blame	Confusion	Impaired hygiene skills
Cranial nerve injury	Emotional lability	Agitation	Impaired dressing skills
Spasticity	Low self-esteem	Memory deficits/amnesia	Impaired feeding skills
Ataxia/incoordination	Egocentricity	Sequencing difficulty	Fine motor impairment
Balance impairment	Lability	Slowed processing	Sexual dysfunction
Fatigue	Apathy	Impaired judgment	Sleep disorders
Seizures	Impaired problem solving	Speech/language problems	Decreased academic skills

From Taylor HG, Yeates KO, Wade SL, et al. Influences on first-year recovery from traumatic brain injury in children. *Neuropsychology.* 1999;13(1):76–89.

of the surrounding environment. Confusion may persist through most of the rehabilitative process, exacerbated by memory loss. When problems with behavior persist and interfere with participation in therapy, it is important for the rehabilitation team to work together and implement a behavior modification program. Initially, the team must identify the unwanted behaviors and any precipitating factors, including environmental factors, that contribute to the behavior problem. Agitation may be precipitated by factors such as pain, occult fractures, restraints, urinary tract infections, constipation, and overstimulation by staff, family, and friends. Precipitating factors should be addressed before the implementation of the behavior modification program and be removed when possible.

Next, rewards and reinforcements for desired behaviors and a reward schedule should be determined. The child's family may be helpful in identifying rewards that are both motivating and satisfying. The reward schedule must be agreed on by the rehabilitation team to maximize compliance and promote the desired behavior. Once the rewards and schedule have been addressed, the team then moves toward redirecting the child to appropriate actions by praising approximations of the desired actions. Because the team works together to address the behavior problem in a consistent manner, the incidence of inappropriate actions may slowly decrease. Keep in mind that, in some cases, the environment cannot be modified and behavior management is ineffective. In that case, the managing physician may consider pharmacologic management.

MEMORY Memory impairment is the most common cognitive impairment in children with TBI.[85] Trauma to the temporal lobe commonly affects memory in children with TBI. Memory includes the ability to learn and recall new information as well as the ability to recall previously learned information. The presence of memory loss, or amnesia, is an indication that a concussion has occurred. The amnesia may be retrograde, involving a period of time before the accident, or anterograde, extending from the incident forward in time. The combination of time to follow commands and posttraumatic amnesia has been found to be predictive of functional, behavioral, and neurocognitive outcomes.[86]

Memory deficits involve verbal recall and visual recognition. They may appear as the inability to remember the sequence of motor tasks from one treatment session to another or as the unsafe performance of functional skills. The omission of safety-related behaviors when performing functional motor skills, such as transfers and ambulation, can limit independence.

Memory with respect to a child's ability to learn new material is of particular interest to the PT. Although retention of information learned before the TBI may remain unharmed, the memory to learn new information may be problematic. The results of a neuropsychological evaluation of a child's memory skills and capacity for new learning will be helpful in the establishment of realistic functional goals and the development of an appropriate rehabilitation program.[40] Information regarding memory

and the capacity to learn will play a part in the plan to return to school participation as well. Working jointly with the child's family, teachers, and psychologist, the PT may help determine the need for compensatory strategies, assistance, and environmental modification in the educational setting.

LANGUAGE Language deficits in the child with TBI are addressed in depth by speech and language pathologists. It is difficult to determine to what extent a child's language skills will be influenced by a TBI; some impairments do not become evident until the child is in school working to meet academic expectations.[87] Damage to the temporal lobe may result in expressive or receptive language deficits that will impede communication between the PT and the child, thus complicating therapy sessions. Receptive language deficits will impair a child's ability to understand verbal instructions for the performance of a gross motor task. When receptive language impairment exists, determination of the best means of communication may decrease the frustration of the child and the therapist. Expressive language disorders impair a child's ability to communicate with others. Although the child with an expressive language disorder may be able to fully comprehend verbally communicated information and form an appropriate response mentally, a breakdown occurs between the formulation of the response and the verbal or gestural execution of what was intended. Once again, the PT's knowledge of the child's most effective mode of communication may lessen the frustration related to the inability to communicate thoughts and feelings.[38]

EXECUTIVE FUNCTIONS Trauma to the prefrontal regions of the frontal lobes results in impairment of executive functions. Executive functions refer to the ability to show initiative, plan activities, change conceptual sets, solve problems, regulate behavior in social settings, and use feedback to initiate behavioral change and monitor success.[38,88]

Deficits in executive functioning may be demonstrated by impulsive behavior, resulting in failure to observe safety precautions or the inability to recognize when behavior is socially inappropriate.[38] The ability to make decisions with the executive function of decision making can be influenced in a variety of ways, including how the child processes information received from the environment.[88] Mental inflexibility may be demonstrated as perseveration on a task or the inability to change activities without becoming disorganized.[38] Difficulty switching conceptual sets may also influence the ability to perform tasks with alternating patterns or reciprocal movements.[88]

Sensorimotor Status

ABNORMAL MUSCLE TONE

Muscle Spasticity Because of damage to the cerebral cortex, children with TBI may present with muscle spasticity.[89] According to the American Association of

Neurological Surgeons, spasticity is defined as "a condition in which muscles stiffen or tighten, preventing normal fluid movement."[90] The increase in tone is velocity-dependent related. This abnormal increase in tone can be associated with TBI, spinal cord injury, stroke, and other neurologic diagnoses.[91] The degree of spasticity may range from mild to severe, with distribution that may be either unilateral or bilateral. Children who present with unilateral involvement display motor impairment and dysfunction similar to that of children with hemiplegic cerebral palsy. Children who present with bilateral involvement often have asymmetric distribution and movements dominated by primitive reflex activity. Spasticity is frequently assessed with both the Ashworth Scale and Modified Ashworth Scale. Research has shown interrater and intrarater reliability variance depending on the specific muscle and joint characteristics.[9]

Children with spasticity may also present with abnormal posturing of the extremities or the whole body. The upper extremities typically present with flexor synergy posturing. Flexor synergy posturing may interfere with hygiene and functional use of the upper extremity for play, schoolwork, and self-care. The lower extremities commonly present with extensor synergy posturing. Extensor synergy posturing may interfere with bed mobility, hygiene, transfers, and ambulation.

Children with TBI who are severely involved may present with whole-body posturing. Whole-body posturing can be decorticate (flexion of the upper extremities and extension of the lower extremities) or decerebrate (extension in all extremities) in nature and is frequently seen in the early stages of recovery. As the child improves, whole-body posturing is often replaced with more volitional movement, including movement utilizing abnormal synergistic patterns.

Ataxia Because of damage to the cerebellum and basal ganglia, children with TBI may experience ataxia, an incoordination of movement and balance. The distribution of ataxia can be unilateral or bilateral. Ataxia may initially be masked by spasticity in the early recovery period. Timing and execution of movement may be difficult, and oscillations during intention may be present and may worsen with task difficulty. Gait in children with ataxia is characterized by a wide base of support, increased loss of balance, and difficulty maintaining static stance. Ataxia is generally not associated with loss of range of motion (ROM) unless combined with spasticity.

Muscle Performance Impairment

STRENGTH LOSS After a TBI and loss of consciousness, children may remain in bed for a prolonged period. During that time, muscle weakness due to disuse atrophy may be expected.[92] Weakness is seen in both the agonist and antagonist muscle groups of a spastic extremity. Standardized manual muscle testing (MMT) may be difficult to perform, because the child with TBI may be unable to follow instructions for testing. Therefore, the PT must observe active movement in various tasks and judge the child's ability to dynamically move against gravity and statically sustain weight bearing. As cognitive function begins to return, the therapist can give simple commands and assess the ability to move during functional tasks such as sitting at the edge of the bed, rising from a seated position, and reaching overhead. Finally, in children with TBI who are older than 7 years of age, and who are able to follow directions, MMT using a handheld dynamometer can yield excellent within-session intrarater reliability for LE strength testing, whereas precision grip strength testing can be accurately used in children older than 5 years of age.[93,94]

IMPAIRED ENDURANCE Children with TBI often present with an overall state of lethargy. Fatigue in a child with TBI may be due to both physical and mental activities associated with motor planning. Both impair the child's ability to participate in activities of functional mobility and self-care. Scheduled rest breaks within sessions and rest between different therapies may help the child with TBI to sustain participation and build endurance. Education and incorporation of energy conservation techniques may help address endurance concerns during therapy and upon return home.

RANGE OF MOTION LOSS Because of the immobilization and stereotypic abnormal movement patterns used, such as synergistic patterns, children with TBI who present with spasticity are at risk for loss of active ROM and joint contracture development. Joints particularly at risk include the elbows, wrists, fingers, knees, and ankle–foot complex. ROM loss can occur quickly, and early management is the key to effective prevention.

BALANCE AND POSTURAL CONTROL LOSS After a TBI, a loss of balance is present in most children. Postural control may be affected by neurologic impairments, sensory disorganization, or biomechanical constraints. Research has shown that even in children with a mild TBI,[78] a loss of balance may prohibit safe participation in preinjury activities for 12 weeks or more postinjury.[95] Care must be taken to thoroughly reevaluate a child for postural control and tolerance of perturbations before allowing the child to safely return to the activity. Common functional tools include the Bruininks–Oseretsky Test of Motor Proficiency,[78] Pediatric Clinical Test of Sensory Interaction for Balance,[78] Postural Stress Test,[78] Modified Functional Reach test,[96] the Berg Balance Scale,[97] and the Timed Up and Go (TUG) test.[98-100]

Sensory Deficits

HEARING Hearing loss is also common in children with TBI.[101] All children with moderate to severe TBI should have a thorough audiologic evaluation to determine the presence of hearing loss. Audiologists may find children who have sustained a TBI to have ear aches, tinnitus, sound sensitivity, and hearing impairments. When hearing loss is present, hearing aids, a frequency modulated (FM) transmitter, or preferential classroom seating may be indicated.[68]

VISION Visual disturbances in children with TBI are common. These deficits may include decreased visual acuity, disturbances of visual pursuit and accommodation, visual field deficits, reduced depth perception, diplopia, transient cortical blindness, and retinal hemorrhages.[68] When visual problems exist, eye patching, glasses, or preferential classroom seating may help alleviate the difficulty.[68] Another option would be the implementation of vision therapy to aid the child in developing eye musculature and skills related to visual input processing, which may use such items as prisms, glasses, and high-contrast environments, to assist with vision.

Cortical blindness occurs in a healthy looking eye with damage to the neural occipital lobe. Transient cortical blindness lasting no longer than 30 days has been associated with nearly complete recovery of vision.[68] However, cortical blindness lasting more than 30 days generally carries a poor prognosis for children with TBI. Retinal hemorrhages in young children with TBI are strongly suggestive of child abuse.[102]

VISUOSPATIAL SKILLS Problems with vision are associated with changes in perception and visuospatial function. Such deficits are frequently associated with lesions in the temporal or occipital lobes of the brain. Visuospatial and perceptual deficits may impair gross motor performance and functional mobility skills, limiting the potential for functional independence. A figure-ground deficit, or the inability to distinguish a given form from the background, may make noting a change in terrain depth during gait training more difficult. Visuospatial deficits may also make activities of daily living, such as donning an orthosis, more difficult. A child with deficits in visuospatial memory may demonstrate difficulty developing a mental map of a familiar environment and consequently may have difficulty moving independently from place to place.[38]

Orthopedic Complications

HETEROTOPIC OSSIFICATION Heterotopic ossification (HO), the formation of mature lamellar bone in soft tissue, can occur in children and adolescents following a TBI.[103] The risk of incidence of HO is reported to be 20% and identified risk factors include age older than 11 years of age and a longer duration of coma.[103] HO commonly occurs at the elbow, shoulder, hip, and knee joint regions. Early signs of HO include decreased joint ROM and pain with movement, swelling, erythema, and increased warmth near the involved joint.

The use of physical therapy in the treatment of HO is controversial. Some studies have associated physical therapy and aggressive ROM exercises with HO formation as a result of local microtrauma and hemorrhage to the tissue.[104] In general, gentle but persistent ROM exercises and management of muscle spasticity with medications or nerve blocks

are imperative.[104] When HO results in significant functional impairment, surgical excision of the bone from the soft tissue is indicated. HO rarely results in functional impairment in younger children.[103] HO in older children and adults is associated with a poorer functional outcome.[105]

FRACTURES Fractures in the pelvis and lower extremities are commonly associated with the traumatic events causing pediatric TBI, yet surgical repair of fractures may be delayed until the child is medically stable. Postsurgical care may also be complicated by the decreased cognitive status of the child, especially when the child is alert, but confused and unable to follow a specific protocol. Therefore, the child must be closely monitored to ensure that proper alignment and weight-bearing status are maintained during functional activities.

Although radiographs identify major trauma to the extremities, care should be exercised by the PT in evaluating additional musculoskeletal complaints, because there is potential for minor trauma and occult fractures that were unidentified during the initial examination to be identified during the acute recovery phase. Particular attention should be given to persistent complaints and activities that are poorly tolerated.

Functional Measures

Early examination of function is difficult because of the compromised cognitive status of the child with TBI. As the child becomes more alert and appropriate in interactions in the clinic, the use of standardized measures, especially those that have shown sensitivity in measuring functional change, may be helpful. In infants, the Alberta Infant Motor Scale (AIMS) can assess gross motor function in children 0 to 18 months old,[106] whereas the Peabody Developmental Motor Scales can assess function in toddlers and preschoolers.[107] The WeeFIM (Functional Independence Measure)[108] can assess the development of functional independence in children with disabilities, including TBI, between the ages of 6 months and 7 years. The WeeFIM measures six domains of function: self-care, sphincter control, mobility, locomotion, communication, and social cognition. The adult FIM can be used with older children. The Bruininks–Oseretsky Test of Motor Proficiency[109] is also used to assess gross and fine motor functioning. It is standardized for children from 4.5 to 14.5 years old, but its use in younger children is questionable.

The Gross Motor Function Measure (GMFM) is designed to evaluate changes in motor performance over time. Although it is more commonly used in children with cerebral palsy and Down syndrome, there is evidence that it is valid in children after TBI.[110] As an alternative to the GMFM in children 8 to 17 years of age, early research indicates that the Acquired Brain Injury-Challenge Assessment (ABI-CA)[111] demonstrates challenges in gross motor activities that are beyond what the GMFM examines and can be used in children 7 years and older.[111] Specific use, however, has not been validated.

The PEDI[112] has also been developed as a functional assessment tool for children. It measures both capability and performance in the domains of self-care, mobility, and social function. The PEDI can be used in children between the ages of 6 months and 7.5 years. The ABI-specific PEDI subscales were constructed from the mobility, self-care, and caregiver assistance scales of the PEDI, and are being used to measure functional change in children with TBI. The Caregiver Assistance Self-Care subscale was more sensitive to measuring change than was the generic PEDI.[113] When interpreting changes in scores using the PEDI, it has been noted that change scores of approximately 11% appear to indicate meaningful clinical difference, and can be used in interpreting positive changes in group or individual scores on the PEDI.[114]

Children with severe TBI have been reported to exhibit a significantly reduced range of walking speeds (73 to 154 cm per seconds) when compared to typically developing peers (54 to 193 cm per seconds).[115] Periodic examination of walking speed should be performed during rehabilitation to monitor progress and to better understand the energy cost of walking. Specific measures such as the 2-minute walk test[116] and the shuttle walk–run[117] tests are helpful in examining children with higher functional levels, specifically for endurance during gait.

>> Evaluation, diagnosis, prognosis, and plan of care

Evaluation

After the examination is complete, the PT must consider all of the data collected and make judgments that will lead to the development of a plan of care. The therapist must weigh the evidence of observed impairments in body structures and function and activity limitations while considering the pathophysiologic condition of the brain injury and other physiologic processes associated with the trauma. In addition, the therapist should consider the environmental and personal factors that impact participation, such as the child's social support, school environment, and home environment. Evidence supports the notion that good family support can positively impact recovery and outcome.[56] Finally, the PT should consider the amount of time that has passed since the injury, interventions received, and progress made.

Diagnosis and Prognosis

Children with TBI and with long acute and rehabilitation stays and low functional gains are associated with greater levels of disability.[118] It has been found that LE hypertonicity, brain injury severity, and LE injury combined were critical predictors of ambulation ability after TBI.[119] In addition, dysautonomia (diagnosis based on fever, hypertension, tachycardia, dystonia, and/or diaphoresis) in children with TBI is associated with the need for prolonged rehabilitation and less improvement in motor scores during recovery.[52]

Plan of Care

On the basis of the physical therapy diagnosis, the PT should determine a plan of care for the child with TBI. The plan of care includes the prescribed treatment interventions, and long- and short-term goals designed to help the child achieve the desired outcomes. Goals should be written on the basis of identified impairments and limitations. Goals should be measurable and expressed in functional terms. Each short-term goal should be written as a component that leads to the accomplishment of the long-term goal. Time frames in which the goals will be achieved are dependent on consideration of the child's cognitive and behavioral status as well as projected length of stay and the care environment. Length of stay depends on a variety of factors, including rehabilitation intensity, FIM score at admission, length of acute care stay, and medical complications such as orthopedic injuries or brain bleeds.[120]

>> Management/interventions

Rehabilitation of children with TBI is different from that of adults with TBI in that the interventions used by the PT must incorporate age-appropriate gross motor challenges at the appropriate level of cognitive function. A number of rehabilitation approaches such as those used with adults post a stroke or children with cerebral palsy may be applied to children with TBI. Although the efficacy of various rehabilitation programs is not known, research is indicative of a positive trend in the benefit of rehabilitative services.[121]

Acute Medical Management

Early medical management of the child with TBI focuses on preservation of life, determination of injury severity, and prevention of secondary brain damage.[33] Once the vital signs are stabilized, the child will undergo a general assessment for potential injuries and a neurologic examination. These tests may include radiographic examination of the skull and cervical spine, CT scan of the head, and the use of the GCS.

Acute medical intervention in children with TBI may include emergency surgery, the use of mechanical ventilation, and the use of pharmacologic agents.[122] If a subdural or intracerebral hematoma is present, immediate neurosurgery is indicated.[34] A delay in performing the surgery can be life threatening, because it helps decrease ICP and reduce pressure-related secondary brain injuries.[34] Surgical interventions could include craniotomy and decompressive craniectomy.[123]

Mechanically assisted ventilation at a rate greater than normal or hyperventilation is used to temporarily reduce ICP.[38] In addition to hyperventilation, pharmacologic agents are also used to decrease cerebral edema and minimize secondary brain damage. Drugs commonly used in the management of edema include mannitol and corticosteroids.[38] Medications may also be used to induce paralysis when the child's body movements interfere with the stability of vital signs and the administration of further medical interventions.[38,122]

Physical therapy in the acute stage may be deferred until the child is medically stable. Once the child is stable, the PT can use the child's current level of cognitive functioning as a guide in planning interventions. It is important for the PT to remember that the cognitive levels of recovery serve only as a general guideline for recovery. Not all children will experience each level of cognitive recovery or progress through recovery in a strict hierarchical sequence. Either the Rancho Scale or the Pediatric Rancho Scale may assist with identification of current cognitive status, help track progression and changes in cognitive status, and help identify potential concerns for the future.

Acute Physical Therapy Management: Prevention

Physical therapy management for children with TBI functioning at low cognitive levels (Rancho Levels I to III and Pediatric Levels V to III) is aimed at the prevention of complications from prolonged inactivity and sensory deprivation. Common complications of prolonged inactivity may include skin breakdown, respiratory complications, and contracture development.

Contracture Management

The importance of preventing soft-tissue contractures in the acute recovery phase cannot be overemphasized. Dystonia is defined as a "movement disorder characterized by sustained or intermittent muscle contractions causing abnormal, often repetitive, movements, postures or both."[124] Dystonic extensor muscle overactivity is a major contributor to progressive ankle contractures, and the development of contractures will delay functional independence and lead to the need for additional therapy or even surgery later in the rehabilitative phase.[54] In a recent study, ROM, prolonged stretch through weight bearing in a standing frame, or tilt table combined with reeducation of functional movement patterns is effective in reducing contractures.[54] In addition to the use of a positioning program, ROM and the application of splints and casts may help improve LE function and prevent soft-tissue contractures.[54]

Contractures in prepubertal children who are not forcefully posturing may be successfully managed with positioning and splinting alone because of the child's smaller size and relative weakness.[66] Coordination of a wearing schedule is a key to enhancing the effectiveness of splinting. Wearing tolerance may be gradual, and the child must be monitored for signs of skin breakdown. In a larger child who is not forcefully posturing, serial casting followed by bivalved fiberglass cast splints may be used to manage contractures.

For children with severe extensor posturing who do not respond to a positioning program, splints, or bivalved casts, serial casts are warranted (Fig. 11.1).[66] These casts must be changed initially every 3 to 5 days to prevent skin breakdown

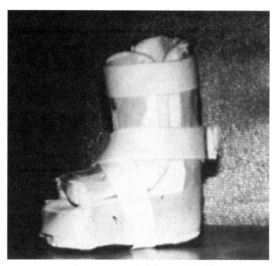

FIGURE 11.1. An example of a bivalved inhibitive cast.

and to allow for ROM monitoring.[54,125] Once it is determined that the child will tolerate the casts without skin breakdown, the casts can be worn for up to 3- to 4-week intervals until posturing diminishes and volitional control increases. Bivalved fiberglass cast splints may then be used at night to maintain ROM. If used during the day, an alternating schedule may be helpful before discontinuing use.[54,125] Continuous use of serial casts in a child who is alert and moving actively should not exceed 2 months to avoid deterring the child's independent mobility and self-care.

Serial casts may be used in conjunction with oral or injectable medications to manage spasticity. Oral medication, such as dantrolene (Dantrium), although useful in decreasing spasticity, is often undesirable because of its sedating properties.[72] Diazepam (Valium) can also be used for treating spasticity, but may be associated with increased agitation in children who are emerging from coma.[72] As an alternative, nerve and motor point blocks, such as phenol and Botox A injections, may be more desirable in the management of spasticity in children, because there are no sedating and cognitive side effects.[72,89] When injections are combined with traditional physical therapy, in some cases, pain levels decreased and functional gains were also noted in gait, transfers, grasping, and releasing.[125] Botox injections vary in how long they have an effect, but average about 3 to 6 months.[89]

Positioning

A positioning program will assist with improving pulmonary hygiene, increasing alertness, maintaining skin integrity, preventing contractures, and providing support for body alignment and movement. Positioning should be implemented with the assistance of the nursing staff and the family. Changes in position for the child confined in bed should be made every 2 hours. When the child is sitting, pressure relief procedures should be performed every 30 minutes, such as readjusting the body position, tilting the wheelchair seat backwards, or reclining the back of the chair.

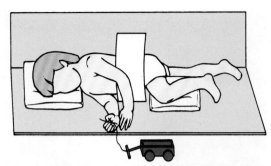

FIGURE 11.2. Child positioned in a side-lyer. Note that the head is maintained in line with the trunk, the upper extremities are in midline, and the lower extremities are dissociated. Gravity is eliminated, and the influence of primitive reflexes is minimized.

When designing a positioning program, the PT should take into consideration any orthopedic and neurologic positioning precautions as well as the influence of abnormal muscle tone and primitive reflexes on posture. Positioning in side-lying (Fig. 11.2) may be preferred to positioning in supine or prone because it is helpful to decrease the influence of abnormal primitive reflexes. Positioning in supine should incorporate strategies to reduce the influence of the tonic labyrinthine reflex and extensor tone. Positioning in prone, although allowable, will seldom be carried out at this phase of recovery because it interferes with accessibility for adequately monitoring the child's vital signs and medical status.

Upright positioning, even at an early stage of recovery, may be achieved with the use of a customized wheelchair (Figs. 11.3 and 11.4). The custom wheelchair may incorporate a tilt-in-space or reclining seating system with postural

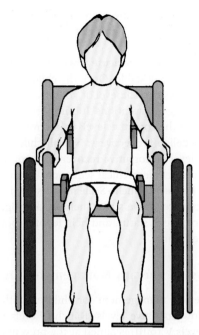

FIGURE 11.4. Child is sitting in a wheelchair with hip blocks and lateral trunk supports for assistance with postural control.

support (including lateral trunk supports and a pelvic strap) to assist the child in maintaining an upright position while preventing overfatigue. A removable headrest can be used to encourage head control when the child is alert and allow for support when the child is fatigued.

Low-Cognitive-Level Physical Therapy Management: Stimulation

Coma Stimulation Program

Coma stimulation programs were developed on the premise that structured stimulation could prevent sensory deprivation and accelerate recovery. However, controversy exists regarding the efficacy of stimulation used in the care of a comatose child.[126] The first step is to select appropriate sensory stimuli. Sensory input may be provided through the vestibular, visual, tactile, auditory, and olfactory systems (Display 11.6).[127] The rehabilitation team should involve the family in the selection of meaningful items to be used for stimulation to individualize the program. Emphasis should be placed on selecting items that reflect the child's age and development, culture, personality, likes/dislikes, hobbies, significant relationships, and pets. In addition, items that are selected should be reevaluated periodically, so that ineffective stimuli can be eliminated.

The next step in program development is to determine an appropriate schedule for stimulation. The PT needs to determine the time of day at which alertness is optimal to conduct therapy and modify the child's schedule as necessary. If this is not possible, the PT will need to modify the treatment goals within a given session and attempt to engage the child at the current level of arousal and attention.[38]

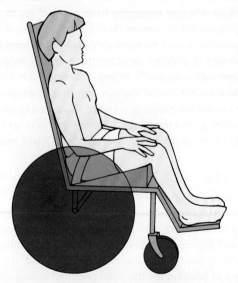

FIGURE 11.3. Child is supported in a wheelchair with a tall back and a seat wedge to maintain hip flexion. The back may be designed to sit upright and either recline or tilt in space to accommodate fatigue in the child.

DISPLAY 11.6	Sources of Sensory Stimulation			
Auditory	**Visual**	**Olfactory**	**Tactile**	**Vestibular**
Verbal orientation	Photographs	Vinegar	Hand holding	Turning
Music	Penlight	Spices	Rubbing lotion	Range of motion
Bells	Familiar objects	Perfume	Heat/cold	Sitting in chair
Familiar voice	Faces	Potpourri	Cotton balls	Tilt table
Tuning fork	Flashcards	Orange/lemon	Rough surfaces	
Clapping	Picture books		Familiar objects	

From Sosnowski C, Ustik M. Early intervention: coma stimulation in the intensive care unit. *J Neurosci Nurs.* 1994;26:336–341.

Before implementation, the PT will need to educate the family on the appropriate levels of sensory stimulation. An environment that is stimulating but not physiologically over-stimulating or noxious is ideal. Decreasing extraneous auditory and visual activity in the child's room or treatment area (such as fluorescent lighting or beeping monitors) may help elicit a response related to specific treatment stimuli.

At the beginning of the session, the PT should orient the child with TBI to who is conducting the session, the surroundings, and the current date and time. Stimulation should be brief and be implemented using one or two sensory modalities at a time while slowly presenting meaningful items. For the child who is unresponsive or responds only to pain, the initial goal of input is to elicit any type of response to stimuli. The PT should be patient and allow time for the child to respond because processing of sensory input may be delayed. A variety of responses may occur depending on the stimulation used (Display 11.7).[127] Precautions should be taken to ensure that the child's medical status remains stable following stimulation. Unfavorable responses to stimulation include agitation, the development of seizure activity, and sustained increases in heart rate, blood pressure, and respiratory rate.[127]

Once the child becomes more alert, the therapist should focus on increasing the consistency, duration, and quality of the child's response. If the vitals are stable, the program should be conducted in a supported sitting or standing position to improve alertness. Initial adjustment to upright may require blood pressure monitoring to avoid complications with orthostatic hypotension. As vital signs stabilize, all team members and the family should document the stimuli utilized and the child's response to note progress and assist with carryover.

As the child continues to attend in therapy and develop strength and endurance, the PT can work on the development of head and trunk control. Treatment progression could include one-step motor commands working to spontaneous upper extremity and LE movement patterns, such as reaching or stepping. The PT should monitor the child for signs of physiologic overload during treatment and make adjustments accordingly. Response should then be channeled into purposeful activity and functional skills, such as bed mobility and transfers. Family education about future recovery phases and possible treatment techniques should be incorporated into therapy.

Vegetative State

A vegetative state is characterized by an absence of response to external stimuli and an absence of attempts to communicate needs to others. Children in a vegetative state may have periods of eye-opening, sleep–wake cycles, and primitive reflexive movement of the limbs, but they do not demonstrate a response to pain or have self-awareness.[128,129] Families often have difficulty distinguishing between coma and persistent vegetative state because the outward presentation is similar. Persistent vegetative state is due to primary brain damage; therefore, the focus of care shifts from promoting functional movement to spasticity and contracture management, as noted earlier in acute care management.

DISPLAY 11.7	Common Responses to Stimulation			
Auditory	**Visual**	**Olfactory**	**Tactile**	**Vestibular**
Startle reaction	Eye blink	Grimacing	Posturing	Spasticity/movement
Localization	Visual localization	Tearing	Withdrawal	Assisted range of motion
Turn toward sound	Visual tracking	Head turning	Localization	Head righting
Follow commands	Visual attention	Sniffing	General response	

From Sosnowski C, Ustik M. Early intervention: coma stimulation in the intensive care unit. *J Neurosci Nurs.* 1994;26:336–341.

Mid-Cognitive-Level Physical Therapy Management: Structure

When the child has emerged from a coma (Rancho Levels IV and V and Pediatric Level II) and begins to participate in functional activities, other cognitive deficits may become evident. Selection of appropriate activities by the PT should be based on cognitive and physical demands, keeping in mind that the progression of cognitive and physical function can proceed at different rates. Children may progress or plateau during recovery, making the establishment of a prognosis difficult. This variability necessitates frequent reevaluation of the child post TBI and the services provided to ensure an appropriate match of cognitive ability and functional performance.

The Agitated Patient

Initially, agitation is in response to poor regulation of stimulation and internal confusion. Common factors that may contribute to agitation include overstimulation by staff, parents, and friends; restraints; confusion from amnesia; occult fractures; pain; constipation; and urinary tract infections. Agitation may be expressed as bizarre or aggressive behaviors. Clinicians should attempt to determine what stimuli increase agitation and attempt to reduce or eliminate the stimuli when possible. A child in a confused and agitated state requires the use of a highly structured environment to decrease the number of behavioral outbursts and prevent overstimulation and distraction. The PT may need to give verbal reassurance to the child with TBI because some agitated behaviors can be related to fear.

In the management of agitation, it is important to utilize a team approach that includes the family. Common management strategies include limiting distractions and noise, which could include having a quiet room with no television or telephone, limited visitors, and planned rest periods as needed. The child's family may resist suggestions to decrease visitors and stimuli, believing that talking loudly and turning on lights, television, and electronic device can help increase the child's alertness and participation in therapy. Staff should reinforce appropriate levels of stimulation during family education, educating the family in the process.

It is important to protect the child who is agitated from potential injury. Environmental evaluation is important to ensure a safe setting for the child. Restraints should be removed when appropriate because they may cause further agitation. If the unrestrained child is at risk for falling out of bed, it may be necessary to modify the room by placing the mattress on the floor or switch to an enclosed protective bed. Other protective devices include alarm devices, such as pressure-detecting seat cushions and doormats and monitor bracelets used for a child or adolescent who is ambulatory and may wander away from supervision.

During the agitated phase, treatment should include activities that are familiar to the child to enhance participation and cooperation. Appropriate tasks and activities include ROM exercises to the child's tolerance and functional gross motor activities such as rolling, transitioning to sit, standing up, and walking. Considering age appropriateness for the child may help guide selection of simple and complex activities to practice, from stacking blocks to navigating a simple obstacle course. It is important for the PT to work within the child's tolerance level on previously learned skills and to anticipate little to no carryover for new learning during this phase of recovery.

The child with TBI is often very unpredictable during the agitated phase, so the therapist should be prepared with several activity options. Choices of activities should be offered to the child when possible, helping provide the child with a sense of ownership in the rehabilitation process. When the child is uncooperative with familiar or routine activities, the PT should try to redirect the child to another therapeutic activity. If unsuccessful, the PT may need to resort to involving the child in any activity in which he or she is willing to participate. Therapy of this nature is still beneficial to the child with TBI because it may serve to increase alertness, attention span, and activity level.

For the child who is extremely difficult to manage, co-treatment with other team members and shortened therapy sessions may be necessary to help limit increasing the child's agitation. As attention span and endurance gradually increase, the PT can reinforce longer periods of attention and direct the child with TBI back to more challenging tasks.

The Confused Patient

Although no longer internally agitated, the child with TBI who is confused will require continued behavior management and structure during the therapy session to perform optimally. Structure may include decreasing the complexity of instructions, simplifying the environment with limited distractors, or simplifying the motor task (Figs. 11.5 and 11.6). The primary goal of therapy during the confused phase of recovery is to enhance successful participation in functional tasks.

In addition, the PT should give the child as much structure and assistance as necessary to allow for success. In children with serious deficits, partial weight-bearing locomotion shows promise for establishing an upright posture during the early stages of gait training.[130] As performance improves, structure can be decreased, and the child can be challenged to perform in a more complex environment.

When the child is confused, it is helpful to work on familiar activities so that the need for verbal instruction is reduced. When giving verbal instruction, the PT should keep directions simple. The PT should pause to allow for delays in processing verbal instructions. In addition, the PT may need to demonstrate new tasks or provide hand-on-hand guidance instead of providing the child with verbal explanations to enhance understanding.

Orientation is very important during the confused phase of recovery. The PT should remember to orient the child to his or her surroundings frequently and establish a familiar routine. Thus, the child may begin to work on recall skills

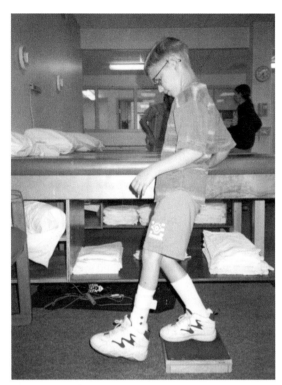

FIGURE 11.5. Stepping down off a small bench facilitates improved eccentric control of the lower extremity during knee extension.

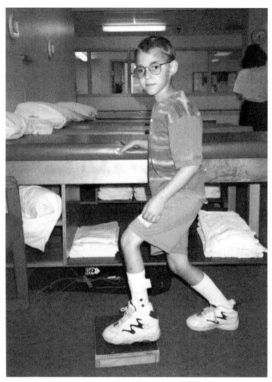

FIGURE 11.6. Lunges on the involved lower extremity enhance balance and may help improve hip and knee control.

and begin to anticipate what is going to happen next in the day. Familiarity and routine are calming and reassuring, and may assist with behavior management as well. Items such as a calendar, clock, and picture schedule may assist with orientation. In addition, the therapist may need to assist the child with topical orientation to his or her surroundings, including environmental scanning and assessment.

Encouraging the child to rely on his or her own memory for sequencing of movement or safety rules will challenge the child to become more independent. The use of a therapy journal or verbal and mental rehearsal may help improve the child's memory. However, the therapist should be careful not to frustrate the child who has difficulty remembering. Instead of a continued open line of questioning, the therapist may offer choices and see if the child can recognize the right response. For example, a child who is learning to transfer from a wheelchair may be asked whether he or she should scoot forward in the chair or lock the brakes first.

Although new learning is still limited, the PT can begin to integrate principles of motor control and motor learning with principles of therapeutic exercise to treat focal deficits, body structure impairments, and activity limitations. Types and scheduling of feedback and the structure of the activity (does it include manipulation, variability, whole-body movement?) integrates motor learning options into therapy. It is the PT's responsibility to select developmentally appropriate functional skills that are motivating and challenging, with the correct spatial and temporal demands for the child's

abilities. The PT should also focus on selecting functional activities that incorporate the use of both cognitive and physical skills. For example, an activity involving maneuvering a walker through an obstacle course addresses memory for verbal commands, motor planning, and mobility skills.

An essential element in motor learning is the opportunity for practice. The child with TBI should be allowed to experience movement with assistance as necessary, make mistakes, and make corrections as his or her ability levels dictate. Practice should encourage active participation in a meaningful play activity within the current capabilities of the child. Repeated practice will be necessary for the child to learn new or previously mastered gross motor tasks. Practice should be monitored to ensure that it is not the source of excessive frustration for the child. Current research suggests that the intensity of training is an important consideration in achieving positive outcomes in return of movement and increased PEDI mobility scores.[131] Although more intense programs often yield better return and higher scores, this must be balanced with awareness that children with TBI may display reduced endurance and increased fatigue with intense training both physically and cognitively. The therapist may need to provide rest breaks for the child both within the therapy session and in between therapies to maximize learning.

Determining the type of feedback to be used during therapy is another important consideration in promoting learning. The PT must make choices regarding the timing, precision, and frequency of feedback. In addition, the child's cognitive and sensory function will provide a guideline for determining the appropriate feedback mode. The types of feedback and scheduling are knowledge of results, knowledge of process, or blocked feedback. The more remedial the child is in the motor learning process, the more feedback the child may require from an external source. If a child is not aware of one side of his or her body, kinesthetic feedback may not be helpful to enhance learning, whereas visual and verbal feedback may be more appropriate (Fig. 11.7). Likewise, if a child is aphasic, the therapist will need to facilitate learning using visual and kinesthetic information.

As the child with TBI improves, the PT must modify the task and the environment to continue to engage the child actively in therapy. If persistent behavioral problems exist, it may be necessary for the PT to continue to use behavior modification techniques to increase compliance in therapy. At this stage of recovery, the child's judgment will be impaired, so it will be important to continue to protect the child from injuring himself or herself.

During both the agitated and the confused phases of recovery, the PT should continue the use of positioning, resting splints, and casting as needed to prevent contractures and maintain full ROM. Orthoses for standing and gait activities may also assist with control for balance and gait. The PT should be cautious to not overbrace or support, which may prevent strength development.

High Cognitive-Level Physical Therapy Management: School/Community Reintegration

Although research suggests that mobility outcomes achieved during the early stages of recovery are sustained and additional gains may be made within 6 months of returning home, it is important for the PT to remember that not all children will reach a high level of cognitive function (Rancho Levels V to VIII and Pediatric Level I) and have complete physical recovery.[131] Toward the end of the inpatient rehabilitation phase, persistent losses of cognitive and physical function become more apparent, and plans must be made to reintegrate the child with TBI back into the home and/or school setting with continued therapies. The family, medical rehabilitation team, and the school district must work together and jointly plan for reentry into the school setting. The PT may need to evaluate the child for orthoses, assistive devices, and mobility devices necessary for function in the child's home and at school. The child's family and teachers will need to be educated on the use of the recommended assistive and mobility devices. In addition, the PT may assist with recommendations regarding any environmental modifications to the child's home or school to help promote a safe environment that the child can function in as independently as possible.

For the child with TBI who does reach the higher stages of cognitive recovery, the PT will begin to wean the child

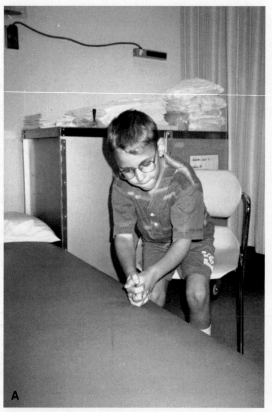
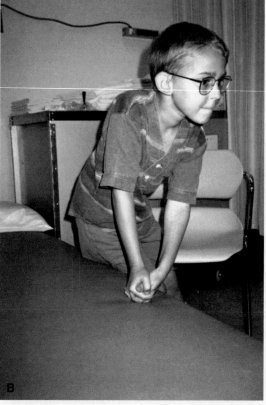

FIGURE 11.7. A, B: Verbal and visual cues to use hands in midline during transfers may enhance the awareness of the involved side and improve safety during movement.

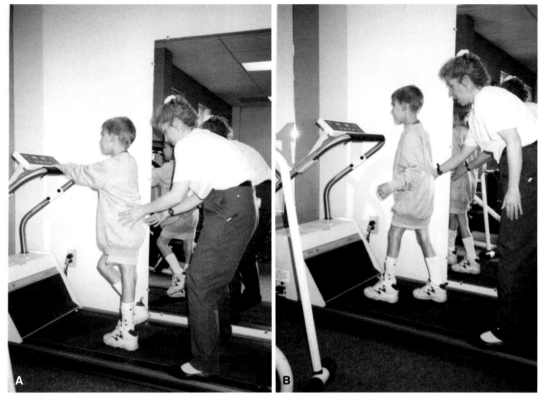

FIGURE 11.8. The use of a treadmill in gait training may facilitate control at various speeds. Training may be performed both with **(A)** and without **(B)** upper extremity support to challenge balance on a dynamic surface.

from the cues and structure previously used to enhance independence at home and/or school. Owing to the tendency of TBI to affect vision and hearing, memory, concentration, impulse control, and organizational skills, the classroom environment may be particularly difficult for the child with TBI.[66] Care should be taken to not remove the structure too early from complex environments because memory retention and generalization of learning in new settings occur at slower rates.

The PT should also continue to focus on treating any residual motor deficits that interfere with the child's development of typical motor skills and functional independence at home or in school. For some children, this will mean continued training with assistive devices and physical assistance for basic motor skills, such as transfers and gait[132] (Figs. 11.8 and 11.9). For others, contemporary treatments may be considered, such as body weight–supported treadmill training (BWSTT),[132,133] or constraint-induced movement therapy that shows promise for improving upper extremity function in children with TBI.[134]

Finally, for children who experience only subtle problems with balance and speed, coordination, timing, and rhythm of movement, participation in challenging physical activities such as balance exercises on a balance board or therapy ball (Figs. 11.10 and 11.11), obstacle course navigation, carrying objects, running, jumping, hopping, skipping, or recreational

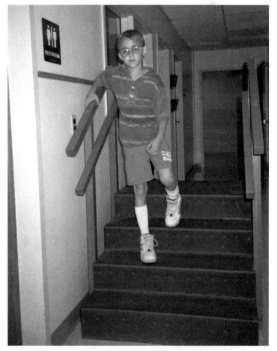

FIGURE 11.9. In gait training on the stairs, note the increased support at the right forearm and the mild internal rotation of the right hip during descent. Verbal cues for upper extremity support and visual cues for lower extremity alignment may improve skill.

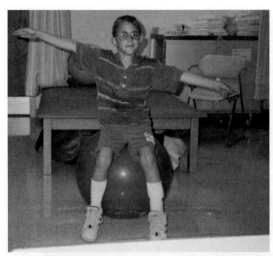

FIGURE 11.10. The therapy ball can be used to challenge dynamic sitting balance and coordination. In addition to moving his arms, the child could also practice alternating forward placement of his feet, practice pelvic tilts while seated on the ball, or move the arms and legs in rhythmic patterns.

activities may be beneficial in improving activity levels. In addition to the problems of motor control and function, children who have experienced moderate or severe brain injury often have difficulty maintaining an appropriate level of fitness (Figs. 11.12 and 11.13). The PT should design a fitness

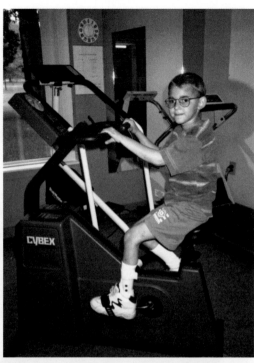

FIGURE 11.12. Bicycling on standard exercise equipment can be used to promote aerobic exercise and lower extremity range of motion (ROM). It can also be done as part of training before returning to riding a standard child's bike.

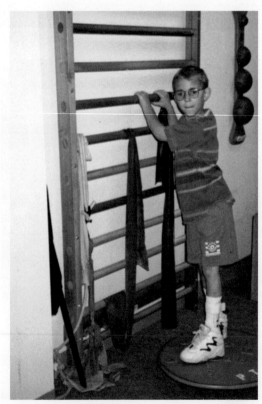

FIGURE 11.11. A BAPS (biomechanical ankle platform system) board can be used to enhance balance and coordination of the lower extremities to maintain balance. The BAPS board can be used both in sitting and standing positions.

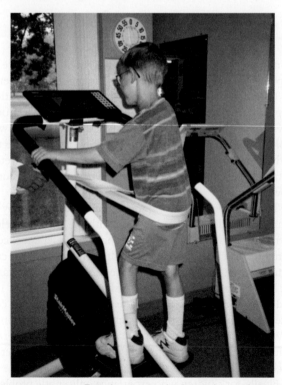

FIGURE 11.13. Exercise on standard exercise equipment improves strength, range of motion (ROM), and endurance. Additionally, the stair stepper improves control in hip extensors and abductors, knee extensors, and ankle plantar flexors. The strap at the hips provides a cue to maintain hip extension and to increase weight bearing on the more involved side.

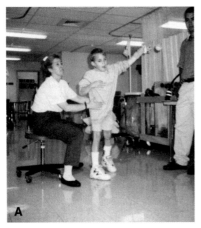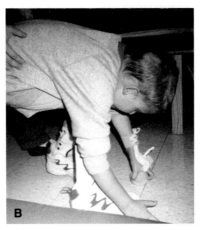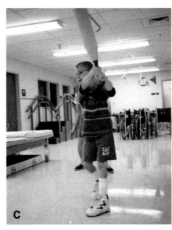

FIGURE 11.14. Sports can be incorporated into therapeutic activities or adaptive physical education to enhance coordination, balance, and motor planning. A game of baseball can incorporate gross motor tasks of **(A)** throwing with the involved arm, **(B)** picking up a ground ball, and **(C)** batting.

program that can be continued after discharge from therapy to address wellness and health. The PT can also work with the physical education teacher in designing an adapted physical education program for the child with TBI (Fig. 11.14). Adapted physical education programs can help encourage participation of the children with their peers and help with social development as well.

School Issues

The Individuals with Disabilities Education Act (IDEA) recognizes brain injury as a separate category of impairment in children, and the school curriculum must be adapted for qualifying children with a TBI. In addition, the educational services the child receives may provide accommodations and physical assistance for activities of daily living, mobility, and motor tasks, such as writing, to assist the child with achieving academic success. Section 504 plans are written to ensure that a child with a disability attending public school, in regular education, is provided the necessary support to succeed and access the typical educational environment.[135] A 504 plan is different from an Individual with Education Plan (IEP) that establishes individualized goals for children needing further supports and special education services under IDEA.[135]

» Prevention

Prevention is the key to decreasing the annual incidence of TBI. Effective prevention involves improving technology to decrease the intensity of impact on the brain during collision, increasing awareness and use of safety measures, and mandating protective laws. Children younger than 12 months are at significant risk for head injury, and much of the risk can be prevented by increased parental supervision or improved home safety devices.[4]

Helmets

The consistent use of helmets can decrease the incidence of injury, because unhelmeted riders are more likely to have a brain injury than are helmeted bicyclists.[136,137–139] Fit of the helmet is important, because poor fit has been associated with an increased risk of TBI in children, especially in boys.[140] Use of helmets can potentially prevent brain injuries from occurring in sports and recreational activities, including baseball, football, horseback riding, rollerblading, skateboarding, hockey, roller skating, skiing, and sledding.[4,84] Barriers to helmet use include the lack of awareness of recreational risks and the effectiveness of helmets, cost, and negative peer pressure. Increasing the use of helmets may be accomplished by advocating for educational programs, discount coupons, helmet subsidies, role modeling by parents, athletic regulation change, and mandatory legislative change.

Playground Equipment

Prevention should also include preventing falls from playground equipment onto hard surfaces. The severity of the injuries can be remarkably decreased if the height of equipment does not exceed 5 feet and materials such as sand, pea gravel, rubber mulch, or wood chips are used under the playground equipment.[84] Surface materials must be continually maintained if they are to be effective. Addition of railings and barriers to prevent falls off of playground equipment can decrease the number injuries sustained.

Traffic Behavior

The inability of a child younger than 11 years old to assess distances and speeds combined with immaturity and typical levels of impulsiveness results in unsafe traffic behavior. Even after training programs, the majority of young children still exhibit risky behavior, and parents should be cautious of younger children crossing the street alone. More effective community approaches should focus primarily on decreasing the traffic speed, enforcing laws governing pedestrian–motor vehicle interaction, and separating the pedestrian from the traffic[84] (see Case Study).

Car Restraints

The use of occupant seat belt restraints is clearly an effective strategy for preventing injury during a crash. The placement of the child in the back seat of the car and the correct use of car seats with proper restraints can prevent up to 90% of serious and fatal injuries to children younger than 5 years of age.[68] Unfortunately, misuse of child seats is still a common problem. In older children and adolescents, the use of lap and shoulder belts can prevent approximately 45% of serious and fatal injuries.[68] Proper restraint laws do vary state to state. According to the American Automobile Association (AAA), Arizona requires children younger than 16 years old to be restrained, children aged 5 to 8 years old and 57 inches or less to be in a booster seat, and child restraints for children younger than 5 years old.[141] For example, the state of Delaware requires that children under 65 inches or younger than 12 years of age do not ride in the front passenger seat of a car that is equipped with an airbag, children younger than 8 years old and under 65 lb must be restrained in a child safety seat or booster seat.

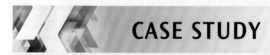

CASE STUDY

JUSTIN: PATIENT CLIENT MANAGEMENT

Element of Patient/ Client Management	Application for a Child with Acquired TBI
Examination	*Examples of history:* Age of child, past medical history, prior functional status, medications *Examples of systems review:* Blood pressure fluctuations, bruising, abrasion or other problem with skin integrity, inability to make needs known *Examples of tests and measures:* Postural observation, FIM, WeeFIM, PEDI, ROM, muscle strength testing, gait analysis
Evaluation	*Synthesis* of observed impairments with *interpretation* from functional examination tools commonly used, such as the FIM and PEDI
Diagnosis	Physical therapy diagnosis based on *impairments and functional limitations*
Prognosis and plan of care	Prognosis and plan of care are based on PT evaluation, including identified problems, comorbidities, and etiology.
Intervention	*Examples of coordination, communication, and documentation:* Case management, patient/client family meetings, outcome data *Examples of topics for patient/client-related instruction:* Current condition, plan of care, fitness program, risk factors, transitions across settings *Examples of procedural interventions:* Balance training, flexibility exercises, postural stabilization, neuromotor development training, gait training, device and equipment use, biofeedback, passive ROM
Outcome	Use the *anticipated goals and expected outcomes* to assist with monitoring progress and documentation

Justin is an 8-year-old boy who experienced a TBI secondary to a pedestrian–MVA. He was unconscious at the scene of the accident and was life flighted to the nearest pediatric trauma center. On arrival at the ER, he had a GCS of 2, and his pupils were fixed and dilated. Justin was in a coma. Diagnostic studies revealed diffuse right intracranial hemorrhage, a right pneumothorax, fracture of the left orbit, and multiple contusions. An ICP monitor, chest tubes, and tracheostomy tube were required for acute management.

Justin lives at home with his parents and a 6-year-old sister in a two-story home with 5 steps to enter and 12 steps to the second floor of the house. His bedroom and bathroom are on the second floor. His past medical history is unremarkable. Justin is a second-grade student at Jones Elementary.

The rehabilitation team was consulted 3 days after admission, and Justin was determined to be at a Rancho Los Amigos Scale Level II at the time of the evaluation. The team implemented a coma stimulation program. Caution was taken when implementing the program owing to Justin's multiple injuries, monitors, and tube placements. In addition, the PT initiated an inhibitory casting program to manage Justin's left ankle plantar flexion posturing, which was measured at 45 degrees before casting.

Justin slowly emerged from the coma over a period of 2 weeks. Subsequent treatment focused on increasing tolerance to the upright position on the tilt table, motor control/strength of the neck and trunk during supported sitting, and contracture management. During the next 2 weeks, Justin's medical condition stabilized, and he progressed to a Rancho Los Amigos Scale Level V. Owing to the severity of his brain injury and the presence of multiple impairments, the team anticipated that Justin would require additional care in the long term, including in an acute rehabilitation setting, an outpatient setting, and additional services at his school setting.

As Justin awoke, his ventilatory status stabilized and the tracheostomy was removed, and he was transferred to a pediatric rehabilitation center. The WeeFIM and the PEDI were used to examine his status upon admission and to determine his projected goals for improvement during his stay. Inhibitory casting, with weekly changes, was continued for the left ankle plantar flexion contracture, which was now measured at 20 degrees plantar flexion. Justin was given a high-back wheelchair for mobility with a custom-fit modular seating system for postural control. Justin began to work on transfers from supine to sit and from the wheelchair to a mat with moderate assistance. He also engaged in supported standing activities and gait training. Decreased motor control and hemiplegia on the left were more evident as he increased his activity level with activities of increasing complexity. Justin moved in synergistic patterns in both the upper and lower extremities on the left. General strength on the right side of the body was good. Balance and coordination in upright positions was impaired, and he required maximal assistance for standing activities.

As rehabilitation progressed, Justin's condition improved, and he began to follow commands consistently and showed some recall of newly learned tasks. His parents participated regularly in family conferences and family education. His parents were instructed on how to assist Justin during tasks of functional mobility and how to perform the prescribed exercises. At the time of discharge from rehabilitation, Justin was able to propel himself in a lightweight wheelchair using his right extremities. He was able to transfer from the wheelchair to the mat with supervision and was able to walk short distances with a forearm crutch on the left. He was still limited in his mobility by the left-sided spasticity. Justin had been evaluated for orthotics and was to receive a left dynamic ankle–foot orthosis (AFO). Neuropsychological testing was completed before discharge and revealed deficiencies in short-term memory, attention span and focus, judgment, and agility to learn new material.

By 4 months after the injury, Justin was transitioning back into his school. His school program was modified for a half-day of inclusion in his regular classroom and a half-day of specialized classroom instruction. Justin would continue to receive physical therapy, occupational therapy, and speech therapy through the school setting. He was independent in his transfers and was ambulating with the left forearm crutch and the dynamic AFO more consistently. Justin used the lightweight wheelchair only for community mobility.

REFERENCES

1. Keenan HT, Bratton SL. Epidemiology and outcomes of pediatric traumatic brain injury. *Dev Neurosci.* 2006;28(4-5):256-263.
2. Atabaki SM. Pediatric head injury. *Pediatr Rev.* 2007;28(6):215-224.
3. Greenwald BD, Burnett DM, Miller MA. Congenital and acquired brain injury. 1. Brain injury: epidemiology and pathophysiology. *Arch Phys Med Rehabil.* 2003;84(3)(suppl 1):S3-S7.
4. Centers for Disease Control and Prevention. *Traumatic brain injury & concussion.* 2019. Accessed July 18, 2020. https://www.cdc.gov/traumaticbraininjury/get_the_facts.html
5. Langlois JA, Rutland-Brown W, Thomas KE. The incidence of traumatic brain injury among children in the United States: differences by race. *J Head Trauma Rehabil.* 2005;20(3):229-238.
6. Kraus JF. Epidemiology of head injury. In: Cooper PR, Golfinos J, eds. *Head Injury.* 4th ed. McGraw-Hill Companies, Inc; 2000:1-25.
7. Faul M, Xu L, Wald MM, et al. Traumatic brain injury in the United States: national estimates of prevalence and incidence, 2002–2006. *Injury Prev.* 2010;16(suppl 1):A268.
8. Mazzola CA, Adelson PD. Critical care management of head trauma in children. *Crit Care Med.* 2002;30(11)(suppl):S393-S401.
9. Gedeit R. Head injury. *Pediatr Rev.* 2001;22(4):118-124.
10. Schneier AJ, Shields BJ, Hostetler SG, et al. Incidence of pediatric traumatic brain injury and associated hospital resource utilization in the United States. *Pediatrics.* 2006;118(2):483-492.
11. Marik PE, Varon J, Trask T. Management of head trauma. *Chest.* 2002;122(2):699-711.
12. Koepsell TD, Rivara FP, Vavilala MS, et al. Incidence and descriptive epidemiologic features of traumatic brain injury in King County, Washington. *Pediatrics.* 2011;128(5):946-954.
13. Bazarian JJ, McClung J, Shah MN, et al. Mild traumatic brain injury in the United States, 1998–2000. *Brain Inj.* 2005;19(1):85-91.
14. Brehaut JC, Miller A, Raina P, et al. Childhood behavior disorders and injuries among children and youth: a population-based study. *Pediatrics.* 2003;111(2):262-269.
15. Gerring JP, Grados MA, Slomine B, et al. Disruptive behaviour disorders and disruptive symptoms after severe paediatric traumatic brain injury. *Brain Inj.* 2009;23(12):944-955.
16. Ponsford J, Willmott C, Rothwell A, et al. Cognitive and behavioral outcome following mild traumatic head injury in children. *J Head Trauma Rehabil.* 1999;14(4):360-372.
17. Guskiewicz KM, Valovich McLeod TC. Pediatric sports-related concussion. *PMR.* 2011;3(4):353-364, quiz 364.
18. Kraus JF, Rock A, Hemyari P. Brain injuries among infants, children, adolescents, and young adults. *Am J Dis Child.* 1990;144(6):684-691.
19. Guerrero JL, Thurman DJ, Sniezek JE. Emergency department visits associated with traumatic brain injury: United States, 1995–1996. *Brain Inj.* 2000;14(2):181-186.
20. Kraus JF, Fife D, Cox P, et al. Incidence, severity, and external causes of pediatric brain injury. *Am J Dis Child.* 1986;140(7):687-693.
21. Crowe LM, Catroppa C, Anderson V, et al. Head injuries in children under 3 years. *Injury.* 2012;43(12):2141-2145.
22. Chadwick DL, Chin S, Salerno C, et al. Deaths from falls in children: how far is fatal? *J Trauma.* 1991;31(10):1353-1355.
23. Centers for Disease Control (CDC). Factors potentially associated with reductions in alcohol-related traffic fatalities—United States, 1990 and 1991. *MMWR Morb Mortal Wkly Rep.* 1992;41(48):893-899.
24. Kraus JF. Epidemiological features of brain injury in children: occurrence, children at risk, causes and manner of injury, severity, and outcomes. In: Bromon SH, Michel ME, eds. *Traumatic Head Injury in Children.* Oxford University Press; 1995.
25. Rivara FP. Epidemiology of violent deaths in children and adolescents in the United States. *Pediatrician.* 1983;12(1):3-10.
26. Koh JO, Cassidy JD. Incidence study of head blows and concussions in competition taekwondo. *Clin J Sport Med.* 2004;14(2):72-79.
27. Yue J, Winkler E, Burke J, et al. Pediatric sports-related traumatic brain injury in United States trauma centers. *Neurosurg Focus.* 2016;40(4):E3.
28. Kaufman BA, Dacey RG Jr. Acute care management of closed head injury in childhood. *Pediatr Ann.* 1994;23(1):18-20, 25-28.
29. Araki T, Yokota H, Morita A. Pediatric traumatic brain injury: characteristic features, diagnosis, and management. *Neurol Med Chir.* 2017;57(2):82-93.
30. Bonadio WA, Smith DS, Hillman S. Clinical indicators of intracranial lesion on computed tomographic scan in children with parietal skull fracture. *Am J Dis Child.* 1989;143(2):194-196.
31. Hahn YS, McLone DG. Risk factors in the outcome of children with minor head injury. *Pediatr Neurosurg.* 1993;19(3):135-142.
32. Griffith ER, Rosenthall M, Bond MR, et al, eds. *Rehabilitation of the Child and Adult with Traumatic Brain Injury.* 2nd ed. F.A. Davis; 1990.
33. Almasi SJ, Wilson JJ. An update on the diagnosis and management of concussion. *WMJ.* 2012;111(1):21-27, quiz 28.
34. Marion D. Pathophysiology and initial neurosurgical care: future directions. In: Horn LJ, Zasler ND, eds. *Medical Rehabilitation of Traumatic Brain Injury.* Hanley & Belfus, Inc; 1996.
35. Blinman T, Houseknecht E, Snyder C, et al. Postconcussive symptoms in hospitalized pediatric patients after mild traumatic brain injury. *J Pediatr Surg.* 2009;44(6):1223-1228.

36. Kaufmann P, Hofmann G, Smolle KH, et al. Intensive care management of acute pancreatitis: recognition of patients at high risk of developing severe or fatal complications. *Wien Klin Wochenschr.* 1996;108(1):9-15.

37. McGrath A, Taylor R. *Pediatric Skull Fractures.* StatPearls. StatPearls Publishing; 2020. Accessed July 18, 2020. https://www.ncbi.nlm.nih.gov/books/NBK482218/

38. Kautz-Leurer M, Rotem H. Acquired brain injuries: trauma, near-drowning, and tumors. In: Campbell S, ed. *Physical Therapy in Children.* W.B. Saunders; 2012:679-701.

39. Graham DI, Gennarelli TA. Pathology of brain damage after head injury. In: Golfinos J, Cooper PR, eds. *Head Injury.* 4th ed. McGraw-Hill Companies, Inc; 2000.

40. Mysiw JW, Fugate LP, Clinchot DM. Assessment, early rehabilitation intervention, and tertiary prevention. In: Horn LJ, Zasler ND, eds. *Medical Rehabilitation of Traumatic Brain Injury.* Hanley & Belfus, Inc; 1996.

41. Mesfin F, Gupta N, Hays Shapshak A, et al. *Diffuse Axonal Injury (DAI).* StatPearls. StatPearls Publishing; 2020. Accessed July 22, 2020. https://www.ncbi.nlm.nih.gov/books/NBK448102/

42. Kukreti V, Mohseni-Bod H, Drake J. Management of raised intracranial pressure in children with traumatic brain injury. *J Pediatr Neurosci.* 2014;9(3):207-215.

43. Bonow R, Oron A, Hanak B, et al. Post-traumatic hydrocephalus in children: a retrospective study in 42 pediatric hospitals using the pediatric health information system. *Neurosurgery.* 2018;83(4):732-739.

44. Hu Q, Di G, Shao X, et al. Predictors associated with post-traumatic hydrocephalus in patients with head injury undergoing unilateral decompressive craniectomy. *Front Neurol.* 2018;9:337.

45. Munakomi S, Das J. *Brain Herniation.* StatPearls. StatPearls Publishing; 2020. Accessed July 15, 2020. https://www.ncbi.nlm.nih.gov/books/NBK542246/

46. Robertson CS, Contant CF, Narayan RK, et al. Cerebral blood flow, AVDO2, and neurologic outcome in head-injured patients. *J Neurotrauma.* 1992;9(suppl 1):S349-S358.

47. Konotos HA. Oxygen radicals in central nervous system damage. *Chem Biol Int.* 1989;72:229-255.

48. Fullerton LD. Diagnosis and management of intracranial complications in TBI rehabilitation. In: Horn LJ, Zasler ND, eds. *Medical Rehabilitation of Traumatic Brain Injury.* Hanley & Belfus, Inc; 1996.

49. National Institute of Neurological Disorders and Stroke. *Hydrocephalus fact sheet.* 2020. Accessed July 1, 2020. https://www.ninds.nih.gov/Disorders/Patient-Caregiver-Education/Fact-Sheets/Hydrocephalus-Fact-Sheet#3125_2

50. Statler Bennett K, DeWitt P, Harlaar N, et al. Seizures in children with severe traumatic brain injury. *Pediatr Crit Care Med.* 2018;18(1):54-63.

51. Weiner HL, Weinberg JS. Head injury in the pediatric age group. In: Golfinos J, Cooper PR, eds. *Head Injury.* Vol 4. McGraw-Hill; 2000.

52. Kirk KA, Shoykhet M, Jeong JH, et al. Dysautonomia after pediatric brain injury. *Dev Med Child Neurol.* 2012;54(8):759-764.

53. Acerini C, Tasker R, Bellone S, et al. Hypopituitarism in childhood and adolescence following traumatic brain injury: the case for prospective endocrine investigation. *Eur J Endocrinol.* 2006;155(5):664-669.

54. Conine TA, Sullivan T, Mackie T, et al. Effect of serial casting for the prevention of equinus in patients with acute head injury. *Arch Phys Med Rehabil.* 1990;71(5):310-312.

55. Teasdale G, Jennett B. Assessment of coma and impaired consciousness. A practical scale. *Lancet.* 1974;2(7872):81-84.

56. Ghaffarpasand F, Razmkon A, Dehghankhalili M. Glasgow Coma Scale Score in pediatric patients with traumatic brain injury; limitations and reliability. *Bull Emerg Trauma.* 2013;1(4):135-136.

57. Calculated Decisions. *Pediatric Glasgow Coma Scale/PECARN pediatric head injury-trauma algorithm. Pediatric emergency medicine practice.* CD1-CD5. 2018. Accessed June 29, 2020. https://www.ebmedicine.net/media_library/files/Management-of-Multiply-Injured-Pediatric-Trauma-Patients-in-the-Emergency-Department-Trauma-CME-Calculators.pdf

58. Reilly PL, Simpson DA, Sprod R, et al. Assessing the conscious level in infants and young children: a paediatric version of the Glasgow Coma Scale. *Childs Nerv Syst.* 1988;4(1):30-33.

59. Asikainen I, Kaste M, Sarna S. Predicting late outcome for patients with traumatic brain injury referred to a rehabilitation programme: a study of 508 Finnish patients 5 years or more after injury. *Brain Inj.* 1998;12(2):95-107.

60. Macpherson V, Sullivan SJ, Lambert J. Prediction of motor status 3 and 6 months post severe traumatic brain injury: a preliminary study. *Brain Inj.* 1992;6(6):489-498.

61. Wilson B, Vizor A, Bryant T. Predicting severity of cognitive impairment after severe head injury. *Brain Inj.* 1991;5(2):189-197.

62. Bijur PE. Cognitive outcomes. *J Dev Behav Pediatr.* 1996;17(3):186.

63. Jaffe KM, Fay GC, Polissar NL, et al. Severity of pediatric traumatic brain injury and neurobehavioral recovery at one year—a cohort study. *Arch Phys Med Rehabil.* 1993;74(6):587-595.

64. Lieh-Lai MW, Theodorou AA, Sarnaik AP, et al. Limitations of the Glasgow Coma Scale in predicting outcome in children with traumatic brain injury. *J Pediatr.* 1992;120(2, pt 1):195-199.

65. Gagnon I, Forget R, Sullivan SJ, et al. Motor performance following a mild traumatic brain injury in children: an exploratory study. *Brain Inj.* 1998;12(10):843-853.

66. Ewing-Cobbs L, Levin HS, Fletcher JM, et al. The Children's Orientation and Amnesia Test: relationship to severity of acute head injury and to recovery of memory. *Neurosurgery.* 1990;27(5):683-691, discussion 691.

67. Katz DI, Alexander MP. Traumatic brain injury. Predicting course of recovery and outcome for patients admitted to rehabilitation. *Arch Neurol.* 1994;51(7):661-670.

68. Cockrell J. Pediatric brain injury rehabilitation. In: Horn LJ, Zasler ND, eds. *Medical Rehabilitation of Traumatic Brain Injury.* Hanley & Belfus, Inc; 1996:171-196.

69. Lah S, David P, Epps A, et al. Preliminary validation study of the Sydney Post-Traumatic Amnesia Scale (SYPTAS) in children with traumatic brain injury aged 4 to 7 years old. *Appl Neuropsychol Child.* 2019;8(1):61-69.

70. Konigs M, Kieviet J, Oosterlaan J. Post-traumatic amnesia predicts intelligence impairment following traumatic brain injury: a meta-analysis. *J Neurol Neurosurg Psychiatry.* 2012;83:1048-1055.

71. Malkmus D, Booth B, Kodimer C. *Rehabilitation of Head Injured Adult: Comprehensive Cognitive Management.* Los Amigos Research and Education Institute, Inc; 1980:2.

72. Professional Staff Association of Rancho Los Amigos Hospital. *Rehabilitation of the Head Injured Child and Adult: Pediatric Levels of Consciousness, Selected Problems.* Rancho Los Amigos Medical Center, Pediatric Brain Injury Service and Los Amigos Research and Education Institute, Inc; 1982:5-7.

73. Anderson V, Jacobs R, Spencer-Smith M, et al. Does early age at brain insult predict worse outcome? Neuropsychological implications. *J Pediatr Psychol.* 2010;35(7):716-727.

74. Kuhtz-Buschbeck JP, Stolze H, Gölge M, et al. Analyses of gait, reaching, and grasping in children after traumatic brain injury. *Arch Phys Med Rehabil.* 2003;84(3):424-430.

75. Kuhtz-Buschbeck JP, Hoppe B, Gölge M, et al. Sensorimotor recovery in children after traumatic brain injury: analyses of gait, gross motor, and fine motor skills. *Dev Med Child Neurol.* 2003;45(12):821-828.

76. Crowe LM, Catroppa C, Babl FE, et al. Executive function outcomes of children with traumatic brain injury sustained before three years. *Child Neuropsychol.* 2013;19(2):113-126.

77. Stancin T, Drotar D, Taylor G, et al. Health-related quality of life of children and adolescents after traumatic brain injury. *Pediatrics.* 2002;109(2):e34.

78. Gagnon I, Swaine B, Friedman D, et al. Children show decreased dynamic balance after mild traumatic brain injury. *Arch Phys Med Rehabil.* 2004;85(3):444-452.

79. Dumas HM, Haley SM, Ludlow LH, et al. Functional recovery in pediatric traumatic brain injury during inpatient rehabilitation. *Am J Phys Med Rehabil.* 2002;81(9):661-669.

80. Williams GP, Schache AG. Evaluation of a conceptual framework for retraining high-level mobility following traumatic brain injury: two case reports. *J Head Trauma Rehabil*. 2010;25(3):164-172.

81. Haley SM, Dumas HM, Rabin JP, et al. Early recovery of walking in children and youths after traumatic brain injury. *Dev Med Child Neurol*. 2003;45(10):671-675.

82. Taylor HG, Yeates KO, Wade SL, et al. Influences on first-year recovery from traumatic brain injury in children. *Neuropsychology*. 1999;13(1):76-89.

83. Rivara JB. Family functioning following pediatric traumatic brain injury. *Pediatr Ann*. 1994;23(1):38-44.

84. Rivara FP. Epidemiology and prevention of pediatric traumatic brain injury. *Pediatr Ann*. 1994;23(1):12-17.

85. Levin HS, Eisenberg HM. Neuropsychological outcome of closed head injury in children and adolescents. *Childs Brain*. 1979;5(3):281-292.

86. Davis K, Slomine B, Salorio C, et al. Time to follow commands and duration of post-traumatic amnesia predict GOS-E Peds scores 1-2 years after TBI in children requiring inpatient rehabilitation. *J Head Trauma Rehabil*. 2017;31(2):E39-E47.

87. Lang B. Pediatric traumatic brain injury: language outcomes and their relationship to the arcuate fasciculus. *Brain Lang*. 2013;127(3):388-398.

88. Levin H, Hanten G. Executive functions after traumatic brain injury in children. *Pediatr Neurol*. 2005;33(2):79-93.

89. Enslin J, Rohlwink U, Figaji A. Management of spasticity after traumatic brain injury in children. *Front Neurol*. 2020;11(126).

90. AANS. *Spasticity*. 2020. Accessed July 1, 2020. https://www.aans.org/Patients/Neurosurgical-Conditions-and-Treatments/Spasticity

91. National Institute of Neurological Disorders and Stroke. *Spasticity information page*. 2019. Accessed July 1, 2020. https://www.ninds.nih.gov/Disorders/All-Disorders/Spasticity-Information-pag

92. Bloomfield SA. Changes in musculoskeletal structure and function with prolonged bed rest. *Med Sci Sports Exerc*. 1997;29(2):197-206.

93. Katz-Leurer M, Rottem H, Meyer S. Hand-held dynamometry in children with traumatic brain injury: within-session reliability. *Pediatr Phys Ther*. 2008;20(3):259-263.

94. Golge M, Muller M, Dreesmann M, et al. Recovery of the precision grip in children after traumatic brain injury. *Arch Phys Med Rehabil*. 2004;85(9):1435-1444.

95. Aitken ME, Jaffe KM, DiScala C, et al. Functional outcome in children with multiple trauma without significant head injury. *Arch Phys Med Rehabil*. 1999;80(8):889-895.

96. Bartlett D, Birmingham T. Validity and reliability of a pediatric reach test. *Pediatr Phys Ther*. 2003;15(2):84-92.

97. Franjoine MR, Gunther JS, Taylor MJ. Pediatric balance scale: a modified version of the berg balance scale for the school-age child with mild to moderate motor impairment. *Pediatr Phys Ther*. 2003;15(2):114-128.

98. Williams EN, Carroll SG, Reddihough DS, et al. Investigation of the timed "up & go" test in children. *Dev Med Child Neurol*. 2005;47(8):518-524.

99. Zaino CA, Marchese VG, Westcott SL. Timed up and down stairs test: preliminary reliability and validity of a new measure of functional mobility. *Pediatr Phys Ther*. 2004;16(2):90-98.

100. Baque E, Barber L, Sakzewski L, et al. Test-re-test reproducibility of activity capacity measures for children with an acquired brain injury. *Brain Inj*. 2015;9:1143-1149.

101. Fligor BJ, Cox LC, Nesathurai S. Subjective hearing loss and history of traumatic brain injury exhibits abnormal brainstem auditory evoked response: a case report. *Arch Phys Med Rehabil*. 2002;83(1):141-143.

102. Forbes BJ, Rubin SE, Margolin E, et al. Evaluation and management of retinal hemorrhages in infants with and without abusive head trauma. *J AAPOS*. 2010;14(3):267-273.

103. Hurvitz EA, Mandac BR, Davidoff G, et al. Risk factors for heterotopic ossification in children and adolescents with severe traumatic brain injury. *Arch Phys Med Rehabil*. 1992;73(5):459-462.

104. Djergaian RS. Management of musculoskeletal complications. In: Horn LJ, Zasler ND, eds. *Medical Rehabilitation of Traumatic Brain Injury*. Hanley & Belfus, Inc; 1996.

105. Johns JS, Cifu DX, Keyser-Marcus L, et al. Impact of clinically significant heterotopic ossification on functional outcome after traumatic brain injury. *J Head Trauma Rehabil*. 1999;14(3):269-276.

106. Piper MC, Pinnell LE, Darrah J, et al. Construction and validation of the Alberta Infant Motor Scale (AIMS). *Can J Public Health*. 1992;83(suppl 2):S46-S50.

107. Darrah J, Magill-Evans J, Volden J, et al. Scores of typically developing children on the Peabody Developmental Motor Scales: infancy to preschool. *Phys Occup Ther Pediatr*. 2007;27(3):5-19.

108. Rice SA, Blackman JA, Braun S, et al. Rehabilitation of children with traumatic brain injury: descriptive analysis of a nationwide sample using the WeeFIM. *Arch Phys Med Rehabil*. 2005;86(4):834-836.

109. Deitz JC, Kartin D, Kopp K. Review of the Bruininks-Oseretsky Test of Motor Proficiency, second edition (BOT-2). *Phys Occup Ther Pediatr*. 2007;27(4):87-102.

110. Linder-Lucht M, Othmer V, Walther M, et al. Validation of the Gross Motor Function Measure for use in children and adolescents with traumatic brain injuries. *Pediatrics*. 2007;120(4):e880-e886.

111. Wong R, McEwan J, Finlayson D, et al. Reliability and validity of the acquired brain injury challenge assessment (ABI-CA) in children. *Brain Inj*. 2014;28(13-14):1734-1743.

112. Feldman AB, Haley SM, Coryell J. Concurrent and construct validity of the Pediatric Evaluation of Disability Inventory. *Phys Ther*. 1990;70(10):602-610.

113. Kothari DH, Haley SM, Gill-Body KM, et al. Measuring functional change in children with acquired brain injury (ABI): comparison of generic and ABI-specific scales using the Pediatric Evaluation of Disability Inventory (PEDI). *Phys Ther*. 2003;83(9):776-785.

114. Iyer LV, Haley SM, Watkins MP, et al. Establishing minimal clinically important differences for scores on the pediatric evaluation of disability inventory for inpatient rehabilitation. *Phys Ther*. 2003;83(10):888-898.

115. Katz-Leurer M, Rotem H, Keren O, et al. The effect of variable gait modes on walking parameters among children post severe traumatic brain injury and typically developed controls. *NeuroRehabilitation*. 2011;29(1):45-51.

116. Katz-Leurer M, Rotem H, Keren O, et al. The relationship between step variability, muscle strength and functional walking performance in children with post-traumatic brain injury. *Gait Posture*. 2009;29(1):154-157.

117. Vitale AE, Jankowski LW, Sullivan SJ. Reliability for a walk/run test to estimate aerobic capacity in a brain-injured population. *Brain Inj*. 1997;11(1):67-76.

118. DeWall J. Severe pediatric traumatic brain injury. Evidence-based guidelines for pediatric TBI care. *EMS Mag*. 2009;38(9):53-57.

119. Dumas HM, Haley SM, Ludlow LH, et al. Recovery of ambulation during inpatient rehabilitation: physical therapist prognosis for children and adolescents with traumatic brain injury. *Phys Ther*. 2004;84(3):232-242.

120. Arango-Lasprilla JC, Ketchum J, Cifu D, et al. Predictors of extended rehabilitation length of stay after traumatic brain injury. *Arch Phys Med Reabil*. 2010;91:1495-1504.

121. Kramer ME, Suskauer SJ, Christensen JR, et al. Examining acute rehabilitation outcomes for children with total functional dependence after traumatic brain injury: a pilot study. *J Head Trauma Rehabil*. 2013;28(5):361-370.

122. Shah S, Taylor Kimberly W. The modern approach to treating brain swelling in neuro ICU. *Semin Neurol*. 2016;36(6):502-507.

123. Karibe H, Hayashi T, Hirano T, et al. Surgical management of traumatic acute subdural hematoma in adults: a review. *Neurol Med Chir (Tokyo)*. 2014;54(11):887-894.

124. Illowsky KB, Alter K. Muscle selection for focal limb dystonia. *Toxins*. 2018;10(1):20.

125. Verplancke D, Snape S, Salisbury CF, et al. A randomized controlled trial of botulinum toxin on lower limb spasticity following acute acquired severe brain injury. *Clin Rehabil.* 2005;19(2):117-125.

126. Lombardi F, Taricco M, De Tanti A, et al. Sensory stimulation for brain injured individuals in coma or vegetative state. *Cochrane Database Syst Rev.* 2002(2):CD001427.

127. Sosnowski C, Ustik M. Early intervention: coma stimulation in the intensive care unit. *J Neurosci Nurs.* 1994;26(6):336-341.

128. Ashwal S. The persistent vegetative state in children. *Adv Pediatr.* 1994;41:195-222.

129. Latour JM. Caring for children in a persistent vegetative state: complex but manageable. *Pediatr Crit Care Med.* 2007;8(5):497-498.

130. Dumas HM, Haley SM, Carey TM, et al. The relationship between functional mobility and the intensity of physical therapy intervention in children with traumatic brain injury. *Pediatr Phys Ther.* 2004;16(3):157-164.

131. Dumas HM, Haley SM, Rabin JP. Short-term durability and improvement of function in traumatic brain injury: a pilot study using the Paediatric Evaluation of Disability Inventory (PEDI) classification levels. *Brain Inj.* 2001;15(10):891-902.

132. Brown TH, Mount J, Rouland BL, et al. Body weight-supported treadmill training versus conventional gait training for people with chronic traumatic brain injury. *J Head Trauma Rehabil.* 2005;20(5):402-415.

133. Damiano DL, DeJong SL. A systematic review of the effectiveness of treadmill training and body weight support in pediatric rehabilitation. *J Neurol Phys Ther.* 2009;33(1):27-44.

134. Karman N, Maryles J, Baker RW, et al. Constraint-induced movement therapy for hemiplegic children with acquired brain injuries. *J Head Trauma Rehabil.* 2003;18(3):259-267.

135. U.S. Department of Education. *Protecting students with disabilities.* 2020. Accessed July 2, 2020. https://www2.ed.gov/about/offices/list/ocr/504faq.html#interrelationship

136. Kaushik R, Krisch IM, Schroeder DR, et al. Pediatric bicycle-related head injuries: a population-based study in a county without a helmet law. *Inj Epidemiol.* 2015;2(1):16.

137. Kiss K, Pinter A. Are bicycle helmets necessary for children? Pros and cons. *Orv Hetil.* 2009;150(24):1129-1133.

138. Coffman S. Bicycle injuries and safety helmets in children. Review of research. *Orthop Nurs.* 2003;22(1):9-15.

139. Cassidy JD, Carroll LJ, Peloso PM, et al. Incidence, risk factors and prevention of mild traumatic brain injury: results of the WHO Collaborating Centre Task Force on Mild Traumatic Brain Injury. *J Rehabil Med.* 2004;(43)(suppl):28-60.

140. Rivara FP, Astley SJ, Clarren SK, et al. Fit of bicycle safety helmets and risk of head injuries in children. *Inj Prev.* 1999;5(3):194-197.

141. American Automobile Association. *Child passenger safety.* 2020. Accessed February 23, 2021. https://drivinglaws.aaa.com/tag/child-passenger-safety/

Spinal Cord Injury

Alison Kreger

≫ Introduction

Treatment of a child with a traumatic or atraumatic spinal cord injury (SCI) can be challenging, demanding attention to the child's current age-specific needs and consideration of the child's physical, cognitive, and emotional development. SCI can lead to a lifelong disability, having a profound effect on both the child and his or her family. A physical therapist (PT) has the unique opportunity to be not only a teacher, a guide, and an advocate but also a coach who empowers his or her patients to live life to their fullest potential. Children with SCIs commonly need episodic care throughout their lifetime. PTs have the responsibility to anticipate the variety of challenges a child will encounter as he or she grows and develops into early adulthood.

The National Spinal Cord Injury Association (NSCIA) defines pediatric SCI as an acute traumatic lesion of the spinal cord and nerve roots in children—from newborn through 15 years of age.[1] The National Spinal Cord Injury Statistical Center notes that there are an estimated 54 new SCI cases per one million people in the United States, resulting in 17,730 new cases a year.[2] The estimate of the number of people living in the United States with an SCI is 291,000, with numbers ranging from 249,000 to 363,000 people. The average age of injury has increased to 43 years, with 78% of new SCI cases being reported in the male population. The overall incidence of pediatric SCI is 1.99 injuries per 100,000 children in the United States.[3]

People who sustain an SCI can be separated into two groups, those with traumatic SCI and those with atraumatic SCI. The mechanism of injury for traumatic SCI is different between pediatric and adult populations. The most common mechanisms of traumatic spinal injury in the adult population include flexion/extension, axial loading, burst, and compression fractures. The immaturity and flexibility of a child's skeleton result in different mechanisms of injury. These immature features can predispose a child under 11 years of age to an upper cervical spine injury at the level of C-3 or above.[4] Ligamentous laxity, disproportionately large head size, and relatively horizontal facet joints can create a fulcrum for a sagittal force and allow a large amount of translatory movement. A child over 11 years of age has a greater tendency toward injury to the lower cervical spine (C-3 and below) as opposed to the adult population.[4] The ring apophysis in the growing pediatric spine can slip or separate into the spinal canal from an axial traumatic force and mimic the symptoms of a herniated intervertebral disk.[4] Finally, the ligamentous laxity in the pediatric spinal column can allow the vertebra to stretch and recoil during a force to the spine or head. This movement causes the relatively inflexible spinal cord inside to stretch as well. This stretching can cause distraction or ischemia to delicate neuropathways and cause an invisible SCI that is not picked up on radiographic assessment as there is no obvious fracture or dislocation. This phenomenon is known as spinal cord injury without radiographic abnormality (SCIWORA) and can present as a complete or incomplete injury. SCIWORA is a prevalent manifestation that has been reported in 13% to 19% of all children who experience SCI.[5] Owing to the increased potential for neurologic devastation, SCIWORA can also have a delayed onset, so all medical staff, including the PT, should carefully monitor the child's clinical presentation. All children who have experienced a trauma should have both head injury and SCIWORA ruled out.

Some causes of traumatic SCI include motor vehicle accident, violence, falls, and sports. The causes of SCI that are unique to pediatrics include birth trauma, child abuse, and motor vehicle lap belt injuries.[5] Motor vehicle restraints are designed to dissipate force over bony areas of the body to prevent injury during a crash. Small children are improperly positioned in a car with the lap belt riding higher than the pelvis, causing a fulcrum of force in the thoracic or lumbar spine and severe pressure on the abdomen.[5] Children with this type of injury often have a burn mark across the abdomen and may have significant visceral injury as well.[4,6]

Atraumatic SCI includes all other spinal cord dysfunction such as myelopathies, cancer, and stroke. Clinically, atraumatic SCI often presents similarly to either a complete or an incomplete SCI. Myelopathies include both compressive and inflammatory disorders. Compressive myelopathies are often caused by an underlying structural abnormality (stenosis, spondylolisthesis) combined with some antecedent trigger such as a fall or a car accident, with resultant compression on the spinal cord. Chiari malformations and protruding disks also have the potential to cause compression on the spinal cord.[7] Inflammatory myelopathies include an entire spectrum of neuroinflammatory disorders, including acute transverse myelitis (ATM), Guillain–Barré syndrome (GBS), multiple sclerosis (MS), acute disseminated encephalomyelitis (ADEM), and neuromyelitis optica (NMO).[8]

ATM affects both children and adults and has the potential to be significantly disabling.[9] The cause of transverse myelitis is not clearly defined, although more information is becoming available about its neuropathology and possible treatments. An underlying systemic inflammation or autoimmune disorder can trigger the development of any inflammatory myelopathy, including transverse myelitis.[8-10] In addition, infection is also considered in these disorders and may initiate the cascade of events resulting in spinal cord dysfunction. There is some documentation relating the onset of transverse myelitis with vaccination, although the benefits of vaccination still far outweigh the risks.[8,10] There is also a high incidence of an antecedent infection (respiratory, gastrointestinal, systemic) prior to the development of transverse myelitis. It is thought that this antecedent infection

initiates a cascade of cellular and immune-mediated events that ultimately result in attack of the spinal cord. A specific protein by-product in this cellular reaction (interleukin-6) has a unique affinity for the spinal cord and has been demonstrated to kill spinal cord cells. Additionally, the spinal cord itself responds differently than other internal organs in how it responds to autoimmune dysfunction.[8-10] Although it is still unknown why a specific transverse segment of the spinal cord is targeted, increased knowledge about the immunopathogenesis of transverse myelitis is leading to better treatment options.

Atraumatic SCI can also be caused by cancer. This may be a primary tumor with focal dysfunction or it could be in the form of metastases with more diffuse dysfunction; 0.5% to 1% of central nervous system neoplasms are within the spinal cord.[11] Nonetheless, the physical effects can include progressive motor weakness, progressive scoliosis, gait disturbances, sensory changes, and muscle tone changes.[11] This can be difficult to identify because of the vague and varied nature of the clinical presentation.

Another form of atraumatic SCI is stroke. This can be caused by arterial or venous ischemia, watershed infarct, arteriovenous malformation (AVM), or a dural arteriovenous fistula. Onset can be either sudden or gradual, depending on the type of bleed. The overall course of recovery may vary as well.[12]

Although traumatic and atraumatic injuries can present similarly, understanding the exact nature of the injury can assist the clinician in formulating a hypothesis that will guide the examination, evaluation, diagnosis, prognosis, intervention, and ultimately outcome that the child achieves.

» Examination

History

The PT begins with a thorough history taken from all available resources. This may include any or all of the following.

History of Present Illness

- Mechanism and date of injury
- Any loss of consciousness at the time of injury or potential brain injury
- Any other injuries sustained at the time of injury
- Any acute medical treatment received (spinal stabilization, steroids, etc.)
- Description of onset and progression of symptoms if atraumatic
- Any medical tests, labs, procedures, or films relating to the injury (specifically neuroimaging tests such as magnetic resonance imaging [MRI] that have been correlated with prognosis)
- Any complications or comorbidities apparent during the hospital stay
- Medications for current or any other condition

Medical History

- All other pertinent medical information, including hospitalizations, injuries, or procedures
- Birth history, if applicable to mechanism or onset of injury

Developmental History

- Developmental history, including prior level of function and achievement of developmental milestones
- Any previously owned adaptive equipment and reason for usage

Social History

- Cultural beliefs and behaviors
- Primary caregivers, family, and community resources
- Learning style of child and caregivers
- Current living situation, including living environment, community characteristics, and projected discharge destination
- Social interactions, activities, and support systems
- Current and prior school situation (services received, individualized education plan, individual family service plan)
- Leisure activities/sports/dreams for the future
- Availability of accessible transportation

Systems Review

Guided by the history and initial information, the PT proceeds to the examination.

Cardiovascular/Pulmonary Systems

Vital signs such as blood pressure, heart rate, and respiratory rate are taken before, during, and after activity, including bed mobility, transfers, and transitions. Examining tolerance for the upright position can sometimes be a slow process as those with SCI are at risk for orthostatic hypotension. Compression stockings and abdominal binders are helpful to aid in vascular support. Children with a lesion above T-6 are also at risk for autonomic dysreflexia, a serious complication of SCI involving the sympathetic nervous system (Display 12.1).

Children post-SCI may demonstrate neuromuscular weakness, which can lead to decreased respiratory efficiency. Quality of cough should be noted, and breathing pattern and chest and diaphragmatic excursion measurements should be taken. Collaboration with medical, nursing, and respiratory staff can help in assessing the respiratory potential. Pulmonary function tests such as vital capacity and forced expiratory volume are helpful. For those on ventilators, parameter settings should be noted. Measurements may need to be repeated, especially if the child is weaning off ventilatory support. In some practice settings, PTs have an active role in airway clearance interventions, including postural drainage, percussion, and vibration. Therefore, a complete examination of the pulmonary system is necessary.

DISPLAY 12.1 Autonomic Dysreflexia

Autonomic dysreflexia is the body's response to lack of sympathetic input during noxious stimuli. The noxious stimulus may include kinked catheter tubing, constipation, muscle spasm, ingrown toenail, or even ROM exercises. Symptoms vary but most often include elevated blood pressure, diaphoresis, headache, and bradycardia and require immediate attention. Treatment requires removal of the noxious stimulus, positioning to decrease blood pressure, and pharmacologic intervention if needed. If left untreated, autonomic dysreflexia may progress to a life-threatening situation.

Integumentary

The skin of a child with an SCI must be fully examined. This includes color, integrity, bruising, and the presence of any scar formation. Neurovascular signs such as pulses, skin temperature, and edema should also be assessed regularly. Decubitus ulcers can be a chronic problem for children with SCI. Regular pressure relief and proper skin care are the only way to prevent this problem. Education regarding position changes, pressure relief, and skin inspection should begin during the initial examination (Displays 12.2 and 12.3).

Musculoskeletal System

Range of motion (ROM), muscle tone, strength, anatomic symmetry, and posture are examined. In the acute phase, muscle tone may initially be flaccid and ROM full, secondary to spinal shock. Special precautions are required to prevent loss of flexibility. Spasticity can begin quickly and interfere with the child's flexibility goals. ROM examinations should be performed with overall diagnosis and prognosis in mind. Depending on functional goals, flexibility is desired in some areas, whereas inflexibility may be ideal in others. For example, overlengthening of certain muscle groups, such as the hamstrings and shoulder internal rotators, may be desirable to assist with functional skills using the upper extremities,

---

DISPLAY 12.2 Nutrition

It is important for any person with a new SCI to have a full nutritional workup in order to ensure that caloric intake is meeting new energy demands and that there is a healthy balance between intake and output. Patients with SCI are at risk for lowered immunity and decreased nutritional status.[64] Unfortunately, both of these issues can delay wound healing, so it is important for the PT to discuss the nutritional status with the patient's physician and nutritionist if there is any disruption in skin integrity. The PT may also refer a patient with an SCI to a nutritionist at any point along the continuum of care to promote a healthy and balanced diet that is individualized for that patient's unique needs.

12.3 Latex Allergy

Patients with significantly increased exposure to latex products, such as children with myelomeningocele or SCI, can develop an allergy to latex. To decrease their exposure to latex, products that are latex free should be used whenever possible. Owing to the need for catheterization supplies and gloves, over the course of a lifetime, many institutions now advocate a "latex-free" environment in which health care workers and other caregivers utilize latex alternatives to provide care. Many products commonly found in both the home and the hospital environment contain latex and have the potential to cause a reaction in the child. Care must be taken to ensure that the child does not encounter latex if he or she already has an allergy to it or to prevent one from occurring. Products that contain latex include Thera-Band, Ace wraps, catheters, many toys, balloons, and even Band-Aids. Many companies offer a latex-free substitute for therapeutic modalities.

12.5 Modified Ashworth Scale[93]

0 = No increase in tone
1 = Slight increase in muscle tone, manifested by a catch and release or by minimal resistance at the end of the ROM
1+ = Slight increase in muscle tone, manifested by a catch, followed by minimal resistance throughout the remainder (less than half) of the ROM
2 = More marked increase in muscle tone through most of the ROM, but the affected part is easily moved
3 = Considerable increase in muscle tone, passive movement is difficult
4 = Affected part is rigid

whereas slight tightening of the heel cords may be desirable to provide stability at the ankle joint for standing transfers.

Spasticity is due to upper motor neuron damage, resulting in velocity-dependent increase in muscle stretch reflexes that lead to an increase in muscle tone.[13] Examination of spasticity is most widely performed using the Modified Ashworth Scale while noting any clonus or spasms (Displays 12.4 and 12.5).[14,15] Other examination tools include the Visual Analog Scale, the Wartenberg Pendulum Test, and the Penn Spasm Frequency Scale. Surface electromyography and isokinetic dynamometry are also used to examine spasticity in people with SCIs.[15] It is important to remember that spasticity may vary throughout the day, sometimes depending on the patient's general health, stress level, or the climate. It is important to remember that spasticity can be useful in some functional situations. For example, someone with significant lower extremity weakness may rely on his or her spasticity for stability in weight bearing for transfers or ambulation. Some children can even learn to trigger a spasm in order to help their lower extremity move in a certain way. Conversely, excessive spasticity can lead to problems with ROM, positioning, or comfort. Excessive spasticity in the hip adductor muscles could cause difficulty with personal hygiene.

12.4 Advantageous Muscle Imbalances

Allowing shortening of the long finger flexors can allow a tenodesis grasp for someone who is able to extend his or her wrist but is unable to actively grasp. It can also allow someone who cannot extend his or her wrist to use his or her hand as a hook.

Tightening of low back extensors can improve sitting stability and assist in moving the lower part of the body in someone with paraplegia.

Excessive shoulder extension and external rotation can combine to substitute for absent triceps, and a straight leg raise of 120 degrees is imperative to allow floor-to-wheelchair transfers.

Children with incomplete SCIs can demonstrate a mix of intact sensory and motor function. Spasticity can mask underlying neuromuscular recovery or weakness; however, it may be necessary for functional activities. A thorough knowledge of the child's spasticity and movement patterns will assist the therapist in understanding the child's process of recovery. Medical management often requires a balance between decreasing and increasing spasticity based on the child's goals and functional needs. Therapists should have a thorough understanding of the medical management of spasticity in order to provide educated recommendations to the physician in order to maximize the child's function.

For strength examinations in the pediatric population, performing manual muscle testing can provide valuable information if the child is able to fully participate in the examination. Games such as "Simon Says" can be useful in helping the child understand the task. For the very young or those with cognitive impairments, functional strength testing can be examined through observation, noting whether the child has the ability to move against gravity or against any resistance (i.e., reaching for a toy in different planes of movement or lifting/kicking against something with force). In the case of working with a child with an SCI, the therapist should note both gross and individual muscle strength and muscle substitutions utilized by the child. It is important for the PT to examine the motor abilities at all spinal levels as this information will have significant impact for the physical therapy diagnosis and prognosis. Examination of muscle strength should be performed on a regular basis in the early phases of recovery as the period of spinal shock can produce different results. Recognizing the use of muscle substitution can help identify functional compensation to help determine if the muscle substitutions should be allowed or discouraged.

Sensory examination includes a thorough screen of all sensory spinal tracts and further individualized testing when warranted. Light touch, temperature, pinprick, and proprioception are important indicators of spinal function. The PT can further pinpoint where the breakdown occurs using a dermatomal chart indicating spinal level.

The presence or absence of any sensory or motor function in the lowest sacral segment is an aspect of the prognosis and should not be overlooked in the examination process.

DISPLAY
12.6   **Heterotopic Ossification**

Patients with upper motor neuron lesions such as SCI are at risk for the development of heterotopic ossification (HO). Primary areas affected are large joints such as the hip, shoulder, knee, and elbow joints. Patients are most at risk during the first 1 to 4 months after injury. There is no acute treatment for the pediatric population because medications that are used for the prevention of HO in adults have not been approved for use with the pediatric population. HO can be surgically excised, but only after the abnormal bone formation is completely mature, usually 1 to 2 years after onset. Current best practice advocates the use of gentle ROM to affected joints and avoiding immobilization or aggressive ROM.[21,22] The entire team should be vigilant in screening for the development of HO because it can be a major setback for the child.

DISPLAY
12.7   **Traumatic Brain Injury**

Because of the high velocity and trauma often associated with SCI, there is an increased risk of associated traumatic brain injury, which may be as high as 24% to 59%.[25] Consequently, cognition should always be screened, and neuropsychologic testing may be indicated with any person who has sustained an SCI in order to rule out any mild cognitive deficits.

Often this information is obtained by the examining physician; however, in some practice settings, a PT may also perform this examination. Sensory information should be examined regularly, as should strength, to note changes in recovery and status.

Position, posture, and alignment must be evaluated in children with SCI. Children with muscular weakness and imbalances may be at risk for developing spinal deformities and scoliosis. Proper positioning is a crucial component to maintaining proper alignment. Examination of the core musculature and the position of the pelvis and spinal column are important in the evaluation of a child's positioning and alignment. Muscle imbalance can lead to the development of flexible scoliosis. Radiographic films of the bones and joints can assist the therapist in determining the child's skeletal alignment (Display 12.6).

Neuromuscular System

In the examination of the neuromuscular system, the PT evaluates all functional movements. Functional movements are related to available ROM, muscle tone, and strength. Although the therapist may strive to assist the child to achieve the most normal movement pattern, it may be more important to the child to be able to perform the activity in any way possible to enable as much functional independence as possible. Neuromuscular evaluation also includes gross coordinated movements, including functional mobility, transfers and transitioning, locomotion, balance, and coordination. In the acute stages of a new SCI, functional movement may be limited to bed mobility and sitting balance on the edge of the bed because of medical restrictions determined by the physician. When the injury is no longer acute, the patient may be able to withstand a more rigorous examination. Functional movement evaluations should occur regularly to monitor progression of recovery and to note use of compensatory movements. This portion of the examination includes wheelchair mobility and skills such as transfers, propulsion, and utilization of wheelies, as appropriate. In these cases, the wheelchair is considered as an extension of the person's body, enabling mobility and independence.

The PT also examines the child's communication, affect, cognition, language, and learning style. Understanding the child's learning style enables the PT to structure educational activities to best suit the unique learning characteristics of the child. This includes the level of consciousness; orientation to person, place, and time; ability to make his or her needs known; expected emotional and behavioral responses; and learning preferences (for both the child and the caregiver). If the child has sustained a traumatic brain injury as a result of the accident, the PT should also consider examination techniques commonly used with that population (Display 12.7). A knowledge of normal cognitive development will assist the therapist in determining what may be a new cognitive deficit versus a deficit that was present prior to the onset of the SCI. A PT awareness of a child's learning style (and that of the caregivers) will allow the educational materials and instructions to be designed and delivered in a manner that is most appropriate for the people involved.

Tests and Measures

The PT has a wide variety of tests and measures to further characterize and quantify the information gathered during the examination. These include but are not limited to:

- Aerobic capacity and endurance
- Anthropometric characteristics
- Assistive and adaptive devices and usage
- Arousal, attention, and cognition
- Circulation
- Cranial and peripheral nerve integrity
- Environmental, home, and work (job/school/play) settings and barriers
- Ergonomics and body mechanics
- Gait, locomotion, and balance (including wheelchair usage)
- Integumentary integrity
- Joint integrity and mobility
- Motor function (motor control and motor learning)
- Muscle performance (including strength, power, tone, and endurance)
- Neuromotor development and sensory integration
- Orthotic, protective, and supportive devices
- Posture
- ROM (including muscle length)
- Reflex integrity (both typical and pathologic reflexes)
- Self-care and home management (including activities of daily living [ADLs] and instrumental ADLs [IADLs])

- Sensory integrity
- Ventilation and respiration
- Work (job/school/play), community, and leisure integration or reintegration (including IADLs)

» Evaluation, diagnosis, and prognosis

During the evaluation process, the PT synthesizes the information that was discovered during the history, systems review, and tests and measures. He or she then formulates a physical therapy diagnosis and prognosis. In the case of SCI, the type and severity of the injury is central to establishing a prognosis and a plan of care.

Standards for neurologic and functional classification of SCI were identified by the American Spinal Injury Association (ASIA) in 1982.[16] This multidisciplinary group of experts established common terminology and a standard classification system for the medical field. It was last revised in 2019, entitled "American Spinal Injury Association: International Standards for Neurologic Classification of Spinal Cord Injury (ISNCSCI)."[17] This document serves to standardize the examination of myotomes and dermatomes among clinicians. Using the information from the examination and the guidelines set forth on the ISNCSCI form, the clinician can determine a sensory and a motor diagnostic level for both the right and left sides of the body. Furthermore, this classification scheme states whether the injury is complete or incomplete. The clinician can then assign an ASIA level of impairment and ASIA Scale (Display 12.8) for classification.

DISPLAY 12.8   ASIA Impairment Scale[17]

A = Complete. No sensory or motor function is preserved in sacral segments S-4 to S-5.

B = Incomplete. Sensory but not motor function is preserved below the neurologic level and extends through the sacral segments S-4 to S-5. Also, no motor function is preserved more than three levels below the motor level on either side of the body.

C = Incomplete. Motor function is preserved at the most caudal sacral segments for voluntary and contraction (VAC) or the patient meets the criteria for sensory incomplete status (sensory function preserved at the most caudal sacral segments [S4 to S5] by light touch [LT], pin prick [PP], or deep anal pressure [DAP]) and has some sparing of motor function more than three levels below the ipsilateral motor level on either side of the body. This includes key or non-key muscle functions to determine motor incomplete status. For ASIA C—less than half of key muscle functions below the single neurologic level of injury have a muscle grade ≤3.

D = Incomplete. ASIA D defined as ASIA C, with at least half or more of key muscle functions below single neurologic level of injury having a muscle grade >3.

E = Normal. If sensation and motor function as tested with the ISNCSCI are graded as normal in all segments and the patient had prior deficits, then the ASIA grade is E.

DISPLAY 12.9   ASIA Clinical Syndromes[17]

Central cord syndrome presents with greater weakness in the upper extremities than the lower extremities and presents with sacral sparing

Brown–Sequard syndrome presents with ipsilateral proprioceptive and motor loss and contralateral loss of pinprick and temperature

Anterior cord syndrome presents with variable loss of motor function and sensation to pinprick and temperature and has sparing of proprioception

Conus medullaris syndrome presents with areflexic bladder, bowel, and lower extremities and may show preserved bulbocavernosus and micturition reflexes

Cauda equina syndrome presents with areflexic bladder, bowel, and lower extremities

---

Some spinal cord lesions present as a clinical syndrome, as described in Display 12.9, and this terminology can also be used universally when discussing the child's presentation with other health care professionals. Although the ASIA has not yet published a specific worksheet for children and youth, current studies support the use of the tool in children older than 6 years who can follow the directions for pinprick and light touch when applied to their cheek.[18,19]

A physical therapy diagnosis for this population may include the following: decreased strength, decreased ROM, decreased endurance, decreased airway clearance and respiratory efficiency, decreased functional mobility, and decreased independence in the home, school, or community because of SCI. The process for making a diagnosis includes the identification of the child's impairments and functional limitations. After establishing a physical therapy diagnosis, the PT can prognosticate the optimal level of function the child may achieve. The amount and intensity of physical therapy services required to achieve that level of function can be discussed as well as future episodes of care that may be needed over the course of the child's lifetime. Formulating a physical therapy prognosis incorporates information from the examination and should include evidence from current scientific literature. The PT is also guided by the medical prognosis in developing goals that the child may be able to achieve. Prognoses for someone with a complete injury and someone with an incomplete injury can be very different based on neurologic potential for recovery. Ongoing reassessment of the child using the ASIA Impairment Scale is critical not only to understand the patient's current status and potential ability but also to monitor for possible change. The most significant recovery is expected in the first year after injury, but some children show improvement for up to 5 years.[20] Studies suggest that some individuals with SCI may skip to the next level on the ASIA Impairment Scale during the period of neurologic recovery.[20-23]

Although the principles of examination, evaluation, and diagnosis are similar to those of children with traumatic injuries, atraumatic SCIs can be more unpredictable in their outcomes. As an example, transverse myelitis involves inflammation of the spinal cord[24] and can have varying functional outcomes.[24] Approximately 30% of those afflicted have full recovery, 30% have partial recovery, and another 30% have little to no recovery.[25] There are some medical factors that help prognosticate recovery, including the speed of onset, amount of paralysis, and the speed of recovery in the first month, but these are never certain. Early treatment with corticosteroids is considered the first-line treatment and has been shown in case studies and research with those with MS to improve functional outcomes.[26] Published research also demonstrates that a high level of interleukin-6 in the cerebrospinal fluid (CSF) correlates with poor functional outcomes.[10,16] The potential for a large amount of neurologic recovery can alter the entire focus of physical therapy from goals of learning to compensate with the remaining intact musculature to a goal for recovering lost function.

Atraumatic SCI caused by a tumor may present with similar clinical symptoms to a traumatic SCI, but cancer treatment such as radiation and chemotherapy can have profound effects on the child's functioning, physical therapy treatment, and the family as a whole. Radiation has been found to alter spinal alignment, leading to the development of a scoliosis or kyphosis.[27] This can greatly impact the child's prognosis.

When considering the child's prognosis, the PT should keep in mind both the potential for neurologic recovery and the functional outcomes that can be realistically achieved. The accepted outcome measures used for adults with SCI include the Modified Barthel Index (MBI), the Functional Independence Measure (FIM), the Quadriplegic Index of Function (QIF), and the Spinal Cord Independence Measure (SCIM).[28] These outcome measures have not been standardized in the pediatric population. The Pediatric Spinal Cord Injury Activity Measure (PEDI-SCI AM) assesses general mobility, daily routines, wheeled mobility, and ambulation.[29] The Pediatric Quality of Life Inventory Spinal Cord Injury (PedsQL SCI) is being developed to assess various domains including daily activities, mobility, bladder function, bowel function, muscle spasms, pressure injury, pain, orthostatic hypotension, autonomic dysreflexia, participation, worry, and emotions.[30] The PT can identify anticipated functional outcomes on the basis of both the adult SCI literature and myelodysplasia literature. The general functional expectations by level of involvement are discussed in Table 12.1.[18]

TABLE 12.1. Functional Expectations by Level of Involvement

Level of Injury	Mobility	Transfers	Activities of Daily Living
C-1–C-4	• Sipping or blowing to independently control a power wheelchair, power-tilt mechanism, and environmental controls	• Dependent for all transfers	• Dependent for dressing, bathing, and bowel and bladder management
C-5: addition of biceps and deltoids	• Can propel a manual wheelchair with hand rims for short distances on level surfaces • Power wheelchair for longer distances	• Able to assist with transfers and bed mobility	• Able to assist with feeding, grooming with adaptive equipment and setup • Dependent for dressing and bathing
C-6: addition of pectorals	• Able to independently use manual wheelchair with projections on the hand rims	• Independent with self-care with equipment • Independent with upper extremity dressing, assists with lower extremity • Independent with bowel program, needs assistance with bladder program • Can drive with a specially adapted van	• Assists with sliding board transfers
C-7–T-1: addition of triceps	• Able to independently propel a manual wheelchair on level surfaces	• Independent with adaptive equipment • Can drive a car with hand controls	• Independent transfers with or without sliding board
T-4–T-6: addition of upper abdominal	• Can ambulate with RGOs for short distances with a walker	• Independent for grooming, bowel and bladder, dressing and bathing	• Independent transfers with or without sliding board
T-9–T-12: addition of lower abdominals	• Household ambulation with RGOs or HKAFOs and assistive device	• Independent for grooming, bowel and bladder, dressing and bathing	• Independent transfers with or without sliding board
L-2–L-4: addition of gracilis, iliopsoas, and quadratus lumborum	• Functional ambulation with KAFOs with crutches	• Independent for grooming, bowel and bladder, dressing and bathing	• Independent transfers with or without sliding board
L-4–L-5: addition of hamstrings, quadriceps, and anterior tibialis	• Able to ambulate with AFOs with or without assistive device	• Independent for grooming, bowel and bladder, dressing and bathing	• Independent transfers with or without sliding board

AFO, ankle–foot orthosis; HKAFO, hip–knee–ankle–foot orthosis; KAFO, knee–ankle–foot orthosis; RGO, reciprocating gait orthosis.

Understanding the child's prognosis for functional outcomes leads the PT to develop a plan of care that includes specific interventions and the frequency, intensity, and duration of those interventions. It also incorporates anticipated goals, expected outcomes, and discharge plans. When working in an interdisciplinary model, the plan of care may involve other health care professionals in both establishing interdisciplinary goals and providing the intervention to achieve them. For example, a child working on transfers in the hospital should have the opportunity to practice these transfers in a variety of environments and situations that incorporate the family, nurses, and other therapists and to help simulate the situations the child will encounter after discharge. Incorporating recommendations from the various professionals working with the child can help with carry over postdischarge and the continuation of work toward goal achievement.

Standardized outcome measures performed prior to and after physical therapy intervention are useful in measuring the progress the child has made over the course of an episode of care. Some outcome measures used with the pediatric population include the WeeFIM, Pediatric Evaluation of Disability Inventory (PEDI), and Gross Motor Function Measure (GMFM).[31] When the test or measure cannot be done in the standard way, creativity may sometimes be useful in modifying existing outcome measures for a child with paralysis. For example, the 9-minute walk/run can be modified into a 9-minute "wheelchair run" to measure endurance. The PT should be familiar with all available outcome measures in order to choose the most appropriate one for a particular child. Standardized outcome measures can help the therapist pinpoint weaknesses as well as focus and modify the plan of care. Standardized outcomes used as a repeated measure can help track progress and change throughout the episode of care.

» Intervention

Medical Intervention

Surgery

MUSCLE TRANSFERS Recent advances in surgical techniques have allowed for the transfer of muscle function from one group to another. If there is sufficient remaining muscle strength in two or more muscle groups that work together to perform a movement, one of the muscles can be transferred biomechanically to perform another movement. There is little or no adverse effect on the original motion. Most commonly, elbow joint extension is achieved by transferring the posterior deltoid muscle to the triceps. There are, however, promising results with a biceps-to-triceps transfer for elbow joint extension to achieve overhead function.[32] Similarly, wrist joint extension is achieved by transferring the brachioradialis to the extensor carpi radialis. Active grasp is achieved by transferring the brachioradialis and using it as a thumb flexor.[33]

Processes such as tenodesis, arthrodesis, tendon lengthening, rerouting, releases, and tendon transfer have the capacity to restore function to persons with tetraplegia. All these surgeries require not only careful surgical technique but also comprehensive postoperative physical and occupational therapy. There is an abundance of literature on these procedures in the adult population. Although there are fewer studies performed on children, the results are similar.[33]

MUSCLE SPASTICITY Muscle spasticity is the clinical manifestation that accompanies upper motor neuron disease or involvement. A muscle displays an increased resistance to passive motion that results from the hyperactivity of the spinal and brainstem reflexes. In SCI, acutely, there is usually muscle flaccidity, then flexor muscle spasticity presents, and then finally extensor muscle spasticity. Muscle tone may plateau at any point along the process, presenting with varying degrees of spasticity.

Conservative interventions to address spasticity include removing the noxious stimuli, stretching the muscle, repositioning the involved limb, using orthotics, biofeedback, or electric stimulation. All these, however, have short-term effects. When conservative interventions are not enough, there are other options that have been shown to reduce muscle spasticity.[34] Oral baclofen, intrathecal baclofen, botulinum toxin, and neurologic and orthopedic surgery are options. Pharmacologically, baclofen acts as a γ-aminobutyric acid (GABA) analog at the site of the spinal cord. Common side effects seen with oral baclofen use are sedation, fatigue, and hepatotoxicity.[35] Obtaining the appropriate dose (via titration) is important to maximize the drug's benefit while minimizing the side effects. Baclofen administered through a surgically implanted intrathecal pump acts directly on the spinal cord with less risk of drowsiness and weakness than oral baclofen. There is risk of infection with the pump insertion.[34] Dantrolene sodium is a medication that acts on the muscle to inhibit the release of calcium from the sarcoplasmic reticulum. This medication carries the same effects of drowsiness and fatigue and can damage liver function. Clonidine, via the oral route or patch, acts centrally as an α-agonist. Clonidine can lead to hypotension; however, its side effects are commonly limited to dry mouth and drowsiness. Diazepam (Valium) acts on the limbic system. Adverse reactions can include drowsiness and fatigue, and its use can lead to drug dependency.[34]

Other pharmacologic interventions include chemical nerve blocks, which work at the motor point. Different chemicals are used depending on the individual and the intended result. Lidocaine is a short-acting agent, whereas phenol can last up to 6 months, but high concentrations of phenol can cause permanent damage to the nerve associated with muscle spasticity. Botulinum toxin (Botox) is so specific that it goes straight to the muscle to treat focal spasticity and its effects last about 3 to 4 months.[35]

PAIN The adult literature has shown that those with SCI experience many different complaints of pain.[34,36,37] Studies of chronic pain reported by children are few, but these studies do report the same results. They report that pain associated with pediatric-onset SCI is common. Reports of nociceptive pain were greater than neuropathic pain.[38] Data suggest that although it is common, chronic pain in childhood SCI has a significantly smaller impact on daily activities than that reported in the literature for adult-onset SCI.[38]

Studies have looked at multiple interventions for pain, including medications, physical therapy, psychotherapy, and spinal cord stimulators. There is consistency in the reports of pain in adults with SCI; the reports of pain continue through the postacute stage, with 60% of those with an SCI reporting pain at 6 and 12 months postinjury.[34] The International Association for the Study of Pain has proposed a scheme for characterizing SCI. It classifies pain into two types: neuropathic and nociceptive. Nociceptive pain is musculoskeletal and visceral. It is characterized by dull, aching, movement-related pain that is eased by rest and responds to opioids. Neuropathic pain is classified as above the level, at the level, or below the level of injury. Neuropathic pain is usually described as sharp, shooting, burning, and electrical with abnormal sensory responsiveness (hyperesthesia or hyperalgesia). Antidepressants and anticonvulsants are typically used in the management of people with SCI; however, neither is particularly effective for SCI pain. Recent reports have shown promise for opioids and α-adrenergic antagonists, as well as baclofen, a GABA-b agonist, when there is muscle spasticity interfering with function.[39]

Sodium channel blockers, such as lidocaine and tetracaine hydrochloride, have been shown to decrease allodynia (pain from a stimulus that is not usually painful). Opioids have been shown to help neuropathic pain as well as nociceptive pain.[39] Intrathecal clonidine in combination with morphine has been shown to have an analgesic effect in those with SCI.[34]

SURGICAL PROCEDURES Surgical procedures such as cordectomy, cordotomy, and myelotomy are most effective for spontaneous lancinating or shooting pain. They are not effective for burning or aching pain. Complications associated with these procedures include contralateral pain, bowel and bladder dysfunction, loss of sexual function, and development of spasms.[34]

SPINAL CORD STIMULATORS Spinal cord stimulators were first used in the 1970s to manage severe pain such as reflex sympathetic dystrophy (RSD). Spinal cord stimulators inhibit spinal transmission of pain through electrical stimulation via the Gate Control Theory of Pain. One to two leads are placed in the epidural space of the spinal cord, and a small electric current is sent through the electrodes. A receiver or battery pack is placed under the skin in the abdomen.[40] Research is finding that neurostimulation can help with pain management, functional motor/sensory recovery, bladder/bowel function, and cardiovascular autonomic dysregulation.[41] It has been shown to be most effective in those with incomplete pain or postcordotomy pain[34] and less effective in those with a complete SCI. Complications may include infections, allergic reaction, electrode migration, CSF leak, and bleeding. Deep brain stimulation was also used in the 1970s and 1980s; however, it has not been used recently because the Food and Drug Administration (FDA) has not approved it for any pain indications.[34]

Therapeutic and Functional Interventions

When working with a child or adolescent with an SCI, physical therapy interventions are similar to those used with adults with SCI, but the approach may be different.

The PT provides interventions that consist of a variety of procedures and techniques that are individualized for each child with the child's goals in mind. These should produce changes in the child's overall function and help make progress toward maximizing independence and function. The therapist should always be reevaluating the child's response to interventions and modifying them as needed, evaluating for changes in muscle strength, movement, and sensation. There are some differences when working with children with SCIs, including noting that some children who sustain an SCI may still be growing and learning new motor skills. Interventions will be discussed as generalizations, though some specifics to the type and level of SCI will also be mentioned.

Therapeutic Exercise

Therapeutic exercise should include ROM for specific areas of limitations (Fig. 12.1). Special attention should be given to the areas where muscle tone is abnormal. Hamstrings, heel cords, and hip joint adductors often develop contractures early. In some cases, however, contractures can facilitate function. An example is allowing a shortening of the long finger flexors to achieve finger flexion when the wrist joint is extended. Some children can use this active tenodesis for a functional grip. There are other situations where excessive ROM is necessary. Demonstrating increased hamstring flexibility will allow a child with an SCI to be able to perform lower extremity dressing independently. This motion does require some supervision, as overlengthening hamstrings can overstretch the low back, which could impact wheelchair positioning.

The implementation of therapeutic exercise in children is similar to that in other populations. Some muscle groups may not be able to be strengthened or improved owing to complete denervation from the SCI. In contrast, some muscle groups may require greater than normal strength to compensate for other muscle groups that are no longer functioning. When considering the child, age-appropriate

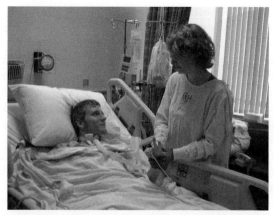

FIGURE 12.1. Physical therapy begins in the intensive care unit with positioning, passive and active range of motion, and family education.

interventions and activities (such as play-based therapy) will be more motivating and likely provide greater success. For example, it is unlikely that a 4-year-old will perform biceps curls with a free weight as instructed; however, he or she may engage in pulling against resistance in a tug-of-war activity. With play-based therapy, it is possible to incorporate therapeutic exercises into play while remaining focused on the goals. In other situations, a child may perform traditional sets of strengthening exercises but may need to be rewarded with a fun and equally therapeutic play activity such as shooting basketballs with wrist cuff weights attached to his or her wrists. Other therapeutic interventions to provide may include:

- Aerobic and endurance conditioning or reconditioning (e.g., playing tag, riding a bike, propelling a manual wheelchair)
- Balance, coordination, and agility training (e.g., navigating an obstacle course, playing Simon Says)
- Body mechanics and postural stabilization (e.g., playing Simon Says, balancing on a physioball)
- Flexibility exercises (e.g., yoga)
- Gait and locomotion training (e.g., walking on a variety of surfaces, moving through an obstacle courses)
- Relaxation (e.g., yoga, relaxation breathing)
- Strength, power, and endurance training for head, neck, limb, pelvic floor, trunk, and ventilatory muscles[42,43] (e.g., blowing bubbles, crab walking)

Therapeutic exercises as described can be performed in a land or aquatic environment. Aquatic therapy can be very useful as the buoyancy and temperature of the water can play a part in muscle relaxation, muscle facilitation, and neuromuscular reeducation in children with neurologic disorders.[44] For some children, supported buoyancy in water allows independent mobility and play that they do not achieve on land. An aquatic environment can also be fun for children, and they often perform more work while having more fun.

Functional Training in Self-Care and Home Management (Including ADLs and IADLs)

Devices and adaptive equipment for children with SCI include wheelchairs, standers, seating systems, braces, and ADL devices. The PT may provide the following types of interventions:

- ADL training with and without assistive devices
- Devices and equipment use training, including donning and doffing equipment, proper positioning, and equipment usage
- Functional training programs, including mobility and function in various environments such as home, school, and community
- IADL training with and without assistive devices
- Injury prevention or reduction, including education on energy conservation and proper positioning to prevention further injury

For an adult, IADLs include caring for dependents, home maintenance, household chores, shopping, and yard work. For children, IADLs include participation in school, family, and play activities. Play is an integral part of a child's life and is necessary for both physical and cognitive development and maturation. Training a child to utilize new movement patterns while playing an age-appropriate game or sport is a very important aspect of a child's life. Other IADLs may include performing basic household chores and eventually prevocational and vocational training.

Adaptations for driving make it possible for some people with SCI to operate a vehicle. Adolescents who are candidates for driving should be referred to rehab centers for driving evaluation and training (Fig. 12.2). Learning to drive with adaptation provides adolescents with independence in the community and more freedom in their lives.

Collaboration with the other providers of services (e.g., occupational therapists) and caregivers is important in ensuring that the goals and strategies to achieve those goals are appropriate and consistent.

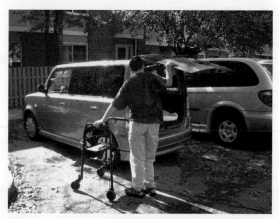

FIGURE 12.2. Adolescents can attend special automobile driving classes for people with disabilities and learn what modifications they may need to safely drive a vehicle.

MOBILITY A wheelchair may be the primary means of locomotion for a child with an SCI. Children as young as 12 to 18 months can independently propel a wheelchair. Early wheelchair mobility can begin with adaptive devices such as Bella's Bumbo or Scoot. Introducing early mobility and enabling a child who sustained an injury to regain independent mobility can help the child in a variety of ways. Mobility can help facilitate exploration of the environment, socialization, and development of cognitive skills.[45] The appropriate wheelchair should be a part of the team evaluation. The team should include the child, the child's parents, therapist, and an assistive technology practitioner. Manual wheelchairs come in many varieties, including lightweight frames, folding frames, and solid frames. Reclining-back wheelchairs can be used to accommodate braces when sitting at a right angle is difficult. Seating principles such as distribution of weight, propulsion, cardiovascular endurance, maintenance of posture, safety, and environmental controls should be considered with children with SCI (Fig. 12.3).

Braces and Ambulation

RECIPROCATING GAIT ORTHOSES VERSUS HIP–KNEE–ANKLE–FOOT ORTHOSES The reciprocating gait orthosis (RGO) is a bracing system composed of a bilateral hip, knee, and ankle orthosis (HKAFO) with the right and left sides connected by a posterior cable. There is also a version designed

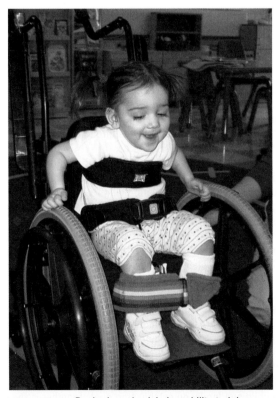

FIGURE 12.3. Beginning wheelchair mobility training as early as possible allows the child to experience a sense of freedom and explore his or her environment for learning opportunities.

to be cableless (isocentric RGO [IRGO]).[46] The cableless connection allows one side of the orthosis to flex when the other extends. The user biomechanically extends one side by weight shifting onto one side while extending his or her trunk. This unweighting mechanism allows the opposite side to flex at the hip allowing for the leg to swing forward. Repeating this action on the contralateral side simulates the gait pattern. Some IRGO models allow hip abduction to occur for the purpose of self-catheterization. Physical therapy and rehabilitation training for RGOs involve evaluation for appropriateness.[47]

There are many things to consider when recommending RGOs. To use RGOs, children should present with significant lower limb weakness with the inability to control the knees and hips. Additionally, the children need to have sufficient upper extremity strength and coordination to assist with weight bearing and advancing an assistive device such as forearm crutches or a walker/gait trainer. Children must be free of significant lower extremity contractures and be able to sit comfortably with their hips and knees flexed to at least 90 degrees. Children should also be cognitively able to follow directions and be motivated to do activities that will allow them to use the RGO system. Prior to the RGO fitting, special attention should be paid to upper extremity strengthening and stabilization activities, especially in the upright position. With RGOs, weight shifting is key to adequate advancement of the lower extremities. This weight shift consists of a diagonal weight shift, push-down through upper extremities, and unweighting of the contralateral side while extending the trunk. No active hip flexion is required to use RGOs.

Training for RGO use begins in the parallel bars. Mirrors can help provide visual feedback for this motion. Hands-on facilitation of the weight shifting by the PT can provide mechanical and tactile feedback to help the child learn the movement. The therapist should be aware of any substitutions, particularly lateral trunk movement and the urge to pull the limbs through using the abdominals. This is usually very typical for those child who have learned a swing-through pattern prior to using RGOs or for those who have sustained a spinal cord impairment after they were independently ambulating. In addition to ambulation, other functional skills such as donning and doffing the braces, skin inspection after removing the braces, coming to and from standing to sitting, and negotiating all levels and uneven surfaces, elevations, and inclines must also be learned (Figs. 12.4 and 12.5; Display 12.10).

LOCOMOTOR TRAINING Locomotor training for children with SCI has received significant attention and acceptance in the rehabilitation community in recent years. By utilizing the concept of activity-based plasticity and automaticity, locomotor training creates a stimulus for the spinal cord network below the level of the lesion to experience repeated sensory input with the goal of generating a learned response in spinal cord circuitry to take steps.[48-50] The Christopher & Dana Reeve Foundation NeuroRecovery Network® (NRN)[51]

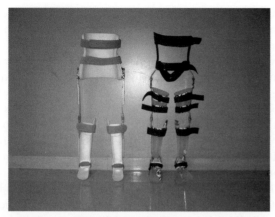

FIGURE 12.4. Braces. **A:** Reciprocating gait orthoses. **B:** Hip–knee–ankle–foot orthoses.

has led the way for large multisite trials exploring the effects of locomotor training in persons with SCI, and the results thus far have been compelling.[43,44] Body weight–supported systems can be used suspended over stationary treadmills and over ground to move freely. By using repeated practice stepping on a treadmill with both body weight support and manual facilitation with progression to overground training, some persons with SCI have demonstrated significant changes in functional ability, including gait speed and balance.[50,52-54] Research is finding that body weight–supported treadmill training has positive effects on the cardiovascular and pulmonary systems.

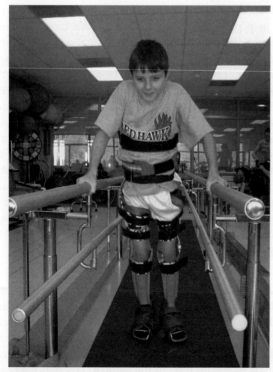

FIGURE 12.5. Ambulation training requires excellent upper body strength and endurance and begins in the parallel bars until the child is ready to progress to an assistive device.

One of the first questions a child or caregiver will ask when first faced with an SCI is, "Will I/he/she ever walk again?" Although many PTs will defer to the physician on this difficult topic, the therapist inevitably will discuss walking at some point with the child and should be well prepared to answer the question before it is asked. For some children with SCI, walking *is* a possibility. This "walking" may require long leg bracing, implantable electric stimulation, and/or assistive devices; however, it may not be the type of walking the child is expecting. The PT should always be honest in what current best practice can achieve, and the child and family can then make an informed decision about whether walking is a goal they want to pursue. Walking as exercise, even with bracing and assistive devices, has benefits that are not only physical but emotional.[88] Walking can also improve the quality of life for children as they can be on an eye-to-eye level with their peers. Many studies have been performed looking at energy expenditure with ambulation and wheelchair use in the population of people with spina bifida, but little research has been done on the pediatric SCI population. Generally, as a child grows and becomes larger, it becomes increasingly difficult to keep up with peers while ambulating. Often, the child ends up choosing a wheelchair as his or her primary means of mobility. The most important concept is that the child is choosing that means of mobility for him- or herself.

During the process of rehabilitation, it is the PT's responsibility to help the child deal with his or her body in its current condition and to help the child achieve the highest level of independence possible. Striving for independence also requires reintegration back into the community and connecting the child with others in the community. One of the most valuable things a therapist can give his or her patient is to put him or her in a situation that challenges him or her to think and solve problems. The therapist can show the patient all the things that he or she can do—the way he or she is now—and provide support as the patient goes through the emotions of losing the way he or she used to be.

A therapist can also provide hope for the future. For a child with an incomplete or atraumatic injury, the period of recovery can last up to 5 years. Being realistic while allowing some hope can help focus and motivate the patient and sustain him or her through this difficult period. The child should come to understand that even though something is not probable does not always mean it is not possible. A child with a complete injury should learn all of the skills necessary as though he or she is going to be a primary wheelchair user. The opportunity for ambulation with an assistive device should be provided if the patient and family desire and if there is potential. To walk or not to walk is not an easy question. It requires careful consideration of the child's diagnosis and prognosis, the known functional potentials based on the literature, and input from the child and family. Being realistic while hopeful and working with the child and family on establishing goals together is the essence of family-centered care.

Another option for children with paraplegia is the use of mobile standers. These devices allow the child's hips, knees, and ankles to be held in a standing position. Although the assistive device allows the child to stand securely, there are wheels that the patient uses to propel forward. In this position, weight bearing is permitted with independent mobility in those without adequate strength to stand independently. Mobile standers help provide an option for children to participate in home and school.[55]

Power mobility is another option for children who cannot propel a manual chair. For those individuals with SCI resulting in C-4 tetraplegia, active functional upper extremity movement is limited to shoulder shrug. Assistive technology such as joysticks, sip and puff, and head arrays assists these children with modified independence with communication and power mobility. Options for self-care are limited for those with this level of injury. There are robotic devices becoming available to assist this patient population (such as robotic arms), but these are expensive and difficult to fund. Some children who have retained shoulder retraction may be able to use mobile arm supports; however, these have shown little promise for those with cervical injury because of decreased control of the glenohumeral joint.[56]

FUNCTIONAL ELECTRIC STIMULATION Functional electrical stimulation (FES) uses surface electrode stimulation to produce functional movements in specific muscles of the upper and lower extremities.[57] Grasping, wrist flexion and extension, and elbow extension have been used with voice activation systems.[58] Intramuscular stimulation systems have also been used to achieve flexion and extension with sip-and-puff control activators.[58] Researchers at Shriners Hospital have shown that the combination of FES and surgical reconstruction provided active palmar and lateral grasp and release in a laboratory setting. The study also showed that FES systems increased pinch force, improved the manipulation of objects, and typically increased the independence in six standard ADLs as compared with pre-FES hand function. Subjects also reported preferring the FES system for most of the ADLs tested.[56] Studies have shown that FES generally provides equal or greater independence in seven mobility activities as compared with long leg braces, provided faster sit-to-stand times, and was preferred over lower leg braces in a majority of cases.[59] FES can be used to simulate the use of orthoses to facilitate anterior tibialis muscle contraction during the swing phase of gait to clear the foot for leg progression. This promotes a more natural gait pattern.

FES during cycling is also being explored as a therapeutic intervention for children with chronic SCI.[60,61] Preliminary results suggest that children with SCI who receive electrically stimulated exercise can experience changes in muscle strength and/or muscle hypertrophy, which could lead to various health benefits such as improved cardiovascular health and decreased risk of diabetes.[60] Other potential benefits from FES cycling may include a slower rate of bone mineral density loss, but more study is warranted.[62]

» Coordination, communication, and documentation

Coordination, communication, and documentation are very important when working with a child with an SCI during the acute and postacute phases of recovery. Specifically, the child's school setting and special education requirements should be considered in treatment planning.

The PT plays an integral part in the health care team and may assist in coordinating care between disciplines and care settings. One of the goals of family-centered care is to ensure a smooth transition for children and families across professionals and institutions. Communication is critical with the PT often participating in case conferences, patient care rounds, and family and school meetings. The therapist may need to make referrals to other sources and communicate with other providers if practicing in an interdisciplinary program. The PT will play an active role in admission and discharge planning and coordination with other professionals when necessary. Discharge planning includes the need to communicate a patient's care and needs among equipment suppliers, community resources, and other appropriate health professionals. Discharge planning includes the identification and utilization of available funds to obtain needed assistive technology. The rehabilitation team may need to guide the family in pursuing or accessing alternative funding sources for assistance. Planning for reentry into the school and the community requires ongoing open communication and coordination of care with the entire team (Fig. 12.6).

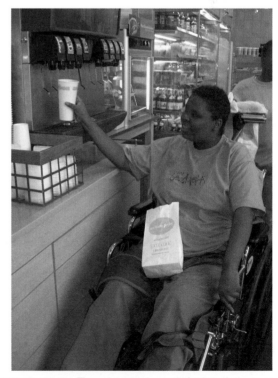

FIGURE 12.6. Therapists can focus their plan of care to assist their children in returning to activities enjoyed prior to their injury.

Documentation should follow the American Physical Therapy Association's Guidelines for Physical Therapy Documentation. It is imperative for the profession as a whole to have a consistent and reliable means of documenting patient status, response to treatment, changes in function, changes in interventions, elements of patient/client management, and outcomes of intervention.

Education

Caregiver instruction is as important as patient education when working with children with SCI. Caregivers must be independent with all aspects of the home program, such as the execution of therapeutic exercises and making or acquiring the appropriate home modifications to facilitate the child's independence.

A key aspect in all physical therapy intervention should be patient and family education. By incorporating the child and family goals into the plan of care, the therapist creates a plan that seeks to educate the child and family according to their learning styles to help them make progress toward their goals, with the ultimate goal being reintegration into the community.

Education begins in the earliest stages of rehabilitation and includes basic education about the child's diagnosis, the role of physical therapy and other involved health professions, the child's prognosis, the plan of care, and what is needed for the family to help the child achieve his or her goals. Tasks such as performing ROM, bed and wheelchair positioning, pressure relief maneuvers, and donning/doffing splints and equipment begin in the acute phases of treatment. Often, the family members are thankful to be able to start doing something for their child and to be involved in their child's care. It is important for the child and his or her family to receive education about skin integrity, autonomic dysreflexia, positioning, assistive technology, therapeutic exercise, and stretching, repeatedly over the course of the admission. As the child advances through the phases of rehabilitation, he or she and his or her family will gradually become more active in the treatment activities. Families must learn and demonstrate all aspects of the child's care, and the child needs to learn how to teach others how to care for him or her. Caregivers of children with an SCI often need support to prevent burnout as care and assistance are needed throughout the life span. The PT may be the health care professional referring the caregiver to a support group, respite care, or mental health professional. Some children perform better in physical therapy when family members are present, but other children may not. In cases when caregivers are asked to step out of a session to enable the child to become a more active participant, the therapist should follow up with a brief education session and explain what the child was able to do and what they can practice at home. Children often demonstrate increased motivation for their personal exercise programs if there is some sort of reward associated with it. Recognizing what motivates a child and incorporating this information into the treatment planning can help increase the child's participation in designed treatment plans. Parents and pediatric psychologists can be extremely useful in helping to determine a plan to increase desirable behaviors and active participation by the child to help support his or her physical therapy goals.

Discharge Planning

Education of the child, the parent, and the child's teacher is critical prior to discharge planning. School visits by a team member may be helpful to provide input regarding school accessibility and assistive technology. Medical issues must be stressed with the school staff, including neurogenic bladder, bowel and skin integrity, autonomic dysreflexia, orthostatic hypotension, and thermoregulation. Ensuring the appropriate school staff is educated regarding the child's medical condition, limitations, precautions, and capabilities will help establish a safe environment for the child.

School Reentry

All children are entitled to a free and appropriate education under the Family Educational Rights and Privacy Act (FERPA).[63] Related services include transportation and developmental, corrective, and other supportive services to assist the child in learning and benefiting from an education. Children with SCI and mobility impairments may need extra time to move between classes or use a peer buddy system to help them manage their school environment. Community resources available to the child and family include counseling, respite care, financial support, legal rights, and advocacy. There are national, state, and local government agencies that are sources of support and information, some of which include the NSCIA, the National Parent Network on Disabilities, and the Family Resource Center on Disabilities.

» Illness prevention and wellness

Fitness

It is important for the child with an SCI to remain active (Fig. 12.7). Lack of activity can lead to a child becoming overweight, and children with an SCI are at increased risk for becoming overweight.[64] Aerobic and endurance conditioning should be performed to improve cardiorespiratory status. Children with lower extremity paralysis can perform upper extremity activity with ergometers, arm bikes, seated yoga and dance, and wheelchair sports. There are a variety of wheelchair sports such as track and field, basketball, and tennis. Studies support that physical training has a positive influence on respiratory muscle strength and thoracic mobility, as well as quality of life, especially in subjects with quadriplegia.[65] Participation in wheelchair sports also provides an opportunity for socialization. Remaining active can reinforce the treatment plan recommended by the rehabilitation team, encouraging maintenance of appropriate ROM and strength needed for independence and function.

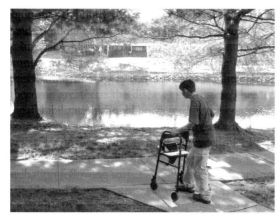

FIGURE 12.7. Teens with a spinal cord injury often have to problem-solve how to access things that they enjoy.

Circulation

Although deep vein thrombosis (DVT) and pulmonary embolism are rare in children, in order to prevent circulatory problems, children with SCI are often placed on prophylactic blood anticoagulation agents. Precautions against injury should be maintained as these children may be at risk for increased bruising. Regular position changes and participation in physical activity will help prevent DVT development.

Dysreflexia/Hyperreflexia

For children with an SCI above T-6, interventions to prevent and monitor for autonomic dysreflexia are extremely important. It is important to teach children who are at risk for autonomic dysreflexia to identify its signs and symptoms as well as educate caregivers about its treatment. Symptoms include severe headache, visual disturbances, nausea and vomiting, excessive diaphoresis above the level of injury, and piloerection above the level of injury.[66] This can be triggered by a noxious stimulus, ranging from a full bladder or catheter bag, urinary tract infection, or pressure ulcer. Treatment includes immediate resolution of the noxious stimulus. Studies show that there is a similar prevalence of dysreflexia in children with pediatric-onset SCI compared with adult-onset SCI. Dysreflexia is diagnosed less commonly in infants and preschool-aged children, and these two populations may present with more subtle signs and symptoms.[67]

Growth Abnormalities

Hip Joint Subluxation

There is a high incidence of hip joint subluxation/dislocation in children with SCI.[68,69] The rate is significantly higher among children with onset of injury before 10 years. Decreased muscle tone that occurs with the onset of paraplegia makes the hip prone to subluxation/dislocation because of the lack of soft tissue support. Children and families should be educated to recognize signs and symptoms of potential hip subluxation/dislocation such as inguinal pain with movement and atypical protrusion of the greater trochanter.[70]

Scoliosis

The incidence of progressive paralytic scoliosis subsequent to acquired SCI has been reported to range from 46% to 98% in children injured before their adolescent growth spurt.[71] Age at injury has been shown to be a critical factor influencing the development of paralytic scoliosis. Some studies have shown that early bracing in children whose curve is less than 20 degrees may slow the progression of the curvature or prevent surgery. Newer research is looking at the effectiveness of the Schroth method in treating scoliosis, either to correct minor curvatures or to strengthen postural muscles in conjunction with bracing.[72] Children whose curve ranges from 20 to 40 degrees should undergo a trial of bracing with the goal to delay surgery. In children with large curves greater than 41 degrees, the use of bracing is ineffective and may actually lead to skin breakdown and hindrance of ADLs so surgery for spinal alignment correction is recommended.[69,71] Children whose curvature falls into this range may be considered for surgical correction of the curvature with bone fusion and growing rods.

Bowel and Bladder Management

Good bowel and bladder management is important for prevention of renal disease in a children who sustained an SCI.[73] Urogenic hygiene education is very important as well. There are many traditional options for handling bowel and bladder incontinence. There is reflex voiding and pressure voiding, where voids are timed and facilitated manually by increasing external pressure on the bladder. Catheterization is another means of emptying the bladder. There are a variety of types of catheters, including indwelling, condom, and straight catheters. Another option is wearing pads or absorbent underpants. The overall goal for these is to avoid infection and to use antibiotics sparingly owing to the development of resistant organisms.

Rehabilitation professionals work together to afford children and young adults as much independence as possible. A child must have the ability to comprehend and the fine motor skills to be able to independently use the equipment for self-catheterization, to have the understanding of when and how to use the equipment, and to realize when a complication has arisen. The typical age that a child begins to understand is around 2 to 3 years. Total independence with toileting is expected by 5 years of age whether or not the child has SCI.

The goal for bowel continence is to control constipation, be convenient, and to allow for independence in personal hygiene. Diets rich in fiber with adequate fluid and exercise are the best way to achieve these goals. Training the bowels is done by habitual voids (e.g., every other day). Digital stimulation and the use of suppositories and enemas can assist with the process. For bowel and bladder incontinence, it is important that orthoses do not interfere with the ability to void or to self-catheterize. Some brace options allow for hip joint abduction to eliminate the need for donning and doffing the braces for catheterization.

Skin Integrity

The importance of skin inspection and pressure relief is increased in those with decreased sensation. Children can be taught to do independent pressure relief, which may include wheelchair tilts, sitting push-ups off the seat, or unweighting each side in the wheelchair. It is recommended that pressure relief be completed regularly, on average about every 15 to 30 minutes. It is important that children and family learn to complete regular skin inspection and recognize signs of impaired skin, such as changes in color, bruising, and chaffing.

Bone Density

Owing to decreased weight bearing, children with an SCI are at risk for osteopenia, especially those with a thoracic- and lumbar-level injury. Children who have spinal cord neoplasm may also develop osteopenia owing to their chemotherapy regimens. Supported standing programs are one intervention used to maintain bone health. Children with an SCI can complete supported standing to achieve weight bearing through the lower extremities. A variety of pieces of assistive technology can be used for weight bearing to address bone density, including RGOs, HKAFOs, mobile standers, prone standers, and supine standers. Care should also be taken when performing ROM, positioning, and sometimes transfers and ambulation because of the potential for fractures as a result of osteopenia and/or osteoporosis. Additionally, there is some support for the improvement in bone density in children with and without disability with the use of lower extremity cycling, with and without the use of electrical stimulation.[74]

Anticipatory Planning

This intervention involves planning for things that a child or adolescent may encounter in life, preparing for transition into adulthood. Often these are normal things that are encountered by children and adolescents even without an SCI.

Sex Education/Reproduction

Adolescents with SCI often have questions about their fertility and sexual function, and they should be appropriately educated on this topic. Boys should learn about fertility options. Male fertility significantly decreases after SCI owing to the inability to ejaculate and poor sperm quality. Males with incomplete, lower-level injuries may experience either psychogenic erections from erotic thoughts or visions.[51] Males who have sustained an SCI but have an intact S2 to S4 pathway may experience reflex erections secondary to physical contact.[51] Ejaculation has been found to happen in about 70% of males after incomplete and 17% after complete lower-level injuries.[51] There are options for those men who want to father a child, including intravaginal and intrauterine insemination and in vitro fertilization. In a woman with an SCI, fertility is not affected. Women should understand that they are still able to conceive and bear a child with the proper medical care and should understand the implications of a pregnancy.[75]

Higher Education/Job Training

When an adolescent begins to think about his or her life goals, there are many things to consider. Attending college in a manual wheelchair may not be the best option for a patient, even if the upper extremities are not involved. There is an increased risk of upper extremity dysfunction or overuse syndromes. Adolescents should consider campus accessibility and design, as well as the use of the institution's disability office and services. Additionally, those entering the workforce should understand their rights under the Americans with Disabilities Act and other services available through the state's vocational rehabilitation program. Understanding their rights, regarding accessibility and equal opportunity, is important for self-advocacy and self-determination.

» Outcomes

When determining appropriate adult outcomes, important milestones in the life of an adult are considered. In today's culture, these milestones for young adults include moving away from parents, achieving an education or training, obtaining a job, becoming financially independent, establishing significant relationships, and forming a family.[76] Generally, it is a young adult's goal to keep pace with his or her peers and achieve these outcomes at the same rate. This has an impact on the individual's quality of life. Understanding an individual's personal goals provides the PT with information about potential motivators and interventions appropriate for this specific individual.

One study that looked at outcomes of pediatric-onset SCI showed that adults with pediatric SCI are not equivalent to their peers.[77] When compared with the general population of the same age, those with SCI have equivalent education levels but demonstrate lower levels of community involvement, employment, income, independent living, and marriage. They also report lower life satisfaction and perceived physical health. Additionally, there are reports that despite similar education, there is difficulty for adults with SCI to obtain jobs. When they do obtain a job, they are not paid similarly to their peers.[77] This presents a challenge for health care providers to work toward transitioning their young adults to adult roles. Self-advocacy education is important to promote equality and fairness in society.

There is also evidence that adults who were injured as children have better outcomes than adults who were injured as adults. The assumption is that those who were injured at a younger age are enabled to develop the career goals and educational preparation that facilitated their entry into the adult workforce. The most highly correlated items to a positive outcome were education, functional independence, and decreased number of medical complications.[76,77]

Vocational Outcomes

A long-term follow-up study of adults who sustained SCIs as children or adolescents showed that there was a high rate of unemployment as compared with the general population. Predictive factors of unemployment included education, community mobility, functional independence, and decreased medical complications. The variables that were positively associated with employment included community integration, independent driving, independent living, and higher income and life satisfaction. Although studies have identified the importance and positive impact of returning to work after sustaining an SCI, only 38% of individuals return to work after SCI.[78] This provides insight into areas to target during the rehabilitation process.[76,79]

Refining the vocational rehabilitation process to include individual placement and follow-up, and increasing the number of suitable jobs are ways to improve the employment outcomes.[80] Providing appropriate assistive technology to facilitate functional independence and improve accessibility assists this goal of participation as an adult.

Psychological Outcomes

Many of those with SCI often experience frustration, loss, and depression. This is especially important to remember with children with SCI because they are in the midst of developing their personality, discovering their place and role in the family and in the community. Adolescent control, anger, fear, and loss of dignity all contribute to psychological implications for the child with an SCI.[81]

Life Satisfaction Outcomes

In a study of long-term outcomes and life satisfaction of adults who had pediatric SCIs, life satisfaction was associated with education, income satisfaction with employment, and social and recreational opportunities. Life satisfaction was inversely associated with some medical complications. Life satisfaction was not significantly associated with level of injury, age at injury, or duration of injury.[81]

>> Future directions

Prevention

There is currently no cure for SCI, traumatic or atraumatic. Prevention and public awareness are clearly the best means to avoid the lifelong disability associated with SCI. Many accidents involving SCI can be avoided with knowledge and education. Along with car seat guidelines for infants and toddlers, the National Highway Traffic Safety Administration (NHTSA) recommends that children from ages 4 to 8 years and under 57 inches in height be placed in a booster seat until they can be properly positioned with a passenger seat belt.[82] The shoulder harness and lap belt together provide

DISPLAY 12.11 Prevention Websites

www.thinkfirst.org
www.safekids.org
www.nhtsa.dot.gov

the safest protection for passengers and have decreased the incidence of SCI caused by lap belt alone. Other prevention measures include protective gear in sports and the prohibition of certain full-contact maneuvers such as "spearing" that carry more risk for SCI. Sports found more commonly related to SCI in children include diving, rugby, horseback riding, skiing, football, cycling, gymnastics, and baseball.[83] Fall prevention for children should include window and stair guards and railings. Violence prevention has taken on many forms in public education as well as legislation at both the community and federal levels. Education about prevention can be found extensively on the Internet and can be focused toward children, teenagers, parents, and teachers. Vehicle safety, water and diving safety, bike safety, playground and sports safety, and gun safety all play a large role in avoiding injury (Display 12.11).

Research

Although there is no cure at the present time, there is hope for the future. There are a number of experimental therapies in human clinical trials that offer promise for improving outcomes in SCI. These include the acute administration of therapeutic agents such as minocycline, riluzole, and magnesium. Also, systemic hypothermia has gained public attention.[84] Similarly, improved knowledge about the neuropathology of transverse myelitis has given physicians clues about what medications to administer during certain points in the cascade of events. Although this is not yet curative, it may help the final outcome. It is important to note that most of these clinical trials are with adults.

One of the most exciting areas of research is the use of stem cells for spinal cord regeneration in both traumatic and atraumatic injuries.[85,86] In motoneuron-injured adult rats, stem cells have been shown to not only survive in the mammalian spinal cord but also send axons through spinal cord white matter toward muscle targets.[87,88] With the addition of certain factors and developmental cues, Deshpande et al. have shown these axons not only reach their muscle targets but also form neuromuscular junctions and become physiologically active, allowing partial recovery from paralysis in adult rats. This groundbreaking research is the first time scientists have shown that stem cell axons can form neuromuscular junctions and synapses within a living body's overall neural circuitry.[89] Further research will continue to expand upon these principles with the ultimate goal to one day become a successful treatment for humans with paralysis.[66] The complexity of the original nervous system will unlikely be completely recreated, but rather the new growth axons will find their way to a muscle in a more primitive manner. Therefore, the plasticity and self-regulation of the nervous system will likely prune and select advantageous motor pathways that will allow for function. This selection process requires appropriate external stimulation such as instructed activities and exercise.[90] Physical therapy will play a key role as stem cell studies advance toward human trials and will be instrumental in this revolution of knowledge, treatment, and recovery.

Summary

This chapter has detailed the examination, intervention, evaluation, prognosis, and care planning for children who have acquired an SCI. Specific attention was given to functional implications in both evaluation and treatment. It is important to keep in mind that although there are common themes that emerge with all patients, each child and family is unique. Keeping a family-centered approach to treatment will ensure the most optimal outcomes for each and every child.

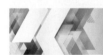 **CASE STUDIES**

MARK

Mark is a 15-year-old boy who developed transverse myelitis of his cervical spine (C-2 to C-5), which resulted in full quadriplegia and ventilator dependency within the first 24 hours. Over the course of the first month of hospitalization, Mark made very little recovery and could only demonstrate trace to poor movement in the right wrist and right ankle muscles. He was transferred to an inpatient respiratory rehabilitation unit with the goal of providing family education for a safe discharge home. Prior to his illness, he lived with his mother in a two-story condominium. His father recently died from cancer and there was no other family nearby to provide support. Mark was an honor student and wanted to become a pilot for the U.S. Air Force. His past medical history was significant for depression.

Examination

Mark initially presented with 0/5 strength throughout except minimal right ankle dorsiflexion and minimal right wrist extension. Sensation was absent from the neck down, and he was dependent for all mobility. He was unable to tolerate sitting out of bed in a chair owing to anxiety and discomfort, and was unable to hold up his head. His muscle tone was flaccid from the neck down and passive ROM was within normal limits throughout. He was dependent on a ventilator for all breathing, and he was unable to produce a cough.

Evaluation

Mark presented with the following problems: decreased strength, decreased sensation, decreased mobility, decreased airway clearance, and respiratory insufficiency. In addition, he had immense needs for caregiver education. His initial goals for physical therapy included tolerating sitting out of bed in a wheelchair for 8 hours to prepare for return to school, manipulate power mobility on level surfaces with supervision, and caregiver education regarding all aspects of dependent care.

Physical Therapy Diagnosis

Impaired strength and decreased functional mobility because of transverse myelitis.

Physical Therapy Prognosis

Good potential to achieve the identified goals with caregiver assistance. Ambulation not likely due to medical prognostic factors of quick speed and severity of onset, slow rate of neurologic recovery, and complicating factors such as ventilator dependency. Mark did have good potential to use a power wheelchair with a head array or sip-and-puff mechanism in the community.

Physical Therapy Interventions and Reexamination

Interventions were initially aimed at maintaining ROM and skin integrity through positioning, pressure relief, and family education. Out-of-bed tolerance was increased with the use of a tilt-in-space wheelchair with elevating leg rests, an abdominal binder, and compression stockings to provide vascular support. Strengthening of available muscle groups was performed using traditional therapeutic exercises as well as biofeedback and neuromuscular electric stimulation (NMES). As the weeks went on, Mark began to experience neurologic recovery, and it was crucial to reexamine and reevaluate and adjust goals and interventions as necessary. A time line is provided below to illustrate the highlights of his medical and physical therapy course in rehabilitation:

September: Onset of illness, full quadriplegia, and vent dependency in first 24 hours

October: Began standing program using a tilt table, sitting edge of mat with maximal assistance; development of grip on right upper extremity, development of increased muscle tone (Modified Ashworth Scale 2 to 3) throughout all extremities

November: Began stand-pivot transfers with moderate to maximal assistance; developed gross flexion/extension of right knee, minimal right elbow flexion (brachialis), and bilateral elbow extension

December: Began ambulation training in partial weight-bearing walker (knee immobilizer and dynamic ankle–foot orthosis [AFO] on left lower extremity); developed right biceps strength; started weaning from the ventilator; received power wheelchair for mobility

January: Began walking with platform rolling walker with standby assist; rolling supine to prone independently; moved left leg for first time (knee flexion/extension, great toe extension); tracheostomy capped during the day and bilevel positive airway pressure (BiPAP) at night

February: Decannulated with no external support and was transferred from the respiratory rehabilitation program to the neuro rehabilitation program to achieve new goals of increasing independence with transfers and ambulation

March: Started performing bed mobility, sit to stand, and transfer board transfers with supervision only; ambulating with
standard walker and supervision only; starting to propel
lightweight wheelchair over level surface with minimal assistance; received Botox injections to bilateral hip adductors
and left hamstrings

April: Ambulating with forearm crutches; stood with quad cane
for 30 seconds; moved left ankle for first time; discharged
from inpatient setting to outpatient setting

Currently: Primary power wheelchair user in community using a joystick for control; uses walker at home and for short
distances; Mark is now working toward long-term goal of
independent ambulation in the community

Owing to Mark's unexpected but definite neurologic recovery,
it was crucial to constantly reexamine and reassess his goals and
the effectiveness of the interventions. It was also important to
communicate his changes with the family and the team and to
advocate for more time in intensive rehabilitation. Finally, it became very important to Mark, his mom, and the team to return
Mark to home and school before the end of the school year, to
assimilate back into the community, and to reestablish peer relationships before the summer.

A constant theme during his physical therapy program included the periodic reexamination of strength in his upper and
lower extremities and the neck and trunk. This also required
careful evaluation and a good working knowledge of Mark's
fluctuating spasticity and subsequent communication with the
medical team who adjusted his antispasticity medications, as
needed. Interventions were progressed to work on Mark's current strengths and to challenge his weaknesses. Gait training
and orthotic and assistive device evaluations were also ever-
changing, and a variety of bracing options were tried to correct his left knee alignment and control. Mark was able to flex
and extend his left hip and knee, but he felt unstable in the
late stance phase of gait. An articulating AFO did not achieve
the stability he needed, so he trialed a stance-control knee–
ankle–foot orthosis on loan from a local vendor. He had difficulty making the mechanism work properly for him, so he
continued with the current program and continued to use a
dynamic AFO on his left ankle. Another constant theme in his
physical therapy course was the consideration of the factors
associated with the World Health Organization (WHO) International Classification of Functioning, Disability and Health (ICF)
framework of health (Display 12.12).[91] Although addressing
Mark's impairments and functional limitations was critical in
the achievement of his goals, considering the impact of his
disability in other aspects of his life was also very important to
him. Physical therapy played a definite role in assisting Mark
and his mother to become advocates for themselves, both to
his school and to the community.

Update: 18 months after his initial diagnosis, Mark remains
a primary power wheelchair user in the community and uses
a walker at home and for short distances. He is now working
toward his long-term goal of independent ambulation in the

DISPLAY 12.12 Using the ICF Framework for Patients with Spinal Cord Injury

The WHO describes health and functioning using the ICF.[91]
The ICF incorporates body, individual, and societal perspectives of function and shifts the focus from disability
to positive capabilities. It integrates the interplay of health
condition, body structures/functions (impairments), activities (abilities and limitations), and participation (abilities and
restrictions) and also considers the facilitators and barriers
in a person's internal and external environment that impact
a person's overall functioning. Evaluating and integrating all
of these factors help to create patient and family-centered
goals and identify areas of prioritization. Most often physical
therapy interventions are aimed at impairments and activity limitations, but a truly holistic approach considers the
meaningful participation and environmental factors as well.
Although improving impairments and activity limitations
were important to help Keith become more independent,
becoming involved in an activity such as sled hockey helped
him to overcome some of the participation restrictions that
he faced. Giving him and his mom the tools and community
resources to start a team in their area taught them valuable
lessons in advocacy that they can continue to use throughout their lifetime. For Mark, finding ways to contribute to
society was a primary goal for him. Independence in power
mobility was the first step, and accessing favorite activities
in the environment can promote meaningful participation,
which can be an ongoing collaborative effort. Considering all
aspects of the ICF model will enable the PT to ensure best
practice and family-centered care.

community and is beginning to take independent steps with a
quad cane. Socially, he is active in extracurricular activities and is
on the honor role at his school. He currently works for an airplane
museum, where he is able to enjoy his love of aviation. He continues to work hard and is looking forward to attending college
to study engineering.

This case is an example of the diversity PTs encounter in patient populations. Although all factors indicated a poor outcome,
Mark's determination and hard work helped him to achieve goals
no one dreamed possible. PTs have a responsibility to balance
being realistic about expected outcomes while also challenging
their patients to achieve their fullest potential. Working together
as a team with patients and families, amazing and life-changing
things can be accomplished.

KEITH

Keith is an 11-year-old boy who was involved in a motor vehicle
accident. He was an unrestrained rear-seat passenger and was
ejected from the car when it struck a tree. He had loss of consciousness and was intubated at the scene. In the emergency
room, he was noted to have no movement in both lower extremities, and computed tomography revealed a T-6 fracture with spinal cord infarct. Other injuries he sustained included left epidural
hematoma, occipital fracture, bilateral pulmonary contusions,

and right iliac fracture with retroperitoneal hematoma. During this time, he received acute-care physical therapy to address ROM, positioning, pressure relief/skin protection, elevating the head of the bed to increase upright tolerance, and caregiver education. Once Keith was extubated and stabilized, he was admitted to an inpatient rehabilitation program. Socially, he lived with his mother and two younger siblings in a two-story house with his bedroom and bathroom on the second floor and 2 steps to enter and 12 steps to the second floor. His father was the driver of the vehicle, and his parents were in the process of a divorce. He attended the local public school and was extremely involved in athletics.

Examination

Keith presented with 4/5 muscle strength above the level of T-6 and 0/5 strength and no sensation below T-6. He was wearing a thoracic–lumbar–sacral orthosis (TLSO) for fracture stabilization and was not yet cleared for lower extremity weight bearing. His muscle tone was grossly 2 on the Modified Ashworth Scale throughout his lower extremities, with three beats of clonus in each ankle and occasional flexor spasms in his left lower extremity when touched. His passive ROM was within normal limits throughout, with bilateral straight leg raise to 90 degrees. He was able to roll with minimal to moderate assistance using bed rails and transferred wheelchair to a level surface with a transfer board, push-up blocks, and moderate assistance. He required minimal assistance to sit upright and moderate assistance to reach outside his base of support.

Evaluation

Keith presented with decreased strength, decreased endurance, decreased flexibility, decreased bed mobility, decreased transfers, decreased functional mobility, and need for family education. Goals established at that time to be achieved during the inpatient rehabilitation admission included:

1. Roll independently supine to prone without a bed rail
2. Transition side-lying to sit with minimal assistance for lower extremities only
3. Transfer between level surfaces with a transfer board and contact guard assistance
4. Transfer to uneven surfaces with a transfer board and minimal assistance
5. Transfer floor-to-wheelchair with assistance only for lower extremities
6. Stand in parallel bars with bracing as needed and contact guard for 5 minutes with vital signs stable
7. Ambulate 25 feet with a wheeled walker and bracing as needed and contact guard assistance
8. Independent wheelchair mobility on level surfaces for 3000 feet without fatigue
9. Ascend and descend a 2-inch curb in his wheelchair with a spotter
10. Independence with wheelchair push-ups for pressure relief every 30 minutes
11. Patient independent with self-ROM

12. Caregiver independent with passive ROM, knowledge of skin checks, safeguarding for all levels of functional mobility, and all adaptive equipment management

Physical Therapy Diagnosis

Decreased strength and functional mobility because of ASIA A T-5 SCI.

Physical Therapy Prognosis

Excellent potential to achieve above goals because of current physical status, motivation, and family support. On the basis of the evidence, Keith has the potential to ambulate household distances with bracing and an assistive device but will most likely be a primary wheelchair user in the community.

Interventions

Increasing Upright Tolerance

Utilized compression stockings, abdominal binder to help prevent orthostatic hypotension. Increased time out of bed in wheelchair on tilt table working toward standing in parallel bars using knee immobilizers and solid AFOs for stability of the lower extremities in the weight-bearing position.

Increasing Strength

Worked with interdisciplinary team on increasing upper extremity muscle strength. Activities included progressive resistive exercises, trunk strengthening, and upper extremity dynamic activities.

Increasing Flexibility

Performed ROM and stretching exercises to the lower extremities, which were carried out by family members as a bedside exercise program under the supervision of nursing staff. Keith was eventually taught to perform self-ROM. Special care was taken to allow enough hamstring flexibility to allow future floor-to-chair transfers and to maintain length in hip flexors and heel cords to allow for stability in standing and assisted ambulation.

Increasing Balance

Keith initially worked on improving sitting balance and reaching outside his base of support with his TLSO, but later learned to sit without the TLSO when it was discontinued owing to fracture stability and healing.

Increasing Endurance

Worked on increasing periods of aerobic activity, including dynamic activities, wheelchair propulsion, upper body ergometer (UBE) work, and recreational activities.

Maintaining Skin Integrity

Keith was instructed in performing wheelchair push-ups to provide adequate pressure relief. He was also instructed in performing daily skin checks to all insensate areas. He maintained a positioning program in bed and used a gel cushion on his wheelchair.

Improving Bed Mobility and Transfers

Keith was instructed in the head–hips relationship and was taught how to move his body without creating shear forces on his buttocks. He initially used a transfer board to perform transfers, but eventually was able to transfer with no equipment and use a transfer board only for car transfers. He was also trained in techniques for floor-to-chair transfers, scooting along the floor, and bumping up and down steps.

Ambulation

Keith initially began standing in the parallel bars using knee immobilizers, temporary solid ankle orthoses, and his TLSO. He attempted to learn how to hang on his Y ligaments, but this was very difficult with the TLSO. Once the TLSO was no longer necessary for fracture stabilization, Keith was able to align and position himself in a standing position in the parallel bars. He was extremely motivated to walk using any assistive device or bracing necessary despite the knowledge of its difficulties. He started with a pair of RGOs, and after much practice preferred to swing through rather than utilize the reciprocating mechanism, which he thought was slower and made him more fatigued. He was transitioned to a pair of lightweight single upright THKAFOs (trunk–hip–knee–ankle–foot orthoses) and was trained in donning, doffing, and ambulation.

Improving Wheelchair Skills

Keith was trained in propulsion, wheelies, ascending and descending curbs and ramps, and wheelchair recoveries. He was also trained in basic wheelchair maintenance.

Equipment

Keith received multipodus boots to wear in bed, molded AFOs to wear while in his wheelchair, THKAFOs for standing and walking, forearm crutches, a rigid-frame lightweight wheelchair, a transfer board, a commode, and bath equipment.

Family Education

Keith's mother was trained and independent with safeguarding at all levels of functional mobility, all adaptive equipment management, and coaching Keith with his home exercise program. Keith was independent in pressure reliefs, skin checks, his home exercise program, and training others how to safely assist him when needed. With the aid of the interdisciplinary team, Keith and his family were provided with basic knowledge of SCI and strategies for functioning and living with a disability.

Reexamination

Keith was reexamined during several points of his admission, but most notably when he had a change in medical status. Once his spinal fractures were adequately healed and he no longer required the use of the TLSO for fracture stabilization, Keith's entire center of gravity changed, and he needed to learn to use his body in a different way. He was reexamined at the time of discharge from the inpatient setting, with his identified needs to be addressed on an outpatient basis.

The Interdisciplinary Team

As is the case with most inpatient rehabilitation settings, Keith had a full team of professionals working closely on his case to achieve his family goal of safe discharge back to home. Although various disciplines have specific roles in caring for a child with an SCI, the team must communicate and work closely together. There is often overlap between professionals, and all team members should carry over the teaching of others to provide optimal family-centered care. Keith had a physiatrist overseeing his medical course with consulting medical services as needed such as orthopedics and urology. He also had nurses who primarily focused on skin, education, bowel and bladder program, and carrying over day-to-day skills such as ADLs and transfers. Psychosocial support came from a psychologist, child life staff, social worker, and the hospital chaplain. Educational needs were covered by the education coordinator, teacher, and neuropsychologist. He received speech therapy initially to work on increasing speaking volume and intensive occupational therapy to achieve goals of independence in ADLs. Physical therapy, occupational therapy, and nursing worked closely together so that Keith had the opportunity to practice new skills in a variety of environments. Together, the team, Keith, and his mother were able to achieve his family goal of successful reintegration back to home, school, and the community.

Discharge Planning

In order to ensure successful reintegration back to home, school, and the community, discharge planning began from the first day of admission. His family learning styles and needs were evaluated and barriers to successful reintegration into the community were identified. First, owing to Keith's mild traumatic brain injury, he was fully evaluated by the hospital education staff and neuropsychologist to identify any new cognitive or learning needs upon return to school. Several meetings were set up with the staff at his school to problem-solve and determine an appropriate educational plan and to remove any physical barriers. To prepare Keith to go home, the physical and occupational therapists performed a home evaluation with both Keith and his mother present. Measurements were taken and the basic layout was assessed in order to make appropriate home modification recommendations, but Keith and his mom also had the opportunity to practice transfers and mobility under the direction of the therapists. The therapists were then able to identify any new physical or occupational needs and those areas that still required more practice in the hospital environment prior to discharge home. Child life and psychology services were instrumental in working with Keith's psychosocial issues regarding transition back into the community, but physical therapy played a large role in helping Keith to identify what types of leisure activities he may enjoy. Previously an athlete, Keith was very interested in pursuing adaptive sports, including wheelchair basketball. Physical therapy introduced him to the idea of sled hockey, and Keith soon found it to be his favorite activity. The therapist had a loaner roller sled for Keith to try out while still an inpatient and helped him and his mom connect with community resources so that he could join a team upon discharge. Keith was thrilled at the idea of playing sports again, making contacts with peers and adult athletes with SCIs, and stated that his new goal was to play sled hockey for the U.S. Paralympic team. This illustrates the importance of considering the entire disablement spectrum in order to treat patients holistically. Follow-up services were established, and Keith had a series of scheduled appointments with physicians trained to follow the needs of a person with SCI through the life span. Keith and his mom were given the tools needed to be advocates for themselves in both the health care and school systems as well as community resources to provide help along the way.

The Continuum of Care

Keith was recommended to be followed by outpatient physical therapy closer to his home to continue work on progressing wheelchair and ambulation skills to achieve his ultimate long-term goal of becoming as independent as possible. A recent study noted that patients with SCI who achieve a higher level of independence have improved quality of life and smoother transition to adulthood.[92] Keith may present with new pathologies, impairments, functional limitations, or disabilities as he grows and develops throughout his lifetime and may require future episodes of care from a PT. Emphasis should be placed on resolving those new problems and returning the patient to self-sufficiency, wellness, and a healthy lifestyle (Fig. 12.8).

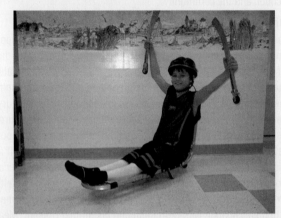

FIGURE 12.8. Adaptive sports such as sled hockey can help fulfill a child's need for peer interaction and participation in the community.

REFERENCES

1. The National Spinal Cord Injury Association (NSCIA). *Spinal cord injury statistics.* http://www.spinalcord.org/. Accessed March 27, 2013.
2. National Spinal Cord Injury Statistical Center. *Spinal Cord Injury: Facts and Figures at a Glance.* Birmingham, England: The University of Alabama at Birmingham; 2018.
3. Parent S, Mac-Thiong JM, Roy-Beaudry M, et al. Spinal cord injury in the pediatric population: a systematic review of the literature. *J Neurotrauma.* 2011;28(8):1515-1524.
4. Segal LS. Spine and pelvis trauma. In: Dormans JP, ed. *Pediatric Orthopedics and Sports Medicine: The Requisites in Pediatrics.* St. Louis, MO: Mosby; 2004.
5. Atesok K, Tanakn N, O'Brien A, et al. Posttraumatic spinal cord injury without radiographic abnormality. *Adv Orthop.* 2018. doi:10.1155/2018/7060654.
6. Shepherd M, Hamill J, Segedin E. Paediatric lap-belt injury: a 7 year experience. *Emerg Med Australas.* 2006;18(1):57-63.
7. National Institute of Neurological Disorders and Stroke. *Chiari Malformation Fact Sheet.* 2020. https://www.ninds.nih.gov/disorders/patient-caregiver-education/fact-sheets/chiari-malformation-fact-sheet. Accessed August 14, 2020.
8. Kerr DA, Ayetey H. Immunopathogenesis of acute transverse myelitis. *Curr Opin Neurol.* 2002;15(3):339-347.
9. Tavasoli A, Tabrizi A. Acute transverse myelitis in children, literature review. *Iran J Child Neurol.* 2018;12(2):7-16.
10. Kerr DA, Calabresi PA. 2004 Pathogenesis of rare neuroimmunologic disorders, Hyatt Regency Inner Harbor, Baltimore, MD, August 19th 2004–August 20th 2004 [Congresses]. *J Neuroimmunol.* 2005;159(1-2):3-11.
11. Huisman T. Pediatric tumors of the spine. *Cancer Imaging.* 2009;9(Special Issue A):S45-S48.
12. Sheikh A, Warren D, Childs A, et al. Pediatric spinal cord infarction—a review of the literature and two case reports. *Childs Nerv Syst.* 2016;33(4):671-676.
13. Elbasiouny S, Moroz D, Bakr M, et al. Management of spasticity after spinal cord injury: current techniques and future directions. *Neurorehabil Neural Repair.* 2010;24(1):23-33.
14. Harb A, Kishner S. *Modified Ashworth Scale.* Treasure Island, FL: StatPearls Publishing; 2020. https://www.ncbi.nlm.nih.gov/books/NBK554572/. Accessed August 14, 2020.
15. Alexander MS, Anderson K, Biering-Sorensen F, et al. Outcome measures in spinal cord injury: recent assessments and recommendations for future directions. *Spinal Cord.* 2009;47(8):582-591.
16. Kirshblum S, Burns SP, Biering-Sorensen F, et al. International standards for neurological classification of spinal cord injury (revised 2011). *J Spinal Cord Med.* 2011;34(6):535-546.
17. American Spinal Injury Association. *(New) ISNCSCI 2019 revision released.* 2020. https://asia-spinalinjury.org/isncsci-2019-revision-released/. Accessed August 14, 2020.
18. Chafetz R, Gaughan JP, Vogel LC, et al. The international standards for neurological classification of spinal cord injury: intra-rater agreement of total motor and sensory scores in the pediatric population. *J Spinal Cord Med.* 2009;32(2):157-161.
19. Mulcahey MJ, Gaughan JP, Chafetz RS, et al. Interrater reliability of the international standards for neurological classification of spinal cord injury in youths with chronic spinal cord injury. *Arch Phys Med Rehabil.* 2011;92(8):1264-1269.
20. Kirshblum S, Millis S, McKinley W, et al. Later neurologic recovery after traumatic spinal cord injury. *Arch Phys Med Rehabil.* 2004;85(11):1811-1817.
21. Linan E, O'Dell MW, Pierce JM. Continuous passive motion in the management of heterotopic ossification in a brain injured patient. *Am J Phys Med Rehabil.* 2001;80(8):614-617.
22. Van Kuijk AA, Geurts AC, Van Kuppevelt HJ. Neurogenic heterotopic ossification in spinal cord injury. *Spinal Cord.* 2002;40(7):313-326.
23. Smith JA, Siegel JH, Siddiqi SQ. Spine and spinal cord injury in motor vehicle crashes: a function of change in velocity and energy dissipation on impact with respect to the direction of crash. *J Trauma.* 2005;59(1):117-131.
24. National Institute of Neurological Disorders and Stroke. *Transverse Myelitis Fact Sheet.* 2020. https://www.ninds.nih.gov/Disorders/Patient-Caregiver-Education/Fact-Sheets/Transverse-Myelitis-Fact-Sheet.
25. Sommer JL, Witkiewicz PM. The therapeutic challenges of dual diagnosis: TBI/SCI. *Brain Inj.* 2004;18(12):1297-1308.
26. Fronmon E, Dean W. Transverse myelitis. *N Engl J Med.* 2010;363:564-572.
27. Gawade P, Hudson M, Kaste S, et al. A systematic review of selected musculoskeletal late effects in survivors of childhood cancer. *Curr Pediatr Rev.* 2016;10(4):249-262.
28. Anderson K, Aito S, Atkins M, et al. Functional recovery measures for spinal cord injury: an evidence based review. *J Spinal Cord Med.* 2008;31(2):133-144.
29. Slavin M, Mulcahey M, Calhoun C, et al. Measuring activity limitation outcomes in youth with spinal cord injury. *Spinal Cord.* 2016;54(7):546-552.
30. Hwang M, Zebracki K, Vogel L, et al. Development of the pediatric quality of life inventory spinal cord injury (PedsQL SCI) module: qualitative methods. *Spinal Cord.* 2020. doi:10.1038/s41393-020-0450-6.

31. Lollar DJ, Simeonssonn RJ, Nanda U. Measures of outcomes for children and youth. *Arch Phys Med Rehabil.* 2000;81(12 suppl 2):S46-S52.

32. Kozin SH, D'Addesi L, Chafetz RS, et al. Biceps top triceps transfer for elbow extension in persons with tetraplegia. *J Hand Surg Am.* 2010;35(6):968-975.

33. Mulcahey MJ, Betz R, Smith B. A prospective evaluation of upper extremity tendon transfers in children with cervical spinal cord injury. *J Pediatr Orthop.* 1999;19(3):319-328.

34. Burcheil KJ, Hsu FP. Pain and spasticity after spinal cord injury: mechanisms and treatment. *Spine (Phila Pa 1976).* 2001;26(24 suppl):S146-S160.

35. Chang E, Ghosh N, Yanni D, et al. A review of spasticity treatments: pharmacological and interventional approaches. *Crit Rev Phys Rehabil Med.* 2013;25(1):11-22.

36. Warms C, Turner J, Marshall H. Treatments for chronic pain associated with spinal cord injuries. Many are tried, few are helpful. *Clin J Pain.* 2002;18(3):154-163.

37. Yap EC, Tow A, Menon EB, et al. Pain during in-patient rehabilitation after traumatic spinal cord injury. *Int J Rehabil Res.* 2003;26(2):137-140.

38. Jan F, Wilson P. A survey of chronic pain in the pediatric spinal cord injury population. *J Spinal Cord Med.* 2004;27(suppl 1):S50-S53.

39. Wooler A, Hook M. Opioid administration following spinal cord injury: implications for pain and locomotor recovery. *Exp Neurol.* 2013;247:328-341.

40. Forest DM. Spinal cord stimulator therapy. *J Perianesth Nurs.* 2006;11(5):349-352.

41. Chari A, Hentall I, Papadopoulos M, et al. Surgical neurostimulation for spinal cord injury. *Brain Sci.* 2017;7(2):18.

42. Sheel AW, Reid WD, Townson AF, et al. Effects of exercise training and inspiratory muscle training in spinal cord injury: a systematic review. *J Spinal Cord Med.* 2008;31(5):500-508.

43. Roth EJ, Stenson KW, Powley S, et al. Expiratory muscle training in spinal cord injury: a randomized controlled trial. *Arch Phys Med Rehabil.* 2010;91(6):857-861.

44. Kelly M, Darrah J. Aquatic exercise for children with cerebral palsy. *Dev Med Child Neurol.* 2005;47(12):838-842.

45. Lobo M, Harbourne R, Dusing S, et al. Grounding early intervention: physical therapy cannot be about motor skills anymore. *Phys Ther.* 2013;93(1):94-103.

46. Arazpour M, Samadian M, Mardani M, et al. Effect of Orthotic Rehabilitation with Isocentric Reciprocating Gait Orthosis on Functional Ambulation in Patients with Spinal Cord Injury. *Journal of Prosthetics and Orthotics.* 2017;29(2):80-87. doi: 10.1097/JPO.0000000000000122. Accessed January 19, 2021.

47. Vogel LC, Lubicky JP. Ambulation in children and adolescents with spinal cord injuries. *J Pediatr Orthop.* 1995;15(4):510-516.

48. Behrman AL, Harkema SJ. Locomotor training after human spinal cord injury: a series of case studies. *Phys Ther.* 2000;80:688-700.

49. Roy RR, Harkema SJ, Edgerton VR. Basic concepts of activity-based interventions for improved recovery of motor function after spinal cord injury. *Arch Phys Med Rehabil.* 2012;93(9):1487-1497.

50. Harkema SJ, Hillyer J, Schmidt-Read M, et al. Locomotor training: as a treatment of spinal cord injury and in the progression of neurologic rehabilitation. *Arch Phys Med Rehabil.* 2012;93(9):1588-1597.

51. Christopher & Dana Reeve Foundation. *About the NeuroRecovery Network.* https://www.christopherreeve.org/research/our-rehabilitation-network/about-nrn. Accessed August 30, 2020.

52. Harkema SJ, Schmidt-Read M, Lorenz DJ, et al. Balance and ambulation improvements in individuals with chronic incomplete spinal cord injury using locomotor training-based rehabilitation. *Arch Phys Med Rehabil.* 2012;93(9):1508-1517.

53. Buehner JJ, Forrest GF, Schmidt-Read M, et al. Relationship between ASIA examination and functional outcomes in the NeuroRecovery Network Locomotor Training Program. *Arch Phys Med Rehabil.* 2012;93(9):1530-1540.

54. Alajam R, Abdulfatah A, Liu W. Effect of body weight-supported treadmill training on cardiovascular and pulmonary function in people with spinal cord injury: a systematic review. *Top Spinal Cord Inj Rehabil.* 2019;25(4):355-369.

55. Yu Covert S. Promoting pediatric participation: the right stander, gait trainer, or stroller can help children to better fulfill their roles in the family and community. *Rehab Manag.* 2019;32(7):20-23.

56. Smith B, Mulcahey MJ, Betz RR. Development of an upper extremity FES system for individuals with C-4 tetraplegia. *IEEE Trans Rehabil Eng.* 1996;4(4):264-270.

57. Gater D, Dolbow D, Tsui B, et al. Functional electrical stimulation therapies after spinal cord injury. *NeuroRehabilitation.* 2011;28:231-248.

58. Mulcahey MJ, Betz R, Smith BT. Implanted functional electrical stimulation hand system in adolescents with spinal injuries: an evaluation. *Arch Phys Med.* 1997;78(6):597-607.

59. Moynahen M, Mullin C, Chohn J, et al. Home use of a functional electrical stimulation system for standing and mobility in adolescents with spinal cord injury. *Arch Phys Med Rehabil.* 1996;77(10):1005-1013.

60. Johnston TE, Modlesky CM, Betz RR, et al. Muscle changes following cycling and/or electrical stimulation in pediatric spinal cord injury. *Arch Phys Med Rehabil.* 2011;92(12):1937-1943.

61. Mayson T, Harris S. Functional electrical stimulation cycling in youth with spinal cord injury: a review of intervention studies. *J Spinal Cord Med.* 2014;37(3):266-277.

62. Lai CH, Chang WH, Chan WP, et al. Effects of functional electrical stimulation cycling exercise on bone mineral density loss in the early stages of spinal cord injury. *J Rehabil Med.* 2010;42(2):150-154.

63. Individuals with Disabilities Education Act (IDEA). *20 U.S.C.* 1400.

64. Liusuwan A, Widman L, Abresch RT, et al. Altered body composition affects resting energy expenditure and interpretation of body mass index in children with spinal cord injury. *J Spinal Cord Med.* 2004;27(suppl 1):S24-S28.

65. Moreno MA, Samuner AR, Paris JV, et al. Effects of wheelchair sports on respiratory muscle strength and thoracic mobility of individuals with spinal cord injury. *Am J Med Rehabil.* 2012;91(6):470-477.

66. Allen K, Leslie S. *Autonomic Dysreflexia.* Treasure Island, FL: StatPearls Publishing; 2020. https://www.ncbi.nlm.nih.gov/books/NBK482434. Accessed August 14, 2020.

67. Hickey K, Vogel L, Willis K, et al. Prevalence and etiology of autonomic dysreflexia in children with spinal cord injuries. *J Spinal Cord Med.* 2004;27(suppl 1):S54-S60.

68. McCarthy J, Chavetz R, Betz R. Incidence and degree of hip subluxation/dislocation in children with spinal cord injury. *J Spinal Cord Med.* 2004;27(suppl 1):S80-S83.

69. Powell A, Davidson L. Pediatric spinal cord injury: a review by organ system. *Phys Med Rehabil Clin N Am.* 2015;26(1):109-132.

70. Dawson-Amoah K, Raszowki J, Duplantier N, et al. Dislocation of the hip: a review of types, causes, and treatment. *Ochsner J.* 2018;18(3):242-252.

71. Mehta S, Betz R, Mulcahey MJ. Effect of bracing on paralytic scoliosis secondary to spinal cord injury. *J Spinal Cord Med.* 2004;27(suppl 1):S88-S92.

72. Weizz H. The method of Katharina Schroth—history, principles, and current development. *Scoliosis.* 2011;6:17.

73. Merenda L, Brown JP. Bladder and bowel management for the child with spinal cord dysfunction. *J Spinal Cord Med.* 2004;27(suppl 1):S16-S23.

74. Lauer RT, Smith BT, Mulcahey MJ, et al. Effects of cycling and/or electrical stimulation on bone mineral density in children with spinal cord injury. *Spinal Cord.* 2011;49(8):917-923.

75. Deforge D, Blackmer J, Garrity C. Fertility following spinal cord injury: a systematic review. *Spinal Cord.* 2005;43(12):693-793.

76. Anderson CJ, Vogel LC, Betz RR, et al. Overview of adult outcomes in pediatric-onset spinal cord injuries: implications for transition to adulthood. *J Spinal Cord Med.* 2004;27(suppl 1):S98-S106.

77. Anderson CJ, Vogel LC. Employment outcomes of adults who sustain spinal cord injuries as children or adolescents. *Arch Phys Med Rehabil.* 1998;79(12):1496-1503.

78. Lidal IB, Huynh TK, Biering-Sørensen F. Return to work following spinal cord injury: a review. *Disabil Rehabil.* 2007;29:1341-1375.

79. Lemley K, Bauer P. Pediatric spinal cord injury: recognition of injury and initial resuscitation, in hospital management, and coordination of care. *J Pediatr Intensive Care.* 2015;4(1):27-34.

80. Sinden KE, Ginis KM; SHAPE-SCI Research Group. Identifying occupational attributes of jobs performed after spinal cord injury: implications for vocational rehabilitation. *Int J Rehabil Res.* 2013;36(3):196-204.

81. Vogel LC, Klaas SJ, Lupicky JP. Long-term outcomes and life satisfaction of adults who had pediatric spinal cord injury. *Arch Phys Med Rehabil.* 1998;79(12):1496-1503.

82. United States Department of Transportation. *Car seats and booster seats.* 2020. https://www.nhtsa.gov/equipment/car-seats-and-booster-seats. Accessed August 14, 2020.

83. Chan C, Eng J, Tator C, et al; Spinal Cord Injury Research Team. Epidemiology of sport-related spinal cord injuries: a systematic review. *J Spinal Cord Med.* 2016;39(3):255-264.

84. Kwon BK, Sekhon LH. Emerging repair, regeneration, and translational research advances for spinal cord injury. *Spine.* 2010;35(215):263-270.

85. Mothe AJ, Tator CH. Advances in stem cell therapy for spinal cord injury. *J Clin Invest.* 2012;122(11):3824-3834, 3867.

86. Gazdic M, Volarevic V, Harrell C, et al. Stem cells therapy for spinal cord injury. *Int J Mol Sci.* 2018;19(4):1039.

87. Harper JM, Krishnan C, Darman JS, et al. Axonal growth of embryonic stem cell-derived motoneurons in vitro and in motoneuron-injured adult rats. *Proc Natl Acad Sci USA.* 2004;101(18):7123-7128.

88. Kerr DA, Llado J, Shamblott MJ, et al. Human embryonic germ cell derivatives facilitate motor recovery of rats with diffuse motor neuron injury. *J Neurosci.* 2003;23(12):5131-5140.

89. Deshpande DM, Kim YS, Martinez T, et al. Recovery from paralysis in adult rats using embryonic stem cells. *Ann Neurol.* 2006;60(1):32-44.

90. Ramer LM, Ramer MS, Steeves JD. Setting the stage for functional repair of spinal cord injuries: a cast of thousands. *Spinal Cord.* 2005;43:134-161.

91. World Health Organization. *International Classification of Functioning, Disability and Health (ICF).* https://www.who.int/standards/classifications/international-classification-of-functioning-disability-and-health. Accessed November 27, 2020.

92. Anderson CJ, Vogel LC, Willis KM, et al. Stability of transition to adulthood among individuals with pediatric-onset spinal cord injuries. *J Spinal Cord Med.* 2006;29(1):46-56.

93. Bohannon RW, Smith MB. Inter-rater reliability of a modified Ashworth scale of muscle spasticity. *Phys Ther.* 1987;67:206-207.

Muscular Dystrophy

Allan M. Glanzman, Jennifer Jones, and Jean M. Flickinger

» Introduction

Children with neuromuscular disorders have a lifelong challenge to maintain function. That challenge can be met with the help of a knowledgeable physical therapist. In this chapter, the term *neuromuscular disease* refers to disorders whose primary pathology affects any part of the motor unit from the anterior horn cell out to the muscle itself. Common to all of these disorders is muscle weakness, which may be produced by pathology at any part of the motor unit. When characterizing neuromuscular disorders and their pathology, it is convenient to consider the various anatomic divisions of this motor unit: the anterior horn cell, the peripheral nerve, the neuromuscular junction, and the muscle.

Neuromuscular diseases of the muscle may be either hereditary or acquired and are variously classified as myopathy or dystrophy, in which the cause of the muscle weakness is attributable to pathology confined to the muscle itself. Similarly, neuropathy, in which the muscle weakness is secondary to an abnormality of the anterior horn cell, peripheral nerve, or myelin sheath, can be differentiated as axonal or demyelinating in its subcategories.

The term *muscular dystrophy* describes a group of muscle diseases that are genetically determined and have a progressive degenerative course and characteristic degenerative features on microscopic examination of the muscle. Further classification of the muscular dystrophies is based on their clinical presentation, including the distribution of weakness, mode of

inheritance, and pathologic findings. In the past two decades, much has been discovered in the area of molecular biology to help us better understand and classify childhood muscular dystrophies. After the cloning of the gene for Duchenne muscular dystrophy (DMD) in 1987,[1,2] more has been learned about the relationship between the different dystrophies and how they relate to the dystrophin–glycoprotein complex (DGC), found within the muscle cell membrane (Fig. 13.1). The DGC is a group of proteins that links the subsarcolemmal cytoskeleton and extracellular matrix with the contractile apparatus of the muscle and gives stability to both skeletal and cardiac muscle cell membranes.[3] When different proteins in the DGC are deficient or made incorrectly, structural abnormalities in the muscle can be identified, and different corresponding muscular dystrophies become phenotypically apparent. For example, when dystrophin is deficient, the result is DMD or Becker muscular dystrophy (BMD). When one of the sarcoglycan proteins is deficient, other limb-girdle muscular dystrophies (LGMDs) result. A deficiency of merosin results in one specific type of congenital muscular dystrophy (CMD).

Some of these dystrophies are categorized by the deficiency of proteins that characterize and often name the corresponding disorder. DMD and BMD are also known as *dystrophinopathies* because dystrophin is deficient in these conditions. Some of the LGMDs are also known as *sarcoglycanopathies* because one of the sarcoglycan proteins is deficient in these conditions. Similarly, merosin-negative CMD is the result of a deficiency of merosin.

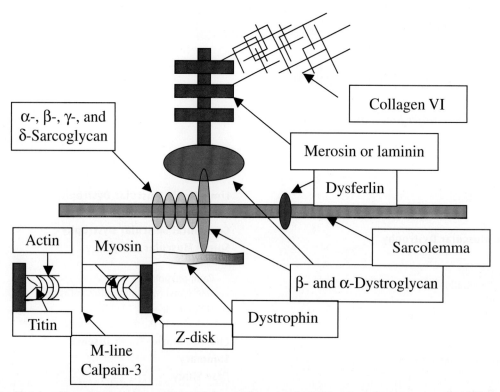

FIGURE 13.1. Muscle cell membrane and associated protein complexes implicated in muscle disease.

The term *spinal muscular atrophy (SMA)* refers to neurogenic disorders whose underlying pathology affects spinal interneurons and, as a result, the anterior horn cell,[4,5] as in the SMAs. The term *Charcot–Marie–Tooth (CMT)* disease refers to neurogenic disorders whose underlying pathology affects the peripheral nerve. Further classification of CMT is based on clinical presentation and mode of inheritance.

The neuromuscular disorders vary significantly in their presentation, pathology, and progression, but are linked with regard to physical therapy intervention by their common characteristic of muscle weakness leading to loss of function and physical deformity. A physical therapist with an understanding of these disorders can help identify, predict, intervene, and, possibly, ameliorate unnecessary complications throughout the course of each disorder. The purpose of this chapter is to provide an overview of select neuromuscular diseases, including clinical presentation, pathology, diagnosis, disease progression, medical treatment, and physical therapy intervention.

Because DMD is one of the most common and best known of the dystrophies affecting children, much of this chapter is devoted to a discussion of this disorder. Physical therapy interventions and principles that apply to the management of weakness and deformity in children with DMD are also applicable to other neuromuscular diseases that present with similar symptoms and complications, with the exception of strengthening strategies. Knowledge of the various disorders will allow appropriate decisions to be made about the

suitability and timing of various physical therapy interventions. Other neuromuscular diseases that are reviewed in this chapter include BMD, myotonic dystrophy (DM), LGMD, congenital myopathy, CMD, SMA, and CMT disease.

» Duchenne muscular dystrophy

DMD, also known as pseudohypertrophic muscular dystrophy or progressive muscular dystrophy, is one of the most prevalent and severely disabling of the childhood neuromuscular disorders, occurring in approximately 1 in 3,500 live male births.[6] It is a dystrophinopathy in which the child becomes weaker and usually dies of respiratory insufficiency and/or heart failure due to myocardial involvement in the second or third decade of life.[6] There is an X-linked inheritance pattern to DMD whereby male offspring inherit the disease from their mothers, who are most often asymptomatic. Advances in molecular biology has shown the defect to be a mutation at Xp21 in the gene coding for the protein dystrophin.[1,7]

Diagnosis

The clinical presentation gives the first clues to the diagnosis, which is confirmed by the results of laboratory studies. Laboratory findings include an abnormally high serum creatine kinase (CK) level, which is 50 to 200 times the normal level[8] and usually ranges from 15,000 to 35,000 IU per L (normal

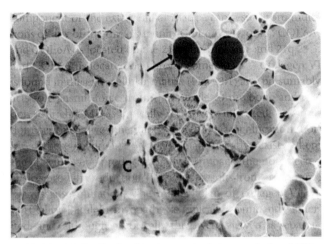

FIGURE 13.2. Dystrophic changes include a marked variability in fiber size; dark, "opaque" fibers (*arrow*); and abnormal quantities of fibrous connective tissue (*C*) (Trichrome, ×300). (Maloney FP, Burks JS, Ringel SP, eds. *Interdisciplinary Rehabilitation of Muscular Dystrophy and Neuromuscular Disorders*. J.B. Lippincott; 1984:203.)

<160 IU per L).[9] Electromyogram (EMG) findings show non-specific myopathic features with normal motor and sensory nerve velocities and no denervation. A muscle biopsy may be performed to confirm the diagnosis; and it shows degenerating and regenerating fibers, inflammatory infiltrates, and increased connective tissue and adipose cells (Fig. 13.2), which can be seen when compared to normal muscle (Fig. 13.3). Immunohistologic staining of the tissue reveals the absence of dystrophin along the muscle cell membranes.[10]

Advances in genetic testing have allowed diagnosis by the type of mutation present in DMD and BMD. With the decrease in the cost of genetic analysis, this is often the first line of testing when the phenotypic presentation and high CK is consistent with that of DMD or BMD. Approximately 65% of children with DMD and BMD have gross deletions of the dystrophin gene, which results in either the complete absence of dystrophin in DMD or some levels of truncated protein in BMD.[11] One-third of DMD cases are caused by very small point mutations.[11] There is also a high frequency of new mutations occurring in approximately one-third of the cases of DMD, which may in part be secondary to the very large size of the dystrophin gene.[2] With the availability of genetic analysis, all male family members may be screened for the disorder, and all female family members may be screened for their carrier status once a mutation is identified in the proband.

Pathophysiology

The absence of dystrophin leads to a reduction in all of the dystrophin-associated proteins in the muscle cell membrane and causes a disruption in the linkage between the subsarcolemmal cytoskeleton and the extracellular matrix. The exact cause of muscle cell necrosis is unknown. However, lack of dystrophin is thought to cause sarcolemmal instability and an increased susceptibility to membrane microtears, which may be exacerbated by muscle contractions. This causes increased calcium channel leaks, and an increase in reactive oxygen species. The activation of this signaling pathway from membrane stress results in an increase in intracellular calcium levels, leading to muscle cell necrosis.[2,12]

The following describes the clinical features of DMD. BMD also follows a similar pattern of muscle degeneration, but at a much slower and variable rate.

Clinical Presentation and Progression

The onset of the disorder is insidious, usually resulting in motor symptoms between 2 and 5 years of age, with more rapid progression of the disease observed around age 7; however, symptoms may not be noticed until the weakness is more pronounced and a Gowers sign is identified when the child begins to rise from the floor through plantigrade. The disease may be misdiagnosed as developmental delay for years.[8]

Earliest symptoms include muscle weakness, but motor and sensory neurons are undamaged, and bowel and bladder control typically remains intact. As weakness progresses, an abnormality in the pattern of the child's walking, running, and/or jumping may be observed. Similarly, the child may develop a delay in appropriate motor skill attainment. A compensated Trendelenburg, falling, difficulty getting up off the floor, toe-walking, clumsiness, or an increase in the size of the gastrocnemius muscles all may be the initial signs noted by the therapist. This "pseudohypertrophy" of the gastrocnemius is marked by a firm consistency of the muscle when palpated (Fig. 13.4).

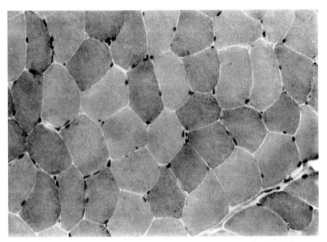

FIGURE 13.3. Normal adult muscle. Muscle fibers are cut in a plane transverse to their long axis and appear to have a polygonal tightly packed appearance. One or more darkly stained nuclei are seen at the edge of most fibers (Trichrome, ×300). (Maloney FP, Burks JS, Ringel SP, eds. *Interdisciplinary Rehabilitation of Muscular Dystrophy and Neuromuscular Disorders*. J.B. Lippincott; 1984:203.)

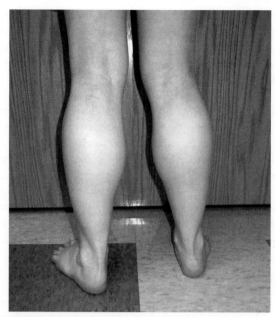

FIGURE 13.4. Ten-year-old with Duchenne dystrophy. Pseudo-hypertrophy of the calf.

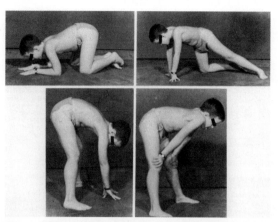

FIGURE 13.5. Gowers sign. This series of maneuvers is necessary to achieve an upright posture, and it occurs with all types of pelvic and trunk weakness. The child "climbs up the legs" when rising from the floor. (From Lovell WW, Winter RB, eds. *Pediatric Orthopaedics.* 2nd ed. J.B. Lippincott; 1986:265.)

The weakness is steadily progressive, with proximal muscles tending to be weaker earlier in the course of the illness and to progress faster. Weakness of the hip and knee extensors often results in an exaggerated lumbar lordosis that is characteristic of the early stages of the disease. The lordosis occurs in response to the attempt to align the center of gravity anterior to the fulcrum of the knee joint and posterior to the fulcrum of the hip joint. This realignment gives maximum stability at both joints. The child attempts to broaden the base of support during walking, and thus develops a compensated Trendelenburg gait that resembles waddling. The child may develop gastrocnemius, iliopsoas, and iliotibial band (ITB) contractures, which are made worse by, as well as compensated for, in this wide-based stance. As the weakness progresses, the child rises from the floor by "climbing up the legs." This maneuver, known as Gowers sign, is indicative of proximal muscle weakness (Fig. 13.5).

As the disease progresses, there is a tendency to develop contractures. These contractures typically result in plantar flexion at the ankle, with inversion of the foot being the earliest contractures to develop and flexion at both the hips and knees typically becoming more noticeable with the onset of wheelchair dependence.

The proximal weakness along with this early loss of range of motion (ROM), noted first in the heel cords and later in the hamstrings, hip flexors, and ITBs, limits stance and ambulation. The result is that children find it difficult to maintain the alignment necessary to hold themselves in an upright posture, with their weight line anterior to the knee using their weak musculature.[13] As these boys spend more time sitting, an increasing degree of contracture is seen at the hips and knees, and upper extremity (UE) contractures begin to develop in the elbows, shoulders, and long finger flexors.

Functional activities may be performed more slowly by children with DMD than by typically developing children, but most of those affected are able to walk, climb stairs (Fig. 13.6), and stand up from the floor without too much difficulty until 6 or 7 years of age. At this time, a relatively rapid decline in function has been documented, which generally results in a loss of unassisted ambulation at 9 to 10 years of age in the natural history, with various medical interventions, the most common being corticosteroid ambulation by 2 or 3 years. By convention, for a child to fit the DMD categorization of a dystrophinopathy, loss of ambulation should be by the age of 13, after which the child

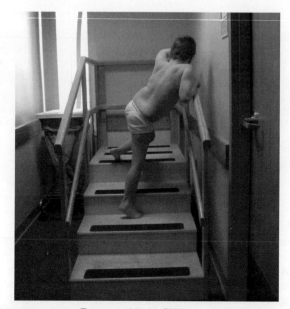

FIGURE 13.6. Ten-year-old with SMA type III. Notice the use of the upper extremities to assist climbing the steps. This posture and the use of a hand to extend the knee are the two most typical patterns noted with proximal weakness.

would be considered to have either BMD or an intermediate phenotype. Some children will choose to use long leg braces and continue to walk as an exercise ambulator for an additional year or so, but will need help getting to and from standing.[14] A partial weight-bearing walker or stander may also be used at this stage. These functional activity milestones represent significant points in disease progression and can be used as guideposts in treatment planning. Arm grades were developed by Brooke and associates[15,16] (Table 13.1), and leg grades are based on a scale proposed by Vignos et al. (Table 13.2).[17]

The mildest of the X-linked progressive dystrophies resulting from abnormalities of dystrophin has been termed *Becker muscular dystrophy* (BMD). This classification applies to individuals who maintain independent ambulation until 16 years of age. The type of mutation on the dystrophin gene

TABLE 13.1.	Functional Grades: Arms and Shoulders
Grades	**Functional Ability**
1	Standing with arms at the sides, the child can abduct the arms in a full circle until they touch above the head.
2	The child can raise the arms above the head only by flexing the elbow (i.e., by shortening the circumference of the movement) or using accessory muscles.
3	The child cannot raise hands above the head, but can raise an 8-oz glass of water to the mouth (using both hands if necessary).
4	The child can raise hands to the mouth, but cannot raise an 8-oz glass of water to the mouth.
5	The child cannot raise hands to the mouth, but can use the hands to hold a pen or to pick up pennies from a table.
6	The child cannot raise hands to the mouth, and has no useful function of the hands.

TABLE 13.2.	Functional Grades: Hips and Legs
Grades	**Functional Ability**
1	Walks and climbs stairs without assistance
2	Walks and climbs stairs with the aid of a railing
3	Walks and climbs stairs slowly (elapsed time of more than 12 sec for four standard stairs) with the aid of a railing
4	Walks unassisted and rises from a chair, but cannot climb stairs
5	Walks unassisted, but cannot rise from a chair or climb stairs
6	Walks only with assistance or walks independently with long leg braces
7	Walks in long leg braces, but requires assistance for balance
8	Stands in long leg braces, but is unable to walk even with assistance
9	Is in wheelchair
10	Is confined to bed

typically causing BMD allows for some dystrophin to be produced. The dystrophin produced is insufficient in quantity and quality, causing muscle breakdown to occur at a slower rate than in DMD. Boys with BMD will usually present with symptoms between 5 and 15 years of age, although onset is variable and may not occur until as late as the third or fourth decade.[2] The course of BMD is much less predictable than that of DMD; however, people with BMD usually live at least until their fourth or fifth decade.[2]

Brooke and colleagues[18] describe children with an intermediate form of dystrophinopathy as outliers when describing the population of boys who, when compared with the DMD population's usual pattern of disease progression, fall outside the usual limits. These outliers, by convention, are classified by the fact that they retain the ability to ambulate until age 13 but lose this ability by 16 years of age.[2] Antigravity neck flexion is also relatively preserved early on in the disease process in these children[2] as well as in BMD, whereas one of the earliest signs of weakness in the untreated DMD population is neck flexor weakness. The heterogeneity with regard to DNA mutations and gene modifiers, and the resulting dystrophin expression, is complex and can result in varying levels of clinical severity associated with DMD.[17–19]

Scoliosis

Scoliosis develops as the age of the untreated child with DMD increases; significant curves are generally not noticed until about 2 years following wheelchair dependence after 11 years of age.[20] This scoliosis tends to progress as the back muscles become weaker and as the child spends less time standing and more time sitting, resulting in a positional scoliosis, which, over time, becomes fixed. Treatment with corticosteroids decreases or delays the likelihood that scoliosis will develop to the point of needing surgical correction, and treatment with bracing has not been shown to be effective in this population.[21–23]

Respiratory Involvement

In addition to the voluntary muscles, DMD affects other body systems as well. Respiratory muscle weakness results in an ineffective cough, and pulmonary infections become more frequent and pulmonary function decline is marked by a forced vital capacity (FVC) decline of 5% per year.[24] This decline is delayed somewhat by corticosteroid treatment.[25,26] The final cause of death in those with DMD can be related to progressive pulmonary decline; however, now it is more commonly related to cardiac failure.[27,28] The major cause of respiratory complications in DMD is the progressive weakness and contracture of the muscles of respiration. The first signs and symptoms of respiratory insufficiency are seen with the onset of nocturnal hypoventilation, typically in the second decade of life. These symptoms include excessive fatigue, daytime sleepiness, morning headaches (secondary to increased carbon dioxide levels), sleep disturbances (nightmares), or feeling the need to strain to "gulp for air" upon arousal during the night.

Gastrointestinal System

The muscles of the gastrointestinal (GI) tract are also affected, causing constipation and the risk of acute gastric dilation or intestinal pseudo-obstruction, which can cause sudden episodes of vomiting, abdominal pain, and distension. If not treated properly, this requires medical attention and can lead to death.[2]

Cardiac Issues

Heart muscle is also affected by a deficiency of dystrophin, resulting in dilated cardiomyopathy, arrhythmia, and congestive heart failure.[27] In DMD, the posterobasal portion of the left ventricle is affected more than are other parts of the heart. In DMD, heart muscle involvement generally occurs later than is skeletal muscle involvement, and may not present until the late second decade.[28] In BMD and female carriers of the dystrophin mutation, cardiac involvement can occur later and may sometimes require heart transplantation.[28] Monitoring of these children should begin early in the second decade for DMD and BMD, and for female carriers of the dystrophin mutation in the third decade.[28]

Cognition

A high rate of intellectual impairment[29] and emotional disturbance has been associated with DMD.[30] Intellectual disability, autistic spectrum disorder, and attention deficit disorder are present in about 30% of children.[31]

Intelligence quotient (IQ) scores fall approximately one standard deviation below the mean[32] and affect verbal scores greater than performance scores, and some have learning disabilities without intellectual disability. Despite these challenges, many children are not cognitively delayed and function at age-appropriate levels.[2] When cognitive delay is noted, this is not progressive; but this intellectual deficit may hinder the child's development and may make a physical evaluation of the child difficult.[33]

Treatment

Although definitive treatment is lacking, proper management[34] can prolong the maximum functional ability of the child. This program of management begins once the diagnosis is established, and it is initiated concurrently with referral for parental counseling in an attempt to mitigate the guilt, hostility, and fear commonly experienced by the parents should this be desired.

The clinician can propose a positive approach on the basis of the following: (1) Some of the complications that magnify the functional disability of DMD are predictable and preventable; (2) an active program of physical therapy may prolong

ambulation and more closely approximate the normal independence of later childhood; and (3) as specific treatments become available, those in optimal physical condition are most apt to benefit.[35]

Medical Treatment

The first established pharmaceutical treatment for DMD was corticosteroids,[35,36] including prednisone and deflazacort. The increase in strength noted results in improved functional ambulation from 6 months to up to 2 years in children with DMD.[37,38] Further investigation has shown that prednisone, despite its many side effects, keeps those affected by DMD "stronger for longer."[39,40] Adverse effects of prednisone include excessive weight gain, cushingoid appearance, behavioral abnormalities, and excessive hair growth.[36] Deflazacort has similar effects, with a slightly different side effect profile and may result in less weight gain and bone demineralization, but perhaps a higher risk of cataracts with equivalent strength and functional benefits to prednisone.[41]

Creatine monohydrate, a naturally occurring substance, often used by body builders to increase muscle performance, is sometimes recommended for boys with DMD.[42] When healthy subjects take oral creatine for 1 to 4 weeks, the result is increases in muscle levels of creatine and improvements in maximal exercise performance and recovery from exercise.[43] Boys with DMD showed increases in fat-free mass (FFM), strength, and subjective reports of improvement after creatine supplementation.[42]

Since the discovery of the genetic defect and identification of the dystrophin protein, there has been a significant interest in the development of medical therapies for children with DMD. These efforts fall into a number of broad groups that include gene therapy, cell therapy, mutation-specific medication, modulation of utrophin expression, modulation of blood flow to the muscle, and treatments to address fibrosis.[44] Eteplirsen (Exondys 51) is the first of the mutation-specific exon-skipping medications designed to create a shortened form of dystrophin without exon 51. The resulting dystrophin expression results in a milder phenotype. To date, there is not an approved therapy to cure the disease; however, viral micro- or minidystrophin delivery via a gene therapy approach is in late-stage trials as are additional exon-skipping products and the nonsense mutation read through therapy. Ataluren has conditional approval in the European Union.[45,46]

Orthopedic Treatment

Spinal fixation is generally recommended for boys with DMD if their scoliosis begins to progress rapidly and their spinal curve becomes greater than 30 degrees, usually once boys are no longer ambulatory.[47] The goals of spinal surgery should include providing a stable spine, maximally correcting scoliosis, correcting pelvic obliquity, and providing sagittal-plane alignment for improved comfort and function.[48,49] Spinal stabilization should be segmental from T2 or T3 at the upper end and attaching into the body of the ilium or sacrum at the lower end, and should attempt to correct pelvic obliquity and provide a lumbar lordosis.[49] The abovementioned surgery allows for immediate postoperative mobilization, often without an orthosis. Timing of surgery is critical because the risks of surgery become greater as the disease progresses. The decision for spinal stabilization should be viewed in the context of the child's pulmonary function because this relates to the child's ability to tolerate the rigors of surgical correction. FVC below 30% or 35% is related to higher complication rates.[22] Failure of extubation following surgery is also an important postoperative risk, and some centers will use bilevel positive airway pressure (BiPAP) as a way to transition following extubation immediately after surgery should this be necessary.

Other orthopedic surgeries include Achilles tendon or gastroc-fascial lengthening, Yount fasciotomies, tibialis posterior transpositions, and percutaneous tenotomies in an attempt to increase joint ROM for prolongation of ambulation. Besides surgery, orthopedic intervention is required in the event of a fracture. There is an increased risk of low-energy fractures in boys diagnosed with DMD and BMD, as well as in children with SMA types II and III compared to controls. Many lower extremity (LE) fractures lead to a permanent loss of function resulting in loss of ambulation. Some have recommended aggressive therapy, including open reduction and internal fixation with early remobilization in lower limb fractures where ambulation is fragile.[50] Maintenance of flexibility through stretching, splinting, and early reintroduction of standing and walking are essential.[51] Use of partial weight-bearing support treadmills and gait trainers as well as aquatic therapy can be utilized in the rehabilitation process to allow earlier mobilization in a safe environment once cleared by the orthopedic physician for weight bearing.

Pulmonary Treatment

A child with DMD will need to be followed up by a pulmonologist beginning from diagnosis for regular monitoring of pulmonary status, initially focusing on evaluation for nocturnal hypoventilation.[52]

If the history and pulmonary function test results suggest that the lungs are not being adequately ventilated, the pulmonologist will need to discuss options for assisted ventilation; typically, this is not until the beginning of the second decade. Nasal BiPAP ventilation may be used at night to assist breathing and to provide a rest for overworked respiratory muscles.[53] An adjustment period is often necessary when this type of ventilation is used, but after a period, the child often derives the benefits of improved sleep and increased energy and alertness in the daytime. Ventilatory assistance might be required both day and night for children with advanced respiratory failure.[54] Ventilators are typically compact, battery-driven devices that can be attached to an appropriately modified wheelchair, and breaths can be delivered by tracheostomy or by a mouthpiece that can be held in the mouth when it is needed or by nasal or mask interface. The pulmonologist and therapist can also recommend various airway clearance techniques and medications to improve pulmonary health, including percussion and postural drainage during illness and the use of a coughalator for airway clearance and to maintain rib cage and lung flexibility.

Cardiac Treatment

Regular cardiac magnetic resonance imaging (MRI), echocardiogram (ECHO), and electrocardiogram monitoring by a cardiologist are necessary for boys with DMD or BMD.[55] Female carriers also need periodic monitoring due to an increased risk of cardiac disease.[56] Cardiac medications for arrhythmias and ventricular function may be necessary. Children with BMD also may eventually need heart transplantation for dilated cardiomyopathy, and the cardiac phenotype may be more severe than is the motor phenotype.

Gastrointestinal/Nutrition

A GI specialist can help with constipation issues and monitor for intestinal pseudo-obstruction. A nutritionist can help prevent weight gain, and assist with diet recommendations in the early years and with weight loss and nutritional support in later life when self-feeding becomes difficult and aspiration becomes more of a risk.

Osteoporosis Management

Osteoporosis is common in boys with DMD, especially with glucocorticoid treatment. This is evident by the high rate of vertebral and long bone fractures.[57]

Early diagnosis and management is crucial because fractures can lead to deformity and loss of function. Spine imaging should be completed because of the high risk of compression factors for impaired bone health in individuals with DMD. Bisphosphonate therapy may be considered to address bone mineral density.[58]

Physical Therapy Examination

The role of the physical therapist in treating DMD and BMD is an important one, and requires a solid understanding of both the unique features and the natural history of the disease in addition to a delicate approach to the issues related to treating a progressive and fatal disorder. When discussing examination and treatment of the child with DMD, it is helpful to categorize the disease into general life stages: early, middle, and late ambulatory phases, and early and late nonambulatory phases.[59,60]

Each child with DMD should undergo a physical therapy examination. Such an examination involves the gathering of information that contributes to the development of a plan of care.[61] That care plan will be based largely on the functional significance of the therapist's findings in the context of the natural history of the disease.

History

A thorough history should be taken and should include family history; birth and developmental history; a review of systems, including cardiac, pulmonary, GI, integumentary, and musculoskeletal systems; functional mobility; social history and environmental barriers; and current durable medical equipment. The primary concerns of the child and family should also be understood before examining the child.

Family History

Understanding the child's family history is important. The child and family may already know someone with the disease and may have a different perspective than has someone diagnosed with no family members with the disease who is unfamiliar with the characteristic phenotypic course. If the child's mother or sisters are carriers, they will need to understand both their risks of cardiomyopathy as well as implications for future family planning.

Developmental History

The physical therapist should gather information regarding the child's birth and development. Often, boys with DMD are late walkers, may never gain the ability to jump, and lag behind their peers in gross motor skills. Parents often report frequent falling or clumsiness as boys develop weakness. It is common for boys to have a lower IQ, and they may have learning disabilities that need to be addressed in school; however, this is only a subset of the population, and many boys are cognitively normal.

Review of Systems

Pulmonary

A good pulmonary history is required to determine whether the child has any pulmonary issues that require treatment or referral to a pulmonologist. Does the child have a strong cough, and is it a productive cough? Can the child clear his own secretions? Does the family currently perform percussion and postural drainage with intercurrent illness or use any devices to aid in airway clearance to maintain pulmonary health? Does the child exhibit any symptoms of respiratory insufficiency or nighttime hypoventilation? If the child demonstrates these symptoms, the child must be referred to a pulmonologist for evaluation for nocturnal hypoventilation.

Other systems, including cardiac, GI, integumentary, and musculoskeletal systems will also need to be reviewed to determine whether referral to a specialist is necessary.

Tests and Measures

Functional Ability

Systematic and serial recording of standard tasks shows that the child with DMD is in one of two general phases: stable performance or declining performance. During the stable phase, which may continue for several years, the child may demonstrate normal performance of various tasks during the serial evaluations, despite a continuing decline in strength.

The use of timed testing during examinations in the clinical setting is useful for monitoring child function and for predicting loss of ambulation. Activities that are frequently timed include transferring from supine to standing, running or walking a distance of 10 m, transferring from sitting to standing, and climbing up four steps. Qualitative description along with timing adds useful information in monitoring function and level of fatigue. For example, it is helpful to note during the floor-to-stand transfer whether a Gowers maneuver is present and whether the child requires the use of one or both hands on knees to complete the transfer. When climbing the steps, it is helpful to describe how many rails are required, the pattern or sequence of steps used (reciprocal vs. step to), and whether use of UEs is required to push on knees or to pull up on the rail to ascend steps (see Display 13.1).

Timed function tests can be useful in predicting loss of ambulation. When the time to ambulate 10 m is greater than 9 seconds, this is predictive of loss of ambulation within 2 years. A 10-m timed test of greater than 12 seconds is predictive of loss of ambulation within 1 year. When a child is no

---

DISPLAY 13.1 Timed Function Tests and Functional Method Grading

Time taken to
1. Stand from a supine position
2. Run/walk 10 m
3. Climb four standard-sized stairs
4. Descend four standard-sized stairs

Standing from a Supine Position
1. Unable to stand from supine, even with use of a chair
2. Assisted Gowers—requires furniture for assist in arising from supine to full upright posture
3. Full Gowers—rolls over, stands up with both hands "climbing up" the legs to above the knees to achieve full upright posture
4. Half Gowers—rolls over, stands up with one-hand support on lower legs
5. Rolls to the side and/or stands up with one or both hands on the floor to start to rise
6. Stands up without rolling over or using hands

Running or walking 10 m
1. Unable to walk independently
2. Unable to walk independently, but can walk with support from a person or with assistive device (full-leg calipers [knee–ankle–foot orthoses, KAFOs] or walker)
3. Highly adapted gait, wide-based lordotic gait, cannot increase walking speed
4. Moderately adapted gait, can pick up speed but cannot run
5. Able to pick up speed, but runs with a double stance phase (i.e., cannot achieve both feet off the ground)
6. Runs and gets both feet off the ground (with no double stance phase)[18]

longer able to attain standing from floor, it is predicted that loss of ambulation is likely to occur within 2 years.[61]

It has been demonstrated that, although functional ability appears to remain at a constant stage in many children for a period, actual muscle strength still declines, and walking speed continues to remain stable even when compared to normative data.[62–65] Brooke and coworkers[66] and Florence and associates have presented a clinical evaluation protocol for DMD—measuring strength, pulmonary function, and functional tasks in combination—that has been demonstrated to be reliable in documenting the disease course in children with DMD.[67] In addition, the protocol is able to detect not only the therapeutic effect of pharmaceutical intervention but also the time course and differences in various dose levels of such intervention.[67,68]

However, many centers also use the 6-minute walk test, and the 100-m timed test has been shown to also be reliable in this population. Instrumented strength measurement such as handheld myometry (HHM) in combination with a gross motor assessment designed for DMD such as the North Star Ambulatory Assessment have been determined to be as reliable tools for individuals with DMD.[69,70]

Muscle Testing

Measurement of muscle strength by way of manual muscle testing (MMT) remains a valid approach to evaluating the progression of disease in children with DMD.[71] MMT has been shown to be both reliable[72] and sensitive to changes in strength in children with DMD.[72]

Because muscle weakness is characteristic of muscle disease, MMT must be a routine part of the physical therapy examination of the child with a dystrophy or a myopathy. The longitudinal results of MMT in children with DMD show linearity in the decline in muscle strength.

By the time the child reaches 7 years of age, or with serial strength scores recorded for 1 year, it is possible to estimate the rate of progression as either rapid (10% deterioration per year), average (5% to 10% deterioration per year), or slow (5% deterioration per year). There is a variation in the rapidity of progression. MMT, along with performance of functional tasks, helps determine when bracing or wheelchairs will be needed.

HHM has been used to better quantify muscle strength in boys with DMD.[73,74] HHM and grip and pinch dynamometers can be useful in obtaining more objective and specific muscle strength data. HHM and dynamometry have been found to be reliable and valid in people with weakness.[73–75]

Range of Motion

Standard examination of joint motion with goniometry should be done periodically. Loss of full ankle dorsiflexion, ankle eversion, knee extension, and hip extension, with resultant contractures, occurs commonly in children with DMD. Measurement of ankle dorsiflexion, knee extension, hip extension, and ITB tightness are the most important aspects of goniometric testing. Measurement of the popliteal angle

is useful in monitoring hamstring flexibility. Special tests, including the Thomas test and Ober test,[76] can also be useful in monitoring hip flexor and ITB tightness.

Physical Therapy Intervention

The primary problems encountered by children with DMD include the following:

1. Weakness
2. Decreased active and passive ROM
3. Ambulation dysfunction
4. Decreased functional ability
5. Decreased pulmonary function
6. Emotional trauma—individual and family
7. Progressive scoliosis
8. Pain

After a physical examination of the child, the physical therapist can identify current problems and, on the basis of a thorough understanding of the natural history of the disease process, should be able to predict the trajectory of functional decline. On the basis of the specific areas of concern for each family, it is possible to identify five major goals of management common to all children with DMD:

1. Prevent deformity.
2. Prolong functional capacity.
3. Improve pulmonary function.
4. Facilitate the development and assistance of family support and support of others.
5. Control pain, if necessary.

As the preceding five goals are accomplished, so also is the goal for all individuals with neuromuscular disease: helping them be as independent and comfortable as possible within the limits of their disability.

ROM exercises and stretching, orthotics and splinting, examination and management of adaptive equipment, and appropriate positioning. Prolonging functional capacity of ensuring safety while functioning may require the prescription of specific orthotics or adaptive equipment can all be helpful in addressing the goals of preventing deformity and prolonging function are important interventions for children with nueromuscular disorders.

A multidisciplinary approach that includes support for the family is vital to optimal care: family education with regard to the disease process and its implications; referral to the Muscular Dystrophy Association (MDA), where they would have access to other families facing similar problems; and the educational, social, financial, and medical care opportunities offered by the MDA. The child and family may be aided by appropriate timing of referral to other associated medical personnel, including orthotist, occupational therapist, nutritionist, adaptive equipment clinic, social worker, or medical specialists, including orthopedic surgeon, pulmonologist, GI specialist, or cardiologist.

Pain control may or may not be necessary, and is often dependent on how successful stretching and bracing strategies were in the child's earlier years. Appropriate stretching, fit and positioning in wheelchairs, cushions, alternating pressure pads, or specialized mattresses and hospital beds can go a long way in assisting the control of discomfort in these children.

Home Program

Because much of the responsibility for daily treatment must be assumed by the family or friends of the child with DMD, an effective program of care at home is essential. Although sustaining enthusiasm and adherence with the home program may be difficult, the likelihood of success can be improved by giving simple instructions, requesting a limited number of exercises and repetitions each day, and offering extensive feedback and positive reinforcement to people in the support system. Physical therapy once or twice each week at times may be indicated with the primary goal of instructing family members in an appropriate home program, providing safe guidelines for exercise, and monitoring of orthotic or splinting needs. Outpatient physical therapy and aquatic therapy may also be indicated in the event of a fracture. Early-intervention physical therapy may be indicated for the younger child if diagnosed early, with a transition to physical therapy in the school setting when the child reaches school age. Periodic reevaluation, retraining, and motivation sessions for parents are recommended.

Preventing Deformity

The tendency for development of plantar flexion contractures is usually the earliest problem.[77]

Daily stretching of the Achilles tendons should slow down the development of this deformity. The use of night splints in combination with heel-cord stretching has been shown to play a significant role in preventing the equinovarus deformity associated with DMD.[18] Use of night splints has been shown to be more effective in preventing deformity of the Achilles tendon than is stretching alone.[77] Boys with DMD who used night splints early on (before the loss of ambulation) walked independently longer than did boys who did not use splints.[78,79]

No studies are available on which to base a passive stretching prescription, but regimen options include standing on a wedge with one's back to a support or a runner's stretch in a stride position or a manual stretch of static holds of at least 15 seconds, performed at least once, and preferably twice, daily.[80]

As soon as the physical therapist sees any change in the length of the hamstring muscles during a periodic evaluation, hamstring stretching should be added to the home program. The ITB, hip flexors, and ankle inverters are other structures that must be monitored carefully for loss of ROM, which usually occurs in all these structures as a result of either weakness or static position.

If plantar flexion contractures and the resultant knee, ITB, and hip flexion contractures are allowed to continue unchecked, the child will progress much sooner than necessary to the late ambulation stage and will lose the ability to ambulate at an earlier age than with intervention. At least 2 to 3 hours of standing or walking is recommended daily in addition to stretching and night splinting to help prevent contracture formation.[81] Therefore, a stander may be considered to aid in the prevention of contractures once ambulation becomes tenuous.

Serial casting to manage plantar flexion contractures has also been used successfully without loss of function in ambulatory boys with DMD.[82] Careful selection of appropriate candidates with good ambulatory ability (able to rise from the floor) and no more than moderate contractures is essential to this success. Functional tasks between cast changes should be monitored, and the boys should always be able to walk comfortably in the casts.

Minimizing Spinal Deformity

As the child's sitting time increases, so does kyphoscoliosis. Previous clinical observations have documented that the convexity will likely be toward the dominant extremity.[83] A lateral support and viscous fluid–filled or air-filled cushions in wheelchairs have been used in an attempt to provide appropriate pressure relief and spinal positioning while the child is seated in the wheelchair, but no studies are available to prove their clinical efficacy. Typically, spinal orthoses are not used in children with DMD because they have not been shown to delay the development of the spinal curve and might increase the work of breathing.[74,84]

The increasing sophistication of spinal instrumentation within the field of orthopedics has made spinal fixation an option for children with DMD. Physical therapy plays an important role in getting these children "up and moving" within days of surgery, depending on their medical status. Additional postoperative concerns specifically for the physical therapist to consider relate to the rigidity of the trunk following fusion. Children will be taller, and entrance into their van as well as other areas need to be considered. Difficulty with self-feeding resulting from the limitation in trunk flexibility also needs to be considered. Many children will benefit from a preoperative evaluation for a mobile arm support so that they can continue to be independent with self-feeding following surgery. The other concern is seating and positioning. The head rest and back of the wheelchair will need to be adjusted following surgery to accommodate the increased trunk length, and if surgical correction results in a pelvic obliquity and asymmetric weight bearing, accommodation within the wheelchair cushion might be necessary. Typically, an air-filled cushion with special setup to control pressure in different areas of the cushion is optimal; however, some will find the instability that comes with this type of cushion unacceptable, and an asymmetric base below a pressure-relieving viscous fluid–filled cushion might be preferable. Typically, foam or gel cushions provide insufficient pressure relief in this population.

Initially, referrals for spinal stabilization were attempts to improve or stabilize a child's respiratory function to alleviate the mechanical disadvantage the kyphoscoliosis placed on the already weak respiratory muscles, and to prevent the potentially deleterious effect of this scoliosis on respiratory function. Recent studies have demonstrated no salutary effect of segmental spinal stabilization on respiratory function based on either short- or long-term follow-up, but all studies have documented improved sitting comfort, appearance, and stabilization, or improvement of kyphoscoliosis.[79,85,86]

Activity Level/Active Exercise

Normal, age-appropriate activities for a young boy with DMD are encouraged. The family should be instructed to allow the child to self-limit his activities and allow rests when needed. Care should be taken to avoid overusing muscles and causing fatigue. Signs of overuse weakness include feeling weaker 30 minutes postexercise or excessive soreness 24 to 48 hours after exercise.[87] Other signs include severe muscle cramping, heaviness in the extremities, and prolonged shortness of breath.[87] In general, eccentric muscle activities, such as walking or running downhill, and closed-chain exercises, such as squats, should be avoided if possible because they tend to cause more muscle soreness. Resistive muscle strengthening is not recommended in boys with DMD because of the risk of contraction-induced muscle injury.

Strengthening

Strength training in boys with DMD has been a subject of controversy. Research on strength training and exercise programs in human subjects with DMD has been limited and has had mixed outcomes. There are few well-controlled, randomized studies, and most have had heterogeneous groups of subjects that include different forms of muscular dystrophies with very different pathologies and clinical presentations. Most of the studies looked at short-term strength gains in individual muscles, but few looked at long-term effects and functional benefits after exercise regimens.

In an early study in 1966, Vignos and Watkins found improvements in weight-lifting capacity in subjects with various forms of muscular dystrophy over a 1-year training period. The strength benefits plateaued in the subjects with DMD after approximately 4 months, and results were less sustainable than in children with other dystrophies.[88,89] Little functional benefits were found in the subjects with DMD, although greater strength gains and functional benefits were found in subjects with limb-girdle and fascioscapulohumeral forms of muscular dystrophy.[88] In 1979, de Lateur and Giaconi found that isokinetic submaximal strength training minimally improved strength in four boys with DMD without negative side effects.[90] Scott et al.[90] also found absence of deterioration with mild to moderate exercise in the short term. Most of the researchers recommended that exercise programs should be started early on in the course of the disease because individuals with the least amount of muscle impairment benefited the most from training programs.[92,93] There is very little research on exercise in nonambulant children with DMD.[94]

There is no evidence in humans that increased activity or resistive exercise caused physical deterioration[94]; however, there are ethical issues related to studying this in boys because studies of the mdx mouse, a dystrophin-deficient mouse, have indicated damage to muscle cell membranes, which increases during exercise.[95] Eccentric exercise, in particular, may induce muscle cell damage, as was demonstrated in a downhill treadmill running protocol with mdx mice.[96] Connolly et al. showed 40% to 45% fatigue when comparing the first two and last two pulls when measuring repetitive grip strength of mdx mice.[97] Various other mdx mice studies have contributed to the theory of contraction-induced muscle cell damage. Lack of dystrophin increases susceptibility to muscle cell damage. Microtears in the muscle cell membrane increase with muscle contractions and cause an increase in calcium leak channel activity, which in turn causes an increase in intracellular calcium. This increase causes calcium-dependent proteolysis, which eventually leads to cell death.[95,98]

Endurance exercise, such as swimming, has been found to be beneficial in mdx mice by increasing the resistance to fatigue in muscles by increasing the proportion of type I (slow oxidative) fibers, and ergometer training has been shown to preserve function of early-stage DMD when compared with ROM exercises only.[99,100]

Care must be taken in interpreting and transferring data from the mdx mouse model to humans. The muscle sizes and forces experienced by muscle groups vary, and the stance of the mouse is quite different from that of humans. In addition, the natural history of the mdx mouse is different from the course of DMD in humans.[99]

More research is needed in the area of strength training; however, given the current research on mice and humans, general recommendations can be made. Avoidance of maximal resistive strength training and eccentric exercise is recommended in boys with DMD. Submaximal endurance training such as swimming or cycling may be beneficial, especially in the younger child with DMD.[101,102]

Prolonging Ambulation

As children with DMD become weaker, their gait pattern is altered in an attempt to improve stability during walking. Stride length decreases, and the width of the base of support increases to provide a more stable base. The ITB accommodates to the new, shortened position associated with the wider base of support. Weakness in the gluteus medius becomes more pronounced, and the child assumes the typical waddling gait associated with a compensated Trendelenburg.

The lordotic curve increases with progressive weakness of the gluteus maximus. As that muscle weakens, the child attempts to increase stability, moving the center of gravity posterior to the fulcrum of the hip joint by pulling the arms back and by exaggerating the lordosis. Stability at the hip joint during standing is now provided passively by structures anterior to the hip joint, primarily the iliofemoral ligament. The presence of a mild knee flexion contracture or the application of an ankle–foot orthosis (AFO) with its angle set in too much dorsiflexion would make ambulation difficult or impossible because of the impact of the weight line and position of the joint axis of the child. In the ambulatory phase, orthotic devices above the ankle joint are not recommended because of the biomechanical disadvantage to gait efficiency.

Treatment programs combining passive stretching and LE bracing at night have demonstrated a reduction in the rate of progression of LE contractures and have prolonged ambulation.[81,103] Various surgical interventions—including Achilles tendon lengthening and Yount fasciotomies,[104] tibialis posterior transpositions,[105] and percutaneous tenotomies[106,107]—in combination with vigorous physical therapy and orthotic intervention (bilateral knee–ankle–foot orthosis [KAFO]), have been reported to improve and prolong ambulation.[108–110]

Whatever the surgical methods, a vigorous postoperative physical therapy program should aim to get the child up and standing and walking as soon as possible. Active joint stretching will help maintain, and may even increase, ROM at those muscles that have been released. The goal of the postoperative physical therapy program is independent ambulation with a minimum of 3 to 5 hours per day of standing and/or walking. Even when no steps are possible, the child is asked to stand at least 1 hour a day (in a stander if necessary). Optimal stance is with the back in extension so that the center of gravity falls behind the hip joint.

Before any lengthening surgery is considered, families must thoroughly weigh the benefits and risks involved with surgical intervention. When children are still ambulatory, an overcorrection of a heel-cord contracture may result in immediate loss of ambulation[79,81] or may result in ambulation with long leg braces only, which may be cumbersome and not very functional. With the increased use of corticosteroids, many boys are reaping the benefit of prolonged ambulation without the risks of surgical intervention, and many centers do not recommend orthopedic intervention uniformly for all children with DMD.[38] An alternative to surgical correction for those children with contractures at the ankle that are limiting ambulation is serial casting. This is best reserved for children who have developed early contractures and are still good ambulators and able to rise from the floor independently. It is vital to ensure that the child is able to ambulate in the cast, and the casts should be changed either weekly or twice a week to ensure that the period of casting is as short as possible.[82]

Wheelchair Use

When ambulation becomes more difficult, falling becomes more frequent, and the child with DMD is unable to get to the places he needs without undue fatigue, it is time to consider the use of a wheelchair for a primary means of mobility. Ideally, this will be in advance of a total loss of ambulation, and the child will be able to use the chair for longer distances

initially. Because of the rapid decline in function and the fatigue induced by pushing a manual wheelchair, a powered wheelchair or scooter is generally recommended for a first wheelchair option. Because of the time it takes to order and get insurance approval for a powered wheelchair, the therapist will need to estimate when a child will no longer be able to ambulate. According to clinical guidelines developed by Brooke et al.[18] for predicting loss of ambulation, ambulation ceased 2.4 years (range = 1.2 to 4.1 years) after the child could no longer climb four standard (6-inch) steps in less than 5 seconds and 1.5 years (range, 0.6 to 2.2 years) after more than 12 seconds were needed.[111]

Some boys with DMD and their families initially resist a powered wheelchair and feel that a powered scooter is more acceptable socially; however, most scooters do not provide sufficient seating support later in the course of the disease, and can be difficult to transport on a bus compared with powered wheelchairs. Most school buses are able to transport a wheelchair, but not a scooter. A scooter can be a nice transitional piece of equipment to be used while the child is still ambulatory, but requires assistance for longer distances. It is important to consider the timing of this purchase, however, because most insurance companies only reimburse for power mobility every 3 to 5 years. A boy with DMD can quickly decline in function and strength, and may require a more supportive wheelchair before funding is available again. It is important to discuss these factors to help children and their families through the decision-making process.[112]

Initially, a powered wheelchair with a conventional joystick and pressure-relieving cushion is usually sufficient to meet the needs of the first-time wheelchair user. As scoliosis develops, a lateral support on the convexity of the scoliotic curve is recommended. Bilateral lateral supports are often not used because this may limit the child's ability to shift weight and perform functional tasks in the chair. Children with DMD often use neck and trunk motions to compensate for trunk weakness in their daily activities; therefore, a seating device that is too stable may restrict a person's ability to perform these maneuvers.[111] A proper pressure-relieving seat cushion is also recommended. Potential pressure areas and/or areas of pain or discomfort can vary depending on the type of spinal deformity present.[111] Children with scoliosis or kyphoscoliosis complained of pain on the lateral thoracic area and ischial area on the convex side of the curve. In children with extended spines, pain was reported on bilateral posterior aspects of thighs and bilateral ischial areas. In children with kyphotic spines, pressure was felt on the sacrum.[111] This should be considered when selecting a pressure-relieving seat cushion.

Once a child undergoes a spinal fusion, some adaptations to the wheelchair and seating components are usually indicated because the child will, in effect, become taller and less able to compensate for antigravity UE movements. The spinal deformity will now be corrected partially, and pressure areas may change as a result. Adjustments in the fit and placement of laterals, headrests, and footrests may need to be made, as well as modifications made to the seat cushion. An adjustable mobile arm support may be indicated to support the upper arm in a position to allow the elbow to move in a gravity-eliminated plane to assist with activities such as eating or brushing teeth because the child will no longer be able to compensate for weakness with trunk flexion. Success with this type of device is often dependent on the child's ability to overcome the antigravity assist provided and pull the arm down.

As the disease progresses, power tilt-in-space capability will be necessary to provide pressure relief and relaxation as neck and trunk musculature weaken. This may also be required for pressure relief following spinal fusion if a residual pelvic obliquity is present. Additional features such as ventilator adaptations will need to be added on as respiratory status declines. As hand strength becomes more markedly impaired, a change in the power control may be indicated, with the first choice for adaptation being a proportional mini-joystick.

In a recent study by Pellegrini et al., adults with DMD who had lost their ability to drive a powered wheelchair without restriction using a conventional joystick were able to regain unrestricted driving once they changed to an alternative control system including mini-joystick, isometric mini-joystick, finger joystick, or pad.[109] In some drivers, the position of the control needed to be modified and also the device, such as using an isometric mini-joystick with the chin or lips. The study also found that restricted ability to drive a powered wheelchair correlated significantly with a decrease in key pinch strength.[109]

Power mobility, although often resisted initially, can provide boys with DMD a positive sense of independence and important means of independent mobility. Careful discussion of power mobility options and provision of adapted mobility early on in the disease process for long distances, while the boy is still ambulating, can help boys with DMD and their families come to accept the positive aspects of power mobility with confidence when the need for such assistance arises.

Weight Control

The need to guard against obesity is especially important now that the use of corticosteroids in children with DMD has become more prevalent, because weight gain is a significant side effect. Weight management for the ambulatory child is now equally as important as it is for the child who is limited to a wheelchair. Despite good use of transfer techniques and proper body mechanics by others, excessive weight gain can reduce the child's ability to get transferred and may restrict both mobility and social activity. Moreover, excessive weight gain in the child with neuromuscular disease may not only reduce mobility but may also have a deleterious effect on self-esteem, posture, and respiratory function.

Edwards and associates have demonstrated that controlled weight reduction in obese children with DMD is a safe and practical way to improve mobility and self-esteem.[112] However, it is probably easier to prevent excessive weight gain in the young, ambulatory child than to initiate dietary restriction in an obese, seated adolescent. It has been proposed that this philosophy of weight control be promoted early for children with neuromuscular disease (taking into account the need for fat intake in early development). Normal growth charts make no allowance for the progressive loss of muscle in DMD, so if the child continues to gain weight according to normal standards, accumulation of fat tissue may occur because there is muscle wasting in boys with DMD.

Typically, many boys with DMD are overweight at the outset of their teen years, and by the end of their teenage years, a large portion are underweight as a result of feeding and GI difficulties.[113] Griffiths and Edwards studied the relationships between body composition and breakdown products of muscle that provide data on ideal weight guidelines for weight control in boys with DMD.[114] The physical therapist can play a major role in promoting this weight control philosophy with the child and family. Despite efforts focused on weight control, often boys become too big for their parents to lift, and use of a hydraulic lift becomes necessary. One or more family members must be trained in the safe and proper use of such a lift that ideally allows the divided leg sling to be removed following the transfer so adequate pressure relief can be attained from the wheelchair cushion.

Facilitating Sleep

Air or memory foam mattresses or commercial flotation pads often improve sleeping comfort for children with advanced deterioration who have difficulty positioning themselves or changing position at night. These devices also provide relief for family members who might otherwise be up three to five times per night to turn the child. A hospital bed may be useful in the later stages of disease to assist with positioning and transfers, as well as to elevate the head of the bed.

Activities of Daily Living

The physical therapist should routinely evaluate the child's ability to perform activities of daily living (ADLs). The child's ability to feed himself, turn pages in a book, and do necessary personal hygiene tasks must all be monitored periodically. The physical therapist may choose to request an occupational therapy consultation. A home visit is most helpful in determining adaptive equipment needs and accessibility.

Respiratory Considerations

The physical therapist's role in the pulmonary care of children with DMD will vary depending on each individual practice setting. All physical therapists working with boys with DMD, however, should be aware of the importance of maintaining good pulmonary health, whether directly or indirectly involved with their respiratory care.

As the diaphragm, trunk, and abdominal muscles weaken, tidal volume and the ability of the child to effectively clear secretions decreases. Spontaneous periodic deep breaths, as occurs with sighs and yawns, which help to reinflate zones of atelectasis and spread surfactant, become absent.[115] A good history and periodic sleep studies and pulmonary function testing with the child in both the seated and supine positions are the most effective means of monitoring respiratory insufficiency. In addition, family members should be trained in the techniques of bronchial drainage, chest percussion, and cough assist.[116]

Use of inspiratory and expiratory aids has been shown to prolong survival and decrease hospitalizations significantly when following an intensive protocol.[117] In this study by Bach et al., children with DMD used noninvasive intermittent positive pressure ventilation (IPPV), manually assisted cough, and mechanically assisted cough (using a mechanical insufflation–exsufflation cough assist). They used these techniques when needed, as indicated by an oximeter, to maintain oxyhemoglobin saturation (SaO_2) greater than or equal to 95%. The protocol subjects required fewer hospitalizations and days in the hospital when compared to subjects who were conventionally managed with tracheostomy and IPPV alone.[117] Pulmonary function after the performance of inspiratory muscle training has been shown to improve in boys with DMD.[118] Wanke et al. found improvements in respiratory muscle strength in 10 out of 15 boys with DMD, and improvements remained at 6 months after inspiratory muscle training had ended. The five subjects who did not show improvements after 1 month of training had less than 25% predicted vital capacity; therefore, the authors concluded that inspiratory muscle training was beneficial in the early stage of DMD.[119] In a study of the long-term effects of respiratory muscle training (RMT) in 21 subjects with DMD and SMA type III, the authors concluded that despite the rapidly reversible RMT-induced strength benefits, long-lasting improvements in respiratory load perception persisted after 12 months.[120]

Facilitating Family Support

The physical therapist plays an important role in providing support, motivation, and training for the child with DMD and his family members. Successful family support depends on the early involvement of the physical therapist in helping the family understand the natural history and opportunities that exist to impact progression of the disease with a home program that is monitored and adapted appropriately. Assessment of the social situation and compliance of the family should be part of each visit.

The mild to moderate intellectual impairment found in some of these young boys often imposes both educational and emotional stressors, in addition to the obvious physical changes accompanying DMD. The child learns that the disease will continuously erode the quality and quantity of his existence, and the resultant reliance and dependence on others frequently give rise to stress within the family. Although not a psychotherapist, the physical therapist must be aware of the emotional factors involved with the illness and must provide strong emotional support to optimize the child and family's ability to function as a team, with the goal of optimizing the boy's function and quality of life. A healthy emotional environment for the family and the child with DMD is at least as important to the child as the prevention of contractures.

Management of Pain

Most of the pain that occurs in these disorders is of three types. First, some boys complain of muscle pain that is often reflective of overuse and delayed muscle soreness. Second, some older children will develop an impingement syndrome at the shoulder from being lifted for transfers. Finally, when the ability to perform independent pressure relief diminishes, some children have pain related to pressure either in the wheelchair or in bed at night. If pain becomes a problem, routine methods of treatment aimed at addressing the cause of the pain may be helpful. Sometimes, making the child aware of the cause of muscle aches will allow them to self-limit. Other times, medical treatment with creatine can be helpful. Instruction in lifting techniques and proper positioning of the hands so as not to overstress the shoulder during lifting or to support the arm in the wheelchair properly can be helpful. Finally, proper wheelchair and bed positioning can aid in adequately distributing the pressure and diminishing the pain.

Summary

A successful treatment program focused on maintaining flexibility and ameliorating functional limitation through the use of assistive technology should optimize quality of life and maintenance of the maximal functional independence allowed by the child's level of strength (see Case Study A.M., 10-year-old Caucasian with DMD).

» Myotonic dystrophy

Myotonic dystrophy type I (DM1) is an autosomal dominant disorder occurring in 1 in 2,500 births. The gene location (dystrophia myotonica protein kinase [DMPK]) is on chromosome 19, with the myotonic dystrophy type II gene being found on the third chromosome.[121] DM presents with a continuum of severity from the severe congenital presentation to parents who are identified only because their children present with weakness[122] and are identified. In the most typical form of DM1, the symptoms are first noticed during adolescence and are characterized by myotonia, a delay in muscle relaxation time, muscle weakness, and cataracts.[123] The typical presentation to the clinic is with complaints of weakness and stiffness. Stiffness, which is often the major complaint, is characteristic of the myotonia. Children often have a characteristic physical appearance that includes a long, thin face with temporal and masseter muscle wasting; frontal balding; and weakness and wasting of the sternocleidomastoids. The pattern of weakness in DM1 presents first with distal wasting and weakness, manifested by a foot drop and difficulty opening jars, whereas type II MTD presents primarily with a phenotype of proximal weakness. In type I, proximal muscle weakness occurs in the later stage of the disease. The most severe form of DM1 is congenital in onset and is associated with generalized muscular hypoplasia, mental retardation, and a high incidence of neonatal mortality. Children with congenital DM1 are typically born to mothers who express the disorder phenotypically. DM1 demonstrates anticipation, with each generation being more severely affected than the prior generation. Because DM1 is inherited in an autosomal dominant pattern, an individual with the disease has a 50/50 chance of each offspring having the disease. The severe congenital form of DM1 is characterized by maternal transmission only. The most severe congenital presentation is characterized by intellectual disability, speech disturbances, delayed motor milestones, distal weakness, and spinal deformities. With survival to adulthood, these individuals follow the pattern of the classic course of the disease, in which cataracts and cardiac conduction abnormalities are common. There is involvement not only of skeletal muscle but also smooth muscle, and cardiac conduction defects (first-degree heart block) can require cardiac pacing. There may be associated infertility, decreased respiratory drive, and endocrine findings. The causative genetic defect is one of a triple repeat expansion that results in a widespread splicing abnormality resulting from the sequestration of RNA binding proteins. The result of this splicing abnormality is the mis-splicing of a wide spectrum of proteins throughout various tissues that are incorrectly sliced or retain a fetal pattern of splicing and do not function properly.[123] Therapeutic strategies have emerged, and they are in clinical trials to target and break down the RNA that instigates the splicing abnormalities in MTD.[123]

Death in these individuals is usually caused by heart block or problems secondary to decreased respiratory drive. The respiratory complications may be severe, and, once mechanically ventilated, these children are very difficult to wean. The congenital forms of DM1 may be accompanied by severe developmental delays, in which case intervention that employs various motor development approaches may be beneficial.

>> Limb-girdle muscular dystrophy

Limb-girdle muscular dystrophy (LGMD) is the term used to refer to a group of progressive muscular dystrophies that primarily affect the proximal musculature. The initial presentation can be quite variable, extending from early childhood into adulthood. Unlike DMD, the underlying pathology of LGMD is quite heterogeneous. There is an ever-growing list of distinct LGMD genes identified. These have been labeled 1A through H representing the dominant forms, and 2A through Q representing the recessive forms.[124] With the elucidation of the underlying genetic and biochemical defects that can cause LGMD, it has become apparent that each of these defects is associated with specific phenotypic patterns. It is helpful to consider grouping the patterns by function or area of the muscle cell or extracellular environment that the protein defect can be localized to as a way to organize one's thoughts about phenotypic commonalities.[125] It is, however, beyond the scope of this chapter to discuss all of the forms of LGMD here; however, we discuss the more common ones that present typically in childhood and may present for treatment in pediatric practice.

The sarcoglycanopathies (LGMD C, D, E, and F) represent those forms of LGMD that most closely resemble the progression of Duchenne. The sarcoglycanopathies are recessively inherited, with a significant number of cases presenting sporadically.[126] These four forms of LGMD are caused by a deficiency of a group of muscle membrane proteins (Fig. 13.1). The sarcoglycan proteins are coded for on four different chromosomes: γ-sarcoglycan at 13q12, α-sarcoglycan at 17q21.1, β-sarcoglycan at 4q12, and δ-sarcoglycan at 5q33. A deletion of any one of these proteins as the primary defect results in problems incorporating the entire complex, or portions of the complex, into the membrane. In almost half the cases, this results in incomplete incorporation of dystrophin in the membrane.[127] As a result, there is a great degree of phenotypic overlap between these muscular dystrophies in addition to a similarity between the sarcoglycanopathies and DMD.

Findings on medical evaluation include elevated serum CK to anywhere from 5 times to 100 times the normal.[127] The EMG examination is marked by myopathic findings similar to those seen in DMD. Muscle biopsy has been needed in the past to determine the diagnosis, although this changing with the advent of inexpensive genetic panels. Muscle biopsy findings should show a dystrophic pattern with a variation in fiber size, degenerating and regenerating fibers, and central nuclei. When stained by immunohistochemical techniques with monoclonal antibodies to the specific sarcoglycan proteins, the specific pathologic basis of the impairment can often be identified. When biopsy is able to identify the protein abnormality, genetic testing can also be used to finalize the diagnosis.[128]

Children with sarcoglycanopathies have an increased risk of dilated cardiac myopathy. Politano et al.[129] found a 40% rate of presymptomatic cardiomyopathy in these children in addition to signs of hypoxic myocardial insults. The children with dilated cardiomyopathy had primarily γ- and δ-sarcoglycanopathies, and those with hypoxic damage had β-, γ-, and δ-sarcoglycanopathies.[130]

These four proteins, α-, β-, γ-, and δ-sarcoglycan, are closely associated with dystrophin, the defective protein in DMD, and share much of the clinical phenotype. LGMD, in general, and sarcoglycanopathies, in particular, can present with a similar, albeit somewhat more variable, phenotype when compared with DMD. The distribution of muscle weakness is marked by a proximal-to-distal gradient; and in sarcoglycanopathies, the abductors and extensors of the hip are the most severely and first involved. Other muscles of the UE that become involved include the deltoids, pectoralis major, rhomboids, and infraspinatus, and a significant number of children demonstrate a progressive lordosis and anterior pelvic tilt.[121]

A second form of LGMD, type 2A or calpainopathy, is also recessively inherited and is caused by the absence of calpain-3 that results from a deletion on chromosome 15q15.1–15.3.[123] Calpain-3 is the first enzyme that was identified as the causative defect through a Ca+-dependent sarcomeric remodeling during muscle regeneration.[131,132] Calpain-3 can also be reduced in children with LGMD 2B and 2J because, presumably, calpain acts together with dysferlin and connectin (titin) in the membrane repair process and interacts with myosin light chain following exercise and are the primary protein defects in these forms of LGMD (Fig. 13.1).[123,133]

Clinical presentation of LGMD 2A includes a typically elevated CK and muscle biopsy findings with degenerating and regenerating fibers, central nuclei, and a variation in fiber size. The EMG will have typical myopathic features. Children show no intellectual deficits, and cardiac defects have not been reported at increased rates in LGMD 2A.[134] Unlike other muscular dystrophies, there seems to be no direct correlation between the amount of protein identified on biopsy and the severity of clinical presentation,[135] and the age at presentation, which ranges from childhood to middle age, does not necessarily provide guidance for the timing of ambulation loss.[136] However, children with in-frame genetic defects on both alleles tend to have a later onset of symptoms and a later diagnosis as compared with those with heterozygous or homozygous null mutations. Ambulation typically continues throughout childhood, with the average child losing ambulation in the late teens or early 20s; however, there can be a significant variability between children and within families, with some continuing to ambulate into middle age and others losing ambulation in early childhood.[136]

LGMD 2A has a wide variation in the severity of presentation and in the course of the disease.

Typically, the presentation is in the second decade of life, initially with proximal atrophy. This is most commonly expressed as scapular winging. Weakness of the elbow flexors can also be present. The wrist extensors are typically weaker than are the flexors; and the hip adductors are more affected, whereas the abductors are preserved long into the disease process. The knee extensors typically remain stronger than do the flexors, and the ankle evertors are typically weaker than are the invertors. Contractures are typically found in the calf muscles along with atrophy of this muscle in most European children; however, in Brazilian children, hypertrophy can be found in the calf. Finger-flexion and elbow-flexion contractures may also be present early on in the disease process. These muscle imbalances correspond with a typical standing posture of hip abduction, knee hyperextension, and inversion at the ankle that is preserved long into the disease process. Children with LGMD 2A typically remain able to stand with support far into the disease process because of this pattern of contracture and muscle involvement.[136,137]

The last form of LGMD discussed here is LGMD 2I. LGMD 2I is recessively inherited and caused by a mutation in the fukutin-related protein (FKRP) gene. This gene is also the cause of some forms of CMD, which is discussed later. The gene is found on chromosome 19q (Table 13.3),[138] and the

TABLE 13.3.	Limb-Girdle Muscular Dystrophy	
Disease Name	Gene, Inheritance	Protein Product
LGMD2A Calpainopathy	15q15.1 Recessive	Calpain-3
LGMD2B Dysferlinopathy	2p13.2 Recessive	Dysferlin
LGMD2C γ-Sarcoglycanopathy	13q12.12 Recessive	γ-Sarcoglycan
LGMD2D α-Sarcoglycanopathy	17q21.33 Recessive	α-Sarcoglycan
LGMD2E β-Sarcoglycanopathy	4q12 Recessive	β-Sarcoglycan
LGMD2F δ-Sarcoglycanopathy	5q33.3 Recessive	δ-Sarcoglycan
LGMD2G Telethoninopathy	17q12 Recessive	Telethonin
LGMD2H	9q33.1 Recessive	TRIM32
LGMD2I KRP	19q13.32 Recessive	Fukutin-related protein (FKRP)
LGMD2J Titinopathy	2q24.3 Recessive	Titin
LGMD2K Disorder of glycosilation	9q34.13	O-mannosyltransferase 1
LGMD2L	11p14.3	Anoctamin 5
LGMD2M Disorder of glycosilation	9q31.2 Recessive	Fukutin
LGMD2N Disorder of glycosilation	14q24.3 Recessive	O-mannosyltransferase 2
LGMD2O Disorder of glycosilation	1p34.1 Recessive	O-mannose beta-1,2-N-acetylglucosaminyl-transferase
LGMD2P	3p21.31 Recessive	Dystroglycan 1
LGMD2Q	8q24.3 Recessive	Plectin 1f
LGMD1A Myotilinopathy	5q31.2 Dominant	Myotilin
LGMD1B Laminopathy	1q22 Dominant	Lamin A/C
LGMD1C Caveolinopathy	3p25.3 Dominant	Caveolin-3
LGMD1D (OMIM) (HUGO: LGMD E)	2q35 Dominant	Desmin
LGMD1E (HUGO: LGMD E)	7q36.3 Dominant	DNAJ/HSP40 homolog, subfamily B, member 6
LGMD1F	7q32.1–32.2 Dominant	
LGMD1G	4p21 Dominant	
LGMD1H	3p25.1–p23 Dominant	

Mitsuhashi S, Kang PB. Update on the genetics of limb girdle muscular dystrophy. *Semin Pediatr Neurol.* 2012;19(4):211-218; Neuromuscular Disease Center. Limb-Girdle Muscular Dystrophy (LGMD) syndromes. Accessed February 22, 2013. http://neuromuscular.wustl.edu/musdist/lg.html#lgmd1f

encoded protein, FKRP, is a glycosyltransferase that aids in the O-glycosylation of α-dystroglycan. As a result of its absence, α-dystroglycan does not form properly.[139] α-dystroglycan is located in the extracellular space and is associated with the dystrophin complex that spans the membrane, and proper glycosylation is required for its association with laminin-α2.[138]

Diagnosis is established first by clinical presentation, which is marked by weakness. EMG shows a typical myopathic pattern and an elevated serum CK, which is typically is in the thousands. Muscle biopsy is typically characterized by a variation in fiber size with type 1 predominance, degenerating and regenerating fibers, an increase in central nuclei, and increased connective tissue.[139] Immunohistochemistry in these children can be variable, with the most common finding being a reduction in laminin α-2; reductions in α-dystroglycan can also be found.[140]

Clinical presentation of children with LGMD 2I can vary somewhat, with initial onset of symptoms typically in the first two decades of life. A significant number of children present with a limb-girdle phenotype. In these children, onset is typically in the preschool years. The pattern of weakness is characterized by proximal weakness predominating and gastroc/soleus contracture and hypertrophy most pronounced. However, in the more severely involved children, the shoulder girdle is more involved than is the pelvic girdle. In the milder cases, the opposite is true. In the more severely involved children, respiratory function can become an issue as the disease progresses. Most children with LGMD 2I typically maintain fairly good respiratory function throughout the first two decades of life.[141,142] Cardiac defects are a common characteristic of LGMD 2I.[143] Males with heterozygous mutations are at increased risk for developing dilated cardiac myopathy when compared with females or those with homozygous mutations,[144,145] and, as a result, these children need to be monitored more closely by their physician.

Clinical care for children with LGMD revolves around anticipating the development of contractures and conservative management with the use of dynamic or static resting splints to maintain muscle length. ROM exercises and exercise to optimize muscle endurance such as swimming can be considered, but because this is a dystrophic process, strengthening exercise, especially of the eccentric variety, should be avoided.

» Congenital myopathy

Congenital myopathy describes a group of diseases, including nemaline myopathy, central core myopathy, and centronuclear (myotubular) myopathy. The three broad categories are based on the microscopic appearance of the muscle; centronuclear myopathy is marked by an abnormal predominance of central nuclei as compared to the normally peripherally placed nuclei of the muscle cell, central core myopathy is marked by the presence of central clearing, or cores, within the cytoplasm, and nemaline myopathy is characterized by nemaline rods that can be seen by electron microscopy. These and the other congenital myopathies typically result from abnormalities of the sarcomeric proteins. These diseases are characterized by weakness and muscle atrophy that typically presents at birth. There are, however, less common forms that can present later in life. The congenital myopathies represent a group of disorders that are less well characterized when compared with the other disorders we have discussed thus far. The broad diagnostic classifications are based on morphologic characteristics found on muscle biopsy, with subtyping based on clinical features. In each broad category, there are a number of genetic mutations that can be the causative factor; however, there is significant clinical variability that can be seen. Here, we discuss two of the most common congenital myopathies, nemaline myopathy and central core myopathy.

Nemaline myopathy has a wide range in the severity of clinical presentation and heterogeneity of genetic causes.[146] Nemaline is a genetically heterogeneous myopathy with mutations in the genes that code for actin, nebuline, or tropomyosin (β-2 and -3) and other proteins. The inheritance pattern is most often sporadic, but can also be dominant or recessive. Pathologically, on muscle biopsy, there are cytoplasmic inclusions visible on light microscopy and called either *rods* or *nemaline bodies*, seen by electron microscopy, that represent deposits of z-line proteins.[147–149]

Nemaline myopathy has been divided into seven different forms on the basis of severity and other factors by the European Neuromuscular Center. These types include the typical or classic form, the severe form, the intermediate form, the mild form, and the adult-onset form. In addition, there is a severe Amish type with neonatal onset and a category for other forms. The typical form of nemaline myopathy presents at birth or early infancy with respiratory insufficiency being an issue, especially at night. These children often become ambulatory; however, some will need wheeled mobility. The severe form is characterized by weakness from birth. Often, in this type of nemaline myopathy, no spontaneous movement is evident. These children can have arthrogryposis and fractures at birth. Lack of respiratory effort and the resulting respiratory insufficiency and ventilator dependence often lead to death in the first year of life. The intermediate form presents in infancy or at birth. Children are able to breathe on their own by a year, and either do not ambulate at all or progress and develop contractures over time and lose the ability to ambulate by 11 years of age. The mild form presents in childhood, often with a history of normal developmental milestones. This form is often slowly progressive, and in the later stages, this form can be clinically indistinguishable from the classic or typical presentation. The adult form tends to be more progressive, and can also demonstrate inflammatory change on biopsy as well as cardiomyopathy.[150,151] The most common form is the classic or typical form, representing 43% of cases in one series.[150] The intermediate and severe congenital forms represent 20% and 16%, respectively, with the less severe form with childhood and adult-onset representing the remaining cases.

Central core myopathy is named for the presence of histologic cores on muscle biopsy. If the cores appear centrally and are large, the name *central core myopathy* is used, and if there are multiple small cores, the term *multiminicore myopathy* is used. Despite the use of these two terms, these only represent a pathologic description and may represent different stages in the same disease process in some cases. Family members with, presumably, the same disease process may have both central and multiminicores, and one with multiminicores may later in the disease process present with central cores.[152] These cores are areas within the muscle that contain no mitochondria, are negative for oxidative enzymes, and contain a collection of proteins that include many cellular proteins. One of the most common genes identified as being responsible for central core disease is found on 19q13; it codes for the ryanodine receptor 1 protein (RYR1) and controls the release of calcium from the sarcoplasmic reticulum.[148,152,153] RYR1-related central core myopathy can be either the result of a dominant or recessive mutation depending on the characteristics of the defect.

Clinically, central core myopathy can be relatively static or mildly progressive over long periods; and phenotype/genotype correlations are emerging surrounding the specific calcium channel abnormality that a given mutation yields, with some variability also being based around the existence of dominant versus recessive inheritance.[154] The pattern of weakness typically with recessive presentation includes facial weakness, neck flexor weakness, and proximal weakness, with the legs being more involved than are the arms.[152] However, a dominant distal calf phenotype also has been described.[155] The other clinical feature of children with dominant gain of function RYR1 mutations is the susceptibility to malignant hyperthermia, which is a severe reaction to anesthesia, and rhabdomyolysis, both of which may be present in the absence of weakness.[155,156] There is a spectrum of children with central core myopathy, and more severe forms have been noted.[157]

Centronuclear (myotubular) myopathy is the other main category of congenital myopathy and results primarily from an abnormality in the *MTM1* gene, which is X-linked and codes for the protein myotubularin. However, other genes also contribute to a portion of children who present with central nuclear myopathy. Clinical presentation typically is more severe, with ventilator and wheelchair dependence being common. Functionally, children typically have myopathic facial muscles with ophthalmoplegia, and a relative preservation of quadriceps strength are a common occurrence.[145] The classic form presents recessively, with carriers often demonstrating asymmetry of skeletal and muscle phenotype and a variable severity of symptomatology.[158]

>> Congenital muscular dystrophy

CMD can be divided into those CMDs with CNS involvement and those without CNS involvement. Fukuyama CMD, Walker–Walburg syndrome, and muscle–eye–brain disease represent the group of CMDs with CNS involvement, and all typically demonstrate muscle, brain, and eye abnormalities. The typical brain abnormalities include a cobblestone lissencephaly with cerebral and cerebellar cortical dysplasia secondary to a neuronal migration abnormality. Eye and vision abnormalities span a wide range of possible abnormalities and vary from one disease to the other, but may include structural abnormalities of the eye as well as myopia and retinal detachment.[159] The muscle abnormalities are based on abnormal glycosylation of α-dystroglycan resulting from the absence of various enzymes that facilitate the process of glycosylation. Glycosylation is the addition of glycans to a protein to form a glycoprotein. As a result of the common pathophysiology, there is significant overlap in the clinical presentation of these diseases and the pathologic findings encountered during the diagnostic workup. All present congenitally in the typical case, although there are also milder limb-girdle phenotypes. Walker–Warburg syndrome is the most severe of the CMDs, and children typically die by 3 years of age. Muscle–eye–brain disease has a variable clinical picture, and presents in infancy. The more mildly involved children may ambulate for a period during childhood; however, their functional abilities are limited by spasticity and ataxia resulting from the brain abnormalities as well as the muscle weakness. Most children with Fukuyama CMD will achieve standing, and some can take steps in early childhood. Typically, in the second decade, respiratory failure becomes a problem, beginning with nocturnal hypoventilation. This can progress, limiting the life expectancy of these children to the third decade of life. Cardiomyopathy is also a feature commonly seen in these children, and they should be periodically followed up by cardiology.

Merosin (laminin)-negative CMD (also known as LAMA2-related CMD or MDC1A) is the most common CMD, representing half of all cases of CMD. The absence of merosin in the extracellular matrix of the muscle (Fig. 13.1) results from an abnormality of the *LAMA2* gene found on chromosome 6q2.[160] Merosin-negative CMD also shows CNS involvement in the form of abnormalities of the periventricular and subcortical white matter including occipital polymicrogyria and cortical heterotopias. To better anticipate the clinical course, it is important to subdivide the group by the presence or total absence of merosin and partial absence, with complete absence predicting a more severe phenotype. The clinical course of this disorder is characterized by severe weakness at birth or in early infancy and the development of contractures, particularly at the ankle and eventually at the knee and elbow. The severe weakness can improve over time, and most children will sit by 2 or 3 years of age and upward of 25% will stand or walk with bracing. Muscle strength can be stable over time, although extraocular muscle involvement can be seen and is often slowly progressive. Nocturnal hypoventilation may also be a problem for many of these children, typically by the second or third decade of life, and a third may have seizures or cardiac abnormalities.[159,160]

Ullrich CMD results from the abnormalities of collagen VI. Collagen VI is composed of three associated proteins that form a triple helix. Abnormalities of collagen VI, also a component of the extracellular matrix, can result from mutations of any of the three subunits COL6A$_1$, A$_2$, or A$_3$. COL6A$_1$ and COL6A$_2$ is located on the 21st chromosome and 21q 23.3, and COL6A$_3$ is located on chromosome 2q37.[160] Collagen VI is found in the extracellular matrix (Fig. 13.1) and presumably acts to transmit force from the muscle to the bone and tendon. Ullrich CMD is typically recessively inherited; however, dominant negative inheritance represents a significant minority of these children.[161,162] A dominant negative exists where the affected gene product negatively impacts the nonaffected allele's protein production. This often results from an in-frame or missense mutation. The milder form of collagen VI abnormality, Bethlem myopathy, is typically dominantly inherited, and, although historically they were viewed as separate conditions, the phenotype is one of a continuous spectrum. There is a movement toward referring to these disorders as COL6-related myopathy. On muscle biopsy, findings can range from mild myopathic to dystrophic in the more severe cases; however, it is rare to see necrotic and regenerating fibers. Classically, findings include variation in fiber size and infiltration of the muscle by fatty and fibrotic tissue. Children with Ullrich CMD typically have weakness at birth in all but the mildest cases. There is an increased risk of congenital hip dislocation and also of torticollis and arthrogryposis; the latter two of these typically improve with stretching. Gross motor skills are typically delayed; however, there are improvements seen in motor skills in the first few years of life, and children typically gain the ability to sit independently and stand with bracing. A significant number of children also gain the ability to ambulate independently. Contractures of pectoral muscles and shoulder internal rotators, in addition to the hips, knees, and elbows, are typical and are combined with hyperlaxity of the distal joints. In children who achieve ambulation, the ability to walk is most often limited by progressive knee flexion contractures or planovarus contracture at the ankle. Respiratory insufficiency can be a problem for the more severely affected children as they age, and can be found in those who are still ambulatory.[162]

Physical therapy intervention in CMD and congenital myopathy needs to take into account the natural history of the specific disorder, and realistic goals need to be planned on the basis of the natural history of the disease. A focus on the maintenance of flexibility with stretching and appropriate bracing or serial casting as needed is important. Bracing may be needed for nighttime positioning, for standing or ambulation, and also for those who are not ambulatory. Standers and wheelchairs as well as bathroom adaptations may provide practical assistance. Even in those children who have some household ambulation, power mobility may be necessary for community mobility or for longer distances at school and in the community.

» Spinal muscular atrophy

SMA is a disorder that is manifested by interneuron abnormality and a loss of anterior horn cells. This results in a phenotypic spectrum of disease states that have been divided into three types of SMA on the basis of a functional classification system.

Three categories of SMA occur in childhood:

1. SMA type I (Werdnig–Hoffman disease)
2. SMA type II
3. SMA type III (Kugelberg–Welander disease)

The classification of a child with SMA into one of these types is based solely on the child's maximal functional abilities. The child who is so weak that they have never learned to sit is diagnosed with SMA type I. Those children who learn to sit but never learn to walk without an assistive device have type II SMA, and the children who walk independently are diagnosed with SMA type III. Some will also include a more severe type 0 with onset of weakness at birth and a less severe group with adult-onset weakness. Other authors will include all motor-only neuropathies in this category, whereas others will include these in their categorization on CMT disease.[163]

In recent years, pharmacologic therapies have emerged, first with the introduction of Spinraza[164] and then Zolgenzma,[165] which have fundamentally altered the natural history of SMA from one of variable onset followed by slow insidious progression to that of a motor neuron disease characterized by consistent strength gains that occur over time and are limited by existing contracture and established weakness in those treated remotely from the onset of weakness. With earlier treatment, motor progress is more robust, and the limitations imposed by contracture less pronounced.

Genetics

SMA is inherited as an autosomal recessive disorder, and here we focus our discussion only on 5q SMA. The underlying genetic defect is located on chromosome 5q13, where the survival motor neuron (SMN) gene is located and the SMN protein is coded for.[166–168] In this region of the chromosome, there are two paralogous genes, *SMN1* and *SMN2*, that code for the SMN protein. Typically, there is one copy of SMN1 and multiple copies of SMN2. SMN1 produces most of the protein that the body uses, and when there is a homozygous deletion, the *SMN1* gene produces no protein and the *SMN2* gene must be relied on to produce the SMN protein. Most (85% to 90%) of the SMN protein that *SMN2* produces is missing exon 7 and is not functional. The total amount of SMN produced in children with SMA, therefore, depends on how many copies of *SMN2* the child has. The number of SMN2 copies also correlates with how severe the phenotypic presentation of the disease is.[167]

Pathophysiology

SMN plays a role in the function of all cells, mediating the assembly of a set of proteins that associate with RNA and function as part of the splicing machinery in every cell. The interneurons and alpha motor neuron are most impacted by the diminished levels of SMN. Abnormalities in mitochondrial biogenesis[166] also contribute to the fatigue of SMA.

As a result of the loss of motor neurons, EMG results will be characterized by diminished compound motor unit action potentials (CMAPs) that are often of short duration; the diminished CMAP will track the course of the disease. Positive sharp waves and fibrillations are also found, and, typically, conduction velocities and sensory studies are normal.[166] The number of motor units are also diminished in children with SMA. The number of remaining motor units can be estimated by EMG using motor unit number estimation (MUNE). The MUNE reflects the number of lower motor neurons that innervate a given muscle. In addition to CMAP, the MUNE can be used to monitor the progress of the underlying pathologic process affecting the motor neuron.[170]

Typically, the histopathology found on muscle biopsy is characterized by groups of small atrophic fibers interspersed with groups of large hypertrophic fibers (Fig. 13.7). This type of grouped atrophy is characteristic of a neurogenic process. The groups of atrophic fibers are the result of lack of innervation to that motor unit. Children with SMA will typically have absent deep tendon reflexes; however, this is not completely uniform. About half of the children will have fasciculations that can be seen in the tongue as spontaneous small muscle contractions[170]; these can be seen on muscle ultrasound at times even if they are not visible on the tongue. Because only the lower motor neuron is affected, sensation is typically intact as is cognitive function in children with SMA. Because this is a lower motor neuron disease, no upper motor neuron signs should be noted.

SMA Type I (Werdnig–Hoffman Disease)

SMA type I in the untreated condition is typically noted within the first months of life before the onset of sitting.

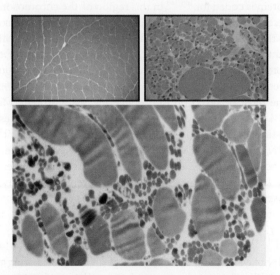

FIGURE 13.7. Neuropathic changes associated with spinal muscular atrophy (SMA) as compared with normal (*upper left*). Note the hypertrophic changes and grouped atrophy.

However, the diagnosis may not be made for a number of months. Depending on severity, decreased movement may be noted during pregnancy or within the first weeks or months of birth. Axial hypotonicity is often the first symptom noted, and difficulty feeding is often a concern shortly after the onset of weakness. Muscle wasting is often severe, and spontaneous movement are infrequent and of small amplitude. On examination, the symptomatic infant with SMA type I will present with a head lag on pull-to-sit and will drape over the examiner's hand when a landau is performed. The infant will be dominated by gravity. In supine, the legs will be abducted and flexed and more impaired than are the arms, which will move primarily with the elbows on the surface; and if they can be brought to midline, this will be with difficulty. In the most severely affected infants, axial strength will be so diminished that in supine the head will not be able to be maintained in midline. Prone position is poorly tolerated because of respiratory limitation, and prone skills will be similarly limited. Infants with SMA type I will not be able to prop and typically cannot turn their heads from side to side in prone. In vertical, some infants will demonstrate tenuous head control, whereas most will not be able to maintain their heads erect.

Infants with SMA type I typically develop significant oral motor weakness that makes feeding progressively more difficult.[171] These infants have difficulty taking in sufficient calories to gain weight and thrive. Medical options for supplemental feeding in these children include nasogastric feeding or the surgical placement of a gastrostomy tube with Nissan fundoplication to diminish the potential for gastroesophageal reflux and aspiration.

Children with SMA type I also have limited respiratory function and develop a paradoxic pattern of breathing, with the diaphragmatic muscles playing the primary role in ventilation. In these infants, inspiration is diaphragmatically initiated, and because negative pressure develops in the thoracic cavity, the intercostals and other thoracic muscles that typically stabilize the ribcage fail; and the ribcage collapses with each breath, eventually creating a parasol deformity. Typically, the belly also rises as the diaphragm lowers, allowing for the creation of negative intrathoracic pressure and inspiration. In the weakest infants, the chest and the abdomen will be directly out of phase, characteristic of a paradoxic breathing pattern. In the infants who are a bit stronger, the chest will stabilize or expand briefly with the abdomen before collapsing; this is in contrast to the normal condition of almost simultaneous abdominal and thoracic expansion. Pulmonary infections are common in infants with SMA type I, and pulmonary management is an important facet of care for these children. Both the inability to take a deep breath and the lack of an effective cough can cause serious respiratory complications, including atelectasis and pneumonia. Percussion and postural drainage should be recommended for use when the infant has upper respiratory infections to move the secretions from the small airways. These infants may also be treated with a mechanical in-exsufflator or coughalator that delivers a positive pressure insufflation followed by an expulsive exsufflation that simulates a cough as an additional means of airway clearance[172] and as a way of maintaining flexibility of the lungs and ribcage. Approximately half of the children with infantile SMA do not survive beyond 2 years of age without medical treatment with one of the SMN-modulating therapies now available or with the assistance of mechanical ventilation.[173] For those who do choose to have tracheostomies or use non-invasive ventilation, the life span can be extended significantly beyond this in the absence of SMN-modulating therapy, with half of children with SMA type 1 surviving to 10 years of age in one trial where proactive respiratory management and nutritional support was commonly applied.[8,174] That said, a new natural history of SMA is now emerging. Treatment with medications that upregulate SMN production fundamentally alters the progression of disease even in the most severe groups of children.[174]

Children with SMA type I have such severe weakness without medical treatment that it is difficult for them to participate in play activities, and lightweight toys may be appropriate. Younger infants may benefit from a sling-and-spring setup that can be made from TheraBand tubing and Velfoam cuffs attached to the infant carrier or PVC frame to aid in antigravity leg movement and to promote active movement and facilitate strength. With existing medical therapies, many children show progress in their motor skills following treatment initiation. Treatment considerations include the maintenance of flexibility at the knee and ankle through the use of bracing and ROM/stretching for both the UEs and LEs. Once children are at the age where standing typically develops, standers and bracing for standing become options, and various mobility options should be considered. The approach to physical therapy for these children must be aimed at quality of life for both the child and the family.[175]

SMA Type II

Type II SMA also affects infants, but is less severe than is SMA type I. However, with medical treatment, there is now considerable overlap between SMA types, and age of presentation is less tightly correlated with ultimate functional skill attainment because it was in the absence of SMN-modulating therapies. Initial presentation is typically later in the first year of life when the child is noted to not be pulling to stand. These children are characterized by proximal weakness. Fasciculations are common on examination of the tongue in these children. There is also often a fine resting tremor when the child attempts to use the limbs. This is not an intention tremor, but has been referred to as a *minipolymyoclonus*.[8]

In children with SMA type II, there is a delay in the acquisition of motor skills that is somewhat variable between children. Approximately one-third of children with SMA type II will sit by the normal time of 6 months, and 90% will be able to sit by their first birthday.[176] Some children may continue to gain skills throughout the second year, even in the absence of SMN-modulating therapy, but there is typically a peak after which a slow decline in skills ensues, the rapidity of which

depends largely on the underlying disease severity. Prompt early treatment ensures the optimal functional outcome, and should not be delayed. Of those children who become independent sitters, and are diagnosed with SMA type II, 75% will remain independent sitters until 7 years, and half will remain sitting at 14 years of age without SMN-modulating intervention.[176] Motor skills that employ a long lever arm are most difficult for these children, and as a result, prone and quadruped skills are most delayed because it is difficult to maintain head control in these positions. Transitions to and from sit will also be difficult because of the weight of the head during the transition. With medical treatment, a slow overall improvement in function is noted as these children grow up.[177] In the absence of treatment, there is a slow functional decline in school-age children that occurs over years, despite a lack of detectable loss in strength.[177]

The pattern of weakness in the natural history seen in the extremities is most notable for the relative strength in the distal muscles as compared with the proximal muscles. On average, strength in children with type II and III SMA falls between 20% and 40% of predicted, depending on age. Quadriceps strength tends to be the most diminished, averaging 5% of normal. However, in children with SMA who ambulate, the variation in quadriceps strength can be three-fold as compared with children who do not ambulate.[178,179]

Contracture formation is also an issue in the management of children with SMA type II. Limitations of the hip and knee flexors and ankle plantar flexors are frequently the most significant contractures in the LE, and contractures of the elbow flexors and wrist flexors are the most significant in the arm. For the hands, resting hand splints are appropriate for night use, and for the legs, KAFO, as discussed in the next section, will aid in maintaining ROM. In addition, a daily stretching program will help maintain the child's flexibility.

By definition, these children do not ambulate independently; however, some of these children may learn to walk with bracing or an assistive device.[180] However, the ambulation is often not functional. Nonetheless, it is important to encourage standing in children with SMA type II. Standing will act to maintain joint mobility, maintain bone stock, prevent problems associated with long-term wheelchair sitting, and attempt to keep the child's back as straight as possible for as long as possible. These children often require KAFOs for standing initially, and as they become stronger with SMN modulation, the height of the bracing may be reduced. The proximal portion of the KAFO may be shaped for ischial weight bearing to improve comfort and control of the proximal femur (Fig.13.8). For children who do not attain independent standing, a transition to a more traditional stander becomes appropriate if contractures allow; and bracing may be only necessary to stabilize the foot and ankle, with the stander providing the remaining support. For those children who can continue in a standing program, there are a number of options, some that will accommodate flexion contractures and others that assist in the transfer, alleviating some of the burden on the parent.

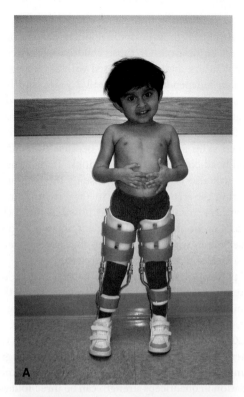

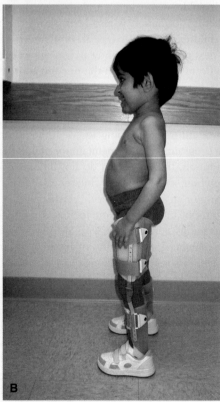

FIGURE 13.8. Anterior–posterior **(A)** and lateral view **(B)** of a 3-year-old with type II spinal muscular atrophy (SMA) wearing ischial weight-bearing knee–ankle–foot orthoses.

and may not gain weight well, and require supplemental feeding to maintain optimal body weight.

These children, even in the absence of SMN-modulating therapy, often survive into adulthood, but are vulnerable to pulmonary infection and may require mechanical ventilation either at night secondary to nocturnal hypoventilation or full time. This vulnerability is significantly improved by SMN-modulating therapy as are their hospitalizations. The use of a mechanical in-exsufflator in this population is also helpful in airway clearance, as is percussion and postural drainage during intercurrent illness, because these children also lack the muscle strength to produce a strong cough and clear secretions that develop with illness.[172]

Children with SMA type II are predisposed to kyphoscoliosis, similar to that which affects other children with neuromuscular weakness. Spinal bracing has been characterized as not preventing progression of the spinal curve,[181] and when spinal bracing is worn, pulmonary function may be limited by the external restriction.[182] However, as a practical matter for children who have pain or postural instability and scoliosis as well, a soft spinal orthosis can provide support for the trunk and allow improved tolerance in sitting until fusion.[183–186] Typically, scoliosis in this population and in children with type III SMA has been treated surgically with segmental spinal fusion once skeletally mature and with either a vertical expandable prosthetic titanium rib (VEPTR) or magnetic-controlled growing rods for younger children.[187,188] This prevents the inevitable progression of the curve, which can be more rapid once the child is in a wheelchair full time.[189] However, there is a downside to spinal fusion. Fusion can be associated with some loss of functional skill. When the flexibility of the spine is taken away, some tasks can become more difficult, especially in marginal skills. Ambulatory children (with SMA type III) are also at risk for functional decline following a fusion because spinal and pelvic flexibility is diminished, and a fusion that maintains pelvic mobility might be preferable in this population.[190] Despite this, typically, the benefits of preventing the inevitable progression of the scoliosis and the associated pulmonary and functional decline outweigh the risks associated with the surgery, and children report improved comfort and sitting balance following surgery.[191]

SMA Type III (Kugelberg–Welander Disease)

SMA type III is characterized by symptoms of progressive weakness, wasting, absent reflexes, and fasciculations. Age of presentation can vary from the toddler years into adulthood, the latter of which some would classify as type IV. Proximal muscles are usually involved first, and because of the age and pattern of presentation, this disease may be confused with the muscular dystrophies. Deep tendon reflexes are decreased, but contractures are unusual, and progressive spinal deformities are less common as long as the child remains ambulatory. Diagnosis is established on

Feeding and swallowing difficulties are seldom a problem early in the course of the disease for children with type II SMA, although some children may have oral motor concerns

the basis of the clinical picture and the results of diagnostic laboratory studies, including an EMG and muscle biopsy, which show denervation as in the other forms of SMA. In addition, genetic testing will show a deletion of the *SMN* gene on the fifth chromosome.

Prognosis in children with SMA type III can be aided by a good developmental history. Children who have symptoms that begin before 2 years of age have a relatively poorer prognosis when compared with children who have symptoms that begin after the age of 2. Russman et al.[178] followed up 159 children with SMA and found that in those with SMA type III, if symptoms began after 2 years of age, on average, children continued to ambulate until 44 years of age, whereas in those who began to have symptoms before 2 years of age, ambulation was maintained until an average of 12 years of age.[189] Montes was able to quantify this slow insidious decline in walking speed and show measurable declines over a year.[192] Similar to type I and type II SMA, treatment with SMN-modulating therapy improves this course, and children demonstrate gains in their ambulatory ability and fatigue.[191–193]

Treatment from a physical therapy standpoint is focused primarily on the maintenance of strength, function, and flexibility.[194,195] Children need to be braced appropriately while they are ambulating and for standing if they are not ambulating. Once it becomes more difficult to handle in braces for standing, sit-to-stand standers can be used, where the child is aided to standing from a sitting position. This can be helpful to maintain flexibility and bone stock by allowing weight bearing through the long bones.

» Charcot–Marie–Tooth disease

CMT disease, also known as hereditary motor and sensory neuropathy (HMSN), is a slowly progressive neuropathy that affects peripheral nerves causing sensory loss, weakness, and muscle wasting primarily in the distal musculature of the feet, lower legs, hands, and forearms. It is the most frequently inherited peripheral neuropathy affecting 1 in 2,500 persons.[196] There are four different types and now more than 100 subtypes of CMT, depending on the specific gene defect, inheritance pattern, age of onset, and whether the primary defect results in an abnormality of the myelin or axon of the nerve. CMT1, a demyelinating form, is the most common form of CMT and often is characterized by an autosomal dominant inheritance, and the typical onset of symptoms is in childhood or adolescence.[197,198] In the most common subtype, CMT1A, a duplication of the *PMP22* gene or peripheral myelin protein 22 gene on chromosome 17 is present.[198] CMT2 shares the inheritance pattern and time of onset of CMT1, although often with a somewhat more severe course. CMT1 primarily affects the axon of the nerve and CMT2 affects the myelin sheath of the nerve.[145] CMT3, also known as Dejerine–Sottas (DS) disease, is often not used as a separate category any longer,[198] and had been used to define an autosomal dominant congenital hypomyelinating neuropathy with onset

in infancy and more severe weakness.[196] CMT4 is autosomal recessive and may also be referred to as AR-CMT2.[196] There are other forms of CMT, including an X-linked form (CMTX) and a mild congenital form as well as motor-only forms that some group with SMA.

CMT is diagnosed by physical examination, genetic testing, EMG, and nerve conduction velocity (NCV) tests. Symptoms of weakness usually begin in the feet and ankles, as is characteristic of length-dependent neuropathies, with a foot drop. Later in the course of the disease, weakness of the hands and forearms can be appreciated. Many people with CMT develop contractures in the feet, causing cavovarus deformity involving the forefoot, hindfoot, midfoot, and toes (Fig. 13.9).[199] Contractures in the long finger flexors may also develop. Decreased sensation to heat, touch, pain, and, most prominently, vibration is also present distally.

A physical therapy program can benefit individuals with CMT by improving strength, ROM, and functional activities.[200] Orthotic examination and prescription can greatly improve the gait and functional mobility of a person with CMT by preventing contracture formation and providing a more stable base for ambulation.[201–203] It has also been proposed that custom braces may improve aerobic performance and decrease energy expenditure in children with CMT.[204,205] There is limited data to guide the specific choice of brace type in CMT, but the therapist should be guided by a few underlying principles in selecting appropriate bracing. First, given that children have significant weakness, the brace weight is an important issue, and a lighter brace will decrease the tendency for the child's gait pattern to be dominated by poor lower leg deceleration at the end of swing. Carbon fiber or laminate braces with a posterior leaf spring design to prevent foot drop often provide sufficient dorsiflexion assist for the more mild cases where there is not significant fixed deformity. However, these provide

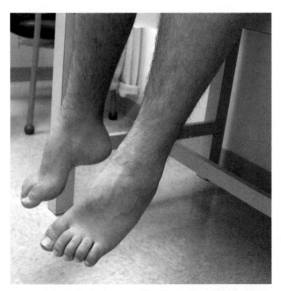

FIGURE 13.9. Sixteen-year-old with Charcot–Marie–Tooth (CMT). Notice the high arch and hammertoes on both feet as well as the varus position of the ankle.

limited deformity accommodation or control, and a carbon fiber brace may require the use of a foot orthotic insert; or if greater control is required, an articulating AFO can be used and a varus control strap added. Stretching, night splints, and serial casting can also improve ROM, but if a fixed deformity develops, orthopedic surgery to correct the deformity may be necessary to produce a plantigrade foot.

A resistance training program can improve strength[206] and ADLs in children with CMT. The addition of creatine monohydrate has been investigated as an adjunct to exercise.[207,208] Resistance training has also been found to be helpful with respect to strength and function, with improvement noted after a home-based strengthening program.[209–211] The therapist should always consider the natural history of the disease and relationships of various functional tasks and impairments when designing an exercise program.[201,212]

Summary

The disorders discussed in this chapter are all characterized by weakness and wasting of the skeletal musculature, progressive deformity, and increasing disability. The physical therapist plays an important role in the management of these disorders. The therapist's role centers on the maintenance of function, both through the management of what is often a progressive process and the provision of assistive technology to compensate for functional limitations. This may be as simple as recommending bath equipment to make transfers more manageable or as involved as prescribing power mobility to compensate for the loss of ambulation. The therapist is also in a position to provide teaching surrounding the natural history and act as a resource for outcome measurement both for monitoring of individual children and as part of a clinical trial team. Finally, the therapist can work together with the psychosocial members of the team to facilitate the necessary emotional support for the affected child and family.

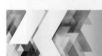

CASE STUDY

A.M., 10-YEAR-OLD CAUCASIAN WITH DUCHENNE MUSCULAR DYSTROPHY

A.M. is a 10-year-old Caucasian boy with a diagnosis of DMD. He was diagnosed at 4 years of age when it was noted that he was slow getting up off the floor after story time at preschool and appeared unable to keep up with his schoolmates. He has been followed up periodically by physical therapy since that time for family education in ROM and active stretching exercises and for monitoring the status of his muscle strength, function, and joint contractures.

At 4 years of age, the family had been instructed in stretching of the heel cords to be performed on a daily basis, and A.M. had been fitted with night splints to maintain a neutral position at his ankles during sleep. (He was encouraged to wear his "moon boots" throughout the night, but if it was only 2 to 3 hours at neutral before he took them off, this shorter period was considered beneficial.) A.M. was started on prednisone by his neurologist, and became somewhat stronger and was able to run better. These functional gains, however, came with a price. A.M. initially gained some weight, but because his parents knew to watch for this, his weight gain was not as great as it could have been. In addition, A.M. was somewhat more active and inattentive in school. Despite the side effects, his parents chose to keep him on the medication because they felt the benefits outweighed the side effects. At 5 to 6 years of age, the stretching of hip flexors and ITBs had been added to the daily stretching regimen because he had developed mild flexion and abduction contractures.

At this time, A.M. comes to physical therapy with the chief complaint of an increased number of falls (approximately four per day), increased difficulty rising from a chair and ascending and descending stairs, and no longer being able to get off the floor without the use of "furniture" along with his Gowers maneuver.

Strength in the UEs graded in the "good" range (4 out of 5), with the LEs grading "fair" (3 out of 5) to "poor" (2 out of 5) in the proximal muscle groups.

Measurements of joint contractures revealed hip flexors that measured −10 degrees bilaterally, ITBs at 0 degrees bilaterally, knees at neutral, and −10 degrees at the right ankle and −8 degrees on the left. In the UE, ROM was within normal limits bilaterally and functionally still independent.

Stretching exercises were reviewed and emphasized with the family. Contracture releases were also discussed with the family as an option, and a future referral to the orthopedic surgeon was discussed. A.M. and his family were instructed to return to physical therapy in conjunction with being fitted by the orthotist with the long leg braces should they opt for surgery. The need for a wheelchair, only to be used for long-distance transport and on uneven terrain, was addressed, and because it had been discussed at previous visits, they were ready to order this and chose a powered wheelchair. They had a "buggy" that they used for long distances, but it was clear that this did not provide the independence that A.M. wanted, especially outdoors with his friends.

Contact was made with the treating physical therapist in the school district for his or her suggestions or comments regarding power mobility, and issues related to home and school accessibility were discussed with the family and therapist, in terms of both transport and access.

A.M. became a full-time wheelchair user at 12, and despite the lateral support on his chair, he developed scoliosis, which required fusion when it reached 40 degrees. Following the fusion, A.M. had trouble feeding himself and was ordered a mobile arm support, and he also began to use the tilt feature on his most recent powered chair not only for pressure relief but also to clear the door while entering his adapted van since he grew 3 inches following the surgery.

As A.M. got older, the focus of therapy shifted to maintaining hand function, and resting hand splints and ROM for the long finger flexors and elbow flexors were taught.

At 22, A.M. was having increasing difficulty driving his chair. He was unable to drive in reverse and could no longer reposition his arm when he went over bumps. In addition, through further discussion, it became apparent that he had been having trouble accessing his computer and had not discussed this at previous clinic visits. A.M. was ordered a mini-joystick to drive his wheelchair and a mouse emulator so he could access the computer with his wheelchair control. In addition, he was referred for evaluation for an on-screen keyboard word prediction software and a dictation program.

REFERENCES

1. Koenig N, Hoffman EP, Bertelson CJ, et al. Complete cloning of the Duchenne muscular dystrophy (DMD) cDNA and preliminary genomic organization of the DMD gene in normal and affected individuals. *Cell.* 1987;50:509-517.
2. Tsao CY, Mendell JR. The childhood muscular dystrophies: making order out of chaos. *Semin Neurol.* 1999;19:9-23.
3. Parvatiyar MS, Brownstein AJ, Kanashiro-Takeuchi RM, et al. Stabilization of the cardiac sarcolemma by sarcospan rescues DMD-associated cardiomyopathy. *JCI Insight.* 2019;5:e123855.
4. Behrman RG, Kleigman R, Jenson HB. *Nelson Textbook of Pediatrics.* 16th ed. WB Saunders; 2000.
5. Brooke MH. *Clinicians' View of Neuromuscular Disease.* 2nd ed. Williams & Wilkins; 1986:117-159.
6. Mercuri E, Bönnemann CG, Muntoni F. Muscular dystrophies. *Lancet.* 2019;394(10213):2025-2038. doi:10.1016/S0140-6736(19)32910-1
7. Hoffman EP, Brown RH, Kunkel LM. Dystrophin: the protein product of the Duchenne muscular dystrophy locus. *Cell.* 1987;51:919.
8. Crisp DE, Ziter FA, Bray PF. Diagnostic delay in Duchenne's muscular dystrophy. *JAMA.* 1982;247:478-480.
9. Blake DJ, Weir A, Newey SE, et al. Function and genetics of dystrophin and dystrophin related proteins in muscle. *Physiol Rev.* 2002;82:291-329.
10. Khairallah RJ, Shi G, Sbrana F, et al. Microtubules underlie dysfunction in Duchenne muscular dystrophy. *Sci Signal.* 2012;5(236):ra56.
11. Roselli F, Caroni P. A circuit mechanism for neurodegeneration. *Cell.* 2012;151(2):250-252.
12. Wendy I. SMN is required for sensory-motor circuit function in Drosophila. *Cell.* 2012;151(2):427-439.
13. Sutherland DH, Olshen R, Cooper L, et al. The pathomechanics of gait in Duchenne muscular dystrophy. *Dev Med Child Neurol.* 1981;23(1):3-22.
14. Magri F, Govoni A, D'Angelo MG, et al. Genotype and phenotype characterization in a large dystrophinopathic cohort with extended follow-up. *J Neurol.* 2011;258(9):1610-1623.
15. Brooke MH, Fenichel GM, Griggs RC, et al. Clinical investigations in Duchenne dystrophy: Part 2. Determination of the "power" of therapeutic trials based on the natural history. *Muscle Nerve.* 1983;6:91-103.
16. Tuffery-Giraud S, Béroud C, Leturcq F, et al. Genotype-phenotype analysis in 2,405 patients with a dystrophinopathy using the UMD-DMD database: a model of nationwide knowledgebase. *Hum Mutat.* 2009;30(6):934-945.
17. Vignos PJ, Spencer GE, Archibald KC. Management of progressive muscular dystrophy of childhood. *JAMA.* 1963;184:89-96.
18. Brooke MH, Fenichel G, Griggs R, et al. Duchenne muscular dystrophy: patterns of clinical progression and effects of supportive therapy. *Neurology.* 1989;39:475-481.
19. Bello L, Pegoraro E. The "Usual Suspects": genes for inflammation, fibrosis, regeneration, and muscle strength modify duchenne muscular dystrophy. *J Clin Med.* 2019;8(5):649. https://www-ncbi-nlm-nih-gov.proxy.library.upenn.edu/pubmed/3108342. doi:10.3390/jcm8050649
20. Dooley JM, Gordon KE, MacSween JM. Impact of steroids on surgical experiences of patients with Duchenne muscular dystrophy. *Pediatr Neurol.* 2010;43(3):173-176.
21. Colbert AP, Craig C. Scoliosis management in Duchenne muscular dystrophy: prospective study of modified Jewett hyperextension brace. *Arch Phys Med Rehabil.* 1987;68(5 pt 1):302-304.
22. Cambridge W, Drennan JC. Scoliosis associated with Duchenne muscular dystrophy. *J Pediatr Orthop.* 1987;7(4):436-440.
23. Karol LA. Scoliosis in patients with Duchenne muscular dystrophy. *J Bone Joint Surg Am.* 2007;89(suppl 1):155-162.
24. Sonia K, Ramirez A, Aubertin G, et al. Respiratory muscle decline in Duchenne muscular dystrophy. *Pediatr Pulmonol.* 2013. doi:10.1002/ppul.22847
25. Villanova M, Brancalion B, Mehta AD. Duchenne muscular dystrophy: life prolongation by noninvasive ventilatory support. *Am J Phys Med Rehabil.* 2014;93(7):595-599.
26. Machado DL, Silva EC, Resende MB. Lung function monitoring in patients with Duchenne muscular dystrophy on steroid therapy. *BMC Res Notes.* 2012;5(1):435.
27. Judge DP, Kass DA, Thompson WR, et al. Pathophysiology and therapy of cardiac dysfunction in Duchenne muscular dystrophy. *Am J Cardiovasc Drugs.* 2011;11(5):287-294.
28. McNally EM, Towbin JA. Cardiomyopathy in muscular dystrophy workshop. 28–30 September 2003, Tucson, Arizona. *Neuromusc Disord.* 2004;20:1-7.
29. Nardes F, Araújo AP, Ribeiro MG. Mental retardation in Duchenne muscular dystrophy. *J Pediatr (Rio J).* 2012;88(1):6-16.
30. Leibowitz D, Dubowitz V. Intellect and behavior in Duchenne muscular dystrophy. *Dev Med Child Neurol.* 1981;23:577-590.
31. Vicari S, Piccini G, Mercuri E, et al. Implicit learning deficit in children with Duchenne muscular dystrophy: evidence for a cerebellar cognitive impairment? *PLoS One.* 2018;13(1):e0191164. doi:10.1371/journal.pone.0191164
32. Prosser JE. Intelligence and the gene for Duchenne muscular dystrophy. *Arch Dis Child.* 1969;44:221-230.
33. Battini R, Chieffo D, Bulgheroni S, et al. Cognitive profile in Duchenne muscular dystrophy boys without intellectual disability: the role of executive functions. *Neuromuscul Disord.* 2018;28(2):122-128. doi:10.1016/j.nmd.2017.11.018
34. Bushby K, Finkel R, Birnkrant DJ, et al. Diagnosis and management of Duchenne muscular dystrophy, part 2: implementation of multidisciplinary care. *Lancet Neurol.* 2010;9:177-189.
35. Ziter FA, Allsop K. The diagnosis and management of childhood muscular dystrophy. *Clin Pediatr.* 1976;15(6):540-548.
36. Brooke MH, Fenichel G, Griggs R, et al. Clinical investigation of Duchenne muscular dystrophy. Interesting results in a trial of prednisone. *Arch Neurol.* 1987;44:812-817.
37. Angelini C, Peterle E. Old and new therapeutic developments in steroid treatment in Duchenne muscular dystrophy. *Acta Myol.* 2012;31(1):9-15.
38. Manzur AY, Kuntzer T, Pike M, et al. Glucocorticoid corticosteroids for Duchenne muscular dystrophy. *Cochrane Database Syst Rev.* 2004;(2):CD003725.
39. Drachman DB, Tokya RV, Meyer E. Prednisone in Duchenne muscular dystrophy. *Lancet.* 1974;2:1409-1412.
40. DeSilva S, Drachman D, Mellits D, et al. Prednisone treatment in Duchenne muscular dystrophy. Long-term benefit. *Arch Neurol.* 1987;44:818-822.
41. Fenichel G, Florence J, Pestronk A, et al. Long-term benefit from prednisone therapy in Duchenne muscular dystrophy. *Neurology.* 1991;41:1874-1877.
42. Banerjee B, Sharma U, Balasubramanian K, et al. Effect of creatine monohydrate in improving cellular energetics and muscle strength

in ambulatory Duchenne muscular dystrophy patients: a randomized, placebo-controlled 31P MRS study. *Magn Reson Imaging.* 2010;28(5):698-707.

43. Chetlin RD, Gutmann L, Tarnopolsky MA, et al. Resistance training exercise and creatine in patients with Charcot-Marie-Tooth Disease. *Muscle Nerve.* 2004;30:69-76.

44. Fairclough RJ, Bareja A, Davies KE. Progress in therapy for Duchenne muscular dystrophy. *Exp Physiol.* 2011;96(11):1101-1113.

45. Alfano LN, Charleston JS, Connolly AM, et al. Long-term treatment with eteplirsen in nonambulatory patients with Duchenne muscular dystrophy. *Medicine (Baltimore).* 2019;98(26):e15858.

46. Shimizu-Motohashi Y, Komaki H, Motohashi N, et al. Restoring dystrophin expression in Duchenne muscular dystrophy: current status of therapeutic approaches. *J Pers Med.* 2019;9(1):1. doi:10.3390/jpm9010001

47. Bushby K, Bann CM, Apkon SD, et al; for the DMD Care Considerations Working Group. Diagnosis and management of Duchenne muscular dystrophy, part 1: diagnosis, and neuromuscular, rehabilitation, endocrine, and gastrointestinal and nutritional management. *Lancet Neurol.* 2018;17(3):251-267.

48. Bentley G, Haddad F, Bull TM, et al. The treatment of scoliosis in muscular dystrophy using modified Luque and Harrington-Luque instrumentation. *J Bone Joint Surg Br.* 2001;83(1):22-28.

49. Miller F, Moseley CF, Koreska J. Spinal fusion in Duchenne muscular dystrophy. *Dev Med Child Neurol.* 1992;34:775-786.

50. Huber H, Andre G, Rumeau F, et al. Flexible intramedullary nailing for distal femoral fractures in patients with myopathies. *J Child Orthop.* 2012;6:119-123.

51. Yildiz S, Glanzman AM, Estilow T, et al. Retrospective analysis of fractures and factors causing ambulation loss after lower extremity fractures in Duchenne Muscular Dystrophy. *Am J Phys Med Rehabil.* 2020;99(9):789-794.

52. Huberclaut V, Haroun D, Bezzou K, et al. Motor and respiratory heterogeneity in Duchenne patients: implications in clinical trials. *Eur J PaediatrNeurol.* 2012;16:149-160.

53. Leger P, Jennequin J, Gerard M, et al. Home positive pressure ventilation via nasal mask for patients with neuromuscular weakness or restrictive lung or chest-wall disease. *Respir Care.* 1989;34:73-79.

54. Bach J, O'Brien J, Krotenberg R, et al. Management of end-stage respiratory failure in Duchenne muscular dystrophy. *Muscle Nerve.* 1987;10:177-182.

55. James KA, Gralla J, Ridall LA, et al. Left ventricular dysfunction in Duchenne muscular dystrophy. *Cardiol Young.* 2020;30:171-176.

56. Florian A, Rosch S, Bietenbec M, et al. Cardiac involvement in female Duchenne and Becker muscular dystrophy carriers in comparison to their first-degree male relatives: a comparative cardiovascular magnetic resonance study. *Eur Heart J Cardiovasc Imaging.* 2016;17:326-333.

57. Alqahtan FF, Offiah AC. Diagnosis of osteoporotic vertebral fractures in children. *Pediatr Radiol.* 2019;49(3):283-296.

58. Larson CM, Henderson RC. Bone mineral density and fractures in boys with Duchenne muscular dystrophy. *J Pediatr Orthop.* 2000;20:71-74.

59. Birnkrant DJ, Bushby K, Bann CM, et al. Diagnosis and management of Duchenne muscular dystrophy, part 2: respiratory, cardiac, bone health, and orthopaedic management. *Lancet Neurol.* 2018;17(4):347-361. doi:10.1016/S1474-4422(18)30025-5

60. Birnkrant DJ, Bushby K, Bann CM, et al Diagnosis and management of Duchenne muscular dystrophy, part 1: diagnosis, and neuromuscular, rehabilitation, endocrine, and gastrointestinal and nutritional management. *Lancet Neurol.* 2018;17(3):251-267.

61. Florence J, Brooke M, Carroll J. Evaluation of the child with muscular weakness. *Orthoped Clin North Am.* 1978;9(2):421-422.

62. Henricson E, Abresch R, Han JJ, et al. Percent-predicted 6-minute walk distance in Duchenne muscular dystrophy to account for maturational influences. Version 2. *PLoS Curr.* 2012;4:RRN1297.

63. McDonald CM, Abresch RT, Carter GT, et al. Profiles of neuromuscular diseases. Duchenne muscular dystrophy. *Am J Phys Med Rehabil.* 1995;74(5)(suppl):S70-S92.

64. Ziter FA, Allsop KG, Tyler FH. Assessment of muscle strength in Duchenne muscular dystrophy. *Neurology.* 1977;27:981-984.

65. Allsop KG, Ziter FA. Loss of strength and functional decline in Duchenne dystrophy. *Arch Neurol.* 1981;38:406-411.

66. Brooke MH, Griggs R, Mendell J, et al. Clinical trial in Duchenne dystrophy. I. The design of the protocol. *Muscle Nerve.* 1981;4:186-197.

67. Florence JM, Pandya S, King W, et al. Clinical trials in Duchenne dystrophy. Standardization and reliability of evaluation procedures. *Phys Ther.* 1984;64:41-45.

68. Griggs R, Moxley RT 3rd, Mendell JR, et al. Prednisone in Duchenne dystrophy. A randomized, controlled trial defining the time course and dose response. *Arch Neurol.* 1991;48:383-388.

69. Scott E, Eagle M, Mayhew A, et al. Development of a functional assessment scale for ambulatory boys with Duchenne muscular dystrophy. *Physiother Res Int.* 2012;17(2):101-109.

70. Alfanoa NL, Miller NF, Berry KM, et al. The 100-meter timed test: Normative data in healthy males and comparative pilot outcome data for use in Duchenne muscular dystrophy clinical trials. *Neuromuscul Disord.* 2017;27:452-457. doi:10.1016/j.nmd.2017.02.007

71. Stuberg W, Metcalf W. Reliability of quantitative muscle testing in healthy children and in children with Duchenne muscular dystrophy using hand held dynamometers. *Phys Ther.* 1988;68(6):977-982.

72. Brussock C, Haley S, Munsat T, et al. Measurement of isometric force in children with and without Duchenne's muscular dystrophy. *Phys Ther.* 1992;72(2):105-114.

73. Kilmer DD, McCrory MA, Wright NC, et al. Hand-held dynamometry reliability in persons with neuropathic weakness. *Arch Phys Med Rehabil.* 1997;78:1364-1368.

74. Hyde SA, Steffensen BF, Fløytrup I, et al. Longitudinal data analysis: an application to construction of a natural history profile of Duchenne muscular dystrophy. *Neuromuscul Disord.* 2001;11(2):165-170.

75. Mathur S, Lott DJ, Senesac C, et al. Age-related differences in lower-limb muscle cross-sectional area and torque production in boys with Duchenne muscular dystrophy. *Arch Phys Med Rehabil.* 2010;91(7):1051-1058.

76. Magee DJ. *Orthopedic Physical Assessment.* 2nd ed. WB Saunders; 1992.

77. Kiefer M, Bonarrigo K, Quatman-Yates C, et al. Progression of ankle plantarflexion contractures and functional decline in Duchenne muscular dystrophy: implications for physical therapy management. *Pediatr Phys Ther.* 2019;31(1):61-66. doi:10.1097/PEP.0000000000000553

78. Hyde SA, Floytruuup I, Glent S, et al. A randomized comparative study of two methods for controlling Tendo Achilles contracture in Duchenne muscular dystrophy. *Neuromusc Disord.* 2000;10:257-263.

79. Scott OM, Hyde SA, Goddard C, et al. Prevention of deformity in Duchenne muscular dystrophy. *Physiotherapy.* 1981;67:177-180.

80. Nishizawa H, Matsukiyo A, Shiba N, et al. The effect of wearing night splints for one year on the standing motor function of patients with Duchenne muscular dystrophy. *J Phys Ther Sci.* 2018;30(4):576-579. doi:10.1589/jpts.30.576

81. McDonald CM. Limb contractures in progressive neuromuscular disease and the role of stretching, orthotics, and surgery. *Phys Med Rehabil Clin N Am.* 1998;9:187-209.

82. Glanzman AM, Flickinger JM, Dholakia KH, et al. Serial casting for the management of ankle contracture in Duchenne muscular dystrophy. *Pediatr Phys Ther.* 2011;23(3):275-279.

83. Johnson E, Yarnell S. Hand dominance and scoliosis in Duchenne muscular dystrophy. *Arch Phys Med Rehabil.* 1976;57:462-464.

84. Miller F, Moseley C, Koreska J, et al. Pulmonary function and scoliosis in Duchenne dystrophy. *J Pediatr Orthop.* 1988;8:133-137.

85. Miller R, Chalmers A, Dao H, et al. The effect of spine fusion on respiratory function in Duchenne muscular dystrophy. *Neurology.* 1991;41:37-40.

86. Alexander WM, Smith M, Freeman BJ, et al. The effect of posterior spinal fusion on respiratory function in Duchenne muscular dystrophy. *Eur Spine J.* 2013;22(2):411-416.

87. Carter GT. Rehabilitation management in neuromuscular disease. *J Neurol Rehabil.* 1997;11:69-80.

88. Vignos P, Watkins M. The effect of exercise in muscular dystrophy. *JAMA.* 1966;197:121-126.

89. Ansved T. Muscle training in muscular dystrophies. *Acta Physiol Scand.* 2001;171:359-366.

90. de Lateur B, Giaconi RM. Effect on maximal strength of submaximal exercise in Duchenne muscular dystrophy. *Am J Phys Med.* 1979;58:26-36.

91. Scott OM, Hyse SA, Goddard C, et al. Effect of exercise in Duchenne muscular dystrophy. *Physiotherapy.* 1981;67(6):174-176.

92. Eagle M. Report on the muscular dystrophy campaign workshop: exercise in neuromuscular diseases Newcastle, 2002. *Neuromusc Disord.* 2002;12:975-983.

93. McCarter GC, Steinhardt RA. Increased activity of calcium leak channels caused by proteolysis near sarcolemmal ruptures. *J Membrane Biol.* 2000;176:169-174.

94. Brussee V, Tardif F, Tremblay J. Muscle fibers of mdx mice are more vulnerable to exercise than those of normal mice. *Neuromusc Disord.* 1997;7:487-492.

95. Connolly AM, Keeling RM, Mehta S, et al. Three mouse models of muscular dystrophy: the natural history of strength and fatigue in dystrophin-, dystrophin/utrophin-, and laminin α2-deficient mice. *Neuromusc Disord.* 2001;11:703-712.

96. Alderton JM, Steinhardt RA. How calcium influx through calcium leak channels is responsible for the elevated levels of calcium-dependent proteolysis in dystrophic myotubes. *Trends Cardiovasc Med.* 2000;10:268-272.

97. Hayes A, Lynch GS, Williams DA. The effects of endurance exercise on dystrophic mdx mice I. Contractile and histochemical properties of intact muscles. *Proc Biol Sci.* 1993;253:19-25.

98. Alemdaroğlu I, Karaduman A, Yilmaz ÖT, et al. Different types of upper extremity exercise training in Duchenne muscular dystrophy: effects on functional performance, strength, endurance, and ambulation. *Muscle Nerve.* 2015;51:697-705. https://doi-org.proxy.library .upenn.edu/10.1002/mus.24451

99. Markert CD, Ambrosio F, Call JA, et al. Exercise and Duchenne muscular dystrophy: toward evidence-based exercise prescription. *Muscle Nerve.* 2011;43:464-478.

100. Markert CD, Case LE, Carter GT, et al. Exercise and Duchenne muscular dystrophy: where we have been and where we need to go. *Muscle Nerve.* 2012;45(5):746-751.

101. Harris SE, Cherry DB. Childhood progressive muscular dystrophy and the role of physical therapy. *Phys Ther.* 1974;54:4-12.

102. Archibald DC, Vignos PJ Jr. A study of contractures in muscular dystrophy. *Arch Phys Med Rehabil.* 1959;40:150-157.

103. Spencer GE. Orthopaedic care of progressive muscular dystrophy. *J Bone Joint Surg Am.* 1967;49:1201-1204.

104. Roy L, Gibson DA. Pseudohypertrophic muscular dystrophy and its surgical management: review of 30 patients. *Can J Surg.* 1970;13:13-20.

105. Siegel IM. Management of musculoskeletal complications in neuromuscular disease. Enhancing mobility and the role of bracing and surgery. In: Fowler WM Jr, ed. *Advances in the Rehabilitation of Neuromuscular Diseases: State of the Art Reviews.* Vol 4. Hanley & Belfus; 1988:553-575.

106. Ziter FA, Allsop KG. The value of orthoses for patients with Duchenne muscular dystrophy. *Phys Ther.* 1979;59:1361-1365.

107. Heckmatt JZ, Dubowitz V, Hyde SA, et al. Prolongation of walking in Duchenne muscular dystrophy with lightweight orthoses. Review of 57 cases. *Dev Med Child Neurol.* 1985;27:149-154.

108. Vignos PJ. Management of musculoskeletal complications in neuromuscular disease: limb contractures and the role of stretching, braces and surgery. In: Fowler WM Jr, ed. *Advances in the*

Rehabilitation of Neuromuscular Diseases: State of the Art Reviews. Vol 4. Hanley & Belfus; 1988:509-536.

109. Pellegrini N, Guillon B, Prigent H, et al. Optimization of power wheelchair control for patients with severe Duchenne muscular dystrophy. *Neuromusc Disord.* 2004;14:297-300.

110. Bach JR, Campagnolo DI, Hoeman S. Life satisfaction of individuals with Duchenne muscular dystrophy using long-term mechanical ventilatory support. *Am J Phys Rehabil.* 1991;70:129-135.

111. Liu M, Kiyoshi M, Kozo H, et al. Practical problems and management of seating through the clinical stages of Duchenne's muscular dystrophy. *Arch Phys Med Rehabil.* 2003;84:818-824.

112. Edwards RHT. Weight reduction in boys with muscular dystrophy. *Dev Med Child Neurol.* 1984;26:384-390.

113. Martigne L, Salleron J, Mayer M, et al. Natural evolution of weight status in Duchenne muscular dystrophy: a retrospective audit. *Br J Nutr.* 2011;105(10):1486-1491.

114. Griffiths R, Edwards R. A new chart for weight control in Duchenne muscular dystrophy. *Arch Dis Child.* 1988;63:1256-1258.

115. Perez A, Mulot R, Vardon G, et al. Thoracoabdominal pattern of breathing in neuromuscular disorders. *Chest.* 1996;110:454-461.

116. Birnkrant DJ, Bushby KM, Amin RS, et al. The respiratory management of patients with Duchenne muscular dystrophy: a DMD care considerations working group specialty article. *Pediatr Pulmonol.* 2010;45(8):739-748.

117. Bach JR, Ishikawa Y, Kim H. Prevention of pulmonary morbidity for patients with Duchenne muscular dystrophy. *Chest.* 1997;112(4):1024-1028.

118. Topin N, Matecki S, Le Bris S, et al. Dose-dependent effect of individualized respiratory muscle training in children with Duchenne muscular dystrophy. *Neuromuscul Disord.* 2002;12(6):576-583.

119. Wanke T, Toifl K, Merkle M, et al. Inspiratory muscle training in patients with Duchenne muscular dystrophy. *Chest.* 1994;105:475-482.

120. Gozal D, Thiriet P. Respiratory muscle training in neuromuscular disease: long-term effects on strength and load perception. *Med Sci Sports Exerc.* 1999;31(11):1522-1527.

121. Udd B, Krahe R. The myotonic dystrophies: molecular, clinical, and therapeutic challenges. *Lancet Neurol.* 2012;11(10):891-905. doi:10.1016/S1474-4422(12)70204-1

122. Kirschner J, Bonnemann CG. The congenital and limb-girdle muscular dystrophies: sharpening the focus, blurring the boundaries. *Arch Neurol.* 2004;61:189-199.

123. Johnson NE. Myotonic muscular dystrophies. *Continuum (Minneap Minn).* 2019;25(6):1682-1695. doi:10.1212/CON.0000000000000793

124. Wicklund MP. The limb-girdle muscular dystrophies. *Continuum (Minneap Minn).* 2019;25(6):1599-1618. https://neuromuscular. wustl.edu/. doi:10.1212/CON.0000000000000809

125. Khadilkar SV, Patel BA, Lalkaka JA. Making sense of the clinical spectrum of limb girdle muscular dystrophies. *Pract Neurol.* 2018;18(3):201-210. doi:10.1136/practneurol-2017-001799

126. Khadilkar SV, Singh RK, Katrak SM. Sarcoglycanopathies: a report of 25 cases. *Neurol India.* 2002;50:27-32.

127. Ferreira AF, Carvalho MS, Resende MB, et al. Phenotypic and immunohistochemical characterization of sarcoglycanopathies. *Clinics (Sao Paulo).* 2011;66(10):1713-1719.

128. Reddy K, Jenquin JR, Cleary JD, et al. Mitigating RNA toxicity in myotonic dystrophy using small molecules. *Int J Mol Sci.* 2019;20(16):4017. doi:10.3390/ijms20164017

129. Politano L, Nigro V, Passamano L, et al. Evaluation of cardiac and respiratory involvement in sarcoglycanopathies. *Neuromusc Disord.* 2001;11:178-185.

130. Fayssoil A, Nardi O, Annane D, et al. Left ventricular function in alpha-sarcoglycanopathy and gamma-sarcoglycanopathy. *Acta Neurol Belg.* 2014;114(4):257-259. doi: 10.1007/s13760-013-0276-5

131. García Díaz BE, Gauthier S, Davies PL. Ca^{2+} dependency of calpain 3 (p94) activation. *Biochemistry.* 2006;45(11):3714-3722.

132. Angelini C, Fanin M. Calpainopathy. In: Adam MP, Ardinger HH, Pagon RA, et al, eds. *GeneReviews®* [Internet]. University of Washington, Seattle; 1993-2019.

133. Richard I, Roudaut C, Saenz A, et al. Calpainopathy—a survey of mutations and polymorphisms. *Am J Hum Genet.* 1999;64:1524-1540.

134. Han R. Muscle membrane repair and inflammatory attack in dysferlinopathy. *Skelet Muscle.* 2011;1(1):10. doi:10.1186/2044-5040-1-10

135. Zatz M, de Paula F, Starling A, et al. The 10 autosomal recessive limb-girdle muscular dystrophies. *Neuromusc Disord.* 2003;13:532-544.

136. Angelini C, Nardetto L, Borsato C, et al. The clinical course of calpainopathy (LGMD2A) and dysferlinopathy (LGMD2B). *Neurol Res.* 2010;32:41-46.

137. Pollitt C, Anderson LVB, Pogue R, et al. The phenotype of calpainopathy: diagnosis based on a multidisciplinary approach. *Neuromusc Disord.* 2001;11:287-296.

138. Driss A, Amouri R, Hamida B, et al. A new locus for autosomal-recessive limb-girdle muscular dystrophy in a large consanguineous Tunisian family maps to chromosome 19q3. 3. *Neuromusc Disord.* 2000;10:240-246.

139. Brockington M, Blake DJ, Prandini P, et al. Mutations in the fukutin-related protein gene (FKRP) cause a form of congenital muscular dystrophy with secondary laminin α-2 deficiency and abnormal glycosylation of α-dystroglycan. *Am J Hum Genet.* 2001;69:1198-1209.

140. Alhamidi M, Kjeldsen Buvang E, Fagerheim T, et al. Fukutin-related protein resides in the Golgi cisternae of skeletal muscle fibres and forms disulfide-linked homodimers via an N-terminal interaction. *PLoS One.* 2011;6(8):e22968. doi:10.1371/journal.ponc.0022968

141. Poppe M, Cree L, Bourke J, et al. The phenotype of limb-girdle muscular dystrophy type 2I. *Neurology.* 2003;60:1246-1251.

142. Mercuri E, Brockington M, Straub V, et al. Phenotypic spectrum associated with mutations in the fukutin-related protein gene. *Ann Neurol.* 2003;53:537-542.

143. Poppe M, Bourke J, Eagle M, et al. Cardiac and respiratory failure in limb-girdle muscular dystrophy 2I. *Ann Neurol.* 2004;56:738-741.

144. Pane M, Messina S, Vasco G, et al. Respiratory and cardiac function in congenital muscular dystrophies with alpha dystroglycan deficiency. *Neuromuscul Disord.* 2012;22(8):685-689. doi:10.1016/j.nmd.2012.05.006

145. Nance JR, Dowling JJ, Gibbs EM, et al. Congenital myopathies: an update. *Curr Neurol Neurosci Rep.* 2012;12(2):165-174. doi:10.1007/s11910-012-0255-x

146. Clarkson E, Costa CF, Machesky LM. Congenital myopathies: diseases of the actin cytoskeleton. *J Pathol.* 2004;204:407-417.

147. Goebel HH. Congenital myopathies at their molecular dawning. *Muscle Nerve.* 2003;27:527-548.

148. Bönnemmann CG, Laing NG. Myopathies resulting from mutations in sarcomeric proteins. *Curr Opin Neurol.* 2004;17:1-9.

149. Sanoudoud D, Beggs AH. Clinical and genetic heterogeneity in nemaline myopathy—a disease of skeletal muscle thin filaments. *Trends Mol Med.* 2001;7:362-368.

150. Wallgren-Pattersson C, Laing NG. Report of the 70th ENMC International Workshop: Nemaline Myopathy 11–13 June 1999, Naarden, the Netherlands. *Neuromusc Disord.* 2000;10:299-306.

151. Ryan MM, Schnell C, Strickland CD, et al. Nemaline myopathy: a clinical study of 143 cases. *Ann Neurol.* 2001;50:312-320.

152. Zhang Y, Chen HS, Khanna VK, et al. A mutation in the human ryanodine receptor gene associated with central core disease. *Nat Genet.* 1993;5(1):46-50.

153. Quane KA, Healy JM, Keating KE, et al. Mutations in the ryanodine receptor gene in central core disease and malignant hyperthermia. *Nat Genet.* 1993;5(1):51-55.

154. Jokela M, Tasca G, Vihola A, et al. An unusual ryanodine receptor 1 (RYR1) phenotype: mild calf-predominant myopathy. *Neurology.* 2019;92(14):e1600-e1609. doi:10.1212/WNL.0000000000007246

155. Knuiman GJ, Küsters B, Eshuis L, et al. The histopathological spectrum of malignant hyperthermia and rhabdomyolysis due to RYR1 mutations. *J Neurol.* 2019;266(4):876-887. doi:10.1007/s00415019-09209-z

156. Helbling DC, Mendoza D, McCarrier J, et al. Severe neonatal RYR1 myopathy with pathological features of congenital muscular dystrophy. *J Neuropathol Exp Neurol.* 2019;78(3):283-287. doi:10.1093/jnen/nlz004

157. Cocanougher BT, Flynn L, Yun P, et al. Adult MTM1-related myopathy carriers: classification based on deep phenotyping. *Neurology.* 2019;93(16):e1535-e1542. doi:10.1212/WNL.0000000000008316

158. Jungbluth H, Sewry CA, Muntoni F. Core myopathies. *Semin Pediatr Neurol.* 2011;18(4):239-249. doi:10.1016/j.spen.2011.10.005

159. Mohassel P, Foley AR, Bönnemann CG. Extracellular matrix-driven congenital muscular dystrophies. *Matrix Biol.* 2018;71-72:188-204. doi: 10.1016/j.matbio.2018.06.005

160. Muntoni F, Voit T. The congenital muscular dystrophies in 2004: a century of exciting progress. *Neuromusc Disord.* 2004;14:635-649.

161. Demir E, Ferreiro A, Sabatelli P, et al. Collagen VI status and clinical severity in Ullrich congenital muscular dystrophy: phenotype analysis of 11 families linked to the COL6 Loci. *Neuropediatrics.* 2004;35:103-112.

162. Baker NL, Morgelin M, Peat R, et al. Dominant collagen VI mutations are a common cause of Ullrich congenital muscular dystrophy. *Hum Mol Genet.* 2005;14:279-293.

163. Morales RJ, Pageot N, Taieb G, et al. Adult-onset spinal muscular atrophy: an update. *Rev Neurol (Paris).* 2017;173(5):308-319. doi:10.1016/j.neurol.2017.03.015

164. Finkel RS, Mercuri E, Darras BT, et al; ENDEAR Study Group. Nusinersen versus sham control in infantile-onset spinal muscular atrophy. *N Engl J Med.* 2017;377(18):1723-1732. doi:10.1056/NEJMoa1702752

165. Mendell JR, Al-Zaidy S, Shell R, et al. Single-dose gene-replacement therapy for spinal muscular atrophy. *N Engl J Med.* 2017;377(18):1713-1722. doi:10.1056/NEJMoa1706198

166. Calucho M, Bernal S, Alías L, et al. Correlation between SMA type and SMN2 copy number revisited: an analysis of 625 unrelated Spanish patients and a compilation of 2834 reported cases. *Neuromuscul Disord.* 2018;28(3):208-215. doi:10.1016/j.nmd.2018.01.003

167. Voit T. Congenital muscular dystrophies: 1997 update. *Brain Dev.* 1998;20:65-74.

168. Bertini E, D'Amico A, Gualandi F, et al. Congenital muscular dystrophies: a brief review. *Semin Pediatr Neurol.* 2011;18(4):277-288. doi:10.1016/j.spen.2011.10.010

169. Guillian T, Brzustowicz L, Castilla L, et al. Genetic hemogeneity between acute and chronic forms of spinal muscular atrophy. *Nature.* 1990;345:823-825.

170. Hamilton G, Gillingwater TH. Spinal muscular atrophy: going beyond the motor neuron. *Trends Mol Med.* 2013;19(1):40-50. doi:10.1016/j.molmed.2012.11.002

171. van der Heul AMB, Wijngaarde CA, Wadman RI, et al. Bulbar problems self-reported by children and adults with spinal muscular atrophy. *J Neuromuscul Dis.* 2019;6(3):361-368. doi:10.3233/JND190379

172. Chatwin M, Simonds AK. Long-term mechanical insufflation-exsufflation cough assistance in neuromuscular disease: patterns of use and lessons for application. *Respir Care.* 2020;65:135-143. doi:10.4187/respcare.06882

173. Lomen-Hoerth C, Slawnych MP. Statistical motor unit number estimation: from theory to practice. *Muscle Nerve.* 2003;28(3):263-272.

174. Mercuri E, Finkel RS, Muntoni F, et al; SMA Care Group. Diagnosis and management of spinal muscular atrophy: part 1: recommendations for diagnosis, rehabilitation, orthopedic and nutritional care. *Neuromuscul Disord.* 2018;28(2):103-115. doi:10.1016/j.nmd.2017.11.005

175. Iannaccone ST, Brown RH, Samaha FJ, et al; DCN/SMA Group. Prospective study of spinal muscular atrophy before age 6 years. *Pediatr Neurol.* 1993;9:187-193.

176. Oskoui M, Levy G, Garland CJ, et al. The changing natural history of spinal muscular atrophy type 1. *Neurology.* 2007;69(20):1931-1936.

177. Rudnik-Schoneborn S, Hausmanowa-Petrusewicz I, Brokowska J, et al. The predictive value of achieved motor milestones assessed in 441 patients with infantile spinal muscular atrophy types II and III. *Eur Neurol.* 2000;45:174-181.

178. Russman BS, Bucher CR, Shite M, et al; DCN/SMA Group. Function changes in spinal muscular atrophy II and III. *Neurology.* 1996;47:973-976.

179. Iannaccone AT, Russman BS, Browne GH, et al; Prospective analysis of strength in spinal muscular atrophy. DCN/Spinal Muscular Atrophy Group. *J Child Neurol.* 2000;15:97-101.

180. Merlini L, Bertini E, Minetti C, et al. Motor function-muscle strength relationship in spinal muscle atrophy. *Muscle Nerve.* 2004;12:561-566.

181. Di Pede C, Salamon E, Motta M, et al. Spinal bracing and lung function in type 2 spinal muscular atrophy. *Eur J Phys Rehabil Med.* 2019;55(4):505-509. doi:10.23736/S1973-9087.18.05046-3

182. Morillon S, Thumerelle C, Cuisset JM, et al. Effect of thoracic bracing on lung function in children with neuromuscular disease [Article in French]. *Ann Readapt Med Phys.* 2007;50(8):645-650.

183. Tangsrud SE, Carlsen KC, Lund-Petersen I, et al. Lung function measurements in young children with spinal muscle atrophy; a cross sectional survey on the effect of position and bracing. *Arch Dis Child.* 2001;84(6):521-524.

184. Doany ME, Olgun ZD, Kinikli GI, et al. Health-related quality of life in early-onset scoliosis patients treated surgically: EOSQ scores in traditional growing rod versus magnetically controlled growing rods. *Spine (Phila Pa 1976).* 2018;43(2):148-153. doi:10.1097/BRS.0000000000002274

185. Nossov SB, Curatolo E, Campbell RM, et al; Children's Spine Study Group. VEPTR: are we reducing respiratory assistance requirements? *J Pediatr Orthop.* 2019;39(1):28-32. doi:10.1097/BPO.0000000000000986

186. Granata C, Cornelio F, Bonfiglioli S, et al. Promotion of ambulation of patients with spinal muscular atrophy by early fitting of knee-ankle-foot orthoses. *Dev Med Child Neurol.* 1987;29(2):221-224.

187. Shapiro F, Specht L. Current concepts review. The diagnosis and orthopaedic treatment of childhood spinal muscular atrophy, peripheral neuropathy, Friedreich ataxia, and arthrogryposis. *J Bone Joint Surg Am.* 1993;75A:1699-1714.

188. Tangsrud SE, Lodrup Carlsen KC, Lund-Petersen KC, et al. Lung function measurements in young children with spinal muscle atrophy: a cross sectional survey on the effect of position and bracing. *Arch Dis Child.* 2001;84:521-524.

189. DP, Roye DP, Farcy JPC, et al. Surgical treatment of scoliosis in a spinal muscular atrophy population. *Spine.* 1990;15:942-945.

190. Tsirikos AI, Chang WN, Shah SA, et al. Preserving ambulatory potential in pediatric patients with cerebral palsy who undergo spinal fusion using unit rod instrumentation. *Spine (Phila Pa 1976).* 2003;28(5):480-483.

191. Montes J, McDermott MP, Mirek E, et al. Ambulatory function in spinal muscular atrophy: age-related patterns of progression. *PLoS One.* 2018;13(6):e0199657. doi:10.1371/journal.pone.0199657

192. Montes J, Dunaway YS, Mazzone ES, et al; CS2 and CS12 Study Groups. Nusinersen improves walking distance and reduces fatigue in later-onset spinal muscular atrophy. *Muscle Nerve.* 2019;60(4):409-414. doi:10.1002/mus.26633

193. Montes J, Garber CE, Kramer SS, et al. Randomized, controlled clinical trial of exercise in ambulatory spinal muscular atrophy: why are the results negative? *J Neuromuscul Dis.* 2015;2(4):463-470.

194. Salazar R, Montes J, Dunaway YS, et al. Quantitative evaluation of lower extremity joint contractures in spinal muscular atrophy: implications for motor function. *Pediatr Phys Ther.* 2018;30(3):209-215. doi:10.1097/PEP.0000000000000515

195. Rodillo E, Marini ML, Heckmatt JZ, et al. Scoliosis in spinal muscular atrophy: review of 63 cases. *J Child Neurol.* 1989;4: 118-123.

196. Muscular Dystrophy Association. Charcot-Marie-Tooth disease and Dejerine-Sottas disease. Accessed May 1, 2005. www.mdausa.org

197. Patzkó A, Shy ME. Update on Charcot-Marie-Tooth disease. *Curr Neurol Neurosci Rep.* 2011;11(1):78-88.

198. Shy ME, Patzkó A. Axonal Charcot-Marie-Tooth disease. *Curr Opin Neurol.* 2011;24(5):475-483. doi:10.1097/WCO.0b013e32834aa331

199. Azmaipairashvili Z, Riddle EC, Scavina M, et al. Correction of cavovarus foot deformity in Charcot-Marie-Tooth Disease. *J Pediatr Orthop.* 2005;25:360-365.

200. Shy ME, Blake J, Krajewski K, et al. Reliability and validity of the CMT neuropathy score as a measure of disability. *Neurology.* 2005;64:1209-1214.

201. El Mhandi L, Millet GY, Calmels P, et al. Benefits of interval-training on fatigue and functional capacities in Charcot-Marie-Tooth disease. *Muscle Nerve.* 2008;37(5):601-610. doi:10.1002/mus.20959

202. Ramdharry GM, Day BL, Reilly MM, et al. Foot drop splints improve proximal as well as distal leg control during gait in Charcot-Marie-Tooth disease. *Muscle Nerve.* 2012;46(4):512-519.

203. Guillebastre B, Calmels P, Rougier PR. Assessment of appropriate ankle-foot orthoses models for patients with Charcot-Marie-Tooth disease. *Am J Phys Med Rehabil.* 2011;90(8):619-627. doi:10.1097/PHM.0b013e31821f7172

204. Bean J, Walsh A, Frontera W. Brace modification improves aerobic performance in Charcot-Marie-Tooth disease: a single subject design. *Am J Phys Med Rehabil.* 2001;80:578-582.

205. Sackley C, Disler PB, Turner-Stokes L, et al. Rehabilitation interventions for foot drop in neuromuscular disease. *Cochrane Database Syst Rev.* 2009;8(3):CD003908.

206. Chetlin RD, Mancinelli CA, Gutmann L. Self-reported follow-up post-intervention adherence to resistance exercise training in Charcot-Marie-Tooth disease patients. *Muscle Nerve.* 2010;42(3):456. doi:10.1002/mus.21705

207. Chetlin RD, Gutmann L, Tarnopolsky M, et al. Resistance training effectiveness in patients with Charcot-Marie-Tooth disease: recommendations for exercise prescription. *Arch Phys Med Rehabil.* 2004;85:1217-1223.

208. Burns J, Raymond J, Ouvrier R. Feasibility of foot and ankle strength training in childhood Charcot-Marie-Tooth disease. *Neuromuscul Disord.* 2009;19(12):818-821. doi:10.1016/j.nmd.2009.09.007

209. Lindeman E, Spaans F, Reulen J, et al. Progressive resistance training in neuromuscular patients. Effects on force and surface EMG. *J Electromyogr Kinesiol.* 1999;9(6):379-384.

210. Kilmer DD. The role of exercise in neuromuscular disease. *Phys Med Rehabil Clin N Am.* 1998;9(1):115-125.

211. Cornett KMD, Menezes MP, Shy RR, et al; CMTPedS Study Group. Natural history of Charcot-Marie-Tooth disease during childhood. *Ann Neurol.* 2017;82(3):353-359. doi:10.1002/ana.25009

212. Estilow T, Glanzman AM, Burns J, et al; CMTPedS Study Group. Balance impairment in pediatric Charcot-Marie-Tooth disease. *Muscle Nerve.* 2019;60(3):242-249. doi:10.1002/mus.26500

Pain and Regional Pain Disorders

Lori Kile and Jamie Bradford

magine waking up one morning with excruciating whole body pain that cannot be explained. Think about how frightened one would be to start with, and then following a visit to a physician, tests are conducted and all findings are negative. The physicians can't explain the pain. This is an all-too-common scenario for children and adolescents who find themselves in the beginning of their battle with one of the many forms of amplified musculoskeletal pain syndrome (AMPS).

The prevalence of AMPS in children and adults is steadily rising, causing a growing number of youth to miss out on school, extracurricular activities, and time with friends and family. Those afflicted with AMPS vary in how they present, ranging from minimally dysfunctional to completely incapacitated by their pain. Because of the fact that the presentation can vary and there is no definitive test for it, many of those suffering from AMPS feel that no one understands or believes them, including their family, friends, and the medical professionals. This often leads to a long course of overmedication as well as social isolation of the individual.

» Nomenclature

Pain, according to the International Association for the Study of Pain, can be defined as an unpleasant sensory and emotional experience with actual or potential tissue damage, or described in terms of such damage. This definition, however, underscores the fact that pain is subjective and that pain can present without a specific, identifiable, or a preceding traumatic event. Furthermore, chronic pain is defined as recurrent or persistent pain lasting longer than normal tissue healing time, which is generally agreed upon to be 3 months or longer.[1]

AMPS is an umbrella term for a group of pain disorders that involve central and/or peripheral sensory amplification. It encompasses all types of pediatric chronic musculoskeletal pain. AMPS is broken down into several subtypes as follows: those with overt autonomic signs (also known as complex regional pain syndromes [CRPSs] type I and II); those without autonomic signs (diffuse, idiopathic, and localized pain); or those with tender points or widespread pain and associated symptoms that categorize them as juvenile fibromyalgia.[2] It is important to note that in a diagnosis of AMPS, the pain can be present for less than 3 months, so long as the child's history and examination are consistent with the diagnosis.

» Incidence and etiology

Approximately 20% to 30% of children and adolescents around the world report some form of chronic pain and 5.1% of youth report moderate pain with decreased physical and psychosocial function.[3–5] With regard to amplified pain, the average age of onset is 12 to 17 years. Approximately 75% to 80% of those diagnosed are female,[2,6] of whom the majority (86%) are Caucasian.[5,7] Individuals come from a variety of socioeconomic backgrounds and often have a family history of pain conditions. Additionally, those diagnosed with amplified pain also tend to be people pleasers; suffer from anxiety, depression, and decreased self-esteem; and are often high achievers and/or perfectionists.[4]

Although the exact etiology is unknown, there are commonalities among those diagnosed with amplified pain. Some children experience pain after a major injury such as a fracture or surgery, an illness, or a milder injury such as a sprain or bumps/bruises. Still others report no injury and that the pain started seemingly out of nowhere. It is widely thought that in addition to the above-named physical causes, there is a strong correlation with psychological stressors, personality tendencies, and family history. These play a role in who will develop amplified pain after an injury, surgery, or illness and who won't. AMPS can also be found in individuals who have other comorbidities that in themselves may be painful, such as arthritis, sickle cell, and other inflammatory diseases.[8]

» Pathophysiology

To better understand the mechanism behind AMPS, an understanding of nociception and how pain is processed in the central nervous system is necessary. Nociception refers to the peripheral and central nervous systems processing information about the internal and external environment of the body in response to the activation of nociceptive fibers. In the presence of a noxious stimuli, the nociceptors, which are present in the peripheral system, are activated, sending afferent information through the dorsal horn of the spinal cord to the brain stem and ultimately the cerebral cortex. It is in the cerebral cortex that the perception of pain is generated. Once the signal is processed, efferent signals are sent from the central nervous system to the area that is experiencing the noxious stimuli. These signals are a direct attempt to avoid tissue damage, including the withdrawal reflex, release of epinephrine and norepinephrine, and vasoconstriction of blood vessels.[9]

In amplified pain syndromes, the reflex functions abnormally. The literature suggests that though the cause and

pathogenesis are widely unknown in children, the pathophysiology of this condition is likely multifactorial, involving the central and peripheral nervous systems, and likely linked to genetic factors.[10–12] However, the majority of the literature is based on the adult population; therefore, it is challenging to determine if the pathophysiology and evidence are the same in pediatrics.

Central Sensitization

Central sensitization is a maladaptive neuroplastic change in the central nervous system that is characterized by hyperexcitability of neurons. In acute injury or illness, damaged or inflamed tissues release growth factors and other proinflammatory neuromediators, which similarly occurs in the spinal cord. This activates and upregulates certain phenotypes in the spinal glia, altering their activity and leading to an increase in excitability. This state of dysregulated nociception is the hypothesized mechanism for exaggerated responses to painful (hyperalgesia) and nonpainful (allodynia) stimuli.[11,13]

Neurochemical Factors

Increased levels of neurotransmitters, such as glutamate and substance P, which are noted to be pronociceptive, may increase pain sensitivity in amplified pain syndromes. A decrease in inhibitory neurotransmitters, such as serotonin and noradrenaline, appears to limit the body's ability to diminish the pain response. Together, this may account for the increase in pain sensation in this population.[11,13]

Neuroendocrine Factors

The vulnerability of developing amplified or chronic pain may be modulated by alterations in the brain networks responsible for reward, motivation, learning, and descending modulatory control. These can be affected in children, particularly exposed to trauma or stress. The descending pain modulatory system helps to regulate nociceptive processing in the dorsal horn of the spinal cord, influencing the experience of pain. The amygdala, hypothalamus, and the anterior cingulate gyrus are part of the descending pain modulatory system. These systems aid in the connection of emotional and cognitive variables to interact with afferent nociceptive input, allowing for the resultant pain experience. Multiple studies indicate that early life injury, trauma, or exposure to stress can lead to an imbalance in the descending pain modulatory system, which in turn leads to inappropriate inhibition or facilitation of pain signals.[11,13]

Other Potential Perpetuating Factors

The literature that exists for chronic and amplified pain syndromes continues to illuminate the complexities of pain. In addition to what has been discussed, the role of the sympathetic nervous system, genetics, inflammatory cytokines, and psychosocial factors has been reviewed extensively. Sympathetically mediated pain is most commonly linked to CRPS; however, the same principles can be applied to other pain conditions. The sympathetic nervous system, our fight-or-flight system, works under stressful situations, and chronic stress (whether it be a precursor to pain or a direct impact of pain) exists in this population. Although it is not clearly known, sympathetic hyperfunction or hypofunction may play a role in pain amplification.

Genetics has been widely studied in this population, with a strong association noted among family members in twin and population-based studies. However, clear modes of inheritance have yet to be described. Epigenetics has been a growing field of interest, noting the potential for understanding a link between pain experience and previous exposure from medications or adverse social experiences.[11,13]

Psychosocial Factors

Quite possibly, psychosocial factors that play a role in the development and continuation of such pain are most important in the mechanism of AMPS. Cognitive, emotional, and behavioral factors significantly influence pain. Such factors include fear and avoidance of pain, maladaptive coping strategies, depressive and anxiety symptoms, and parental behaviors regarding pain. Additionally, it has been found that many children with a diagnosis of amplified pain syndrome often have older relatives with chronic pain syndromes and thus have learned maladaptive skills in managing their pain. Many children with amplified pain also carry confounding diagnoses of depression and/or anxiety, which is debated whether this is premorbid to their pain or secondary to their pain. Early exposure to traumatic life events may influence the development of amplified pain. In studies of children with posttraumatic stress disorder (PTSD), it was found that those with PTSD were at higher risk of developing amplified pain compared to adults with PTSD. This is possibly due to developmental changes in the brain that cause increased duration of stress.[11,13]

Key Points in Pathophysiology

Clearly, pediatric chronic and amplified pain syndromes are multifactorial and multidimensional. Though it can be challenging to understand all of the various pain literature that exists in the adult and pediatric world, the most important thing to understand and teach children is the philosophy of what happens with pain and AMPS. A good way to describe this is as follows: in a typical pain response, as in stepping on a tack, nerve fibers send a message to your brain indicating pain; your brain reflexively reacts, sending

descending messages through the spinal cord to the tissues and muscles to contract to move away from the painful stimuli in order to avoid damage to the tissue; the same nerves send messages to your blood vessels to constrict in order to prevent excessive bleeding, but this leads to a decrease in oxygen to the tissue and an increase in lactic acid, which directly leads to pain. However, in AMPS, the nervous system short-circuits like a computer, and these nerve fibers overfire to the point where the pain response occurs without direct tissue damage and can occur with something as little as someone brushing the skin incidentally. In order to treat this amplification of pain, one needs to expose their nervous system to what is felt to be painful stimuli in order to reconfigure the system to understand what is truthfully tissue damaging in nature versus what is not.

≫ Specific diagnoses

Fibromyalgia

The previous diagnostic criteria for fibromyalgia in children was based on those set forth in adults and not validated in children although the criteria themselves were slightly adjusted for children in that it required 5 instead of 11 tender points and a history of chronic widespread pain. Because of the unreliability of tender points in children and adolescents,[14] in 2010 the American College of Rheumatology revised the diagnostic criteria eliminating the tender point examination and added a checklist of 41 associated symptoms, diagnostic measures of a widespread pain index (WPI), and a symptom severity (SS) scale. Further changes were made in 2016, which changed the minimum number of the WPI and SS scales for diagnosis. Additionally, it looks at pain in 4/5 areas including the left and right upper body, right and left lower body, and axial portion of the body. It also removed the exclusion of other painful diagnoses, thus recognizing that fibromyalgia can be present with other pain-causing comorbidities. Also added in 2016 was the fibromyalgia symptom (FS) or polysymptomatic distress (PSD) scale as criteria. The last change in 2016 was removal of self criteria and using physician-only criteria.[14]

Complex Regional Pain Syndrome

In CRPS, the pain is typically found in a single area or limb of the body and does not follow typical dermatomes or nerve distribution. Often, CRPS presents as what is often thought of as the "cold, blue foot or hand"; however, it does not always present as such. When considering this as a diagnosis, it is important to acknowledge that and use the current diagnostic criteria to guide diagnosis and treatment. The diagnostic criteria for CRPS has also undergone some changes over time, and currently the most widely used are those outlined in the Budapest criteria (Table 14.1). Although it can at times

TABLE 14.1.	Budapest Criteria		
Continuing Pain, Which is Disproportionate to Any Inciting Event; There are No Other Diagnoses That Better Explain the Signs and Symptoms			
Symptoms: **Must report at least one symptom in the following categories**	Sensory	Reports of hyperesthesia and/or allodynia	
	Vasomotor	Reports of temperature asymmetry and/or skin color changes and/or skin color asymmetry	
	Sudomotor/edema	Reports of edema and/or sweating changes and/or sweating asymmetry	
	Motor/trophic	Reports of decreased range of motion and/or motor dysfunction (weakness, tremor, dystonia) and/or trophic changes (hair, nail, skin)	
Signs: **Must display at least one sign in two or more of the following categories**	Sensory	Evidence of hyperalgesia (to pinprick) and/or allodynia (to light touch and/or temperature sensation and/or deep somatic pressure and/or joint movement)	
	Vasomotor	Evidence of temperature asymmetry ($>1°$ C) and/or skin color changes and/or asymmetry	
	Sudomotor/edema	Evidence of edema and/or sweating changes and/or sweating asymmetry	
	Motor/trophic	Evidence of decreased range of motion and/or motor dysfunction (weakness, tremor, dystonia) and/or trophic changes (hair, nail, skin)	

still be a diagnosis of exclusion, there are definitive signs and symptoms that must be present to receive the diagnosis of CRPS.[15–17]

Diffuse and Localized Idiopathic Musculoskeletal Pain

This term is used for individuals who have one or more areas of pain or total body pain; however, they do not meet the criteria for juvenile fibromyalgia or CRPS. Included, as well, in this group are a subset of those who also demonstrate intermittent pain that can come and go randomly or at times of higher or lower stress. In order to be diagnosed with these types of amplified pain, there are criteria that must be considered. Psychosocial factors that play a role in the development and continuation of such pain may be the most important mechanism of AMPs. For localized pain, children must demonstrate the following three criteria: pain localized to one limb persisting 1 week with medically directed treatment or 1 month without medical treatment; an absence of prior trauma that could reasonably explain their symptoms; as well as the exclusion of other disease processes that could reasonably explain their symptoms.[18]

It is important to note that the above types of AMPS often overlap and individuals may experience more than one type over time or even concurrently. In addition to those often overlapping types of pain, another diagnosis that is often seen in conjunction is functional neurologic disorder (FND; formerly known as conversion disorder).

Children with diffuse, localized, and intermittent pain also tend to experience other associated symptoms such as irritable bowel syndrome (IBS), mood difficulties, reports of cognitive challenges, chronic fatigue, dizziness, and brain fog/dyscognition.[19,20]

» Examination

The initial examination of a child with any form of AMPS plays a critical role in diagnosis, treatment, and prognosis. Research suggests that earlier diagnosis leads to better outcomes overall in this population. Additionally, findings in the evaluation can assist diagnosing amplified pain syndromes versus organic causes of pain, especially in the direct access setting. In this section, common findings and important aspects of the physical therapy examination will be discussed.

Common Findings from Past Medical History/ History of Present Illness

When chart reviewing and organizing questions to be asked as a part of the examination, it is common to find that these children present with pain that increases over time. For example, a typical ankle sprain, once immobilized and treated, will improve over time; however, in this population, it is frequently reported that an increase in pain with immobilization occurs. Additionally, these children may note a history of poor healing with previous injuries and illnesses. Lastly, they will likely report failed attempts at traditional therapies, such as rest, ice, and progressive mobilization. Ensuring to inquire about these will aid a clinician in forming a diagnosis of an amplified pain syndrome.[21]

Common Findings from Social History

When moving onto a child's social history, some very common findings are noted within this population. Children will report a coexistence of development of pain with a life event. These life events can include, but are not limited to, a change in the family (death, divorce, etc.), a change in school, or a move to a new location. A large percentage of these children will report a role model of pain within their home or life, such as a parent with chronic low back pain. Secondary to this, these children develop ineffective coping strategies and methods to manage their pain. Typically, when asked, these children or their families will report personality styles of perfectionism, anxiousness, and people-pleasing. Because of these personality traits, a child will usually agree to try any activity within the examination, like putting their foot on the ground despite 10/10 pain complaints.[21,22]

Impact of Pain

Just as in any typical initial examination, a clinician would inquire about a child's home, school, and community setup. Specific to this population, the impact of pain on their daily routine is imperative to examine. Listed below are examples of questions that can be asked alongside the common "who do you live with" social history questions. Additionally, there are examples of some typical narrative that a child may report in response.[21]

* What is your home setup—asking how a one does the stairs or if stair avoidance occurs? *I live in a two-story home. My bedroom/bathroom is on the second floor. On my bad pain days, I will either avoid going up/down the stairs or butt scoot to get to my room when I need to.*
* Are you doing anything different in getting ready for the day—assessing if they are sitting/standing to dress, shower, groom or if anyone is helping them to do this? *I stand to take a shower, but on bad days, I will sit. I typically sit to get dressed because it is less painful.*
* What kind of school do you attend—inquiring about missed days; late arrivals/early dismissals; accommodations in school (504, IEP, no gym, etc.); has school setup changed because of pain? *I attend 9th grade in a public school; because of my pain, I have a 504 that allows me to skip gym, use the elevator, and leave class when necessary. I have missed probably 10 to 15 days of school.*
* What do you like to do for fun—has this changed because of pain? *I don't do much now. I previously was very active, playing multiple sports and hanging out with my friends. Because of my pain, I now prefer to stay home and spend a lot of time in my room.*

Those are just some examples of questions that can be asked; however, as a child is responding, a clinician can develop further questions that will help to drive treatment overall. The ultimate goal of evaluating the impact of pain on this population is to learn what their previous level of function was, what they are currently limited to, and what their goal is. This is critical because some children may never wish to return to their previous level of intensity in extracurricular activities. However, as physical therapists (PTs), the goal is to assist them back into what is typical for their age (i.e., return to school, chores, normalized movement

patterns) and to develop ways to push through their pain in order to ultimately diminish it entirely. By learning what is important to the child, the PT can work together with them to achieve this.[21]

Examining Pain

The examination of pain in this population is a lengthy, yet important, aspect to their overall care moving forward. Just as in any standard evaluation, it is important to ascertain the location of a child's pain; the current level; the lowest/highest levels; the quality of their pain; the frequency and duration of the pain; and what aggravates and alleviates the pain. It can also be helpful to have a child fill out a pain diagram, as displayed in Figure 14.1. A child in this population may state that "everything hurts," but when filling out a diagram, they are more specific to where that pain is located. This tool is also a helpful visual for children as they progress in treatment, especially at the time of discharge to see how exactly their pain report has changed. Additionally, utilizing the visual analog scale (VAS) to measure pain may demonstrate a discrepancy in pain report, as some children become stuck on a numeric value for their pain.[21]

These children often present with allodynia. As central sensitization occurs, one of the features is typically the presence of sensory changes, also known as dysesthesia, with areas of hyperalgesia. This is thought to be due to heterotopic facilitation in the dorsal horn of the spinal cord. Included in these changes are allodynia, hyperalgesia, and hyperesthesia.[23] Allodynia is the type we typically see in children with various forms of amplified musculoskeletal pain. It can be present in any area of the body affected by amplified pain syndromes and can present in a variety of forms such as to light or deep touch, temperature, and even sounds or light. Often, the exact borders of allodynia are variable, and it is not uncommon for the location or intensity to change over the course of the child's treatment. When examining a child for allodynia, a clinician may need to physically provide light touch, deep touch, and vibratory sensation to determine the presence.

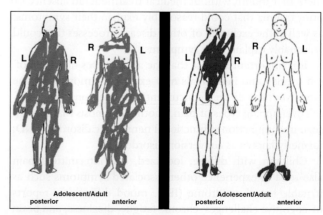

FIGURE 14.1. Pain diagram.

Systems Review

Most commonly in this population, the use of a musculo-skeletal examination template is most appropriate to utilize for in-depth information. However, a brief screen of all of the body systems should be completed and could draw some additional insight to the child's diagnosis. Listed are some important aspects to touch on in each system:

1. Cardiopulmonary
   a. Presence of asthma—children may report exercise-induced asthma, but this can also be from anxiety, so determining the cause can guide need for medications within session.
   b. Heart rate/blood pressure—some children will complain of dizziness or tachycardia with changes in position; however, this can be anxiety related or secondary to deconditioning, not necessarily a true cardiac issue.
2. Integumentary
   a. Presence of scarring—some children may have a history of self-injurious behaviors or may currently have such behaviors; checking skin can keep them safe.
   b. Autonomic changes in skin—presence of color, temperature, or trophic changes indicates CRPS (Figs. 14.2 and 14.3).
3. Neuromuscular
   a. Quick screen of coordination and motor control—is movement limited by pain or conversion symptoms?

Tests and Measures

At the time of the physical examination of a child, the clinician should have a good picture in their head as to what to prioritize in the examination. If a child is specifically sensitive to touch or movement in one part of their body, it may be important to work up to that area, that is, starting with examining the upper extremities (UEs) if the lower extremities (LEs) are the chief complaint. However, it is ultimately necessary to examine, whether briefly or in-depth, all movements of

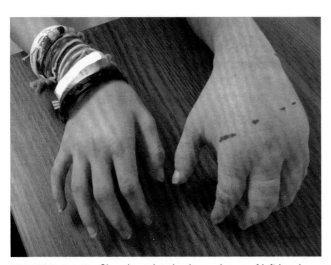

FIGURE 14.2. Chronic regional pain syndrome of left hand.

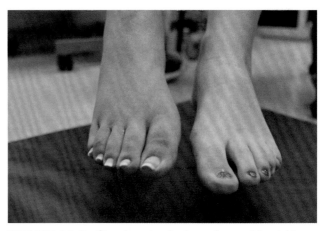

FIGURE 14.3. Chronic regional pain syndrome of the right foot. Noted are color changes, trophic skin changes, and edema of the foot.

the body in order to determine impairments and any potentials to barriers to treatment.

Range of Motion

Beginning with active range of motion (AROM), examination of all UE and LE joints should be completed. Allowing a child to move actively initially allows the clinician to assess willingness to move through pain. Passive ROM should also be measured, regardless of whether or not restriction is present in AROM. Passive ROM examination allows the clinician to ascertain areas of limitation secondary to muscle tightness, muscle guarding, or capsular restrictions. Therapists should be aware that in children with high sensitivity to touch, ROM examination may be limited by the child's acceptance of pressure to the skin and should document this clearly as the restriction. Additionally, examination of cervical and trunk ROM should be completed, especially in patients with reports of head, neck, back, and/or abdomen pain. Documenting pain behaviors, such as facial grimacing, pulling away from clinician, crying, or screaming, should be completed at the time of both the initial and discharge examination in order to help determine progress.

Strength

Utilizing standardized manual muscle testing (MMT) for UE and LE strength testing helps to determine children's strength in open chain positions as well as their willingness to move through painful motions. Of note, children may "break" out of the position secondary to pain rather than true muscle weakness. Depending on areas of reported pain, a quick screen versus an in-depth look at strength can be completed (i.e., in a child with complaints of LE pain, the PT can do a quick screen of UE strength and then take the child through all antigravity positions of LE strength testing). If a child presents with wrist or hand pain, fine motor strength, like grip and pinch, should be tested. Once again, documentation of pain behaviors, such as facial grimacing, pulling away from clinician, crying, or screaming, should be completed at the time of initial and discharge examination in order to help determine progress.

Joint Laxity

A common comorbidity in this population is hypermobility or reports of Ehlers–Danlos syndrome (EDS), which may or may not have been properly diagnosed. Utilizing the Beighton Scale depicted in Table 14.2, a screen of a child's joint laxity can be completed. This is not necessary to confirm or deny a potential diagnosis of hypermobility or EDS, but rather is used to assist a clinician in determining any potential modifications that should be taken into consideration when creating a safe treatment plan for a child.

Balance

Examination of a child's balance in sitting and standing should be completed along with questions about these positions. Sustaining static positions, such as sitting at a school desk or standing in line, may present as a challenge for this population; therefore, inquiring about tolerance to such positions can aid in developing treatment goals. Additionally, examining the posture of a child in these positions is critical. The answers to the following questions can be helpful in this examination:

- Is the child that complains of a constant headache sitting with forward head and rounded shoulders?
- Is the child that complains of right leg weakness standing with all of their weight on their left leg?
- Is the child willing to stand in single leg stance on their painful leg?

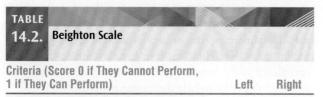

TABLE 14.2.	Beighton Scale		
Criteria (Score 0 if They Cannot Perform, 1 if They Can Perform)		Left	Right
1. Extension of fifth metacarpophalangeal beyond 90° (in sitting, elbow extended and forearm pronated)			
2. Apposition of thumb to flexor aspect of forearm (in sitting, elbow extended and forearm pronated)			
3. Hyperextension of elbow >10° (shoulder abducted to 90°, elbow extended, hand supinated)			
4. Passive hyperextension of the knee >10° (patient in standing, passive knee extension)			
5. Active forward flexion of the trunk with the knees fully extended and palms resting flat on the floor			

Mobility

Examining movement patterns in this population can provide critical information for the clinician. Observing the way in which a child transfers, ambulates, and completes the stairs will allow the clinician to note compensations that are present secondary to pain and/or weakness. In particular, a child with CRPS of an LE will likely avoid use of or weight bearing on their affected extremity and may even use an assistive device. Attempting to have the child mobilize without an assistive device will provide information on readiness for treatment.

Functional Strength Testing

Examining a child's strength in functional movements such as squats, lunges, planks, push-ups, and agility activities as appropriate can provide a clinician with what the child's current abilities and disabilities are secondary to their pain. Ensuring that a child utilizes proper form in closed chain activities, such as avoiding genu valgum, will confirm that the child does not have pain from organic reasons and is able to progress during treatment.

Utilizing standardized assessments and self-reported outcome measures, such as the Bruininks–Oseretsky Test of Motor Proficiency, Second Edition (BOT-2), and Functional Disability Inventory (FDI), can assist in developing a plan of care based on objective findings as well as in developing functional goals.

Evaluation of Findings

Synthesizing the information obtained in the initial examination of a child with amplified pain syndrome determines the most appropriate level of care required for treatment. A range of intervention options from consultative PT services to intensive daily programs exist for this population. Regardless of the level of service required, prioritizing findings in the examination and developing a targeted PT plan of care to treat impairments and functional limitations are imperative. The treatment of children in this population will be discussed in-depth; however, it is important to note here that the children who are most successful in treatment are those that follow the recommendation of physical therapy, desensitization, and cognitive behavioral therapy (CBT). The synthesis of findings will lead to a clear plan of care that is based on restoration of function in the individual.

» Treatment

Treatment for children and adolescents with AMPS is a complicated algorithm and one not without controversy and varying approaches. Treatment for AMPS, regardless of which type the child is presenting with, takes many forms depending on where treatment is sought. There are many centers that take a strictly medical treatment approach using multitudes of pain medicines, spinal cord stimulators, and implantable pain pumps. The majority of studies on those more invasive and medical-based techniques show some limited improvement, and most of the data are related to adults with minimal data in pediatric populations.[24,25]

Over the past two decades, many research articles calling for a standardized treatment have been published.[26] This includes systematic and Cochrane reviews of the current literature and those published between 2001 through 2016; yet no consensus has still been achieved.[26] The majority of articles agree on the need to incorporate physical therapy into the treatment regimen in order to provide the best functional outcomes.[6,11,13,26] Although physical therapy is an integral piece, those who have proposed specific treatment approaches have suggested that physical therapy alone is not an effective approach to the treatment of AMPS. Instead, it is important to have a multimodal and multidisciplinary approach that is focused on function, changing beliefs about pain, and addressing the child's fear of pain.[6,12,26–29]

This approach involves addressing the treatment for and the impact of biologic, psychological, environmental, and social issues.[6] Studies have shown that when a child in the household has pain, it has a negative effect on the siblings and the overall functioning of the household.[6] Additionally, research also shows a correlation between higher disability levels with increased numbers of pain medications.[24] It is common for individuals with AMPS to see themselves as more disabled, often demonstrating a decreased ability and decreased willingness to move because of pain catastrophizing. Miro et al. have shown that children are unwilling to move their body because of fear of pain and injury, which then leads to increased pain catastrophizing, increased pain intensity, and increased disability.[30] Research has shown that movement therapy with moderate and greater intensity of aerobic and functional activities provides more functional improvements and better reduction in pain than rest and passive modalities.[31,32] Passive and manual therapies only serve to maintain or increase pain intensity and disability and do not provide long-term functional improvements.[6,31,32]

It is important to note that active participation from the child is crucial for successful treatment in this population, and often it involves having the right care at the right time in the right place and with the right providers.[6] The child needs to be an active participant in their treatment including goal development, moving their body, not avoiding painful areas and/or activities, ownership for their wellness, and exercise program.[30,33] The ideal combination of treatments involves active movement-based physical therapy combined with CBT to address fear of movement as well as pain and life-related stressors. During treatment, focusing on functional improvements and not on pain levels or pain relief is important as research has shown that function returns prior to seeing pain relief in the vast majority of cases.[27] Additionally, Low et al.[34] have demonstrated that, particularly in CRPS, quicker diagnosis and earlier treatment lead to decreased recovery time and overall improved outcome.

Although most research is limited in the descriptions of the specific PT interventions, there are themes that occur across the board, including functional activities and neuromuscular retraining, overall strengthening, weight bearing, aerobic conditioning, desensitization, plyometrics, and sports-specific training.[11,13,28,29,35]

» Intervention

Complex Regional Pain Syndrome

This form of amplified pain presents with its own challenges with regard to treatment as it is common for individuals with CRPS to be avoidant of using the extremity, performing tasks with the uninvolved arm when UE is involved, or using assistive devices with LE involvement. Once the child is fully weight bearing and overall functional with extremity, treatment can also incorporate the focus and ideas presented in the localized treatment section.

Lower Extremity

When CRPS is present, pain and edema are typically seen and therefore many children present with disuse atrophy because of the use of assistive devices, bracing, and avoidance of the extremity. The main tenets of treatment therefore are ROM, weight bearing, strengthening, and gait training.

When beginning treatment for CRPS, it is important to remember that function will always return before pain relief is seen. Additionally, it is not uncommon for pain to initially rise with the start of desensitization and mobilization. Because of the importance of restoring function, early and often weight bearing is crucial to progress and the overall success in the treatment of CRPS. The longer an assistive device or bracing is used, and the child is allowed to avoid use of the extremity, the longer one can expect before full function and eventually pain relief can be achieved.[7,36] See Table 14.3 for an overview on assistive device and activity progression. The starting place for treatment will be determined by how the child presents at initial evaluation and also by their willingness to participate in therapy. All children should begin a home program of active ankle, foot, and toe ROM and progress to resisted exercises as soon as possible. Particularly important is gastrocnemius strengthening as this will help with toe-off during functional mobility once they are ambulating.

Initially, if they are not placing their foot on the ground, increasing their tolerance of pressure is an important first step. This can be done in sitting or standing to start; however, it should progress quickly to standing and then with just tapping or placing the foot on flat ground, progressing to resting the foot on the ground and standing with weight on their foot. In order to track progression of early weight bearing, using a nondigital scale will give you a tool to monitor and quantify how much pressure the child is placing on their foot and also a way for the therapist to set goals for the child to reach in each subsequent trial in a session. Increasing both

TABLE 14.3. Assistive Device Progression in CRPS of LEs			
Starting in Wheelchair	**Starting on Walker**	**Starting on Crutches**	**No Assistive Device**
• Standing with assistance • Touching foot to floor • Resting foot on floor when sitting • Shoes and socks on • Working on weight bearing on scale • Standing and taking steps with walker and, if possible, crutches or handheld assist • Can attempt without upper extremity support • Child leaves session with least restrictive assistive device.	• Walking with foot full contact to floor • Resting foot on floor in standing and sitting • Shoes and socks donned • Standing without upper extremity support • Taking steps with crutches or handheld assist. Can also try without upper extremity assistance • Working on weight bearing on scale, weight-shifting activities, and general weight bearing • Leaves session with least restrictive device possible	• Walking with foot full contact to floor • Resting foot on floor at all times • Weight-shifting and weight-bearing activities • Shoes and socks donned • Standing without upper extremity support • Gait training with one crutch and/or no crutches • Gait mechanics • Start ankle dorsiflexion/plantarflexion exercises. • Leaves session with one or no crutches	• Full foot contact • Gait training to encourage heel strike, toe-off, and normal dorsi- and plantarflexion • Weight-shifting and weight-bearing activities • Normalizing gait • Reciprocal stairs with no railing • Shoes on for outside of therapy • Perform many exercises barefoot to watch for compensations and proper form. • Do not go backward with assistive devices if their function declines.

CRPS, complex regional pain syndrome; LE, lower extremity.

the time and the amount of pressure is important and can be done over time in the same session.

As the child is able to maintain foot contact on the ground for longer periods of time, other weight-shifting exercises become valuable. Start with activities that encourage basic weight shifting over to the affected side and progress to having unaffected extremity up on a surface in order to assist with increased amounts of weight on the affected side. Although engaging in weight-shifting activities, it is important to watch for compensations and avoidance of weight on the affected extremity, such as altered body positioning or leaning on hands. Some examples of structuring the exercises to limit the ability to perform compensations are as follows: (1) Limit UE support to none or just a few fingers and try to have that support at a higher height so they are unable to place all of their weight on UEs. (2) When on bilateral LEs watch for body compensations that will shift weight off the extremity, especially hip positioning. It is not uncommon for the child to hold the hip of their affected leg in a posterior and rotated position to decrease weight on the extremity. (3) If utilizing a support surface for the unaffected extremity, use a higher or dynamic surface, placing it more forward or laterally to decrease the amount of pressure that can be placed on it.

Ambulation should begin early and be progressed as quickly as possible. It is important to not wait for gait to be normal without assistive device in order to eliminate it. It is possible that you may see gait worsen without assistive device; however, it is important to continue to not use the assistive device and continue working on gait training and weight bearing because returning to the assistive device will only serve to decrease the weight on the affected extremity. It often makes subsequent attempts to remove any assistive device more difficult as well. As increased weight is tolerated on the affected extremity, more specific gait mechanics

including heel strike and toe-off can be worked on while reminding the child that normalizing their gait is the first step toward full function. Plantarflexion during gait and performing toe-off is often the last functional piece to return. There are also times where the child is completing toe-off and then stops. If this happens during treatment for a period of time, continue strengthening and plantarflexion strengthening exercises. It may also help to just focus on strength and decrease the focus on those specific mechanics during functional mobility if that temporary plateau is reached.

Once general weight shifting to the affected side is no longer the primary issue, ideally after just a few sessions, the focus of treatment should then be on exercises and activities, which include strengthening and total body endurance as well as agility, plyometric training, when they are ready, and sport-specific training.[6,26] Throughout this remaining piece of treatment, it is important to monitor form and watch for compensations that may not be due to weakness but rather due to habit and/or avoidance of pain.[30,32,33]

When determining discharge from physical therapy, there are several considerations that need to be taken into account. You want to examine not only whether or not they have achieved their functional goals but also if they have not met their goals, that is, if they have met a treatment plateau. There are times where a child may need to be discharged with residual weakness or gait deviations and continue to progress over time. In those cases, it is important for the child to continue to take ownership for their function and continue to participate fully in life in order for that remaining piece of functional mobility and strength to return. Another important piece of this path of treatment as with all treatments is the continuation of psychotherapy. This often leads to full recovery on their own in this final phase of treatment. Occasionally, children will need to revisit physical therapy for fine-tuning or sport-specific training if they play at a higher level of sport, but this is not often the case.

Upper Extremity

CRPS in the UE presents with its own individual challenges and likewise the amount of disability often depends on location in the extremity. An additional consideration for the UE is whether it is on their dominant or nondominant side, which can also affect the ease of compensations and avoidance.

When CRPS is present in the UE, it is common to see moderate amounts of edema and disuse atrophy because of its consistently dependent position and ease of avoidance. To address the edema, you can start with tubular stretch bandaging if available or ACE™ wrapping to help with control when not in therapy sessions; however, the best way to control and eliminate the edema is through active muscle movement and muscular contraction through normal use of the extremity and exercise.

Often it is easier to develop compensatory movements and avoidance of the affected UE because of the ability to just use the opposite extremity for functional tasks. Use of the affected extremity both inside and outside of therapy sessions is crucial and should not be avoided as it will only serve to prolong the course of treatment. This is true not only during the child's activities of daily living but also in positioning the arm during the day and while sleeping at night. This can mean a variety of activities depending on whether it is the child's dominant or nondominant hand, ranging from carrying objects, opening doors, holding weights during exercises, to name a few examples.[7,36]

Closed chain exercises and activities are also important for those with UE CRPS. This will not only help provide proprioceptive feedback to the extremity but also serve to strengthen the extremity in preparation for functional activities that involve weight bearing.

To target allodynia in those with UE CRPS, you can incorporate clothing with sleeves in various textures or think about short-sleeved apparel if brushing against textures or wind exacerbates their allodynia.[11]

Fibromyalgia/Localized/Diffuse Pain

The other forms of amplified pain are all treated similarly in philosophy, with the differences being based more in the individual's areas of pain and goals. It is important to note that juvenile fibromyalgia tends to be different than adult fibromyalgia in that it is more responsive to treatment and is curable/manageable.[2]

When planning activities, exercises, and recommendations for this population, one should consider what was learned from their examination including pain location, what elicits pain (moving slowly or quickly, specific motions, being still after movement, or just being still in general), and what keeps them from being functional in their daily life. Also, it is important to know if they have allodynia, if it's light or deep touch, and if they have dizziness, brain fog, and/or noise sensitivity. The answers to those questions are going to steer the interventions and recommendations for outside of therapy sessions as well as ensure the best outcome possible.[21]

Based on the examination, treatment should be focused on strengthening exercises targeting the specific areas of pain as well as endurance building, total body strengthening, closed and open chain exercises, plyometric activities, agility and sport-specific exercises if they are looking to return to sports.[2,11,21,27] See Table 14.4 for suggested activities for

TABLE 14.4.	Nontraditional Interventions for Targeting AMPS
Abdominal pain	• Core strengthening • Snacks, eating avoidant foods • Plyometric activities • Prone over textures during exercises to incorporate desensitization
Dizziness/brain fog	• Quick up and down from mat tables or floor • Varying exercise positions: one on the floor, then one standing, and then another on the floor • Performing rolling, spinning, or exercises that involve bending over • Combine exercises with memory tasks, word searches, or other cognitive tasks
Difficulty being still after moving	• Exercises in short bursts rather than long periods of time • Alternate strengthening or endurance exercises (one or two exercises or 2–5 minutes of endurance) with short amounts of time (3–5 minutes) of sitting, standing, or laying down
Difficulty moving slowly	• Have patient move slowly through exercises • Slow, exaggerated movements • Holding various portions of exercise for a number of seconds to assist with slowing down
Noise/light sensitivity	• Loud music in treatment area or on headphones • Use noise apps on phone such as alarms, sirens, static, etc. • Use noisemakers as part of therapy such as tambourine, answer buttons, bells, etc.

AMPS, amplified musculoskeletal pain syndrome.

those symptoms and impairments that may not be helped by general exercise alone.

Timed Activities

As discussed previously, the focus on treatment, no matter the form of amplified pain, should be on return to full function as that is typically the first piece to return and pain relief is rarely seen prior to the child being fully functional in their daily life.

Often, at the beginning of treatment, when taking an exercise- and function-based philosophy, it is not uncommon for the child's pain to rise, for them to demonstrate or complain of increased pain, new pain, somatic symptoms, and/or symptoms consistent with FND. New pain should be examined to ensure it is not of an orthopedic nature, but once cleared, return to the original treatment plan is necessary. The somatic pain and FND symptoms should be worked through and is not a reason to stop or alter treatment whenever possible. Some of the more common somatic symptoms seen are dizziness, nausea, vomiting, and visual disturbances, whereas some of the more common FND symptoms are difficulty moving their body or an extremity, not being able to see, and/or shaking of one or more extremities.[37]

To help children work through those symptoms and ensure they are making continual progress despite the challenges they may face, it is often helpful to utilize the performance of individualized timed activities. Through having the child meet the requirement of beating their time each session in the outpatient setting or daily in the rehabilitation setting, it helps to ensure that there is continual

functional progress. It also educates the child that they can choose to work through those other symptoms with the use of encouragement and/or coping strategies (specifics of coping strategies will be discussed in another section). Many children with amplified pain have perfectionistic tendencies and seek approval from those around them, which, in moderation, can be positive characteristics; however, when these are present in overwhelming levels, it can be more difficult for the child to cope with everyday challenges. By having the child work through the idea of having to continually increase function with repeated trials, if needed, a variety of coping strategies are built, which can benefit all aspects of life. Many of these children have a history of difficulty working through challenging situations and exercises as they often have been rescued by family, teachers, and friends when faced with adversity and therefore have never built up a variety of coping strategies in order to help them be able to move forward in situations where they lack perfection or need to work at the problem to succeed. Learning to work through these situations helps the child regain power and control over their emotions, body, and life, and it can provide for important breakthroughs in their ability to function in life regardless of pain.[30,33]

Which ones and how many timed activities chosen to have the child perform is flexible, and among the factors to be considered are the environment they are treated in, how often they are seen in therapy, the length of sessions, where pain and deficits are, as well as any comorbidities or restrictions that exist. See Table 14.5 for a description of a wide variety of examples, but remember these are not the only timed activities that can be used, and being creative to

TABLE 14.5.	Timed Activities
Animal Walks	
Kangaroo	Standing on bilateral lower extremities with hands on hips. Hop forward making sure to use both legs equally and not compensating through leaning on one leg or galloping
Inchworm	Starting with hands and feet close together with buttocks in the air. Then walk hands forward until in full plank position on hands with hips fully extended. Next, step legs forward one at a time until feet are close to hands and buttocks up in the air. Keep repeating this for chosen distance.
Three-Legged Puppy	Starting with bilateral upper extremities and one lower extremity on the ground with hands and foot 6–12 inches from each other. Then bring hand forward (at the same time if possible, but in cases of hypermobility may need to move them one at a time) 6–12 inches and then hop foot forward, making sure that shoulders are not forward of their hands. This forward position unweights their lower extremity and is a common compensation seen in those with lower body pain. Typically will have them go a distance and turn, returning on opposite extremity
Crab Walk	While sitting on the floor, reach back with upper extremities and place on the floor. Next bend knees and place feet flat on the floor. Now lift body off the floor supporting weight with arms and left. Move forward and backward on a "walking" fashion as able.
Frog	From standing, lower into a full squat with heels close and toes/knees spread apart. Place bilateral upper extremities on ground with hands flat and arms between knees. Next step is to place bilateral upper extremities forward, lean on them, and hop forward using a manner that elicits contraction of abdominals and use of feet more than quadriceps so that the buttocks do not raise up high during the hop. Continue that for set distance.
Hallway Sprint	If you have a hallway that will allow a sprint, this is a good way to work on having them run and to increase the pace of that run.
Leg Step-Ups	On a standard size step, without using a railing, step up with one foot then the other and the foot that went on step first is the first foot to step down. Complete a certain number (typically between 20 and 40) with one leg leading then repeat on opposite leg with separate times for each leg.

TABLE 14.5.	Timed Activities (*continued*)
Arm Step-Ups	Using a 4-inch step, have them in modified push-up position (can have knees on a chair but making sure only half or less of the thigh is supported). They then step up similar to the description of leg step-ups above, however typically smaller reps such as 20–30 and using arms rather than legs. Make sure they maintain a tight core and do not let their back sag.
Box Carry	Holding some sort of box or basket with 5–10 lb of weight inside, have child step forward 2–3 feet, then squat and place box on ground, stand up then squat again to pick box up. Repeat for 3–8 stops, can use cones as marks to stop and squat.
Laundry Carry	If you have a full-sized stairway in your treatment area, can have child ascend and descend stairs while carrying a laundry basket. Can have them complete 3–5 sets for the time using a reciprocal pattern
Tub Step Ins	If you have a tub in your treatment space or a hurdle that is tub height, can have child complete this timed activity. It is done typically with bilateral upper extremities on a wall, then step over one foot at a time into tub or other side of hurdle and then back. Complete as many as possible in 60 seconds.
Socks and Shoes On/Off	If it is difficult for patient to perform single leg stance can work on this functionally by having them doff/don socks and shoes in standing without leaning on a surface for a certain number of repetitions for time
Floor to Stand	Floor-to-stand transitions through half-kneeling is another activity that can have a certain number of repetitions completed on each leg for time and is a functional way to incorporate timed activities.

find the right ones for a particular child and situation is important.

When completing timed activities, it is important to monitor form and look for compensations that may be due to pain and not deconditioning based on the location of the child's pain. When a child first starts working on their timed activities, depending on the distance they are traveling and their level of function, they may not be able to complete the whole distance without a rest. This is okay and the timer should remain running when they take a break; as they regain strength, endurance, and function, the need for rest breaks will decrease and it will also be reflected in their overall time. As their times increase and get faster, eventually it is better to discontinue the timed activities and continue with strengthening and functional activities.

There are some children with amplified pain who struggle more with moving slowly through space, whereas it is easy to move quickly through their exercises and timed activities. For this cohort of children, it is often more beneficial to slow down all of their exercises including their timed activities in order to continue to challenge their pain. They should go slower daily on their timed activities until they reach a time of up to several minutes, then discontinue and focus more on strengthening and functional activities.

Allodynia

All forms of amplified pain may or may not present with one or more forms of allodynia, and it is treated through various forms of desensitization, which typically involves the use of an unpleasant stimulus to the area of increased sensitivity. Some demonstrate light touch allodynia to the skin, which can include any part of the body from scalp to toes; some require more of a moderate touch or even a deep touch to the body to feel the sensitivity. Children with amplified pain may have one or more of the aforementioned types of allodynia or some do not have any. The stimuli that

evoke pain tend to be things that the body may be routinely exposed to and do not elicit pain responses when applied to nonaffected areas of the body. Even though some of those stimuli may be slightly uncomfortable to nonaffected areas, they are not normally painful, and it is important to remember that they are not harmful or damaging. Although not always considered to be true allodynia, other types of sensitivity may also be present such as to noise, temperature, smells, and light. These should be treated the same as other types of sensitivity and challenged in similar manners rather than avoided.

Desensitization can be an intervention on its own or incorporated into exercises and activities of daily living depending on the needs of the child and the amount of time able to be dedicated to it in a session. Some common equipment that can be used for desensitization include, but are not limited to, massagers and massage mats of all sizes and intensities, surgical scrub brushes and loofa, textured disks and other sensory equipment, ice massage or ice immersion, warm water immersion, and contrast baths.[11] Table 14.6 shows some examples of how desensitization can be used as its own intervention and as an adjunct to therapy.

Coping Strategies

As discussed previously, in most of the children who develop amplified pain, one of the biggest factors that play a role is stress and their inability to cope with normal and/or abnormal amounts of life stressors. In the majority of children with amplified pain, this stress is brought on by and comprises everyday stressors of school, family, community as well as self-imposed stress brought on by personality tendencies for pleasing and perfection. The goal of coping is not to take away the pain but rather to take attention away from the pain. Research has shown that the more attention is focused toward the pain, the more likely a child is to feel it and rate it

TABLE 14.6. Desensitization Activities		
As Intervention	**In Conjunction with Exercises**	**During ADLs**
• Various types of massagers • Ice massage or immersion • Warm water soaks • Rubbing skin with various textures • Laying on textures such as bumpy pads, tennis balls, etc. • Lotion massage • Audible tapping • Retrograde massage	• Barefoot on various textures during standing • Hands on various textures for closed chain exercises • Exercises in prone/supine on textures • Wind through fan during session • Soft textures brushed against skin during exercise • Strings/feathers, etc. hanging on arms/legs	• Towel rubs after shower/bathing • Varying temperature of water during showering or hand washing • Lotion massage while applying lotion after shower • Using textured sponge in shower • Varying pressure of shower head • Audible taps during commercials of favorite show • Hugs from family members • Long/short sleeves • Tight/loose clothing

ADLs, activities of daily living.

at a higher number. However, with distraction and taking the focus off the pain, their ratings tend to be lower and they are able to remain in a more calm state.[38]

In order to help children with amplified pain learn to face their fears, anxieties, and difficult activities, it is important to assist the child with learning to identify and use coping strategies. These strategies can take many forms and often what works in one situation may not work in another. This is why it is important to learn a variety of techniques rather than just trying one and evaluating whether coping works based on that one experience. By building up their variety of coping strategies, children with amplified pain can build a virtual "coping tool box" where they can pull out various strategies depending on the situation and what is needed or appropriate in the moment. Learning these techniques will serve them in working through not only their amplified pain but also in other areas in life such as school, jobs, and relationships throughout their lifetime.

Among the most popular of techniques are distraction, which can be done via conversation, word games, music, or videos; mantras such as saying what you are doing, for instance, "hand, hand, foot, foot," positive affirmations such as "I'm strong I can do this" or "the faster I go, the faster I'm done" or "if I've already done x, I can certainly do y"; grounding and deep breaths, for example, naming things in the room, taking a certain number of deep breaths, or squeezing something in their hand. As these techniques are used and practiced, they become easier to use and eventually can become automatic and take less thought process to remember to use.

Cognitive Behavioral Therapy

In addition to learning and practicing coping strategies in therapy sessions, another important place to learn them is through talk therapy with a psychologist. Using talk therapy

and specifically a cognitive behavioral approach (CBT) in conjunction with physical and/or occupational therapy (OT) is the most evidence-based treatment to overcome amplified pain. It takes working hard in both of those areas to fully recover and decrease the likelihood of pain and loss of function returning. Although PTs and PT assistants will not be providing the CBT, it is important to understand the basic tenets of it and incorporate pieces of it into therapy sessions.[39–41]

Stress is a normal part of life and regardless of where those stressors originate from, there is a connection between thoughts and feelings and behaviors or actions. CBT is a type of talk therapy that is aimed at using this relationship between thoughts, feelings, and behaviors to make more educated choices in life through altering thought patterns away from negative statements and instead developing more healthy statements and balance thoughts.[42,43]

One example of the relationship between thoughts and actions is the fear-avoidance model. This model predicts that increased anxiety about pain then causes avoidance of activity and use of extremity, which then causes more pain from disuse and therefore more anxiety about movement and even greater decrease in function. This in turn often leads to increased disability and depression.[44,45]

Using CBT helps break this fear-avoidance cycle by helping child focus on increasing the flexibility of their thoughts and therefore use them in an adaptive rather than maladaptive manner. Through CBT, children learn to utilize adaptive coping strategies such as distraction, reframing negative thought patterns into more positive or action-oriented ones, relaxation, decreased catastrophic thought patterns, and problem-solving skills. Being able to catch those thought patterns early and work on changing them before they lead to the fear-avoidance cycle not only can help children when they are recovering from pain but also leads to increased confidence and skills they can use throughout life to adapt to ever-changing stressors.[43]

Studies have shown that CBT results in neurologic changes in many areas of the brain and its network connections, which leads to the thought that this may be one of the reasons for its efficacy in the treatment of pain. Functional magnetic resonance imaging (fMRI) has shown that after receiving CBT, there is an increase in activation of the prefrontal cortex, which is the area of the brain thought to be related to acute pain. This area of the brain is also involved in the ability to process and anticipate pain events as well as regulate the emotions around this pain. Normalization of the abnormal connections in the sensorimotor network and increased connectivity have also been noted on follow-up imaging. Posttreatment with CBT, fMRI results also have shown that children had reduced dorsal posterior cingulate cortex activity. This is thought to lead to decreased pain ratings and anxiety related to pain as well as improvements of thoughts surrounding pain.[46] Additionally, in a randomized controlled study, CBT was found to demonstrate greater clinically significant improvements in functional disability and depression than controls who had standard talk therapy; those improvements were still evident at 6 months follow-up. Learning the skills associated with CBT not only helps children while they are participating in treatment for AMPS or other conditions but also leads to adaptive behaviors, increased confidence, and a greater sense of control over their lives that can be taken and used in other facets of daily life and over the course of their lifetime.[43]

Outcomes

The literature suggests that the most optimal outcomes in this population derive from a multidisciplinary, non-pharmacologic treatment approach. CBT was the first evidence-based treatment approach that was found to be effective in pain symptoms; however, it was not associated with improved functional outcomes. Once CBT was combined with neuromuscular exercise, greater reductions in pain scores as well as improved functional outcomes were noted.[40] The Center for Amplified Pain at The Children's Hospital of Philadelphia published data in 2015 in the *Journal of Pediatrics* that further support this notion. It was found that children receiving 5 to 6 hours of intensive PT/OT as well as 4 hours a week of psychosocial services (psychology, music therapy, art therapy, social work) demonstrated significantly decreased pain scores from 65/100 VAS to 25/100 VAS, and one-third of children reported no pain at their 1-year follow-up appointment. More importantly, their functional progress was noted in improved scores on the BOT-2 scores and the FDI, indicating a return to normalized function.[27] As one part of the multidisciplinary treatment approach, PTs can encourage children to participate in all aspects of treatment as well as educating other medical professionals on the AMPS diagnosis in order to provide the best care to this unique population.

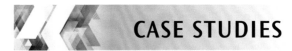

CASE STUDIES

CASE STUDY #1

History as of clinic visit: Jenny was overall a healthy child until approximately 2 years prior to treatment. The first incident that was possibly the start of her amplified pain was on a trip to Europe where she walked a lot and developed pain in her left foot. She was unable to place her foot on the ground, but she saw orthopedics and took ibuprofen and was fine in approximately 3 days. One year prior to treatment for amplified pain, Jenny was hit by a door at a friend's house and sustained a concussion. After her concussion, she received outpatient PT for concussion-related issues for approximately 8 months off and on. The day after discharge from outpatient PT, she attended a pool party with lots of diving and swimming and did not report any injury to her foot. Two days later, however, she developed pain in her left foot over the lateral aspect and by the next day her left foot was inverted. She had a normal radiograph but because of pain they placed her in a Controlled Ankle Motion (CAM) boot and recommended return to outpatient PT. She attended five sessions of PT, but her foot pain became worse and she began limping more. At that time, her radiographs were repeated and she also had MRI, and both studies were normal. She began to complain of weakness in her left leg, so her doctor ordered electromyograph (EMG) and nerve conduction studies as well as a lumbar MRI; again all studies were normal. Because of her progression of symptoms, she also visited the emergency department at her local children's hospital where they recommended discontinuation of the CAM boot as it was not relieving her pain, continuation of physical therapy, and referral to the Amplified Musculoskeletal Pain Clinic. Her pain at this time was along the inner aspect of her left foot to palpation and with dorsiflexion. Two months after the pool party, she is unable to ambulate without assistance and uses two crutches and is electively non–weight bearing on her left LE. Her foot is held in a position of inversion and plantarflexion and she refuses to place her foot on the ground or wear a shoe and/or sock.

Previous imaging: All normal (MRI of lumbar spine, left ankle, brain; radiograph of lumbar spine)

Examination: Jenny rated her pain as 4/10 at rest and a highest pain level of 9/10. She describes her pain as constant, pressurizing, and throbbing. Jenny states that nothing makes it better, and the pain is made worse by activity, touching, and in the evening/nighttime. Because of her pain she cannot do chores, socialize, walk long distances, participate in sports, and play the piano because of not being able to push the pedals or get comfortable. In addition, she has headaches, muscle spasms, and an inability to move her left ankle.

Functional Disability Inventory (60 signifying worst): Patient FDI: 35/Parent FDI: 35

Physical examination: She is unable to touch her left foot to the ground, and while it is held in an inverted and plantar-flexed position, she can achieve neutral ankle dorsiflexion. She has allodynia from her knees to her toes, and her lower leg is cold and bluish. She is resistant to attending PT sessions as well talk therapy. Recommendation from clinic was that she attend counseling sessions, desensitize to work on her allodynia, and practice weight bearing so she can wean herself off the crutches and also return to school full time.

PT evaluation (3 months postclinic evaluation): Her current pain score is 6/10, with the best being a 4/10 and the worst level rated at a 10/10. The location of her pain at this time was left posterior ankle, left mid foot up to left calf and occasionally left knee. Jenny stated that it feels like "you are hitting something really hard" and that the pain was constant. Jenny states that bike riding, pressure or weight bearing, tight shoes, and sitting longer than 20 minutes all make her pain worse, and sometimes ice makes it better. She reports that she was doing scrubbing in shower for desensitization and occasionally ice.

Social history: Jenny lives with her twin sister and both parents in a two-story house with three steps to enter. Her bedroom is on the second floor; however, her parents have arranged a room downstairs for her so she could avoid using stairs inside the house. Jenny is in fifth grade and attending school; however, she is not attending recess or gym class.

Activity level: Jenny ambulates with bilateral axillary crutches, non–weight bearing on left LE, and reports she has been so for several months. Jenny has not been as active as she previously was. She currently is not hanging out with friends as much because of pain and fatigue, she does not sit on the floor with her friends (stands instead), and feels as though she does not get to participate in fun things at school. She was going to outpatient PT; however, she did not find it helpful and stated that during those sessions, she was attempting to put foot on ground but just hopping on right LE, riding different types of bikes, and rubbing her foot on various textures.

Strength/range of motion: Bilateral UEs and right LE: Full ROM and strength grossly 5/5 MMT. Left LE: Full ROM to knee and hip with strength in those areas 4+/5 MMT. Ankle ROM noted for positioning into inversion and plantarflexion able to actively achieve neutral positioning with moderate pain behaviors. Passive ROM and strength of left foot was unable to be assessed because of maximal pain behaviors and muscle co-contraction because of guarding and child pulling away when foot was touched.

Gait: Child ambulates with bilateral forearm crutches, maintaining non–weight bearing on left LE and performing swing-through gait.

Stairs: Jenny is able to ascend and descend two flights of stairs with one crutch and one railing while maintaining non–weight bearing on her left LE.

Standardized testing: Not performed because the child was unable to use left LE in a functional manner.

Short-Term PT Goals (Time Frame: 3 to 4 Weeks)

1. Jenny will participate in 30 minutes of continuous moderate-level cardiovascular activity with no to minimal pain behaviors and compensations.
2. Jenny will participate in 25 minutes of total body strengthening with no to minimal pain behaviors and compensations.

3. Jenny will independently ambulate community distances on even and uneven terrain, demonstrating age-appropriate gait speed, no to minimal pain behaviors and compensations.
4. Jenny will reciprocally negotiate a full flight of standard height stairs independently without handrails needed, demonstrating no to minimal pain behaviors and compensations.
5. Jenny will participate in 25 minutes of dynamic standing balance activities, demonstrating no to minimal pain behaviors and compensations.
6. Jenny will participate in 20 minutes of sports-specific activities (running and fencing), demonstrating no to minimal pain behaviors and compensations.

First Week of Therapy

Session 1: This session was spent encouraging Jenny to place increased amounts of weight on her foot through weight-shifting exercises and placing her foot on an analog scale to measure the pounds of pressure on her foot. She was able to achieve up to 20 lb of pressure. Gait training was the other focus of this session, working on placing her foot flat on the ground and using a three-point gait with bilateral crutches and weight bearing as tolerated as well as two-point gait with one crutch. She demonstrated maximal pain behaviors throughout the session of crying, avoidance of use of her foot, and attempting to bargain activities down. She was allowed to take both crutches home that day with encouragement to work on using one crutch at home in preparation for removal of one crutch at the next session.

Session 2: Focus continued to be placed on weight shifting to the left, and among the techniques used were video games on a balance board, standing with opposite foot on a higher surface to complete UE activities, standing on bilateral LEs and reaching outside base of support toward her left. Gait training and weaning of crutches continued and she was required to walk in sessions without crutches. Her gait consisted of wide base of support with most of her weight shifted to the right side, minimal weight bearing on the left as demonstrated by a shorter step length with the right leg and UEs held in high guard. She was allowed to take one crutch home with the understanding that at the next session that crutch would then be removed. She continued to demonstrate maximal pain behaviors of crying, occasional refusals of activities, and attempts to bargain activities down and moderate avoidance of her left LE. She required maximal support to assist with coping with the pain and anxiety surrounding activities. We worked on using distraction, name games, and explanation of the importance of why we are doing the activities.

Session 4: She was refusing to participate in session and required maximal support and talking through the importance of using her foot and rationale for activities. She eventually agreed to participate in session, demonstrated decreased weight shift to the left and bearing weight on the lateral border of her foot at the start of the session; however, by the end of session, she demonstrated increased use of entire foot as the day progressed. Timed activities of step-ups and a 90-foot walk were started to assist with maintaining functional gains of each session.

Session 5: She demonstrated increased investment in completing activities and was able to demonstrate increased weight shift to the left. She was able to briefly complete single leg stance and began working on LE strengthening with specific focus on gastrocnemius, soleus, as well as foot intrinsic muscles. Those areas tend to be the weakest in children with the chronic regional pain syndrome type of amplified pain. She demonstrated decreased pain behaviors, mostly through facial grimacing and occasional bargaining of activities. She was no longer crying and screaming in sessions.

Second week of sessions: We increased the number of timed activities she was completing in order to continue increasing functional demands. Focus continued to be placed on ankle and foot strengthening, single leg stance, and single leg balance activities. Each activity was structured in a way that she would be required to use her left leg in order to be successful. She continued to vary in her levels of participation in the program as well as her ability to cope with activities. She would vary in her demonstration of pain behaviors from minimal to maximal and her affect would vary from engaged and laughing to crying and attempting to avoid activities. We continued to focus on building her variety of coping strategies.

Third week of sessions: Jenny demonstrated decreased pain behaviors this week and increased focus on decreasing compensations. She was able to ambulate on the treadmill at moderate speeds with noticeably decreased compensations in gait mechanics at higher speed walking. She continued to work on single leg stance activities as well as gastrocnemius strengthening and activities to work on increasing push-off with her forefoot. She worked on heel walking for desensitization and toe walking for strengthening and began to be able to run toward the end of the week.

Fourth week of sessions: This week, Jenny worked on helping choose some of what she wanted to work on in preparation for discharge. Strengthening work continued as per the other weeks, and in addition Jenny worked on sport-specific exercises and drills for preparation to return to soccer and possibly start fencing lessons. She worked on running and jumping although during both of those tasks we continued to see compensations, but this week they were more because of weakness than pain behaviors. She was discharged at the end of the week with recommendations to continue being an active child, but was not given specific home exercise program. This is to keep with the philosophy of normalizing life after the program and immersing herself in activities she enjoys and continue gaining strength in that manner. Because it is more meaningful to her, she would be more likely to complete those activities and continue strengthening in a more functional manner.

Discharge: Pain level was rated at a 7/10, with best being 6/10 and worst being 10/10. She was still reporting increased pain when jumping and running; however, she was able to identify that distraction and other coping strategies helped decrease her pain. She was demonstrating no pain behaviors. Jenny's pain location was left knee and foot, with allodynia to her foot that was sensitive to vibration and cold only. She demonstrated no color or temperature changes to her foot and no swelling was noted.

Strength/range of motion: Bilateral UEs and Right UE: Full ROM; Strength 5/5 MMT. Left LE: Full ROM; Strength 5/5 grossly overall except for left ankle 4−/5. ROM was within normal limits (WNL) in left LE.

Gait: Jenny is able to ambulate at an age-appropriate speed with minimal compensations noted. Those consisted of decreased weight shift to the left, decreased plantarflexion, and decreased toe-off on left LE.

Stairs: Jenny is able to ascend and descend two full flights of stairs without handrail with reciprocal pattern, noted for altered mechanics of decreased weight shift to the left and decreased forward reach with left toes onto lower step when descending.

Evaluation: Despite struggling to cooperate at times and difficulty with utilizing coping strategies, Jenny left the program fully functional with minimal deficits. Even though she was not reporting decreased pain, which is normal at the functional stage she was currently in, research has shown that pain does not normally decrease until full function returns. Although her pain rating had not changed, her pain behaviors had changed dramatically, going from not being able to use her foot at all and crying/screaming throughout sessions to being able to run and jump while still laughing and engaging in conversations with staff. The main goal of treatment is not to keep the child as a patient until they are pain free but make them functional and able to engage fully in life rather than see themselves as a sick or nonfunctional child. Research has shown that as they continue to engage in a normally functioning life, their pain will decrease over time.[27]

CASE STUDY #2

History from initial clinic visits: Mary was well until about 3.5 years ago when she developed head pain after sustaining a whiplash while snow tubing. At that time, she was diagnosed with occipital and trigeminal neuralgia, which was unresponsive to medication including nerve blocks. Over the past few years, she has attended appointments on average twice yearly with a chiropractor after which she notes temporary relief. Over time, her pain has spread to her back and the joints of her LEs, which in turn has caused her to continue to seek medical evaluation and subsequently was diagnosed with AMPS after which she started physical therapy. Mary was attending outpatient PT three times a week at a standard PT clinic without AMPS experience. She states that despite therapy her pain is about the same and her joints hurt when they are touched. At the time of this evaluation, she has continuing pain in her lower back, hips, knees, and hands and will get random tremors to her fingers. She also, at times, feels weak and will drop whatever she is holding. Occasionally, her legs go numb, especially when she ascends/descends stairs. She will often have to sit when descending stairs and use the railing when ascending. She does not always associate this with pain, but states it is very hard for her to describe. Clothing and undergarments hurt and when she is at home, she wears only a large sweatshirt or T-shirt. She also states she has to sit in the shower. She describes her pain as intermittent but occurs daily and is becoming more frequent. Mary states that at times her legs will turn blue, feel cold, and look modeled. Mary feels as though she sweats a lot and associates this with feeling over-whelmed with anxiety that especially happens when she takes a shower. She is also dealing with anxiety and depression.

Imaging: All normal (radiograph of lumbar spine, left ankle; MRI of lumbar spine, left ankle, brain; MR angiogram of neck)

Examination: Presently she has 4/10 pain. Her pain goes as high as 8/10 and as low as 0/10. She is in pain daily, but the pain is in-termittent with exacerbations of severe pain lasting as long as 10 minutes and as short as seconds (with pain peaking at 8/10). Her pain is made worse by touching, weather, stress, cold, and being still. Her pain is made better by medication (meloxicam), heat, and moving. Overall, her pain is getting worse. She describes her pain as shooting, stabbing, tingling, stiff, and gnawing. Be-cause of her pain, she cannot walk long distances, play sports, write a long time, or get comfortable. In addition, she has muscle spasms, dizziness, and visual disturbances—like cotton over her eyes or she will look at a page but not be able to recognize words. She complains of having dyscognition (unable to comprehend) but is still making good grades.

Functional Disability Inventory (60 signifying worst): Patient FDI: 17/Parent FDI: 26

Physical examination: Tender to palpation chest, back, right hip, and fingers right 2nd and left 5th, 4th, and 2nd (not fingertips). Pain up to 7/10 without withdrawal or pain behaviors. No color or temperature changes. Incongruent affect. Axial loading and passive rotation negative. Straight leg raise test negative. She did not guard her back when getting up off the table. Her left foot is slightly edematous. Heart rate: supine (5′) 89 bpm; standing—1′: 94 bpm; 3′: 94 bpm; 5′: 103 bpm

Clinic follow-up 2 months later: Mary has been struggling since her last clinic visit. Overall, her pain has decreased, but she has had an increase in her level of dizziness. She was feeling quite dizzy when lying down and she was worried so she went to the emergency department 1 month ago. Mary stated she is wor-ried she has multiple sclerosis. She also was noted by her PT to have upbeat nystagmus, but this was not noted by the neuro-ophthalmologist and she had normal vestibular testing. She gets very dizzy after physical therapy so she was discharged. Mary is now stating that she believes her dizziness goes back to approxi-mately 8 months prior on Christmas Eve. She states her pain still comes intermittently and becomes quite severe for a second or two or can last hours, but at a generally lower level than severe. Mary continues to have allodynia to her chest and right hip, her hands and knees still hurt, but are better and she still gets swell-ing to the top of her left foot. Mary continues to complain of difficulty concentrating but still makes good grades. She states she sees spots and at times the visual image lags behind her eye movement. She has constipation and urinary incontinence and a host of symptoms and states she is worse with changes

in weather, especially rain. Despite her symptoms, she is able to work as a cashier at a food store without having to miss work. She is in counseling with a new counselor who believes that she is demonstrating signs and symptoms consistent with anxiety and obsessive/compulsive disorder (OCD) but does not think she has attention-deficit/hyperactivity disorder (ADHD) as was previ-ously thought. She is particular about areas being clean, but is not endorsing any OCD rituals.

Examination: Presently Mary has 5/10 pain with allodynia to her right hip at the anterior superior iliac spine, chest (spares her breasts), and back lower ribs—half-way to spine with variable border as well as pain issues with her hands and knees with hy-perbolic behaviors. Her pain goes as high as 9/10 and as low as 0/10. She is in pain most of the day and is better on meloxicam.

Functional Disability Inventory (60 signifying worst): Patient FDI: 29/Parent FDI: 25

Other symptoms: In addition to the above pain, she has fatigue, muscle spasms, dizziness, visual disturbances, edema, constipa-tion, urinary incontinence, tinnitus, modeled skin, and dyscogni-tion. Romberg test was normal, normal finger to nose with eyes closed, normal tandem walking forward and backward, mostly reporting dizziness with eyes closed. Intermittent and mild lateral nystagmus. Axial loading and passive rotation negative, straight leg raising negative. Somewhat pressured speech.

Impression: Diffuse amplified musculoskeletal pain—less pain overall but still with allodynia to her chest, lateral ribs, right hip, and now severe dizziness and dyscognition. Her examination is normal, suggesting these are conversion-like symptoms, and additionally she is hyperfocused on her symptoms and physical complaints. Mary endorsed 21 symptoms and rated her level of function in the severely disabled range with an FDI of 29, but also said she was normally functional and that she just pushes through. It was discussed with the patient that she should not keep going for testing, that rather than putting her anxiety of a serious illness out of her mind it is instead increasing her anxiety.

PT examination (6 weeks post last clinic visit): Mary's current pain level is zero, with her best level being 0 and her worst be-ing 4—all on a 0–10 scale. She describes it as intermittent and is worst in hips (right greater than left), shoulders, hands, chest (allodynia), joints (allodynia) and that it feels as though it is burn-ing, gnawing, sharp, shooting. She states that it is irregular in frequency and duration, does not occur daily during summer but does in winter. Mary states that prolonged positioning, sitting for a long time, standing up too quickly all exacerbate her pain, while heat and exercise alleviate her pain. She has allodynia of deep touch to chest and joints.

Other symptoms: Mary endorses vision changes including spots, opaque areas.

Social history: Mary lives with her mother, father, and one younger sibling in a split-level home with stairs to her bedroom. She is able to drive and got her license a few months ago. She attends public school, is going into grade 12, and does not miss days because of pain.

Activity level: Mary has a heavy activity level and enjoys being busy. Her activities include maintaining independent functional mobility and hiking; she works at a natural food store, likes to engage in embroidery, sings in jazz band at school, and is on tech crew for the school play.

Strength/range of motion: Bilateral UEs and LEs: 4–5/5 MMT throughout. Cervical spine AROM: grossly WNL into flexion/extension, right/left rotation, and right/left lateral flexion. Trunk AROM: grossly WNL into flexion/extension, right/left rotation, and right/left lateral flexion.

Gait: Patient ambulates greater than 500 feet over even surfaces, independent; gait remarkable grossly unremarkable except for bilateral pes planus

Stairs: ascends full flight of stairs with reciprocal gait pattern, independent; descends full flight of stairs with reciprocal gait pattern, independent

Standardized Testing

BOT-2 Balance and Coordination: 18th percentile
BOT-2 Running and Strength Subtest: 50th percentile
Bruce Treadmill Protocol: 14 minutes 28 seconds

Short-Term PT Goals (Time Frame: 2 to 3 Weeks)

1. Mary will participate in 30 minutes of cardiovascular activity with minimal to no compensations and minimal to no pain behaviors.
2. Mary will participate in 30 minutes of total body strengthening with minimal to no compensations and minimal to no pain behaviors.
3. Mary will participate in 30 minutes of sports/activity-specific training (hiking, tech crew) with minimal to no compensations and minimal to no pain behaviors.
4. Mary will participate in 45 minutes of static positioning activity while engaged in cognitive challenge with minimal to no compensations and minimal to no pain behaviors in order to simulate return to school.

First Week of Therapy

Mary was begun on timed activities; however, she showed no difficulty with completing. Much of the focus this first week in her sessions was on total body strengthening, especially core and LEs. She also completed activities in various cold temperatures in room and also standing exercises in ice water. This was due to patient stating that she experienced great difficulty functioning in cold temperatures and that her decline in function would last for hours after exposure. When in PT, however, she was able to complete high-level exercises and activities for several hours after cold exposure without accommodations. She also worked on static standing activities in preparation for return to her job working at food store where she stands still for several hours at a time. She had described previously having moderate to maximal difficulty with this but showed none to minimal pain behaviors in session.

Second Week

Mary was able to discontinue timed activities because of her ability to perform them at a maximal effort and speed. Among the activities completed this week were total body strengthening

exercises, agility and plyometric exercises. Mary also worked on standing while completing UE tasks for extended lengths of time in preparation for return to work after discharge from the program. She was demonstrating no pain behaviors with those activities. Early in the week, Mary was still complaining of brain fog and dizziness, so additional exercises that incorporated quick change of position, 180 degree turns, and jumping alternated with cognitive tasks were incorporated in her sessions and she demonstrated no more than normal amounts of dizziness.

Discharge

Strength/range of motion: All strength was measured to be 5/5 except bilateral hips, which measured at 4/5. All ROM was WNL. She met all her goals that were set during evaluation at admission. Plan was for patient to return to school full time and work part-time as well as extracurricular activities. No home exercise program was given and patient was instructed to participate in active things that she enjoys participating in.

Standardized Testing

BOT-2 Balance and Coordination Subset: 58th percentile
BOT-2 Running and Strength: 86th percentile
Bruce Treadmill Protocol: 16 minutes

Clinic Follow-up (6 Weeks Postdischarge)

Upon follow-up to clinic, Mary presented with no pain or motor conversions. She was no longer complaining of dizziness or brain fog and was attending school and work without missing days. She demonstrate normal ROM, and strength in all body areas was 5/5. She was not in counseling and reported her stress as high, so it was recommended she seek a provider. She was staying normally active through participating in clubs, activities, and hiking.

REFERENCES

1. Cohen M, Quintner J, Rysewyk S. Reconsidering the International Association for the Study of Pain definition of pain. *Pain Rep.* 2018;3(2):1-7.
2. Gmuca S, Sherry DD. Fibromyalgia: treating pain in the juvenile patient. *Paediatr Drugs.* 2017;19(4):325-338.
3. Gmuca S, Xiao R, Urquhart A. Role of patient and parental resilience in adolescents with chronic musculoskeletal pain. *J Pediatr.* 2019;210:118-126.
4. King S, Chambers CT, Huguet A, et al. The epidemiology of chronic pain in children and adolescents revisited: a systematic review. *Pain.* 2011;152(12):2729-2738.
5. Neville A, Jordan A, Beveridge J, et al. Diagnostic uncertainty in youth with chronic pain and their parents. *J Pain.* 2019;20(9):1080-1090.
6. Stinson J, Connelly M, Kamper S, et al. Models of care for addressing chronic musculoskeletal pain and health in children and adolescents. *Best Pract Res Clin Rheumatol.* 2016;30:468-482.
7. Bialocerkowski A, Daly A. Is physiotherapy effective for children with complex regional pain syndrome type 1? *Clin J Pain.* 2012;28:81-91.
8. Laxer RM, Sherry DD, Hashkes PJ. *Pediatric Rheumatology in Clinical Practice.* 2nd ed. Springer-Verlag; 2016:241-255.
9. Dubin A, Patapoutian A. Nociceptors: the sensors of the pain pathway. *J Clin Invest.* 2010;120(11):3760-3772.
10. Marinus J, Lorimer Moseley G, Birklein F, et al. Clinical features and pathophysiology of complex regional pain syndrome. *Lancet Neurol.* 2011;10:637-648.

11. Hoffart C, Wallace D. Amplified pain syndromes in children: treatment and new insights into disease pathogenesis. *Curr Opin Rheumatol.* 2014;26:592-603.

12. Weissmann R, Uziel Y. Pediatric complex regional pain syndrome: a review. *Pediatr Rheumatol.* 2016;14(29):1-10.

13. Landry B, Fischer P, Driscoll S, et al. Managing chronic pain in children and adolescents: a clinical review. *PM&R.* 2015;7(11): S295-S315.

14. Sanctis V, Abbasciano V, Soliman A, et al. The juvenile fibromyalgia syndrome (JFMS): a poorly defined disorder. *Acta Biomed.* 2019;90(1):134-148.

15. Harden NR, Bruehl S, Perez RS, et al. Validation of proposed diagnostic criteria (the "Budapest Criteria") for Complex Regional Pain Syndrome. *Pain.* 2010;150(2):268-274.

16. Bruehl S. An update on the pathophysiology of complex regional pain syndrome. *Anesthesiology.* 2010;113(3):713-725.

17. Abu-Arafeh H, Abu-Arafeh I. Complex regional pain syndrome in children: incidence and clinical characteristics. *Arch Dis Child.* 2016;101:719-723.

18. Sherry DD, Malleson P. The idiopathic musculoskeletal pain syndromes in childhood. *Rheum Dis Clin North Am.* 2002;28: 669-685.

19. Tian F, Guittar P, Moore-Clingenpeel M, et al. Healthcare use patterns and economic burden of chronic musculoskeletal pain in children before diagnosis. *J Pediatr.* 2018;197:172-176.

20. Caes L, Fisher E, Clinch J, et al. Current evidence-based interdisciplinary treatment options for pediatric musculoskeletal pain. *Curr Treatm Opt Rheumatol.* 2018;4:223-234.

21. Clinch J, Eccleston C. Chronic musculoskeletal pain children: assessment and management. *Rheumatology.* 2009;48:466-474.

22. Sorensen K, Chritiansen B. Adolescents' experience of complex persistent pain. *Scand J Pain.* 2016;15:106-112.

23. Maracle E, Hung L, Fell S, et al. A comparison of the sensitivity of brush allodynia and Semmes-Weinstein Monofilament Testing in the detection of allodynia within regions of secondary hyperalgesia in humans. *Pain Pract.* 2017;17(1):16-24.

24. Guite J, Sherry D, Jarvis E, et al. Medication use among pediatric patients with chronic musculoskeletal pain syndromes at initial pain clinic evaluation. *Pain Manag.* 2018;8(1):15-25.

25. Rodriguez M, Fernandez-Baena M, Barroso A, et al. Invasive management for pediatric complex regional pain syndrome: literature review of evidence. *Pain Physician.* 2015;18:621-630.

26. Pons T, Shipton EA, Williman J, et al. A proposed clinical conceptual model for the physiotherapy management of complex regional pain syndrome (CRPS). *Musculoskelet Sci Pract.* 2018;38:15-22.

27. Sherry DD, Brake L, Tress J, et al. The treatment of juvenile fibromyalgia with an intensive physical and psychosocial program. *J Pediatr.* 2015;167(3):731-737.

28. Rabin J, Brown M, Alexander S. Update in the treatment of chronic pain within pediatric patients. *Curr Probl Pediatr Adolesc Health Care.* 2018;47(7):167-172.

29. Logan DE, Carpino E, Chiang G, et al. A day-hospital approach to pediatric complex regional pain syndrome: initial functional outcomes. *Clin J Pain.* 2012;28(9):2-22.

30. Miro J, Castarlenas E, de la Vega R, et al. Pain catastrophizing, activity engagement as and pain willingness as predictors of the benefits of multidisciplinary cognitive behaviorally-based chronic pain treatment. *J Behav Med.* 2018;41:827-835.

31. Michaleff ZA, Kamper SJ, Maher CG, et al. Low back pain in children and adolescents: a systematic review and meta-analysis evaluating the effectiveness of conservative interventions. *Eur Spine J.* 2014;23:2046-2058.

32. Chatzitheodorou D, Kabitsis C, Malliou P, et al. A pilot study of the effects of high-intensity aerobic exercise vs. passive interventions on pain, disability, psychological strain, and serum cortisol concentration in people with chronic low back pain. *Phys Ther.* 2007;87:304-312.

33. Simons L, Logan D, Chastain L, et al. Engagement in multidisciplinary interventions for pediatric chronic pain: parental expectations, barriers, and childhood outcomes. *Clin J Pain.* 2010;26:291-299.

34. Low AK, Ward K, Wines AP. Pediatric complex regional pain syndrome. *J Pediatr Orthop.* 2007;27(5):567-572.

35. Gmuca S, Xiao R, Weiss P, et al. Opiod prescribing and polypharmacy in children with chronic musculoskeletal pain. *Pain Med.* 2019;20(3):495-503.

36. Katholi B, Daghstani S, Banez G, et al. Noninvasive treatments for pediatric complex regional pain syndrome: a focused review. *PM&R.* 2014;6:926-933.

37. Popkirov S, Hoeritzauer I, Colvin L, et al. Complex regional pain syndrome and functional neurological disorders—time for reconciliation. *J Neurol Neurosurg Psychiatry.* 2019;90:608-614.

38. Walker LS, Williams SE, Smith CA, et al. Parent attention vs distraction: impact on symptom complaints by children with and without chronic functional abdominal pain. *Pain.* 2006;122(1-2):43-52.

39. Black WR, Kashikar-Zuck S. Exercise interventions for juvenile fibromyalgia: current state and recent advancements. *Pain Manag.* 2014;7(3):143-148.

40. Kashikar-Zuck S, Black WR, Pfeiffer M. Pilot randomized trial of integrated cognitive-behavioral therapy and neuromuscular training for juvenile fibromyalgia: the FIT Teens program. *J Pain.* 2018;19(9):1049-1062.

41. Lee BH, Scharff L, Sethna NF, et al. Physical therapy and cognitive-behavioral treatment for complex regional pain syndromes. *J Pediatr.* 2002;141(1):135-140.

42. Lynch-Jordan AM, Sil S, Peugh J, et al. Differential changes in functional disability and pain intensity over the course of psychological treatment for children with chronic pain. *Pain.* 2014;155(10):1955-1961.

43. Kashikar-Zuck S, Sil S, Lynch-Jordan AM, et al. Changes in pain coping, catastrophizing, and coping efficacy after cognitive-behavioral therapy in children and adolescents with juvenile fibromyalgia. *J Pain.* 2013;14(5):492-501.

44. Fisher E, Keogh E, Eccleston C. Adolescent's approach-avoidance behaviour in the context of pain. *Pain.* 2016;157(2):370-376.

45. Crombez G, Eccleston C, Damme SV, et al. Fear-avoidance model of chronic pain: the next generation. *Clin J Pain.* 2012;28(6):475-483.

46. Urits I, Hubble A, Peterson E, et al. An update on cognitive therapy for the management of chronic pain: a comprehensive review. *Curr Pain Headache Rep.* 2019;23(8):57.

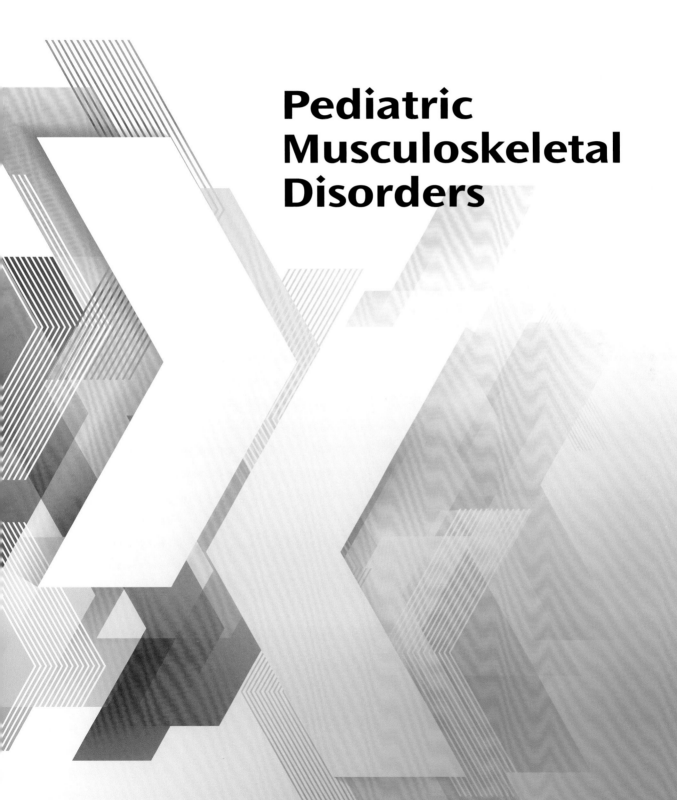

Pediatric Musculoskeletal Disorders

IV

Pediatric Musculoskeletal Disorders

Orthopedic Conditions

Karen A. Josefyk and Jessica Laniak

Chapter Outline

» Introduction

The term *orthopedics* in pediatric physical therapy is often used to refer to a specific group of pediatric diagnoses. Within the profession of physical therapy, *orthopedics* refers to a subspecialty of practice. As the profession has increased its focus on specialization and board certification, pediatric orthopedics has begun to emerge as a subspecialty within a specialty. Many pediatric medical professionals have a tendency to compartmentalize their profession and the children they see by body systems, such as children with orthopedic disabilities or children with neurologic disabilities. This practice lends itself to specialization or the development of clinical expertise in a well-defined area. However, this practice may also fragment the care of children and even the thinking of the professionals involved treating those children.

The various systems of the body are intertwined, and normal or atypical influences on one system almost always have an impact on other body systems. This is especially true of a young child whose musculoskeletal system is immature and susceptible to external and internal influences. The action of muscles working within a normal neurologic system is necessary for the development of joints and the shape and contour of a child's bones. When the neurologic or muscular systems are altered or impaired, secondary skeletal impairments often develop.

This chapter discusses the growth and development of a child's musculoskeletal system and pediatric musculoskeletal examination. It also introduces a classification system based on morphogenesis as well as provides an overview of pediatric orthopedic diagnoses commonly encountered by pediatric physical therapists. It is important to remember that the effects of normal and atypical forces on an immature musculoskeletal system and the secondary impairments that may develop, as well as the discussion of the components of a pediatric musculoskeletal examination, can be applied to many children seen in pediatric physical therapy. For example, most children with a primary diagnosis of neurologic origin will present with impairments of their musculoskeletal system that may impact their overall function.

» Musculoskeletal development

The initial formation of the musculoskeletal system occurs during the embryonic period (second to eighth week post conception). This system develops sequentially and follows a specific outline that is defined by the earliest embryonic or germinal layers. The limb buds arise from mesenchymal cells and appear during the fourth week, with the upper limb developing 2 days ahead of the lower limb. Mesenchymal cells begin to differentiate into cartilage within 4 to 5 days of the formation of the limb bud. The formation of a cartilaginous skeletal template occurs rapidly and is completed during the first fetal month (3 months from conception). The cartilaginous template then begins to be replaced by bone with the appearance of primary ossification centers in the diaphysis of the long bones. Secondary ossification centers appear near the end of fetal development and remain until puberty, when skeletal growth is complete.[1,2]

The initiation of joint formation begins as the cartilaginous template is being formed. An area of flattened undifferentiated cells forms between two areas of cartilage. The flattened area transforms into three layers, and the peripheral layers maintain contact with the cartilage and eventually become the joint capsule. The middle layer cavitates and forms the joint cavity. The original cartilage at the interface of the joint capsule remains and becomes the articular cartilage.[1,2]

The developing musculoskeletal system is vulnerable to external influence at various stages of its pre- and postnatal development. The extremities are susceptible to major morphologic abnormalities during the embryonic period when the limb buds are developing. For example, exposure of the embryo to pharmacologic agents while the limb buds are forming may result in congenital limb deficiencies. During the fetal period, structures increase in size, and cartilage begins to be replaced by bone formation; however, minimal bone remodeling occurs. During this time, the fetus is more susceptible to minor morphologic abnormalities that are the result of position constraints and abnormal mechanical forces.[2] For example, torticollis or clubfeet may result from position constraints late in the pregnancy. Postnatally, bone remodeling occurs at a rapid rate of 50% annually in the infant and toddler and gradually slows to the adult rate of 5% annually.

There are two types of bone growth that are present in a growing child, bone growth in length and bone growth in diameter. Bone grows in length through the continuation of the process of endochondral ossification begun during the fetal period. *Endochondral ossification* is often referred to as epiphyseal growth because longitudinal growth occurs at the epiphyseal plate. Increases in the diameter of bone or bone thickness occur through appositional growth or the laying down of new bone on top of old bone. These two types of bone growth respond differently to mechanical loading and the forces associated with weight bearing and muscle pull. Appositional bone growth is stimulated by increased compressive forces. Increased weight bearing results in increased thickness and density of the shaft of long bones.[3,4] However, decreased weight bearing, as seen with immobilization, results in atrophy of the bone.[3]

The response of epiphyseal growth to mechanical forces is dependent on the direction, magnitude, and timing of the force. Intermittent compressive forces applied parallel to the direction of growth cause longitudinal bone growth; however, constant compressive forces of excessive or high magnitude retard bone growth.[5] A compressive force may be applied unevenly across the physis, resulting in slowing of growth on one side only. The uneven growth produces an angulation of the physis and changes the direction of growth.[3] Mechanical loads or forces that are applied perpendicular to the longitudinal growth of the bone result in a change of direction or deflection of bone growth. New growth is deflected and results in displacement of the epiphysis if the load is maintained. A torsional stress to the physis deflects columns of cartilage around the circumference of the physis in either a clockwise or a counterclockwise direction. New bone then grows away from the physis in a spiral pattern, resulting in a torsional deformity.

In summary, the growth and development of the musculoskeletal system is dependent on the normal interplay of multiple factors, including hormones, nutrition, and mechanical forces.[5,6] The immature musculoskeletal system is vulnerable to abnormal mechanical forces and pressures; alterations in the timing, direction, or magnitude of forces may have a deleterious effect on the growing and developing musculoskeletal system. Congenital deformities and secondary musculoskeletal impairments that are seen in children with or without neurologic diagnoses are examples of the vulnerability of the immature musculoskeletal system to abnormal extrinsic forces. However, the immaturity of a child's musculoskeletal system can also be an advantage and is often used as the rationale for many treatment interventions that will be discussed throughout this chapter.

>> Musculoskeletal examination

A thorough musculoskeletal examination should be part of a comprehensive evaluation of a child seen by a physical therapist. Depending on the history or diagnosis, certain aspects of the musculoskeletal examination should be performed, whereas other aspects may be omitted. However, for those children with a diagnosis that includes multiple joint or system involvement, a complete musculoskeletal examination should be performed, beginning as a postural screen with a more in-depth examination dependent on the findings of the initial screening. The examination should be completed in a timely and organized manner in the order outlined in the following sections. The order may be altered depending on the comfort and interaction of the child.

History

A thorough history should be obtained from the caregivers and the child if the child is able to convey the information to the examiner. The history should include information about onset of the presenting complaint; whether pain is present; what aggravates or alleviates the pain; any changes in alignment, activity, or participation noted; and a comparison with normal routines. While talking with the parents, the physical therapist should be observing the child's posture, play, spontaneous movements, and activities relating to the child's posture, noted asymmetries, and difficulty with age-appropriate skills. For older children, questions regarding sexual maturation, including Tanner staging for males and females as well as age at onset of menstruation should be considered to provide information related to bone age and development.[7]

Postural Screen

During the postural screen, the therapist examines skeletal alignment in a variety of positions, including anterior, posterior, and sagittal views, depending on the age of the child. This process should include head, spinal, and lower extremity alignment, limb length, and upper extremity position. These are best completed with good visualization of the area being examined, which can be accomplished by wearing a bathing suit to examine the torso and pelvis and removing bracing and shoes from the lower extremities. The therapist evaluates torso posture for typical upright head, cervical lordosis, thoracic kyphosis, lumbar lordosis, pectus excavatum or carinatum, and anterior or posterior pelvic tilt relative to the age of the child from a sagittal view. From the posterior view, the physical therapist visually notes symmetry of shoulder, scapulae, pelvic height, and lateral rib asymmetries, such as a rib hump, that would indicate a rotational deformity of the spine. An anterior view can help identify asymmetries in nipple height, lateral rib position, and pelvic height.

Lower extremity alignment should also be screened from an anterior, posterior, and sagittal view. The therapist looks at symmetry of pelvic height; rotational variations of the lower extremities, such as the knees or feet pointing in or out; and a valgus or varus position of the knees, forefoot, or hindfoot. From a sagittal view, the physical therapist examines pelvic position and alignment of the hip, knee, and ankle.

Limb length should be reviewed in both a weight-bearing and non-weight-bearing position using the accepted bony landmarks of the anterior superior iliac spine and the medial malleolus. The posterior superior iliac spine may also be included to determine the presence of innominate bone rotation. On the basis of the postural screen, the physical therapist will know where to focus the next portion of a more in-depth musculoskeletal examination.

Range of Motion

Although the goniometric techniques used to measure active or passive joint range of motion (ROM) in children and adults are similar, several factors must be kept in mind when evaluating ROM in children. Age-related differences exist in ROM values between adults and an infant or skeletally immature child. The knowledge of the child's skeletal development stage as well as any anticipated environmental or positional postures will assist the physical therapist in identifying whether the ROM is appropriate or abnormal. For example,

a full-term newborn will exhibit flexion contractures of the hips and knees secondary to intrauterine positioning.

Before any goniometric measurement is taken, it must be ensured that the child is relaxed and remains calm. The therapist's movements of the child should be slow and deliberate so as to limit anxiety and to avoid eliciting a stretch reflex in children with increased muscle tone or guarding postures. This also applies if pain is present or suspected and for those children who may have more brittle bones or recent injuries. Giving examples of what ROM looks and feels like to the child on their uninvolved extremity first or allowing them to explore and play with the therapist's tools used for measurement will encourage the child to be more compliant with the examination.

Reliability studies of goniometry in children should guide physical therapists in their use of goniometric measures to document ROM. Several researchers have investigated the reliability of goniometric measurement of the hip, knee, and ankle of children with cerebral palsy. High intrarater reliability was present in those studies, but interrater reliability was variable from moderate to high throughout the studies.[8–11] Improved reliability is observed with strict measurement protocols and when the same therapist measures changes in ROM over time.

Muscle length tests that focus on flexibility should also be included in the overall joint motion examination. Specific tests and their procedures do not differ from standard procedures used with the adult population. Hip flexor muscle length is examined using the Thomas test or the prone hip extension test. Hamstring length is usually examined in adults using the straight leg raise test; however, the popliteal angle (PA) measurement is commonly used in pediatrics (Fig. 15.1). The PA measurement can be used in the presence of a knee flexion contracture; therefore, it is useful for children who present with involvement of multiple joints.[12] Ankle dorsiflexion should be measured with the knee flexed and extended to determine soleus and gastrocnemius contributions to limitations. Care should be taken to maintain subtalar joint neutral

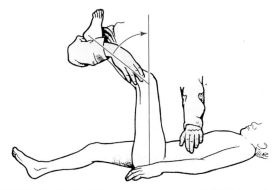

FIGURE 15.1. Popliteal angle measurement. Child is supine, hip is flexed to −90 degrees, and the knee is slowly extended until resistance is felt. The angle between the anterior aspect of the lower leg and a vertical line corresponding to the thigh is recorded as a measure of hamstring contracture.

during the measurement to minimize midfoot dorsiflexion contributing to an overestimated hindfoot measurement.

Overall joint mobility should be measured using techniques such as the Beighton score to determine the presence of generalized joint hypermobility.[13]

Strength

An accurate examination of strength requires careful consideration in the pediatric population but yields important information regarding deficits and changes over time. A variety of methods to examine strength are available, and their use may depend on the age and ability of the child. For infants and children younger than 3 or 4 years, examination of strength is most often accomplished through observation of movement, developmental skill achievement, and age-appropriate functional skill evaluation. An example of functional strength evaluation would be observing whether or not a child is able to transfer from the floor to standing through half-kneel on both sides. Compensatory movement, poor dynamic alignment, or asymmetric movement between sides may be indicative of muscle weakness.

A child must be able to follow the directions of the testing procedure to ensure accurate results using either manual muscle testing (MMT) or dynamometry.[14] Strength may also be reliably measured using isokinetic machines with some positioning modification to accommodate for small size or the use of pediatric extremity attachments, as seen in the Biodex System 4.[15,16]

MMT has the same inherent weaknesses with the pediatric population as with the adult population. The grades of "good" and "normal" are very subjective and do not account for any changes that may occur in a child over time, secondary to maturation. Isometric handheld dynamometry (HHD) has been found to be a reliable and sensitive method of measuring strength in various populations of children.[15–17] Gajdosik determined that HHD could be used reliably with typical developing children between 2 and 5 years old as long as they could follow the directions and understand the command to push as well as agree to participate in the process.[18] Hébert et al. have established normative reference values for isometric testing using HHD of both the upper and lower limb in children 4 to 17 years old, which can be a helpful reference tool.[19] Therapist training and standardized procedures for completing HHD must be established and followed for reliability to be established.

Strength may also be reliably measured using isokinetic machines with some positioning modification to accommodate for small size or the use of pediatric extremity attachments, as seen in the Biodex System 4.[20,21] Normative and percentile values for isokinetic knee extension and flexion strength have been published by multiple authors for children aged 6 to 13 years.[22,23] The normative data that is presented in the literature are usually determined from testing typically developing children, and the physical therapist should take care to compare those measurements with children who have an atypical neurologic system. Along with functional performance, these strength measures provide additional objective data to consider when determining a child's readiness to return to recreational or competitive sports.

Lower Extremity Alignment (Rotational and Angular)

Normal skeletal development includes rotational or torsional and angular changes of bones and joints. Any therapist working with children will need to develop an understanding of the timeline for these structural milestones. This knowledge is imperative to determine whether the child's alignment is typical or atypical for the child's age. These normal developmental processes may then be altered secondary to injury, abnormal muscle pull or weight-bearing forces. Consequently, the result of the abnormal forces on a developing skeletal system often creates alterations in typical alignment that have the potential to create impairment in functional skill and development. The bones remain susceptible to deforming forces until growth is complete; therefore, the impairments may increase in severity over time.

Rotational Profile

Many children with orthopedic and neurologic diagnoses in pediatrics can present with a variation of lower extremity rotational profile. The understanding of the rotational presentation in a typical development structure is essential to then be able to analyze the congenital diagnoses that may be superimposed on that structure. Rotational profile is always prominent in planning for operative procedures and can be assisted with computed tomography (CT) or radiographs as well.[24] The static alignment will then need to be compared with the gait evaluation to see how the child functions.

Staheli et al. have developed a rotational profile to assess lower extremity alignment in a clinic setting and assist in determining which component of the lower extremity contributes to the rotational variation. The rotational profile consists of six measurements: (1) foot progression angle (FPA), (2) medial rotation of the hip, (3) lateral rotation of the hip, (4) thigh–foot angle (TFA), (5) angle of the transmalleolar axis (TMA), and (6) configuration of the foot. Normal values have been established for the first five measurements and can be used to determine whether the variation falls within the wide range of normal or whether intervention is indicated.[25] The procedures listed in the following sections assist the clinician in identifying the contributing factors to the overall rotational profile of the child.

FOOT PROGRESSION ANGLE The *FPA* is defined as the angle between the longitudinal axis of the foot and the line of progression of the child's gait. This is not to be confused with the TFA, which will be discussed later. The FPA provides an overall summation of the child's rotation during gait but does not identify the contributing factors. A positive sign denotes out-toeing, and a negative sign in-toeing. The FPA can be measured objectively using a variety of footprint measures, including ink or chalk on the feet or more expensive commercially available gait mats. Often in the clinic, the FPA is administered subjectively to give the clinician an overall view of the child's rotation during gait (Fig. 15.2A).

HIP ROTATION Medial and lateral hip rotation in prone are measured in order to determine femoral torsion. Femoral torsion is the rotation of the femoral shaft on the neck of the femur. The child is in prone with hips in neutral and knees flexed to 90 degrees, and medial and lateral hip rotation measurements are then taken with a goniometer. Soft tissue limitations may influence the final measure of hip rotation as well as the degree of femoral torsion. Normal medial hip rotation is less than 60 to 65 degrees (Fig. 15.2B and C).

The literature also describes a test to determine the degree of femoral torsion referred to as the *Ryder method* in some resources as well as the *Craig test* in others. The child lies prone with knees flexed to 90 degrees at the edge of a table. The greater trochanter is palpated while rotating the leg. When the greater trochanter is palpated most laterally, which should correspond to the femoral neck being parallel to the examining table, the angle of hip rotation (typically medial) is measured with a goniometer. The measure of medial hip rotation should correspond to the degree of femoral anteversion, although data compared with CT suggest that the test may underestimate the measurement by up to 20 degrees.[8,26]

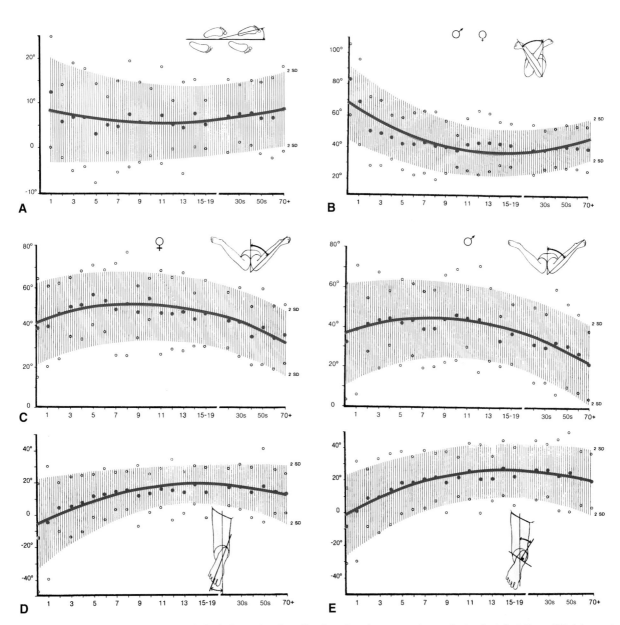

FIGURE 15.2.   The five measurements in Staheli rotational profile plotted as the mean values ±2 standard deviations (SDs) for each of the age groups. The dark line indicates the mean values as they change with age, and the shaded areas indicate the normal ranges. **A:** Foot progression angle (FPA). **B:** Lateral rotation of the hip in males and females. **C:** Medial rotation of the hip in females and males (separate). **D:** Thigh–foot angle (TFA). **E:** Angle of the transmalleolar axis.

THIGH–FOOT ANGLE The *TFA* is defined as the angle that exists between lines that bisect the longitudinal axis of the thigh and the longitudinal axis of the foot. The child is in the prone position with the hips in neutral flexion/extension, the knee flexed to 90 degrees, and the foot in a natural resting position. There should not be an attempt to align the foot. The stationary arm of the goniometer is positioned along the axis of the thigh with the fulcrum at the center of the heel; the movement arm is then directed along the axis of the foot, and the angle is measured. This TFA is used to determine rotational variation of the tibia and the hindfoot. If the foot is in an out-toeing position, the value is positive; if the foot is in an in-toeing position, the value is negative (Fig. 15.2D).

TRANSMALLEOLAR AXIS The TMA is a measure of torsion of the tibia compared with the frontal plane of the lower leg. The child is positioned in prone, as previously described with the hip in neutral and knee flexed to 90 degrees. A line perpendicular to the axis between the lateral and the medial malleoli is established. The angle formed between this perpendicular line and a line established through the medial and lateral condyles of the femur is measured. This angle examines the contribution of the distal tibia to the rotational profile (Fig. 15.2E).

CONFIGURATION OF THE FOOT The contribution of the foot must also be included and considered when examining rotational variations. Identifying the alignment of the hindfoot and forefoot in subtalar joint neutral will determine whether hindfoot or forefoot varus or valgus deviations, hindfoot equinus with midtarsal hypermobility, or metatarsus adductus is contributing to the FPA. Consideration should be made in determining the variations in presentation of the foot when comparing alignment in weight-bearing or non-weight-bearing positions.

Angular Alignment

If the initial postural screening revealed suspected lower extremity alignment deviations, such as a varus or valgus posture, an objective angular measurement should be performed. Expected values for genu varus and valgus will differ depending on the age of the child. Genu varum is measured with the child in supine with legs extended and the patella facing upward and the medial malleoli touching. The distance between the femoral condyles is measured. Genu valgum is measured in the same position but with the knees touching. The distance between the malleoli is measured.[27] The contribution of angular variations must be delineated from rotational variations.

Muscle Tone, Sensation, Developmental Skills

Additional areas that may be included in the musculoskeletal evaluation include examination of muscle tone, sensation testing, and developmental skill level. An examination of muscle tone may reveal hypertonicity or hypotonicity of specific muscle groups and an imbalance of muscle forces around specific joints. These unbalanced muscle forces may produce changes in the alignment of the body and could cause impairments over time that result in pain or interfere with the child's functional abilities.

Sensation testing is performed with children just as with adults and incorporates the same rationale for inclusion of testing. Sensory testing is indicated when nerve involvement is suspected, such as with fractures or after an amputation or application of an external fixator.

Evaluation of a child's developmental level is indicated if the orthopedic condition is suspected of delaying or interfering with motor development. Developmental skills can be evaluated through general clinical observation as well as standardized testing (both criterion- and norm-referenced tools). Alterations in functional strength and alignment can become more apparent and further focus testing and plan of care. For the ambulatory child, the developmental evaluation also includes an examination of gait. Observing gait is an excellent opportunity to evaluate how the static alignment measurements obtained with the previous testing interact with function and movement. Gait evaluation is similar to that of an adult and can be performed through systematic clinical observation or with more objective measures, ranging from video analysis to an instrumented gait laboratory. The age of the child must be considered when examining gait, and knowledge of the characteristics of early walking must be incorporated into the evaluation.

» Classification of errors of morphologic development

The terminology adopted by the World Health Organization's (WHO) International Classification of Functioning, Disability, and Health (ICF)[28] will be utilized in this chapter when discussing various diagnoses and their impact on the functional ability of the child. The ICF model also includes environmental and personal factors that will differ from one child to another and are unrelated to the child's diagnosis or health condition but may impact his or her activity or participation levels.

To illustrate the ICF model, a child with osteogenesis imperfecta (OI) will be used as an example. For a child with OI, the pathophysiology is the abnormality in the connective tissue at the cellular level. One of the impairments that results is fragile bones susceptible to deforming forces and fracture. The child may sustain multiple lower extremity fractures that result in misalignment, short stature, weakness, and a slow labored gait. The slow labored gait is an activity limitation that may hinder the child from keeping up with his or her peers during play or at school. Participation restrictions may include not permitting the child to attend a day care with age-matched peers or to play outside at recess owing to a fear of increased risk of fractures.

Environmental factors such as a teacher's fear or a crowded recess area may have contributed to the child's ability to participate.

Spranger's classification of morphogenesis will also be used to introduce and discuss a multitude of diagnoses that fall under the category of pediatric orthopedics. This classification system provides a framework within which to understand the pathophysiology resulting in a particular diagnosis, the impairments that may develop as the child grows, the impact of the impairments on the child's activities and participation levels, and the role of physical therapy. An understanding of the pathophysiology enables one to identify impairments that may be present or that may develop and the impact of physical therapy on preventing or limiting the impairments, with the ultimate goal of minimizing the activity limitations and participation restrictions for the child.

Spranger's classification of disorders of morphogenesis consists of four divisions: malformations, disruptions, deformations, and dysplasias.[29] Malformations are morphologic defects of an organ or body part from an intrinsically abnormal developmental process. Because the abnormality is intrinsic from the moment of conception, the organ or body part never had the potential to develop normally. Longitudinal limb deficiencies are an orthopedic example of malformations, whereas other examples would include cleft lip and palate as well as septal defects of the heart.[29]

Disruptions are morphologic defects of an organ or body part resulting from the extrinsic breakdown of an originally normal developmental process. Normal development is interrupted at the cellular level by an external factor such as a teratogen, trauma, or infection. Transverse limb deficiencies historically seen with the use of thalidomide or as seen with amniotic band syndrome are an example of a disruption.[29]

Deformations are abnormalities in form, shape, or position of a body part caused by mechanical forces. The deforming forces may be extrinsic to the fetus, such as intrauterine constraint, or intrinsic to the fetus, such as fetal hypomobility resulting from a neuromuscular defect. Examples of deformations include torticollis, metatarsus adductus, and clubfoot. Deformations can be delineated into prenatal and postnatal deformities versus pathologic processes. Examples of postnatal deformities include tibial varum or Blount disease and rotational variations. Pathologic processes are usually deformities resulting from an insult to the physis or other area of the bone. These processes include the diagnoses of Legg–Calvé–Perthes disease, slipped capital femoral epiphysis, and limb length discrepancies resulting from insults or abnormal forces to the growth plate. Deformations can often be ameliorated with the application of forces in the opposite direction of the deforming mechanism through medical and therapeutic management. The application of forces must be timed correctly with expected maturation of the musculoskeletal system to allow for normal growth and remodeling to occur.[29]

The final division in Spranger's classification is dysplasia. Dysplasias result from an abnormal organization of cells into tissues, leading to abnormal tissue differentiation. OI and Ehlers Danlos Syndrome (EDS) are examples of dysplasias. Dysplasias usually involve whole systems of the body with multiple impairments present that will lead to activity limitations and possibly participation restrictions.[29]

» Malformations and disruptions: congenital limb deficiencies

Using the International Society for Prosthetics and Orthotics (ISPO) classification system, congenital limb deficiencies are described as either longitudinal or transverse (Fig. 15.3A and B).[30] Longitudinal limb deficiencies are described as reduction or absence of an element or elements within the long axis of the limb. There may be normal skeletal elements distal to the affected bone or bones.[30] A longitudinal limb deficiency is an example of a malformation in which a morphologic defect of an organ or larger region of the body occurs when normal organogenesis is interrupted. Any combination of skeletal limb involvement is possible, but certain distinct entities are more commonly seen than others. For this chapter, congenital longitudinal deficiency of the radius, also referred to as *radial club hand*, will be used as an example of upper extremity involvement and proximal femoral focal deficiency (PFFD) as an example of a lower extremity longitudinal limb deficiency. Both are examples of congenital malformations and are more frequent in their incidence. These diagnoses are also examples of children with limb deficiencies that are typically seen by therapists.

Longitudinal deficiency of the radius is the most common upper extremity limb deformity. There are reports of variable incident rates for this diagnosis, showing anything from 5.25 per 10,000 to 1 per 100,000 live births.[31] A radial deficiency presents 67% of the time with a medical or musculoskeletal anomaly such as hematologic abnormalities, cardiac, or renal diagnosis.[32] *Radial deficiencies* can be defined as the failure of formation of parts or deficiencies on the radial side of the upper extremity, including the radius, carpals, metacarpals, and phalanges of the first ray and thenar musculature.[33,34] Heikel as well as Bayne & Klug classified radial deficiencies into four types, ranging in severity from type I (consisting of delayed appearance of the distal radial physis) to type IV (involving complete absence of the radius).[35,36] Type IV is the most common presentation.[27,37] Clinically, children with type IV radial deficiency present with a shortened forearm of no greater than 50% of the length of the contralateral forearm, an elbow extension contracture, and radial deviation of the hand with an absent or deficient thumb. James et al. updated the classification of radial deficiency further, on the basis of six common presentations, ranging from hypoplasia of the thumb to absence of the radius and portions of the hand distal to the humerus.[37]

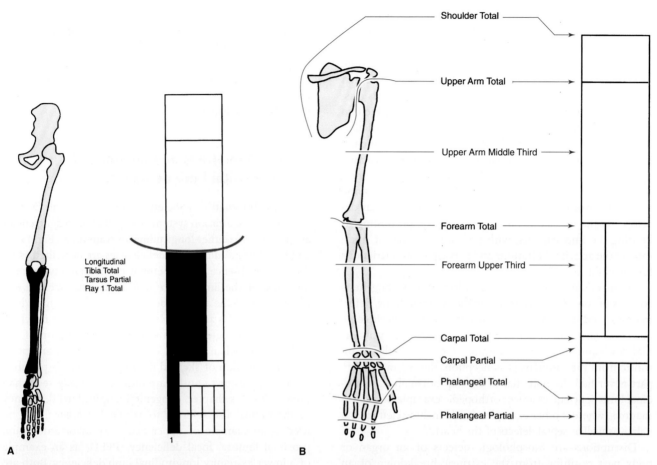

FIGURE 15.3. A: Example of a longitudinal deficiency of the lower extremity. **B:** Example of transverse deficiencies at various levels of the upper extremity.

The incidence of PFFD is 1 per 50,000 live births and is bilateral in 15% of children with PFFD.[38] Aitken first described and classified four classes of severity of PFFD, with class A exhibiting the least involvement and class D being the most severe (Fig. 15.4).[39] PFFD includes absence or hypoplasia of the proximal femur with varying degrees of involvement of the acetabulum, femoral head, patella, tibia, fibula, cruciate ligaments, and the foot. Clinically, infants with PFFD present with an abnormally short thigh held in hip flexion, abduction, and external rotation (Fig. 15.5). Hip and knee flexion contractures are often present along with anteroposterior instability of the knee and a significant leg length difference, with the foot of the involved leg often at the height of the opposite knee.

In comparison, in a child with transverse limb deficiencies, the limb develops normally up to a particular level, beyond which no skeletal elements exist.[30] Transverse limb deficiencies are an example of a disruption using Spranger's classification of morphogenesis and appear similar to a residual limb after surgical amputation. Most transverse deficiencies are unilateral, frequently occurring as a transverse forearm deficiency (Fig. 15.6).[33] This type of transverse deficiency occurs more frequently in females and exhibits a 2:1 left-sided predominance.[40]

Surgical and Nonsurgical Management of Congenital Limb Deficiencies

Children with longitudinal limb deficiencies often require multiple surgical procedures to obtain maximal function of the involved limb. Surgical procedures for the upper extremity may include tendon transfers, realignment or repositioning of the hand and/or fingers, and osteotomies. Surgical intervention for the lower extremity most commonly includes amputation, fusion, limb lengthening, limb and foot realignment, muscle and tendon lengthening, and osteotomies. Surgical correction is rarely required for children with transverse limb deficiencies, unless terminal limb shape causes prosthetic fit to be problematic or terminal bony overgrowth causes protrusion into soft tissues, resulting in pain and skin breakdown.

Upper Extremity: Longitudinal Radial Deficiency

Shortly after birth, the child's hand should be serially splinted or casted to stretch the shortened soft tissues and realign the hand as centrally as possible over the distal forearm. At the same time, therapy goals should also focus on increasing elbow ROM, especially elbow flexion.

TYPE		FEMORAL HEAD	ACETABULUM	FEMORAL SEGMENT	RELATIONSHIP AMONG COMPONENTS OF FEMUR AND ACETABULUM AT SKELETAL MATURITY
A		Present	Normal	Short	Bony connection between components of femur

Femoral head in acetabulum

Subtrochanteric varus angulation, often with pseudarthrosis |
| B | | Present | Adequate or moderately dysplastic | Short, usually proximal bony tuft | No osseous connection between head and shaft

Femoral head in acetabulum |
| C | | Absent or represented by ossicle | Severely dysplastic | Short, usually proximally tapered | May be osseous connection between shaft and proximal ossicle

No articular relation between femur and acetabulum |
| D | | Absent | Absent

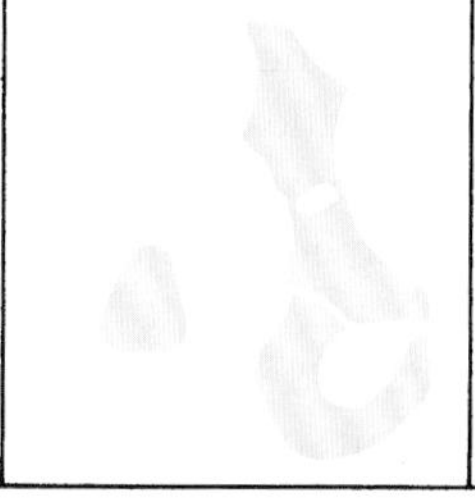

Obturator foramen enlarged

Pelvis squared in bilateral cases | Short, deformed | (none) |

FIGURE 15.4. Aitken classification of PFFD.

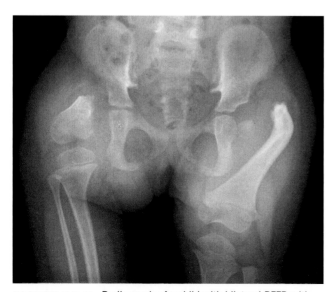

FIGURE 15.5. Radiograph of a child with bilateral PFFD with asymmetric involvement of each femur, tibia, and fibula.

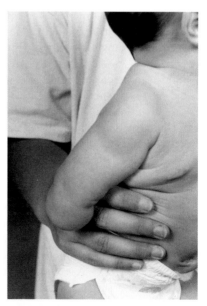

FIGURE 15.6. Child with congenital transverse below-elbow limb deficiency.

Stretching of the soft tissues is necessary before any surgical procedures. Between 6 months and 1 year of age, surgical centralization of the hand by an orthopedic surgeon is often performed. The goal of centralization is a stable wrist centered on the distal ulna while maintaining functional wrist motion.[36]

After the initial centralization procedures, the child's hand is splinted in the newly aligned position on the distal ulna. Compliance with wearing of the splint is crucial for long-term success of the surgical centralization. The splint should be worn throughout the day and night during the healing phase. After the initial healing phase is complete, a splint should be worn at night until skeletal maturity is achieved. By skeletal maturity, the ulna has undergone epiphyseal adaptation to accommodate the centralized carpus to ensure stability of the wrist position, no longer necessitating the use of a night splint.[36]

Centralization of the hand is contraindicated in older children or adolescents who have adapted to their hand position, when severe deformity of the hand is also present that would limit hand function and when elbow flexion is less than 90 degrees. Adequate elbow flexion is needed prior to surgery so that when the hand is realigned, the child can still bring his or her hand to the mouth.

Lower Extremity: Proximal Femoral Focal Deficiency

Surgical intervention for children with PFFD is varied, must be individualized, and can include any combination of amputation, reconstruction with pelvic and femoral osteotomy, fusion, or limb-lengthening procedures. Surgery addresses the unstable hip joint and the inequality of limb lengths, the two issues that interfere with the child's overall functional abilities. Many children require multiple surgical procedures; thought must be given early to develop a long-term surgical plan for family education and to condense surgeries into one procedure when possible. Surgery is generally not recommended for children with bilateral PFFD, because their limb length is equal or near equal and they are able to ambulate with or without extension prostheses.[27,41,42]

Surgical options can be divided into those that involve amputation and reconstruction for eventual prosthetic fitting and those that involve limb-lengthening and reconstruction techniques. Three typical surgical scenarios include foot amputation with proximal reconstruction, rotationplasty, and limb lengthening. Following foot amputation with proximal reconstruction, the child's limb resembles and functions as an above-knee amputation requiring prosthetic use and intervention. For children with unilateral involvement, using an extension prosthesis on an existing residual limb is a nonsurgical approach to treatment that has been found more satisfactory than amputation-type procedures.[43] A rotationplasty, or the turnabout procedure, is a surgical technique that allows

the child to function similarly to a child with a below-knee amputation. This complex procedure involves significant limb reconstruction, including 180-degree realignment of the lower leg. As a result, the child's ankle then functions as a knee joint, with ankle plantar flexion acting as knee extension and ankle dorsiflexion acting as knee flexion (Fig. 15.7).[27,44] Limb lengthening may be indicated when more than 60% of predicted femoral length is present[41,45] or the discrepancy in femoral length is predicted to be less than 15 cm. An in-depth description of limb-lengthening procedures is provided later in this chapter under the section "Limb Length Discrepancies."

Prior to any surgical intervention, physical therapy should be initiated in early infancy to improve ROM at the involved hip, promote developmental activities (including symmetry of skills and weight bearing at the age-appropriate times), and assist with the development of age-appropriate balance and transfer skills (Fig. 15.8).

Postoperatively, acute physical therapy interventions will depend on the procedure and will involve improving or maintaining ROM, strength, gait training with appropriate assistive device, splinting, positioning, balance, and prosthetic training. For example, following a rotationplasty, ROM and stretching activities of the ankle (now the functioning knee) are essential to ensure proper prosthesis movement and functional lower extremity alignment. Maximum plantar flexion range is needed to promote knee extension in the prosthesis. Sitting and other activities involving knee flexion will require close to 20 degrees of ankle dorsiflexion. Strengthening of these muscle groups is also important; ankle plantar flexion and dorsiflexion strength provide stability in stance and power the prosthesis during gait. Recent literature has reported good long-term functional and quality-of-life outcomes but with persistent gait deviations following rotationplasty procedures.[46]

» Prenatal deformations

According to Spranger's classification, deformations are normal responses of the tissue to abnormal mechanical forces that may be extrinsic or intrinsic to the fetus. Intrauterine constraint is an example of an extrinsic force, whereas fetal hypomobility secondary to a nervous system impairment such as myelomeningocele is an example of an intrinsic force. If the deforming force is removed, normal development or maturation of the body part would be expected to occur.

This section discusses congenital muscular torticollis (CMT) as an example of an extrinsic deformation and clubfeet as an example of either an extrinsic or intrinsic deformation. Both of these diagnoses may also have other causative factors; abnormal mechanical forces are only one of the possible contributing factors. Developmental dysplasia of the

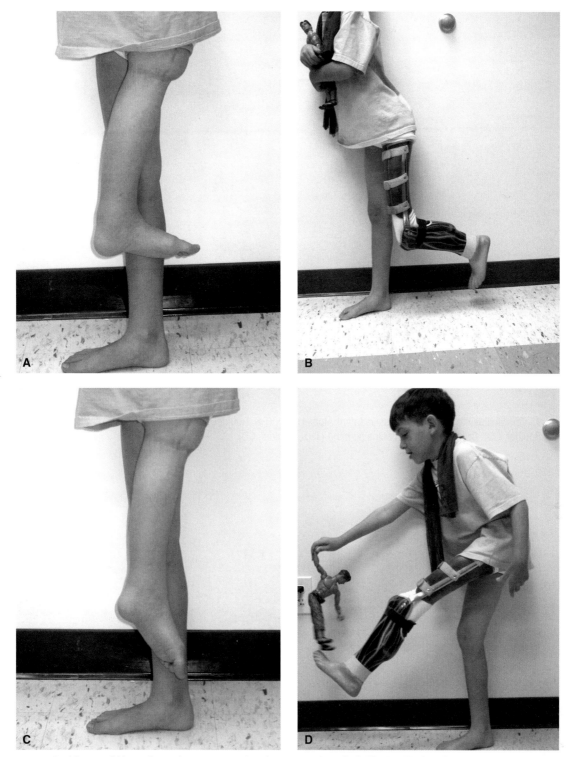

FIGURE 15.7. An 11-year-old boy who underwent a rotationplasty procedure. **A:** Ankle dorsiflexion. **B:** Ankle dorsiflexion produces prosthetic knee flexion. **C:** Ankle plantar flexion. **D:** Ankle plantar flexion produces prosthetic knee extension.

hip (DDH) is an example of a deformation that probably begins prenatally, continues to progress if the deforming forces are not altered, and may not be recognized until much later in postnatal life. Lastly, this section discusses arthrogryposis

as an example of an intrinsic deformation that begins very early in fetal development and consequently results in significant deformations at birth and throughout later life (Figs. 15.9 and 15.10).

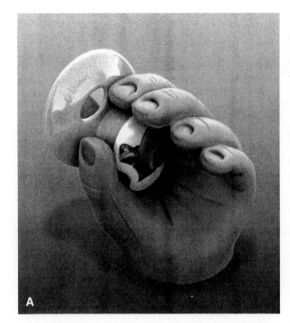
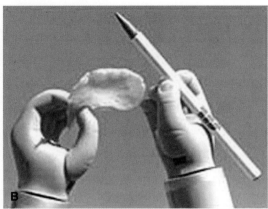
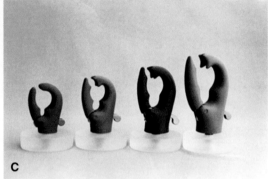

FIGURE 15.8. Terminal device options. **A:** Passive Infant Alpha Hand (TRS, Boulder, CO). **B:** L'il E-Z Hand promotes grasping when thumb is moved (TRS, Boulder, CO). **C:** ADEPT voluntary closing hand (TRS, Boulder, CO).

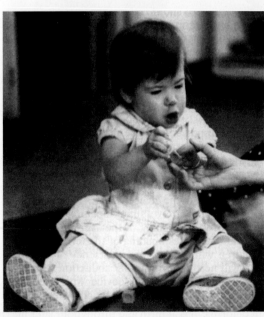

FIGURE 15.9. Child is wearing a left below-elbow prosthesis with an ADEPT voluntary closing hook. Therapist assisting child to operate the terminal device.

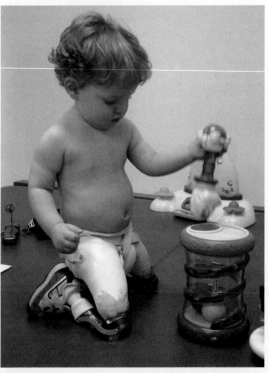

FIGURE 15.10. Toddler wearing bilateral transfemoral prosthesis with knee joint to promote age-appropriate ambulation skills and play activities on the floor.

Congenital Muscular Torticollis

The term *torticollis* comes from the Latin for twisted neck. CMT is a common diagnosis involving a unilateral shortening of the sternocleidomastoid (SCM) muscle. The infant with CMT typically presents with ipsilateral cervical lateral flexion toward the shortened SCM, resulting in a head tilt, with contralateral cervical rotation away from the shortened SCM. Cranial and facial asymmetry caused by plagiocephaly (flattening of the skull) often develop secondary to the persistent asymmetric positioning of the head. Table 15.1 summarizes the typical clinical presentation found in the head, neck, and face with CMT on each side. Although the SCM may be the primary muscle involved, secondary shortening of other cervical muscles such as scalenes, levator scapulae, or upper trapezius occurs (Fig. 15.11).

CMT is usually noted in the first 2 to 3 weeks after birth, with a reported incidence of 0.4% to 1.9%.[47] The etiology of CMT is uncertain. A mass or fibrotic pseudotumor can be observed or is palpable within the belly of the SCM muscle and appears within the first few weeks after birth and then gradually disappears. The exact cause of the fibrotic mass within the SCM muscle is not known. Researchers have hypothesized that occlusion of blood vessels with resultant anoxic injury to the SCM muscle may produce the fibrotic changes observed within the muscle. Intrauterine malposition and birth trauma have been hypothesized as causative factors.[48] Infants with CMT have a higher incidence of breech presentations[49] and associated congenital musculoskeletal diagnoses, such as hip dysplasia and foot deformities.[49,50]

Historically, authors have proposed that fibrosis of the SCM muscle is present in all children with CMT and ranges on a continuum of no palpable mass to a firm palpable mass.[49,50] Consequently, CMT is often classified into three clinical groups: (1) sternocleidomastoid tumor (SMT), when a definitive mass or tumor is palpable within the SCM muscle, (2) muscular torticollis (MT), when contracture of the SCM muscle is present but no palpable mass is present, and (3) positional torticollis (POST), when both contracture of

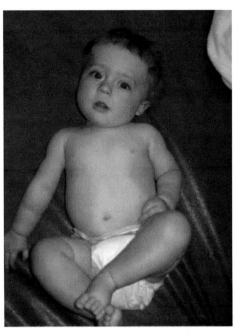

FIGURE 15.11. Infant with left congenital muscular torticollis. Note the facial asymmetry in the region of his mandible. (Used with permission from Taylor JL, Norton ES. Developmental muscular torticollis: outcomes in young children treated by physical therapy. *Pediatr Phys Ther*. 1997;9(4):173–178.)

the SCM muscle and a palpable mass are absent but the alteration in resting head position exists.[51,52]

The "Back to Sleep" program, initiated by the American Academy of Pediatrics in 1992 to reduce the incidence of sudden infant death syndrome (SIDS), recommended sleeping in supine for infants.[53] Since the inception of this program, SIDS rates have declined more than 50%, but the incidence of plagiocephaly and POST has increased dramatically.[54–56] The torticollis associated with positional plagiocephaly develops as a secondary impairment from the plagiocephaly. Not only can there be a difference in resting head position, but ROM restrictions can develop over time owing to positional shortening. This is the direct opposite of what is seen with CMT, where the plagiocephaly develops secondary to the persistent asymmetric positioning of the head because of the muscle imbalance. Ultimately, the treatment for POST would follow an approach very similar to that for other forms of CMT.

Most recently, in 2018, the American Physical Therapy Association (APTA) has developed and updated the first pediatric Clinical Practice Guideline (CPG). The first version of the CPG was published in 2013. This guideline describes and grades the severity of the torticollis on a scale of 1 to 8. In order to grade the severity, the CPG incorporates the age of the child when the condition was recognized, the age the child presents at the time of physical therapy evaluation, the degree of cervical ROM restriction, and whether or not there is a mass in the SCM. Best practice and first choice interventions are recommended on the basis of the most current and

TABLE 15.1.	Head and Neck Features of CMT	
Left SCM Torticollis		**Right SCM Torticollis**
Left	Cervical lateral flexion	Right
Right	Cervical rotation	Left
Right	Frontal bossing	Left
Right	Occipital flattening	Left
Left	Occipital bossing	Right
Left	Jaw retraction	Right
Right	Anterior ear shift	Left
Right	Anterior cheek and orbit displacement	Left

SCM, sternocleidomastoid muscle.

strongest level of research. Supplemental interventions are also described with reference to these standards.[57]

A full systems review and a developmental screen are vital during the initial examination to rule out nonmuscular causes of torticollis. Almost 20% of cases of torticollis involve a more serious underlying condition, so it is important to consider an expanded differential diagnosis.[58] Physician specialist collaboration and diagnostic imaging may be necessary to rule out atlantoaxial rotatory instability, hemivertebrae, cervical subluxation, posterior fossa tumors, Chiari malformations and other neurologic conditions, ocular and vestibular abnormalities, gastrointestinal disorders, and Grisel syndrome related to recurrent nasopharyngeal infection.

Conservative Management

Conservative management of CMT is generally recommended for infants aged 12 months and under. The CPG recognizes the complexity of older children presenting to physical therapy for the first time and encourages a team collaboration and referrals to other specialists for medical intervention if needed. According to the research compiled by the APTA, first choice intervention provided by a physical therapist includes cervical PROM, including prolonged passive stretching of the SCM muscle; active exercises to improve cervical and trunk ROM with subsequent strengthening exercises; and symmetric developmental activities (both passive and active) to correct the infant's head, neck, trunk, and extremity position. Teaching families how to add towel rolls to support a child in a midline position in a car seat would be an example of a passive activity. The final first choice intervention, consistent caregiver education and a home exercise program (HEP), is essential to success.[57]

Passive ROM and SCM stretching can be achieved through a variety of positioning and handling techniques.[49,50] Stretching should be gentle and low grade and gradually increase in duration to prevent microtrauma and further fibrosis.[52,59] Pain responses such as crying may indicate stretching intensity that is too high. Shoulder stabilization should be considered for the side of the involved SCM to address other cervical muscle involvement when stretching.

Active cervical ROM exercise, including rotation to the involved side, may be introduced in children younger than 3 to 4 months old who can visually track objects or respond to stimuli to attend to the involved side. For children older than 4 months, active cervical ROM and strengthening should also include via equilibrium and righting reactions[49,50] and developmental play promoting upper extremity weight bearing, weight shifting, and reaching. Intensity may be progressed by gradually increasing active head movement against gravity and duration or amount of unilateral upper extremity weight bearing during facilitation of play. Midline position for head and trunk should be emphasized as the child progresses from supine and prone skills through the transition to supported sitting, independent sitting, and standing. Neutral shoulder girdle alignment should also be promoted with progression from supported to independent prone, quadruped, and reaching activities.

A strong emphasis should be placed on caregiver education during each session, including time for observation and caregiver practice of HEP activities. *Tummy time* is the term used to encourage play in a prone position to facilitate active cervical movement and developmental play. Positional activities to promote active ipsilateral rotation, contralateral righting, midline head and trunk orientation as well as stretching recommendations should be addressed and incorporated into daily activities such as diaper changes, feeding, naps, play, and use of equipment such as car seats, infant swings, and feeding chairs. For example, caregivers who bottle-feed should be encouraged to do so on the side that promotes rotation to the involved side; gentle prolonged stretching may be better achieved while an infant is asleep.

The prognosis for creating a treatment plan and resolution of torticollis is guided by current research as well. Cheng reported and the CPG reinforces that the most important predictors of successful response to manual stretching and resolution of symptoms are the clinical group, neck rotation deficit, and age at initial presentation.[51] The POST type, neck rotation deficits of less than 15 degrees, and presentation at less than 1 month of age were associated with increased success of stretching protocols. Several other studies, including the literature compiled to create the CPG, have demonstrated the success of conservative management during the first year.[49,50,57,59] None of these studies included a control group who did not receive physical therapy intervention to assist with determining the extent of time and maturation on the resolution of the CMT. Multiple authors have suggested treatment strategy algorithms based on age and cervical ROM in order to improve outcomes and create consistency of care.[52,60]

Persistent facial asymmetry, intermittent head tilt with fatigue or illness, and functional asymmetry resembling hemiplegia but with a normal neurologic examination have been observed in children with full resolution, indicating the complexity of this disorder as well as possible long-lasting implications.[49]

Orthotic Devices

The treatment for plagiocephaly and torticollis should be addressed simultaneously. Head shape can impact the presentation and resolution of symptoms of torticollis. If repositioning techniques are not successful in the early treatment of plagiocephaly, the alterations in head shape can be treated with a cranial orthosis aimed at correcting the cranial–facial asymmetry. A few band and helmet devices are available commercially and through local vendors and certified orthotists, such as the Symmetry Through Active Remolding (STARband®) orthosis, the Dynamic Orthotic Cranioplasty system (DOC band®), and other custom-molded helmets (Fig. 15.12). The cranial remolding devices apply pressure

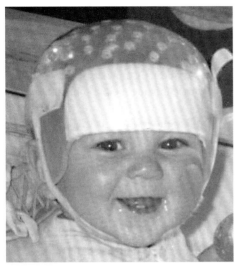

FIGURE 15.12. Infant wearing a STARband cranial orthosis to correct plagiocephaly. (From Kyle T, Carman S. *Essentials of Pediatric Nursing*, 3rd ed. Philadelphia: Wolters Kluwer, 2017.)

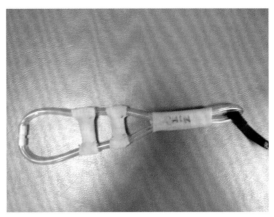

FIGURE 15.13. TOT collar. Notice addition of moleskin to prevent skin breakdown.

to the anterior and posterior prominences of the cranium but allow growth in the flattened areas. A cranial orthosis is generally recommended between ages 3 and 4 months but not for children older than 12 months. The band or helmet is initially worn for 23 to 24 hours a day and then only while sleeping once symmetry has been achieved.

It is difficult to draw conclusions for the use of helmets or cranial remolding orthoses to correct plagiocephaly because the population is not always defined and the studies often do not differentiate between plagiocephaly resulting from CMT and positional plagiocephaly.[61,62] Variability is evident in the length of time for helmet versus no helmet intervention and outcome measurements and scores. There is agreement that helmets achieve cranial remolding more quickly compared with conservative interventions without a helmet, although long-term benefit may not outweigh the excessive cost associated with the devices. Cranial orthoses are not consistently covered by insurance and can be a significant out-of-pocket expense for families.

A cervical orthosis may be beneficial for infants and young children with torticollis that is not responding to conservative treatment. An orthotic device is intended to help maintain cervical ROM or limit the ability to tilt toward the involved side. The TOT collar (tubular orthosis for torticollis) is a soft tubular collar with rigid struts of varying lengths that are positioned to elongate targeted muscles and limit motion in the opposite direction (Fig. 15.13). The TOT collar is recommended for infants at least 4 months old who have a consistent head tilt of 5 degrees or greater for more than 80% of the day and perform all movements with a head tilt. Appropriate candidates for use of the TOT collar must also exhibit a minimum of 10 degrees of lateral neck flexion toward the uninvolved side or demonstrate the ability to laterally flex the head away from the involved side[63] (Fig. 15.14A and B). Fabricated or modified foam soft collars may be used

for infants that are unable to fit into a TOT collar. Cervical orthotic devices should be used only when the child is awake and supervised.

Surgical and Medical Management

Surgical treatment is indicated for infants with CMT that does not respond to conservative treatment even after 6 months, who present with a residual head tilt, and who exhibit deficits of passive rotation and lateral flexion of the neck greater than 15 degrees and have a tight band or tumor.[51] Surgical treatment is typically not indicated without

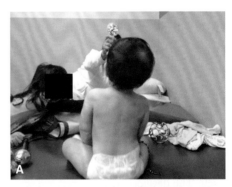

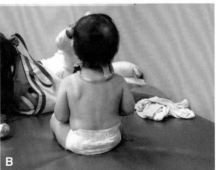

FIGURE 15.14. A: Child with right torticollis showing natural resting head and trunk position in sitting. **B:** Same child wearing TOT collar. Notice improvement in midline alignment of head and trunk.

residual ROM restriction. The need for surgical intervention can also be predicted on the basis of classification of CMT, neck rotation deficit, and age at initial presentation. Cheng and colleagues followed 821 infants with CMT classified as SMT, MT, and postural torticollis (PT). Surgery was needed for 8% of the infants in the SMT group, 3% in the MT, and none in the PT group. Infants with greater than 15 degrees of neck rotation deficit and older ages at presentation were more likely to need surgery.[51]

Surgical intervention usually involves release of the muscle distally at one or both of the heads, depending on the severity; excision of a portion of the muscle may also be indicated.[27] Splinting is required postoperatively; the use of a pinless cervical halo or custom orthotic splinting is common in order to maintain the SCM in a lengthened position that opposes the presenting torticollis posture. Postoperatively, physical therapy is indicated for achieving and maintaining cervical ROM and for strengthening musculature to maintain newly achieved alignment of the head.

An alternative treatment to surgical release for resistant torticollis that has also been found to be effective is the injection of botulinum toxin in conjunction with physical therapy treatment.[64] The injection or injections would be conducted by the physician into the restricted SCM. Then the child would undergo a physical therapy plan of care similar to previous treatment strategies mentioned previously. In Limpaphayom's study, the infants underwent PT two times per week for 6 to 8 weeks as well as a focused home stretching program as caregivers performed cervical stretches multiple times a day. In this particular study, none of the infants required surgical intervention following this treatment.[64]

Overall, torticollis is an extremely common orthopedic diagnosis that pediatric therapists will treat in multiple settings. ROM that fails to improve, worsening cranial asymmetry, and children older than 9 months at the time of presentation are all cause for concern during treatment programs. If left untreated, CMT may lead to increased facial and cranial asymmetries secondary to abnormal growth of soft tissues, including the SCM muscle and surrounding fascia and vessels. The development of a cervical scoliosis with compensatory thoracic curvature as well as ocular and vestibular impairments has been reported in cases of unresolved CMT.[27,48]

Congenital Metatarsus Adductus and Clubfoot Deformity

Metatarsus adductus is characterized by adduction of the forefoot in relation to the midfoot and hindfoot. The lateral border of the foot is convex, with the curve beginning at the base of the fifth metatarsal, resulting in the classic bean shape.[65] Metatarsus adductus is an example of a deformation caused by intrauterine positioning and is associated with other positional deformations, such as CMT and dysplasia of the hip.[66]

Metatarsus adductus is classified as mild Grade I with clinical correction of the foot beyond the lateral border, moderate Grade II with correction of the foot to a straight lateral border, or severe Grade III that does not correct to midline.[67] Severe metatarsus adductus may also be referred to as *metatarsus varus* and may include medial subluxation of the tarsometatarsal joint.[27]

Grades I and II metatarsus adductus, accounting for about 95% of cases, resolve spontaneously without treatment by 4 to 6 months of age, until when monitoring is generally recommended.[68–70] Infants with moderate or severe metatarsus adductus should be treated with serial casting until a flexible forefoot with proper alignment is achieved.[68] The height of the serial cast may need to extend above the knee to control any tibial rotation.

Clubfoot, or congenital talipes equinovarus, is a complex deformity involving ankle plantar flexion, hindfoot varus, and forefoot adduction and pronation. The incidence is 1 per 1,000 live births, but the etiology is unclear.[65] Intrauterine positioning may be a causative factor in milder forms or when a primary neuromuscular impairment, such as myelomeningocele or arthrogryposis, is present. In the latter cases, decreased or absent fetal movement secondary to the primary neuromuscular impairment could lead to prolonged abnormal fetal positioning and the resultant clubfoot deformity at birth.

In the severe forms of congenital talipes equinovarus, pathologic deformities in the anatomy and alignment of the bony and cartilaginous structures of the foot are present. The muscles are also hypoplastic, giving an overall smaller appearance to both the foot and the lower leg on the involved side. The etiology may be a defect in the mesenchymal cells forming the template for the cartilaginous model of the hindfoot structures, indicating a dysplasia rather than a deformation.[27] More recently, the genetic and chromosomal abnormality links to idiopathic clubfoot are being uncovered.[71,72] The comparison of genetic findings in children with syndromes associated with club foot is providing a much better understanding of the causes of the diagnosis in isolated cases when children have no other known causes.[73]

The goal of treatment for congenital clubfoot is to restore alignment and correct the deformity as much as possible and to provide a mobile foot for normal function and weight bearing. Initial treatment is begun shortly after birth. The Ponseti treatment method has demonstrated considerable success in reducing or eliminating the need for extensive corrective surgery.[74] It consists of serial casting with manipulation to correct the forefoot adduction and pronation and hindfoot varus along with percutaneous Achilles tenotomy to correct equinus. The cast extends above the knee to address medial tibial torsion that usually accompanies the foot deformity. Casting should continue until the foot achieves approximately 70 degrees of hyper abduction and should be followed by 3 additional weeks to allow the Achilles tendon to heal. Long-term postcorrection brace use for up to 4 years is necessary to maintain correction.[74] Children treated with the Ponseti method demonstrate minimally delayed achievement of gross motor milestones, including ambulation.[75]

Initial surgical correction is usually performed before 6 months of age to limit the extent of development of secondary deformities. Other surgical procedures are dependent on the age of the child and the severity of the deformity, previous treatment, and history of recurrence, but typically include soft tissue releases of the tight structures or an anterior tibialis transfer to promote realignment of the foot and ankle. The role of the physical therapist in the treatment for clubfoot varies depending on the facility the therapist works in and his or her training. Therapists may assist with casting the child's foot, provide education to families, and treat the short-term and long-term impacts of clubfoot such as gait training and developmental skill progression.

Developmental Dysplasia of the Hip

DDH is a term used to cover a broad spectrum of hip anomalies in infants and young children that result from abnormal growth and development of the joint. The etiology of DDH most likely includes multiple factors, such as malposition and mechanical factors in utero such as a small intrauterine space, hormone-induced ligamentous laxity, genetics, and cultural or environmental factors. The greatest risk factors for DDH are a breech position, female gender, first-born child, and a positive family history for DDH. The incidence of DDH is highly variable and dependent on environmental factors, age of diagnosis, and inclusion criteria for its diagnosis.[27] However, the incidence of DDH increases in infants with other congenital deformities, such as torticollis or metatarsus adductus.[66,76] A thorough history and review of imaging is important for physical therapists to consider all possible diagnoses and for awareness of increased incidence in order to make appropriate referrals.

During early fetal development, the acetabulum is very deep, and the femoral head is spherical. Consequently, the femoral head is well covered by the acetabulum, and the hip is a stable joint. With fetal growth and development, the acetabulum increases in diameter and becomes shallower, providing less coverage for the femoral head. The shallow acetabulum, less rounded femoral head, and increased femoral anteversion values present normally in infants at birth and result in a very unstable hip. In the immediate postnatal period, the depth of the acetabulum increases relative to diameter, producing a more stable ball-and-socket joint. The increased room for movement available to the newborn outside the uterus creates modeling forces that deepen the acetabulum as growth occurs. The most significant acetabular growth occurs during the first 18 months, and minimal acetabular growth after 3 years of age.[2]

Any interference with the normal growth and development of the hip joint may result in DDH. Interference can include abnormal forces resulting from positioning and confined space in utero, positioning that restricts normal kicking movements postnatally, and abnormal or absent muscle

TABLE 15.2.	Classification of Newborn Infant's Hips
Classification	**Criteria**
Normal	No instability of hip joint
Subluxatable	Femoral head within the acetabulum but can be partially displaced out from under the acetabulum
Dislocatable	Femoral head within the acetabulum but can be fully dislocated using the Barlow maneuver
Subluxed	Femoral head rests partially out of the acetabulum but can be reduced
Dislocated	Femoral head is completely out of the acetabulum

pull in utero and postnatally. The timing of these factors impacts the severity of the joint changes. DDH that results from malpositioning late in the last trimester shows fewer anatomic changes and responds more quickly to intervention than in the case of an infant whose hip development was affected early in fetal life. DDH in a newborn can be classified as subluxatable, dislocatable, subluxed, or dislocated (see Table 15.2).

Examination

Newborn screening for DDH includes the Ortolani test and the Barlow maneuvers (Fig. 15.15A and B). Both of these tests are more reliable before 2 months of age and when the infant is calm and not crying to facilitate soft tissue relaxation. As the infant grows, the unstable hip remains either in the acetabulum through normal development or outside the acetabulum and is prevented from relocating. Therefore, the Ortolani and Barlow maneuvers are much less reliable for infants older than 2 to 3 months of age.[27,68] Additional signs that may be noted in the newborn period include asymmetry of thigh or gluteal folds, limitation of hip abduction ROM or asymmetric hip abduction ROM, and apparent unequal femoral lengths, referred to as *Galeazzi sign*. These signs become strong indicators of DDH in the older infant when the Ortolani or Barlow maneuvers are no longer reliable. In older children who are ambulatory, DDH is usually diagnosed by an abnormal gait pattern. Children with unilateral DDH exhibit a positive Trendelenburg sign, and children with bilateral DDH walk with a waddle.[27,68]

When DDH is suspected from your examination, the infant should be referred back to the physician for an ultrasound or radiography, depending on his or her age. Ultrasound is used for young infants when ossification of the femoral head is minimal and would not be detected on radiography. Any time an infant is referred for physical therapy, regardless of diagnosis, hip stability should be examined. If risk factors are present, such as breech presentation or other congenital deformities, and the evaluation is normal, the infant may still benefit from a referral for imaging to confirm that DDH is not present.

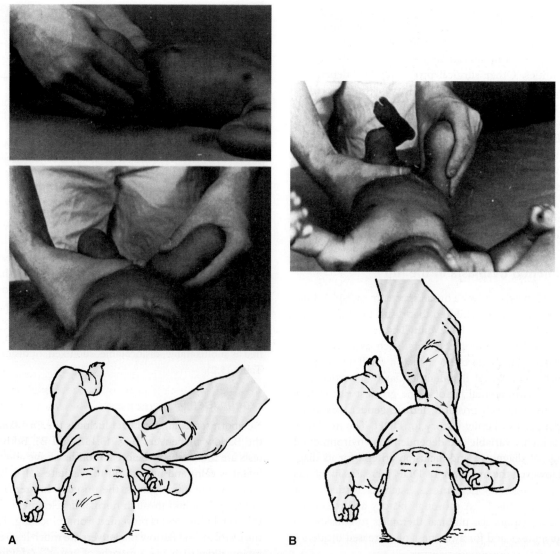

FIGURE 15.15. A: The Ortolani maneuver. From a flexed and adducted position, the hip is abducted; the examiner feels a clunk as the femoral head moves into the socket. The examiner's other hand stabilizes the infant's pelvis. **B:** The Barlow test. The examiner holds the infant's hip in flexion and slight abduction. The infant's hip is adduced while applying pressure in a posterior direction. Dislocation of the femoral head with pressure indicates an unstable hip.

Management

The aim of treatment is to return the femoral head to its normal relationship within the acetabulum and to maintain this relationship until the abnormal changes reverse.[76] The earlier the treatment is initiated, the fewer abnormal changes are present in the structures of the hip joint and the less time is needed for the structures to return to their normal relationship. Treatment regimens will vary slightly between facilities and preference of the physician, but the same general concepts are followed in the management of infants and children with DDH.

NEWBORN TO 6 MONTHS The goal of treatment is to maintain the femoral head within the acetabulum. An orthosis, typically the Pavlik harness, is used to maintain the infant's hips in a flexed and abducted position.

The Pavlik harness consists of a shoulder harness with two anterior and two posterior straps, stirrups for the legs, and booties to secure the feet (Fig. 15.16). In the Pavlik harness, the infant's hips are flexed 90 to 100 degrees, which locates the femoral head in the acetabulum. With the infant in supine, the hips are allowed to fall into abduction; they are not forced into abduction. The abducted position stretches the hip adductor muscles and allows the femoral head to slide over the posterior rim into the acetabulum. The anterior and posterior straps permit active hip flexion and abduction but limit hip extension and adduction. Therefore, the Pavlik harness has a dynamic component that promotes active movement and modeling of the hip joint.

The Pavlik harness is worn 23 to 24 hours a day until the hip is stable; full-time use of the harness is continued after stability is achieved, and then a period of weaning out of the

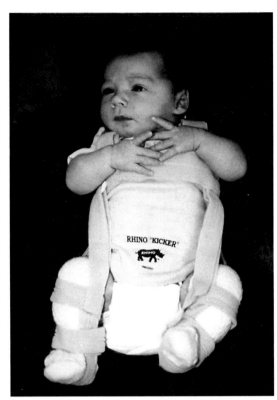

FIGURE 15.16. The Pavlik harness maintains the infant's hips in flexion and allows active movement of the hips into abduction. (Photo courtesy of RhinoPediatric Orthopedic Design, Inc.)

harness is instituted. The child's progress must be closely monitored to detect complications or determine alternative treatments if hip stability is not developing.

Complications that can develop with the use of the Pavlik harness include avascular necrosis of the femoral head, femoral nerve palsy, and inferior dislocation.[27,77] These complications can be avoided through regular monitoring of the child's hips, parent or caregiver education, and proper fit of the harness. At many centers, the physical therapist works with the orthopedic team and instructs the family in proper donning and doffing of the Pavlik harness. In an outpatient facility, an infant being treated for another impairment may be wearing a Pavlik harness. The physical therapist must be knowledgeable in the fitting of the Pavlik harness and recognize signs of ill-fit when he or she is working with these infants. Another consideration for a physical therapist for a child at this age is the impact of the use of the harness on the development of prone skills. It is important to educate families on positioning and modifications to promote these skills.

6 TO 12 MONTHS After 6 months of age, it may become more difficult to relocate the femoral head in the acetabulum. Traction for a certain period may be attempted to relocate the hip and then institute wearing of the Pavlik harness. If the child is ambulatory, an abduction orthosis may be more practical than a Pavlik harness. Closed reduction under anesthesia may be required with the application of a hip spica cast to maintain the hip in the located position.[27]

AFTER 12 MONTHS The child's hip is only rarely able to be relocated without surgical intervention. Conservative methods, such as home traction followed by closed reduction, may be attempted before a surgical procedure. Surgical correction may include release of tight soft tissue structures or osteotomy of the proximal femur to allow the femoral head to move into the acetabulum. Older children may require the removal of a portion of the femoral shaft to reduce the forces on the femoral head when it is relocated in the acetabulum, femoral osteotomy, or acetabular osteotomy to aid in relocating the femoral head.[27,68] Following these more extensive surgical procedures, a physical therapist will work with the child to regain ROM after postsurgical casting, gait training, and strengthening.

Arthrogryposis Multiplex Congenita

Arthrogryposis multiplex congenita (AMC), also referred to as *multiple congenital contracture* (MCC), is a nonprogressive disorder characterized by multiple joint contractures and muscle weakness or imbalance. The reported incidence of AMC varies from 1 in 3,000 to 1 in 4,000 live births.[78,79] The disorder is related to a paucity of movement early in fetal development, leading to multiple contractures at birth. The exact etiology is unknown but is probably multifactorial with genetic mutation causes currently being uncovered. AMC is associated with multiple neurogenic or myopathic disorders that exhibit a defect in the motor unit, including the anterior horn cells, roots, peripheral nerve, motor end plates, or muscle, resulting in weakness and decreased fetal movement early in development. Fetal immobility results in multiple joint contractures, fibrosis of muscles, and fibrosis of the periarticular structures.[79,80]

There is much variability among infants with AMC; however, common clinical features are generally present and include the following: (1) featureless extremities that are often cylindrical in shape with absent skin creases, (2) rigid joints with significant contractures, (3) dislocation of joints, especially the hips, (4) atrophy and even absence of muscle groups, and (5) intact sensation, although deep tendon reflexes (DTRs) may be diminished or absent.[79] The infant's contractures are usually symmetric and typically include shoulder internal rotation, elbow flexion or extension, wrist flexion with ulnar deviation, hip flexion with either internal rotation or a frog-legged posture, knee flexion or extension, and equinovarus deformities of the feet (Fig. 15.17).[27]

Management

Intervention throughout childhood should be conducted as a team and involves multidisciplinary work sharing the same goal and timeline. The goal of intervention is to achieve the maximum functional level for each child. Treatment techniques include passive stretching through positioning, casting and splinting, strengthening activities, developmental skills, surgical procedures, and the use of adapted or rehabilitation equipment. The family is crucial in planning the

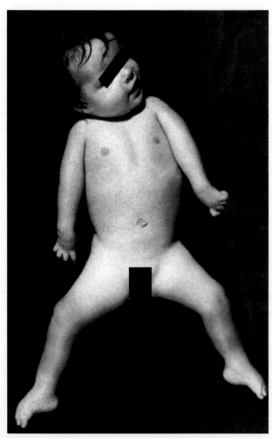

FIGURE 15.17. Arthrogryposis multiplex congenita in an infant. The shoulders are internally rotated and adducted, and the elbows and wrists are extended. The hips are flexed, externally rotated, and abducted, and the feet demonstrate talipes equinovarus.

long-term goals for the child and assisting with the carryover of activities.

INFANCY Positioning and passive stretching exercises should begin shortly after birth. Serial casting begins in the first few months for foot deformities (see section "Congenital Metatarsus Adductus and Clubfoot Deformity"), knee flexion contractures, and wrist flexion contractures. Caution must be used to stretch only to the end range and maintain the stretch with a cast or a splint. Forceful, aggressive stretching of a rigid joint can damage the joint capsule and surrounding soft tissue.[27] Any gains in ROM must be maintained with a splint or positioning device, or the contracture will recur.

Usually between 6 and 12 months of age, residual contractures at the feet and knees will be surgically corrected.[68] Surgical correction involves release of the tight joint capsule and soft tissues. Surgical correction is maintained by splinting, strengthening exercises, and active functional movement. For example, a child who had a bilateral release of posterior structures of the ankle to correct an equinovarus deformity should have a splint fabricated to maintain the ROM as well as begin a standing program with the use of a standing device or ambulation aid depending on his or her age.

The goals of intervention for the child's upper extremities must be well planned. For optimum function and independence with self-care skills, the child should be able to flex and extend the elbows. If this is not possible, treatment should aim to ensure that one elbow is able to flex for feeding activities and that the other elbow is able to extend for reaching and toileting activities.

During this age range, the child should develop some mobility skills. Rolling is often difficult secondary to the lower extremity contractures. Some children may learn to scoot on the floor on their belly or their back initially. Most children can learn to sit but have difficulty getting into the sitting position independently. From sitting, floor mobility should be encouraged. Creeping on hands and knees is often difficult, and children often learn to scoot on their bottom. Pulling to stand may be limited by contractures of the lower extremity. Surgical techniques should be timed to prepare the child to stand when he or she is developmentally ready. Preambulation activities should begin before 1 year of age. Supportive splinting may be required such as AFOs and knee, ankle foot orthoses (KAFOs) with specific strategies to adjust for angular deformity in order to allow for full foot contact with the floor. For example, wedging may be added to the bracing or shoe to adjust for a heel cord contracture that is still present.

12 MONTHS THROUGH PRESCHOOL The goal of treatment during this age range is to develop the maximum level of independence with mobility and self-care skills. Ambulation is possible for many children with AMC and should be considered a viable goal until proven otherwise. Recent reviews have shown that ambulation potential in certain types of AMC can be predicted by lower extremity position at birth and muscle strength[81] and can be helpful to guide a therapist's choice of bracing support and assistive device needs for this population. Upper extremity skills focus on feeding and dressing activities. Maintenance of acquired ROM is crucial, as are continued gains in ROM. Strengthening exercises through age-appropriate activities, as well as specific mobility training, are incorporated into the program.

SCHOOL AGE The school-age period often highlights the functional impairments that may exist for a child with AMC. The child's ambulation speed may be slow compared with his or her peers, and fine motor difficulty may interfere with writing speed and clarity. Adaptive and rehabilitation equipment may be necessary to assist the child with functioning independently in the school setting and maintaining social interaction with his or her peers.

» Postnatal deformations

Deformations can also occur postnatally secondary to the immaturity of the musculoskeletal system of a growing and developing child. The effect of growth on the musculoskeletal system can be used to correct prenatal deformities, such as those seen in the treatment rationale for CMT or metatarsus adductus. However, the effect of growth can also produce additional deformities postnatally if a force is abnormal or unopposed.

Rotational Deformities

The variation of a child's rotational profile that occurs with normal growth and development produces many questions for parents and subsequent visits to an orthopedic specialist or a physical therapist. The child with a rotational variation presents with either an in-toed or out-toed gait. Clarification on what is a true normal rotational variation, when the rotation becomes a deformity and appropriate examination and intervention are necessary to answer parents' questions, recognize true problems, and possibly impact those problems. The causative factors of the in-toeing or out-toeing must be evaluated and the rotational components measured using Staheli rotational profile outlined earlier in the chapter. Staheli rotational profile includes FPA as an overall measure, hip rotation ROM in combination with the Ryder method or the Craig test to examine femoral torsion, TFA to examine tibial torsion and the hindfoot, angle of the TMA to examine the distal tibia, and the configuration of the foot. The measurements can then be compared with the normative values to determine whether the child falls within the range of normal for his or her age and which component or components of the lower extremity are contributing to the in-toed or out-toed gait pattern (see Fig. 15.2).

FPA shows the greatest variability in infancy before leveling off to a mean of 10 degrees with a range of −3 to 20 degrees in childhood. Hip rotation ROM is divided into medial and lateral rotation of the hip and is a clinical measure to assist in examining femoral torsion. The sum of medial and lateral hip rotation is approximately 100 degrees and slightly more in infants.[82] Lateral rotation of the hip is greater than medial rotation in infants secondary to tightness of soft tissues from intrauterine positioning. Femoral anteversion is present in infancy but is not as noticeable because of the infant's position of lateral rotation. Femoral anteversion is usually noticeable in young children but continues to decrease from infancy through childhood. Persistent femoral anteversion may be classified as a rotational deformity when the following values exist: mild if medial rotation is 70 to 80 degrees and lateral rotation is 10 to 20 degrees, moderate if medial rotation is 80 to 90 degrees and lateral rotation is 0 to 10 degrees, and severe if medial rotation is greater than 90 degrees and no lateral rotation is present.[25,82] The TFA increases from a negative angle in infancy to a positive angle throughout childhood. The angle of the TMA also increases from infancy through childhood. The tibia is medially rotated in infancy secondary to intrauterine positioning. De-rotation of the tibia toward the normal lateral tibial torsion values in adulthood occurs normally through growth and development.

Infants and young children exhibit greater femoral anteversion and medial tibial torsion that gradually decrease through normal growth and development. An in-toeing gait is most common during the second year after the child begins to walk. If the measured values fall outside the two standard deviation values for normal, a rotational deformity exists. Intervention is necessary only if the deformity interferes with function or has the potential to interfere with function or development, such as a child tripping over their feet.[82] However, if a rotational deformity is cosmetically unappealing for the child, adolescent, or parent, intervention may also be considered, although not medically necessary.[82]

Previously, treatment has included exercise, bracing, shoe modifications, and orthopedic correction. Shoe modifications are ineffective in correcting in-toeing problems, and devices such as the Denis Browne bar or twister cables may actually cause secondary deformities at the knee as well.[25,69] Hip, knee, ankle foot orthoses (HKAFO) and knee, ankle foot orthoses (KAFO) constructed of newer light polymer material shell and multiplane movement joints may have clinical benefits, but evidence so far has been no more than anecdotal. Orthopedic surgery consisting of a femoral or tibial rotational osteotomy may be indicated for children who exhibit deformities greater than three standard deviations from the normal values (i.e., femoral anteversion >50 degrees) and when the deformity interferes with function or is a cosmetic concern.

» Dysplasias

A dysplasia is an abnormal organization of cells into tissue that leads to abnormal tissue differentiation.[6,33] Children born with a dysplasia exhibit widespread involvement because the abnormal tissue differentiation is present wherever the tissue is present.

Osteogenesis Imperfecta

OI is a congenital disorder of type I collagen synthesis that affects all connective tissues in the body. The reported incidence is dependent on criteria used for OI and ranges from 1 in 15,000 to 1 in 100,000.[83,84] The musculoskeletal involvement is diffuse and includes osteoporosis with excessive fractures even at birth, bowing of long bones, spinal deformities, muscle weakness, and ligamentous laxity.[83–86] In addition to the musculoskeletal involvement, other clinical features of children with OI may include blue sclera in the eyes, dentinogenesis imperfecta, hearing loss, growth deficiency, cardiopulmonary abnormalities, easy bruising, excessive sweating, and loose or dislocated joints (Fig. 15.18).[83,84]

In 1979, Sillence first described OI Types I through IV based on genetic, clinical, and radiographic findings without regard for molecular involvement.[83,87] Recently, the genetic complexity of OI has been becoming more transparent, and approximately 2,000 different type I collagen mutations have

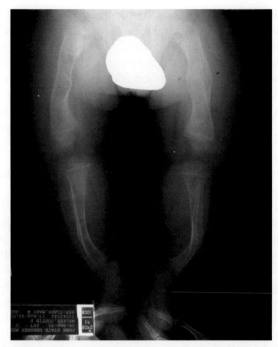

FIGURE 15.18. Radiograph of a 13-month-old child with type III OI. Note the poor bone density, previous fracture sites, bowing of the bones, and the length of the femurs in relation to the tibias.

been identified.[87] The International Skeletal Dysplasia Society has recommended utilizing Sillence typing to classify the severity of OI or phenotypic presentation. In addition, these classifications should not include direct molecular reference to eliminate typing that only reflects newly discovered genetic variants that have few distinguishing features in the clinic.[88] Table 15.3 outlines the specific characteristics for OI Types I through VIII.

Binder et al.[86] developed a classification system based on body size and limb proportions and their expected functional outcomes (Table 15.4). Consequently, physical therapy interventions can then be aimed at potential musculoskeletal deformities that presently interfere with the child's expected functional abilities or at preventing those deformities from developing.

Management

PHARMACOLOGIC Several pharmacologic and vitamin supplements have been studied in an attempt to decrease the fragility of the bones of children with OI. Agents such as calcitonin, fluoride, hormones, and vitamins C and D have all been shown to be ineffective in preventing fractures.[89] Calcium and vitamin D may be ineffective alone but can

TABLE 15.3. Classification of Osteogenesis Imperfecta

Type*	Severity	Inheritance	Characteristics	Mobility Status
I	Mildest form of OI	Autosomal dominant	Blue sclera, dentinogenesis imperfecta, fewer bone fractures and progressive deformity, mild short stature or normal height	Ambulatory—may use an orthotic device
II	Lethal in perinatal period	Autosomal dominant	Severe bone fragility with multiple rib and long bone fractures at birth. Bones are "crumpled"; ribs may be beaded	Not applicable
III	Severe form	Autosomal dominant or recessive	Blue or normal sclera, dentinogenesis imperfecta, variable bone fragility but often severe, progressive skeletal deformity, scoliosis, very short stature	Variable; may be ambulatory with assistive device and orthotic devices, may use wheelchair for all or partial mobility
IV	Moderate	Autosomal dominant	Gray or normal sclera, dentinogenesis imperfecta, moderate fragility of bones, scoliosis, moderate short stature	Often independent at home and community, with or without assistive device
V	Moderate	Autosomal dominant	Normal sclera and teeth, frequent dislocation of radial head and calcification of forearm interosseous membrane, moderate-to-severe bone fragility, mild-to-moderate short stature	Ambulatory
VI	Moderate	Autosomal recessive	Normal sclera and teeth, vertebral compression fractures often seen, more fractures than seen in type IV but at birth, scoliosis, moderately short stature	May be ambulatory or use wheelchair
VII	Moderate	Autosomal recessive	White sclera, normal teeth, moderate bone fragility with fractures at birth, very short humeri and femurs with coax vara, mild short stature	May be ambulatory or use wheelchair
VIII	Severe to lethal in perinatal period	Autosomal recessive	Severe growth deficiency and bone demineralization	Variable to not applicable

*Types I to IV are based on Sillence classification system. Types V to VIII are expanded types clinically distinguishable by bone histology or recessive inheritance.
OI, osteogenesis imperfecta

TABLE 15.4.	Functional Classification for Osteogenesis Imperfecta and Focus of Rehabilitation		
Type	Physical Characteristics	Functional Expectations	Focus of Rehabilitation Interventions
A	Most severely involved group Large head relative to body, very short stature, bowing of long bones with joint contractures and weakness May have severe scoliosis and/or vertebral compression fractures	Dependent for ADLs except for feeding May use manual wheelchair; more likely to use power wheelchair	Positioning, including molded seating systems, therapeutic water activities Soft tissue mobilization to increase shoulder and MCP joint ROM and soft tissue mobilization techniques to alleviate back pain
B	Severe short stature, high incidence of femoral bowing, scoliosis, hip flexion contractures Strength generally at least 3/5	Stand and/or ambulate with assistive devices and braces Partial independence with ADLs Contractures of hips and shoulders and limited forearm supination interfere with function	Posture and active ROM exercises aimed at limiting contractures Strengthening with emphasis on abdominals, hip extensors and abductors, and quadriceps Endurance through swimming and biking, developmental activities through normal sequence Many children will not crawl but scoot in sitting
C	Less growth deficiency, poor LE alignment, including hip abduction and external rotation contractures Joint laxity with LE valgus and pronation of the feet Strength of 3/5 or greater, poor endurance	Community ambulation with or without orthotic devices Independent with ADLs	Strengthening exercises with weights *proximal* on limb Conditioning exercise to improve endurance and long-distance ambulation May use orthotic devices for alignment, but all orthotic devices should be articulated

ADLs, activities of daily living; LE, lower extremity; MCP, metacarpophalangeal; ROM, range of motion.

From Binder H, Conway A, Gerber LH. Rehabilitation approaches to children with osteogenesis imperfecta: a ten-year experience. *Arch Phys Med Rehabil.* 1993;74:386–390.

support greater efficacy in conjunction with bisphosphonate drug therapies.[87]

Medications from the bisphosphonate family such as pamidronate, alendronate, and zoledronic acid have been administered to children and adults with OI to improve their bone density. Bisphosphonates inhibit osteoclast activity and have been used in postmenopausal women to decrease osteoporosis. They can be administered orally or intravenously at cyclic periods. Intravenous (IV) administration has been found to be effective in improving bone density, especially vertebral body; decreasing fracture rate; decreasing back pain; improving sense of well-being; and improving grip strength, mobility, self-care skills, and ambulation.[90–93] Maximum bone density benefits are realized with pamidronate in the first 2 to 4 years of treatment, but maintenance therapy is suggested until bone growth is finished.[87] Oral administration may not be as effective as IV administration. However, there is significant evidence for the effectiveness of oral administration of bisphosphonates in improving bone density.[91,94,95] Moderate-to-strong evidence supports oral bisphosphonate efficacy in reducing the fracture rate, improving the functional status of some subjects, and improving quality of life in children with OI Types I, III, and IV.[89,91,94] Future study of bisphosphonates should include further analysis of how long the child should receive the medications, whether the results are reversed if the medication is stopped, and which groups should receive which medications. Other novel approaches currently under investigation include the efficacy of gene therapy to silence allele mutations, bone marrow transplant, and selective mesenchymal stem cell transplant to treat OI.

ORTHOPEDIC Fractures are managed with a soft splint or fiberglass cast for immobilization. The period of immobilization is kept short to minimize the bone demineralization that normally occurs with inactivity. Frequent fractures can lead to further demineralization, refractures, and bony deformity, specifically bowing of the long bones as well as possible nonunion of the fracture site. Muscle pull on long bones can also cause significant anterior bowing of the long bones of the lower extremity. Osteotomy, flexible intramedullary nails, and telescoping intramedullary rod fixation may be used to correct bowing deformities or stabilize fractures.[83,87] Surgical corrections of these deformations facilitate improved alignment to allow orthotic use and standing programs and also provide support to the bones, decreasing the fracture rate.

Rehabilitation

Several practitioners from the Children's Hospital Medical Center, Washington, DC, and the National Institutes of Health have developed and revised a rehabilitation protocol for children with OI.[85,86,96] Much of this information is now published in a book with clear explanations of exercises from early infancy through gaining independence for adolescents.[97] In view of wide variability among children with OI, the protocol is meant to serve as a guideline and must be individualized for each child and family. The goals for the child with severe OI include the following: (1) prevent deformities of the head, spine, and extremities, (2) avert cardiorespiratory compromise by avoiding constant positioning in supine, and (3) maximize the child's ability to move actively.[85] These goals are based on the theory that muscle strengthening and weight-bearing programs for upper and lower extremities promote active earlier use of the extremities and may lead to increased bone mineralization and less severe musculoskeletal deformities.[85,96]

It is crucial to provide instruction in handling of an infant with OI to all parents and caregivers. The infant should be held with the head, trunk, and extremities fully supported. For infants with severe OI, caregivers may initially be more comfortable holding the child on a pillow. Careful positioning of an infant with OI should begin in the first few days after birth with instruction from a knowledgeable physical therapist. Positioning aims to align the infant's head, trunk, and extremities and to protect the infant from hitting hard surfaces with activity. Emphasis is on midline orientation of the head and trunk and position changes to prevent the development of cervical malalignment and a misshapen skull. Active movement is encouraged as beginning strengthening exercises. Careful handling activities can be performed in straight frontal or sagittal plane movements. Rotary movements should be avoided to prevent rotational fractures. Care should be taken to avoid grasping, applying traction or passively moving extremities through extreme ROM during play or daily care activities such as changing clothing and diapering.

Strengthening activities progress from active movement to playing with lightweight toys and rattles. Active movement can be further encouraged in water either at bath time or in a swim program with the parent present. Standard active-assistive and resistive exercises can be incorporated as the child grows a little older. Emphasis is also placed on the development of head control and head righting in a variety of positions because children with OI often have a very large head. Developmental activities such as prone skills and rolling are encouraged. Independent sitting is encouraged when developmentally appropriate, as is some type of floor mobility. Those children who do not have the ability to develop independent sitting skills should be fitted for a custom-molded seat to promote head and trunk alignment and afford the child the opportunity to play in an upright position. Proper positioning will also assist in avoiding compressive forces on the spinal vertebrae owing to the risk of developing vertebral body wedging, compression fractures, and complications resulting from poor spinal alignment. Throughout the developmental progression, increasing or maintaining ROM and strength, especially of the pelvic girdle, is incorporated into activities.

Children should be fitted with lower extremity orthoses when they have developed independent sitting skills and balance and are beginning to pull to stand. Those children who cannot sit independently but have developed head control should be fitted for a standing frame. Recent standing equipment design advances may eliminate the need for custom-molded frames. The orthoses recommended in the protocol are containment or clamshell HKAFOs.[85,97] Clamshell orthoses are similar to standard HKAFOs except that a contoured anterior shell is present to support the thigh and lower leg. Gait training begins with an assistive device and may or may not progress to independent ambulation without an assistive device. With ambulation and upright positioning, attention must be directed to the pelvic girdle. Hip flexion contractures often develop, and children with OI typically require ongoing strengthening of their hip extensors and abductors.[97]

Children who do not develop independent functional ambulation should be fitted with a manual or power wheelchair as appropriate. Positioning remains key with any seating system, and attention is given to head and trunk alignment.

In a 10-year follow-up report, Binder and colleagues emphasized the need for rehabilitation to focus on the child's functional needs.[86] These key rehabilitative strategies are outlined in Table 15.4. Binder et al. reported progress with functional skills in all groups of children with OI, ranging from improved head control to community ambulation. Progress appears related to severity of the disease but should be expected for all children with OI if the goals address functional needs. Factors that impair independence include joint contractures and muscle weakness for those children with severe forms of OI and endurance capabilities for children with less severe forms of OI.

Recent studies show that children with OI can participate in physical therapist-supervised exercise programs and demonstrate improved aerobic and muscle performance with decreased fatigue.[98] Detraining observed following the completion of these programs emphasizes the need for safely monitored exercise programs developed by the therapist as part of a weekly routine. The use of whole body vibration (WBV) systems has been incorporated into training programs to improve muscle strength and power in healthy and motor-impaired adults, demonstrating results beyond that of training without WBV.[99,100] WBV has shown promising results in improving mobility and function and decreasing support devices needed for children with OI.[100] Changes in bone strength were not observed in a study by Högler et al. utilizing the same type of vibration equipment in isolation of physical therapy intervention despite a 5-month regimen of vibration intervention in children who were described to have limited mobility at baseline.[101] Current equipment costs make treatment outside of the clinical or research setting prohibitive, but further technological or home gaming system development will likely change this.

Joint Hypermobility Syndromes

EDS is another disorder of collagen synthesis, primarily type V, with an incidence of 1:10,000.[102,103] It is a clinically and genetically heterogeneous group of connective tissue disorders characterized by joint hypermobility, skin hyperextensibility,

TABLE 15.5. Ehlers Danlos Syndrome Classifications		
Current Classification	Prior Classification	Clinical Presentation
Classic	EDS I and EDS II	Joint hypermobility Skin hyperextensibility Atrophic scars Smooth velvety texture
Hypermobile	EDS III	Joint hypermobility Mild skin hyperextensibility ± smooth velvety texture
Vascular	EDS IV	Thin skin Easily bruised Pinched nose Appearance of premature aging Rupture of medium and large arteries within uterus and bowel
Kyphoscoliotic	EDS VI	Joint hypermobility Progressive scoliosis Scleral fragility with rupture Tissue fragility Aortic dilation Mitral valve prolapse (MVP)
Arthrochalasia	EDS VII A EDS VII B	Severe joint hypermobility Joint subluxations Congenital hip dislocation Skin hyperextensibility Tissue fragility
Dermatosparaxis	EDS VII C	Severe skin fragility Decreased skin elasticity Easily bruised Hernias Premature rupture of fetal membranes
Unclassified	EDS V EDS VIII EDS X, EDS XI EDS IX EDS, Progeroid form	Classic features Classic features and peri-odontic disease Mild classic features, MVP, joint instability Classic features, occipital horns, premature aging

EDS, Ehlers Danlos Syndrome.

and tissue fragility.[102–104] There are now seven accepted general classification types of EDS, as against 14 distinct variations formerly[103] (Table 15.5). However, the classic and hypermobility type account for 90% of all cases and involve mostly orthopedic complaints.[104]

In 1967, Kirk et al. first described a similar condition known as benign joint hypermobility syndrome (BJHS), which is also characterized by generalized joint laxity with musculoskeletal complaints. It is called "benign" owing to the absence of a specific genetic, musculoskeletal or rheumatic disorder.[105] Examination and treatment approaches to EDS and BJHS are indistinguishable.

Examination

Examination procedures for children with EDS and BJHS should include a hypermobility scale and lower extremity rotational profile as well as ROM measurements of extremities. Multiple hypermobility scales exist, but the Beighton score is frequently used in clinical settings. The Beighton score is a component of the full Beighton Criteria used to diagnose hypermobility syndromes[106] (Table 15.6). Other areas of specific concern include the shoulders, ankles, and feet, which are not specifically incorporated into the Beighton score. Complaints of hypermobility are often accompanied by diffuse muscle and joint pain and general fatigue along with hand pain and fatigue with prolonged handwriting.

Management

Intervention focus and strategies will depend on the child's age and severity of joint involvement. Most programs should include a combination of the following four areas: targeted therapeutic exercise, self-care and home management, including joint protection training, functional training for recreation, school, or work, and orthoses or adaptive equipment.[13]

TABLE 15.6. Beighton Criteria for Joint Hypermobility	
Major Criteria	A Beighton score of 4/9 or more (either current or historic) Joint Pain for more than 3 mo in four or more joints
Minor Criteria	A Beighton score of 1, 2, or 3/9 (0, 1, 2, or 3 if aged 50+) Joint pain (>3 mo) in one to three joints or back pain (>3 mo), spondylosis, spondylolysis/spondylolisthesis. Dislocation/subluxation in more than one joint, or in one joint on more than one occasion. Soft tissue inflammation >3 lesions (e.g., epicondylitis, tenosynovitis, bursitis). Marfan-like symptoms (tall, slim, span/height ratio >1.03), upper: lower segment ratio >0.89, arachnodactyly (positive Steinberg thumb/Walker wrist signs). Abnormal skin: striae, hyperextensibility, thin skin, papyraceous scarring Eye signs: drooping eyelids, nearsighted or antimongoloid eye slant Varicose veins or hernia or uterine/rectal prolapse
Beighton Score	1, 2—Passive 5th MCP extension >90 degrees (Right and Left) 3, 4—Passive thumb apposition to forearm (Right and Left) 5, 6—Elbow hyperextension >10 degrees (Right and Left) 7, 8—Knee hyperextension >10 degrees (Right and Left) 9—Standing trunk flexion with knees extended, palms flat on floor
Positive Diagnosis Criteria	2 major criteria 1 major and 1 minor criteria 4 minor criteria

Therapeutic Exercise

Therapeutic exercise programs should include a combination of strengthening, neuromuscular education, neuromuscular stabilization, and stretching usually of the hindfoot only. Focused stretching of lower extremity muscle groups such as hamstrings, gastroc/soleus complex, and hip flexors may be necessary during periods of rapid growth. Care should be taken to avoid extreme joint end ranges of motion while stretching these muscle complexes. Glenohumeral joint and scapular stabilization and strengthening are important to combat recurrent subluxations. This reduction in subluxations also improves proximal stability to facilitate functional use of the hand and arm without recurrent pain. However, this level of achievement may be difficult for younger children, and goals for improvement may be delayed until a child can follow more complex instruction. Foot and ankle strengthening will promote stability and preserve foot function. Full hindfoot ROM should be achieved, as Achilles tightness usually develops owing to midfoot and hindfoot breakdown, as noted with ligamentous laxity in the foot and ankle complex. Abdominal and trunk strengthening for overall proximal and lumbar stabilization is frequently necessary because low back pain is a common complaint. Wrist and hand work should focus on small intrinsic muscle strengthening without joint hyperextension to facilitate hand use in fine motor tasks, especially for school and work.

Self-Care

Children require to be educated about the need for joint stability and protection. End-range positions such as leaning on hyperextended elbows and standing for long periods with hips and knees hyperextended for comfort should be avoided.[13] Children with hypermobility also commonly demonstrate joint "tricks" such as contortion or shoulder popping. However, these movements can result in microtrauma of joints and ligamentous structures, which further exacerbate pain symptoms. Gym class limitations include allowance for rest periods and no somersaults, push-ups, arm hanging activities, timed exercises, or unsupervised stretching, which often occur in large classes. Aside from these, activity modification rather than elimination should be considered.

Functional Training

Children with EDS and BJHS are at increased risk for ligamentous and repetitive use injuries because muscles constantly perform double duty as joint stabilizers and movers.[107] Training will vary with the age of the child but can include recreational or organized play, school or work activity. Examination of specific functional tasks with recommendations for modification, optimization of good body mechanics, and exercise prescription for injury prevention is required.

Orthoses and Adaptive Equipment

Primary equipment and device needs are related to the hands, patella, ankles, and feet. Children benefit from wider grip pens and pencils or regular ones with grip-widening foam attached to them. Some children benefit from early use of the computer or laptop for note-taking. More widespread academic use of electronic tablets may provide even more hand symptom relief.

The foot and ankle should be protected as early as possible to prevent structural deformity associated with excessive pronation. A biomechanical foot exam should be performed with the foot in subtalar joint neutral to ensure that the hindfoot mobility is accurately measured before an orthotic or orthosis is prescribed. A bracing device should provide the maximum support with the minimal degree of anatomic control to facilitate maximal muscle activity and bone development. Children with EDS and BJHS do well with custom and semicustomized shoe orthotics and University of California Biomechanics Lab (UCBL)-type orthoses for mild-to-moderate foot hypermobility and lightweight supramalleolar orthoses in severe cases.

» Pathologic processes

Pathologic processes are a broad category of abnormal conditions and may impact the developing and growing musculoskeletal system of a child. These processes are of varied origin and may include vascular, infectious, metabolic, mechanical, traumatic, or structural causes.

Legg–Calvé–Perthes Disease

Legg–Calvé–Perthes disease is a self-limiting disease of the hip initiated by avascular necrosis of the femoral head. The precise cause of the avascular necrosis that disrupts blood flow to the capital femoral epiphysis is unknown. Microtrauma, transient synovitis, infection, insulin-like growth factor I pathway abnormalities, congenital or developmental vascular irregularities, and thrombotic vascular insults have all been theorized as producing the avascular necrosis, but there is strong recent evidence for the role of vascular abnormalities and dysfunction.[108,109] The disease typically occurs between 3 and 13 years of age, boys being affected three to five times more frequently than girls. However, Legg–Calvé–Perthes disease is most commonly seen in boys between 4 and 10 years of age who are active yet small for their age. Bilateral presentation is seen in 10% to 20% of children with the disease.[27]

Legg–Calvé–Perthes disease progresses through four clearly defined stages: (1) initial, (2) fragmentation, (3) reossification, and (4) healed.[110] During the initial phase, a portion or all of the femoral head becomes necrotic, and bone growth ceases. The necrotic bone is resorbed and fragmented; at this time revascularization of the femoral head is initiated. During this second stage, the femoral head often becomes deformed, and the acetabulum becomes flattened in response to the deformity of the femoral head. With revascularization, the femoral head begins to reossify. As the femoral head grows, remodeling of both the femoral head and the acetabulum occurs.[108,110] The stage of the disease when diagnosed, gender of the child, and age at onset impact the final outcome and congruency of the hip joint.

There are several classification systems that aim at assisting with the prediction of outcomes of children with Legg–Calvé–Perthes disease. Kim and Herring developed a classification system based on the involvement of the lateral aspect of the femoral head. They found this lateral pillar classification to demonstrate good-to-excellent reliability among users.[110] The original A, B, C classification, progressing from least to most lateral pillar deterioration, is the most widely used. Modifications to include a fourth B/C border category have not demonstrated the same reproducibility.[111]

Clinically, children with Legg–Calvé–Perthes disease present with a limp and pain referred to the groin, thigh, or knee.[27,112] If the condition is undetected, hip ROM limitations may develop with restrictions in hip internal rotation and abduction, a hip flexion contracture may be present, and a Trendelenburg-type gait is frequently observed.[112] Muscle spasm of the hip adductors and iliopsoas may also be noted. Children who present to a physical therapist with the preceding symptoms and unknown etiology should be referred to a pediatric orthopedist.

Management

The goals of treatment are to relieve the symptoms of pain and muscle spasm, prevent or minimize femoral head deformity, contain the femoral head in the acetabulum while bone remodeling occurs, and restore ROM. Treatment for relief of pain includes anti-inflammatory medications, traction, and partial weight bearing with the use of crutches. Deformity may be minimized and the femoral head contained through the use of traction; orthotic devices such as a Petrie cast, Scottish-Rite orthosis, or A-Frame orthosis (Figs. 15.19 to 15.21); or surgical procedures such as a femoral or innominate osteotomy.

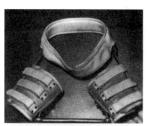
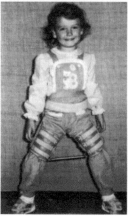

FIGURE 15.20. Scottish-Rite orthosis. The abduction bar contains a swivel joint that allows reciprocal motion of the legs.

If an orthotic device is used to achieve femoral head containment, it may be required for a prolonged period, up to 1 or 2 years. While wearing the orthosis and after healing, physical therapy is often warranted to address ROM limitations and strength deficits. After the orthotic device has been removed, children may continue to walk with a Trendelenburg-type gait because of weakness of their hip

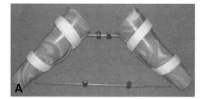
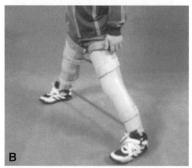

FIGURE 15.21. A-Frame Orthosis. Custom-molded in: **A:** approximately 30 degrees of bilateral hip abduction and **B:** slight knee flexion. (From Rich MM, Schoenecker PL. Management of Legg–Calvé–Perthes disease using an A-frame orthosis and hip range of motion: a 25-year experience. *J Pediatr Orthop.* 2013;33:112–119.)

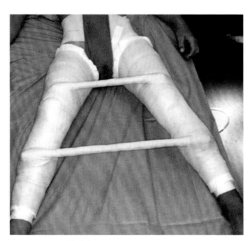

FIGURE 15.19. Petrie cast.

extensors and hip abductors. Physical therapy after surgical intervention focuses on gait training and restoration of hip ROM, muscular flexibility, and strength. Knee and ankle strength and ROM should also be continually addressed owing to long-term immobility.

Although multiple treatment methods exist for Legg–Calvé–Perthes disease, decision making and outcomes are more correlated with certain factors such as age at onset, total amount of femoral head involvement, Herring lateral pillar classification, and the disease stage at the time of diagnosis. Children under 6 years do well regardless of treatment protocol, and surgery may not be necessary.[112–114] Children who are under 8 years of age at the time of onset and have minimal involvement of the lateral aspect of their femoral head have very favorable outcomes regardless of the type of treatment received.[113,114] However, children who are over the age of 8 years at the time of onset and have moderate involvement of the lateral aspect of the femoral head have improved outcomes with surgical intervention.[113] Children who have complete collapse of the lateral aspect of their femoral head, more total femoral head involvement, or who are in later stages of the disease at diagnosis typically have poor outcomes.[112–114]

Recent literature suggests a specific protocol that demonstrated excellent outcomes over a 25-year period.[115] This protocol included an adductor tenotomy as needed to achieve 35 to 40 degrees of hip abduction, Petrie casting for 6 weeks, followed by donning of a custom A-Frame orthosis for 20 hours a day for up to 3 years, and a hip ROM HEP performed twice a day. Of 240 hips studied having congruency, good spherical hip congruency was developed with an overall rate of 93%. This included 78% of the more involved B and C Herring Classification hips as well. During the bracing period, children were permitted to ambulate while wearing the brace, and they maintained a normal school schedule, thereby demonstrating minimal limitations to daily living participation.

Slipped Capital Femoral Epiphysis

Slipped capital femoral epiphysis (SCFE) is typically described as occurring when the femoral head slips, or is displaced, from its normal alignment with the femoral neck. However, it is actually caused by displacement of the femoral neck usually anteriorly and superiorly.[116] Weakness of and excessive stresses on the growth plate are thought to contribute to the displacement of the femoral head. Increased shear forces are commonly caused by obesity and structural problems such as femoral retroversion and physeal obliquity.[116,117] Testosterone in boys and hormonal imbalances in boys and girls, and growth spurts may contribute to growth plate weakness or instability.[116,117] SCFE is the most common hip problem of adolescence, but the incidence of SCFE varies according to age, gender, and race. The incidence is higher in males and the African American population and is often associated with the onset of puberty.[116,117] Bilateral occurrence has been reported in at least 50% of young adolescents.[116–118]

SCFE is classified by weight-bearing ability, duration of symptoms, and radiographic findings. In the Loder Classification, adolescents with stable SCFE (representing greater than 90% of cases) are able to bear weight with or without support, but those with unstable SCFE cannot bear weight even with an assistive device owing to pain.[116,117] When classifying based on the duration of symptoms, an *acute SCFE* is defined as a sudden onset of painful symptoms of less than 3 weeks' duration, whereas chronic SCFE is characterized by a gradual onset of symptoms for greater than 3 weeks. The third type is acute-on-chronic SCFE with a history of mild pain for greater than 3 weeks and a recent sudden exacerbation of symptoms.[117] Classification according to the severity of the displacement of the femoral head is defined as follows:

a. Grade I, displacement of the femoral head up to one-third of the width of the femoral neck;
b. Grade II, greater than one-third but less than one-half displacement;
c. Grade III, displacement greater than one-half (Fig. 15.22).[27,116]

Clinical presentation of young adolescents with SCFE includes pain in the groin, medial thigh, or knee; limping; external rotation of the leg; and limited hip ROM, especially flexion, abduction, and internal rotation.[69,116] External rotation is noted with attempts to flex the affected hip. With an acute onset, pain is often severe, and the adolescent is unable to bear weight on the affected lower extremity. History may include a traumatic or gradual onset. If an undiagnosed young adolescent presents to physical therapy with the preceding symptoms, the therapist should consider immediate referral to a pediatric orthopedic specialist for further workup.

Management

The goals of treatment include growth plate stabilization to prevent further displacement and prevention of complications, including avascular necrosis, chondrolysis, and early osteoarthritis.[27,116,117] Physeal stabilization is achieved through surgical pin fixation in situ.[118,119] This may also include prophylactic fixation of an uninvolved hip, especially in younger children.[116,118] Additional arthroscopic osteochondroplasty may be utilized to treat femoral acetabular impingement, which occurs in every hip with SCFE.[119] More significant procedures such as osteotomies are required for advanced and complicated cases. Nonsurgical treatment, including bed rest, traction, and casting, is not successful; long-term outcomes may include limited hip ROM, pain, and surgical procedures necessitated by early osteoarthritis.

Physical therapy includes gait training with an assistive device postoperatively; usually, a non-weight-bearing status is recommended during the acute recovery period, but often increases within 4 to 6 weeks. Bilateral strength and ROM throughout the lower extremities should be maintained

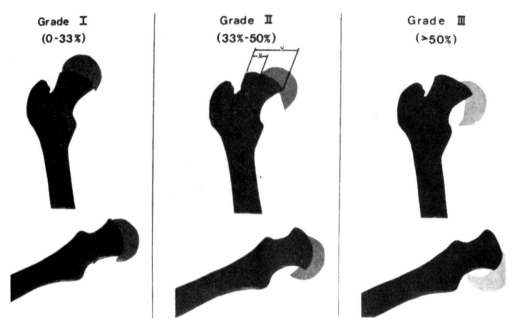

FIGURE 15.22. Classification of the three grades of SCFE.

through open chain exercises and stretching, respectively, during the non-weight-bearing phase. Care should be taken to maintain full knee and ankle ROM, which can decrease from minor amounts of lower extremity immobility and previous surgery. In view of the association with obesity, strengthening of the abdominal and trunk musculature is important preparatory work prior to return to bilateral weight-bearing activities and gait training post acutely. After weight-bearing advances, interventions should focus on increasing lower extremity strength to restore proper gait patterns and functional activity. Strengthening progress may be slow and complicated by excess weight or by a premorbidly decreased activity level. Consideration can be given to closed chain activities and gait training in a gravity-lessened environment such as during aquatic therapy or the use of gravity-lessening overhead sling systems such as the Zero-G®. This will allow for closed chain activities with less stress on the surgical site.

Tibia Vara (Blount Disease)

Tibia vara, or Blount disease, is a growth disorder of the medial aspect of the proximal tibia, including the epiphysis, physis, and metaphysis.[27,120] Tibia vara is classified as three types, related to the age of onset:

1. Infantile—less than 3 years of age is the most common;
2. Adolescent—between ages 6 and 13 years is often related to partial growth plate closure after trauma or infection;
3. Late onset between the ages of 6 and 15 years, seen primarily in obese, black males.[121]

Diagnostic radiographic changes include sharp varus angulation in the metaphysis, beaking of the medial tibial metaphysis, wedging of the medial epiphysis, widening of the growth plate, and the presence of cartilage islands in or near the metaphyseal beak (Fig. 15.23A and B).[122,123] This growth disturbance is thought to be the result of asymmetric and excessive compressive and shear forces across the proximal tibial growth plate.[27]

The child with tibia vara presents with a bow-legged stance. Infantile tibia vara, which is typically bilateral, must be distinguished from normal physiologic genu varum and medial tibial torsion. Physiologic genu varum gradually decreases until a genu valgus alignment is present between 2.5 and 3 years of age. Toddlers with tibia vara are often obese, are often early walkers, and may exhibit a lateral thrust of the knee during stance.[27,123,124] Tibia vara increases in severity, whereas physiologic genu varum decreases as the child grows and develops. Other diagnoses that must be ruled out include various skeletal dysplasias, rickets or vitamin D deficiency, or a fracture that involved the growth plate of the proximal medial tibia. Juvenile or adolescent tibia vara may also result from infection or trauma that disrupted growth of the proximal medial tibia.

Management

Treatment is dependent on the age of the child and the stage of the disease. Langenskiöld differentiated tibia vara into six stages, with guidelines for prognosis and intervention.[122] Stage I occurs between 18 months and 3 years of age and is characterized by beaking of the medial metaphysis and delay in growth of the medial epiphysis of the tibia. The stages progress in severity until stage VI. Stage VI is seen between 10 and 13 years of age and is characterized by fusion of the medial aspect of the physis while growth continues laterally.[27,122]

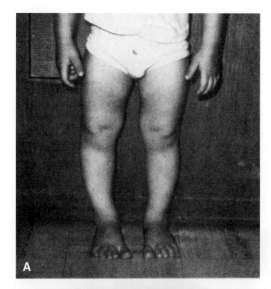

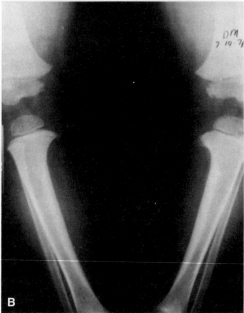

FIGURE 15.23. A: A 2-year-old child with varus on weight bearing. **B:** Same child at 2 years of age and progression of the Blount disease; note the varus angulation and beaking of the medial tibial metaphysis.

Treatment options include orthotic devices or surgical procedures. Orthotic intervention is recommended for children under 2 to 3 years of age, with radiographic findings consistent with stage I or II.[123,125] Of this group, children with smaller angular deformity and unilateral disease often respond better to bracing.[125] An HKAFO or KAFO used in full knee extension is recommended primarily while the child is weight bearing.[123,125] Proper fit and valgus correction adjustment should be evaluated every 2 to 4 months. Physical therapy intervention may include family instruction in orthosis donning, doffing, wearing schedule, as well as skin inspection during brace use. Gait training with or without an assistive device may be warranted.

After the age of 4 years, surgical options produce better outcomes than orthotic devices.[120,123,124] Despite disease severity, stage, and age of presentation, there are ultimately two tibial osteotomy surgical categories[124]: tibial osteotomy with full angular correction using internal or external fixation; or tibial osteotomy with gradual angular correction using a multiaxial correction (MAC) monolateral external fixator device, or a circular device such as a Taylor Spatial or Ilizarov frame (see Fig. 15.24).[120,124] Gradual corrections are performed by the child and family actually being responsible to turn the screws on external fixation devices at a set daily rate to correct angular deformities. MAC devices have demonstrated comparable outcomes to circular frame devices but with easier application and improved ROM and decreased interference with general mobility.[120] Guided growth procedures such as lateral hemiepiphysiodesis,

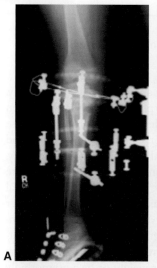
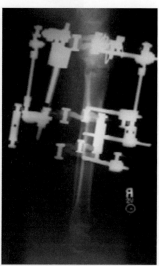
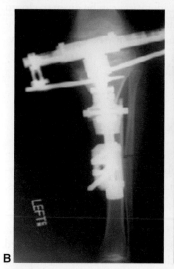
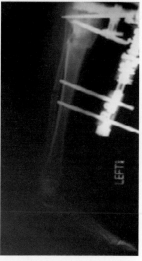

FIGURE 15.24. A: Ilizarov placement on right lower extremity. **B:** Left tibia with MAC device. (Used with permission from Clarke SE, McCarthy JJ, Davidson RS. Treatment of Blount disease: a comparison between the multiaxial correction system and other external fixators. *J Pediatr Orthop.* 2009;29:103–109.)

stapling, or tension band plate ("8-plate") placement are not indicated for correction of angular deformity related to Blount disease.[126]

Physical therapy intervention following surgical correction includes lower extremity strengthening, knee and ankle ROM, stretching, and gait training. Loss of knee flexion, terminal extension, and ankle dorsiflexion ROM can slow progress with functional activities during gradual correction procedures if consistent stretching is not performed in an HEP. Infection of the pin sites is one of the most common complications following application of external correction devices.[120] Children and families will need education in skin and pin care when external fixator devices are used to prevent pin site infections as well as tissue mobility. The recommendations for skin care may vary depending on physician preference as well as current resources available to families. ROM and strengthening interventions may be complicated for the obese child who presents with limited premorbid joint mobility and muscle strength.

Limb Length Discrepancy

A limb length discrepancy may be caused by shortening or overgrowth of one or more bones of the leg. Inequality of leg lengths may result from congenital conditions such as limb deficiencies or hemihypertrophy, infections or fractures that injure the physis, neuromuscular disorders, tumors, or trauma that results in overgrowth and disease processes. Injuries to the physes are often asymmetric and result in angular deformities in addition to the shortening of the affected limb. Leg length differences range from 1 to 10 cm or greater.

Measurements must be taken when a leg length difference is suspected. Functional measurements can be taken by placing blocks of known height under the shorter leg until bilateral pelvic landmarks are level, assuming there is no pelvic deformity. Clinical measurement may be taken with the child supine by measuring from the anterior superior iliac spine to the medial malleolus. Reliability of this measurement is affected by soft tissue asymmetries, excess fat tissue, and identification of bony landmarks.[127] More precise measurements are needed to predict the leg length discrepancy that will be present at maturity, evaluate treatment options, and predict the timing of surgical intervention if necessary. To assist with the prediction of future growth and treatment options, the orthopedist uses radiographic methods to obtain accurate measurements and determine bone age, and growth charts or mathematical prediction models to estimate future skeletal growth of the child.[128] Leg length is generally examined using plain film, computed radiography, or CT scanogram.[127]

Significant leg length discrepancies greater than 2 cm are a cosmetic as well as a functional issue. Gait is less efficient and awkward, and postural compensations of the leg, pelvis, and spine often develop. Postural compensations may not lead to a structural deformity but may cause discomfort in adulthood. Functional compensatory mechanisms include toe walking or foot and ankle supination on the short side or vaulting, circumduction, persistent knee flexion, or foot and ankle pronation on the longer side.[128]

Management

Treatment is dependent on the age of the child, expectation of remaining limb growth, severity of the leg length difference, and preference of the family and child. Intervention is usually not indicated for leg length differences of less than 2 cm.[27] A lift inside the shoe or a custom-fabricated external heel-sole lift may be used for differences of 1 to 2 cm. Surgical treatment options are suggested for discrepancies of greater than 2 to 2.5 cm.[128] These procedures fall into either of two categories: guided growth and growth restriction of the longer limb or lengthening of the shorter limb, but the approaches may be combined. It is less common for a child, unless skeletally mature, to undergo a shortening osteotomy of a long bone.

Guided growth procedures are indicated for leg length discrepancies of 2 to 5 cm.[27,69,128] Lessening the discrepancy is commonly achieved through epiphysiodesis on the longer limb. Permanent physeal ablation methods include percutaneous drilling or curettage through the growth plate. Alternatively, "temporary" methods can be performed by staple or tension band ("8 plate") fixation in the metaphysis and epiphysis across both the medial and the lateral sides of the growth plates of the distal femur and/or the proximal tibia. The medial–lateral "8 plate" approach has not been shown to be as effective as medial or lateral use for angular conditions. Percutaneous transphyseal screw implantation is a newer technique that is becoming a standard approach.[128] Most physicians opt for lengthening the shorter limb when the discrepancy is greater than 5 cm.

If the adolescent has reached skeletal maturity, then epiphysiodesis is not an option. In these cases, shortening of the longer limb is accomplished through osteotomy involving removal of a portion of the bone to equalize leg lengths. The maximum for removal is 5 to 6 cm in the femur and 2 to 4 cm for the tibia. The disadvantages of shortening by osteotomy are that the overall height of the individual is reduced, body proportions may be cosmetically unappealing, the amount of equalization is limited, and the uninvolved leg has undergone surgery, which can impact muscle performance and efficiency.

Limb-lengthening techniques are directed at the involved leg and allow for equalization of discrepancies greater than 5 cm.[27] Limb-lengthening techniques are based on the concept of distraction osteogenesis, which means that new bone is formed as two segments of bone are slowly moved apart. Despite the surgical technique or apparatus used, the procedures are most successful when based on the Ilizarov biologic principles and the Law of Tension Stress.[129] These principles are named after the physician who proposed them and include minimizing bone disturbance, delaying distraction, rate and frequency of distraction, and the number and site of osteotomies.

A corticotomy minimizes bone disturbance by only cutting the cortex of bone while keeping the periosteum and nutrient artery within the medullary cavity intact. Delaying distraction 5 to 10 days after completion of the osteotomy and application of the lengthening device allows the osteogenesis process to sufficiently initiate before the segments are pulled apart. The number of days to delay the distraction is dependent on the age of the child. The rate of distraction is about 1 mm per day, but the process should be broken down into a frequency of 0.25-mm increases every 6 hours to boost the osteogenesis process. The family follows a schedule provided by the physician to adjust the lengthening device applied.

The original Wagner technique, once popular in the United States, did not follow a majority of these principles and had high rates of complication.[129] A complete diaphyseal osteotomy was performed with a monolateral frame external fixator placed. Distraction was immediately initiated at a rate of 1.5 to 2.0 mm per day performed at one interval. After full distraction was achieved, an iliac crest bone autograft was implanted and plated to support the bone gap, and the external fixator was removed. After the graft was incorporated into the bone, the plates were removed. The entire process involved three operative procedures and could not be used to correct angular or rotational deformities.

Ilizarov introduced a circular frame external fixator with telescoping rods to employ his biologic principles during a metaphyseal lengthening procedure (Fig. 15.25).[129] The Ilizarov principles are successfully applied with the use of newer devices previously discussed in relation to Blount disease such as the Taylor Spatial Frame (TSF), Limb Reconstruction System (Orthofix®) and the Multiaxial Correction System (Biomet®). The principles are also applied with the newest limb-lengthening technology using motorized internal lengthening nails such as Precise® Intramedullary Limb Lengthening System and Fitbone®. After the desired length is achieved, the external fixator device is kept in place for approximately 1 month for every 1 cm of distraction until the bone consolidation phase is complete.[129] Typically, the internal lengthening nails are removed after about 1 year. The external frames can accomplish both lengthening and rotational and angular correction, whereas the internal nails are used purely for lengthening. The pins of external frames can be removed in an outpatient procedure. The disadvantages of the Ilizarov and TSF are the multiple pin sites and bulkiness of the apparatus. The overall length of time required to achieve the desired length and keep the fixator in place are disadvantages of all lengthening systems.

Internal limb lengthening has gone through a recent evolution. Originally, the Intramedullary Skeletal Kinetic Distractor (Orthofix®) was an internally implanted device utilized for limb lengthening. The child controls the lengthening process through rotational movements of the lower leg. These systems eliminate the spatial problems and extended duration of external frames, but there have

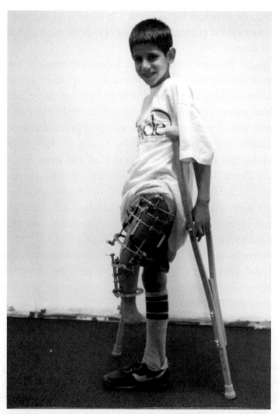

FIGURE 15.25. A 9-year-old boy with a diagnosis of PFFD who is presently undergoing an Ilizarov lengthening. The lengthening will provide a longer lever arm when wearing his prosthesis and bring the height of his knees closer together.

been concerns that this device had many of its own complications, including not achieving the desired length and difficulty to use. Dror Paley introduced the lengthening on nail (LON) procedure, which combines traditional external fixators with an intramedullary nail to decrease the overall duration of external fixator placement and bone healing time.[130] This procedure has been shown to result in a higher incidence of treatable hindfoot equinus likely because of accelerated lengthening.[130] Most recently, the use of motorized intramedullary lengthening such as the Precise® Nail and Fitbone® has revolutionized limb-lengthening procedures. The internal lengthening nail has a small motor that is attached to a receiver, and the child places an external controller over the specific location of the receiver. When the controller is turned on, the nail is able to be lengthened or shortened depending on the programming. Advantages of this type of lengthening procedure include decreased bulk compared with external frames, decreased infection risk caused by lack of external pins, and cosmetic appearance during the lengthening process. Disadvantages include nonfunctioning muscle in the nail resulting in inability to lengthen, fractures, inability to manage angular deformities, and weight-bearing restrictions resulting from lack of nail strength during the distraction phase.[131]

Limb-lengthening procedures bring their own set of problems to the child, family, and professionals involved in the care of the child. Families must be able to make multiple appointments over a period of time, perform daily pin care, and carry out exercise programs. Problems that may be encountered during the course of a lengthening procedure include infection at the pin sites, joint stiffness, subluxation or dislocation (especially of the proximal tibia), nonunion, and fractures. ROM limitations occur secondary to shortening of the soft tissues and the rate of soft tissue growth compared with that of bone.

Physical Therapy

Physical therapy intensity varies with the five phases of the process: latency, distraction, consolidation, fixator removal and healing, and the rehabilitation phase. Immediately after surgery during the latency or delayed distraction period, the physical therapist is involved for gait-training activities and promoting early weight bearing if permitted by physician and surgical precautions. Weight bearing further facilitates bone growth for most children who have undergone a lengthening procedure. Instruction in pin care must also begin immediately postoperatively to prevent infection. Pins can also be wrapped with gauze to provide soft tissue compression, which reduces pain resulting from tissue movement or microtearing around pin sites. Stretching can be initiated to minimize immediate postoperative ROM limitations.

During the distraction phase, physical therapy should be frequent and focused on ROM and stretching along with corresponding strengthening activity. Decreased knee and ankle joint ROM are common and should be addressed consistently. Splinting can be utilized during this phase, especially for the ankle. Hip ROM may become limited to a lesser extent. It is important for the therapist to acknowledge that maintaining the same ROM measurement over the duration of the distraction phase actually represents increased muscle and soft tissue length, and this should be considered successful ROM intervention progress. Therapists should be considerate of fixator pin placement, especially in the thigh and around the knee. Typical lateral pin placement, especially distal on the femur, will contribute to soft tissue impalement of the tensor fascia lata and iliotibial band complex, thereby limiting achievable knee ROM. As a result, progressive ROM losses may occur during the distraction phase. But aggressive intervention is still necessary during the lengthening process. Strengthening can safely include modalities such as electric stimulation and aquatic therapy. Limited motion and muscle atrophy may also contribute to muscle adhesion. Tissue mobilization should be used to facilitate soft tissue movement and improved joint motion.

During the consolidation phase, strengthening and tissue mobilization activities should be continued, whereas previously achieved ROM should be at least maintained. An appropriate physical therapy goal in this phase would be to regain ROM lost during distraction. For children who have undergone internal lengthening, increasing weight-bearing progression

through gait training as well as other activities will be included in the PT program. This phase should include formal program supervision or weekly monitoring by the therapist. However, insurance restrictions may require the use of a comprehensive HEP rather than supervised therapy sessions. Once ossification has reached an appropriate level, a cast or CAM boot is placed following a tibial fixator removal, and a knee immobilizer is placed following a femoral fixator removal to protect the new bone during continued healing. During this phase, an HEP is sufficient to promote continued allowable stretching and strengthening of nonimmobilized joints.

The rehabilitation phase may last up to 1 year. During this phase, aggressive stretching is advanced to achieve as much functional ROM as possible. Flex casting and dynamic splinting are often utilized as a stretching adjunct to address knee flexion or extension and ankle plantar flexion contractures. ROM status often regresses, so the therapist should remain steadfast and utilize soft tissue mobilization techniques to maintain progress. Strengthening activities are progressed as muscles and soft tissue are further lengthened. Functional activities and gait normalization can be implemented as bone healing progresses and muscle strength and ROM increase. Postural reactions and balance training should be addressed as the body accommodates to the new limb length, limits of stability, base of support, and center of gravity.

Scoliosis (Idiopathic)

Scoliosis is a lateral curvature of the spine greater than 10 degrees. Idiopathic denotes that the scoliosis is of unknown origin—the most common form of scoliosis. Idiopathic scoliosis can be further delineated by age of onset: infantile occurs in children from birth to 3 years of age, juvenile between the ages of 3 and 10 years, and adolescent after 10 years of age.[132] This section of the chapter focuses on adolescent idiopathic scoliosis (AIS). However, the pediatric therapist should be mindful that not all scoliosis is idiopathic; therefore, congenital or neurologic causes should be ruled out. The incidence of idiopathic scoliosis greater than 10 degrees is approximately 2%, greater than 20 degrees approximately 1%, greater than 40 degrees 0.4%, demonstrating the uncommon nature of large curves.[133,134]

Scoliosis is defined as either structural or nonstructural. Structural curves are fixed and do not correct with lateral trunk bending or traction. Structural curves have a rotary component that is visible when the trunk is flexed forward. Nonstructural curves correct on lateral trunk bending, and their etiology is often a pelvic obliquity, limb length discrepancy, or medical factors such as a tumor or muscle spasm. Structural scoliosis is further identified by the location and direction of the apex of the curve. For example, a curve with the apex in the thoracic region and convexity toward the right would be labeled a right thoracic curve. Most curves have both a primary and a compensatory curve. The compensatory curve is the body's attempt to keep the head and trunk aligned vertically. In the preceding example of the right

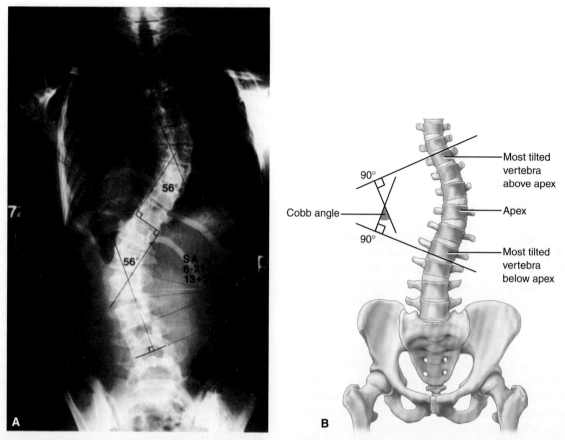

FIGURE 15.26. **A:** Right thoracic, left lumbar scoliosis. **B:** The degree of curvature is measured using the Cobb method. The end vertebrae, or the vertebrae that tilt toward the concavity the most, are identified. Lines are drawn extending the end plate of the top and bottom vertebrae for each curve. Perpendicular lines to the end plate lines are then drawn. The *degree of curvature* is defined as the angle of intersection of the end plate and perpendicular lines.

thoracic curve, there may be smaller compensatory curves in the cervical or lumbar regions with their convexity toward the left (Fig. 15.26A). More than 90% of AIS is right thoracic or left lumbar, and an atypical presentation should be cause for further investigation.[132]

Multiple structural changes occur with scoliosis, and their severity is related to that of the curve.[27] Changes occur in the growing spine in response to compression and distraction forces that are altered in the presence of a curvature. The vertebrae become wedge shaped, higher on the convex side and compressed on the concave side, and muscles on the concave side become shortened. The vertebral body rotates toward the convex side so that the spinous process is rotated toward the concave side. Because the ribs are attached to the thoracic vertebrae, the vertebrae may rotate. The rotation of the ribs produces a posterior rib hump, which is noted on the forward-bend test (Fig. 15.27). Thoracic scoliosis can also decrease normal kyphosis, further exemplifying the three-dimensional nature of the disorder.

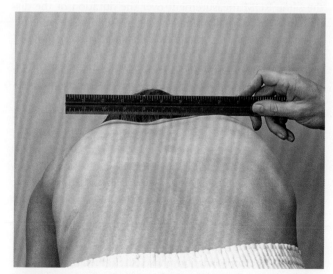

FIGURE 15.27. Forward-bend test. Rib hump is visible on bending forward.

Screening

School-based screenings for scoliosis are mandated in many states but have been a source of controversy with recent conflicting recommendations from two major health policy groups.[132] Screening should be targeted at girls aged 10 and again at 12 years and for boys at 13 or 14 years. A screening should include anterior and posterior views of the trunk with the shirt removed and a forward-bend Adams test (Fig. 15.25).[132] On the anterior and posterior views, the examiner looks for asymmetries in shoulder, nipple, scapular, or pelvic heights; asymmetric inguinal or gluteal folds; and curvature of the spine. The adolescent is then asked to bend over, keeping the knees extended, and allowing the arms to dangle toward the floor. During the forward-bend test, the examiner looks for asymmetries in the contour of the back (classic rib hump), indicating the rotary component of the curvature.

When scoliosis is detected, the adolescent should be referred to an orthopedic specialist. Accurate measurement of the curve is performed through a variety of methods, a common one being a radiograph and the Cobb angle (Fig. 15.24A and B). To limit radiographic exposure, other measurement methods include Moiré topography and the Integrated Shape Imaging System 2 (ISIS2).[135] Moiré topography is a photogrammetric technique that visually depicts shadow patterns that identify asymmetries. ISIS2 utilizes computer images in the transverse, frontal, and sagittal planes to develop contours of the adolescent's trunk.[135] The goal of measurement is to determine a baseline and monitor the progression of the curve.

Management of Scoliosis

Treatment intervention is based on the sex, age, and skeletal maturity of the adolescent and the severity of the curvature.[132,136] Prepubertal children are almost certain to exhibit progression of their curvature, especially when initially presenting with a curve of greater than 20 degrees. Females with a bone age of 15 years and males with a bone age of 17 years with curves less than 30 degrees generally do not require surgical treatment.[132] Curves less than 25 degrees can be observed on a regular basis to monitor progression of the curve. Curves between 25 and 40 degrees should be treated with nonsurgical methods. Adolescents with curves greater than 40 degrees are candidates for surgical intervention.[132,136]

NONOPERATIVE MANAGEMENT The goal of nonoperative intervention is to maintain the curvature during growth, not to correct the curvature, although improved alignment can occur.[136] Nonoperative intervention methods have included exercise, electrical stimulation, and orthoses. Evidence supporting the beneficial effects of therapeutic exercise or electric stimulation in reducing or altering the progression of a curvature is inconsistent and lacks supportive controlled studies.[132] Exercise is still indicated to maintain strength of muscles when an orthosis is used.

Orthosis management has been used in the treatment of scoliosis for many years. A recently published randomized controlled trial was discontinued early owing to the efficacy of bracing.[137] Most orthotic devices operate on the principle of three-point pressure against the apex of the curve and may also incorporate a traction component. The cervicothoracic lumbosacral Milwaukee brace was one of the first orthoses developed for scoliosis. It incorporates a custom-molded trunk shell with metal uprights attached to a collar that supports the chin and occiput. Although it is effective, it is no longer a brace of choice on account of significant cosmetic concerns and individual preferences.

Much slimmer and lighter-weight thoracic–lumbar–sacral orthoses (TLSO) (Fig. 15.28) that eliminate the chin and occiput component of the Milwaukee brace are the gold standard for most curves. The Boston Brace or similar variations are the most common TLSOs used in North America.[137] The pelvic stabilization and lateral pressure pads are present in a TLSO. Adolescents are generally instructed to wear the orthosis until skeletal maturity or unless the curve continues to progress and surgery is indicated. Recommended wear time is at least 18 hours. Published controlled data demonstrate the positive correlation between success rate and increased average wear time.[137]

Instruction in donning and doffing the orthosis, developing a wearing schedule, skin care, and an exercise program to maintain ROM, flexibility, and strength while wearing the orthosis are provided by a physical therapist. Exercise should be focused on maintaining flexibility and muscle strength of the trunk and extremities. Hip flexion contractures can

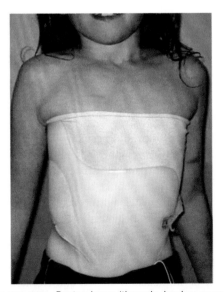

FIGURE 15.28. Boston brace (thoracic–lumbar–sacral orthosis [TLSO]). (From Sponseller PD. Bracing for adolescent idiopathic scoliosis in practice today. *J Pediatr Orthop.* 2011;31:S53–S60.)

develop with the use of the orthosis; routine stretching of the hip flexors should be instituted when orthosis wearing is initiated. Muscle strength must be maintained while wearing the orthosis to prepare the trunk muscles for eventual discontinuation of the orthosis. Exercise should include strengthening for abdominals, gluteal muscles such as squats and lunges, and paraspinal musculature through traditional core and lumbar stabilization programs.

OPERATIVE MANAGEMENT Surgical intervention is warranted if the curve is greater than 40 degrees, the curve is progressing with conservative management, or there is decompensation of the spine or thoracic cavity.[132,136] The goal of surgery is to obtain as much correction as possible and to stabilize the spine and maintain the correction over time. The Lenke Classification, which considers the curve type, relationship between lumbar and sacral alignment, and the sagittal curve profile, was developed to guide operative treatment decisions for orthopedic surgeons.[136]

Two main surgical approaches exist: the anterior and the posterior approach. The anterior approach goes through the chest cavity and has been associated with increased morbidity caused by decreased pulmonary function.[136] The posterior approach is becoming the option of choice for AIS. This option has been further facilitated by the development and progression of pedicle screw technology. Pedicle screws provide solid fixation through most of the vertebrae. The screws are then connected by rods allowing deformity correction in all three planes. That is, the primary curve in the frontal plane, vertebral rotation in the transverse plane, and kyphosis or lordosis restoration or stabilization in the sagittal plane. Recent approaches target surgical correction of the primary structural curve, allowing flexible compensatory curves to self-correct over time.[136] This approach preserves as much natural spinal motion as possible, limiting previous detrimental effects of unnecessary lumbar spine anchoring. Pedicle screws and shorter segment rod fixation have replaced most hook, wire, and Harrington rod procedures with good outcomes and less complication.

Physical Therapy

Ideally, physical therapy has been involved preoperatively with ROM and trunk-strengthening exercises as well as bed mobility and transfer training. Instruction in deep breathing and coughing exercises should be initiated preoperatively and adhered to immediately postoperatively. The adolescent is always encouraged to begin early mobilization, including transfers and gait training, to expedite healing and recovery. Balance, vestibular, and field of vision changes should be considered during gait training because the head position and height may be immediately altered and elevated following spinal straightening. Time frames for early mobilization and ambulation depend on the surgical technique, surgeon's preference, and whether or not a supportive orthosis is needed, but in some cases can begin as early as postoperative day one.

Physical therapy is one of the important interventions for the adolescent with AIS, regardless of whether conservative or surgical care has been employed.

Summary

The growth and development and disorders of a child's musculoskeletal system were discussed in this chapter. The immature musculoskeletal system of a child is susceptible to abnormal forces and stresses. Physical therapists must be alert to those forces and the consequences they may have on the developing musculoskeletal system. Many orthopedic diagnoses that were discussed in this chapter are the result of the effect of abnormal forces on the developing child and morphologic defects occurring during fetal development. However, the examination and intervention principles that were discussed and the evaluation procedures that were outlined can be applied to any child seen by a physical therapist, not just those children with a diagnosis of orthopedic origin. Identifying the underlying causes, estimating the risk of further deformity or disease progression, and developing an evidence-based plan of care based on a complete examination is the challenging, yet rewarding aspect of pediatric physical therapy.

CASE STUDY

M.D., 4-MONTH-OLD CAUCASIAN GIRL WITH RIGHT CONGENITAL MUSCULAR TORTICOLLIS

M.D. was referred to physical therapy for right CMT at the age of 4 months. She was first diagnosed with torticollis at 3 months of age by her pediatrician when she was still presenting with an altered head position. During her initial evaluation, her mother reported that this was her first pregnancy, and the baby was breech until week 39 of gestation, when M.D. then flipped into the head down position. M.D. was delivered at 41 weeks' gestation via vacuum delivery after a 24-hour labor. Her initial Apgar scores were a 10 at 1 minute and a 10 at 5 minutes. M.D. did not require any prolonged stay in the hospital.

Her mother reported her daily routines and M.D.'s developmental milestones. M.D. appropriately responded to voices and visual cues with toys. She was positioned for sleep during the day in a swing or car seat at the day care program but slept in her crib at home. When on the floor, M.D. did not tolerate the prone position, so she was usually positioned supine in a positioning pillow. She was being breastfed but uses a bottle at day care, where she prefers to be held by her caregivers in their right arm with her head rotated to the left.

M.D. preferred to play in supine on an activity mat. She had limited tolerance for playing in the prone position and would cry when placed in that position. Her parents supported her head when they picked her up after diaper changes. M.D.'s preferred position was supine with right lateral flexion and left rotation of her head. Slight flattening of her left occipital area was noted. When encouraged with a toy and visual cues, she could visually track appropriately but had difficulty with cervical rotation to the right. Passive ROM of her cervical spine presented with normal rotation and lateral flexion bilaterally, with the exception in rotation to the right, which measures 25 degrees from midline. Her hip joint screen revealed a positive Ortolani test on her right hip, which resulted in a referral to orthopedics for further examination.

Upon examination of her mobility, she could roll from supine to left side lying but required moderate assistance from supine to right side lying. From side lying to prone, she required the maximum assistance to move her weight-bearing shoulder to unweight it and to prone prop. She required the maximum assistance to move into prone prop and could hold her head in extension for three to five seconds. She was unable to tolerate prone well and could not track toys in prone. Once placed on a 30-degree wedge with maximum support at her shoulders in prone prop, she could hold her head up for 10 seconds in extension. Her pull to sit strength was limited, and she required assistance to perform a chin tuck in a semireclined position with support on her scapulae. This presentation demonstrated a developmental delay in her rolling and pull to sit milestones at 4 months of age, which was attributed to her limited cervical strength and ROM.

Physical therapy was initiated with M.D. once a week to address her impairments in ROM and expression of developmental milestones. Interventions included passive left lateral flexion and right rotation of her cervical spine through manual stretches in supine as well as in a "football hold" position. Visual cues were used to facilitate active ROM. Her caregivers were instructed to limit the use of the car seat or swing for naps throughout the day, because she tended to fall into right lateral flexion when placed without additional support. Facilitating her ability to roll from supine to side lying and from side lying to prone and then maintain her head in extension were her functional play activities. Parental and caregiver instructions were provided for daily stretches and encouragement of active motion of the cervical spine.

In one month, she was able to tolerate the prone position holding her head in extension for 1 minute and started to reach for toys placed in front of her. She demonstrated an improved posture when pulled to sit, using an appropriate chin tuck. Her referral to orthopedics revealed no hip dysplasia, and she no longer presents with any occipital flattening. It was determined to decrease her frequency of services to every other week sessions to continue to address her preferred head position, which continued to present with a right lateral flexed position when she was fatigued.

At her 7-month appointment, M.D. presented with full passive and active ROM of her cervical spine. She can move from side lying or prone to ring sitting independently and play with a toy at midline. Her preference for a right lateral flexed head posture, even in an upright position, has resolved.

Discussion Questions

1. What other diagnoses are often seen with a presentation of torticollis? What special tests could be utilized in the examination?

   Hip dysplasia—Ortolani/Barlow; Plagiocephaly—circumferential measurements

2. What developmental milestones examinations/assessments can be utilized to evaluate a child with torticollis more comprehensively?

   Alberta Infant Motor Scale, Peabody Developmental Motor Scale

3. How would the plan of care have changed if the child had not been meeting appropriate developmental milestones? If her head position had not resolved?

   Milestones—continue to engage the child every week or twice a week to address developmental milestones practice; referral to early intervention services to be able to give the child services at the day care program; potential referral to neurology to screen for other developmental delays. Head position—Consider referral to orthopedics for examination of hemivertebrae and sternocleidomastoid tissue construct for potential surgical options; use of orthoses such as TOT collar for prolonged positioning assistance; if plagiocephaly persists, referral to orthotist for helmet.

REFERENCES

1. Crelin ES. Development of the musculoskeletal system. *Clin Symp*. 1981;33:2–36.
2. Walker JM. Musculoskeletal development: a review. *Phys Ther*. 1991;71:878–889.
3. Arkin AM, Katz JF. The effects of pressure on epiphyseal growth. *J Bone Joint Surg Am*. 1956;38:1056–1076.
4. Storey E. Growth and remodeling of bone and bones. *Dent Clin North Am*. 1975;19:443–454.
5. LeVeau BF, Bernhardt DB. Developmental biomechanics: effect of forces on the growth, development and maintenance of the human body. *Phys Ther*. 1984;64:1874–1882.
6. Dunne KB, Clarren SK. The origin of prenatal and postnatal deformities. *Pediatr Clin North Am*. 1986;33:1277–1297.
7. Puberty and the Tanner Stages. Accessed November 10, 2013. www.childgrowthfoundation.org/CMS/FILES/Puberty_and_theTanner_Stages.pdf
8. Stuberg WA, Metcalf WK. Reliability of quantitative muscle testing in healthy children and in children with Duchenne muscular dystrophy using a hand-held dynamometer. *Phys Ther*. 1988;68:977–982.
9. Allington N, Leroy N, Doneux C. Ankle joint range of motion measurements in spastic cerebral palsy children: intraobserver and interobserver reliability and reproducibility of goniometry and visual estimation. *J Pediatr Orthop Part B*. 2002;11:236–239.
10. McWhirk LB, Glanzman AM. Within-session inter-rater reliability of goniometric measures in patients with spastic cerebral palsy. *Pediatr Phys Ther*. 2006;18(4):262–265.
11. Glanzman AM, Swenson AE, Kim H. Intrarater range of motion reliability in cerebral palsy: a comparison of methods. *Pediatr Phys Ther*. 2008;20(4):369–372.

12. Bleck EE. *Orthopedic Management in Cerebral Palsy.* JB Lippincott; 1987.

13. Russek LN. Examination and treatment of a patient with hypermobility syndrome. *Phys Ther.* 2000;80(4):386–398.

14. Kendall FP, McCreary EK. *Muscles: Testing and Function.* Williams & Wilkins; 1993.

15. Effgen SK, Brown DA. Long-term stability of hand-held dynamometric measurements in children who have myelomeningocele. *Phys Ther.* 1992;72:458–465.

16. Hinderer K, Gutierrez T. Myometry measurements of children using isometric and eccentric methods of muscle testing (Abstract). *Phys Ther.* 1988;68:817.

17. Stuberg WA, Koehler A, Wichita M, et al. Comparison of femoral torsion assessment using goniometry and computerized tomography. *Pediatr Phys.* 1989;1:115–118.

18. Gajdosik CG. Ability of very young children to produce reliable isometric force measurements. *Pediatr Phys Ther.* 2005;17(4): 251–257.

19. Hébert LJ, Maltais DB, Hébert LJ, et al. (2015). Hand-held dynamometry isometric torque reference values for children and adolescents. *Pediatr Phy Ther.* 27(4):414–423.

20. Merlini L, Dell'Accio D, Granata C. Reliability of dynamic strength knee muscle testing in children. *J Sports Phys Ther.* 1995;22:73–76.

21. Tsiros MD, Grimshaw PN, Shield AJ, et al. The Biodex isokinetic dynamometer for knee strength assessment in children: advantages and limitations. *Work.* 2011;39(2):161–167.

22. Holm I, Fredriksen P, Fosdahl M, et al. A normative sample of isotonic and isokinetic muscle strength measurements in children 7 to 12 years of age. *Acta Paediatr.* 2008;97(5):602–607.

23. Wiggin M, Wilkinson K, Habetz S, et al. Percentile values of isokinetic peak torque in children six through thirteen years old. *Pediatr Phys Ther.* 2006;18(1):3–18.

24. Radler C, Kranzl A, Manner HM, et al. Torsional profile versus gait analysis: consistency between the anatomic torsion and the resulting gait pattern in patients with rotational malalignment of the lower extremity. *Gait Posture.* 2010;32(3):405–410.

25. Staheli LT, Corbett M, Wyss C, et al. Lower-extremity rotational problems in children. *J Bone Joint Surg.* 1985;67A:39–47.

26. Cusick BD, Stuberg WA. Assessment of lower-extremity alignment in the transverse plane: implications for management of children with neuromotor dysfunction. *Phys Ther.* 1992;72:3–15.

27. Tachdjian MO. *Pediatric Orthopedics.* 2nd ed. WB Saunders Co.; 1990.

28. World Health Organization. *International Classification of Functioning, Disability, and Health.* World Health Organization; 2001.

29. Spranger J, Benirschke JG, Hall W, et al. Errors of morphogenesis: concepts and terms. *J Pediatr.* 1982;100:160–165.

30. Day HJB. The ISO/ISPO classification of congenital limb deficiency. *Prosth Orthot Int.* 1991;15:67–69.

31. Koskimies E, Lindfors N, Gissler M, et al. Congenital upper limb deficiencies and associated malformations in Finland: a population-based study. *J Hand Surg.* 2011;36(6):1058–1065.

32. Goldfarb CA, Wall L, Manske PR. Radial longitudinal deficiency: the incidence of associated medical and musculoskeletal conditions. *J Hand Surg Am.* 2006;31(7):1176–1182.

33. Wright PE, Jobe MT. Congenital anomalies of the hand. In: Canlae ST, Beaty JH, eds. *Operative Pediatric Orthopedics.* Mosby–Year Book; 1991:253–330.

34. Swanson AB, Barsky AJ, Entin MA. Classification of limb malformations on the basis of embryological failures. *Surg Clin North Am.* 1968;48:1169–1179.

35. Heikel HVA. Aplasia and hypoplasia of the radius. *Acta Orthop Scand.* 1959;39(Suppl):1.

36. Bayne LG, Klug MS. Long-term review of the surgical treatment of radial deficiencies. *J Hand Surg.* 1987;12(2):169–179.

37. James MA, McCarroll HR Jr, Manske PR. The spectrum of radial longitudinal deficiency: a modified classification. *J Hand Surg Am.* 1999;24(6):1145–1155.

38. Morrissy RT, Giavedoni BJ, Coulter-O'Berry C. The limb-deficient child. In: Lovell WW, Winter RB, eds. *Pediatric Orthopedics.* 5th ed. Lippincott Williams & Wilkins; 2001:1217–1272.

39. Aitken GT. Proximal femoral focal deficiency: definition, classification and management. In: *Proximal Femoral Focal Deficiency: A Congenital Anomaly.* National Academy of Sciences; 1969:1–22.

40. Shurr DG, Cook TM. *Prosthetics and Orthotics.* Appleton & Lange; 1990:183–193.

41. Herzenberg JE. Congenital limb deficiency and limb length discrepancy. In: Canale ST, Beaty JH, eds. *Operative Pediatric Orthopedics.* Mosby–Year Book; 1991:187–252.

42. Kruger LM. Lower-limb deficiencies: surgical management. In: Bowker JH, Michael JW, eds. *Atlas of Limb Prosthetics: Surgical, Prosthetic, and Rehabilitation Principles.* Mosby–Year Book; 1981:795–834.

43. Kant P, Koh SH, Neumann V, et al. Treatment of longitudinal deficiency affecting the femur: comparing patient mobility and satisfaction outcomes of Syme amputation against extension prosthesis. *J Pediatr Orthop.* 2003;23:236–242.

44. Krajbich JL. Rotationplasty in the management of proximal femoral focal deficiency. In: Herring JA, Birch JG, eds. *The Child with a Limb Deficiency.* American Academy of Orthopedic Surgeons; 1998:87.

45. Gillespie R. Principles of amputation surgery in children with longitudinal limb deficiencies of the femur. *Clin Orthop Rel Res.* 1990;256:29–38.

46. Ackman J, Altiok H, Flanagan A, et al. Long-term follow-up of Van Nes rotationplasty in patients with congenital proximal focal femoral deficiency. *Bone Joint J.* 2013;95-B:192–198.

47. Suzuki S, Yamamura T, Fujita A. Aetiological relationship between congenital torticollis and obstetrical paralysis. *Int Orthop.* 1984;8:175–181.

48. Bredenkamp JK, Hoover LA, Berke GS, et al. Congenital muscular torticollis. *Arch Otolaryngol Head Neck Surg.* 1990;116:212–216.

49. Binder H, Eng GD, Gaiser JF, et al. Congenital muscular torticollis: results of conservative management with long-term follow-up in 85 cases. *Arch Phys Med Rehabil.* 1987;68:222–225.

50. Emery C. The determinants of treatment duration for congenital muscular torticollis. *Phys Ther.* 1994;74:921–929.

51. Cheng JCY, Wong MWN, Tang SP, et al. Clinical determinants of the outcome of manual stretching in the treatment of congenital muscular torticollis in infants. *J Bone Joint Surg.* 2001;83A(5):679–687.

52. Van Vlimmeren LA, Helders PJM, Van Adrichem LNA, et al. Torticollis and plagiocephaly in infancy: therapeutic strategies. *Pediatr Rehabil.* 2006;9(1):40–46.

53. American Academy of Pediatrics. Changing concepts of sudden infant death syndrome: implications for infant sleeping environment and sleep position. *Pediatrics.* 2000;105:650–656.

54. Kane AA, Mitchell LE, Craven KP, et al. Observations on a recent increase in plagiocephaly without synostosis. *Pediatrics.* 1996;97:877–885.

55. Persing J, James H, Swanson J, et al. Prevention and management of positional skull deformities in infants. *Pediatrics.* 2003;112:199–202.

56. De Chalain TM, Park S. Torticollis associated with positional plagiocephaly: a growing epidemic. *J Craniofac Surg.* 2005;16(3): 411–418.

57. Kaplan SL, Coulter C, Sargent B. Physical Therapy Management of congenital muscular torticollis: a 2018 evidence-based clinical practice guideline from the APTA academy of pediatric physical therapy. *Pediatr Phys Ther.* 2018;30(4):240–290.

58. Ballock RT, Song KM. The prevalence of nonmuscular causes of torticollis in children. *J Pediatr Orthop.* 1996;16(4):500–504.

59. Taylor JL, Norton ES. Developmental muscular torticollis: outcomes in young children treated by physical therapy. *Pediatr Phys Ther.* 1997;9(4):173–178.

60. Christensen C, Landsettle A, Antoszewski S, et al. Conservative management of congenital muscular torticollis: an evidence-based algorithm and preliminary treatment parameter recommendations. *Phys Occup Ther Pediatr.* 2013;33(4):453–466.

61. Vles JSH, Colla C, Weber JW, et al. Helmet versus nonhelmet treatment in nonsynostotic positional posterior plagiocephaly. *J Craniofac Surg.* 2000;11(6):572–574.

62. Lipira AB, Gordon S, Darvann TA, et al. Helmet versus active repositioning for plagiocephaly: a three-dimensional analysis. *Pediatrics.* 2010;126:e936–e945.

63. Jacques C, Karmel-Ross K. The use of splinting in conservative and post-operative treatment of congenital muscular torticollis. *Phys Occup Ther Pediatr.* 1997;17:81–90.

64. Limpaphayom N, Kohan E, Huser A, et al. Use of combined botulinum toxin and physical therapy for treatment resistant congenital muscular torticollis. *J Pediatr Orthop.* 2019;39(5):e343–e348.

65. Hensinger RN, Jones ET. Developmental orthopedics: the lower limb. *Dev Med Child Neurol.* 1982;24:95–116.

66. Dunn PM. Congenital postural deformities. *Br Med Bull.* 1976;32:71–76.

67. Furdon SA, Donlon CR. Examination of the newborn foot: positional and structural abnormalities. *Adv Neonatal Care.* 2002;2(5):248–258.

68. Beaty JH. Congenital anomalies of the lower and upper extremities. In: Canale ST, Beaty JH, eds. *Operative Pediatric Orthopedics.* Mosby–Year Book; 1991:73–186.

69. Staheli LT. *Fundamentals of Pediatric Orthopedics.* Lippincott-Raven; 1992.

70. Hart ES, Grottkau BE, Rebello GN, et al. The newborn foot: diagnosis and management of common conditions. *Orthop Nurs.* 2005;24(5):313–321.

71. Weymouth KS, Blanton SH, Bamshad MJ, et al. Variants in genes that encode muscle contractile proteins influence risk of isolated clubfoot. *Am J Med Genet A.* 2011;155:2170–2179.

72. Alvarado DM, Aferol H, McCall K, et al. Familial isolated clubfoot is associated with recurrent chromosome 17q23.1q23.2 microduplications containing TBX4. *Am J Hum Genet.* 2010;87(1):154–160.

73. Sadler B, Gurnett CA, Dobbs MB. The genetics of isolated and syndromic clubfoot. *J Child Orthop.* 2019;13(3):238–244.

74. Morcuende JA, Dolan LA, Dietz FR, et al. Radical reduction in the rate of extensive corrective surgery for clubfoot using the Ponseti method. *Pediatrics.* 2004;113:376–380.

75. Sala DA, Chu A, Lehman WB, et al. Achievement of gross motor milestones in children with idiopathic clubfoot treated with the Ponseti method. *J Pediatr Orthop.* 2013;33(1):55–58.

76. Hensinger RN. Congenital dislocation of the hip, treatment in infancy to walking age. *Orthop Clin North Am.* 1987;18:597–616.

77. Mubarak MD, Garfin S, Vance R, et al. Pitfalls in the use of the Pavlik harness for treatment of congenital dysplasia, subluxation, and dislocation of the hip. *J Bone Joint Surg Am.* 1981;63:1239–1247.

78. Darin N, Kimber E, Kroksmark A, et al. Multiple congenital contractures: birth prevalence, etiology, and outcome. *J Pediatr.* 2002;140:61–67.

79. Thompson GH, Bilenker RM. Comprehensive management of arthrogryposis multiplex congenita. *Clin Orthop Rel Res.* 1985;194:6–14.

80. Banker BQ. Neuropathic aspects of arthrogryposis multiplex congenita. *Clin Orthop Rel Res.* 1985;194:30–43.

81. Donohoe M, Pruszcynski B, Rogers K, et al. Predicting ambulatory function based on infantile lower extremity posture types in amyoplasia arthrogryposis. *J Pediatr Orthop.* 2019;39(7):E531–E535.

82. Staheli LT. Torsional deformity. *Pediatr Clin North Am.* 1986;33(6):1373–1383.

83. Forlino A, Cabral WA, Barnes AM, et al. New perspectives on osteogenesis imperfecta. *Nat Rev Endocrinol.* 2011;7(9):540–557.

84. Basel D, Steiner RD. Osteogenesis imperfecta: recent findings shed new light on this once well-understood condition. *Genet Med.* 2009;11(6):375–385.

85. Binder H, Hawks L, Graybill G, et al. Osteogenesis imperfecta: rehabilitation approach with infants and young children. *Adv Pediatr.* 1984;65:537–541.

86. Binder H, Conway A, Gerber LH. Rehabilitation approaches to children with osteogenesis imperfecta: a ten-year experience. *Arch Phys Med Rehabil.* 1993;74:386–390.

87. Amor MB, Rauch F, Monti E, et al. Osteogenesis imperfecta. *Ped Endocrinol Rev.* 2013;10(S2):397–405.

88. Cundy T. Recent advances in osteogenesis imperfecta. *Calcif Tissue Int.* 2012;90:439–449.

89. Seikaly MG, Kopanati S, Salhab N, et al. Impact of alendronate on quality of life in children with osteogenesis imperfecta. *J Pediatr Orthop.* 2005;25(6):786–791.

90. Plotkin H, Rauch FH, Bishop NJ, et al. Pamidronate treatment of severe osteogenesis imperfecta in children under 3 years of age. *J Clin Endocrinol Metab.* 2000;85:1846–1850.

91. Castillo H, Samson-Fang L. Effects of bisphosphonates in children with osteogenesis imperfecta: an AACPDM systematic review. *Dev Med Child Neurol.* 2008;51:17–29.

92. Vuorimies I, Toiviainen-Salo S, Hero M, et al. Zoledronic acid treatment in children with osteogenesis imperfecta. *Horm Res Paediatr.* 2011;75:346–353.

93. Land C, Rauch F, Montpetit K, et al. Effect of intravenous pamidronate therapy on functional abilities and level of ambulation in children with osteogenesis imperfecta. *J Pediatr.* 2006;148:456–460.

94. Ward LM, Rauch F, Whyte MP, et al. Alendronate for the treatment of pediatric osteogenesis imperfecta: a randomized placebo-controlled study. *J Clin Endocrinol Metab.* 2011;96:355–364.

95. Sakkers R, Kok D, Engelbert RH, et al. Skeletal effects and functional outcome with olpadronate in children with osteogenesis imperfecta: a 2 year randomized, placebo-controlled study. *Lancet.* 2004;363:1427–1431.

96. Gerber LH, Binder H, Weintrob J, et al. Rehabilitation of children and infants with osteogenesis imperfecta. *Clin Orthop Rel Res.* 1990;251:254–262.

97. Cintas HL, Gerber LH. *Children with Osteogenesis Imperfecta: Strategies to Enhance Performance.* Osteogenesis Imperfecta Foundation Inc; 2005.

98. Van Brussel M, Takken T, Uiterwaal CSPM, et al. Physical training in osteogenesis imperfecta. *J Pediatr.* 2008;152:111–116.

99. Osawa Y, Oguma Y, Ishii N. The effects of whole-body vibration on muscle strength and power: a meta-analysis. *J Musculoskelet Neuronal Interact.* 2013;13(3):342–352.

100. Semler O, Fricke O, Vezyroglou K, et al. Results of a prospective pilot trial on mobility after whole body vibration in children and adolescents with osteogenesis imperfecta. *Clin Rehab.* 2008;22:387–394.

101. Högler W, Scott J, Bishop N, et al. The effect of whole body vibration training on bone and muscle function in children with osteogenesis imperfecta. *J Clin Endocrinol Metab.* 2017;102(8):2734–2743.

102. Mitchell AL, Schwarze U, Jennings JF, et al. Molecular mechanisms of classical ehlers-danlos syndrome. *Hum Mutat.* 2009;30:995–1002.

103. Childs SG. Musculoskeletal manifestations of Dhlers-Danlos syndrome. *Orthop Nursing.* 2010;29(2):133–139.

104. Voermans NC, van Alfen N, Pillen S, et al. Neuromuscular involvement in various types of Ehlers-Danlos syndrome. *Ann Neurol.* 2009;65:687–697.

105. Kirk JA, Ansell BM, Bywaters EG. The hypermobility syndrome. Musculoskeletal complaints associated with generalized joint hypermobility. *Ann Rheum Dis.* 1967;26:419–425.

106. Grahame R. The revised (Beighton 1998) criteria for the diagnosis of benign joint hypermobility syndrome (BJHS). *J Rheumatol.* 2000;27:1777–1779.

107. Wolf JM, Cameron KL, Owens BD. Impact of joint laxity and hypermobility on the musculoskeletal system. *J Am Acad Orthop Surg.* 2011;19:463–471.

108. Kim HKW. Legg-Calve-Perthes disease: etiology, pathogenesis and biology. *J Pediatr Orthop.* 2011;31(2 suppl):S141–S146.

109. Perry DC, Green DJ, Bruce CE, et al. Abnormalities of vascular structure and function in children with Perthes disease. *Pediatrics.* 2012;130:e126–e131.

110. Kim HKW, Herring JA. Pathophysiology, classifications, and natural history of Perthes disease. *Orthop Clin North Am.* 2011;42:285–295.

111. Rajan R, Chandrasenan J, Price K, et al. Legg-Calve-Perthes disease: intraobserver and intraobserver reliability of the modified herring lateral pillar classification. *J Pediatr Orthop.* 2013;33:120–123.

112. Nguyen NT, Klein G, Dogbey G, et al. Operative versus nonoperative treatments for legg-calve-Perthes disease: a meta-analysis. *J Pediatr Orthop.* 2012;32:697–705.

113. Herring JA, Kim HT, Browne R. Legg-Calve-Perthes disease. Part II: prospective multicenter study of the effect of treatment on outcome. *J Bone Joint Surg.* 2004;86A(10):2121–2134.

114. Terjesen T, Wiig O, Svenningsen S. The natural history of Perthes' disease: risk factors in 212 patients followed for 5 years. *Acta Orthop.* 2010;81(6):708–714.

115. Rich MM, Schoenecker PL. Management of Legg-Calve-Perthes disease using an A-frame orthosis and hip range of motion: a 25 year experience. *J Pediatr Orthop.* 2013;33:112–119.

116. Gholve PA, Cameron DB, Millis MB. Slipped capital femoral epiphysis update. *Curr Opin Pediatr.* 2009;21:39–45.

117. Loder RT, Aronsson DD, Dobbs MB, et al. Slipped capital femoral epiphysis. *Instr Course Lect.* 2001;50:555–570.

118. Riad J, Bajelidze G, Gabos PS. Bilateral slipped capital femoral epiphysis: predictive factors for contralateral slip. *J Pediatr Orthop.* 2007;27:411–414.

119. Millis MB, Novais EN. In situ fixation for slipped capital femoral epiphysis: perspectives in 2011. *J Bone Joint Surg Am.* 2011;93(suppl 2):46–51.

120. Clarke SE, McCarthy JJ, Davidson RS. Treatment of Blount disease: a comparison between the multiaxial correction system and other external fixators. *J Pediatr Orthop.* 2009;29(2):103–109.

121. Langenskiold A. Tibia vara: a critical review. *Clin Orthop Relat Res.* 1989;246:195–207.

122. Langenskiöld A. Tibia vara: osteochondrosis deformans tibiae: a survey of 23 cases. *Acta Chir Scand.* 1952;103:1–8.

123. Zionts LE, Shean CJ. Brace treatment of early infantile tibia vara. *J Pediatr Orthop.* 1998;18(1):102–109.

124. Gilbody J, Thomas G, Ho K. Acute versus gradual correction of idiopathic tibia vara in children: a systematic review. *J Pediatr Orthop.* 2009;29:110–114.

125. Richards BS, Katz DE, Sims JB. Effectiveness of brace treatment in early infantile Blount's disease. *J Pediat Orthop.* 1998;18(3):374–380.

126. Wiemann JM, Tryon C, Szalay EA. Physeal stapling versus 8-plate hemiepiphysiodesis for guided correction of angular deformity about the knee. *J Pediatr Orthop.* 2009;29:481–485.

127. Sabharwal S, Kumar A. Methods for assessing leg length discrepancy. *Clin Orthop Relat Res.* 2008;466:2910–2922.

128. Friend L, Widmann RF. Advances in management of limb length discrepancy and lower limb deformity. *Curr Opin Pediatr.* 2008;20:46–51.

129. Birch JG, Samchukov ML. Use of the Ilizarov method to correct lower limb deformities in children and adolescents. *J Am Acad Orthop Surg.* 2004;12:144–154.

130. Sun XT, Easwar TR, Manesh S, et al. Complications and outcome of tibial lengthening using the Ilizarov method with and without a supplementary intramedullary nail: a case-matched comparative study. *J Bone Joint Surg Br.* 2011;93-B:782–787.

131. Dinçyürek H, Kocaoğlu M, Eralp IL, et al. Functional results of lower extremity lengthening by motorized intramedullary nails. *Acta Orthop Traumatol Turc.* 2012;46(1):42–49.

132. Hresko MT. Idiopathic scoliosis in adolescents. *N Engl J Med.* 2013;368:834–841.

133. Yawn BP, Yawn RA, Hodge D, et al. A population-based study of school scoliosis screening. *JAMA.* 1999;282:1427–1432.

134. Rogala EJ, Drummond DS, Gurr J. Scoliosis: incidence and natural history, a prospective epidemiological study. *J Bone Joint Surg Am.* 1978;60:173–177.

135. Berryman F, Pynsent P, Fairbank J, et al. A new system for measuring three-dimensional back shape in scoliosis. *Eur Spine J.* 2008;17(5):663–672.

136. Hoashi JS, Cahill PJ, Bennett JT, et al. Adolescent scoliosis: classification and treatment. *Neurosurg Clin N Am.* 2013;24:173–183.

137. Weinstein SL, Dolan LA, Wright JG, et al. Effects of bracing in adolescents with idiopathic scoliosis. *N Engl J Med.* 2013;369:1512–1521.

Sports Injuries

Elliot M. Greenberg and Eric T. Greenberg

>> Introduction

It is currently estimated that nearly 38 million children and adolescents participate in youth sports each year in the United States.[1] The participation in sports allows children to learn about teamwork, competitiveness, and sportsmanship. At the same time, it helps develop physical fitness, promote improved self-esteem, lay the foundation of a healthy active lifestyle, and, most importantly, allow them to have fun. Participation in any sport carries inherent risk of injury, and with the increased popularity of youth sports has come a concomitant rise in youth sports injuries. Each year, more than 3.5 million children require medical treatment for sports-related injuries.[1] Pediatric and adolescent athletes differ from adult athletes in several ways and require a specialized treatment approach. The goal of this chapter is to familiarize the reader with these differences, describe specific injuries commonly encountered within youth athletes, outline general rehabilitation schemes for these injuries, and identify strategies to promote injury prevention within this population.

>> Anatomic and physiologic differences of the skeletally immature athlete

Bone Composition

The anatomic or physiologic differences between children and adult bone growth and development lead to altered patterns of injuries. The presence of epiphyseal growth plates

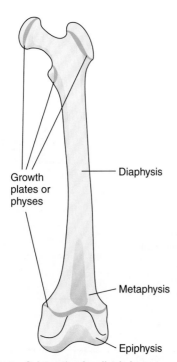

Growth plates or physes

Diaphysis

Metaphysis

Epiphysis

FIGURE 16.1. Schematic of pediatric bone.

DISPLAY 16.1	**Salter–Harris Classification**
Type I	Fracture line extends through the physeal plate
Type II	Fracture line extends through the physeal plate and metaphysis
Type III	Fracture line extends from the joint surface through the epiphysis and across the physis, causing a portion of the epiphysis to become displaced
Type IV	Fracture line extends from joint surface through the epiphysis, physeal plate, and metaphysis causing a fracture fragment
Type V	Crush injury to the growth plate

From Perron AD, Brady WJ, Keats TA. Principles of stress fracture management—the whys and hows of an increasingly common injury. *Stress Fract Manage.* 2001;110(3):115-124.

or physes is unique to the skeletally immature child, and injuries to the physis are common because of its inherent vulnerability (see Fig. 16.1).[2] Physeal fractures are usually caused by falls but can also occur as a result of overuse. These fractures are commonly classified using the Salter–Harris scheme, which describes five distinct types of fractures. A visual schematic and detailed written description are outlined in Figure 16.2 and Display 16.1.

Physeal fractures result in a risk of premature physeal closure, creating a shorter limb or angular limb deformity as the child progresses toward skeletal maturity. Type I and II fractures typically carry a lower risk of growth disturbance; however, close monitoring by an orthopedic physician over time is typically recommended for all physeal fractures.

The presence of secondary growth centers, known as the apophysis, is also unique to the skeletally immature child. An apophysis is a prominence containing growth cartilage that is located on the bones and serves as an attachment site for muscle tendons.[3] Apophyseal injuries occur owing to the large traction forces applied by muscles to the bone complex. In the skeletally immature child, the bone interface is the weaker link of the musculoskeletal complex

and is therefore more prone to injury. An apophysitis results from the cumulative effects of repeated microtrauma to these growth centers, resulting in chronic irritation and inflammation at the bone–cartilage interface.[3] Decreased muscle-tendon flexibility, which commonly occurs during the adolescent growth spurt, has been associated with an increased risk of developing an apophysitis injury.[4] If the tensile force is large enough, it may create an avulsion fracture in which the entire apophysis is separated from the underlying bone.

Physiologic differences also give children an advantage in bone healing when compared with adults. The bones of children are more highly vascularized, which allows for improved availability of healing factors after injury. Furthermore, the periosteum of bone in children is thicker and stronger than in adults, which makes it less likely to be fully disrupted during injury. Both of these factors will lead to improved rates of bone healing after fracture.

Juvenile osteochondritis dissecans (OCD) is a lesion of the subchondral bone that often results in articular cartilage softening, fibrillation, and fragmentation, which may result in loose bodies within the joint. Juveniles with OCD lesions have been shown to have improved healing potential compared with those who have reached skeletal maturity.[5] The pathogenesis of OCD is not fully understood; however, many agree that repetitive stress to the subchondral bone results in cumulative microtrauma in a region with poor blood supply, resulting in damage.[6,7] This hypothesis of pathology is supported by study findings that note increased incidences of juvenile OCD lesions in highly active populations.[5] Males are more affected than females, and the knee is the most commonly affected joint.[8] Treatment of OCD will depend on the lesion severity, location, and degree of skeletal maturity. Conservative treatment will typically consist of a period of prolonged rest or immobilization, followed by rehabilitation and gradual

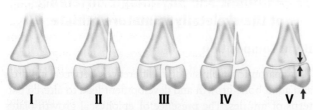

I   II   III   IV   V

FIGURE 16.2. Salter–Harris classification of fractures.

return to sports over a 3-to-6-month period. Surgical treatment is usually recommended for unstable lesions and those that fail conservative treatment.[5] Additionally, adolescent nearing skeletal maturity have decreased healing capacity, and early operative treatment is usually advocated to maintain the integrity of the joint.[8] A variety of surgical techniques have been developed in an attempt to replace the articular cartilage defect. Drilling, abrasion arthroplasty, and microfracture procedures attempt to recruit pluripotential cells from marrow elements. The recruited cells will eventually differentiate in fibrocartilage that restores the articular surface but is weaker than the hyaline cartilage typically found in the joint. Rehabilitation principles specific to the affected joint will be covered in detail later in this chapter.

Muscular Properties

At one point in time, it was suggested that owing to the lack of circulating androgens, prepubescent children would be unable to demonstrate increases in muscular strength in response to a resistance training program. However, recent reports have evidenced that children can demonstrate strength gains with proper training programs. The physiologic mechanism of strength gains in children is different than that of adults. It appears that the strength gains observed in prepubescent children are more related to improving neuromuscular control, such as increased motor unit activation and/ or coordination, than to true muscular hypertrophy.[9] In summary, the scientific literature supports the safety and efficacy of strength training in children, as long as they are properly supervised by adults.

Muscular flexibility has been shown to decrease during the adolescent growth spurt and may result in an increased potential for injury.[4] A regular static stretching program is effective in producing gains in muscle flexibility. It has been advocated that an athlete engage in a dynamic warm-up consisting of generalized movement to increase heart rate and systemic blood flow along with dynamic stretching prior to athletic activity to prepare the body for sports demands, whereas static stretching may be incorporated after activity in order to improve baseline flexibility and reduce the potential for injury in this high-risk group.[10]

» Examination principles

The examination of the pediatric or adolescent athlete will entail history taking, systems review, palpation, muscle performance testing, range of motion (ROM), flexibility, and special testing. Although these are common parts to most orthopedic evaluations, the child athlete examination differs from that of a typical adult examination. Pediatric-specific injuries require selection of alternative tests and measures, whereas differences in emotional maturity will also influence the examination.

History

The history-taking process is very important and serves many functions. Details regarding the mechanism of injury and acute response to injury can give the examiner many clues regarding the nature of injury (overuse vs. trauma), the tissue involved, and help with initiating treatment planning. In addition, the history-taking process can serve as a period to help the child relax and become more familiar with the treating therapist. This may help decrease anxiety and provide for a more effective physical examination. During historical questioning, the child or adolescent will typically forget or gloss over details that may be important for the examiner. Utilizing very specific questioning, with age-specific terminology, is usually helpful in ascertaining a complete history. When available, the parent should be asked to recall injury specifics.

Determination of the athlete's sports-specific history is also important in order to judge possible contributing factors of overtraining and to initiate goal planning for treatment outcomes. The clinician should address what sports they participate in, positions played, level of mastery (recreational or elite), whether they are currently in season, volume of practice, how long they have participated in a certain sport, whether they play year-round, and whether they are currently participating in any other outside training regimens.

Physical Examination

A complete review of all physical examination procedures is beyond the scope of this textbook. The practitioner should be familiar with standardized examination procedures such as ROM, flexibility assessment, manual muscle testing (MMT), handheld dynamometry, and commonly used injury-specific special tests. This section will focus on examination elements specific to the pediatric sports population. Special tests that are specific to pediatric injuries will be covered during the discussion of that injury; however, for detailed descriptions of these tests, the reader is referred to special test-specific texts.

Generalized ligamentous laxity is a condition in which most of the synovial joints of an individual tend to have more than normal ROM.[11] This condition is commonly encountered in the pediatric population and decreases with increasing age. There tends to be a familial predisposition, and females are more commonly affected.[11] Determination of ligamentous laxity is important because it may affect clinical decision making and play a role in injury pathogenesis in certain conditions such as patellofemoral pain, patella dislocations, and shoulder instability. The Beighton–Horan ligament laxity scale is the most frequently utilized assessment scale. The index includes examination of fifth-finger extension, opposition of the thumb to forearm, and trunk and hip flexion. One point is given on the basis of performance of these tasks, with a total of 9 points possible. The composite score gives an understanding of the level of laxity present, and a score of 5 to 9 is typically utilized to indicate a high degree of laxity.[11] Refer to Display 16.2 for a detailed description of each test.

Muscle performance testing for the athletic population requires more detail than that elicited by MMT or dynamometry alone. Functional movement observation during a single-leg squat or lateral step-down will give the examiner much needed information regarding how the neuromusculoskeletal system performs as a unit. In the lower extremity, the biomechanical contributions of femoral internal rotation (IR), femoral adduction, tibial IR, and foot pronation lead to a position of dynamic knee valgus that has been linked to knee injuries, such as anterior cruciate ligament (ACL) tears and patellofemoral dysfunction.[12,13] During functional testing, the clinician observes to determine whether there is proper trunk, pelvic, and lower extremity positioning maintained during the movement (Fig. 16.3). The subject should be able to maintain steady balance with an upright trunk. In the frontal plane, the knee should be kept in alignment with the second metatarsal (i.e., no dynamic valgus). Specific descriptive classification schemes have been developed and have demonstrated adequate reliability.[14] However, in the author's experience written description of the compensatory strategies is often adequate and may even prove more useful in terms of repeat testing to evaluate specific improvement. The clinician should also seek information regarding

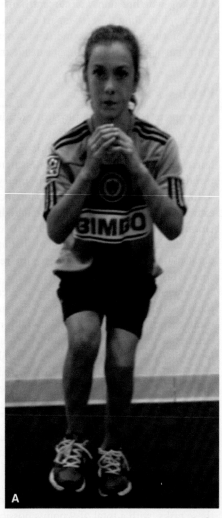
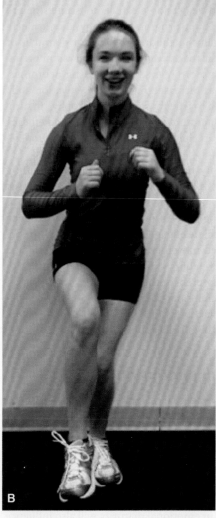

FIGURE 16.3. Functional examination of single-leg squat. **A:** Good lower extremity alignment and neuromuscular control with a single-leg squat. **B:** Poor lower extremity control with femoral adduction, femoral internal rotation, knee dynamic valgus, and foot pronation.

pain associated with movement and whether any mechanical symptoms are present. This data can serve as a comparable sign to help determine improvement throughout the course of rehabilitation.

In athletes with injuries that involve low levels of pain and irritability, more aggressive functional testing may be necessary in order to stress their system adequately to identify impairments. These athletes are typically suffering from overuse syndromes and report the onset of pain after performing activity for several minutes or more. The Drop Vertical Jump is one clinical test that allows for the identification of pathologic lower extremity alignment during a more sports-specific task.[15] For this test, the athlete stands on top of a box approximately 12 inches in height and is instructed to jump directly down off the box and immediately perform a maximal vertical jump raising both arms overhead. The clinician evaluates for symmetrical weight acceptance, the degree of knee valgus, lack of pelvic or trunk control, and overall quality of movement (Fig. 16.4). The Landing Error Scoring System (LESS) is a valid and reliable tool to help qualify biomechanical errors during this activity.[16] This assessment of movement quality has been shown to be predictive in identifying female athletes at risk for ACL injury and may also provide a tool for the identification of more subtle biomechanical faults that may contribute to overuse injuries.[15]

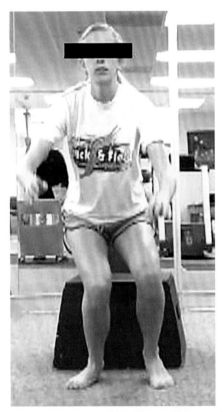

FIGURE 16.4. Drop vertical jump. Poor neuromuscular control, asymmetrical weight acceptance, and right dynamic valgus collapse throughout lower kinetic chain.

Running athletes represent a specialized group of patients and require detailed analysis of running mechanics. Although there is no agreed upon "perfect" style of running, studies have identified biomechanical factors that may predispose a runner to certain injuries. Running analysis is most easily performed on a treadmill. The use of video capture device with a frame rate greater than 100 Hz will permit the accurate evaluation of running gait utilizing slow motion replay. The athlete should be viewed from the front, back, and side. From the side, the clinician should note the athlete's step rate (steps per minute), stride length, foot strike pattern (forefoot, midfoot, rearfoot), trunk position, degree of knee flexion at loading, peak knee flexion and dorsiflexion during stance, tibial and foot inclination angles, and the distance of the foot at ground contact in relation to the body's center of mass (Fig. 16.5). Posteriorly, the clinician should look to identify abnormal trunk lean, pelvic instability during stance phase, presence of dynamic knee valgus (knee window during midstance), excessive crossover, position of the foot at ground contact (degree of supination and relationship to body midline), and the amount and timing of foot pronation that occurs during stance (Fig. 16.6). Abnormalities identified during running analysis may lead to more detailed examination of areas of biomechanical stress and will help guide treatments aimed at modifying running techniques via formal gait retraining strategies.

Upper extremity functional testing allows the clinician to analyze an athlete's performance on specific tasks and determine whether biomechanical flaws exist. Upper extremity testing is generally less defined in the literature. One commonly described test is the Closed Kinetic Chain Upper Extremity Stability Test.[17] In the test, two lines are placed on the ground 36 inches apart. The athlete assumes a push-up position with one hand on each piece of tape. The athlete will have 15 seconds to reach across their body and touch the tape under the opposite shoulder, as many times as they can. The number of touches can be compared with normative data for participants of similar age and sports; however, the volume of normative data available for the pediatric population is not large. The clinician can also utilize this test to look for any compensatory patterns that may indicate weakness in the kinetic chain. The inability to maintain a neutral spine posture while in the push-up position could be related to core weakness. Scapular winging or asymmetries in shoulder positioning are also commonly seen compensatory patterns. Sport-specific functional testing such as throwing for a baseball player can also be included as part of the examination. Owing to the high speeds involved with this motion, video assessment utilizing slow motion replay or motion analysis software may be necessary and useful.

The examination of the entire kinetic chain is required for almost every injury treated by a sports physical therapist. Most sports activities involve the transfer of energy from the lower extremities, through the trunk, to some other distal

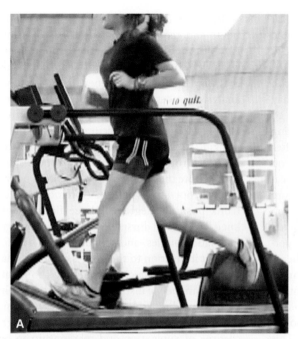
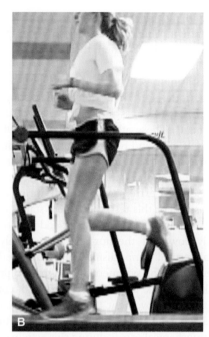

FIGURE 16.5. Running examination lateral view. **A:** Rearfoot strike pattern, over striding and contacting anterior to base of support with knee extended; leaning forward from the hip. **B:** Forefoot strike pattern contacting closer to base of support and greater knee flexion angle; upright posture.

segment such as the hand to throw or the foot to kick a ball. Deficits in kinetic chain function have been linked to a wide array of overuse and traumatic injuries in the upper extremity, lower extremity, and trunk. The comprehensive examination should include evaluation of single-limb balance, core stability, and hip muscle function even if the athlete presents with a seemingly unrelated injury, especially if the injury is of the overuse etiology. Incomplete rehabilitation of any kinetic chain deficits may predispose him or her to repeat injury or suboptimal outcomes.

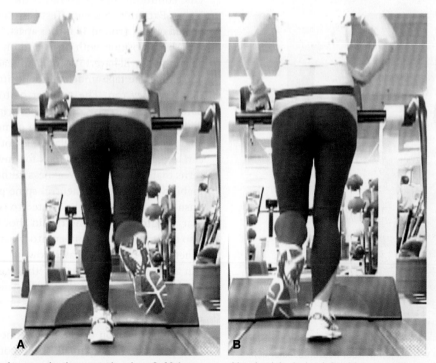

FIGURE 16.6. Running examination posterior view. **A:** Maintenance of level pelvis during left midstance with good lower extremity alignment. **B:** Contralateral left pelvic drop, excessive toe out, and poor lower extremity alignment during right midstance.

» Upper extremity

Examination and Intervention Principles

Generally, the examination of an athlete's shoulder should begin with a detailed postural examination. In particular, the examiner should note resting scapular position, degree of thoracic kyphosis, and general muscular bulk or appearance. An excessive thoracic kyphosis is typically associated with a position of scapular protraction and downward rotation. These factors have been linked to decreased shoulder mobility, increased likelihood of shoulder pathology, and impaired muscle activation.[18] When examining muscular bulk, the clinician may be able to identify areas of muscle atrophy, which may prompt further investigation during specific muscle performance testing. It is important to note that it is not uncommon for the athlete's dominant shoulder to be slightly depressed relative to the contralateral limb. As discussed earlier, the athlete should be screened for generalized ligamentous laxity, and pathology-specific special tests should be utilized to rule in or out specific diagnoses. These tests are outlined in Addendum B.

Scapular dysfunction is a common clinical problem in many athletes, and normal scapular motion and stability are crucial for optimal function of the shoulder.[19] The clinician should observe the athlete from behind while he or she actively elevates and lowers both shoulders. The scapulae should be observed, judging for an abnormal degree of motion or altered pattern of mobility. Several visual observation methods of determining scapular dyskinesis have been described and shown to be reliable in distinguishing normal from abnormal motion.[20-22] If scapular dyskinesia is present, any correlation with pain or symptoms should be noted and the surrounding anatomic structures evaluated in order to determine the cause. This should include examination of thoracic spine mobility and flexibility of the pec minor, latissimus dorsi, and teres major. In addition, isolated muscle performance testing of scapular stabilizing muscles (serratus anterior, middle and lower trapezius) and rotator cuff function should be performed.

Examination of shoulder ROM is also a key concept that must be performed. It has been shown that overhead athletes, particularly pitchers, are likely to develop unique shoulder ROM characteristics. When measured in 90 degrees of abduction, the throwing athlete will typically demonstrate limited IR with an excessive degree of external rotation (ER) when compared with the nonthrowing shoulder. This unique ROM profile is considered normal and reflective of tissue adaptive changes that have occurred owing to the stress of throwing. However, if there is a relative difference of greater than 20 degrees of loss of IR between sides, the athlete is then considered to have developed a pathologic condition, thought to contribute to shoulder injury, known as glenohumeral internal rotation deficit (GIRD). GIRD has been linked to deficits in posterior shoulder tissue length, as well as alterations in bony alignment. The clinician should attempt to identify posterior tissue tightness that may

contribute to this pathology through examination of cross-body adduction, spinal level reached behind the back, and degree of posterior glenohumeral capsular laxity.[18] Additionally, the concepts of total rotational motion (TRM) and horizontal adduction mobility are important. When compared with the nonthrowing shoulder, total arc of motion (IR+ER) deficits of greater than 5 degrees and horizontal adduction deficits of greater than 15 degrees have been associated with an increased risk of throwing-related injuries.[23,24] Any differences greater than these magnitudes should once again prompt further evaluation of anatomic structures to identify the cause of asymmetry.

Examination of the elbow, wrist, and hand should include general ROM, strength measurement, and careful palpation of the involved structures. Injury-specific special testing can help confirm suspected diagnosis and should be conducted toward the end of the physical examination out of respect for the provocative nature of these procedures.

The clinician should be aware that many upper extremity pathologies, both traumatic and overuse, may involve dysfunction at remote anatomic locations that would alter body function and contribute to the athlete's symptoms. This concept is commonly referred to as regional interdependence.[25] For example, the mechanics of throwing involves a transfer of energy from the lower body and trunk to the upper extremity. Owing to the integrated nature of this activity, an inclusive evaluation should also address any limitations in the entire kinetic chain that may alter biomechanics and contribute to injury. Balance, core stability, hip/leg strength, and ROM may all need to be evaluated and addressed in a comprehensive treatment plan.

As with all other areas of physical therapy management, the findings on the initial evaluation will guide treatment decisions. It is important that the athlete be instructed on exercise technique and continually monitored to ensure that he or she is performing the exercises properly. Visual demonstration, tactile cuing, and mirror feedback are all excellent measures to help ensure proper form.

Scapular stabilizing muscles function in an endurance role to provide proper alignment of the scapula for optimal glenohumeral function. Therapists should keep this physiologic role of the muscles in mind while developing rehabilitation programs and implement a scapular stabilization program that emphasizes longer hold times and repetitions, as opposed to high-load exercises. If deficits in posterior tissue tightness are identified during examination, the clinician should implement exercises targeted at the restricted tissue. As demonstrated in Figure 16.7, the sleeper stretch, towel IR stretch behind the back, and cross-body adduction are all effective means of increasing posterior soft tissue flexibility.

The shoulder is required to be utilized overhead for many of the demands of sports. With this in mind, the clinician should progress an athlete's rehabilitation from less provocative positions below 90 degrees of elevation to more sports-specific activities involving overhead activity.

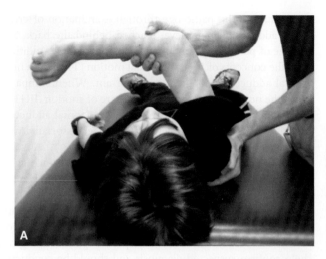

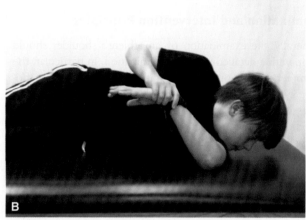

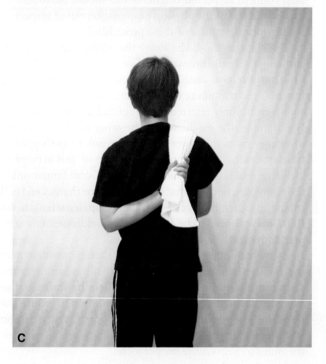

FIGURE 16.7. Methods of stretching posterior shoulder soft tissues. **A:** Shoulder horizontal adduction with scapular blocking, **B:** sleeper stretch, and **C:** towel internal rotation stretch.

Similarly, the exercise program should also be adapted to meet the muscular demands of the imposed stresses of the athlete's sport. For example, the rotator cuff is responsible for deceleration of the shoulder after ball release in throwing. The rehabilitation program should include exercises that focus on eccentric control in similar positions. Working with the athlete to develop a working knowledge of the biomechanical demands of his or her sport or position is important during the late phases of shoulder rehabilitation.

As the throwing athlete regains function, a return-to-throwing program can be initiated. Typically, these programs vary by position, consist of many phases, and progress over several weeks. Typically, they include warm-up, throwing at progressively longer distances, and significant

rest periods between bouts of throwing in a given session. The reader is referred to Axe et al.[26] for a detailed description of a return-to-throwing program.

The Pediatric Throwing Athlete

Baseball is one of the most popular sports among children and adolescents in the United States. Although baseball is inherently a very safe sport, the repetitive nature of throwing and biomechanical stresses placed across the throwing arm predisposes these athletes to specific overuse injuries. The following sections will summarize the most frequently encountered diagnoses in the pediatric thrower. It should be noted that although this section is directed toward throwing athletes, other overhead athletes that participate in activities such as tennis, volleyball, or swimming are also likely to present with these diagnoses.

Little League Shoulder

Little league shoulder is an overuse injury caused by rotational torque and stress across the proximal humeral physis and is typically described as a proximal humeral epiphysiolysis or as a rotational stress fracture of the proximal humeral epiphyseal plate.[1-3,4,7,27-29] Although plain films may show a widening of the proximal humeral physis, this finding is not required for diagnosis. Clinically, the athlete will complain of throwing- or activity-related shoulder pain. The pain may resolve after rest, but quickly return on resumption of activity. The athlete will typically have tenderness to palpation over the physis. The initial treatment for little league shoulder is rest from throwing for 6 to 12 weeks.[30] Physical therapy treatment may begin during this period of relative rest. Rehabilitation should be structured along the continuum, as previously discussed, with the latter phases of rehabilitation, including plyometric exercises and return-to-throwing simulation. Review and education of proper pitching mechanics, suggested pitch types, appropriate rest intervals, and pitching volume limits should be reviewed because these have been identified as risk factors for shoulder injury in youth throwing athletes.[7] The latest recommendations for pitch count, pitch-type progression, and rest intervals are summarized in Tables 16.1 through 16.3.

Superior Labrum Anterior-to-Posterior Lesions

Superior labrum anterior-to-posterior (SLAP) lesions occur in adolescents as a result of trauma and overuse. Traumatic injuries are typically related to a fall onto an outstretched arm or a traction injury. Throwing athletes are particularly vulnerable to overuse SLAP lesions because of the high stresses that repetitive overhead throwing place on the shoulder. Several theories regarding the pathophysiology of SLAP lesions in throwers have been

proposed and likely include a combination of the following: (1) a traction injury from the pull of the biceps tendon on the labrum during the deceleration phase of throwing, (2) contracture of the posterior shoulder capsule, resulting in a posterosuperior migration of the humeral head, and (3) "peel back" mechanism where the biceps tendon imparts torsional forces to the posterosuperior labrum in the late cocking phase of throwing.[31] SLAP lesions can result in laxity of the shoulder because the structural integrity of the shoulder is impaired. Typically, an athlete will complain of vague shoulder pain with overhead or cross-body activities. Complaints of popping, clicking, or catching are also common along with reports of decreased throwing velocity and accuracy. Numerous physical examination tests for detecting SLAP lesions have been described and include O'Brien's active compression test, biceps load I and II tests, anterior slide test, resisted supination ER test, and crank test. Clinical diagnosis of SLAP lesions is challenging because most studies have shown that the clustering diagnostic tests to support or refute a hypothesis will improve both the sensitivity and the specificity.

TABLE 16.2.	Recommended Rest Periods for Youth Pitchers	
Number of Pitches Thrown		Mandatory Days of Rest Between Pitching
Ages 14 and Under	Ages 15–18	Days
1–20	1–30	0
21–35	31–45	1
36–50	46–60	2
51–65	61–75	3
66 and over	76 and over	4

2012 Little League Pitch Count Limits and Mandatory Rest Rules.
Source: https://www.littleleague.org/playing-rules/pitch-count/

TABLE 16.1.	Pitch Count Recommendations for Youth Pitchers
Age (yr)	Maximum Pitches Per Day
7–8	50
9–10	75
11–12	85
13–16	95
17–18	105

2012 Little League Pitch Count Limits and Mandatory Rest Rules.
Source: https://www.littleleague.org/playing-rules/pitch-count/

TABLE 16.3.	Recommended Pitch-Type Progression for Youth Pitchers
Type of Pitch	Age (yr)
Fastball	8 ± 2
Slider	16 ± 2
Changeup	10 ± 3
Forkball	16 ± 2
Curveball	14 ± 2
Knuckleball	15 ± 3
Screwball	17 ± 2

Source: https://www.littleleague.org/playing-rules/pitch-count/

Initial treatment of SLAP lesions typically consists of a period of rest followed by rehabilitation. The rehabilitation program will typically focus on restoring normal scapular mechanics, strengthening of scapular stabilizers and rotator cuff musculature, dynamic stabilization, and proprioceptive awareness. GIRD is typically present with SLAP lesions and should be addressed accordingly. If the athlete is unable to resume his or her previous level of activity after a proper course of conservative treatment, then surgical intervention is indicated because SLAP lesion likely will cause ongoing limitations. There are several surgical techniques described, ranging from simple debridement to labral reattachment.[31] Postoperative rehabilitation will vary depending on the extent of injury and procedure performed. However, the overriding principle that will apply to all SLAP rehabilitation programs is protection of the healing tissue. ROM will be slowly progressed after an initial period of immobilization, and comprehensive rehabilitation activities will progress in a graded fashion.

Elbow Injuries

Injuries to the elbow, especially among pitchers, appear to be on the rise. A recent review of pediatric sports elbow injuries noted that 50% to 70% of adolescent baseball players develop elbow pain yearly, with overuse being implicated as the major causative factor.[32] Poor pitching mechanics and pitching too often with inadequate rest have been implicated as major risk factors for pediatric elbow injuries.[7] Excessive pitching might not occur during a single game but is often the summation of pitches thrown during practice, while at home, or while playing on multiple teams in the same season. The mechanics of the throwing motion place a significant degree of stress across the elbow. During late cocking and early acceleration phases of the throwing motion, valgus tension stresses are placed across the medial elbow, whereas the lateral aspect of the elbow receives compressive forces. During deceleration, shearing forces occur across the elbow as the forearm fully pronates and the elbow extends. Medial elbow injuries commonly encountered in the pediatric thrower include little league elbow, medial epicondyle apophysitis, and medial epicondyle avulsion fractures. Lateral elbow injuries include Panner disease and OCD lesions of the capitellum.

Little League Elbow

Little league elbow is a traction injury to the medial epicondylar physis caused by valgus distraction forces during the late cocking and early acceleration phases of throwing. Players typically complain of medial elbow pain during throwing activities. In hindsight, players or coaches may note a period of decreasing throwing velocity or accuracy prior to symptom onset. In highly irritable elbows, the pain may be present during normal activities such as writing or lifting objects. Radiographs may reveal a widening of the apophysis or an avulsion fracture in more severe cases.

Comparison views of the contralateral limb are usually recommended because of a variation in the size of normal growth centers between individuals.[3] Treatment consists of rest from throwing and activity modification until pain free, which may take 3 to 6 weeks. Rehabilitation focuses on scapular and rotator cuff strengthening and endurance, addressing any limitations in shoulder ROM, localized pain-free wrist and forearm muscle strengthening, strengthening of abdominal and hip musculature, and optimizing throwing mechanics. An interval return-to-throwing program can be initiated after the resolution of all impairments. The athlete should be closely monitored during this period for any return of symptoms, and the program should be adjusted accordingly. As high throwing volumes are the most predominant risk factor for index and repeat elbow overuse injuries, athletes and parents should be counseled on limiting throwing exposure during each season prior to discharge. In addition, the physical therapist should advocate for that athlete to adhere to expert recommendations of 3 to 4 months' rest from strenuous overhead activities in order to reduce the potential for repeat injury.

The influence of pitch type on injury is a topic of significant debate. Recent studies have found the volume of pitching, poor biomechanics, and pitch velocity more highly correlated with an increased risk of elbow injuries rather than the type of pitch thrown.[7] The therapist must emphasize the importance of early instruction in proper pitching mechanics and volumes to the athlete, parents, and coaches. The use of a radar gun to measure pitch velocity should also be discouraged in this population in order to decrease the risk of overthrowing. The fastball should be the foundation for all young pitchers, and the mechanics of this pitch should be mastered early in a pitcher's career.[33] Although there is a common misconception that throwing breaking pitches creates more injurious forces to the throwing arm, recent research has shown that the forces encountered during these pitch types are actually lower than those encountered during fastball throwing and thus may not be more likely to cause injury.[34,35] Nevertheless, the increased volume of practice and breakdown of mechanics that can occur with learning breaking pitches at an early age may place the athlete at higher risk for overuse injuries, and focusing on establishing sound mechanics during fastball pitching should be the main focus of young athletes learning to pitch. The changeup is recommended as a safe secondary pitch that can be added only after fastball mechanics are mastered. The curveball and other breaking pitches can then be added in the later phases of the athlete's baseball participation (see Table 16.3).

Medial Epicondyle Apophysitis

Apophysitis may develop at the medial epicondyle as a result of repetitive tensile forces subjected to attachment of the medial elbow musculature. Symptoms generally consist of pain with activity, pain with resisted muscle testing, and pain with palpation. In the case of medial epicondyle apophysitis, clinical exam is similar to that of little league elbow, and imaging studies may be required for differential diagnosis. Treatment is consistent with previous outlined programs of education regarding throwing volume, activity modification, and progressive resolution of impairments noted on evaluation.

Medial Epicondyle Avulsion Fracture

An acute valgus stress to the medial epicondyle may result in an avulsion fracture.[36] This injury is most often seen in baseball pitchers and gymnasts. Nonoperative management for minimally displaced fractures consists of a period of immobilization followed by rehabilitation. Recently, some reports favor operative management for these injuries owing to an increased understanding of the detrimental effects medial elbow instability may have on high-demand sports.[36]

Elbow Ulnar Collateral Ligament Injury

Ulnar collateral ligament (UCL) tears have typically been an injury of high-level skeletally mature throwing athletes.[36] However, recent reports indicate that UCL tears and surgical reconstruction are being seen with increasing frequency in young athletes.[3,37,38] Evidence regarding this alarming trend incriminates cumulative trauma caused by overuse in the throwing arm of youth pitchers. High pitching volumes, pitching with arm fatigue, and inefficient pitching mechanics appear to place the athlete at the greatest risk of developing UCL injury.[7,39] The athlete will complain of medial elbow pain typically noted during or immediately following a bout of throwing. Valgus stress testing to the elbow joint is provocative, especially at 20 degrees of flexion and may occur in conjunction with increased joint gapping compared with the contralateral limb. A prolonged trial of rest may resolve symptoms initially; however, pain will return immediately on resuming high-velocity throwing. Surgical reconstruction, commonly known as "Tommy John" surgery, is considered only after a failure of at least 6 months of conservative care.[36] Surgical procedures are similar to those used in adults and target return to throwing roughly 6 months postoperatively. Outcomes studies are limited in children, but similar success rates have been noted in adults and high school–age athletes.[40]

Panner Disease

Panner disease occurs generally in younger children aged 4 to 8 years and is a self-limiting avascular necrosis of the developing ossific nucleus of the capitellum.[36] It is associated with degeneration and necrosis of the capitellum, followed by regeneration and recalcification. It is a self-limiting disorder of nontraumatic origin. Treatment consists of rest with avoidance of valgus stress and splinting for pain relief. Outcomes are typically good with resumption of full activity common after treatment.

Osteochondritis Dissecans

OCD of the capitellum typically affects the young adolescent athlete involved in high-demand, repetitive overhead, or weight-bearing activities.[6] OCD is most common in 12- to 17-year-olds involved in baseball, gymnastics, racquet sports, football, or weightlifting.[6] The pathogenesis of OCD is not fully understood but likely results from cumulative injury from repetitive compressive forces and resultant microtrauma in a region with tenuous blood supply.[6,7] During the late cocking and early acceleration phases of baseball throwing, the lateral radiocapitellar joint undergoes significant compressive forces, and repeated exposures may lead to subchondral bone fatigue fracture. The athlete typically complains of localized lateral elbow pain and swelling, decreased ROM, and tenderness to palpation over the radiocapitellar joint on physical examination.

Conservative treatment involves complete elbow rest from offending forces for up to 6 months. Rehabilitation may begin with gentle ROM and strengthening exercises when the athlete is asymptomatic. Repeat imaging studies and clinical examination will help determine readiness to progress back to sports.[6] A gradual return to full activity may occur after 6 to 12 months.[36]

Several operative techniques exist for OCD lesions that fail to respond to conservative measures. Loose fragment removal with or without microfracture or drilling of the lesion are the most commonly seen procedures.[6,36] When microfracture is performed, postoperative rehabilitation typically begins after 6 weeks of immobilization or protected use. Return to sports may begin as early as 3 to 6 months but may be delayed contingent on the achievement of necessary strength, ROM, and muscular endurance goals.

Other Shoulder Pathologies

Multidirectional Instability

Chronic multidirectional instability (MDI) of the shoulder in the young athlete can be caused by an acute traumatic dislocation or an underlying capsular laxity. MDI is typically associated with generalized ligamentous laxity, and bilateral involvement is common. Presenting symptoms usually consist of bilateral shoulder pain with a loose or unstable feeling during activities such as overhead lifting, swimming, tennis, and throwing. The athlete may also note shoulder subluxation during normal activities of daily living such as rolling over in bed or lifting a backpack.

Clinical examination reveals increased glenohumeral translation during passive mobility testing, with a positive sulcus sign and increased anterior–posterior glide during the load and shift test. Imaging is usually not indicated for MDI, except to rule out other possible diagnoses, such as labral pathology.[3] Those with MDI often present with scapular dyskinesis and muscle performance deficits in the scapular stabilizing and rotator cuff muscles. Comprehensive rehabilitation is the preferred initial management strategy for MDI.[41]

Athlete education in regard to avoiding provocative positions and subsequent dislocations is a key component to successful rehabilitation. Exercises should focus on normalizing scapular mechanics, regaining rotator cuff strength and endurance, and dynamic shoulder stabilization activities. These exercises should be performed in both open- and closed-chain positions in order to maximize active control of centration of the humeral head within the glenoid. The athlete should begin these activities with the arm in low-stress positions and limited weight bearing, while the therapist ensures that the scapula is in a desired position. Progression should include higher-demand overhead positions and increased loading in the closed chain while incorporating exercise principles to maximize local muscular endurance. Return-to-sport training should include exercises that replicate the forces and positions the shoulder must endure during sporting activity. For example, throwing athletes would benefit from open-chain plyometric activities, whereas a wrestler's program should include more aggressive closed-chain upper extremity, weight-bearing activities.

Traumatic Shoulder Dislocation

Acute traumatic shoulder dislocations occur most commonly in the anterior direction, male athletes involved in contact sports being most at risk. The typical mechanism of injury is a fall onto the arm or an anteriorly directed force to the shoulder while in an abducted and externally rotated position. Closed reduction is usually performed and radiographs used to rule out associated fracture and confirm relocation. Neurovascular examination should be performed before and after relocation, because secondary injury to vascular or neural structures can occur. A high risk of associated injuries is seen, including Hill–Sachs lesion, glenoid rim fracture, anterior inferior glenoid labrum tear or avulsion (Bankart lesion), and capsular avulsion fracture. Advanced imaging with magnetic resonance imaging (MRI), magnetic resonance angiography (MRA), or computed tomography (CT) scan may be indicated if these injuries are suspected. Identifying associated pathologies and directing proper initial treatment is important as young athletes have been noted to be at high risk for recurrent dislocations, with some studies reporting rates as high as 90%.[42]

Nonoperative management includes rest or sling immobilization for 1 to 3 weeks. Rehabilitation should focus initially on pain management, gentle ROM, and muscle activation. The provocative position of 90 degrees abduction and ER should be avoided until late phases of rehabilitation. Treatment will progress on the basis of symptoms and stability. Principles of progression and return-to-sport training are similar to those discussed with MDI.

Because secondary injuries and recurrent instability are common after first-time dislocation, several open and arthroscopic procedures may be customized to the athletes specific intra-articular pathology. Postoperative treatment will vary depending on the specific procedure performed; however, most protocols share a period of immobilization lasting 4 to 6 weeks. Rehabilitation will progress focusing on progressive restoration of ROM, strength, normalizing scapular movement, and dynamic stabilization of the shoulder. Aggressive ROM techniques are contraindicated because they may violate the stabilization procedure performed and lead to recurrent instability. The athlete progresses slowly to more stressful overhead and 90/90 positions over the course of rehabilitation, using principles already discussed. Return to contact sports typically occurs after 6 months and with a satisfactory clinical exam to ensure adequate strength, ROM, and dynamic stabilization.

Acromioclavicular Joint Separations

Acromioclavicular (AC) joint separations also occur in this population and are often caused by a fall onto the shoulder. These injuries are generally treated nonoperatively with good results.[43] The AC joint may not return to its normal configuration after injury, and a noticeable "bump" may result. This abnormality is cosmetic and will not affect function. Occasionally, this bump may be painful with direct irritation from equipment, such as football shoulder pads. A simple donut pad can be fabricated to relieve pressure. Rehabilitation is fairly uncomplicated and should focus on regaining lost shoulder mobility and progressive total arm strengthening.

Clavicle Fractures

Clavicle fractures usually occur as a result of a fall onto the shoulder. Most clavicle fractures in children remain nondisplaced or minimally displaced on account of the thick periosteum in a child and can be treated nonoperatively.[44] The treatment of displaced clavicle fractures remains controversial; however, recent literature reports indicate that surgeons are favoring surgical fixation for completely displaced, comminuted, or open-type fractures.[44,45] Nonsurgical treatment consists of 2 to 4 weeks of immobilization in a shoulder sling or a figure-of-eight brace, followed by ROM and strengthening exercises. Rehabilitation is usually minimal and return-to-sports activity is usual around 6 to 8 weeks. Following surgical management, the athlete is immobilized in a sling for 3 weeks, after which they may begin progressive ROM and strengthening exercises. Return to sports is allowed at 12 weeks if there is clinical and radiographic evidence of healing.[45]

Other Elbow Injuries

Pediatric athletic elbow injuries include traumatic fractures and dislocations, as well as overuse injuries already discussed. Traumatic injuries usually occur as a result of falling and are common in sports such as gymnastics, snowboarding, and football. An elbow fracture or dislocation may represent a medical emergency in view of the possibility of associated neural or vascular compromise. Commonly encountered injuries will be summarized in the following section.

Supracondylar Elbow Fractures

Supracondylar fractures commonly occur in children and carry a risk of secondary neurovascular damage. This damage can lead to long-term functional deficits in the upper extremity, and, therefore, prompt treatment is required.[46] Treatment is based on the severity of fracture displacement and identification of any associated injuries. Nonsurgical immobilization is typically recommended for nondisplaced fractures, whereas most other injury patterns require surgical fixation.[46] Elbow stiffness and loss of elbow extension is a significant concern after the initial management of supracondylar fractures, and it may take up to 1 year for elbow ROM to approach normal. Athletes with more severe injuries, surgically managed fractures, and younger age have the greatest difficulty regaining motion.[47] The therapist should initiate progressive elbow ROM and upper extremity strengthening exercises when cleared by the surgeon. Care should be taken to avoid aggressive stretching because of the inherent risk of the onset of myositis ossificans. Instead, functional use of the elbow and low load long duration stretching is more effective in regaining elbow ROM. Methods such as dynamic splinting or serial casting may be necessary to regain motion in difficult cases.

Lateral Condyle Fractures

Lateral condyle fractures occur less commonly than supracondylar humeral fractures but have a similar mechanism of injury. Stable, minimally displaced fractures have been treated successfully with cast immobilization; however, surgical fixation is required for most displaced injuries.[48] The healing of lateral condyle fractures is slower than supracondylar fractures, and longer immobilization time may be required. As with supracondylar fractures, elbow stiffness is a serious concern after initial management, and physical therapy treatment will be similar.

Monteggia Fracture

Monteggia fracture dislocations describe a radial head dislocation with concomitant ulnar fracture. This rare injury accounts for fewer than 1% of pediatric elbow fractures.[49] Complications of Monteggia fractures can include posterior interosseous nerve palsy, radial nerve palsy, and ulnar deformity. There is no agreed upon optimal management strategy for Monteggia fractures with regard to surgical versus nonsurgical treatment. Conservative management with closed reduction and immobilization has shown good results; however, open reduction internal fixation (ORIF) may be indicated if anatomic reduction cannot be achieved.[49] Rehabilitation time frames will be directed by the surgeon, based on the method of treatment and healing response.

Forearm, Wrist, and Hand Injuries

Forearm fractures occur as a result of a fall and can occur in the distal, proximal, or midshaft of the radius or ulna. In children, forearm shaft fractures are usually treated with closed reduction and cast immobilization. Indications for surgery include open fractures, unstable fractures, fractures that have failed closed reduction, and sometimes in the management of older adolescents.[50]

Distal Forearm Fractures

Distal forearm fractures occur most commonly in the distal radius owing to bony architecture at the articulation with the wrist. Fractures of the distal radius metaphysis rarely require surgery and are treated with cast immobilization for 4 to 6 weeks.[51] Most injuries of the distal radius physis are of the Salter–Harris type II classification, and nonsurgical treatment is usually successful. Injury to the physis can cause growth arrest with resulting angular deformity, and close monitoring by the physician is required. Torus or Buckle fractures occur at the diaphyseal–metaphyseal junction with impaction of trabecular bone on the dorsal aspect of the radius, creating a characteristic bulge on radiographs.[52] Similarly to other injuries in the forearm, conservative management is the preferred treatment method.

Gymnast Wrist

Wrist pain is a common complaint among gymnasts, and "gymnast wrist" refers to an overuse injury caused by mechanical overload to the distal radius.[53] The wrist is subjected to large amounts of static and dynamic stress in gymnastics owing to the regular use of the upper extremity to support body weight during activities such as handstands and tumbling. Symptoms include pain over the distal radius with wrist extension, especially with weight-bearing positions. Early detection is important in order to prevent physeal injury or premature physeal closure with resulting wrist deformity.[53] Typically, activity modification with restriction of painful activities is required for a period of at least 4 weeks. If pain occurs with normal activities of daily living, bracing may help with pain resolution. Rehabilitation should focus on addressing local and systemic deficits, such as limitations in shoulder elevation, that may impart increased stress across the wrist. The gymnast should be counseled in regard to progressive return to weight-bearing activities and variation of training to reduce the risk of recurrent injury.

Scaphoid Fractures

Scaphoid fractures are the most commonly encountered carpal bone fracture but account for only 0.45% of pediatric upper extremity fractures.[54] The most common mechanism of injury is a fall onto an outstretched hand. Although rare, accurate diagnosis and treatment of scaphoid fractures is important in view of the likelihood of non-union or avascular necrosis with improper treatment.[55] Those with a scaphoid fracture will typically complain of lateral wrist pain, which is increased with radial deviation and wrist extension. Point tenderness is typical with palpation of the scaphoid within the anatomic snuffbox, located between the abductor pollicis longus and the brevis tendons. Treatment typically consists of cast immobilization in a thumb spica cast for 6 weeks, followed by rehabilitation. If the fracture is unstable or if nonunion develops, surgical fixation may be indicated.[56] Scaphoid fractures are sometimes difficult to diagnose because the fracture may not be evident on initial radiographs. Owing to the severe consequences of misdiagnosis, a suspected scaphoid fracture is typically immobilized for 2 weeks followed by repeat examination.[55]

Fracture of the Hook of the Hamate

Hook of the hamate fractures can occur during sports such as baseball, golf, or hockey. The typical mechanism of injury is a mistimed swing that contacts a solid object, translating excessive forces through the hamate.[56] Acute tenderness will exist over the hook of the hamate, and pain will typically be experienced when gripping a racquet or club. Conservative treatment consists of cast immobilization for 6 weeks; however, surgical excision of the fracture fragment may be necessary.[56]

Boxer's Fracture

A boxer's fracture involves the neck of the fifth metacarpal and typically occurs as a result of a closed fist striking an immovable object. Owing to the effect of muscular attachments, there is a resulting volar angulation of the head of the fifth metacarpal.[57] Treatment will typically consist of closed reduction with cast immobilization for 3 to 6 weeks.

Finger Fractures

Finger fractures and tendon injuries to the fingers also occur during sports participation. In general, the majority of finger fractures in children can be treated by closed means with excellent outcomes expected.[58] Mallet finger is an injury in which the extensor digitorum tendon is avulsed from the distal phalynx, causing an inability to extend the distal interphalangeal (DIP) joint of the finger. This typically occurs owing to an unexpected flexion force such as jamming a finger on a ball or with sliding into a base. Jersey finger is an avulsion of the flexor digitorum profundus (FDP) from the distal phalynx. This injury most commonly occurs in the ring finger and may result from the forceful contraction of the FDP when the finger gets caught in another player's jersey. Treatment for these mallet or jersey finger injuries typically consists of continuous splint immobilization.

» Pelvis, hip, and thigh injuries

Examination Principles

Pelvis, hip, and thigh injuries in youth athletes can be a result of isolated traumatic events, overuse, and idiopathic origins. The pelvis is composed of a series of bones, including the ischium, ilium, pubic bone, sacrum and femur, and their articulations. These bones serve as attachment sites for a number of muscles and ligaments. Knowledge of this anatomy is paramount in the understanding and diagnosing of injury. With complaints of hip, pelvis, thigh, or knee pain, careful examination must be performed to rule out pathologic disease processes and other orthopedic and nonorthopedic conditions (Display 16.3).

A detailed history is important in the diagnosis and treatment of injuries to the hip and pelvis. Mechanism of injury, location and description of pain, and aggravating activities will assist in ensuring proper diagnosis and direction of examination. Inspection of diffuse or localized swelling and bruising will help identify locations of trauma. Careful palpation, with attention to localized swelling, pain, and tenderness, is crucial and should include bony landmarks, sites of muscle attachments, and surrounding soft tissues. Active and passive ROM testing of the hip in all planes will help identify provocative positions and any limitations when compared with the contralateral limb. Selective tissue muscle tension testing and tests of muscle performance will help discern involvement of contractile tissues and their ability to function properly. It is important to screen the surrounding joints, including the lower thoracic spine, lumbar spine, and knee to rule out potential distant contributions of hip pain.

Specific Injuries to the Pelvis, Hip, and Thigh

Pelvic Apophysitis

During periods of rapid growth, the immature skeleton of the pediatric athlete is at risk for overuse injuries. Bone

---

DISPLAY 16.3   Differential Diagnoses of Hip Pain

Causes of Hip Pain in Athletes
Apophyseal injury/fracture
Stress fracture
Slipped capital femoral epiphysis, septic/inflammatory arthritis, Legg–Calve–Perthes disease
Femoral acetabular impingement, acetabular labral tears, loose body
Snapping hip syndrome, tendonitis or bursitis
Muscle strain
Traumatic hip dislocation
Osteitis pubis, osteomyelitis, sport hernia
Nerve entrapments
Lumbar radiculopathy

growth exceeds the ability of muscle tissue to sufficiently lengthen and stretch, thus increasing tensile forces across pelvic apophyses, the weakest point in the muscle-tendon unit of a growing athlete.[59] Repetitive contractions and pulling of the muscle along the apophysis will cause microtrauma and progressive weakness and inflammation at the cartilaginous muscular attachment. As the injury progresses, the apophysis widens slightly of and may place the athlete at greater risk for avulsion injury.

The most common sites for pelvic apophysitis are the anterior inferior iliac spine (AIIS), anterior superior iliac spine (ASIS), and ischial tuberosity. The lesser trochanter, iliac crest, and greater trochanter are also possible but less frequently encountered locations for apophysitis.[3] The site of the apophysitis is dependent on the skeletal age and maturity of the athlete as the apophysis will fuse during certain age ranges and will no longer be susceptible to pathology (see Table 16.4). The type of activity performed may predispose athletes to an apophysitis in a particular location. For example, soccer players often experience AIIS apophysitis from ballistic rectus femoris contractions required with repetitive kicking.

Well-localized, dull pain with activity at the involved location is the common complaint with apophysitis. Pain often worsens with increased activity and is alleviated with rest. Progression to pain with daily activities such as walking and stair negotiation, with or without a limp, may occur without adequate rest. Examination will find tenderness at the apophysis with possible inflammation. Tensioning the muscle attachment at the apophysis will reproduce the athlete's symptoms. This can be done either by stretching or forcefully contracting the muscle of interest. Owing to rapid growth, generalized bilateral muscle inflexibility is often noted along with limited ROM on the involved side. Distinction between avulsion fractures can be appreciated on physical exam and diagnostic imaging, because radiographs in the presence of simple apophysitis are generally normal.

TABLE 16.4.	Hip Apophysitis Locations	
Apophysitis Site	**Muscle Attachments**	**Age of Ossification**
ASIS	Sartorius, tensor fascia lata	14–16
AIIS	Rectus femoris	14–16
Ischial tuberosity	Hamstring group	21–25
Iliac crest	Tensor fascia lata, deep abdominal muscles	16–18
Greater trochanter	Gluteus maximus and medius, hip external rotator group	14–16
Lesser trochanter	Iliopsoas	14–16

Treatment of a pelvic apophysitis begins with rest, activity modification, and management of pain and inflammation. Educating the athlete, parents, and coaches about overtraining and excessive sports participation should be paramount. Weight bearing is permitted as long as it is pain free and the athlete demonstrates a nonantalgic gait. In some cases with significant pain, a short course of protected weight bearing with crutches may be needed. Once pain is controlled, the focus of treatment shifts to improving muscle flexibility and ROM. Muscle strengthening to the surrounding lumbopelvic musculature and lower extremity is also of paramount importance to restore pelvic balance and lower extremity control. Return to sport should be in a progressive manner, depending on symptoms and quality of movement and may take up to 6 weeks for full, unrestricted participation.[60]

Pelvic Avulsion Fractures

Avulsion fractures may occur with the progression of an unmanaged apophysitis in the pelvis and are found at similar locations. They occur most commonly in adolescent athletes from 14 to 25 years old, as a result of an acute injury with a distinct mechanism of injury. Strong and violent contraction of a muscle against its apophyseal attachment site, especially during the eccentric phase of a sporting activity where higher forces are generated, contributes to failure and subsequent avulsion.[61]

The athlete will often recall the isolated event and time of injury and will report feeling or hearing a "pop." Symptoms include tenderness and swelling over the site of the avulsion. Weight bearing is usually painful and results in an antalgic gait pattern. Associated bruising is also characteristic of avulsion fractures. As occurred during the injury, pain is elicited on a strong muscle contraction of the associated muscle group. Radiographs can confirm diagnosis on the suspicion of avulsion in most cases. Some smaller avulsions not seen on plain films may be diagnosed with CT scan. MRI is also available for soft tissue injuries and partial avulsions but should be used when other more serious concerns exist.[3,62]

Treatment of pelvic avulsion fractures depends on the degree of widening and displacement of the apophysis. Injuries with less than 2-cm displacement will respond to a conservative course of management. The athlete is placed on relative rest from activity for the first 3 weeks and may include a short course of protected weight bearing. Once pain has subsided and time has been allotted to allow for bony healing, regaining full pain-free motion is of next concern. A short course of muscle strengthening is initiated, and once restored, a progressive return to sports-specific activities may begin 6 to 8 weeks following injury, barring other complications.[61]

Surgical ORIF of the avulsion has been more effective than conservative care when there is evidence of greater than 2-cm or complete displacement of the fragment or when ischial tuberosity is involved.[61]

Snapping Hip Syndrome

Snapping hip syndrome is characterized by audible and/or palpable "popping" of the hip caused by tendons moving over bony prominences. It is usually accompanied by pain and is consistently replicated with certain movements of the hip. Snapping hip syndrome is classified as external and internal. "Intra-articular" snapping hip is no longer considered appropriate nomenclature owing to the improved accuracy, description, and diagnosis of intra-articular hip pathology.[63] Snapping hip is often seen in performing artists, distance runners, and hurdlers.

The friction of the iliotibial (IT) band and/or anterior aspect of the gluteus maximus passing over the greater trochanter causes external snapping hip syndrome. A thickened portion of the IT band, located posterior to the greater trochanter, will pass over the anterior portion of the trochanter with hip flexion. When the hip is extended, the IT band will return to its posterior position, contributing to repetitive snapping and clicking.[63] Between the IT band and the greater trochanter lies the greater trochanteric bursa, which may become inflamed with repetitive snapping, resulting in trochanteric bursitis. Tendinopathy, degeneration, and tears of the gluteus medius tendon are also likely to develop owing to the mechanical irritation at its bony attachment.[63]

External snapping hip syndrome may present in athletes in two different ways. True snapping hip syndrome is characterized by lateral hip pain and tenderness around the greater trochanter and occurs with repetitive hip flexion and extension. The snapping is located along the greater trochanter with standing from a chair, stair climbing, and athletic activities and is often palpable. An athlete may also report snapping with a description of the "hip dislocating." The sensation is often repeatable with pelvic tilting activities and not usually painful. This snapping does not usually contribute to altered athletic participation or performance.[63] Dynamic ultrasound will help identify and confirm the snapping phenomenon.[59]

Treatment of external hip snapping is usually conservative and varies depending on the level of irritability. When snapping is not painful, soft tissue techniques to the tensor fascia lata and gluteal musculature will aid in decreasing pain and modulating muscle tone. Activity modification and pain control are of primary importance in the symptomatic external snapping hip. As the level of irritability in the tissue decreases, stretching to hip flexors and soft tissue techniques can be progressed. In both cases, the normalization of trunk control, pelvic stability, and balance is necessary for full recovery. If initial management is not successful, an ultrasound guided injection into the underlying bursal tissue may be considered to assist with symptomatic relief.[64] With a failed course of conservative management, surgical release may be indicated.[65]

Internal snapping hip occurs commonly in dancers and other performing artists. The snapping phenomenon occurs as the iliopsoas tendon chronically subluxes from lateral to medial while the hip is brought from a flexed, abducted, externally rotated position into extension with IR.[66] Internal snapping hip may be present but asymptomatic in approximately 10% of the population.[63]

An athlete with complaints of symptomatic internal snapping hip describes a deep, often painful and audible clunking sensation in the anterior groin. Symptoms are easily reproduced with repeated flexion and extension or when moving from a position of hip flexion, abduction, and ER to a position of hip extension and IR.[67] Although less likely, symptoms may also be reported as posterior achiness to the buttocks and sacroiliac (SI) region, owing to the origin of the iliopsoas tendon on the lumbar spine. Examination elicits the snapping on anterior hip palpation when performing incriminating motions. When the snapping occurs, the athlete will likely become apprehensive, anticipating the replication of pain. Direct pressure over the iliopsoas tendon may decrease the snapping phenomenon and aid in the diagnosis of internal snapping hip. Dynamic ultrasound of the iliopsoas tendon may identify the snapping phenomenon and any associated pathologic changes of the iliopsoas tendon and its bursa.[68] Although MRA cannot detect the dynamic snapping phenomenon, it may be useful in ruling out intra-articular hip pathology. This may be important because nearly half of those with complaints of internal snapping hip syndrome have an associated intra-articular injury.[69] Treatment of internal snapping hip syndrome is similar in scope to external snapping hip syndrome. Activity modification and pain control is the primary goal to reduce irritability. Physical modalities, medication, and injection may be necessary. Stretching and soft tissue mobilization to the iliopsoas or anterior hip structures is utilized to normalize mobility. Exercises should be directed at improving trunk control, stability, and lower extremity positioning.[63] Again, in case of failure of conservative measures, positive responses have been associated with surgical release and muscle lengthening interventions.[70]

Femoral Stress Fracture

Stress fractures to the femoral neck are frequently associated with physically active athletes and long-distance runners. Abnormal compression stress along the medial aspect of the femoral neck and excessive tensioning along the lateral side represent the two varieties of fractures. Microtrauma during repetitive stress from successive foot strikes in long-distance runners is usually the mechanism for this type of stress fracture. Factors such as poor training regimens, bone composition, vascular supply, and anatomic alignment have been linked with femoral neck stress fractures. Female athletes have up to four times higher risk of bone stress injury than their male counterparts.[71] Females with menstrual abnormalities such as amenorrhea, delayed menarche, disordered eating, and osteoporosis are at even greater risk.[72,73]

Athletes with femoral stress fractures will present with thigh, knee, or groin pain that increases with weight-bearing activities. Symptoms are often decreased or relieved following inactivity and rest. Compensatory gait strategies are often observed with decreased weight acceptance on the involved limb. Tenderness along the proximal femur and groin are consistent findings, along with limitations in hip ROM, especially hip flexion and medial rotation. Plain radiographs may not initially detect stress fractures for the first 2 weeks, although follow-up films may demonstrate sclerosis or evidence of fracture. MRI is more sensitive for early diagnosis.

Treatment of suspected femoral stress fracture with protected weight bearing and crutches should occur immediately, regardless of radiographic evidence. A compression-side fracture is treated conservatively with protective weight bearing. A slow and progressive course of care is expected and should be monitored with frequent repeat imaging. Tension-side fractures are at higher risk for displacement and require surgical intervention and fixation. In the event that treatment is not initiated early, complications of nonunion, avascular necrosis of the femoral head, early-onset arthritis, and deformity are likely. Complete blood workup, nutritional consultation, and psychological interventions are also recommended with suspicions of energy deficits caused by disordered eating.[74] Only after the athlete is pain free, demonstrates evidence of radiographic bone healing, and maintains a satisfactory clinical exam should a gradual running progression or sport-specific activities be initiated. This process will usually take several months.

Femoral Acetabular Impingement and Labral Tears

Femoral acetabular impingement (FAI) syndrome is a diagnosis that has been recognized recently as a source of hip pain and sequelae of hip pathology in the young athlete. FAI syndrome is a motion-related clinical disorder of the hip with triad of symptoms, clinical signs, and imaging findings.[75] It is characterized by the mechanical abutment and approximation of the femoral head or neck with the acetabular rim. This pathology is more likely found in males and has been linked to hip osteoarthritis, slipped capital femoral epiphysis (SCFE), and femoral neck fracture.[76] FAI can be a result of a cam lesion, pincer lesion, or a combination of the two. Cam lesions are a result of an abnormally shaped femoral head repeatedly impinging on an acetabulum that cannot accommodate this altered bone morphology. More commonly found in the young athletic male, resultant increased shearing forces might result in labral and chondral lesions to the anterior superior acetabulum.[77] Pincer lesions occur with excessive coverage of the acetabular rim, resulting in abutment of the femoral head and neck when the hip is flexed. This is most commonly found in the more mature athletic woman and may eventually lead to pathology along the anterior labrum and/or posteroinferior acetabulum. The hip labrum functions more like the meniscus in the knee, and with injury will result in decreased shock absorption, joint lubrication, pressure distribution, and hip joint stability.

In conjunction with evidence of structural findings on diagnostic imaging, associated symptoms and pertinent clinical exam findings are required for the diagnosis of FAI.[75]

Complaints often include deep hip and groin achiness, pain, and associated clicking that is reproduced with isolated or combined movements of hip flexion, adduction, and IR. The athlete will often describe the location of pain by making a "C" with their hand ("C sign"), placing the thumb posteriorly and the remaining fingers anteriorly, surrounding the lateral aspect of the hip. The athlete may complain of pain with prolonged weight bearing, cutting and pivoting, impact activities, and sustained positions of hip flexion, such as sitting. As the condition progresses, the pain will become more constant and debilitating, affecting more of the surrounding tissues including labrum, joint surfaces, and surrounding musculature. Clinical exam will often reveal a limitation in ROM to IR, especially with the hip flexed and adducted. Reproduction of the athlete's pain with combined hip flexion and IR is supportive for anterior hip impingement, whereas posteroinferior hip impingement is examined with hip extension and ER.[78] Although these provocative tests have also been thought to be suggestive of labral hip tears, specific labral stress tests do exist. The anterior labrum is stressed by moving the hip from a position of flexion, ER, and abduction into extension, IR, and adduction. Moving the hip from flexion, adduction, and IR into extension, abduction, and ER is diagnostic of posterior labral tears.[79] Although plain radiographs will be able to detect bony abnormalities and adaptive changes, MRI is more commonly used in the detection of FAI.[80,81] When labral tear or chondral damage is suspected, MRA is the diagnostic test of choice, with the sensitivity and specificity of 90% and 91%, respectively.[82,83]

Although the evidence is variable, conservative treatment is typically recommended as the first-line treatment for FAI. Studies have shown short- and long-term symptom relief and functional improvement similar to surgery; however, further research is needed to fully understand which athletes with FAI would benefit from conservative versus surgical management.[84-86] Conservative treatment includes a period of rest, activity modification, pain and inflammation control modalities, and trunk motor control and strengthening exercises.[87] Attempts are made to regain ROM with joint mobilization and stretching activities; however, with mechanical causes of the pain, surgical measures are more effective in regaining function in the highly active, athletic populations that do not respond to conservative measures. Surgical intervention involves either open or arthroscopic reshaping of the associated lesion and can occur simultaneously with labral debridement, direct repair, osteotomy, and/or chondroplasty. Rehabilitation following surgical interventions is dependent on the performed procedure. In the more simple arthroscopic procedures, such as labral debridement, the athlete may be permitted to weight-bear as tolerated immediately. Initially, focus is placed on pain control, inflammation control, and gait normalization. Progression to exercises and interventions aimed at ROM restoration, muscle functioning, and faulty movement patterns are performed in the subacute phases. Exercises that stress the anterior hip musculature, such as straight leg raises, sit-ups, and lunges, should be avoided early in the rehabilitation process to decrease the likelihood of hip flexor tendinopathy.[88] Gradual and slow return to sport should be initiated once the athlete no longer has significant impairment, asymmetry, or pain with provocative testing on clinical exam.

Muscle Strains

Muscle strains are not commonly seen in young athletes; instead, these athletes tend to incur more apophyseal avulsion injuries. However, in the older adolescent whose apophyses are beginning to ossify, muscle strains should be considered as a possible differential diagnosis. Muscle strains can occur in the same locations as apophyseal injuries. Most common muscle strains to the hip and thigh include adductor, hip flexor, and hamstring strains. Strains are commonly a result of extreme lengthening or forceful eccentric muscle contractions to the involved muscle group, contributing to overload and microtearing.[89] These injuries are often seen in high-velocity sports, including track, football, and soccer, and activities requiring large arcs of motion, such as dancing or kicking. Injuries can occur within the muscle belly or at the musculotendinous junction. Location of the injury has a relationship with expected healing times. For instance, distal strains within the hamstring muscles tend to follow a shorter, more predictable course of recovery than injuries to the proximal tendon.[89] Classification of muscle strains helps determine severity of injury and is based on pain, weakness, and loss of motion. Muscle strains are graded as grade 1 (minimal muscle damage), 2 (moderate amounts of microtears), or 3 (complete muscle rupture). This classification will assist in injury prognosis and management.

Athletes with acute muscle strains will report a sudden onset of pain that can be attributed to a specific activity or event. They may report feeling a pull or a "pop" in the location of the involved muscle-tendon unit. Pain will be present within the muscle or along the musculotendinous junction and will usually limit the athlete from continuing sport participation. Bruising and diffuse swelling over the injured muscle may be present in the more acute and subacute phases. An antalgic gait may also be present in attempts to unload the involved extremity. Physical examination and palpation of the muscle tissue may identify muscle spasm and a palpable defect within the muscle belly. Stressing the tissue with active contraction and extreme lengthening will help confirm the diagnosis. ROM and strength limitations occur commonly from muscle strains. MRI can assist in the diagnosis and help define the extent of the muscle strain but is usually reserved for more severe injury.[89,90] Plain radiographs are usually not indicated but may be helpful in differentiating between avulsion injury and true muscle strain when complaints are in proximity to bony attachment sites. Additional sources of pain must be considered in the suspicion of muscle strains of the thigh, hip, and pelvic musculature. For example, neural irritation and sensitivity along the sciatic

tract, with reoccurring hamstring injuries, can contribute to posterior thigh pain and replicate symptoms of a true hamstring strain. Combined injuries to multiple muscle groups, such as the hamstrings and adductors, are possible owing to their close proximity and related functions.[89] Contusions to the iliac crest or greater trochanter, called "hip pointers," are caused by a direct blow and are common in adolescents approaching skeletal maturity. Therefore, a complete and thorough evaluation is needed to determine the true nature of the athlete's complaints.

There is a high rate of muscle strain recurrence in the athletic population. Recurrence is thought to result from persistent weakness in the injured muscle, reduced extensibility of the muscle-tendon unit, and adaptive changes in the biomechanics and motor patterns of sporting movements following the original injury.[89] The primary objective for the treatment of muscle strains is to return the athlete to the previous level of functioning while decreasing the likelihood of reinjury.

In the more severe, grade 3 complete ruptures, surgical repair or reattachment is warranted. However, most grade 1 and 2 hamstring strains will respond to conservative care. Initial treatment of acute muscle strains should follow a similar course. Historically, the principle of PRICE (protection, rest, ice, compression, and elevation) was utilized to acutely manage most soft tissue injuries, such as muscle strains. However, more contemporary recommendations seek to improve healing by harnessing the benefits of progressive tissue loading via carefully controlled activity in the early phases of healing.[91,92] The acronym POLICE has replaced PRICE and represents protection, optimal loading, ice, compression, and elevation. Protection of the injured muscle is paramount at this time. Muscle stretching to the injured tissue should be avoided to allow for muscle regeneration and decrease the likelihood of scarring. Instead, pain-free ROM activities are encouraged to the associated joint segments. Optimal loading can be achieved by facilitating early functional mobility and gait; however, the athlete may require the use of crutches or alteration of gait (shorter strides with hamstring strain) to avoid overloading the tissue and causing pain. Therapeutic exercises may be initiated to promote hamstring, lumbar–pelvic, hip, and knee musculature, while monitoring loads and activity to avoid pain. As the athlete progresses, attention to normalization of ROM and muscle strength should be of concern. Neuromuscular control, balance, and trunk stability activities also become a focus. Eccentric muscle training should also be encouraged to enhance neuromuscular control and protection during muscle lengthening activities.[89] For example, the inclusion of the Nordic hamstring exercise into injury prevention programs has been effective in reducing the risk of hamstring strains in soccer players.[93] Sports-specific progression can be initiated once the athlete has a satisfactory physical exam without pain during muscle stretching, normal strength based on symmetry to the contralateral limb, and proper control with functional activities.

Corticosteroid injection has been utilized in the adult population for the management of muscle strains without any long-term side effects. This treatment is used mostly in professional athletes but should not be a primary treatment option for the adolescent population.[94]

Traumatic Hip Dislocation

Traumatic hip dislocation is most often seen during high-impact sports such as football, skiing, and motocross. The majority of hip dislocations occur in the posterior direction as a result of a high-energy, posteriorly directed force into a flexed knee. Associated fractures may occur in combination with a dislocation as a result of the abutment of the femoral head against the posterior acetabular wall. With this injury, the athlete will have intense pain with the limb in a position of flexion, adduction, and IR. Weight bearing and limb movements are unlikely because of the severity of pain. Hip dislocation is an emergent situation and warrants immediate medical attention. On-field joint reduction is not often performed owing to the proximity and potential damage to neurovascular structures. Instead, splinting and prompt transport to a medical facility is recommended to allow reduction within a few hours of injury. Standard radiographs will reveal the dislocated hip and should coincide with MRI and/or CT scan to assess the potential of associated injury. After relocation and repeat radiographs, the athlete is treated with non–weight bearing for 6 weeks. Following that time, repeat imaging studies are performed in view of the risk of the development of avascular necrosis or chondrolysis. With an uncomplicated course of recovery including normalization of hip mobility and strength, return to athletics can begin at 12 weeks following satisfactory physical exam.[94]

Slipped Capital Femoral Epiphysis

Slipped capital femoral epiphysis (SCFE) is one of the most prevalent hip disorders seen during adolescence and is rarely associated with distinct traumatic event. SCFE occurs with increased mechanical shearing forces across the physis of the femoral head, resulting in posterior slippage of the proximal epiphysis. SCFE is more prevalent in boys, especially those with an increased body mass index (BMI) and recent rapid growth. In females, the greatest incidence occurs around 9 years of age, whereas in males the peak incidence is at 11 years. Early onset of SCFE usually manifests with an associated endocrine disorder.[95] Despite a keen understanding of the risk factors and symptoms of SCFE, the diagnosis is still frequently overlooked or delayed. Early diagnosis of SCFE helps decrease the likelihood of subsequent hip pathology, including chondrolysis, femoral head avascular necrosis, and osteoarthritis.[96]

SCFE should be considered a differential diagnosis for any adolescent who presents with a significant limp. Pain may be described as insidious and gradual in onset to the groin, thigh, or medial knee, increasing with physical activity. However, a more diffuse hip or thigh ache or complete absence of pain may coincide with SCFE. In acute cases, the limb of interest may assume a resting position of extension, adduction, and ER. In more chronic slips, the limb will likely fall into hip ER with painful and limited combined flexion and IR. Radiographic or clinical evaluation of the contralateral limb may also be indicated because the incidence of bilateral involvement has been reported to range from 20% to 80%.[97]

Treatment of SCFE is surgical with open fixation of the slipped epiphysis immediately following diagnosis. More stable slips tend to fare better postoperatively with less deformity and comorbidity. Following fixation, the athlete is treated with protected weight bearing on crutches for 6 to 8 weeks. Formal rehabilitation is initiated with the goals of maximizing ROM, muscle strength and endurance, balance, and proprioception. Most athletes are permitted a progressive return to sports once they are pain free and demonstrate symmetrical limb strength and function. However, some literature advocates restricting a return to contact sports until the physis has fully fused. More severe cases of SCFE with associated loss of motion, stiffness, and pain may require salvage procedures such as arthrodesis or osteotomy and will have difficulty returning to higher-level sport participation.[98]

Legg–Calve–Perthes Disease

Legg–Calve–Perthes disease (LCPD), or Perthes, is the eponym given to idiopathic osteonecrosis of the capital femoral epiphysis of the femoral head, usually presenting among males 4 to 8 years old. However, bilateral diagnoses are more commonly seen in females and account for 8% to 24% of all cases.[96] The lack of blood flow and subsequent necrosis to the femoral head promotes a cascade of events resulting in impaired growth and development of the hip joint. Early onset, early diagnosis, and early intervention are favorable to allow more time for bone growth and remodeling.

Children with LCPD present with an insidious onset of a limp usually without any associated pain. However, with exercise, mild pain may be reported to the hip, groin, thigh, and/or knee. Limitations in hip IR and abduction mobility are classically associated with LCPD. Complete blood workup and radiographs are helpful in determining the presence of infection and existence and/or degree of disease progression.

The primary goals of LCPD management include maintenance of hip mobility, decreased pain with weight bearing, and containment of the femoral epiphysis within the acetabulum. The treatment remains highly controversial. However, in children with severe disease, surgical intervention appears preferable compared with nonoperative treatment, because surgery improves the shape and sphericity of the femoral head, providing greater acetabular coverage.[96] The two most common surgical methods for containment include femoral varus osteotomy and the Salter innominate osteotomy. Once the femoral head demonstrates signs of healing, the athlete is more than likely able to return to impact activities and sports, although the level of participation may be limited.

» Knee injuries

Examination Principles

As with most other body-specific examination procedures, a detailed history gives the examiner good insight into the injury and guides the differential diagnosis. The mechanism of injury, via traumatic or insidious onset, and resultant forces transferred to the joint during injury offer clues to what knee structure may be involved. The degree and timeline of any edema should also be determined, with more acute swelling indicating injury to a highly vascularized structure. With insidious onset, symptom response to activity should be explored in detail. A child may require more specific questioning regarding pain with activity than an adult, because children typically do not offer many details with open-ended questions. The painful area should be identified, and in cases where the child cannot verbalize the extent of pain, it is sometimes helpful to have them point to the most painful area with one finger. The parents and child should be questioned about any prior orthopedic injuries or predisposing factors, such as W-sitting as a child, which may impact current function.

Physical examination should include special tests to rule in or out specific pathologies, ROM, and muscle testing. As discussed earlier in this chapter, functional testing of the lower extremity to identify poor limb control and impairments in balance or functional strength and gait assessment also provide valuable information. It might be helpful to view gait patterns without children being aware, because they may not walk "naturally" while being watched. Another helpful technique is to distract them by engaging them in conversation, asking them to count backward or tell a story while walking. Gait abnormalities such as trunk shifting/listing, pelvic motion, decreased weight bearing, excessive femoral IR, knee valgus, and abnormal foot movements should all be noted and guide further examination.

Ligamentous Injuries

Anterior Cruciate Ligament Injuries

Anterior Cruciate Ligament (ACL) injuries are among the most severe and frequent activity-related injuries sustained by children participating in cutting and pivoting sports.[4] In the skeletally immature child, failure of the ACL complex can occur at different sites. Intrasubstance tears may occur, but failure may also present as an avulsion fracture at the insertion site of the ACL at the tibial spine. Tibial spine avulsion fractures are rarely seen after skeletal maturity. Some propose that a higher degree of cartilage within the area of the tibial spine, with the bone–tendon interface being weaker than the ligament itself, leads to failure of the bone rather than the ligament.[99] This injury with the loss of continuity of the ACL results in an unstable knee complex. The mechanism of injury is similar to that of ACL tears, with failure typically during a deceleration or pivoting maneuvers

with the knee undergoing valgus, hyperextension, or rotational forces.[100] The athlete will typically present with a large and rapidly developing joint effusion (hemarthrosis), decreased knee ROM, and decreased ability to bear weight. Owing to the resultant loss of integrity of the ACL complex, joint laxity with increased anterior translation of the tibia on the femur may exist, which can be examined utilizing a Lachman or anterior drawer test. Radiographs or MRI may be necessary to classify the injury and determine the extent of any secondary damage.[100]

Treatment is based on the degree of fragmentation or displacement. Minimally displaced fractures can be treated nonoperatively with cast immobilization for 6 to 8 weeks.[99,100] Several options exist for arthroscopic or open surgical fixation and vary depending on injury specifics and surgeon preference. Rehabilitation goals are to restore knee ROM, strength, balance, coordination, and dynamic knee stability in preparation for return to sports.

Intrasubstance ACL tears are encountered with increasing frequency in the skeletally immature population.[101] ACL injury typically occurs during sports or activities that involve running, cutting, jumping, or pivoting maneuvers. Sports that carry a high risk of ACL injury include soccer, basketball, volleyball, and football. The youngster with an ACL tear will have a similar history and physical examination findings of their adult counterparts. They will typically describe a "giving way" sensation of the knee and possibly an audible "pop" at the time of injury. Hemarthrosis, decreased knee ROM, and increased laxity with Lachman or anterior drawer testing are also typical. Specialized devices, such as a KT-1000 arthrometer, may help quantify the degree of anterior translation between the tibia and the femur. Children tend to have more available joint translation than adults, and, therefore, comparison with the uninjured side is necessary for accurate examination.

The natural sequelae of the ACL-deficient knee in the young athlete typically include recurrent knee instability, cumulative intra-articular damage (meniscus tears or osteochondral defects), and decreased activity levels.[99,102] Owing to the ACL's proximity to the physes of the distal femur and proximal tibia, there is a risk of damage when typical adult ACL reconstruction surgical techniques are performed. Damage to the physis could lead to limb-length discrepancy or angular deformity as skeletal growth continues. Pediatric-specific ACL reconstruction techniques minimize this risk and are successful at restoring a stable knee complex. With the development of these innovative techniques, surgeons are more likely to favor operative reconstruction over conservative management.[103-106]

Early postoperative rehabilitation should focus on effusion management, maintaining full knee extension, regaining flexion ROM, and restoration of quadriceps activation. Progression of rehabilitation incorporates open- and closed-chain lower extremity strengthening. Initially, open-chain knee extension should stay within the limits of 90 degrees to 40 degrees of knee flexion to protect the ACL graft from excessive strain but can be progressed to full arc after 8 to 10 weeks. Neuromuscular electrical stimulation (NMES) has been shown to improve quadriceps strength return after surgery[107]; however, some children may not tolerate this modality well, and use should be on a case-by-case basis. Integrated lower extremity activities using balance exercises, perturbation training, and proprioceptive exercises should be incorporated. Additionally, core stabilization and hip strengthening should be included as part of an inclusive rehabilitation program.

Progression to jogging and bilateral jumping activities typically begin around 3 to 4 months postoperatively. Single-leg plyometrics, agility activities, and general conditioning should be progressed after this period, with return-to-sports participation ranging from 6 to 12 months postoperatively.[99,108] A fusion of time-based criterion and functional performance testing has been advocated to determine the athlete's readiness for high-level training and return-to-sports integration.[109] Typical requirements are 90% limb symmetry index in quadriceps strength testing and 90% symmetry with a battery of single-leg hop tests.[99,106,108,110,111]

Recent research has highlighted the importance of ascertaining an athlete's psychological state with regard to fear of reinjury, athletic confidence, and emotional well-being prior to returning to sports. Although there are no psychological measures specifically designed for the youth athlete, the authors recommend using the Anterior Cruciate Ligament–Return to Sport after Injury (ACL-RSI) short form scale. The ACL-RSI has shown good criterion validity, reliability, and responsiveness. This scale is user friendly and may help clinicians identify athletes who may struggle with returning to competitive sports or may be at a higher risk for repeat injury.[112,113]

ACL Injury Risk Reduction

Female adolescent athletes are the highest risk population for a noncontact ACL injury, with injury rates ranging from two to nine times higher than in male counterparts.[109,114,115] Similarly, trends have demonstrated that the risk of ACL injury for any adolescent athlete, regardless of gender, increases steadily from the age of 10 through adolescence.[116] Altered lower extremity movement patterns such as dynamic knee valgus, femoral IR, and limited hip/knee flexion during jumping and cutting motions have been shown to increase stress on the ACL and increase the likelihood of rupture.[12,114] Deficits in strength or neuromuscular control in the growing adolescent, especially females, predispose to these pathologic patterns and a higher risk of injury. This recognition has led to the development of injury risk reduction programs designed to retrain the athlete by improving dynamic limb control. Efficacy of these programs has been studied and proven successful for athletes involved in many high-risk sports.[115,117,118] Several well-designed ACL injury risk reduction programs are readily available, such as the FIFA 11+, Sportsmetrics or Prevent injury Enhance Performance (PEP) programs.

Medial Collateral Ligament Injuries

Medial collateral ligament (MCL) injuries usually occur from a valgus stress to the knee. The mechanism of injury commonly reported is another athlete falling onto the lateral aspect of his or her knee, which occurs frequently in sports like football, soccer, and basketball. The athlete will typically present with a small effusion and tenderness localized to the medial knee, along the MCL.[119] In the young athlete with open physes, the possibility of avulsion of the MCL at its tibial attachment should be suspected. As a general rule, avulsion injuries should be suspected in the younger, more skeletally immature athlete, whereas older adolescents have a higher probability of soft tissue MCL injury.[119] Clinical examination will help discern between these two injuries, but imaging will likely be necessary. The athlete with an MCL injury will have tenderness to palpation along the course of the ligament, whereas the athlete with avulsion injury will be more tender near the distal attachment on the tibia. Special tests, such as the Valgus Stress Test at 30 degrees and 0 degrees flexion, will also help determine the degree of laxity, structures involved, and severity of injury. MCL injuries are graded 1, 2, and 3, depending on the degree of laxity present, end feel, and degree of fiber disruption. This classification system is commonly utilized to grade most ligamentous sprains throughout the body and is detailed in Display 16.4.

Isolated MCL injuries typically respond well to conservative management.[120] A hinged knee brace may be utilized early after injury for protection against valgus forces. Early rehabilitation is advocated with focus on ROM, early and pain-free weight bearing, strengthening, balance, and dynamic stability activities. Grade 1 and 2 injuries typically do not require extended rehabilitation, with an average return-to-sport time of 1 to 3 weeks and 4 to 6 weeks, respectively.[121] Grade 3 injuries are more complex and may require 9 to 12 weeks of rehabilitation.[122]

Posterior Cruciate Ligament Injuries

The posterior cruciate ligament (PCL) serves as the primary restraint to posterior translation of the tibia on the femur. This ligament is typically injured from a direct blow to the anterior aspect of the knee such as falling onto a flexed knee during activity or the knee contacting the dashboard in a car

DISPLAY 16.4	Ligament Sprain Grading Scale
Grade	**Description**
1	Pain with stress testing without associated joint laxity
2	Pain with stress testing with increased joint excursion; presence of distinct end point
3	Complete ligament disruption with excessive excursion; no distinct end point

accident. Isolated injuries to the PCL are not common. The athlete with a torn PCL will demonstrate posterior laxity on physical examination. Special tests, such as the posterior drawer or sag (Godfrey) sign, will help identify instability; the dial test is helpful for determining isolated PCL or multiligament involvement.[123]

Most PCL injuries are treated conservatively. Avoidance of activity is necessary, and a brief period of immobilization may be recommended. Initial rehabilitation focuses on resolving impairments related to the acute injury such as pain, effusion, and gait abnormality. ROM exercises into the extremes of flexion cause increased stress across the PCL and should be avoided until several weeks after injury because this motion may delay healing. Similarly, open-chain hamstring exercises are contraindicated because they may also stress the PCL complex by exerting a posterior translator force on the knee joint.[123] A heavy emphasis is placed on quadriceps strengthening and dynamic stabilization or proprioceptive training. Rehabilitation can range from 2 to 6 months. As with ACL rehabilitation, functional performance measures, such as quadriceps strength and functional hop tests, should be used to determine readiness for sports participation.[124]

Lateral Collateral Ligament Injuries

Lateral collateral ligament (LCL) injuries are rarely seen in the pediatric athlete. An injury to the LCL is usually in conjunction with injury to the entire posterolateral corner (PLC) of the knee and results from a high-energy blow to the medial aspect of an extended knee.[119] Once again, the ligament is not the weakest link in the pediatric athlete, and bony avulsion of the LCL from the fibula can mimic the laxity associated with an LCL injury. Surgery may be necessary to fixate a displaced fracture of this nature.

Intra-articular Injuries

Meniscus Injury

Most meniscal injuries in children under age 10 occur in the setting of a congenital malformation known as a discoid meniscus.[125,126] The discoid meniscus is shaped like a disc, instead of the normal semilunar shape, and is more likely to develop tears. Discoid menisci occur most commonly in the lateral meniscus. The overall prevalence of discoid menisci in the United States has been reported to be between 3% and 5%, with male and female occurrence rates being similar.[126,127] Younger, preschool-aged children with a discoid meniscus may be asymptomatic and complain only of a snapping sensation in the knee. Symptomatic snapping with pain will usually be present in older, elementary-aged children. This pain may be accompanied by intermittent effusion, joint line tenderness, positive McMurray test, and gait abnormalities. The entire meniscus may also be unstable, in which a palpable prominence along the joint line may be seen with knee flexion and extension.

Treatment of the asymptomatic discoid meniscus usually consists of observation only. Although the likelihood

of developing meniscal tears is higher, it is currently unclear whether surgical intervention in this population would lessen this risk.[125] Surgical intervention is recommended for the symptomatic discoid meniscus. Arthroscopic reshaping of the meniscus is typically performed using a procedure called saucerization.[126] Any associated meniscus tears are treated with partial meniscectomy or repair. Stabilization procedures are performed for unstable discoid variants. Rehabilitation programs and expected time for full recovery will vary depending on the procedure performed. A period of limited weight bearing or ROM restrictions may be required and will be directed by the treating surgeon.

Traumatic meniscal tears, absent of congenital meniscus malformation, usually occur in older children or adolescents as a result of a twisting injury in sports. The meniscus of the developing child is more vascular than that of adults and has thus been noted to have better capacity for healing.[125] Clinical diagnosis is sometimes challenging, with physical examination and special tests yielding somewhat limited diagnostic reliability.[128] The most consistent findings during meniscus tear physical examination include history of a twisting injury, joint effusion, and joint line tenderness. Other special tests such as McMurray test, Apley compression or distraction, Thessaly or Ege test may also aid in diagnosis. A detailed injury history and clustering of positive or negative findings with multiple special tests will improve the diagnostic accuracy of the physical examination for meniscal tears. The athlete may complain of the knee becoming "stuck" or "catching" if a fragment of meniscus is blocking motion between the tibia and the femur. An MRI is often obtained to assist in diagnosis; however, it should be noted that the MRI is less accurate in diagnosing meniscus tears in children compared with adults.[125]

Treatment of meniscus tears will vary depending on the location of the tear within the meniscus, tear orientation, and degree of displacement of the torn fragment. As mentioned earlier, certain characteristics of the meniscus of the skeletally immature child allow for more healing potential than adults, and thus most tears in children are managed using repair rather than meniscectomy. Postoperatively, a athlete will typically be treated with non- or partial weight bearing for 4 to 6 weeks with use of hinged knee brace. Knee flexion ROM is also typically limited from 0 to 90 degrees for the first 4 to 6 weeks, with progressive flexion permitted beyond that point. Rehabilitation should continue with addressing deficits in strength, coordination, and limb control. Return to sports usually occurs around 3 to 4 months postoperatively and return of symmetrical limb strength and functional performance.

Osteochondritis Dissecans in the Knee

As discussed earlier, OCD is a condition in which damage to the subchondral bone causes secondary damage to the overlying articular cartilage. The knee is the most commonly involved joint, the lateral aspect of the medial femoral condyle being the most commonly affected site.[8] Children with OCD typically complain of activity-related anterior knee pain. Differential diagnosis should include patellofemoral pain, chondromalacia patella, and plica syndrome, because these may all have similar symptoms. With the knee in varying degrees of flexion, the examiner may note a distinct area of point tenderness at the medial femoral condyle where the lesion is located. Wilson sign is a special test that has been described but may have limited diagnostic value.[129] If the lesion has progressed to being unstable, mechanical symptoms are more likely to be noted, such as crepitus, knee effusion, and an abnormal gait.[130] Plain radiographs are typically part of the initial diagnostic workup of a child suspected to have an OCD lesion. If positive, MRI or other advanced imaging will typically be utilized to gain more information and improve decision making for treatment.[131]

Treatment will vary depending on the age of the athlete and the extent and location of the lesion. Nonsurgical treatment is advocated for the stable lesion. In the classic treatment protocol, the athlete is non–weight bearing with the knee immobilized in a brace for a period of 6 weeks.[130] Recently, some surgeons have advocated that immobilization and weight-bearing restrictions are not necessary. In these cases, the athlete may bear full weight, but should avoid any sports or impact activity for a period of 6 to 8 weeks.[131] In either scenario, adherence is typically an issue, and considerable education regarding the long-term risks associated with improper treatment of OCD may be necessary. After this period of immobilization or activity modification, rehabilitation is initiated and focuses on deficits in strength, ROM, and other kinetic chain deficits that impact lower extremity control. Close communication with the referring orthopedic provider is necessary, because the return to running, jumping, and sports activity is dependent on radiographic examination of lesion healing. That being said, many athletes can usually begin a progressive introduction of these activities around 3 months after diagnosis. When initiating plyometric training, proper lower extremity alignment and impact absorption through the hip, knee, and ankle during jump landing should be emphasized. In addition, the physical therapist will need to closely monitor the athlete for any return of symptoms while undergoing this period of impact loading and sports activity resumption.

Surgical management is typically recommended for unstable lesions or those that do not heal with conservative measures. Several surgical treatment options exist and include antegrade or retrograde drilling procedures, fragment removal, internal fixation, microfracture, autologous chondrocyte implantation, or osteochondral autograft or allograft transplantation.[130,131] Rehabilitation protocols will vary depending on the procedure performed; however, typical protocols will require an early period of immobilization and weight-bearing restrictions. Rehabilitation is similar in scope to most other postoperative knee procedures addressing local deficits about the knee as well as any other noted kinetic chain deficits. Return to sports will typically not occur until 6 to 9 months postoperatively as the athlete demonstrates the attainment of required performance measures in the involved limb.

Acute Patella Dislocations and Osteochondral Fractures

Most acute dislocations of the patella are caused by planting or twisting maneuvers, which usually occur while rapidly changing directions during sports. The athlete will note the knee "giving way" and can occasionally recall seeing the patella located on the lateral aspect of the knee. Relocation may occur spontaneously or is usually accomplished by simply straightening the involved leg. The knee will be swollen, generally tender, and ROM will typically be limited owing to guarding. Lateral displacement of the patella may evoke an apprehension sign. Radiographs or MRI will be necessary to rule out the possibility of osteochondral fractures. If no osteochondral damage is noted, acute patella dislocations are usually treated conservatively with a brief period of immobilization in extension, followed by progressive ROM and rehabilitation. If an athlete continues to experience recurrent patella dislocations, surgical intervention may be indicated. Medial patellofemoral ligament (MPFL) reconstruction is a common surgical option and has been associated with good functional outcomes.[132] Weight bearing is protected early with the knee locked in extension. Early ROM and quadriceps activation are emphasized. Comprehensive rehabilitation after MPFL reconstruction overlaps considerably with the principles discussed after ACL reconstruction with return to sports around 6 to 12 months.

Osteochondral fractures typically occur with an acute lateral patella dislocation and are most frequently located in the medial patella facet and/or lateral femoral condyle. During relocation of the patella, the medial patella surface shears across the lateral femoral condyle/trochlea, damaging the articular surface.[133] Although the frequency of this injury is difficult to quantify, some reports have found occurrence with patella dislocations to be as high as 25% to 75%.[133] The presentation of the child with an osteochondral fracture will be similar to that of an acute patella dislocation; however, there may be palpable crepitus during movement or a mechanical, bony block to motion, owing to a loose body. Plain films may not always detect the lesion, and MRI is typically the image of choice.[133] Surgical treatment is indicated in most cases of displaced osteochondral fractures with arthroscopic fixation or removal of the fragment. A resurfacing procedure, such as microfracture, is performed when the fragment is removed.[133] The microfracture procedure stimulates bone marrow, causing bleeding, and a resulting fibrin clot forms that eventually differentiates into fibrocartilage to repair the defect.[134] To protect the healing tissue, most surgeons recommend a period of protected weight bearing and ROM restrictions postoperatively on the basis of lesion location and procedure performed. Rehabilitation will be similar to other knee disorders previously discussed. The projected time frame for return to sports is 4 to 6 months.[133]

Overuse Injuries

Anterior knee pain is a common complaint among skeletally immature athletes and can stem from a variety of causes, many of them related to overuse. Commonly encountered diagnoses that cause anterior knee pain are patellofemoral pain syndrome (PFPS), Osgood–Schlatter disease (OSD), Sinding–Larsen–Johansson disease (SLJ), inflamed synovial plica, and patella tendinopathy.

Patellofemoral Pain Syndrome

PFPS is a broad diagnosis that refers to pain in the patellofemoral joint and the surrounding structures. PFPS is the most common cause of all knee overuse injuries.[3] Biomechanical alterations in lower extremity function result in abnormal stress across the patellofemoral joint and tissue overload, which results in anterior knee pain. The interaction among several intrinsic and extrinsic factors is thought to be responsible for causing PFPS. Structural abnormalities such as femoral anteversion, femoral trochlea dysplasia, and bipartite patella may contribute to the development of PFPS. Flexibility limitations in the quadriceps, hamstrings, hip flexors, IT band, and gastrocsoleus complex, as well as strength/neuromuscular control deficits in the gluteus medius, gluteus maximus, and quadriceps, have all been implicated as factors related to PFPS.[135] Extrinsic factors related to PFPS include training errors such as inadequate rest, rapid progression of training volume, and improper shoe wear. More recently, some researchers have emphasized that psychological constructs, such as anxiety, depression, fear, and catastrophizing, may play a role in PFPS; however, this has not been researched specifically within the pediatric or adolescent population.[136]

The athlete will usually complain of a dull ache from underneath or around the patella that increases with activities such as squatting, ascending/descending stairs, running, or prolonged sitting. As mentioned previously, proximal and distal factors may contribute to the development of PFPS, and thus a comprehensive physical examination is required. Special attention should be paid to the examination of gluteus medius and gluteus maximus strength and the resulting coordination during closed-chain limb control, because there is a mounting body of evidence that these deficits play a large role in the development of PFPS.[135,137,138] Distal factors such as excessive foot pronation and limited ankle dorsiflexion may also contribute to the pathomechanics involved in PFPS and should be examined accordingly.[139] Limb control can be evaluated utilizing the Eccentric Step Down test, which may help identify limb control deficits. Locally, patella alignment and mobility should be examined looking for evidence of either restricted or excessive patella mobility and abnormal tilting. The articulating surface of the patella should be palpated because it will usually be painful in PFPS. Pain with compression of the patellofemoral joint should also be noted (grind test). Radiographs are not necessary for diagnosing PFPS, but they may be helpful in ruling out any other possible diagnosis or related issues.[3]

Treatment must first focus on removing the offending forces during everyday activities. Relative rest from painful activities during sports should be advocated, and complete rest may be necessary in severe cases. All exercises in physical therapy should be closely monitored and should remain pain free. Increasing load tolerance to the patellofemoral joint through progressive loading and correction of biomechanical problems should be the primary goal of all interventions.[140] Close supervision and feedback are required during functional exercises to ensure proper lower extremity alignment. The multifactorial nature of PFPS dictates a diverse and extensive treatment plan. Strength training, flexibility, balance, core strengthening, and neuromuscular control exercises have all been shown to be helpful in treating PFPS.[135,141] Adjunct treatments such as orthotic intervention, patellofemoral taping, or bracing may be effective for pain relief and may be used to enhance the athlete's ability to participate in therapeutic exercises. If a he or she fails to respond to conservative treatment and symptoms continue to limit function, surgical treatment could be considered. Lateral release with patellar realignment procedures for the correction of PFPS has been described. Rehabilitation from these procedures is usually extensive, and a prolonged absence from sports is required.

Apophysitis

OSD and SLJ are common overuse injuries that will present as anterior knee pain. Both are caused by traction forces from muscle contraction leading to increased stress across the apophysis. These repetitive forces lead to cumulative microtrauma, inflammation, and pain.[3] OSD represents injury at the tibial tubercle, whereas SLJ represents an apophysitis at the inferior pole of the patella. Symptoms typically present between the ages of 9 and 15 years in children who participate in activities that involve excessive running and jumping. The symptoms include achy pain in the anterior knee that is aggravated by activity or with direct pressure, such as kneeling. Tenderness to palpation will exist at the location of apophysitis (tibial tubercle or inferior pole of patella) and will help with differential diagnosis. Contractile testing of the quadriceps will also produce pain. Radiographs are helpful in ruling out any other possible diagnoses such as avulsion fractures.

OSD and SLJ are considered self-limiting processes, because symptoms will resolve at skeletal maturity when the apophysis fuses. Acute management consists of rest from aggravating activities, ice, and possibly nonsteroidal anti-inflammatory drugs (NSAIDs). Treatment should focus on normalizing lower extremity flexibility, especially to the quadriceps and hamstring muscle groups. Strengthening of the quadriceps, hip abductors, and external rotators may help improve lower extremity alignment, efficiency, and load tolerance during functional activities. Exercises should not provoke symptoms. Patella strapping and braces may also help to decrease symptoms and facilitate exercise participation to prevent deconditioning.

Patellar Tendinopathy

Older adolescents with fused growth plates are more likely to develop a tendinopathy with overuse, as opposed to an apophysitis. Patellar tendinopathy or "jumpers knee" is commonly seen in adolescents who play basketball, volleyball, and running. This is a mechanical overuse syndrome resulting from the cumulative effects of repetitive microtrauma within the patellar tendon.[3] Athletes report anterior knee pain aggravated by activity. Contractile testing of the quadriceps will be painful, and tenderness to palpation along the patella tendon is common.

The mainstay of treatment for all lower limb tendinopathies is progressive tendon loading and is based on the athlete's irritability and reactivity. In more painful and reactive tendons, a short period of relative rest, refraining from any aggravating activities, may be warranted. The use of isometric contractions is beneficial in continuing to stress the tendon in a controlled manner to prevent tendon weakening and deconditioning. Regardless of contraction type, heavy loading programs that focus on time under tension have been advocated as tendons become less reactive or irritable[142-144] The single-leg decline squat is a commonly utilized exercise to direct loads to the patella tendon.[145] Owing to the forces associated with sports, rehabilitation of athletes with patella tendinopathy should eventually incorporate activities that stress tendon energy storage and release such as running, plyometrics, and agility training. In conjunction, improving global lower limb flexibility, strength, and neuromuscular control should also be components of a comprehensive treatment plan. Lack of flexibility in quadriceps and hamstrings has been implicated as a risk factor for lower extremity overuse syndromes; therefore, a long-term flexibility program should be advocated for injury prevention.[146]

Plica Syndrome

Plicae are bands of tissue in the synovial lining of the knee that arise from remnants of embryologic knee development.[147] Although plicae can be found at multiple locations, the medial plica is most commonly symptomatic. A medial plica should be considered a normal variant in anatomy, because its presence does not always cause symptoms. A plica can become symptomatic when it rubs across the medial femoral condyle with movement, causing inflammation and subsequent anteromedial knee pain. The athlete will occasionally complain of "pseudo" locking episodes or snapping sensation with flexion/extension of the knee, making diagnosis difficult.[148] Palpation of a symptomatic plica is important for clinical examination, but can be difficult. The plica is usually felt as a painful, taut band, running from the medial patella to the medial femoral condyle and orientated perpendicular to the patella. Treatment is similar to that discussed for PFPS, involving activity modification, inflammation control, patella taping techniques, flexibility restoration, pain-free strengthening, and emphasis on dynamic limb control. If conservative measures fail, arthroscopic excision may be recommended.

» Lower leg injuries

The lower leg refers to the area of the tibia, fibula, and all the surrounding tissues. The term "shin splints" is a nonspecific term to describe pain to the lower leg but can refer to various injuries to the lower leg tissues. The lower leg is susceptible to both traumatic and overuse-type injuries in athletes. Common differential diagnoses of lower leg pain include medial tibial stress syndrome, tibia and/or fibula stress fracture, chronic exertional compartment syndrome, acute compartment syndrome, muscle strains and tendinopathy, and traumatic tibia and/or fibula fracture.

Shin Splints

Medial Tibial Stress Syndrome

Medial tibial stress syndrome (MTSS) is the most common cause of pain to the lower leg. It is characterized by pain and inflammation along the anteromedial plane of the distal to central one-third of the tibia with running and jumping activities. Although not fully understood, MTSS was initially thought to be caused by overuse of the posterior tibialis and/or soleus muscles, contributing to subsequent periosteal reaction along the medial border of the tibia. High, repetitive loads and rapid foot pronation will contribute to microtears at the soft tissue and periosteal attachments. However, an alternative mechanism is that MTSS is caused by bony overload, resulting in an osteopenic cortex and bone marrow edema and not periostitis.[149] Contributing factors to MTSS include decreased hip internal rotation ROM, excessive plantarflexion ROM, excessive midfoot mobility, poor shock attenuation, rapid changes in exercise intensity, weakness or imbalance about the lower leg, and high BMI.[59,149]

An athlete with MTSS complains of pain and tenderness to the distal to central one-third of the lower leg along the posteromedial border of the tibia. Initially, the athlete may report pain with the start of the activity that decreases with continued participation. However, as symptoms worsen, pain will become more consistent and may carry over into other less demanding activities. Physical exam may demonstrate weakness and imbalances about the lower leg muscles, namely, the posterior tibialis and flexor hallucis longus. Biomechanical deformities to the lower kinetic chain that contribute to excessive compensatory foot pronation are also likely. MRI remains the most sensitive and specific test for diagnosing and discerning between an MTSS and stress fracture. Initially, plain radiographs will be normal. Bone scans may confirm the diagnosis of MTSS by showing diffuse longitudinal area of uptake, as opposed to a focal, transverse line that is indicative of a stress fracture.

Treatment for MTSS begins with a period of active rest from painful activities such as running and jumping. Low-impact activities such as swimming, cycling, and other modes of cardiovascular training are recommended to maintain fitness levels and decrease the effects of deconditioning.

Pain control modalities, including ice, compressive taping/wrapping techniques, and NSAID, may be helpful in alleviation of symptoms. A rehabilitation program should consist of flexibility and strength training of the lower leg musculature, with a special focus on the calf musculature. Treatment should also restore balance and dynamic control of the foot and lower kinetic chain and trunk. A thorough functional evaluation should also be performed to identify any contributory factors present during sport-specific movements. Shoes with adequate foot support and/or orthotic intervention may be helpful during the initial phases of treatment to off-load painful structures. With proper management, it may take 6 to 8 weeks before returning to running and impact activities. Return to running is performed with a progressive running program. Increasing running distance, frequency, and intensity should be gradual and not be performed concurrently and should take into consideration athlete fitness level, pain response, and goals.

Tibial Stress Fracture

Tibial stress fractures are common with activities that include repetitive loading to the lower leg, including running, basketball, gymnastics, and dance. Stress fractures are osseous fractures caused by repetitive bony overload and the inability to meet the demands of the levels of force. Contributing factors for tibial stress fracture are unstructured training regimens, impaired bone health, high BMI, abnormally high or low medial longitudinal arch heights, and excessive foot pronation.[150] Owing to the high incidence in distance runners, certain characteristics of running mechanics have been studied and linked to tibial stress fracture. These include high vertical peak loads and loading rates, heel striking at ground contact, increased step length, decreased step rate, and high tibial accelerations.[151-153]

Tibial stress fractures will cause localized, acute, and sharp pain on the tibial surface. This can occur anywhere along the length of the tibia but is usually along the central to upper one-third of the anterior cortex. Focal tenderness and pain is reported along the site of the fracture and may be associated with a palpable thickening. Pain will usually not be present at the start of activity but will gradually worsen as activity continues and may eventually occur at rest. Diagnosis may be confirmed with diagnostic imaging. Initially, plain radiographs may be normal but will eventually demonstrate periosteal healing or callus formation to the area indicative of bony healing. Bone scan is not specific, but will demonstrate a focal uptake along the anterior tibia. MRI is more specific and can better assist in the diagnosis and determine the severity of the tibial stress fracture.

Initial treatment for tibial stress fractures is relative rest and activity limitation to allow for bony remodeling. Pain-free weight bearing, muscle activation, and flexibility activities can be initiated. In cases where weight bearing is painful, a walking boot or restriction of weight bearing with crutches may be warranted for a short period. Once there is evidence of radiographic healing, progressive weight bearing and a more advanced strengthening and flexibility program can be implemented. As strength is progressed and the athlete can tolerate more load-demanding tests, sport-specific training can begin with an emphasis on quality of movement and progressive return. Running gait retraining with the goals of limiting vertical and torsional loading has also been effective in the management of tibial stress fractures.[151,153] When the athlete fails to improve, has a history of multiple stress fractures, or a long history of bone health compromise, a more thorough medical workup may be warranted. This includes blood testing and nutritional consult.

Compartment Syndrome

The lower leg is comprised of four compartments: anterior, lateral, superficial posterior, and deep posterior. Each compartment is comprised of muscle, vascular, and nervous tissues, all encapsulated by a facial membrane.

Acute compartment syndrome is an emergent condition that results from acute trauma to the lower leg. An increase in intracompartmental pressure is caused by soft tissue swelling and contributes to localized pain, parasthesia, and weakness. In suspicion of acute compartment syndrome, immediate attention is required. Fasciotomy is performed to relieve the compartment pressure and prevent permanent tissue damage.

Chronic exertional compartment syndrome (CECS) or exercise-induced compartment syndrome is a transient condition commonly seen in long-distance runners but can be functionally disabling to all athletes. Pain results from muscle ischemia during exercise owing to significantly elevated intracompartmental pressures. During exercise, increased muscle contractions can lead to increased blood flow and volume within the affected lower leg compartment. Normally, the surrounding fascia will adapt and expand to meet the demands of the increased muscle volume. However, in CECS, the containing fascia is unable to accommodate, thereby constricting blood flow and resulting in ischemia. Complaints of pain and tightness result, with or without neurovascular compromise. The location and presentation of symptoms will vary depending on the affected compartment. The anterior and lateral compartments are the most commonly affected; however, any of the four compartments of the lower leg can be involved.

An athlete with CECS will commonly report aching pain, tightness, and/or squeezing sensations about the lower leg in the distribution of the affected compartment. Commonly, the athlete will first report tightness or cramping but may progress to altered sensation and motor weakness. Symptoms are usually predictable, exacerbated by a given exercise intensity and duration, and relieved shortly after cessation of activity. Diagnosis of the syndrome can be confirmed with intracompartmental pressure testing. Conservative treatment of activity modification, soft tissue mobilization and massage, muscle stretching and strengthening, and orthotic prescription have not been very successful in the management of CECS.[154] However, research is emerging regarding the use of the gait retraining technique for the treatment of CECS of the anterior compartment.[155] In the event that conservative treatment fails, surgical fasciotomy of the involved compartments is recommended and often allows the athlete to return to full activity within 8 to 12 weeks.[59]

» Ankle injuries

The ankle is the most common site for athletic injuries, accounting for 20% to 30% of all musculoskeletal injuries.[156] The ankle joint is comprised of three main joint articulations. The talocrural joint is the bony articulation between the distal tibia and fibula and the proximal surface of the talus and is responsible for nearly all of ankle plantarflexion and dorsiflexion. The subtalar joint comprises the talocalcaneal and talocalcaneonavicular joints. Inversion and eversion occur predominately at the subtalar joint. It is important to note that despite the dominance of one motion occurring at a given joint, mobility occurs simultaneously in all three planes of motion owing to joint axis orientation. Therefore, triplanar movement about the ankle is often described as "supination"—or combined plantarflexion, inversion, and adduction—and "pronation," or combined dorsiflexion, eversion, and abduction.

More common differential diagnoses for ankle pain are lateral ankle sprain, syndesmosis sprain, distal physeal fracture, peroneal longus subluxation, osteochondral fracture of the talar dome, Maisonneuve fracture or combination of a distal syndesmosis tear and a proximal fibular fracture, and sinus tarsi impingement.

Ankle Sprains

Stability to the lateral ankle is caused primarily by the lateral ligament complex, consisting of the anterior talofibular ligament (ATFL), calcaneofibular ligament (CFL), and posterior talofibular ligament (PFL). All three ligaments aid in the restriction of excessive ankle inversion, with the ATFL also resisting anterior translation of the talus. The medial ankle ligaments are comprised of the thicker and stronger deltoid ligament and are responsible for restraining ankle eversion, pronation, and anterior displacement of the talus. The tibia and fibula are connected distally by the anterior and posterior distal tibiofibular ligaments and the distal interosseous ligament. Together, they comprise the distal portion of the interosseous membrane that traverses the entire lengths of the tibia and fibular shafts and contributes to lower leg stability and force transmission.

Eighty-five percent of all ankle pathology is caused by acute ankle sprains and most often involve injury to the lateral ligaments. Mechanism of injury is usually excessive inversion and plantarflexion. Deltoid sprains are also known as eversion sprains because of their mechanism of

injury. Syndesmotic sprains, commonly named "high ankle sprains," may occur in conjunction with medial ankle sprains and are caused by forced eversion and ER of the ankle, causing a widening of the distal tibiofibular joint. Injuries to the medial ankle or along the tibiofibular syndesmosis are less common on account of their inherent strength.[157]

In examining an ankle injury, careful inspection of foot position at the time of injury, location of tenderness, and mobility testing aid in the recognition of the injured ligaments. The athlete will often report a distinct injury with a sudden pain or "pop." With more severe sprains, pain will not allow continued participation in athletic activity. The athlete will initially present with pain, swelling, and ecchymosis throughout the ankle and into the foot and toes. It should be noted that because of the dependent position of the foot, swelling and bruising may not always correspond to the site of injury. Weight bearing may also be limited and painful.

Physical exam should include careful palpation along the ankle ligaments to help discern the ligaments involved. ROM will be limited, especially in motions that stress the involved ligament. Isolated ligamentous stress testing may also be beneficial in the diagnosis of ankle instability. Lateral ligamentous stress testing includes the anterior drawer and talar tilt tests. The anterior drawer test tests the stability of the ATFL, whereas the talar tilt test targets the integrity of the CFL. The Kleiger test, or forced foot eversion and ER, and squeeze test stress the medial ankle's deltoid ligament and syndesmosis ligaments, respectively. All tests should be performed bilaterally to compare the amount of excursion, provocation of pain, and appreciation of a distinct end point to the uninjured ankle. In the acute stage, the ankle is often too swollen and painful to perform the tests with accuracy. Resistive muscle testing performed in midrange is usually pain free, except in the case of an associated injury to a musculotendinous unit, such as concomitant peroneal tendon strain with a lateral ankle injury.

Like any acute injury, treatment of ankle sprains initially follows the principles of POLICE: protection, optimal loading, ice, compression, and elevation of the involved extremity (Table 16.5). A few days of active rest and immobilization

TABLE 16.5.	POLICE Principles for Acute Injury Management
Principle	**Management Options**
Protection	Splinting, bracing, walking boot, taping procedures
Optimal loading	Altered weight-bearing, activity modification, cross-training, protective mobility
Ice	Localized ice bath, cold pack, ice massage
Compression	Ace wrap, open basket weave tape application, felt padding, compressive sleeve
Elevation	Elevate injured area above level of heart to promote lymph drainage

may be necessary to allow for pain and swelling to subside; however, early joint mobility and weight bearing has been shown to be more favorable for functional return in comparison with prolonged immobilization.[158]

The severity of ligament disruption will affect the treatment plan design. Grade 1 ankle sprains may respond more quickly than grade 2 or 3 sprains. Owing to the higher chances of the recurrence of ankle sprain following previous injury,[158] a rehabilitation program is recommended for all ankle sprains to assist in the restoration of mobility, proprioception, and muscle performance. ROM activities can begin in the acute phases of injury, starting with ankle dorsiflexion and plantarflexion. Progression to frontal plane inversion and eversion may be initiated in pain-free, limited ranges and monitored by pain response to facilitate tissue remodeling and ligamentous healing. Straight-plane weight-bearing activities should follow a similar progression, with eventually challenging the athlete in multiplanar and unilateral activities on various surfaces. Careful attention to muscle activation, recruitment, and timing should be paramount owing to the associated increase in muscle latency following lateral ankle sprains.[159] In the case of continued ankle instability and impaired function following a rehabilitative course, especially in grade 3 injuries where there is complete ligamentous disruption, surgical reconstruction of ankle stabilizers may be warranted and yields favorable results.

Ankle Fractures

When evaluating the pediatric ankle following acute injury, it is important to discern between ligamentous sprain and growth plate injury owing to the inherent weakness of the physis. Ankle fractures in sports occur with deceleration or rotational forces about a fixed foot. In children under 12 years with an immature skeletal system, a physeal fracture of the distal fibula is highly probable with a lateral ankle injury mechanism.[160] Nondisplaced Salter–Harris type I is the most common fracture of the distal fibular physes. Pain on palpation is over the physeal growth plate, which is located about one finger width above the distal portion of the lateral malleolus (Fig. 16.8). Management is with cast immobilization for 3 weeks followed by a rehabilitation program similar to that of a lateral ankle sprain. Plain radiographs are able to assist in the diagnosis of ankle fracture. The Ottawa ankle rules have been shown to be sensitive in detecting fractures in those over 5 years of age and should be utilized in the clinical decision process and diagnosis of traumatic ankle injuries in children[161,162] (Display 16.5).

Triplane fractures and Tillaux fractures occur as the athlete approaches skeletal maturity, usually around 15 and 17 years in girls and boys, respectively. Both fractures result from partially closed growth plates. The growth plate will first fuse centrally, followed by medial and lateral closures, leaving the lateral portion vulnerable to injury. A triplane fracture occurs in three planes: coronal, sagittal, and transverse.

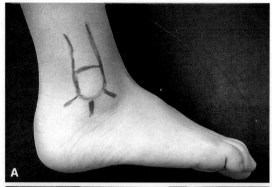

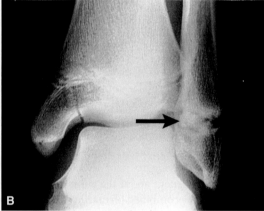

FIGURE 16.8. A: Location of distal fibular physis and lateral ankle ligaments, **B:** distal fibular physis location (arrow) with an associated Salter–Harris II fracture of distal tibia.

A Tillaux fracture is a Salter–Harris type III fracture of the unfused anterolateral segment of the distal tibial epiphysis caused by avulsion of the epiphyseal segment by the ATFL.[160] Forceful ER of the foot is the common mechanism of injury. Both fractures are managed with the athlete non–weight-bearing in a long leg cast for 3 to 4 weeks followed by a short leg walking cast for another 3 to 4 weeks. Once the cast is removed, rehabilitation can be initiated to regain normal strength and mobility to the entire lower extremity.

Osteochondral fractures of the talar dome can result from an ankle sprain if the talus abuts the medial or lateral malleolus during the injury. Injury to the bone and overlying cartilage can produce a free-floating, painful fragment in the joint

DISPLAY

16.5 Ottawa Ankle Rules

An ankle X-ray series is required only if there is any pain in malleolar zone and any of these findings:

1. Bone tenderness at posterior edge or tip of lateral malleolus
2. Bone tenderness at posterior edge or tip of medial malleolus
3. Inability to bear weight both immediately and in emergency room

space and may limit motion. Osteochondral fractures are difficult to diagnose during the acute stage of an ankle sprain, when much of the surrounding tissue is inflamed. Persistent pain after the sprain with continued edema and intermittent clicking or locking may suggest an osteochondral fracture.[160] Casting and orthotic interventions are the treatments of less severe lesions in the younger athletes, to provide a controlled environment for chondral healing. However, more severe lesions may require surgical intervention with either arthroscopic drilling, loose body removal, pinning, or cartilaginous transfer or grafting.

Ankle Impingement

Ankle impingement can be the source of anterior, anterolateral, or posterior pain. Anterior impingement is often seen in football, basketball, and dance and is often caused by the formation of an osteophyte on the distal anterior tibia owing to abnormal ankle joint mechanics. As the ankle is forced into maximal dorsiflexion, the osteophyte contacts the talus and causes pain. Anterolateral ankle impingement is often an area of chronic pain, which persists after an ankle sprain. Possible causes are impingement of the tibiofibular ligament, impingement of the synovium, or osteochondral fracture.[160] Pain is reported in the area between the fibula and the lateral talus, within the sinus tarsi, or near the ATFL. Treatment includes rest, NSAIDs, bracing, joint mobilization, and possible arthroscopic debridement.

Posterior impingement is described as pain in the posterior ankle when the foot is plantarflexed and is commonly experienced by ballet dancers or athletes who repetitively point their foot. The pain is caused by a bony protrusion such as an os trigonum, a small, round bone behind the ankle joint. An os trigonum is found in about 5% to 15% of normal, asymptomatic ankles near the posterior talus. When the os trigonum fails to fuse with the talus, it can impinge on the soft tissue during forced, end-range plantarflexion.[160] Management consists of rest, NSAIDs, and surgical excision of the bony ossicle.

≫ Foot injuries

Overuse Injuries

Sever Disease

The cause of foot and heel pain in the young athlete will vary depending on skeletal maturity. Achilles tendinopathy and plantar fasciopathy are observed more frequently in the skeletally mature athlete. In the skeletally immature athlete, atraumatic pain along the posterior calcaneus is likely caused by Sever disease. Sever disease is a traction apophysitis of the calcaneus at the site of the attachment of the Achilles tendon, plantar fascia, and intrinsic muscles of the foot. This occurs during periods of rapid skeletal growth in athletes 9 to 12 years old.[163] Pain is reported along the heel and will

increase during sports such as soccer, gymnastics, and basketball with repetitive running and jumping. Pain is usually bilateral; however, it can also occur unilaterally and can occur in conjunction with Achilles tendinopathy.

A young athlete with Sever disease will complain of sharp or dull pain along the calcaneal apophysis. A history of any rapid recent changes in activity levels, training errors, recent changes in shoe wear, and rapid skeletal growth will be consistent with Sever disease. Gently squeezing the lateral borders of the calcaneus will often replicate painful symptoms. Musculoskeletal evaluation will often find muscle length restrictions to calf muscle complex, excessive foot pronation, and possible swelling. In more severe cases, weight bearing and walking will also be asymmetric and painful.[3]

Treatment of Sever disease begins with pain control modalities, including activity modification, ice, and NSAIDs. This condition is benign and self-limiting without any long-term consequences. Therefore, continuation with normal athletic activities should be permitted if tolerated. However, the presence of gait and running asymmetries, pain at rest, and persistent debilitating pain following sport should temporarily exclude an athlete's participation in the painful activity owing to the risk of further injury. Rehabilitation interventions are aimed at the restoration of flexibility and strength to calf and foot musculature. The incorporation of a gel heel lift in the athlete's shoe may also be appropriate to unload the Achilles tendon and cushion the heel. In the presence of an excessively dropped medial longitudinal arch, temporary use of prefabricated orthotics may assist in unloading the Achilles tendon and the apophysis. The condition usually resolves within a few weeks or months with proper treatment. Although rare, persistent cases may require casting and immobilization.

Iselin Disease

Iselin disease, similarly to Sever disease, is a traction apophysitis but to the proximal fifth metatarsal. This condition is seen in children 10 to 12 years old. Traction to the insertion site of the peroneus brevis muscle to the lateral aspect of the foot on the proximal aspect of the fifth metatarsal will contribute to inflammation, irritation, and pain in adolescents who participate in sports with repetitive running and jumping.[3]

On examination, the athlete may present with localized swelling and tenderness along the proximal physis of the fifth metatarsal and increase upon weight bearing. Stressing the peroneus brevis with resistive testing into eversion will replicate symptoms, along with positions of end-range plantarflexion, dorsiflexion, and inversion.

Treatment of Iselin disease is similar to that of Sever disease. A short period of activity modification and pain control modalities are the initial treatment options of choice. Treatment should also include ankle flexibility to the evertors and plantarflexors, general ankle strengthening, and proprioceptive activities. In the milder cases, the athlete can return to unrestricted activity within 3 to 6 weeks. However, in those instances where the athlete is not responding and pain continues to limit functional activity, a short period of immobilization may be warranted, thus increasing recovery time.[3]

Tendinopathy and Plantar Fasciopathy

The diagnosis of a tendinopathy, although not as common in the young, skeletally immature athlete, can contribute to pain and disability. Achilles tendinopathy is typically reported as pain along the Achilles tendon just proximal to the superior margin of the calcaneus, often seen in ballet dancers, runners, basketball players, and other field athletes. Causative factors include rapid increases in training duration and intensity, rapid skeletal growth, and excessive foot pronation.[164] Examination should include palpation along the entire length of the tendon, starting proximally and continuing inferiorly to the heel pad, noting the area of maximal tenderness. Swelling, decreased or excessive dorsiflexion ROM, and pain with resisted plantarflexion are common findings. Single-leg heel raise and hopping reproduces pain at the Achilles tendon.

Interventions should begin with relative rest, ice, NSAIDs, gentle activation of the gastrocnemius and soleus muscles. A temporary heel lift or orthotic may aid in tendon unloading and should be discontinued gradually as pain subsides. Stretching of the Achilles tendon should be performed with caution as compressing the tendon against its bony insertion can contribute to increased stress and potential pain. The mainstay of treatment for Achilles tendinopathy is progressive tendon loading and is based on the athlete's irritability and reactivity. In more painful and reactive cases, a short period of relative rest, refraining from any aggravating activities, may be warranted. Slow and heavy loading programs that focus on time under tension have been advocated as tendons become less reactive or irritable.[142-144] Unilateral heel raises performed both with the knee extended and the knee flexed are exercises to introduce load progressively and gradually to the tendon.[165,166] Decisions regarding exercise dose and activity progression are typically guided by a pain-monitoring model. According to the pain-monitoring model, the pain during or after exercise or activity is allowed to reach level 5 on the visual analog scale (VAS) but return athletes to baseline pain level the following morning. Additionally, Achilles tendon pain and stiffness should not increase from week to week.[167] Balance exercise, proprioception, and entire lower extremity and core strengthening are also recommended to control excessive compensatory foot mechanics. Impact activities are added slowly with a graduated return to running and sport-specific training.

Other regions of the foot and ankle are susceptible to tendinopathy. Treatment of the painful tendon follows a similar course, including activity modification, pain control, normalization of mobility, and progressive tendon loading strategies. Activity can be gradually increased in a progressive manner, once symptoms have resolved, on the basis of quality of movement and soreness. Posterior tibialis tendon pain can be seen in running athletes, skaters, and gymnasts. Pain is localized to the posterior aspect of the medial malleolus. Flexor hallucis longus tendinopathy is commonly seen in athletes who repetitively point their toes, such as dancers working "on pointe," gymnasts, and runners. Pain can be reported on the plantar aspect of the foot and/or along the posterior aspect of the medial malleolus. Peroneal tendinopathy is seen in skaters, dancers, and running athletes. Pain is typically located posterior to the lateral malleolus.

Traumatic Injuries

Lisfranc (Midfoot) Injury

The tarsometatarsal joint complex is more commonly known as the Lisfranc joint. This joint aids in the intrinsic, osseus stability of the foot. The middle three metatarsal bases and the cuneiforms form the transverse arch of the foot. Injuries to this joint complex include ligamentous sprains and/or fracture dislocations, with the ligament extending from the base of the second metatarsal to the medial cuneiform being most commonly injured. Although commonly associated with high-energy motor vehicle accidents, Lisfranc injuries are also seen in sports owing to a low-energy axial load on a plantarflexed foot with the knee anchored on the ground. This is often seen in football while a player is lying prone on the ground and another player falls on the athlete's heel. Lisfranc injuries can often occur owing to excessive abduction stress to the midfoot, where the forefoot is abducted around a fixed hindfoot. This mechanism is commonly associated with sports that require the use of a foot stirrup, such as equestrian and windsurfing.[168]

A Lisfranc injury can be difficult to identify because of the often subtle instability. More severe injuries, such as a fracture dislocation, present with noticeable foot deformity. An athlete with a Lisfranc injury often complains of pain to the dorsum of the foot following a specific mechanism of injury. Forefoot edema and bruising along the plantar arch are paramount findings of a Lisfranc injury. Weight bearing is painful and increases when asked to stand on their tiptoes.[169] Physical exam reveals tenderness on palpation along the tarsometatarsal joints and gapping between the hallux and second toe when compared with the contralateral limb. Mobility testing will replicate pain on abduction and pronation of the forefoot, while maintaining a fixed hindfoot. Mobility of the first and second metatarsals in all planes, along with their association with one another, should be examined, noting any pain and/or joint subluxation. It is important to discern between a stable, ligamentous sprain and complete rupture that will contribute to a gross midfoot instability.[168] Radiographs with the athlete standing that stresses the tarsometatarsal joints are helpful in diagnosis, because non–weight-bearing films may not capture a slight instability and may appear normal.[170]

Stable Lisfranc injuries are managed conservatively. The athlete is immobilized with a walking boot for 6 to 10 weeks and allowed to weight-bear according to pain tolerance. Rehabilitation is recommended to aid in restoration of normal gait, balance, mobility, and strength. A full-length insert is often helpful during the transition from the walking boot to a supportive shoe. Complete recovery will take about 4 months, although some injuries may not permit an athlete to return to the prior level of sports participation. Unstable Lisfranc injuries, even subtle ones, are treated surgically.[168]

Bony Abnormalities

Tarsal Coalition

Tarsal coalition is a congenital malformation where two or more of the tarsal bones fail to differentiate, resulting in a cartilaginous, fibrous, or bony union. This often occurs bilaterally, involving the calcaneonavicular and talocalcaneal articulations. Symptoms restricting mid- and hindfoot mobility begin to appear during the second or third decade of life, as the coalition attempts to ossify. Fractures within the coalition will result in pain following fusion of the associated joints.

An athlete presenting with tarsal coalition typically complains of an insidious onset of foot or ankle pain. Pain is often exacerbated with sports requiring cutting, pivoting, changing direction, and running on uneven surfaces. Recurrent and chronic ankle sprains are also reported owing to the lack of available foot mobility, thus stressing the surrounding tissues. Physical exam often reveals a fixed, hyperpronated foot type. Limited accessory joint mobility to the midfoot and/or hindfoot is a paramount finding with tarsal coalition that coincides with the inability to reconstitute the medial longitudinal arch upon heel rise. A suspicion of tarsal coalition can be most accurately confirmed with CT imaging.

Treatment for tarsal coalition is directed at controlling foot motion to decrease stresses about the fusing joints. Orthotics is recommended to help support the foot and unload painful structures. Strengthening for the intrinsic and extrinsic foot musculature is helpful for dynamic support of the foot and ankle complex, as are ankle joint flexibility activities, to decrease compensatory subtalar joint mobility. Advanced pain may respond more favorably to aggressive immobilization in a cast. If conservative treatment fails, referral for surgery prior to joint ossification is recommended and is successful in resolving pain and restoring mobility.

Accessory Navicular

Accessory navicular is the congenital formation of a small ossicle adjacent to the navicular bone or within the tibialis posterior tendon. Also known as an os navicular secundum, this condition is not always asymptomatic on diagnosis. However, when problematic, an athlete will present with localized pain and inflammation along the navicular tuberosity and medial arch. High-impact sports and activities are often painful, especially when wearing tight-fitting shoes or cleats. Pain is often replicated with resistive foot inversion owing to one of the attachment sites of the tibialis posterior muscle. Both plain radiographs and CT scans will help confirm the diagnosis.

Conservative and surgical treatment options are available for an accessory navicular. Activity modification, NSAIDs, and orthotic interventions that support the midfoot are the primary nonsurgical options. However, a period of more aggressive immobilization within a walking boot or cast may be necessary in more painful cases. Padding along the navicular tuberosity within the shoe will also assist in pain control by alleviating direct pressure along the bony prominence. Surgical excision of the ossicle is recommended when pain continues to limit activity following attempts at conservative management.

Forefoot Injuries

Forefoot Fractures

Metatarsal fractures in children are usually a result of direct trauma, with the fifth metatarsal being most frequently injured.[171] Metatarsal stress fractures are rare in children but may be seen in dancers and runners owing to repetitive loading.[172] Sites of fracture include the physes, located distally in metatarsals 2 to 5, metatarsal shafts, and fifth metatarsal styloid. Localized pain, tenderness, and swelling over the fracture site are reported and can include deformity when the fracture is displaced. Plain radiographs of the foot will assist in the diagnosis of acute fractures. The Ottawa foot rules are sensitive in ruling out fractures to the foot in children over 5 years of age and should be utilized in the clinical decision process and diagnosis of traumatic foot injuries in children[161,162] (Display 16.6).

Nondisplaced fractures are treated conservatively with immobilization and closed reduction in a short leg walking cast, boot, or postoperative walking shoe for 4 to 6 weeks. Management of displaced fractures may require surgery. Once there is evidence of bony healing, rehabilitation assists in normalizing gait, improving balance, and managing the adverse effects of prolonged immobilization.

In addition to shaft and physeal fractures, a fracture of the proximal diaphysis of the fifth metatarsal is called a Jones fracture. Owing to a decreased blood supply to this area, there is a greater risk of nonunion and refracture.[173] Athletes

DISPLAY 16.6	Ottawa Foot Rules

A foot X-ray series is required only if there is any pain in midfoot zone and any of these findings:

1. Bone tenderness at the base of the fifth metatarsal
2. Bone tenderness at the navicular
3. Inability to bear weight both immediately and in emergency room

closer to skeletal maturity, ranging from 15 to 21 years of age, are most affected. This injury, often seen in basketball players and track athletes, is caused by hyperinversion of the foot or by high-impact loading along the fifth metatarsal. Symptoms are tenderness to palpation over the proximal shaft of the fifth metatarsal, localized swelling, and decreased ability to bear weight. Management of Jones fractures in athletes has been much debated and will vary depending on the stability of the fracture, the healing process, and the athlete's functional goals. Conservative management is typically longer than management for basic fractures. The athlete is placed in a non–weight-bearing cast for 6 weeks, followed by another 6 weeks in a weight-bearing cast, brace, or orthotic. With nonunion or in high-level athletes, surgical ORIF with various techniques may be indicated.[173,174] Return to sport should be permitted once the athlete demonstrates radiographic healing of the fracture site and has progressed through a comprehensive rehabilitation program.

Turf Toe

Turf toe is a hyperextension injury to the first metatarsophalangeal (MTP) joint, resulting in damage to the plantar capsuloligamentous structures. Mechanism of injury is a forceful hyperextension of the great toe, especially while playing on hard, artificial surfaces as in soccer, basketball, and football. This is a ligamentous sprain, and severity is classified with grades 1 through 3, as previously described. An athlete will present with pain along the plantar surface of the toe along with possible bruising and swelling. Pain is replicated with active or passive great toe extension.

Treatment is initiated with POLICE modalities and will progress on the basis of severity of the injury. Minor sprains can often be taped, allowing the athlete to continue with sports participation with or without a period of rest. More severe grade 3 injuries will often be treated with a few days of crutches and a steel spring plate shoe insert to limit and protect great toe hyperextension. Early mobility of the first MTP joint is recommended owing to the high incidence of long-term mobility loss (hallux rigidus). An athlete may return to play within 6 weeks once there is full, pain-free extension to the great toe and after he or she has been tolerating a functional progression back to activities that load the great toe.

» Spine injuries

Low back pain is a frequent complaint in young athletes. Characteristics of the developing spine predispose these athletes to patterns of injuries that are different than those in adults. While disc-related pathology is commonly seen in adults, it is relatively rare in the youth athlete. Similarly, children are more likely to present with pathology-related repetitive stress injury to the pars interarticularis (spondylolysis), and the presence of growth centers makes them vulnerable to developing apophyseal injuries.[175] Young athletes who present with low back pain are more likely to have structural injuries, and, therefore, full investigation, including imaging studies, will likely be necessary.[175,176]

General Examination

Examination begins with a thorough history via open-ended questions to ascertain whether there was a traumatic onset, specific mechanism of injury, previous injuries, and symptom behavior. The clinician should also question athletes about the sports-specific history including sports in which they participate, level of participation, volume of practice, how long they have participated in a certain sport, whether they play year-round, and outside training regimens. Symptomatic onset, duration, response to certain activities, and training/sports participation history will help the clinician differentiate between possible diagnoses and improve clinical decision making for treatment. A thorough screening is necessary to help discriminate musculoskeletal origin of pain from more sinister pathology. Prompt referral to appropriate medical professionals should be considered when red flags are present.

Posture should be examined from the front, behind, and to the side. The clinician should note postural abnormalities that may contribute to altered biomechanical forces during function. These may include scoliosis, rounded shoulders, excessive thoracic kyphosis, hyperlordotic lumbar spine, or anterior pelvic tilt. ROM should also be measured in all planes of movement (flexion, extension, lateral flexion, and rotation), and the clinician should note not only the range of available motion, but also the quality of the movement and symptomatic response during or after each movement. It is important to measure lower extremity and upper extremity flexibility, because decreased mobility in these structures may predispose the athlete to increased stress across the spine during activity. The clinician should be sure to measure hip and shoulder ROM, flexibility of the hip flexors, quadriceps, hamstrings, and adductors.

Palpation should identify areas of localized tenderness in the spine or SI joints, as well as areas of tenderness or muscle spasm in adjacent soft tissue. Segmental mobility of thoracic and lumbar vertebrae should be examined, looking for areas of hyper- or hypomobility and associated reactivity. Special tests should be utilized to help rule in or exclude certain pathologies that may exist in lumbar spine, SI joints, or hips.

Spondylolysis and Spondylolisthesis

Spondylolysis

Spondylolysis is a fracture in the pars interarticularis of the lumbar spine, with the L5 segment most commonly involved.[177] Spondylolysis is a common injury for young athletes, with one study indicating that 47% of young athletes with complaints of back pain had spondylolysis.[175] Spondylolysis is often referred to as a stress fracture and is typically caused by repetitive stress within an area of spine during hyperextension and rotation. Certain athletes, such as gymnasts, figure skaters, and dancers, are more prone to developing spondylolysis, because the demands of their sport predispose them to these typical injury patterns. The mean age for spondylolysis is 15 to 16 years old. Diagnostic imaging is typically used to determine accurate diagnosis. Radiographs are performed first and may visualize the fracture through the pars interarticularis, which is referred to as a "scotty dog fracture" on the oblique view.[178] However, radiography has shown poor sensitivity in detecting spondylotic injuries, and further diagnostic imaging is usually recommended.[179] Single photon emission computed tomography (SPECT) is a very sensitive but nonspecific imaging procedure that will show increased uptake in areas where there is increased bone metabolism, such as a stress reaction or fracture.[179] CT scan provides good visualization of osseous anatomy and can be used in cases where SPECT is positive in order to provide an accurate diagnosis. CT scan is the most accurate imaging modality for detecting spondylolysis; however, its drawbacks include high exposure to radiation and decreased ability to detect early stress reactions when no fracture line is present. Recent studies have shown improved diagnostic accuracy in the use of MRI for spondylolysis, and many practitioners are favoring the use of MRI as the primary advanced imaging modality for this condition. MRI offers many advantages over CT, including no radiation exposure and earlier identification of prelytic pathology through the ability to visualize bone stress reactions, when an outright fracture line is not visible on CT scan.[180,181]

Spondylolisthesis

Spondylolisthesis describes an anterior slippage of one vertebral body on another. This commonly occurs at the L5–S1 level and is often graded on a I to IV scale representing the amount of anterior displacement relative to vertebral body width (see Display 16.7). Grades I and II spondylolisthesis respond well to conservative management, and sports participation has not been shown to increase the degree of slippage.[182] Sports participation is more controversial in grade III or IV spondylolisthesis.

Clinical examination findings guide treatment of the athlete, and the general examination principles discussed earlier will apply. Additionally, it should be noted that most athletes with spondylolysis or spondylolisthesis will typically demonstrate pain with spinal extension and combined extension–rotation movements. Their pain is often aggravated by activity, especially those that place the spine in an extended position. A "step-off" sign of adjacent spinous processes may be palpated if spondylolisthesis is present. Pain is often replicated ipsilaterally by having the athlete stand on one leg and extend backward.

The mainstay of treatment of spondylolysis and spondylolisthesis revolves around reducing the offending forces so the athlete can become pain free. He or she may utilize a custom-molded TLSO (Thoracolumbar sacral orthosis) or soft corset-type brace to aid pain relief via partial immobilization, protection from spinal extension, or hyperlordotic posturing. Bracing is controversial, but some studies have demonstrated improved rates of bone healing with bracing in early treatment.[183,184] As discussed earlier, the therapist should examine the spine to identify areas of hyper- or hypomobility that may focus the stress of movement to an isolated area. Owing to the effect of restricted lower extremity muscle length on lumbopelvic motion, close examination of flexibility is also required. In addition, the clinician should examine functional movements required by the athletes sport activity and determine whether any dysfunctional movement would correlate with pathologic stress in the spine. Trunk muscle strengthening and endurance training are necessary during rehabilitation, and these principles will be discussed later in this chapter.

Other Spine Pathologies

Posterior Element Overuse Syndrome

Posterior element overuse syndrome refers to a constellation of conditions involving muscle tendons, ligaments, facet joints, and joint capsules that create pain in the lower back.[177] Symptoms may be similar to spondylolysis, and imaging is important in differential diagnosis. Treatment will usually consist of rest, activity modification, and rehabilitation to address flexibility, strength, and motor control deficits. A short trial of bracing may be helpful for pain relief.

Apophysitis

Apophysitis is another common cause of pain in the spine of the young athlete. Clinically, it is marked by mechanical pain that is irritated with repeated motions of the spine and improves with rest. In the spine, the apophysis is a ring at the vertebral end plates and is not palpable. Apophysitis can also occur at the iliac crest. If this occurs, athletes will typically be tender to palpation along this region and may have pain with resisted contraction of the oblique muscles.

Stingers

Injuries to the cervical spine can occur from sports participation. A "stinger" or "burner" is a traction injury of the brachial plexus that usually involves the C-5 and C-6 nerve roots and occurs most commonly in collision athletes.[185]

DISPLAY 16.7	Spondylolisthesis Grading System	
Grade I	0%–25% vertebral body width	
Grade II	25%–50% vertebral body width	
Grade III	50%–75% vertebral body width	
Grade IV	75%–100% vertebral body width	

The athlete will often complain of stinging or burning pain with paresthesias in the affected upper extremity. Muscular weakness in shoulder abduction, ER, and flexion may be present. The symptoms usually resolve quickly and allow the athlete to return to play without significant loss of playing time. If symptoms persist for more than 24 hours, further diagnostic workup, including imaging studies, is recommended. In more severe injuries, treatment consists of supportive rest in a sling and pain relief modalities until the symptoms resolve. After resolution of symptoms, rehabilitation for lost strength is required. The decision to return to sports is based on normal imaging studies and satisfactory clinical strength examination. The role of electromyographic testing is usually minimal because it is not a valid tool for stinger diagnosis or an indicator of recovery for return-to-play decision making.[185]

General Treatment Principles

Many injuries to the spine share common rehabilitation principles. The functional requirements of the spine are somewhat paradoxical. The spine requires a high degree of mobility for the performance of functional tasks but also a concurrent need for dynamic stability. When treating the spine, the therapist must remember these requirements while addressing deficits that may inhibit function in either realm.

Regional interdependence is evident in spine rehabilitation, and deficits in upper extremity or lower extremity flexibility, strength, or neuromuscular control may contribute to an athlete's back pain. Similarly, any areas of hypomobility in the vertebral segments above or below the injury should be examined to ensure adequate contribution of movement throughout the spine as a unit.

Trunk stabilization is an essential component of spine rehabilitation in the young athlete. An inclusive exercise program should be developed to target important stabilizing muscles, such as the multifidus, transversus abdominis, erector spinae, internal/external obliques, and gluteus muscles. The therapist and athlete must incorporate the concepts of trunk stabilization training into functional activities that replicate the sport demands on the athlete. Willardson has advocated that development of trunk muscle endurance, not necessarily strength, be the primary goal of rehabilitation.[186] Lumbar stabilizing muscles are composed mainly of type 1 muscle fibers, and only relatively low loads are needed to improve their performance.[187] Thus, the clinician should incorporate exercises with longer periods of "hold" or higher repetition of movement, as opposed to heavy-weight, low-repetition training. Advancement to higher load activities is warranted to mimic the forces with athletic activities to prepare the athlete for sports participation. Finally, as many sports activities occur in standing or involve single-limb support, balance training should be incorporated as part of an inclusive rehabilitation program.

Guidelines for resuming activity after spinal injury are not easy to generalize owing to the highly variable nature of athletic activities. Generally, resumption of activity should occur in a graded fashion, beginning with less stressful and pain-free activities. Activities can be gradually progressed, monitoring for response to increasing sport demands. Owing to the prolonged nature of many spinal injuries, the athlete may require increased time to return to baseline level of fitness prior to being ready to resume full sports participation.

» Sports-related concussion

Between 1.7 and 3.8 million sports-related concussion injuries occur in the United States each year, accounting for 5% to 9% of all sports injuries.[188,189] Approximately 50% of all concussions go unreported and undiagnosed.[189] Concussion in sports is a growing problem that affects athletes at all ages, and numbers are likely to increase with heightened awareness. Concussion injuries in youth athletes between the ages of 5 and 19 are rising and comprise 30% of all sports-related concussions. Although more common in contact sports, such as football, rugby, soccer, and hockey, all athletes are potentially at risk of a concussive event.

Pathophysiology

The American Medical Society for Sports Medicine (AMSSM) defines concussion, also termed mild traumatic brain injury (mTBI), as a "traumatically induced transient disturbance of brain function, caused by a complex pathophysiological process."[189] It is a less severe form of brain injury and is generally self-limited in duration and symptom resolution. Concussions are caused by a direct blow either to the head, face, neck, or elsewhere on the body, resulting in excessive linear and rotational forces transmitted to the brain. "Coup" injuries define the injuries when a stationary skull is hit by a moving object at high velocity (head being struck by a baseball). Conversely, "countercoup" injuries result from the sudden deceleration of the skull moving at a high velocity (head contacting the ground/floor or goalpost).

When the brain sustains a concussion, microscopic axonal injury occurs in conjunction with a complex cascade of ionic, metabolic, and pathophysiologic events.[189] In order to regain ionic balance and normal brain metabolism, the brain requires increased energy. However, damage to mitochondria and a decrease in cerebral brain flow contribute to a shortage of energy, resulting in decreased overall brain function.[189] If, during this time of decreased function prior to full recovery, there is a second injury, the brain is at even greater risk for cellular metabolic changes and significant cognitive defects. This finding is more pronounced in youth where the immature brain is still developing, thereby placing this population at a greater risk of repeat concussion prior to complete symptom recovery.[189]

Signs and Symptoms

Signs and symptoms of concussion often vary with the individual (Table 16.6). Headache is the most common sign of concussion, followed by dizziness.[189] Loss of consciousness occurs in 10% of concussions but is not a reliable predictor of severity. Most symptoms are not specific to concussion and may mimic other conditions, including but not limited to, cardiac compromise, acute gastroenteritis, attention deficit disorder, and depression. Therefore, it is helpful to determine whether the symptoms were present prior to the concussion injury to allow for more accurate determination of symptom resolution. In 80% to 90% of concussions, symptoms resolve within 10 to 14 days for adults and up to 1 month for children following injury.[189,190] Despite the resolution of subjective concussive symptoms, complete cognitive impairment may still exist with further neuropsychological (NP) testing.

Risk Factors

History of previous concussion puts an athlete at a two to five times greater risk of sustaining another concussion.[189] The more concussions sustained, the greater the severity of the concussion. Duration of symptoms is also a predictor of prolonged recovery. In sports with similar rules, females are at greater risk for concussion than their male counterparts. The type of sport and position is also correlated with an increased risk. For example, athletes who are in frequent high-velocity–contact situations, such as football quarterbacks, running backs, wide receivers, and defensive backs, are at greater risk for injury than other position players such as linemen. History of migraine headaches, learning disabilities, attention deficit disorders, and mood disorders may be associated with increased cognitive dysfunction and a prolonged recovery following a concussion, and could potentially complicate diagnosis and management.[189]

Physiologic differences exist between the adult and the youth brain. When dealing with the immature brain, it is important to understand their inherent increased risk of sustaining a concussion in combination with a catastrophic injury and associated prolonged recovery times. For instance, one study reported that athletes 13 to 16 years of age take longer to return to their baseline levels of symptoms and normal neurocognitive function compared with athletes 18 to 22 years old.[188]

Diagnosis and Assessment Tools

A health care provider specially trained and knowledgeable in recognition and evaluation of concussions is best qualified to make the clinical diagnosis. Concussions are graded retrospectively following symptoms resolution. Therefore, grading a concussion at the time of injury is considered unreliable and is no longer performed. Diagnosis should include thorough physiologic, neurologic, vestibular/balance, oculomotor, and cognitive assessments. A graded symptoms checklist should serve as an objective assessment tool for assessing the symptoms associated with a concussion, while also tracking the severity, longevity, and changes over serial reevaluations. Other assessment tools include baseline symptom scoring, balance testing, sideline evaluation tools, and computerized NP testing. Some commonly used sideline measures include symptom scores, Sports Concussion Assessment Tool (Child SCAT5 and SCAT 5), Maddocks Questions, Standardized Assessment of Concussion (SAC), and the Balance Error Scoring System (BESS).[189] It is important to understand that certain tests are more appropriate at different times during the recovery time period. Balance testing is typically normal after 3 days, making it a useful test for sideline management of an athlete and less useful for later follow-up. Baseline testing prior to sports participation may aid in the identification of high-risk individuals and allow for comparison purposes following injury. This approach is somewhat controversial as the role of preinjury baseline testing remains unclear and has yet to be validated.[189] However, baseline testing may be most beneficial in those with a prior history of concussion, confounding medical conditions, and high-risk sports. Testing should be performed routinely with attempts to control certain variables, including the athlete's age, fatigue level, mood, and testing environment.

Neuropsychologic Testing

NP testing in athletes began in the 1980s, and its role has increased in recent years with the availability of computers. NP tests are objective measures of brain behavior and are more sensitive than clinical exam for subtle cognitive impairment. However, NP testing should be an adjunct to clinical evaluation and one component of a comprehensive concussion management plan and should not be used in isolation. NP testing will evaluate several domains of cognitive function such as memory, cognitive processing speed, and reaction time.[189,191] There are two commonly utilized testing

TABLE 16.6. Concussion Signs and Symptoms		
Physical	**Cognitive**	**Emotional**
Headache	Mentally "foggy"	Irritable
Fatigue, nausea, vomiting	Got "bell rung"	Sadness
Dizziness, balance disturbance	Feeling run down	More emotional
Visual problems	Difficulty concentrating	Nervousness
Sensitivity to light, noise	Impaired memory	
Numbness, tingling	Confusion	
Drowsiness	Slowed responses	
Sleep disturbances	Loss of consciousness	

formats: paper and pencil and computerized. Owing to the ease of administration and cost-effectiveness, there has been a shift toward the use of computerized testing.

NP testing has been shown to have moderate sensitivity in the detection of postconcussive cognitive deficits[192] and is still recommended and used in high-risk athletes with and without prior concussion. NP tests aid in the return-to-sport decision-making process, especially for athletes who deny symptoms with the desire to return to activity sooner than otherwise likely. However, the validity of the tool has yet to be determined because it shows cognitive deficits longer than athletes are symptomatic and should be a monitoring tool in the event of a concussion.[189]

Management and Return to Play

The first step in the management of concussion will usually occur at the time of injury. The level of consciousness should be assessed. In an unresponsive athlete, assessment of airway, breathing, and heart function is of primary concern. Once established, physical evaluation of the cervical spine and other more serious injuries should be performed. On the slightest suspicion of cervical spine injury, the athlete should be immobilized and transferred to the emergency department for advanced imaging and care. Other reasons for immediate emergency transport include deteriorating mental status, focal neurologic findings, and worsening of symptoms. Only when serious cognitive and emergent medical situations are excluded can secondary concussion examination including symptoms, neurologic function, cognition, and balance be initiated.

If sideline testing appears normal and concussion is not suspected, the athlete is permitted to resume playing. Serial evaluations should be performed during and following the event to ensure the decision was correct. When concussion is suspected, the athlete should not return to play on that day. The athlete should be monitored incrementally over a period of time, recognizing deterioration of mental status, cognition, and/or consciousness. It was previously recommended to frequently wake up the concussed athlete throughout the night to ensure consciousness. However, this is no longer recommended because sleep is important in allowing the brain to rest and recover.[189] Because of the theoretical risk of bleeding, aspirin and NSAIDs are generally avoided. Other medications that mask symptoms should also be avoided.

Athletes with concussion should have a medical follow-up by a physician. The primary treatment includes a brief period of physical and cognitive rest. Activities and environments that exacerbate symptoms should be avoided and moderated. Dim, quiet environments assist in moderating headache and symptoms of phonophobia and photophobia. Youth athletes may require accommodations in school, including a reduced workload and extended time to take tests. In most cases, the athlete should be permitted to miss school or only attend part of the day in the initial acute stage.

DISPLAY 16.8 | **Activity Progression Following Concussion**

Stepwise Return-to-Play Protocol

Activity Level	Examples
No activity/rest	Dim environments, school accommodations, no television or radio
Light aerobic activity	Stationary bike, elliptical trainer, brisk walking
Sport-specific exercise	Shoot baskets, swinging a bat, running, submaximal resistance training
Noncontact training drills	Practice drills, complex sports movements
Full contact drills/practice	Incorporate live play and/or contact drills in practice
Return to play	Scrimmages followed by games

Treatment of concussion is multidisciplinary and can include interventions aimed at restoring cognitive ability, balance, oculomotor function, cervical spine movement dysfunctions, and tolerance to aerobic conditioning.

Return-to-play progression should be individualized, gradual, and progressive. The process should begin once the athlete is free of symptoms at rest and demonstrates a normal neurologic exam when compared with baseline measures, including balance and cognitive function. Only then should the athlete begin a medically supervised stepwise return (Display 16.8). The progression may take a few days to a few weeks to complete, depending on the severity of concussion and individualized response to physical demands. If the athlete develops symptoms at any point during the progression, the aggravating activity should be stopped, symptoms allowed to subside, and the previous phase of the progression eventually resumed. A licensed health care provider specifically trained in the management of concussions should be consulted for medical clearance prior to unrestricted activity.

Special Considerations

Second Impact Syndrome

A young athlete who returns to play while experiencing symptoms is at risk for persistent symptoms, more severe concussion, cerebral swelling, and second impact syndrome (SIS). SIS is the loss of autoregulation of the brain's blood supply, leading to vascular enlargement, increase in intracranial pressure, brain herniation, and subsequent coma and/or death.[189] SIS is not fully understood; however, it is seen typically in those under the age of 18. Therefore, concussion in the youth athlete should be managed carefully with the assurance that symptoms have resolved and all brain function has returned to baseline prior to permitting the athlete to return to play.

Persistent Postconcussive Symptoms

Persistent postconcussive symptoms are signs and symptoms of a concussion that persist for longer than the expected time frame, such as weeks or months. Symptoms are similar to those initially following concussion but are often more vague and nonspecific, making the diagnosis complicated. Factors associated with persistent postconcussive symptoms are not fully clear but may include prolonged loss of consciousness, prolonged posttraumatic amnesia, and a history of psychiatric condition; however, compared with other forms of concussion, sports-related concussions are less likely to result in the condition.

Graded return to activity is the paramount treatment for persistent postconcussive symptoms. The use of supervised aerobic exercise programs, such as the Buffalo Concussion Treadmill Test, administered at subsymptom thresholds have been recently advocated to establish a safe aerobic exercise treatment program and desensitize chronically symptomatic athletes to help speed recovery and return to activity.[193] Retesting of the threshold should be performed on a regular basis, with progression being a slow and steady process, symptom permitting. As time progresses and symptoms continue, other multifactorial treatment options may be explored. These include cognitive therapy, integrated neurorehabilitation programs, supervised progressive exercise programs, and sleep disturbance programs.

Prevention

Education and awareness are the hallmarks of concussion prevention. Enforcement of rule modifications, such as number of weekly headers permitted in soccer, to reduce the risk of concussion should be strictly followed. Fair play and respect for opposing players and coaches have been shown to decrease the likelihood of concussion in sports such as hockey.[189] Coaches, parents, educators, and referees should be educated on the signs and symptoms of a concussion to allow for better detection and injury identification. They can also assist in the safety of the youth athlete by teaching correct sport-specific techniques, emphasizing body control and proper movements, education on appropriate athletic behaviors, and limiting the number of contact exposures in practice.

Proper protective equipment should be worn at all times during competition, and athletes should be monitored for correct size and fit. This includes helmets, shoulder pads, and mouthpieces. Despite the lack of data to suggest that the use of these pieces of equipment can minimize the risk of concussion and mTBI, they have been found to be an effective means of limiting scalp lacerations, skull fractures, intracranial bleeds, and dental injuries.[189]

Strengthening of neck musculature has been studied to determine its effectiveness on concussion prevalence. Some believed that increased strength of neck musculature could enable an athlete to better attenuate the acceleration forces associated with a forceful blow to the head. However, because of the unpredictable nature of a sports concussion, no association between neck muscle strength and concussion has been identified.[189]

» The female athlete

Special Considerations

As a female athlete progresses through sexual maturity, physiologic and anatomic changes occur, which leave her vulnerable to injury. Earlier in this chapter, we noted that female adolescent athletes are two to nine times more likely to suffer a noncontact ACL tear than their male counterparts.[109] In addition, female athletes are more likely to suffer other knee pathologies such as patellofemoral syndrome or patella dislocations. A wider pelvis, increased femoral anteversion, increased ligamentous laxity, increased knee valgus positioning, and altered neuromuscular firing patterns have all been suggested as factors related to the increased incidence of knee injuries in females. Measurements of dynamic knee valgus during a jumping task have been shown to be predictive of knee injuries.[12] Neuromuscular retraining programs that focus on reducing dynamic knee valgus, improving knee and hip flexion during landing, and lessening ground impact forces have been effective in reducing this injury risk.[115] The clinician should focus on identifying any female athletes exhibiting the noted biomechanically risky movement patterns and provide instruction and training to help lessen the possibility of injury.

Female Athlete Triad

The *female athlete triad* refers to a constellation of three clinical entities: menstrual dysfunction, low energy availability from diminished caloric intake (with or without an eating disorder), and decreased bone mineral density.[194] Prevalence rates for individual factors involved in the triad vary widely in the athletic population, but studies have shown that 23% to 70% of female athletes can be affected.[194] There is generally a higher rate of presence in sports that require weight classes and those that emphasize aesthetics such as ballet and gymnastics. The term Relative Energy Deficiency in Sport (RED-S) has also been utilized to describe this, because a female athlete need not demonstrate all three factors of the triad in order to suffer negative health sequelae. Additionally, a relative energy deficiency contributing to pathologic bone health and other negative consequences may also be present in male athletes.[195]

Menstrual dysfunction in the athlete includes a wide spectrum of disorders, but amenorrhea is the most commonly discussed. Amenorrhea, defined as the absence of menses for 3 months or more, can be subcategorized into primary or secondary types. Primary refers to a delay in the age of onset of menarche, whereas secondary refers to a loss of menses after menarche inception. Delayed or altered menarche can lead to decreased bone density associated with the

TABLE 16.7.	Signs and Symptoms of Relative Energy Deficiency in Sport (RED-S), Female Athlete Triad, and Disordered Eating	
RED-S	**Female Athlete Triad**	**Disordered Eating**
Decreased muscle strength	Weight loss	Continued dieting in spite of weight loss
Decreased endurance	Absent or irregular periods	Preoccupation with food, weight, and/or exercise
Increased injury risk	Fatigue and decreased ability to concentrate	Frequent trips to the bathroom during and after meals
Decreased training response	Stress fractures with or without significant injury	Use of laxatives
Impaired judgment	Longer healing times	Always wearing baggy clothing
Decreased coordination	Muscle injuries	Brittle hair or nails
Decreased concentration		Cold hands and feet
Irritability		Dental cavities and eroding tooth enamel due to frequent vomiting
Depression		Heart irregularities and chest pain
Decreased Glycogen stores		Low heart rate and blood pressure

female athlete triad. Normally, the greatest accumulation of bone mass occurs during the adolescent years, but compromised bone development during this period can have severe life-long consequences. In the short term, low bone density places the athlete at an increased risk for stress fractures, whereas long-term consequences can include suboptimal peak bone mass acquisition and higher risk of premature osteoporosis.[194]

Energy availability refers to the amount of dietary intake required in order to support the needs of an athlete's caloric expenditure. Low energy availability may result from a diagnosed eating disorder such as anorexia nervosa, bulimia nervosa, or eating disorder not otherwise specified (EDNOS).[194] However, low energy availability can also occur without a diagnosed disorder in cases where the caloric deficit is a result of poor dietary choices or lack of nutritional knowledge. The adverse effects of disordered eating can include cardiac dysfunction, gastrointestinal problems, hair loss, decreased sports performance, and decreased concentration.

Treatment of the female athlete triad involves a multidisciplinary team approach, involving a physician, nutritionist, psychiatrist, team coach, and the athlete's family. A physical therapist or athletic trainer may form part of the treatment team for resolving impairments to help the athlete make a safe return to sports. The primary goals of treatment are to restore normal menstrual cycle, enhance bone mineral density, and improve psychological health related to body image and sports performance.

Prevention of the female athlete triad should be of paramount importance. Early recognition of the female athlete triad allows for timely intervention and limits the resulting damage. Screening for symptoms during regular sports pre-participation physicals is an excellent opportunity for early recognition and should be encouraged. Specific assessment tools have been developed to help identify athletes at risk for the female athlete triad and RED-S.[196] Furthermore, the education of coaches, players, and families in recognizing the signs and risk factors may lead to increased reporting of issues and early treatment (Table 16.7).

Summary

Developing good exercise habits earlier in life establishes healthier lifestyles throughout adulthood. There has been a dramatic increase in youth recreational and competitive sports participation in recent years. The choices are endless for most children, with gymnastics, dancing, swimming, field sports, running, skateboarding, rock climbing, riding a bike, and jumping rope all acting as modes of physical activity. Sports can provide children with psychological, social, and physical benefits; however, it can also heighten the inherent risk of sustaining an injury. Increased exposures, improper training methods, and early sports specialization have all been attributed to athletic injuries in the youth. Proper prevention strategies and education of parents, coaches, and health care providers will allow children and adolescents to participate in sports and recreational activities in a safer and more enjoyable fashion.

Youth athletes will participate in sports similarly to their adult counterparts, but anatomic, physiologic, and psychological differences exist between adults and children. Despite the similar nature of the sporting events, it is important to understand that skeletally immature athletes are vulnerable to sustaining different types of musculoskeletal injuries. The physical therapist working with these children must take these differences into account during rehabilitation of the youth athlete. Awareness of the special needs of the youth athlete will allow a health care provider to diagnose and administer appropriate medical care, increasing the likelihood of a safe return to full and unrestricted sports participation following injury.

REFERENCES

1. Mickalide A, Hansen L. *Coaching Our Kids to Fewer Injuries: A Report on Youth Sports Safety*. Safe Kids World Wide; 2012.

2. Musgrave DS, Mendelson SA. Pediatric orthopedic trauma: principles in management. *Crit Care Med*. 2002;30(11)(suppl):S431-S443.

3. Hoang QB, Mortazavi M. Pediatric overuse injuries in sports. *Adv Pediatr*. 2012;59(1):359-383.

4. Caine D, Maffulli N, Caine C. Epidemiology of injury in child and adolescent sports: injury rates, risk factors, and prevention. *Clin Sports Med*. 2008;27(1):19-50, vii.

5. Wall E, Von Stein D. Juvenile osteochondritis dissecans. *Orthop Clin North Am*. 2003;34(3):341-353.

6. Baker CL 3rd, Romeo AA, Baker CL Jr. Osteochondritis dissecans of the capitellum. *Am J Sports Med*. 2010;38(9):1917-1928.

7. Ray TR. Youth baseball injuries: recognition, treatment, and prevention. *Curr Sports Med Rep*. 2010;9(5):294-298.

8. Kocher MS, Tucker R, Ganley TJ, et al. Management of osteochondritis dissecans of the knee: current concepts review. *Am J Sports Med*. 2006;34(7):1181-1191.

9. Ozmun JC, Mikesky AE, Surburg PR. Neuromuscular adaptations following prepubescent strength training. *Med Sci Sports Exerc*. 1994;26(4):510-514.

10. Carter CW, Micheli LJ. Training the child athlete for prevention, health promotion, and performance: how much is enough, how much is too much? *Clin Sports Med*. 2011;30(4):679-690.

11. Boyle KL, Witt P, Riegger-Krugh C. Intrarater and interrater reliability of the Beighton and Horan joint mobility index. *J Athl Train*. 2003;38(4):281-285.

12. Hewett TE, Myer GD, Ford KR, et al. Biomechanical measures of neuromuscular control and valgus loading of the knee predict anterior cruciate ligament injury risk in female athletes: a prospective study. *Am J Sports Med*. 2005;33(4):492-501.

13. Powers CM. The influence of altered lower-extremity kinematics on patellofemoral joint dysfunction: a theoretical perspective. *J Orthop Sports Phys Ther*. 2003;33(11):639-646.

14. Chmielewski TL, Hodges MJ, Horodyski M, et al. Investigation of clinician agreement in evaluating movement quality during unilateral lower extremity functional tasks: a comparison of 2 rating methods. *J Orthop Sports Phys Ther*. 2007;37(3):122-129.

15. Myer GD, Ford KR, Khoury J, et al. Development and validation of a clinic-based prediction tool to identify female athletes at high risk for anterior cruciate ligament injury. *Am J Sports Med*. 2010;38(10):2025-2033.

16. Padua DA, Marshall SW, Boling MC, et al. The Landing Error Scoring System (LESS) is a valid and reliable clinical assessment tool of jump-landing biomechanics: the JUMP-ACL study. *Am J of Sports Med*. 2009;37(10):1996-2002.

17. Roush JR, Kitamura J, Waits MC. Reference values for the Closed Kinetic Chain Upper Extremity Stability Test (CKCUEST) for collegiate baseball players. *N Am J Sports Phys Ther*. 2007;2(3):159-163.

18. McClure P, Greenberg E, Kareha S. Evaluation and management of scapular dysfunction. *Sports Med Arthrosc*. 2012;20(1):39-48.

19. Ludewig PM, Reynolds JF. The association of scapular kinematics and glenohumeral joint pathologies. *J Orthop Sports Phys Ther*. 2009;39(2):90-104.

20. Kibler WB, Uhl TL, Maddux JW, et al. Qualitative clinical evaluation of scapular dysfunction: a reliability study. *J Shoulder Elbow Surg*. 2002;11(6):550-556.

21. McClure P, Tate AR, Kareha S, et al. A clinical method for identifying scapular dyskinesis. Part 1: reliability. *J Athl Train*. 2009;44(2):160-164.

22. Uhl TL, Kibler WB, Gecewich B, et al. Evaluation of clinical assessment methods for scapular dyskinesis. *Arthroscopy*. 2009;25(11):1240-1248.

23. Wilk KE, Meister K, Andrews JR. Current concepts in the rehabilitation of the overhead throwing athlete. *Am J Sports Med*. 2002;30(1):136-151.

24. Shanley E, Kissenberth MJ, Thigpen CA, et al. Preseason shoulder range of motion screening as a predictor of injury among youth and adolescent baseball pitchers. *J Shoulder Elbow Surg*. 2015;24(7):1005-1013.

25. Wainner RS, Whitman JM, Cleland JA, et al. Regional interdependence: a musculoskeletal examination model whose time has come. *J Orthop Sports Phys Ther*. 2007;37(11):658-660.

26. Axe M, Hurd W, Snyder-Mackler L. Data-based interval throwing programs for baseball players. *Sports Health*. 2009;1(2):145-153.

27. Adams JE. Little league shoulder: osteochondrosis of the proximal humeral epiphysis in boy baseball pitchers. *Calif Med*. 1966;105:22-25.

28. Carson WG Jr, Gasser SI. Little Leaguer's shoulder. A report of 23 cases. *Am J Sports Med*. 1998;26:575-580.

29. Tullos HS, Fain RH. Little league shoulder: rotational stress fracture of proximal epiphysis. *J Sports Med*. 1974;2:152-153.

30. Wasserlauf BL, Paletta GA Jr. Shoulder disorders in the skeletally immature throwing athlete. *Orthop Clin North Am*. 2003;34(3):427-437.

31. Knesek M, Skendzel JG, Dines JS, et al. Diagnosis and management of superior Labral Anterior Posterior tears in throwing athletes. *Am J Sports Med*. 2012;41:444-460.

32. Greiwe RM, Saifi C, Ahmad CS. Pediatric sports elbow injuries. *Clin Sports Med*. 2010;29(4):677-703.

33. Fortenbaugh D, Fleisig GS, Andrews JR. Baseball pitching biomechanics in relation to injury risk and performance. *Sports Health*. 2009;1(4):314-320.

34. Nissen CW, Westwell M, Ounpuu S, et al. A biomechanical comparison of the fastball and curveball in adolescent baseball pitchers. *Am J Sports Med*. 2009;37(8):1492-1498.

35. Grantham JW, Iyengar JJ, Byram IR, et al. The curveball as a risk factor for injury: a systematic review. *Sports Health*. 2015;7(1):19-26.

36. Kramer DE. Elbow pain and injury in young athletes. *J Pediatr Orthop*. 2010;30(2):S7-S12.

37. Fleisig GS, Weber A, Hassell N, et al. Prevention of elbow injuries in youth baseball pitchers. *Curr Sports Med Rep*. 2009;8(5):250-254.

38. Hodgins JL, Vitale M, Arons RR, et al. Epidemiology of medial ulnar collateral ligament reconstruction: a 10-year study in New York state. *Am J Sports Med*. 2016;44:729-734.

39. Fleisig GS, Andrews JR. Prevention of elbow injuries in youth baseball pitchers. *Sports Health*. 2012;4(5):419-424.

40. Petty DH, Andrews JR, Fleisig GS, et al. Ulnar collateral ligament reconstruction in high school baseball players: clinical results and injury risk factors. *Am J Sports Med*. 2004;32(5):1158-1164.

41. Guerrero P, Busconi B, Deangelis N, et al. Congenital instability of the shoulder joint: assessment and treatment options. *J Orthop Sports Phys Ther*. 2009;39(2):124-134.

42. Dumont GD, Russell RD, Robertson WJ. Anterior shoulder instability: a review of pathoanatomy, diagnosis and treatment. *Curr Rev Musculoskelet Med*. 2011;4(4):200-207.

43. Shah RR, Kinder J, Peelman J, et al. Pediatric clavicle and acromioclavicular injuries. *J Ped Orthop*. 2010;30:S69-S72. doi:10.1097/BPO.1090b1013e3181ba1099e1094

44. Caird MS. Clavicle shaft fractures: are children little adults? *J Pediatr Orthop*. 2012;32(suppl 1):S1-S4.

45. Pandya NK, Namdari S, Hosalkar HS. Displaced clavicle fractures in adolescents: facts, controversies, and current trends. *J Am Acad Orthop Surg*. 2012;20(8):498-505.

46. Howard A, Mulpuri K, Abel MF, et al. The treatment of pediatric supracondylar humerus fractures. *J Am Acad Orthop Surg*. 2012;20(5):320-327.

47. Spencer HT, Wong M, Fong YJ, et al. Prospective longitudinal evaluation of elbow motion following pediatric supracondylar humeral fractures. *J Bone Joint Surg Am*. 2010;92(4):904-910.

48. Song KS, Waters PM. Lateral condylar humerus fractures: which ones should we fix? *J Pediatr Orthop*. 2012;32(suppl 1):S5-S9.

49. Leonidou A, Pagkalos J, Lepetsos P, et al. Pediatric Monteggia fractures: a single-center study of the management of 40 patients. *J Pediatr Orthop.* 2012;32(4):352-356.

50. Weiss JM, Mencio GA. Forearm shaft fractures: does fixation improve outcomes? *J Pediatr Orthop.* 2012;32(suppl 1):S22-S24.

51. Stutz C, Mencio GA. Fractures of the distal radius and ulna: metaphyseal and physeal injuries. *J Pediatr Orthop.* 2010;30:S85-S89. doi:10.1097/BPO.1090b1013e3181c1099c1017a

52. van Bosse HJ, Patel RJ, Thacker M, et al. Minimalistic approach to treating wrist torus fractures. *J Pediatr Orthop.* 2005;25(4):495-500.

53. DiFiori JP, Caine DJ, Malina RM. Wrist pain, distal radial physeal injury, and ulnar variance in the young gymnast. *Am J Sports Med.* 2006;34(5):840-849.

54. Elhassan BT, Shin AY. Scaphoid fracture in children. *Hand Clin.* 2006;22(1):31-41.

55. Evenski AJ, Adamczyk MJ, Steiner RP, et al. Clinically suspected scaphoid fractures in children. *J Pediatr Orthop.* 2009;29(4):352-355.

56. Prosser R, Herbert T. The management of carpal fractures and dislocations. *J Hand Ther.* 1996;9(2):139-147.

57. Haughton D, Jordan D, Malahias M, et al. Principles of hand fracture management. *Open Orthop J.* 2012;6:43-53.

58. Cornwall R. Pediatric finger fractures: which ones turn ugly? *J Pediatr Orthop.* 2012;32(suppl 1):S25-S31.

59. Patel DR, Lyne ED. Overuse injuries of the hip, pelvis and thigh. In: Patel DR, Greydanus DE, Baker RJ, eds. *Pediatric Practice Sports Medicine.* The McGraw-Hill Companies; 2009.

60. Soprano JV, Fuchs SM. Common overuse injuries in the pediatric and adolescent athlete. *Clin Pediatr Emerg Med.* 2007;8(1):7-14.

61. Porr J, Lucaciu C, Birkett S. Avulsion fractures of the pelvis—a qualitative systematic review of the literature. *J Can Chiropr Assoc.* 2011;55(4):247-255.

62. Anderson K, Strickland SM, Warren R. Hip and groin injuries in athletes. *Am J Sports Med.* 2001;29(4):521-533.

63. Ilizaliturri VM Jr, Camacho-Galindo J, Evia Ramirez AN, et al. Soft tissue pathology around the hip. *Clin Sports Med.* 2011;30(2):391-415.

64. Yen YM, Lewis CL, Kim YJ. Understanding and treating the snapping hip. *Sports Med Arthrosc Rev.* 2015;23(4):194-199. doi:10.1097/JSA.0000000000000095

65. Provencher MT, Hofmeister EP, Muldoon MP. The surgical treatment of external coxa saltans (the snapping hip) by Z-plasty of the iliotibial band. *Am J Sports Med.* 2004;32(2):470-476.

66. Byrd JWT. Snapping hip. *Oper Tech Sports Med.* 2005;13(1):46-54.

67. Allen WC, Cope R. Coxa saltans: the snapping hip revisited. *J Am Acad Orthop Surg.* 1995;3(5):303-308.

68. Cardinal E, Buckwalter KA, Capello WN, et al. US of the snapping iliopsoas tendon. *Radiology.* 1996;198(2):521-522.

69. Byrd JWT. Evaluation and management of the snapping Iliopsoas tendon. *Tech Orthopaedic.* 2005;20(1):45-51.

70. Taylor GR, Clarke NM. Surgical release of the "snapping iliopsoas tendon." *J Bone Joint Surg Br.* 1995;77(6):881-883.

71. Brunet ME, Cook SD, Brinker MR, et al. A survey of running injuries in 1505 competitive and recreational runners. *J Sports Med Phys Fitness.* 1990;30(3):307-315.

72. Lassus J, Tulikoura I, Konttinen YT, et al. Bone stress injuries of the lower extremity: a review. *Acta Orthop Scand.* 2002;73(3):359-368.

73. Bennell K, Matheson G, Meeuwisse W, et al. Risk factors for stress fractures. *Sports Med.* 1999;28(2):91-122.

74. Goolsby MA, Barrack MT, Nattiv A. A displaced femoral neck stress fracture in an amenorrheic adolescent female runner. *Sports Health.* 2012;4(4):352-356.

75. Griffin DR, Dickenson EJ, O'Donnell J, et al. The Warwick Agreement on femoroacetabular impingement syndrome (FAI syndrome): an international consensus statement. *Br J Sports Med.* 2016;50:1169-1176.

76. Fraitzl CR, Kafer W, Nelitz M, et al. Radiological evidence of femoroacetabular impingement in mild slipped capital femoral epiphysis:

a mean follow-up of 14.4 years after pinning in situ. *J Bone Joint Surg Br.* 2007;89(12):1592-1596.

77. Imam S, Khanduja V. Current concepts in the diagnosis and management of femoroacetabular impingement. *Int Orthop.* 2011;35(10):1427-1435.

78. Philippon MJ, Stubbs AJ, Schenker ML, et al. Arthroscopic management of femoroacetabular impingement: osteoplasty technique and literature review. *Am J Sports Med.* 2007;35(9):1571-1580.

79. Huffman GR, Safran M. Tears of the acetabular labrum in athletes: diagnosis and treatment. *Sports Med Arthrosc Rev.* 2002;10(2):141-150.

80. Crawford JR, Villar RN. Current concepts in the management of femoroacetabular impingement. *J Bone Joint Surg Br.* 2005;87(11):1459-1462.

81. Ito K, Minka MA II, Leunig M, et al. Femoroacetabular impingement and the cam-effect. A MRI-based quantitative anatomical study of the femoral head-neck offset. *J Bone Joint Surg Br.* 2001;83(2):171-176.

82. Ferguson TA, Matta J. Anterior femoroacetabular impingement: a clinical presentation. *Sports Med Arthrosc Rev.* 2002;10(2):134-140.

83. Czerny C, Hofmann S, Neuhold A, et al. Lesions of the acetabular labrum: accuracy of MR imaging and MR arthrography in detection and staging. *Radiology.* 1996;200(1):225-230.

84. Griffin D, Dickenson E, Wall P, et al. Hip arthroscopy compared with best conservative care for the treatment of femoroacetabular impingement syndrome: a randomized controlled trial (UK FASHIon). *Lancet.* 2018;391:2225-2235.

85. Wright AA, Hegedus EJ, Taylor JB, et al. Non-operative management of femoroacetabular impingement: a prospective, randomized controlled clinical trial pilot study. *J Sci Med Sport.* 2016;19(9):716-721. doi:10.1016/j.jsams.2015.11.008

86. Mansell NS, Rhon DI, Meyer J, et al. Arthroscopic surgery or physical therapy for patients with femoroacetabular impingement syndrome: a randomized controlled trial with 2-year follow-up. *Am J Sports Med.* 2018;46(6):1306-1314. doi:10.1177/0363546517751912

87. Samora JB, Ng VY, Ellis TJ. Femoroacetabular impingement: a common cause of hip pain in young adults. *Clin J Sport Med.* 2011;21(1):51-56.

88. Groh MM, Herrera J. A comprehensive review of hip labral tears. *Curr Rev Musculoskelet Med.* 2009;2(2):105-117.

89. Heiderscheit BC, Sherry MA, Silder A, et al. Hamstring strain injuries: recommendations for diagnosis, rehabilitation, and injury prevention. *J Orthop Sports Phys Ther.* 2010;40(2):67-81.

90. Koulouris G, Connell DA, Brukner P, et al. Magnetic resonance imaging parameters for assessing risk of recurrent hamstring injuries in elite athletes. *Am J Sports Med.* 2007;35(9):1500-1506.

91. Glasgow P, Phillips N, Bleakley C. Optimal loading: key variables and mechanisms. *Br J Sports Med.* 2015;49:278-279.

92. Bleakley CM, Glasgow P, MacAuley DC. PRICE needs updating, should we call the POLICE? *Br J Sports Med.* 2012;46:220-221.

93. Attar WSAA, Soomro N, Sinclair PJ, et al. Effect of injury prevention programs that include the nordic hamstring exercise on hamstring injury rates in soccer players: a systematic review and meta-analysis. *Sports Med.* 2017;47:907-916.

94. Cline S. Acute injuries of the hip, pelvis and thigh. In: Patel DR, Greydanus DE, Baker RJ, eds. *Pediatric Practice Sports Medicine.* The McGraw-Hill Companies; 2009.

95. Wells D, King JD, Roe TF, et al. Review of slipped capital femoral epiphysis associated with endocrine disease. *J Pediatr Orthop.* 1993;13(5):610-614.

96. Kocher MS, Tucker R. Pediatric athlete hip disorders. *Clin Sports Med.* 2006;25(2):241-253, viii.

97. Riad J, Bajelidze G, Gabos PG. Bilateral slipped capital femoral epiphysis: predictive factors for contralateral slip. *J Pediatr Orthop.* 2007;27(4):411-414.

98. Uglow MG, Clarke NM. The management of slipped capital femoral epiphysis. *J Bone Joint Surg Br.* 2004;86(5):631-635.

99. Hinton RY, Sharma KM. Anterior cruciate ligament injuries. In: Micheli LJ, Kocher MS, eds. *The Pediatric and Adolescent Knee.* Saunders Elsevier; 2006.

100. Anderson CN, Anderson AF. Tibial eminence fractures. *Clin Sports Med.* 2011;30(4):727-742.

101. Moksnes H, Engebretsen L, Risberg MA. Management of anterior cruciate ligament injuries in skeletally immature individuals. *J Orthop Sports Phys Ther.* 2012;42(3):172-183.

102. Lawrence JT, Argawal N, Ganley TJ. Degeneration of the knee joint in skeletally immature patients with a diagnosis of an anterior cruciate ligament tear: is there harm in delay of treatment? *Am J Sports Med.* 2011;39(12):2582-2587.

103. Wojtys EM, Brower AM. Anterior cruciate ligament injuries in the prepubescent and adolescent athlete: clinical and research considerations. *J Athl Train.* 2010;45(5):509-512.

104. Milewski MD, Beck NA, Lawrence JT, et al. Anterior cruciate ligament reconstruction in the young athlete: a treatment algorithm for the skeletally immature. *Clin Sports Med.* 2011;30(4):801-810.

105. Vavken P, Murray MM. Treating anterior cruciate ligament tears in skeletally immature patients. *Arthroscopy.* 2011;27(5):704-716.

106. Ardern CL, Ekas G, Grindem H, et al. International Olympic Committee consensus statement on prevention, diagnosis and management of paediatric anterior cruciate ligament (ACL) injuries. *Br J Sports Med.* 2018;26:989-1010.

107. Kim KM, Croy T, Hertel J, et al. Effects of neuromuscular electrical stimulation after anterior cruciate ligament reconstruction on quadriceps strength, function, and patient-oriented outcomes: a systematic review. *J Orthop Sports Phys Ther.* 2010;40(7):383-391.

108. Greenberg EM, Albaugh J, Ganley TJ, et al. Rehabilitation considerations for all epiphyseal ACL reconstruction. *Int J Sports Phys Ther.* 2012;7(2):185-196.

109. Logerstedt DS, Snyder-Mackler L, Ritter RC, et al. Knee stability and movement coordination impairments: knee ligament sprain. *J Orthop Sports Phys Ther.* 2010;40(4):A1-A37.

110. Noyes FR, Barber SD, Mangine RE. Abnormal lower limb symmetry determined by function hop tests after anterior cruciate ligament rupture. *Am J Sports Med.* 1991;19(5):513-518.

111. Yellin JL, Fabricant PD, Gornitzky A, et al. Rehabilitation following anterior cruciate ligament tears in children: a systematic review. *JBJS Rev.* 2016;4(1). doi:10.2106/JBJS.RVW.O.00001

112. Webster KE, Feller JA. Development and validation of a short version of the anterior cruciate ligament return to sport after injury (ACL-RSI) scale. *Orthop J Sports Med.* 2018;6(4):2325967118763763.

113. McPherson AL, Feller JA, Hewett TE, et al. Psychological readiness to return to sport is associated with second anterior cruciate ligament injuries. *Am J Sports Med.* 2019;47(4):857-862. doi:10.1177/0363546518825258

114. Myer GD, Chu DA, Brent JL, et al. Trunk and hip control neuromuscular training for the prevention of knee joint injury. *Clin Sports Med.* 2008;27(3):425-448, ix.

115. Hewett TE, Ford KR, Myer GD. Anterior cruciate ligament injuries in female athletes: part 2, a meta-analysis of neuromuscular interventions aimed at injury prevention. *Am J Sports Med.* 2006;34(3):490-498.

116. DiStefano LJ, Blackburn JT, Marshall SW, et al. Effects of an age-specific anterior cruciate ligament injury prevention program on lower extremity biomechanics in children. *Am J Sports Med.* 2011;39(5):949-957.

117. Mandelbaum BR, Silvers HJ, Watanabe DS, et al. Effectiveness of a neuromuscular and proprioceptive training program in preventing anterior cruciate ligament injuries in female athletes: 2-year follow-up. *Am J Sports Med.* 2005;33(7):1003-1010.

118. Hewett TE, Myer GD, Ford KR, et al. The 2012 ABJS Nicolas Andry Award: the sequence of prevention: a systematic approach to prevent anterior cruciate ligament injury. *Clin Orthop Relat Res.* 2012;470(10):2930-2940.

119. Shea KG, Apel PJ, Pfeiffer R. Injury of the medial collateral ligament, posterior cruciate ligament, and posterolateral complex in skeletally immature patients. In: Micheli LJ, Kocher MS, eds. *The Pediatric and Adolescent Knee.* Saunders Elsevier; 2006.

120. Miyamoto RG, Bosco JA, Sherman OH. Treatment of medial collateral ligament injuries. *J Am Acad Orthop Surg.* 2009;17(3):152-161.

121. Derscheid GL, Garrick JG. Medial collateral ligament injuries in football. Nonoperative management of grade I and grade II sprains. *Am J Sports Med.* 1981;9(6):365-368.

122. Indelicato PA, Hermansdorfer J, Huegel M. Nonoperative management of complete tears of the medial collateral ligament of the knee in intercollegiate football players. *Clin Orthop Relat Res.* 1990;(256):174-177.

123. McAllister DR, Petrigliano FA. Diagnosis and treatment of posterior cruciate ligament injuries. *Curr Sports Med Rep.* 2007; 6(5):293-299.

124. Senese M, Greenberg E, Todd Lawrence J, et al. Rehabilitation following isolated posterior cruciate ligament reconstruction: a literature review of published protocols. *Int J Sports Phys Ther.* 2018;13(4):737-751.

125. Kramer DE, Micheli LJ. Meniscal tears and discoid meniscus in children: diagnosis and treatment. *J Am Acad Orthop Surg.* 2009;17(11):698-707.

126. Stanitski CL. Discoid meniscus. In: Micheli LJ, Kocher MS, eds. *The Pediatric and Adolescent Knee.* Saunders Elsevier; 2006.

127. Jordan MR. Lateral meniscal variants: evaluation and treatment. *J Am Acad Orthop Surg.* 1996;4(4):191-200.

128. Konan S, Rayan F, Haddad FS. Do physical diagnostic tests accurately detect meniscal tears? *Knee Surg Sports Traumatol Arthrosc.* 2009;17(7):806-811.

129. Conrad JM, Stanitski CL. Osteochondritis dissecans: Wilson's sign revisited. *Am J Sports Med.* 2003;31(5):777-778.

130. Ganley TJ, Flynn JM. Osteochondritis dissecans of the knee. In: Micheli LJ, Kocher MS, eds. *The Pediatric and Adolescent Knee.* Saunders Elsevier; 2006.

131. Pascual-Garrido C, Moran CJ, Green DW, et al. Osteochondritis dissecans of the knee in children and adolescents. *Curr Opin Pediatr.* 2013;25(1):46-51.

132. Buckens CF, Saris DB. Reconstruction of the medial patellofemoral ligament for treatment of patellofemoral instability: a systematic review. *Am J Sports Med.* 2010;38(1):181-188.

133. Kramer DE, Pace JL. Acute traumatic and sports-related osteochondral injury of the pediatric knee. *Orthop Clin North Am.* 2012;43(2):227-236, vi.

134. Lewis PB, McCarty LP 3rd, Kang RW, et al. Basic science and treatment options for articular cartilage injuries. *J Orthop Sports Phys Ther.* 2006;36(10):717-727.

135. Davis IS, Powers CM. Patellofemoral pain syndrome: proximal, distal, and local factors, an international retreat, April 30-May 2, 2009, Fells Point, Baltimore, MD. *J Orthop Sports Phys Ther.* 2010;40(3):A1-A16.

136. Richard WW, Lisa TH, Christian JB, et al. Patellofemoral pain: clinical practice guidelines linked to the International Classification of Functioning, Disability and Health from the Academy of Orthopaedic Physical Therapy of the American Physical Therapy Association. *J Orthop Sports Phys Ther.* 2019;49(9):CPG1-CPG95.

137. Robinson RL, Nee RJ. Analysis of hip strength in females seeking physical therapy treatment for unilateral patellofemoral pain syndrome. *J Orthop Sports Phys Ther.* 2007;37(5):232-238.

138. Dierks TA, Manal KT, Hamill J, et al. Proximal and distal influences on hip and knee kinematics in runners with patellofemoral pain during a prolonged run. *J Orthop Sports Phys Ther.* 2008;38(8):448-456.

139. Barton CJ, Bonanno D, Levinger P, et al. Foot and ankle characteristics in patellofemoral pain syndrome: a case control and reliability study. *J Orthop Sports Phys Ther.* 2010;40(5):286-296.

140. Willy RW, Meira EP. Currrent concepts in biomechanical interventions for patellofemoral pain. *Int J Sports Phys Ther.* 2016;11(6):877-890.

141. Bolgla LA, Boling MC. An update for the conservative management of patellofemoral pain syndrome: a systematic review of the literature from 2000 to 2010. *Int J Sports Phys Ther.* 2011;6(2):112-125.

142. Peers KH, Lysens RJ. Patellar tendinopathy in athletes: current diagnostic and therapeutic recommendations. *Sports Med.* 2005;35(1):71-87.

143. Larsson ME, Kall I, Nilsson-Helander K. Treatment of patellar tendinopathy—a systematic review of randomized controlled trials. *Knee Surg Sports Traumatol Arthrosc.* 2012;20(8):1632-1646.

144. Beyer R, Kongsgaard M, Hougs Kjær B, et al. Heavy slow resistance versus eccentric training as treatment for Achilles tendinopathy: a randomized controlled trial. *Am J Sports Med.* 2015;43(7):1704-1711. doi:10.1177/0363546515584760

145. de Michelis Mendonça L, Ocarino JM, Bittencourt NFN, et al. The accuracy of the VISA-P questionnaire, single leg decline squat and tendon pain history to identify patellar tendon abnormalities in adult athletes. *J Orthop Sports Phys Ther.* 2016;46(8):673-680.

146. Witvrouw E, Bellemans J, Lysens R, et al. Intrinsic risk factors for the development of patellar tendinitis in an athletic population. A two-year prospective study. *Am J Sports Med.* 2001;29(2):190-195.

147. Bellary SS, Lynch G, Housman B, et al. Medial plica syndrome: a review of the literature. *Clin Anat.* 2012;25(4):423-428.

148. De Carlo M, Armstrong B. Rehabilitation of the knee following sports injury. *Clin Sports Med.* 2010;29(1):81-106, table of contents.

149. Moen MH, Bongers T, Bakker EW, et al. Risk factors and prognostic indicators for medial tibial stress syndrome. *Scand J Med Sci Sports.* 2012;22(1):34-39.

150. Beck BR. Tibial stress injuries. An aetiological review for the purposes of guiding management. *Sports Med.* 1998;26(4):265-279.

151. Crowell HP, Davis IS. Gait retraining to reduce lower extremity loading in runners. *Clin Biomech (Bristol, Avon).* 2011;26(1):78-83.

152. Lieberman DE, Venkadesan M, Werbel WA, et al. Foot strike patterns and collision forces in habitually barefoot versus shod runners. *Nature.* 2010;463(7280):531-535.

153. Heiderscheit BC, Chumanov ES, Michalski MP, et al. Effects of step rate manipulation on joint mechanics during running. *Med Sci Sports Exerc.* 2011;43(2):296-302.

154. Diebal AR, Gregory R, Alitz C, et al. Effects of forefoot running on chronic exertional compartment syndrome: a case series. *Int J Sports Phys Ther.* 2011;6(4):312-321.

155. Diebal AR, Gregory R, Alitz C, et al. Forefoot running improves pain and disability associated with chronic exertional compartment syndrome. *Am J Sports Med.* 2012;40(5):1060-1067.

156. Sharma P, Maffulli N. Tendon injury and tendinopathy: healing and repair. *J Bone Joint Surg Am.* 2005;87(1):187-202.

157. McCollum GA, van den Bekerom MP, Kerkhoffs GM, et al. Syndesmosis and deltoid ligament injuries in the athlete. *Knee Surg Sports Traumatol Arthrosc.* 2013;21(6):1328-1337.

158. Tiemstra JD. Update on acute ankle sprains. *Am Fam Physician.* 2012;85(12):1170-1176.

159. Knight AC, Weimar WH. Effects of previous lateral ankle sprain and taping on the latency of the peroneus longus. *Sports Biomech.* 2012;11(1):48-56.

160. Chambers HG. Ankle and foot disorders in skeletally immature athletes. *Orthop Clin North Am.* 2003;34(3):445-459.

161. Runyon MS. Can we safely apply the Ottawa ankle rules to children? *Acad Emerg Med.* 2009;16(4):352-354.

162. Plint AC, Bulloch B, Osmond MH, et al. Validation of the Ottawa ankle rules in children with ankle injuries. *Acad Emerg Med.* 1999;6(10):1005-1009.

163. Pontell D, Hallivis R, Dollard MD. Sports injuries in the pediatric and adolescent foot and ankle: common overuse and acute presentations. *Clin Podiatr Med Surg.* 2006;23(1):209-231, x.

164. Rowe V, Hemmings S, Barton C, et al. Conservative management of midportion Achilles tendinopathy: a mixed methods study, integrating systematic review and clinical reasoning. *Sports Med.* 2012;42(11):941-967.

165. Alfredson H, Cook J. A treatment algorithm for managing Achilles tendinopathy: new treatment options. *Br J Sports Med.* 2007;41(4):211-216.

166. Malliaris P, Barton CJ, Reeves ND, et al. Achilles tendinopathy loading programmes: a systematic review comparing clinical outcomes and identifying potential mechanisms for effectiveness. *Sports Med.* 2013;43(4):267-286.

167. Silbernagel KG, Thomeé R, Eriksson BI, et al. Continued sports activity, using a pain-monitoring model, during rehabilitation in patients with Achilles tendinopathy: a randomized controlled study. *Am J Sports Med.* 2007;35(6):897-906. doi:10.1177/0363546506298279

168. Watson TS, Shurnas PS, Denker J. Treatment of Lisfranc joint injury: current concepts. *J Am Acad Orthop Surg.* 2010;18(12):718-728.

169. Mantas JP, Burks RT. Lisfranc injuries in the athlete. *Clin Sports Med.* 1994;13(4):719-730.

170. Nunley JA, Vertullo CJ. Classification, investigation, and management of midfoot sprains: Lisfranc injuries in the athlete. *Am J Sports Med.* 2002;30(6):871-878.

171. Zwitser EW, Breederveld RS. Fractures of the fifth metatarsal; diagnosis and treatment. *Injury.* 2010;41(6):555-562.

172. Niemeyer P, Weinberg A, Schmitt H, et al. Stress fractures in the juvenile skeletal system. *Int J Sports Med.* 2006;27(3):242-249.

173. Hunt KJ, Anderson RB. Treatment of Jones fracture nonunions and refractures in the elite athlete: outcomes of intramedullary screw fixation with bone grafting. *Am J Sports Med.* 2011;39(9):1948-1954.

174. Murawski CD, Kennedy JG. Percutaneous internal fixation of proximal fifth metatarsal jones fractures (Zones II and III) with Charlotte Carolina screw and bone marrow aspirate concentrate: an outcome study in athletes. *Am J Sports Med.* 2011;39(6):1295-1301.

175. Micheli LJ, Wood R. Back pain in young athletes. Significant differences from adults in causes and patterns. *Arch Pediatr Adolesc Med.* 1995;149(1):15-18.

176. Rodriguez DP, Poussaint TY. Imaging of back pain in children. *AJNR Am J Neuroradiol.* 2010;31(5):787-802.

177. Purcell L, Micheli L. Low back pain in young athletes. *Sports Health.* 2009;1(3):212-222.

178. Leone A, Cianfoni A, Cerase A, et al. Lumbar spondylolysis: a review. *Skeletal Radiol.* 2011;40(6):683-700.

179. Kim HJ, Green DW. Spondylolysis in the adolescent athlete. *Curr Opin Pediatr.* 2011;23(1):68-72.

180. Rush JK, Astur N, Scott S, et al. Use of magnetic resonance imaging in the evaluation of spondylolysis. *J Pediatr Orthop.* 2015;35(3):271-275. doi:10.1097/BPO.0000000000000244

181. Yamaguchi K Jr, Skaggs D, Acevedo D, et al. Spondylolysis is frequently missed by MRI in adolescents with back pain. *J Child Orthop.* 2012;6(3):237-240.

182. Muschik M, Hahnel H, Robinson PN, et al. Competitive sports and the progression of spondylolisthesis. *J Pediatr Orthop.* 1996;16(3):364-369.

183. Sairyo K, Sakai T, Yasui N, et al. Conservative treatment for pediatric lumbar spondylolysis to achieve bone healing using a hard brace: what type and how long?: clinical article. *J Neurosurg Spine.* 2012;16(6):610-614.

184. Sys J, Michielsen J, Bracke P, et al. Nonoperative treatment of active spondylolysis in elite athletes with normal X-ray findings: literature review and results of conservative treatment. *Eur Spine J.* 2001;10(6):498-504.

185. Weinberg J, Rokito S, Silber JS. Etiology, treatment, and prevention of athletic "stingers". *Clin Sports Med.* 2003;22(3):493-500, viii.

186. Willardson JM. Core stability training: applications to sports conditioning programs. *J Strength Cond Res.* 2007;21(3):979-985.

187. Arokoski JP, Valta T, Airaksinen O, et al. Back and abdominal muscle function during stabilization exercises. *Arch Phys Med Rehabil.* 2001;82(8):1089-1098.

188. Zuckerman SL, Lee YM, Odom MJ, et al. Recovery from sports-related concussion: days to return to neurocognitive baseline in adolescents versus young adults. *Surg Neurol Int.* 2012;3:130.

189. Harmon KG, Drezner JA, Gammons M, et al. American medical society for sports medicine position statement: concussion in sport. *Br J Sports Med.* 2013;47(1):15-26.

190. McCrory P, Meeuwisse WH, Dvorak J, et al. 5th International conference on concussion in sport (Berlin). *Br J Sports Med.* 2017;51(11):837.

191. Ellemberg D, Henry LC, Macciocchi SN, et al. Advances in sport concussion assessment: from behavioral to brain imaging measures. *J Neurotrauma.* 2009;26(12):2365-2382.

192. Fazio VC, Lovell MR, Pardini JE, et al. The relation between post concussion symptoms and neurocognitive performance in concussed athletes. *NeuroRehabilitation.* 2007;22(3):207-216.

193. Leddy JJ, Baker JG, Willer B. Active rehabilitation of concussion and post-concussion syndrome. *Phys Med Rehabil Clin N Am.* 2016;27:437-454.

194. Nazem TG, Ackerman KE. The female athlete triad. *Sports Health.* 2012;4(4):302-311.

195. Mountjoy M, Sundgot-Borgen JK, Burke LM, et al. IOC consensus statement on relative energy deficiency in sport (RED-S): 2018 update. *Br J Sports Med.* 2018;52:687-697.

196. Koltun KJ, Strock NC, Southmayd EA, et al. Comparison of female athlete triad coalition and RED-S risk assessment tools. *J Sports Sci.* 2019;37(21):2433-2442.

17

Juvenile Idiopathic Arthritis and Other Rheumatic Disorders

Courtney L. Ginter and Leslie F. Vogel

>> Introduction

Juvenile idiopathic arthritis (JIA) is the most common of the rheumatic diseases of childhood. Other less common diagnoses occurring in childhood include juvenile dermatomyositis (JDM), chronic recurrent multifocal osteomyelitis (CRMO), systemic lupus erythematosus (SLE), and scleroderma. If not medically managed, these diagnoses can impact multiple body systems, causing physical impairments, activity limitations, and participation restrictions in the growing child.

The purpose of this chapter is to prepare the physical therapist to participate in the medical care and management of children followed up in the pediatric rheumatology clinic.

The first section of this chapter describes the pathophysiology, diagnosis, pharmacologic management, and classification of JIA in some detail. This section also provides a brief introduction to JDM, CRMO, SLE, and scleroderma to identify the differences in pathophysiology that may require modification to the physical therapy plan of care (POC). The second section of this chapter focuses on the role of physical therapy in the evaluation and management of children to maximize their function and increase their participation within their community. Advances in medical management have significantly improved the functional outcomes for most children with JIA and other rheumatic diseases. A case study has been included to illustrate the physical therapist's management of an older child with JIA.

>> Medical management of juvenile idiopathic arthritis

Definition, Incidence, and Prevalence of Juvenile Idiopathic Arthritis

JIA is currently defined as arthritis of unknown etiology occurring in children younger than 16 years and lasting for at least 6 weeks.[1] However, the Pediatric Rheumatology International Trials Organization (PRINTO) has recently recommended expanding the definition to include chronic inflammatory disorders lasting for at least 6 weeks beginning before 18 years of age after other known conditions have been excluded.[2] Redefinition emphasizes that JIA is a group of distinct disorders with several subtypes extending into adulthood.

Arthritis is a medical condition describing inflammation of a joint characterized by warmth, pain, redness, and/or swelling. Inflammation often causes joint stiffness that frequently occurs in the morning upon waking or after periods of immobility. This stiffness may be referred to as *gelling* and makes morning routines more difficult. Chronic joint stiffness and muscle guarding can lead to limited range of motion (ROM), muscle weakness, and, if left untreated, a loss of function.

According to a systematic review of 33 publications, the global annual incidence of JIA ranged from 1.6 to 23 per 100,000 children. The incidence is increased in Caucasians with a pooled rate of 8.2 per 100,000. The incidence is also increased for females (pooled rate of 10.0/100,000) compared to males (pooled rate of 5.7/100,000). The prevalence of JIA is reported as 70.2 per 100,000 or 1 per 1000 children.[3,4]

Pathophysiology

The exact etiology and pathophysiology of JIA is not fully understood. However, there does seem to be some genetic predisposition that may be triggered by viral, bacterial, or environmental factors.[5] The major histocompatibility complex (MHC) consists of various genetic alleles located on chromosome 6 that are associated with autoimmune and inflammatory disease. The human MHC region is also referred to as the *human leukocyte antigen* (HLA) region.[6] Various genetic markers in this HLA region, including HLA-DRB1 and HLA-B27, appear to be associated with JIA subtypes and disease severity.[7] Other genes that may help predict a child's response to specific pharmacologic treatment have been identified.[8]

There is also a familial association when large groups of subjects are studied. Thirteen percent of children with JIA were found to have a family history including siblings and cousins.[9] One study of over 3,000 children with arthritis found there was concordance between siblings with JIA for age at onset, clinical manifestations, and disease course.[10] Mothers of children with JIA had a higher prevalence for autoimmune disease (32.3%) when compared to fathers (11.4%). Maternal second-degree relatives were at higher risk for autoimmune disease than were paternal relatives.[11] Other studies have shown alterations in the gut microbiome in some children with JIA.[12]

As a heterogeneous disease, there is more than one inflammatory pathway. Autoimmunity occurs when the immune system targets one's own antigens, causing an imbalance in the body's immune response. Self-antigens within the joint tissue activate T cells that secrete proinflammatory cytokines including interleukin (IL)-1, IL-6, and tumor necrosis factor-alpha (TNF-α). Other regulatory T cells work to inhibit these cytokines, creating a balance between pro- and anti-inflammatory cells. An increase in proinflammatory cells leads to synovial inflammation and arthritis. Autoimmunity occurs more frequently in females than in males. This type of inflammatory pathway is often genetically linked to specific MHC alleles and features circulating autoantibodies.[13,14]

In other JIA subtypes, there is an autoinflammatory process with activation of an inflammatory response due to a defect in the normal self-inhibitory pathway. Activation of monocytes, macrophages, and neutrophils release proinflammatory cytokines and proteins, causing an inflammatory cascade.[13] These diseases are often associated with rashes and fevers. They occur in equal numbers in males and females and often present at younger ages.[14]

Synovial joints are composed of two bony surfaces covered in hyaline articular cartilage and enclosed within a capsule that is stabilized with muscles and ligaments (Fig. 17.1). Within the joint capsule is the synovial lining that produces synovial fluid which lubricates and supplies nutrients to the intra-articular structures. Synovial fluid is produced by type B synovial cells, and can be excessive in response to inflammation, trauma, as well as bacterial, fungal, or viral infection. Synovial fluid contains hyaluronan, lubricin, proteinase, collagenases, and prostaglandins.[15]

When inflammation is present, there is thickening of the synovial membrane called *panus* and increased secretion of synovial fluid containing inflammatory cytokines. The increased fluid causes joint swelling or effusion. Severe swelling can lead to distension of the joint capsule. There is also increased vascular blood supply that causes the joint to be warm, with occasional erythema. The intra-articular effusion increases the pressure within the joint, stimulating pain receptors. This pressure is increased when a joint is fully extended. An inflamed painful joint can lead to muscle guarding or spasm that limits voluntary movement and maintains the joint in partial flexion to reduce pain. Children report morning joint stiffness that can last for minutes to hours depending on disease activity.

When inflammation is left untreated, children can develop joint contractures. These contractures may initially be associated with muscle spasm and guarding that limit full joint extension and reduce pain. However, in untreated JIA, inflammation and flexor posturing may cause capsular tightness, intra-articular adhesions, fibrosis of tendons and ligaments, as well as soft-tissue shortening.

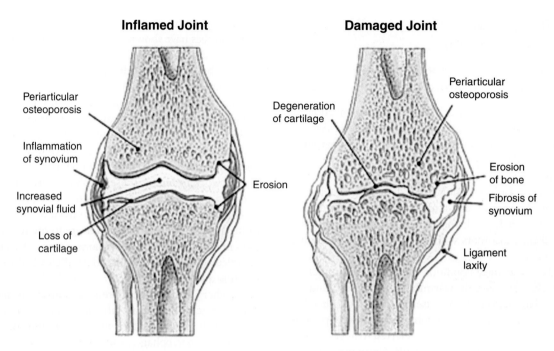

FIGURE 17.1. Changes caused by the inflammatory process within and surrounding the synovial joint.

JIA has negative effects on bone health, causing low bone mineral density (BMD) and decreased bone strength when compared to that in healthy children. Cortical bone thinning and decreased trabecular BMD was seen in all children, initially presenting with more than four active joints. Severe persistent arthritis increases the risk of fracture and failure to achieve optimal peak bone mass in adolescence and young adulthood. Additional risk factors for poor bone development in JIA include delayed pubertal maturation, malnutrition, muscle atrophy, inadequate physical activity and long-term use of glucocorticosteroids.[16]

Prolonged inflammation can cause erosion of the articular cartilage and bony surfaces. Inflammatory cells and enzymes degrade the articular cartilage. Osteophytes degrade the bony surfaces, causing erosion and cysts that can be seen on radiographic images. Smooth articular surfaces become irregular, and joint congruency, alignment, and stability are compromised. Persistent joint destruction causes chronic pain and functional disability. In severe arthritis, the hip joint is at risk from inflammatory bony erosion and avascular necrosis. Joints including the knee or wrist are at risk for subluxation. In the smaller finger joints, severe chronic inflammation can lead to ligament and tendon destruction (i.e., swan-neck deformity).

Younger children with JIA are at risk for skeletal deformity. Bone epiphyses in children are vascularized. Epiphyseal growth plate disturbances are caused by an increase in vascular blood flow to the swollen joint. At the knee, an asymmetric growth plate disturbance can lead to increased genu valgus or varus. A disturbance to the entire growth plate can lead to a leg length discrepancy (LLD).[17] A young child will often maintain their affected knee in flexion to limit pain, but also to compensate for a longer affected limb. Children can also exhibit asymmetric rotational deformities such as tibial torsion. At the wrist, ankle, or subtalar joint, growth disturbances may cause permanent hand and foot deformity.

Severe arthritis can also cause epiphyseal cartilage destruction and premature closure of the growth plate. This is commonly observed at the temporomandibular joint (TMJ), where the center of growth is in the mandibular condyle near the joint space.[18] Arthritic changes at the TMJ may cause asymmetric jaw alignment and poor occlusion when chewing. Premature growth plate closure is also responsible for the micrognathia or smaller retracted lower jaw that had been a common feature for young adults with JIA (Fig. 17.2). Closure of the growth plate can occur at other joints, causing shortening and asymmetry of the limbs.

Children with JIA generally exhibit weakness during active flares of their disease. Lindehammar and Backman reported that children with JIA had a 45% to 65% reduction in peak isometric force values when compared to normative values for muscles located near an inflamed joint.[19] When testing muscles not associated with an inflamed joint, the peak isometric force was 80% to 90% of normal or within the normal range. Periarticular muscles may exhibit arthrogenic muscle inhibition (AMI) in which muscle swelling due to trauma or inflammation causes acute muscle weakness. This has been observed in the quadriceps muscle in adults following joint surgery, where peak extensor torque was decreased by 80% to 90% in the first few days after the procedure.[20] The mechanisms behind AMI are not well understood, but appear to be mediated by spinal reflex pathways. Intra-articular swelling of 20 to 60 mL has been shown to reduce the maximum effort in quadriceps peak torque by 30% to 40% in adults. Joint

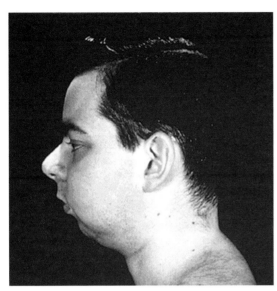

FIGURE 17.2. Micrognathia or undergrowth of the mandible that results from chronic arthritis of the temporal mandibular joint.

aspiration and corticosteroid injections can improve quadriceps peak by 30% in adults with rheumatoid arthritis (RA).

Lindehammar and Sandstedt reported on a 2-year longitudinal study of quadriceps strength that was correlated to joint severity scores at the knee and hip during periods of disease flare as well as improvement.[21] The authors did not identify atrophy of type II fibers or neuropathy, which has been reported in adults with RA.[22] In 2008, Saarinen et al. reported on isometric knee and ankle strength in subjects with inactive JIA disease.[23] They noted a nonsignificant trend toward lower strength values in children with JIA compared to match controls. With a trend toward more aggressive use of biologics to reduce inflammation earlier in the disease process, there may be less muscle weakness. A recent study compared children with JIA on drug therapy to children matched for age and activity. The authors found no difference in muscle structure (muscle thickness, cross-sectional area, or fascicle angle) nor in isometric force production for knee extension between the two groups.[24]

Physician's Examination

Rheumatologists rely on patient history and their clinical examination of each joint starting at the toes and working up to the TMJ. Individual joints and extremities are examined visually for asymmetry in contour, skin color, nail changes, muscle bulk, joint deformity, or limb length. The physician relies on palpation to identify warmth, swelling, and tenderness at the joint. A swollen joint can be related to intra-articular effusion, joint capsule thickness, or bony hypertrophy. The clinician palpates the insertion site of tendons and ligaments to identify the presence of enthesitis. They may also squeeze a small joint such as the metatarsophalangeal joint to identify tenderness known as metatarsalgia. Finally, the rheumatologist moves the joint assessing for limitation due

to pain, spasm, muscle guarding, or contracture.[25] Rheumatologists generally perform a limited strength and gait assessment to assess global function.

Laboratory Assessments

There is not one specific laboratory or genetic test that is conclusive for the diagnosis of JIA. However, the rheumatologist relies on the results of multiple tests to help diagnose and treat children with JIA.[26] New genetic biomarkers are currently being identified and explored; however, they may not yet be part of the routine laboratory panel used by clinicians.[27]

Erythrocyte sedimentation rate (ESR) is used to measure the amount of inflammation present within the body. This test measures the rate of sedimentation of erythrocytes or red blood cells in a sample of blood. Red blood cells settle faster when there are more proteins such as C-reactive protein (CRP) and fibrinogen that are present during inflammation. Similar to other tests, the ESR is not diagnostic of JIA, but may be used along with clinical signs to support a diagnosis. It may also be used in monitoring disease activity, and may be included in several of the validated disease activity scores.

CRP is a protein that is produced in the liver and is elevated in conditions where there is inflammation. Similar to the ESR, this test is not diagnostic of JIA, and can be elevated in other autoimmune diseases or when there is sepsis or infection. A CRP test can also be used to monitor disease activity and response to medications.

Complete blood counts (CBCs) are used to evaluate the number of red blood, white blood, and platelets cells. These cell counts may be increased because of inflammation, but are also used to rule out other conditions caused by infection, anemia, or leukemia.

Antinuclear antibodies (ANAs) are a group of autoantibodies that are produced by the immune system when there is an autoimmune condition. These autoantibodies bind to various components within the nucleus of the cell. ANAs are also found in 15% of healthy children; therefore, their presence is not diagnostic of JIA.[28] They do identify children with JIA who are at increased risk for chronic anterior uveitis. ANAs are also positive in other rheumatologic diseases including SLE and Sjögren syndrome.

Rheumatoid factor (RF) is an immunoglobulin (IG)-M that is produced by our immune system. When this autoantibody is present, it is often suggestive of more erosive and chronic arthritis. Children with a positive RF test finding are often older, with disease similar to that seen in adults. A positive RF finding is not diagnostic for JIA, and can also be present in children with SLE, scleroderma, and other connective tissue disorders.

Anti-citrullinated protein antibodies (ACPAs) are autoantibodies produced by the immune system that are directed against cyclic citrullinated peptides (CCPs). Citrulline is produced in the body as part of the metabolism of arginine, an amino acid. Increased levels of citrulline can trigger an immune response, producing autoantibodies against joint proteins. Children with a positive RF finding and elevated ACPAs are likely to have more aggressive disease activity.[28]

HLA-B27 is a protein found on cell surfaces. The term is also used when describing the gene that codes for the protein. This laboratory test determines whether the protein is located on the surface of a person's white blood cells. The HLAs may help the body's immune system distinguish between its own cells and foreign cells. In the presence of a specific pattern of arthritis, a positive test result for HLA-B27 is suggestive of enthesitis-related arthritis (ERA).[27] However, healthy children may also test positive for HLA-B27, in which case it is not predictive of future arthritic disease. The presence of HLA-B27 is often found in other family members.

A metabolic panel (basic metabolic panel [BMP] or comprehensive metabolic panel [CMP]) is used to rule out other diagnoses and monitor for the side effects caused by medication. A metabolic panel consists of multiple tests to identify abnormalities in the liver, kidney, and in metabolic function. The test monitors sugar and protein levels in the blood, as well as fluid and electrolyte balance.

Synovial fluid analysis may be performed when there is suspected joint infection or septic arthritis. Joint aspiration is commonly performed along with intra-articular injections, where a sample of synovial fluid is removed before the injection of corticosteroid. In cases of significant swelling, the removal of excessive fluid can help reduce pain and improve motion. The joint aspirate can be visually examined or analyzed for white blood cell count, polymorphic nuclear cells, or cultured for the presence of other infectious organisms.

Radiographic Assessments

Radiographic images assist the rheumatologist in creating a differential diagnosis to rule out potential disorders including trauma, tumors, and skeletal dysplasia. Conventional radiographs were previously used to identify irreversible cartilage and bone damage. The emphasis on early treatment to suppress inflammation has encouraged radiographic tools that can identify joint inflammation and early soft-tissue changes. Evaluating radiographic images in children is challenging and requires an understanding of the normal growth-related joint changes. The immature skeleton is characterized by age-related changes to ossification centers, timing of growth plate closures, and alterations in bone shape and contours. These skeletal changes can be affected by acute and chronic inflammation.[29,30]

Conventional radiographs are still the most frequently used imaging tool at the time of diagnosis and provide a good baseline to assess future skeletal changes. A radiograph film can identify skeletal structures and contours, including periarticular osteoporosis, periosteal thickening, development and maturation of epiphyses and ossification centers, as well as ankylosis of spinal vertebrae. Bony changes related to arthritis are often seen late in the disease process and are generally irreversible.[31] Plain radiographs are limited in

their ability to identify active inflammation and changes to soft-tissue structures.[29] Assessment of the articular cartilage is made indirectly by measuring the empty space between two articulating bones (joint space narrowing). Radiographs may identify increased density in periarticular soft tissues that could be suggestive of inflammatory processes. For example, synovial fluid and pannus can be viewed as increased density in the infrapatellar and suprapatellar region of the knee.[29] It is difficult to use adult-validated radiograph scoring methods because the bony epiphyses in children are vascularized, allowing inflammation at the epiphyseal cartilage to spread to the ossification center.[32]

Plain radiographs can identify sites of ossifications and erosions at the site of tendon, ligaments, or capsular insertions onto bone that can suggest enthesis.[33] In children, it is difficult to identify radiographic changes at the spine and sacroiliac (SI) joint because the surface of these joints show little erosive change early in the disease process. Many bony abnormalities are easier to identify when visualizing both extremities simultaneously, which is easier when using plain radiograph.

Musculoskeletal ultrasound (MSUS) is being used increasingly by rheumatologists in the clinic. This procedure is cost-effective and safe when used to assess multiple joints during a clinic visit. In the absence of ionizing radiation, this imaging technique can be repeated frequently to monitor treatment effects. MSUS has been shown to be more accurate in identifying subclinical inflammation when compared to clinical joint assessment.[30,34] Doppler ultrasound can identify the volume of joint effusion and differentiate between hypervascular active synovitis and fibrotic pannus.[29] The ability to measure cartilage thickness is enhanced because of its high water content. Age-related normal standards for hyaline cartilage thickness have been published for several joints.[35] MSUS can also be used to diagnose enthesis and tenosynovitis. In a recent study, MSUS was 90% sensitive and 100% specific in the detection of effusion in active knee joints.[31] It is less sensitive in identifying effusion at the ankle.

Magnetic resonance imaging (MRI) can be used to assess all joint structures including those joints that are difficult to assess clinically (TMJ, hip, and SI joints). Unfortunately, it often requires sedation when used in younger children who are unable to remain motionless. It is more costly, and assessments must be limited to restrict radiation. When enhanced with gadolinium, tissue vascularity and capillary permeability can be quantified and used to discriminate between hypervascular active synovitis and fibrotic pannus.[30] MRI has detected subclinical synovitis in children who have satisfied the criteria set for remission. One benefit of MRI is the ability to identify bone marrow edema, which has been identified as a predictor of severe joint damage and disability in adults with RA. Inflammation within the bone marrow may induce central erosive changes in the trabecular bone. MRI is superior in detecting early erosive damage, but not all bone erosion is pathologic in pediatrics.[29]

Disease Activity Examination Tools

Historically, examination findings were recorded using a joint diagram or homunculus (Fig. 17.3) and also paper chart notes. This diagram became more difficult to use as paper charting moved to electronic formats. The need to track and quantify disease improvement for both clinical and research purposes has encouraged the development of validated outcome measures. There are now validated measures of disease activity, function, and child/parent-reported outcomes specific to JIA.[36]

Juvenile Arthritis Disease Activity Score

The Juvenile Arthritis Disease Activity Score (JADAS) was developed in 2009 as a composite score to track disease activity for use in both clinical and research settings.[37] This composite score includes four measures: physician's global assessment of disease activity measured using a 0 to 10 visual analog scale (VAS); parent global assessment of well-being measured on a 0 to 10 VAS; the ESR normalized to a 0 to 10 scale; and a count of joints with active disease. There are several versions of the JADAS that include different disease counts. The JADAS10 includes a count of any involved joint up to a maximum of 10 joints. The JADAS27 includes of count of the 27 selected joints chosen as a good representation of the disease. The JADAS71 includes 71 joints and was developed to be less restrictive, but does not include the thoracic and lumbar spine or the SI joints. This tool has been validated, and is often cited as an outcome measure in JIA publications.

This JADAS-CRP has been modified to substitute an ESR score with a CRP score.[38] Another modification for clinical use excludes the ESR or CRP, and is referred to as the clinical Juvenile Arthritis Disease Activity Score (cJADAS) or JADAS3-joint count. This modification was made because ESR or CRP may not be measured at each clinic visit.[39]

Criteria have been developed to classify JADAS composite scores into low and high disease activity states. For example, in children with oligoarticular JIA using the JADAS10 composite score, disease activity would be defined as inactive disease (≤1); low disease activity (1.1 to 2.0); moderate disease activity (2.1 to 4.2); and high disease activity (>4.2). For children with polyarticular JIA using the JADAS10 composite score, disease activity would be defined as inactive disease (≤1); low disease activity (1.1 to 3.8); moderate disease activity (3.9 to 10.5); and high disease activity (>10.5). Other disease activity ranges are published for the other JADASs.[36]

JADASs have also been used to define clinical meaningful improvement in disease activity for use in clinical trials. The absolute and percent improvement differs according to the child's baseline level of disease activity. For example, children in the low disease activity group would have an increase in absolute score of 4 or a 41% improvement to be defined as clinically meaningful. For moderate and high disease groups, an increase of 10 and 17 points or percent improvement of 53% and 57%, respectively, are suggestive of a clinically meaningful change.[36]

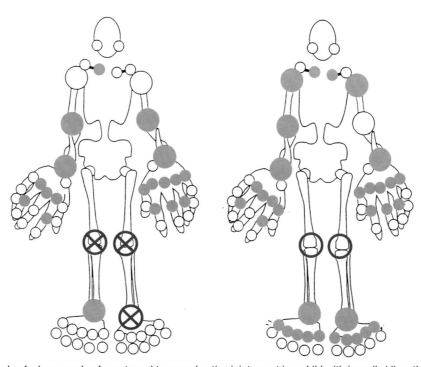

FIGURE 17.3. Example of a homunculus format used to record active joint count in a child with juvenile idiopathic arthritis. The left figure shows joints with an effusion (*solid circle*) or soft-tissue swelling (X). The right figure shows joints with pain or tenderness (*solid*). (From Wright V, Smith E. Physical therapy management of the child and adolescent with arthritis. In Walker J, Helewa A, eds. *Physical Therapy in Arthritis.* W.B. Saunders; 1996:211–244 with permission.)

American College of Rheumatology Criteria— Pediatric Score

The American College of Rheumatology (ACR) developed a set of criteria used to report disease activity in 1997.[40] The criteria include the physician global assessment of disease activity (10-point VAS), parent/child assessment of overall well-being (10-point VAS), functional ability, number of joints with active arthritis, number of joints with limited ROM, and ESR. An ACR Pediatric (Pedi) 30 is defined as at least a 30% improvement from baseline in three of six variables, with no more than one variable worsening by greater than 30%. A similar definition is used for the ACR Pedi 50%, 70%, 90%, and 100% improvement. A JIA disease "flare" is defined as worsening of two variables by at least 40% without improvement in more than one variable by at least 30%.[41] The ACR Pedi 30 criteria is accepted by the U.S. Food and Drug Administration (FDA) as outcome measures to assist the response to medical treatment in phase III clinical trials.

Juvenile Spondyloarthritis Disease Activity Index

The Juvenile Spondyloarthritis Disease Activity (JSpADA) Index was developed for use in 2014 for use in children with spondyloarthritis. Using the International League of Associations for Rheumatology (ILAR) criteria described later in this chapter, this would include children classified within the ERA, psoriatic arthritis, or undifferentiated arthritis groups. The composite score consists of eight items including active arthritis, active enthesitis, pain rating, morning stiffness, clinical sacroiliitis, uveitis, limited back mobility (Schober test <20 cm), and abnormal inflammatory markers. Each abnormal item is assigned a value of 1, making a range of scores from 0 (no active disease) to 8 (severe disease).[42]

Wallace Criteria for Disease Remission

Wallace et al. published a set of criteria to define inactive disease and remission in children with oligoarticular, polyarticular, and systemic juvenile idiopathic arthritis (sJIA; Display 17.1).[43] A child with JIA was defined as having inactive disease if they had no joints with active arthritis or systemic symptoms (fever, rash, serositis, splenomegaly, lymphadenopathy, or uveitis). These children should have a normal ESR and/or CRP. Their physician's global assessment of disease activity needs to indicate no disease activity (best score achievable). The authors also proposed two definitions for clinical remission. Clinical remission on medication was defined as inactive disease for a minimum of 6 continuous months while on medication. Children with clinical remission off medication had to meet the criteria for inactive disease for a minimum of 12 continuous months while off all anti-arthritis or uveitis medication. The criteria were modified in 2011 to improve the definitions of uveitis and ESR and include morning stiffness less than 15 minutes as an additional criterion for inactive disease.[44]

> **DISPLAY 17.1**   **Criteria for Inactive Disease and Disease Remission**
>
> 1. No joints with active arthritis
> 2. No systemic symptoms (fever, rash, serositis, splenomegaly, or lymphadenopathy)
> 3. No active uveitis
> 4. Normal ESR and/or CRP
> 5. Physician's global assessment of disease shows no disease activity.
> 6. Morning stiffness lasting <15 min
>
> **Criteria for Disease Remission**
> 1. Clinical remission on medications: Criteria for inactive disease must be met for a minimum of 6 consecutive months while the patient is on medications.
> 2. Clinical remission off medications: Criteria for inactive disease must be met for a minimum of 12 consecutive months while patient is off all anti-arthritis medications.
>
> Wallace CA, Giannini EH, Huang B, et al. American College of Rheumatology provisional criteria for defining clinical inactive disease in select categories of juvenile idiopathic arthritis. *Arthritis Care Res.* 2011;63:929–936.

Juvenile Arthritis Parent Assessment Index and Juvenile Arthritis Child Assessment Index

The Juvenile Arthritis Parent Assessment Index (JAPAI) and Juvenile Arthritis Child Assessment Index (JACAI) were developed to collect more information from parents and children regarding their JIA disease activity. Both tools include a 10-point visual analog global disease rating scale. Each scale also includes a 10-point visual analog pain rating. Parents are able to report physical function using the Child Health Activity Questionnaire (CHAQ) or the Juvenile Functionality Scale (JAFS), and the Child Health Questionnaire, or the Pediatric Rheumatology Quality of Life (PRQL) Scale, whereas children report on the JAFS and PRQL scales. The scores range from 0 to 30 to 0 to 40 depending on whether one or two physical function tools used.[45]

Juvenile Arthritis Damage Index

The Juvenile Arthritis Damage Index (JADI) was developed to assess articular and extra-articular joint damage in children with JIA using an observational score sheet.[46] *Damage* is defined as changes in the anatomy, physiology, pathology, or function present for at least 6 months, which was caused by active disease or the side effects of medication. The index includes an assessment of articular damage (JADI-A) and extra-articular damage (JADI-E). The JADI-A has a maximum score of 72 using defined deformities of the TMJ, cervical spine, and extremity joints. The JADI-E has a maximum score of 17 and includes defined damage to the ocular, nonarticular musculoskeletal, cutaneous, and endocrine systems. Singh and Aggarwal recommended

- Juvenile Arthritis Disease Activity Score with ESR (JADAS)
- Juvenile Arthritis Disease Activity Score with CRP (JADAS-CRP)
- American College of Rheumatology Criteria (ACR Ped#)
- Juvenile Spondyloarthritis Disease Activity Index (JSpADA)
- Juvenile Arthritis Parent Assessment Index (JAPAI)
- Juvenile Arthritis Child Assessment Index (JACAI)
- Physician global assessment of disease activity on a 10-cm VAS anchored by the words "remission" and "very severe" (MD Global)
- Parent or patient global assessment of overall well-being on a 10-cm VAS anchored by the words "very well" and "very poor" (Parent/Patient Global)
- Number of joints with active arthritis (joint count)
- Juvenile Functionality Scale (JAFS)

modifications to the index to include damage seen in patients with ERA.[47] They proposed inclusion of damage to the tarsal joints and lumbar spine on the JADI-AM and to include symptomatic cardiac dysfunction as part of the JADI-EM (Display 17.2).

Pharmacologic Treatment

Recent advances in medical treatment have significantly improved the prognosis and quality of life (QOL) for children with JIA. There is an emphasis on early and aggressive medical management to control inflammation and encourage disease remission. In this section, we outline the general classifications of medications used to treat children with JIA and describe some common examples. Not all arthritis drugs have been approved by the FDA for the treatment of JIA. We will go into more detail on the use of specific medications and outcomes for treatment when we review the specific JIA subgroups.

Nonsteroidal Anti-inflammatory Drugs

Nonsteroidal anti-inflammatory drugs (NSAIDs) are a class of drugs that block cyclooxygenase (COX)-1 and COX-2 enzymes that produce prostaglandins leading to inflammation. NSAIDs are prescribed to reduce pain, fever, and inflammation. Examples of NSAIDs include ibuprofen, naproxen, and meloxicam. In the past, these drugs were often used as a first line of treatment, especially in children with only a few inflamed joints. Research has now suggested that there is a window of opportunity directly following diagnosis to use disease-modifying drugs or biologics to get control of the inflammation and perhaps induce disease remission. The treatment benefits of using NSAIDs as a stand-alone therapy are minimal, and their chronic use does come with some risk.

Corticosteroids

Corticosteroids are still used for children with a more severe onset of their disease. However, this group of drugs can have significant side effects, especially when used over long periods of time. Corticosteroids are delivered in several forms including intra-articular injections, oral pills, intravenous (IV) pulses, and eye drops. Corticosteroids can be injected into an inflamed joint to avoid systemic side effects and encourage timely inflammatory control. In young children, intra-articular corticosteroids can help prevent LLDs when delivered at the onset of joint inflammation.[48]

Research suggests that triamcinolone hexacetonide (Aristospan) will have a longer effect on controlling inflammation than does triamcinolone acetonide (Kenalog).[49] In younger children, this treatment may require sedation, especially when performing multiple injections. When injecting the hip or TMJ, clinicians often rely on interventional radiology to guide them into the joint space. Immediately after the injection, children should be discouraged from excessive limb movement to avoid pushing the medication out of the joint. Intra-articular injections can cause hypopigmentation and/or atrophy of the subcutaneous fat at the injection site, leaving a noticeable demarcation. Other rare adverse events can include periarticular calcifications and avascular necrosis of the femoral head.[50] Following joint injection, most children feel a rapid and significant reduction in their pain and swelling. These treatment effects can last at least 4 months, buying time for other disease-modifying drugs to take effect.[51]

Chronic use of oral corticosteroids such as prednisolone or prednisone is discouraged secondary to their multiple side effects. These side effects include a cushingoid appearance and weight gain, growth disturbances, osteopenia, high blood pressure, insulin resistance, and behavioral issues. Oral steroids are most often used in cases with severe inflammation to achieve immediate relief of pain and swelling. This drug must be tapered or weaned down at a rate dependent on the duration of treatment to avoid adrenal crisis. Most rheumatologists try to wean children down to the lowest effect dose and try to discontinue steroids as soon as other medications appear to be as effective. Another way to mitigate side effects is to use periodic pulses of IV methylprednisolone. This is most often seen in children with severe disease who are already scheduled to receive other IV therapies. Children with uveitis are often treated with corticosteroid eye drops to reduce eye inflammation while receiving other systemic treatments.

Disease-Modifying Antirheumatic Drugs

The most commonly used treatment for all subgroups of JIA is methotrexate (MTX).[52] This drug is a chemotherapy drug that is used in smaller doses to inhibit inflammatory T-cell activation, downregulate B cells, and inhibit interleukin 1 (IL-1) receptor binding to suppress the immune system. MTX has been used for over 30 years in children with JIA with the goal of disease remission. It often takes

2 to 3 months for this drug to take effect, and may have more benefit when taken for longer periods. Therefore, corticosteroids or NSAIDs may be used in combination to provide some inflammatory control until MTX takes effect. This drug is given orally or by subcutaneous injection. The injection appears to have a better bioavailability with a greater treatment effect, but is often not tolerated by younger children.[53,54] Parents are instructed to give the injection, which is generally placed under the skin of the child's thigh or abdomen. Side effects can include gastrointestinal (GI) upset, and children may require additional nausea medication. Children should be prescribed folic acid to replace their folate production, which is suppressed while on MTX. Frequent monitoring of blood counts and liver enzymes are needed to minimize more significant side effects. New research suggests that children with a genetic SLCO1B1*14 allele may be less responsive to MTX.[8] This suggests that genetic factors may not only play a role in predisposing children to JIA but may also determine who will respond to a specific treatment.

Other disease-modifying antirheumatic drugs (DMARDs) used to treat JIA include sulfasalazine, used less frequently than is MTX, which is more effective in lower doses. Leflunomide has been shown to have effectiveness and safety profile similar to that of MTX, and is often used when the latter is not well tolerated. There are some concerns for the drug's long half-life in children with JIA. Other DMARDS including hydroxychloroquine (Plaquenil), cyclosporine, and azathioprine can be effective, but have increased risk for side effects.[52]

Biologics

Biologics are drugs that have a direct effect on the inflammatory pathway by blocking the effects of specific cytokines or immune cells. This class of drugs has had a significant effect on reducing disability in children and young adults with JIA. These drugs are highly effective and felt to be safe. Children may be asked to have a tuberculosis test before starting a biologic medication. Other contraindications for taking a biologic drug include bacterial, viral, or fungal infection; hepatitis B; HIV; diabetes; or heart disease. Children may need to temporarily discontinue a biologic drug when experiencing a significant infection or when undergoing surgery because these drugs lower the body's immunity. These drugs are not without some risk, including the development of malignancies.[55]

The most commonly used biologic is etanercept or ETN (Enbrel), which is a TNF inhibitor. This was the first biologic therapy approved in 1999 for the treatment of moderate to severe polyarticular disease in children aged 2 and older. The initial study used a drug-withdrawal design in 69 children with treatment-resistant disease.[56] ETN is delivered with a weekly subcutaneous injection and has since been approved for the treatment of other forms of JIA. Research suggests that ETN may be more effective if taken in combination with MTX.[57,58]

Other commercially available TNF inhibitors include adalimumab (Humira) and infliximab (Remicade). Adalimumab is a humanized IgG1 monoclonal antibody that binds to TNF-α. It was approved in 2008 for the treatment of children 2 years of age and older with polyarticular JIA.[59] The drug is delivered via a subcutaneous injection every other week. Similar to ETN, studies have suggested that the adalimumab is more effective in combination with MTX.[60] Infliximab is a chimeric human/mouse monoclonal antibody that binds to and blocks the action of TNF-α. It has not been approved by the FDA for JIA, but was approved for pediatric ulcerative colitis in children older than 6 years of age.[59] This drug is delivered by IV infusion over at least 2 hours every 2 to 8 weeks.[61] Infliximab is often used in combination with MTX for better efficacy.

Abatacept (Orencia) is another biologic that was approved for the treatment of children older than 6 years of age with JIA in 2008. Since that time, it has also been approved in children older than age 2 years. It is a human fusion protein that binds to CD80 and CD86 to inhibit T-cell activation. Initial studies suggested a beneficial response in biologic-naive patients, with less benefit in children who had failed treatment with an anti-TNF therapy. This drug can be taken along with MTX, and is administered by infusion every 2 to 4 weeks.[62]

For children who do not respond to anti-TNF therapy, tocilizumab (Actemra) has been shown to be very effective. It was approved for IV use in sJIA in 2011 and in polyarticular JIA in 2013.[59] Recently, a subcutaneous injection was approved in 2018, which makes this drug easier to administer. It is a humanized anti-human IL-6 receptor monoclonal antibody and, therefore, uses a different pathway to reduce inflammation than do the anti-TNF drugs.[63,64]

IL-1 cytokines are mediators of inflammation, and are significantly elevated in children with sJIA. Two anti-IL-1 receptor drugs have been developed for the treatment of sJIA. Ilaris (canakinumab) is an IL-β inhibitor that was approved in May 2013 for use in children 2 years of age and older with sJIA. It is delivered by a weekly subcutaneous injection. Anakinra (Kineret) is an IL-1 receptor antagonist that has been effective in children with sJIA and adult-onset Still disease. It was approved by the FDA in 2011 for children older than 18 years of age with adult RA.[59] Although it has not yet been approved for use in pediatrics, it has been used in research trials or as an off-label treatment in severe cases of sJIA. It is given daily as a subcutaneous injection and has side effects similar to that of other biologics. Both drugs have been shown to allow for the reduction of high doses of glucocorticosteroids in children with sJIA.[65]

≫ Classification and juvenile idiopathic arthritis subtypes

In 1995, based on expert opinion, the ILAR created a classification system consisting of eight subgroups. This was the first international classification system to define and group the heterogeneous patterns of disease.[1] The ultimate goal of classification criteria is for each disease type to be as homogeneous as possible and mutually exclusive of the other categories. The FDA and European authorities currently recognize these ILAR subgroups. Although these subgroups are currently in use, clinicians and scientists have begun to look more carefully at the genotypic data and biomarkers, as well as the similarities between adult and childhood disease patterns. Currently, the PRINTO is using systematic review and a Delphi panel to develop a new classification system based on updated science.[2] We start by reviewing the current ILAR classifications, which are summarized in Table 17.1. However, we also describe the scientific issues driving the work for future reclassification.

TABLE 17.1.	Classification Criteria, Frequency, Onset Age, and Sex Ratio for the International League of Associations for Rheumatology Categories of Juvenile Idiopathic Arthritis			
JIA Disease Type	Diagnostic Criteria	Frequency	Onset Age	Sex Ratio
Systemic arthritis	Arthritis in one or more joints with or preceded by fever for ≥2 weeks that is documented to be daily for ≥3 days, and accompanied by one or more of the following: 1. Evanescent erythematous rash 2. Generalized lymphadenopathy 3. Enlarged liver or spleen 4. Serositis Exclusions*,a–d	5%–15%	<16 years	F=M
Oligoarthritis	Arthritis in one to four joints during the first 6 months of disease; two categories are recognized: 1. Persistent: affecting no more than four joints throughout disease course 2. Extended: Affecting more than a total of four joints after the first 6 months of disease Exclusions*,a–e	30%–50%	Peak: 2–4 years	F>M (3:1)
Polyarthritis (RF-positive)	Arthritis affecting five or more joints during the first 6 months of disease; IgM RF detected in two or more tests at least 3 months apart during the first 6 months of disease Exclusions:a–c,e	2%–7%	Late childhood to early adolescence	F>M 2:1
Polyarthritis (RF-negative)	Arthritis affecting five or more joints during the first 6 months of disease; test finding for RF is negative. Exclusions:a–e	11%–28%	Early peak: 2–4 years Later peak: 6–12 years	F>M 2:1
Psoriatic arthritis	Arthritis and psoriasis t arthritis plus at least two of the following: 1. Dactylitis 2. Nail pitting or onycholysis abnormalities 3. Psoriasis in a first-degree relative Exclusions:b–e	2%–11%	Early peak: 2–4 years Later peak: 9–11 years	F>M
ERA	Arthritis and enthesitis, or arthritis or enthesitis plus at least two of the following: 1. Presence or history of sacroiliac joint tenderness and/or inflammatory lumbosacral pain 2. Presence of HLA-B27 antigen 3. Onset of arthritis in a male older than 6 years 4. Acute anterior uveitis 5. History of AS, ERA, sacroiliitis with inflammatory bowel disease, Reiter syndrome, or acute anterior uveitis in a first-degree relative Exclusions:a,d,e	15%–20%	Late childhood or adolescence	M: 2 to 1
Undifferentiated	Arthritis that does not fulfill criteria in one of the abovementioned categories or fulfills criteria in more than one category	11%–21%		

*Exclusion criteria reflect the principle of the International League of Associations for Rheumatology (ILAR) classification that all juvenile idiopathic arthritis (JIA) categories are mutually exclusive.
aPsoriasis or a history of psoriasis in the patient or first-degree relative
bArthritis in a human leukocyte antigen (HLA)-B27-positive male beginning after the sixth birthday
cAnkylosing spondylitis (AS), enthesitis-related arthritis (ERA), sacroiliitis with inflammatory bowel disease, Reiter syndrome, or acute anterior uveitis, or a history of one of these disorders in a first-degree relative
dPresence of immunoglobulin M (IgM) rheumatoid factor (RF) on at least two occasions at least 3 months apart
ePresence of systemic JIA in the patient
Source: Zeft A, Shear ES, Thompson SD, et al. Familial autoimmunity: maternal parent-of-origin effect in juvenile idiopathic arthritis. *Clin Rheumatol.* 2008;27:241–244.

Systemic Juvenile Idiopathic Arthritis

sJIA is characterized by systemic manifestations including recurrent spiking fevers that often precede the presence of joint arthritis. Unlike other forms of JIA, the disease is felt to be autoinflammatory rather than an autoimmune disease. Genetic and phenotypic characteristics are not similar to that of other subtypes of JIA, but rather consistent with adult Still disease.[2,65]

sJIA accounts for 5% to 15% of children diagnosed with JIA. There is no specific age of onset; however, it often occurs in children younger than 6 years of age.[66] The median age of onset is reported at 4.7 years, and the disease is evenly distributed between boys and girls.[67] sJIA occurs more frequently in non-Hispanic Caucasians; however, African Americans with sJIA tend to have more severe joint arthritis and longer periods of active disease.

Children with systemic arthritis present with fevers that spike greater than 39°C once or twice a day. These fevers are followed by periods where the child's temperature may drop below normal. The ILAR criteria require this fever to reoccur on at least 3 consecutive days for a minimum of 2 weeks. Children may have a single multiweek episode of spiking fevers before or with the onset of their arthritis, or they may have recurrent periods of fever. Children may also present with an evanescent erythematous rash lasting a few hours on their trunk or extremities. This rash often reoccurs while spiking a fever and then fades. If children do not present with a rash, they must exhibit lymph node enlargement, hepatomegaly, splenomegaly, or serositis to meet the ILAR diagnostic criteria.[1] Arthritis often develops following these systemic symptoms, and may involve one or more joints lasting for at least 6 weeks. Arthritis tends to evolve in a symmetric pattern and often includes the cervical spine, wrists, hips, and ankles. Children with sJIA present with a feeling of general malaise followed by periods of well-being (Fig. 17.4).

There are no conclusive laboratory tests for sJIA; however, CRP is often markedly elevated. Other common laboratory findings include elevation of the ESR and ferritin levels, with a decreased hemoglobin and albumin level. RF, ANAs, and HLAB27 generally return negative results. On initial evaluation, the rheumatologist must rule out systemic infections, malignancies, and other autoimmune conditions.

The disease course is variable, and has been described in four subgroups.[67] Some children have persistent active systemic disease and arthritis (7.5%). Other children have persistent systemic features without joint arthritis (5.1%). Systemic symptoms may subside after several months, leaving children with persistent polyarticular arthritis (32%). With aggressive medical treatment, children can present without systemic and arthritic disease (56%). Research suggests that the presence of increased IL-6 cytokines may be suggestive of more severe joint disease, whereas an increase in IL-18 can be suggestive of greater systemic complications including macrophage activation syndrome (MAS).[68]

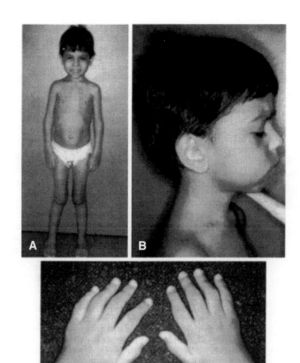

FIGURE 17.4. A: General appearance of systemic juvenile idiopathic arthritis (sJIA). **B:** Temporomandibular arthritis. **C:** Hands of a child with polyarticular arthritis.

Children with sJIA are at risk for developing MAS, an uncontrolled immune response caused by the activation of T lymphocytes and macrophages. This is a life-threatening medical condition that can occur in 7% to 13% of children with sJIA. The syndrome presents with a sustained fever and involves phagocytosis and intravascular coagulation, leading to high ferratin levels causing liver and central nerve system dysfunction.[69] Various triggers have been suggested including viral infection, change in drug treatment, or drug toxicity. Research suggests that children with increased levels of the IL-18 cytokines may be a greater risk for this severe complication.[68] The mortality rate for children with sJIA and MAS may be as high as 6%.[70]

Long-term outcomes for children with sJIA are variable, and children tend to fall into one of three groups. Some children have a self-limiting course or go into remission following medical treatment after one disease episode lasting up to 24 months. Another cohort of children has reoccurring disease flares along with months or years of inactive disease. The last group presents with chronic and persistent joint arthritis, leading to joint space narrowing and physical disability.[71]

If left untreated, sJIA has a poor prognosis, with greater joint erosion leading to more disability. Children diagnosed before 2 years of age or with systemic disease duration longer than 6 months have the poorest outcomes. Historically, children with sJIA have been treated with chronic glucocorticosteroids and suffer from their side effects. These children often have the growth disturbances that may be related to the inflammatory process, nutrition, immobilization, and the effects of steroid treatment. As described previously, inflammation in young children cause epiphyseal plate disturbance and skeletal deformity. Joint space narrowing and erosion can lead to the need for premature joint replacement in teens or young adults with sJIA. Before the development of biologic drugs, about 75% of children with sJIA required a prosthetic joint in young adulthood.[72]

In 2012, the Childhood Arthritis and Rheumatology Research Association (CARRA) published a consensus for treatment of children with sJIA. They proposed four clinical pathways using glucocorticosteroids, MTX, IL-1 antagonists (anakinra), and IL-6 antagonists (tocilizumab).[73] Treatments targeting IL-1 and IL-6 have been shown to be very effective in treating systemic disease. The German Biologics Registry (BIKER) study followed up 245 children with sJIA who had been treated with biologics following early glucocorticosteroids. The authors reported that about 50% of children were in remission at 6 months following treatment with anti-IL drugs. Most of the subjects (about 66%) had minimal or no active disease. Children taking tocilizumab reported more adverse events than those on anakinra or canakinumab. ETN had less effect, with children observed to have a greater number of active joints than those treated with anti-IL therapies.[74]

Early studies using IL antagonists enrolled subjects with chronic sJIA who had failed other forms of treatment. Since that time, several studies have looked at the use of anakinra as a monotherapy. One study of 46 newly diagnosed children initially treated with anakinra reported inactive disease in 60% of children, with only 11% having chronic synovitis.[75] The use of anakinra at the onset of disease in these studies appears to have decreased the percentage of children with chronic unremitting arthritis from 50% to 10% to 30%, while also limiting the need for glucocorticosteroids and their side effects.[76] In 2013, the ACR reviewed the literature and updated their recommendations, suggesting a role for anakinra as an initial therapy in those with at least one active joint.[77]

The ACR review recommends the use of tocilizumab as an option for children with active disease who have not responded to treatment with anakinra or glucocorticosteroids. A phase 3 randomized control trial (RCT) of tocilizumab demonstrated treatment efficacy in children who had not responded to glucocorticosteroids.[64] After 1 year, 48% of these children had no active arthritis and many had discontinued steroid treatment. The authors reported that 80% of these children had at least 70% improvement in their disease scores. There were more infections in the tocilizumab group when compared to the control. More adverse events were also reported in the German BIKER study in subjects on tocilizumab.[74] Remission in children with sJIA who were followed up between 2005 and 2010 was 22% in the first year and 87% at 5 years. Authors calculated the probability of discontinuing all treatment was 0.613 within 5 years of disease onset.[78]

Although sJIA has been described as an autoinflammatory process, Ombrello et al. has recently linked the genetic risk for sJIA to a specific MHC II haplotype on chromosome 6, with an association with two specific alleles of HLA-DRB1*11.[79] This type of linkage is generally related to autoimmune pathways. Nigrovic suggests that sJIA may have a biphasic mechanism, whereby the onset of the disease is driven by autoinflammatory processes causing fever and rashes (systemic phase).[14,76] He hypothesizes that elevated levels of cytokines may eventually push the T-cell regulatory system out of balance, supporting an autoimmune response and chronic arthritis (articular phase). His hypothesis supports the early use of anti-IL drugs to suppress the initial autoinflammatory pathway that could then prevent the development of autoimmunity and chronic arthritis. A better understanding of the genetics and disease pathology will lead to improved treatment strategies for children with sJIA.

Oligoarticular Arthritis

Oligoarticular juvenile idiopathic arthritis (oligoJIA) is defined by the ILAR as arthritis in four or fewer joints during the first 6 months of their disease. In earlier classifications, this subgroup was called *pauciarticular arthritis*. Most children (27% to 56%) diagnosed with JIA have an oligoarticular onset with an asymmetric pattern of lower extremity joint arthritis. The knee is the most common joint (85%) (Fig. 17.5), but children can also present with arthritis at the ankle (33%), wrist (9%), or hand (7%). Children are generally female, with a mean age of onset of 4.9 years.[80] The ILAR criteria recognized two separate groups of children with oligoJIA, persistent and extended.

Children who are younger than 6 years of age and present with arthritis in a single knee generally respond well to treatment, but should also be screened for eye disease (Fig. 17.6). These children comprise 30% to 50% of children with oligoJIA, and often present to a pediatrician orthopedist who must rule out trauma or infection.[81] Children are usually started on NSAIDs before being referred to a rheumatologist.

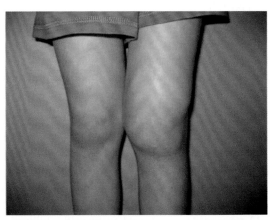

FIGURE 17.5. An older child with asymmetric oligoarticular arthritis.

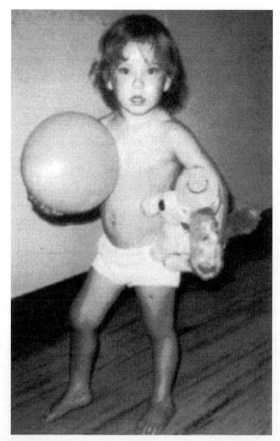

FIGURE 17.6. A younger child with asymmetric oligoarticular juvenile idiopathic arthritis (JIA) resulting in a leg length discrepancy (LLD).

Intra-articular corticosteroid injections along with NSAIDs are the first line of therapy in this subgroup. Early use of steroid injections decreases joint inflammation, inhibits the growth effects at the epiphyseal plate, and reduces the development of contractures.[50] Following intra-articular injections, remission of joint arthritis was reported in 67% to 82% of children followed up at 6-months with inflammatory remission lasting for 10 to 28 months.[50] Children who do not respond to joint injections can have persistent disease and require additional treatment with MTX or ETN.

Other children with an oligoarticular onset (10% to 50%) have disease activity that "extends" into multiple joints after the first 6 months. Children who present with a symmetric joint pattern or have arthritis in a wrist, hand, or ankle joint are at higher risk to extend into a polyarticular course. These children often have elevated inflammatory markers (ESR) and are ANA positive. Extension to a polyarticular course can occur several years after the disease onset. Children with an extended disease course have a poorer outcome, and are often started on a TNF inhibitor along with MTX. Their disease prognosis is similar to that of the polyarticular RF–negative subgroup.

ANA positivity can be used to identify children who are at risk for developing uveitis. One form of this eye condition, chronic anterior uveitis, is identified in 30% of high-risk children and remains asymptomatic. When untreated, this form of uveitis may cause cataracts, glaucoma, or vision loss. Those at higher risk include children with oligoarticular and polyarticular RF–negative arthritis who are ANA positive and younger than 7 years of age at the onset of their disease. The ACR has recommended that high-risk children have an ophthalmic examination using a slit lamp every 3 months.[82] Children in the lower risk category can be screened every 6 to 12 months. Treatment of uveitis includes the use of prednisolone acetate topical drops in addition to the child's disease-modifying therapies including MTX and TNF inhibitors.[52]

Disease remission in children with oligoJIA who were followed up between 2005 and 2010 was 32% in the first year and 94% at 5 years. Authors reported a probability of 0.807 of discontinuing all treatment within 5 years of disease onset.[78] This classification is based on a clinical phenotype, and is currently being challenged on the basis of evolving knowledge of genetics and biomarkers. Genetic HLA associations for HLA-DRB1 are similar in both oligoarticular and RF-negative polyarticular subgroups. Both groups are at risk for uveitis and positive ANA titers. The increased use of ultrasound may identify additional joints with subclinical inflammation that could decrease the incidence of oligoJIA based on joint number classification.[30]

Polyarticular Rheumatoid Factor–Negative Juvenile Idiopathic Arthritis

Polyarticular RF–negative juvenile idiopathic arthritis (PolyRF-JIA) is defined in the ILAR classification as arthritis in five or more joints during the first 6 months of their disease. Children in this group must have a negative RF test finding. Other exclusions include a history of psoriasis, enthesitis, sacroiliitis, ankylosing spondylitis, inflammatory bowel disease, Reiter syndrome, acute anterior uveitis, or a history of one of these disorders in a first-degree relative.[1] Arthritis in an HLA-B27 male older than 6 years of age would also be excluded. This subgroup accounts for 11% to 28% of all children with JIA.

Within the PolyRF-JIA group are two subgroups based on a positive or negative ANA titer. These two groups are reported to be significantly different.[83] PolyRF-negative groups with a positive ANA titer are similar to those with extended oligoJIA disease. These children are generally female, younger than 6 years of age, and are at higher risk for chronic anterior uveitis. They demonstrate an asymmetric pattern of arthritis, often in fewer than 10 joints. Common joints include the knee (90%), ankle (59%), proximal interphalangeal (PIP) joint (30%), and wrist (25%). This ANA-positive subgroup has a genetic association with HLA-DRB1, which is also seen in early-onset oligoJIA.[84] The PRINTO has recommended reclassifying children with a positive ANA titer into their own subgroup regardless of the number of joints involved at disease onset or a family history of psoriasis.[2]

Children with polyRF-JIA having an ANA-negative titer are less likely to be female, and are slightly older than 6 years of age at the onset of their disease. Similar to the ANA-positive groups, these children generally have an asymmetric disease pattern. ANA-negative children often have more joints involved, including the knee (81%), ankle (57%), wrist (47%), PIP joint (41%), metacarpophalangeal (MCP; 31%), hip (30%), and elbow (26%). Forty percent of these children have radiographic joint changes.[83] These ANA-negative children have disease similar to seronegative adults with RA.[84]

CARRA has recommended that children with polyRF-JIA initiate therapy with MTX using intra-articular joint injections in cases of low disease activity. Children with moderate/high disease who do not initially respond to MTX were encouraged to add a biologic. Children who do not respond to a TNF inhibitor could be transitioned to abatacept or tocilizumab.[85] Disease remission in children with polyRF-JIA who were followed up between 2005 and 2010 was 25% in the first year and 86% at 5 years. The probability of discontinuing medical treatment was 0.549 within 5 years of disease onset.[78]

Polyarticular Rheumatoid Factor–Positive Juvenile Idiopathic Arthritis

Polyarticular RF–positive juvenile idiopathic arthritis (PolyRF+JIA) is defined in the ILAR classification as arthritis in five or more joints during the first 6 months. Children in this group must have a positive RF on at least two occasions more than 3 months apart. Children also exhibit positive ACPAs, a highly sensitive test for adults and children with RF-positive arthritis that is correlated with more aggressive disease.[28]

Polyarticular RF–positive arthritis accounts for 2% to 7% of all children with JIA. These children are generally adolescent females with a clinical phenotype similar to that of those with RF with a younger disease onset (16 to 29 years).[7] This disease is characterized by symmetric polyarticular arthritis affecting the smaller joints of the hands and feet along with rheumatoid nodules on the forearm and elbow in about 33% of those.[81] Larger joints and the cervical spine and TMJ can also be involved with more aggressive and erosive disease.

CARRA has recommended early and aggressive treatment for children with polyRF-positive disease. Children with ACPAs may be encouraged to initiate therapy with a biologic and DMARD combination.[85] Historically, drug-free remission in this subgroup was rarely reported, and children were generally transitioned to adult care.[84] Disease remission in children with polyRF+JIA who were followed up between 2005 and 2010 was 31% in the first year and 93% at 5 years. The probability of discontinuing all treatment was 0.078 within 5 years of disease onset.[78]

Enthesitis-Related Arthritis

ERA is defined in the ILAR classification as arthritis with enthesitis, or one of these symptoms in the presence of two of the following: (1) SI tenderness or inflammation; (2) presence of the HLA-B27 antigen; (3) onset of arthritis in males older than 6 years of age; (4) acute anterior uveitis; and (5) history of ankylosing spondylitis, ERA, sacroiliitis with inflammatory bowel disease, Reiter syndrome, or acute anterior uveitis in a first-degree relative.[1] This disease subtype includes children who would have previously been classified as having "juvenile spondyloarthropathy." A larger juvenile spondyloarthritis group includes children with ERA, undifferentiated arthritis, psoriatic arthritis, and inflammatory bowel disease–related arthritis. This larger group is genetically similar to that of adult spondyloarthritis.[84,86]

ERA accounts for 15% to 20% of all children with JIA in the United States. It is the most common subtype (40%) of JIA in Asia.[87] Children are generally boys (60% to 86%), with an age of onset between 8 and 13 years.[86,87] Children often report having enthesitis that is defined as inflammation at the bony attachment site of a tendon, ligament, or joint capsule. Common sites of enthesitis are illustrated in Figure 17.7 and include the patellar ligament insertion at the inferior pole of the patella (50%), as well as the attachment of the Achilles (22%) and the plantar fascia (38%) to the calcaneus. Enthesitis can be confirmed using ultrasound. When untreated, inflammation at the bony insertion can cause erosion, osteopenia, soft-tissue calcification, and bone spurs.[88]

Children with ERA initially present with asymmetric arthritis in less than five joints involving the hips, knees, and ankles. Inflammation of the small joints of the midfoot is also common, although rarely reported in other subtypes. Radiographic evidence of sacroiliitis has been reported in 30% to 50% of children at diagnosis, with the incidence increasing over the duration of the disease. Sacroiliitis is reported as lower back pain and stiffness that improves with activity. Physical examination can identify tenderness on direct palpation or a positive Patrick test finding. Children should be monitored for subtle losses in joint motion and tissue extensibility in the hips and spine. Clinicians may use measurements of lumbar forward or lateral flexion to monitor disease activity. A modified Schober test measures changes in lumbar flexion and is considered abnormal when less than 21 cm (<6 cm of lower lumbar flexion). Ultrasound and MRI are recommended for diagnosis and longer term follow-up of SI and spinal disease. Inflammation can develop into spondylitis and ankylosis of the spinal vertebrae over time.[86]

A positive test finding for HLA-B27 antigens is present in 70% to 80% of children with ERA. However, the presence of this antigen in healthy children is not predictive of future disease. About 20% of these have a family history of HLA-B27–associated disease. Children with ERA are also at risk for acute anterior uveitis, which is symptomatic including pain and photophobia. This form of uveitis occurs in about 30% of children with ERA and is often recurrent.[89]

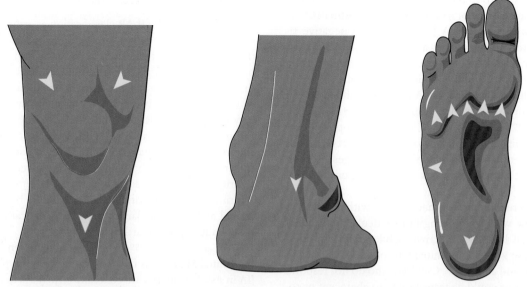

FIGURE 17.7. The most common sites of tenderness associated with enthesitis in the knees, ankles, and feet.

Over time, acute anterior uveitis can lead to cataracts, glaucoma, and visual loss. The influence of abnormalities of the gut biome are also being investigated in children with ERA.[90,91]

CARRA has published recommendations for treatment of children with active sacroiliitis. They have strongly recommended the initial use of NSAIDs. In children who do not respond to NSAIDs, they recommend the addition of a TNF inhibitor. ERA is a diagnosis where the use of sulfasalazine has been recommended as the DMARD of choice over MTX. In some cases, intra-articular glucocorticosteroid injections into the SI or hip joint may be considered as a bridging treatment.[4]

Children with ERA have significant pain intensity and functional limitations when compared to other subtypes.[12] Before the use of biologics, less than 20% of those with ERA were reported to achieve remission.[86] Shih et al. reported a 33% remission rate in their ERA cohort in which 78% of children had been treated with a TNF inhibitor.[88] Disease remission in children with ERA who were followed up between 2005 and 2010 was 37% in the first year and 96% at 5 years. The probability of discontinuing all treatment was 0.712 within 5 years of disease onset.[78]

Psoriatic Arthritis

Psoriatic arthritis is defined in the ILAR classification as arthritis with psoriasis or two of the following: (1) dactylitis (Fig. 17.8), (2) nail pitting or onycholysis, and (3) family history of psoriasis in a first-degree relative.[1] Psoriasis often precedes the onset of arthritis by up to 15 years. Children diagnosed with juvenile psoriatic arthritis (JPsA) account for 2% to 11% of all children with JIA. There is a debate on the homogeneity of this subgroup and whether it should be a

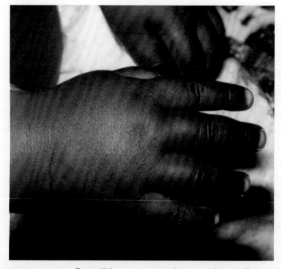

FIGURE 17.8. Dactylitis represents the combined effects of arthritis and tenosynovitis, and is characterized by swelling of one or more digits that extends beyond the joint margins. (Courtesy of Thomas D. Thacher, MD.)

distinct classification. In their 2019 publication, the PRINTO group was unable to reach consensus on how best to classify children with JPsA.[2]

Previous researchers have identified two subgroups differing in the age of disease onset with a peak below age 6 years and another after 10 years of age.[92] A younger cohort consists of females (76%) diagnosed before 6 years of age. Children present with dactylitis (63%), which is a combination of joint arthritis and tenosynovitis. It presents as swelling of a digit that extends beyond the joint margin. Children exhibit polyarticular onset (20%) with a positive ANA titer (64%). An ANA-positive titer increases the risk of chronic anterior uveitis in this young population. This subgroup of children has been compared with those in the oligoJIA and polyRF-JIA subgroup with an ANA-positive titer.[93,94] However, other studies have suggested that the JPsA subgroup is slightly older, with more frequent involvement of the wrist and hand.[95] The second JPsA subgroup has a later onset, with a more even distribution between males and females. They were more likely to exhibit psoriasis (31%), enthesitis (57%), nail pitting (38%), and axial disease (26%).[92]

Children with JPsA are initially treated with MTX, with a TNF inhibitor added if needed for disease control. In a CARRA 1-year follow-up study, 48% of subjects exhibited no active arthritis, whereas the number of subjects with polyarticular disease (62%) decreased to (10%) because they had a reduced number of active joints. Subjects also had improvements in other variables including nail pitting, dactylitis, psoriasis, enthesitis, sacroiliitis, and uveitis. Disease remission in children with JPsA who were followed up between 2005 and 2010 was 37% in the first year and 94% at 5 years. The authors reported the probability of discontinuing all treatment as 0.739 within 5 years of disease onset.[78]

Undifferentiated Arthritis

The ILAR criteria assign children who do not meet the criteria for the previously described subgroups as undifferentiated arthritis. This group includes 11% to 21% of children with JIA.[1,81] Disease remission in children with undifferentiated arthritis who were followed up between 2005 and 2010 was 24% in the first year and 91% at 5 years. The probability of discontinuing all medical treatment was 0.587 within 5 years of disease onset.[78]

» Other rheumatic diseases

Juvenile Myositis and Juvenile Dermatomyositis

Juvenile myositis (JM), JDM, or juvenile polymyositis (JPM) is a series of diagnoses that features inflammation of the muscle tissue and blood vessels of the muscles and skin. Common symptoms feature several types of skin rashes and also muscle weakness, particularly of the proximal muscles (abdominals, hip flexors, neck flexors, shoulder flexors).[96–98] See Figure 17.9 for a description of common skin symptoms. Secondary symptoms include fever, calcinosis, GI complications, contractures, joint pain, and lipodystrophy. This disease is diagnosed in only two to four children per million in the United States each year, and occurs in girls twice as often as in boys. Diagnostic measures include a physical examination, a blood test that looks at muscle enzymes (creatine kinase [CK], aldolase, lactate dehydrogenase [LDH], aspartate aminotransferase [AST], and alanine aminotransferase [ALT])

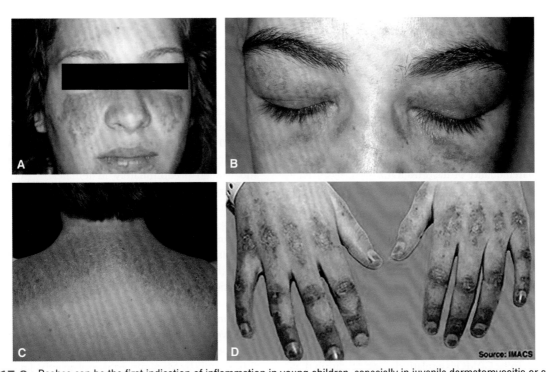

FIGURE 17.9. Rashes can be the first indication of inflammation in young children, especially in juvenile dermatomyositis or systemic lupus erythematosus. Rashes can also indicate disease flares in these individuals. They may be painful or itchy and are worsened with sun exposure. **A:** Malar rash or butterfly rash is a red or purplish rash on the cheeks and bridge of nose. **B:** Heliotrope rash is a red or purple rash often on eyelids that is sometimes accompanied by swelling. **C:** Heliotrope rash can also present on chest or back and is referred to as *shawl sign* or *V-sign*. **D:** Gottron papules are raised bumps that are sometimes scaly. They are generally on fingers, elbows, and sometimes on knees.

as well as ANAs, immune activation, and/or blood vessel damage. MRI or muscle biopsy may also be utilized to look for muscle tissue damage. Recently, myositis-specific antibodies have been identified in 60% to 70% of children with JM.

There is currently no cure for JM, but the disease can go into remission with proper medical treatment. Socioeconomic status and ethnicity were found to be associated with poor outcome and increased functional morbidity.[99] The first line of treatment is often glucocorticosteroids and MTX. The addition of hydroxychloroquine (Plaquenil) is used in the presence of predominant skin disease. For persistent disease, treatment may include intravenous immunoglobulin (IVIG), cyclosporine, or mycophenolate mofetil (MMF).[100] Protection from the sun, specifically ultraviolet B (UVB) rays, is essential, because exposure can trigger an immune response, activate the disease, and will worsen rashes.[98]

A physical therapist evaluating a child with JM should look closely at muscle strength, endurance, and ROM. There are two standardized measures that have been validated specifically in the JM population. One is called the Manual Muscle Test-8 (MMT8), a selection of eight muscles that are most often impacted which are graded on a scale of 0 to 10.[101] The second is the 14-item Childhood Myositis Assessment Scale (CMAS), which includes timed measures graded on the quality of antigravity movements.[102] Other functional assessments, such as a timed run, two-footed jump, or single-leg hop can pick up subtle strength discrepancies. ROM should also be screened for muscle tightness or contractures.

Physical therapists play a valuable role in both notifying the rheumatology team about changes in disease activity and providing children and families with useful tools to increase their PA. Exercise in children with JM is safe; it has been shown to reduce inflammation, combat weakness and contractures, and manage the stress that comes with living with chronic disease.[103–105] Similar to JIA, children with JM can be physically active during both active and nonactive disease periods.[106] They can make improvements in strength, function, aerobic conditioning, bone mass, disease activity, and health-related quality of life (HRQOL).

Chronic Recurrent Multifocal Osteomyelitis

CRMO or chronic nonbacterial osteomyelitis (CNO) is a rare autoinflammatory disease featuring pain and inflammation within one or more bones that is not the result of bacterial infection or malignancy. Pain, tenderness, and, sometimes, swelling are the most common signs and symptoms, and are a result of overactive osteoclasts that are damaging the healthy bone tissue. Secondary symptoms occur as a result of the bone damage and include high risk for fracture, LLD, and bony deformity. CRMO is a relatively rare condition that is not yet well understood. Incidence rates were previously believed to be 0.4 out of 100,000 people per year, but this rate appears to be increasing as medical professions learn more.[107] Diagnosis is one of exclusion, resulting in the need for physical examination, blood examination, and several

sources of imaging or biopsy. Girls are affected more often than are boys, with the average age of diagnosis occurring around 9 or 10 years. CRMO is most common in the long bones, such as in the tibia and femur, as well as in the thoracic spine and clavicle.[108] Clinical examination most often identifies signs and symptoms in the tibia and clavicle. Although there is no cure, CRMO is treated to reduce inflammation, minimize pain, and prevent bone damage. Rheumatologists often begin with an NSAID, but may also prescribe MTX, sulfasalazine, corticosteroids, or TNF inhibitors. In cases where the spine is involved, children may also be treated with bisphosphonates.[109]

As a physical therapist, your role is to minimize disability and maximize function. Similar to other chronic diseases, HRQOL, severity of disability, and degree of deconditioning are closely related to the duration of active disease in an individual.[110] Children with CRMO may require mobility aids, such as a walker or wheelchair, to keep them independent and active during lesion flares. Monitoring of joint mobility and prescription of a home stretching program to prevent contractures secondary to muscle guarding may also be beneficial. Bone-strengthening activities will be essential once lesions have healed, but special caution should be taken to reduce risk for fractures.

Lupus Erythematosus

SLE describes an autoimmune disease where one's body attacks its own organs, resulting in systemic inflammation and multisystem organ dysfunction.[111] Lupus derives from a combination of epigenetic and environmental exposures and risk factors, and can affect many different body systems. Common symptoms include fatigue, fever, joint pain and swelling, malar rash, skin lesions, Raynaud phenomenon, shortness of breath, and headaches.[112,113]

Lupus is diagnosed in children at a rate of 0.3 to 0.9 per 100,000 per year at a median age of onset between 11 and 12 years. SLE primarily impacts non-Caucasian children, and is seen predominately in females.[111] Because of the large array of symptoms and system involvement, physical examination, laboratory values, and other exclusion tests may be required to confirm a diagnosis of SLE. Glucocorticosteroids remain a first line of treatment in SLE; children may also be prescribed hydroxychloroquine, which is effective but has retinal toxicity. Azathioprine is a DMARD used more frequently in SLE than is MTX. Severe disease is treated with MMF, cyclophosphamide, and rituximab (Rituximab).[114]

Lower PA levels, decreased measures of physical fitness, and poor HRQOL have been documented in people with SLE. A study by Margiotta et al. looked at PA levels in children with SLE and found that only 40% met the World Health Organization (WHO) recommendation for PA (150 minutes of moderate-to-vigorous-intensity or 75 minutes of vigorous-intensity activity per week).[115] Sule and Fontaine found that 89% of children with SLE had body fat percentages greater than the recommended value of 30%, with 40% of all participants exhibiting low muscle mass.[116] Pinto et al. compared subjects with SLE to healthy controls and matched them by their inactivity levels, finding that those with SLE had lower levels of aerobic capacity and poorer HRQOL.[117] Fortunately, a systematic review by O'Dwyer et al. proposed exercise as an important and safe intervention in the management of cardiovascular disease, mental health, fatigue, and function in individuals with lupus.[118] Physical therapists play a crucial role in educating children and families on the role of exercise and PA to improve physical function and enhance overall well-being.

Scleroderma

Localized scleroderma (LoS), also known as morphea, is a connective tissue disease in which the immune system malfunctions and causes dysfunction of the fibroblasts. This results in inflammation, abnormal collagen deposition, and fibrosis of the skin and underlying tissues. There are five subtypes of LoS, with linear scleroderma being the most common type seen in pediatrics (65% to 85%).[119] In linear scleroderma, sclerotic plaques are most often seen on the extremities and the head. These plaques can be painful, erythemic, and cause itching when active with dormant lesions, resulting in hair loss, altered pigmentation, and subcutaneous atrophy.[120] Sclerotic skin does not heal as well as healthy skin and has increased risk of developing skin cancer, so extra care is required.[121] Secondary symptoms arise based on the location of these plaques. Common complications include joint contractures, arthritis, and pain. Inflammation and vasculopathy can also affect other systems in the body, such as GI reflux, renal crisis, and dental anomalies.[121]

LoS is diagnosed in 0.4 to 3 per 100,000 children per year, with girls being diagnosed more than twice as often as boys, and Caucasian children being diagnosed significantly more often than any other ethnicity.[122] Children are initially diagnosed around 5 to 9 years of age, and this is done through a detailed history, physical examination, and possible skin biopsy or dermoscopy.[120]

There is no cure for LoS, so treatment is geared toward minimizing inflammation and reducing impairment. Treatment for LoS can involve systemic medications similar to those of other inflammatory diseases (corticosteroids, TX, hydroxychloroquine), but is more often addressed using topical medications and UV light or laser treatments. Typical disease course is 2 to 5 years; however, relapse rate is relatively high.[121] Physical therapy is commonly prescribed for anyone with a lesion that crosses a joint and is beneficial to address muscle weakness, pain, and decreased ROM to minimize functional damage.[122] Physical therapists may also support children following orthopedic or plastic surgery intervention, which may be indicated in severe cases to manage secondary impairments of joint contractures or limb length discrepancy.

» Physical therapy management

The World Health Organization International Classification of Functioning, Disability, and Health (ICF) provides a framework to help the physical therapist synthesize the medical history with the physical therapy evaluation, to identify and prioritize functional problems and impairments, and develop family-oriented treatment goals. Disease type and course, current and anticipated problems, as well as personal and environmental factors are considered. Because few studies provide strong evidence for the effectiveness of any particular intervention, the physical therapist must often draw from literature in other areas to develop the POC.

A top-down approach, beginning with the child's activities and participation, allows the therapist to focus the physical examination on areas that most impact the child's participation in home, school, and community settings. The therapist must be alert to changes in joint mobility and integrity or loss of muscle bulk and strength that signal a disease flare or joint damage. The child's age, cognitive development, and emotional development must also be considered as well as the amount of support and resources available to the family. Figure 17.10 provides an example of examination findings in the context of the ICF model.

Examination of Activities and Participation

The impact of JIA on a child's daily activities and participation depends on disease type, course, and severity. Lower extremity arthritis may cause difficulty in transitional movements, stair negotiation, school and community ambulation, as well as participation in recreational activities. Children with disease onset at a young age may demonstrate subtle motor deficits in balance, coordination, agility, and speed.[123] Chronic arthritis, pain, and stiffness in the cervical spine and upper limbs may cause difficulties with basic activities of daily living (ADLs) including dressing, grooming, and handwriting. The child's personality and drive to be independent, as well as the expectations of caregivers and friends impact the child's functional performance and adaptation to a chronic disease.

Standardized Outcome Measures

Standardized outcome measures are validated tools that can help quantify a child's ability to participate in functional or leisurely activities. Self—or parent—as proxy report questionnaires, including the Childhood Health Assessment Questionnaire (CHAQ), Pediatric Outcomes Data Collection Instrument (PODCI), and the Activities Scale for Kids (ASK) measure the child's capability during a defined period of time (e.g., previous 1 to 2 weeks). The ASK also measures the child's performance (what he or she *actually did* during the defined time period). Only one measure, the Juvenile Arthritis Functional Assessment Scale (JAFAS), assesses the child's functional capacity under standardized conditions. Other outcome tools that may not be specific to JIA may also be useful to monitor functional changes and develop an appropriate therapy POC (Table 17.2).

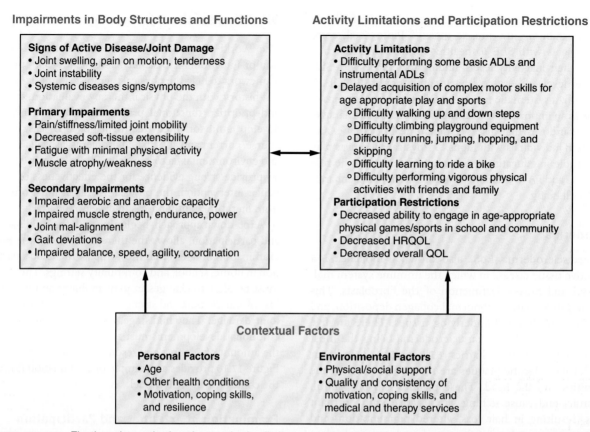

FIGURE 17.10. The therapist synthesizes the examination findings and information from the medical history and interview with the parent and child, analyzes the data, and formulates hypotheses regarding the relationship between disease status, impairments, and activity limitations. ADLs, activities of daily living; HRQOL, health-related quality of life; QOL, quality of life.

Childhood Health Assessment Questionnaire

The CHAQ is the most frequently used validated measure of disability in JIA and has been translated in more than 40 languages as well as adapted for cultural differences.[124] It was originally adapted from the Stanford Health Assessment Questionnaire (Display 17.3)[125]. Limitations of the test include a high ceiling effect, although the revised CHAQ38 has been found to improve this[126] (Display 17.4). The original CHAQ targets children aged 1 to 19 years and includes 30 activities organized into eight categories. Pain intensity over the past week is also assessed, resulting in nine total categories.

TABLE 17.2.	Standardized Assessment Instruments in Juvenile Idiopathic Arthritis		
Level of ICF	Instrument	Outcome Measured	Reference
A&P, I	CHAQ	BADLs and IADLs, pain, overall health status	Singh et al.[125]
A&P	ASK	BADLs, IADLs, play, transfers	Young et al.*
A	JAFAS	BADLs, IADLs (observed performance of activities under standardized conditions)	Lovell et al.[132]
A&P, I	JAQQ	BADLs, IADLs, pain, HRQOL	Degotardi[133]
A&P, I	PedsQL	BADLs, IADLs, pain, HRQOL	Varni et al.[134]
QOL	QOML scale	Overall and HRQOL	Gong et al.[135]
A&P, QOL	PROMIS	BADLs, IADLs, pain, anxiety, fatigue, HRQOL	Brandon et al.[129]

*Available at http://www.activitiesscaleforkids.com/
A, activity; ASK, Activities Scale for Kids; BADLs, basic activities of daily living; CHAQ, Childhood Arthritis Health Questionnaire; HRQOL, health-related quality of life; I, impairment; IADLs, instrumental activities of daily living; ICF, World Health Organization International Classification of Functioning, Disability, and Health; JAFAS, Juvenile Arthritis Functional Assessment Scale; JAQQ, Juvenile Arthritis Quality of Life Questionnaire; P, participation; PedsQL, Pediatric Quality of Life Questionnaire; PROMIS, Patient-Reported Outcomes Measurement Information System; QOML, Quality of My Life Questionnaire.

In this section, we are interested in learning how your child's illness affects his or her ability to function in daily life. Please feel free to add any comments on the back of this page. In the following questions, please check the one response that best describes your child's usual activities (averaged over an entire day) *over the past week*. If your child has difficulty in doing a certain activity or is unable to do it because he or she is too young but NOT because he or she is *restricted by arthritis*, please mark it as "Not Applicable." *Only note those difficulties or limitations that are due to arthritis.*

	Without Any Difficulty	With Some Difficulty	With Much Difficulty	Unable To Do	Not Applicable
Dressing and Grooming					
Is your child able to:					
• Dress, including tying shoelaces and doing buttons?	_____	_____	_____	_____	_____
• Shampoo his or her hair?	_____	_____	_____	_____	_____
• Remove socks?	_____	_____	_____	_____	_____
• Cut fingernails/toenails?	_____	_____	_____	_____	_____
Arising					
Is your child able to:					
• Stand up from a low chair or floor?	_____	_____	_____	_____	_____
• Get in and out of bed or stand up in crib?	_____	_____	_____	_____	_____
Eating					
Is your child able to:					
• Cut his or her own meat?	_____	_____	_____	_____	_____
• Lift a cup or glass to mouth?	_____	_____	_____	_____	_____
• Open a new cereal box?	_____	_____	_____	_____	_____
Walking					
Is your child able to:					
• Walk outdoors on flat ground?	_____	_____	_____	_____	_____
• Climb up five steps?	_____	_____	_____	_____	_____

*Please check any *aids* or *devices* that your child usually uses for any of these activities:

_____ Cane
_____ Walker
_____ Crutches
_____ Wheelchair

Devices used for dressing (button hook,
_____ zipper pull, long-handled shoe horn, etc.)
_____ Built-up pencil or special utensils
_____ Special or built-up chair
_____ Other (specify: _____)

*Please check any categories for which your child usually needs help from another person *because of arthritis*:

_____ Dressing and grooming
_____ Arising

_____ Eating
_____ Walking

	Without Any Difficulty	With Some Difficulty	With Much Difficulty	Unable To Do	Not Applicable
Hygiene					
Is your child able to:					
• Wash and dry entire body?	_____	_____	_____	_____	_____
• Take a tub bath (get in and out of tub)?	_____	_____	_____	_____	_____
• Get on and off the toilet or potty chair?	_____	_____	_____	_____	_____
• Brush teeth?	_____	_____	_____	_____	_____
• Comb/brush hair?	_____	_____	_____	_____	_____
Reach					
Is your child able to:					
• Reach and get down a heavy object, such as a large game or books, from just above his or her head?	_____	_____	_____	_____	_____
• Bend down to pick up clothing or a piece of paper from the floor?	_____	_____	_____	_____	_____
• Pull on a sweater over his or her head?	_____	_____	_____	_____	_____
• Turn neck to look back over shoulder?	_____	_____	_____	_____	_____

(continued)

Grip

Is your child able to:
- Write or scribble with a pen or pencil? _____ _____ _____ _____ _____
- Open car doors? _____ _____ _____ _____ _____
- Open jars that have been previously opened? _____ _____ _____ _____ _____
- Turn faucets on and off? _____ _____ _____ _____ _____
- Push open a door when he or she has to turn a door- _____ _____ _____ _____ _____
  knob?

Activities

Is your child able to:
- Run errands and shop? _____ _____ _____ _____ _____
- Get in and out of car or toy car or school bus? _____ _____ _____ _____ _____
- Ride bike or tricycle? _____ _____ _____ _____ _____
- Do household chores (e.g., wash dishes, take out trash, _____ _____ _____ _____ _____
  vacuum, do yard work, make bed, clean room)?
- Run and play? _____ _____ _____ _____ _____

*Please check any *aids* or *devices* that your child usually uses for any of these activities:

_____ Raised toilet seat   _____ Bathtub bar
_____ Bathtub seat   _____ Long-handled appliances for reach
_____ Jar opener (for jars previously opened)   _____ Long-handled appliances in
                                                bathroom

*Please check any categories for which your child usually needs help from another person *because of arthritis*:

_____ Hygiene   _____ Gripping and opening things
_____ Reaching   _____ Errands and chores

Pain

We are also interested in learning whether your child has been affected by pain because of his or her illness.
- How much pain do you think your child has had because of his or her illness *in the past week*? Place a mark on the line below to indicate the severity of the pain.

No Pain   Very Severe Pain
_____
0   100

Health Status

1. Considering all the ways that arthritis affects your child, rate how your child is doing on the following scale by placing a mark on the line.

_____
0   100
Very Well   Very Poorly

2. Is your child stiff in the morning?   _____ Yes   _____ No
   If YES, about how long does the stiffness usually last (in the past week)?   Hours/Minutes _____

Adapted from Singh G, Athreya B, Fries JF, et al. Measurement of health status in children with juvenile rheumatoid arthritis. *Arthritis Rheum.* 1994;37:1761–1769.

A child aged 9 years or older, or a parent as proxy for a younger child, scores each statement based on item difficulty during the previous week (0 = no difficulty, 1 = some difficulty, 2 = much difficulty, 3 = unable to do). An item is scored as "not applicable" if the child is too young to perform the task. The highest scored item in each section dictates the score for that category; if the respondent reports needing an assistive device or assistance from another person to perform any task in that category, the minimum score for the category is 2. The global Disability Index (DI), calculated as the average of the eight functional category scores, has a range of 0 to 3, with higher scores indicating greater disability. Some studies employ a range of DI scores to categorize levels of disability: 0 = no disability, 0 to 0.5 = mild, 0.6 to 1.5 = moderate, and greater than 1.5 = severe.[125] The CHAQ-DI scores have been shown to correlate highly with disease activity

DISPLAY
17.4   **Eight Additional Items Included in the CAT$_{CHAQ38}$ and the VAS$_{CHAQ38}$**

1. I think I could have done climbing activities by myself.
2. I think I could have played team sports with others in my class.
3. I think I could have played some sports by myself.
4. I think I could have played team sports in competitive leagues.
5. I think I could have kept my balance while playing rough games.
6. I think I could have done activities I usually enjoy for a long time without getting tired.
7. I think I could have run a race.
8. I think I could have worked carefully with my hands.

From Shimzu M, Nakagishi Y, Inoue N, et al. Interleukin-18 for predicting the development of macrophage activation syndrome in systemic juvenile idiopathic arthritis. *Clin Immunol*. 2015;160:277–281

during active flares with poor correlation during periods of remission.[127] Dempster et al. found that a minimum decrease of 0.13 in the DI was correlated with a parent's assessment of clinical improvement in the child's functional abilities, whereas a minimum increase of 0.75 correlated with parents' assessment of decline in function.[128]

Patient-Reported Outcomes Measurement Information System

The Patient-Reported Outcomes Measurement Information System (PROMIS) was recently developed by the National Institutes of Health (NIH) as a collection of generic questionnaires across physical, mental, and social health domains. Questions are relevant for children aged 5 to 17, with parents serving as proxy for children younger than 8 years of age. Pediatric domains include anxiety/fear, cognition, depression, fatigue, mobility, pain, upper extremity function, well-being, and relationships. A short form consists of four to ten items per domain. The first clinical validation for the PROMIS in children with JIA was conducted by Brandon et al.[129] The only domain that did not discriminate between active and inactive disease was the upper extremity function, which is relevant in JIA. Morgan et al. reported that clinical relevance varied by severity, domain, and reporter.[130] Clinicians tended to report smaller changes as being clinically relevant when compared to children and parents. More research is needed to determine whether the PROMIS will be a useful tool in understanding outcomes in JIA.

Juvenile Arthritis Functional Assessment Scale

The JAFAS is the only measure of physical capacity for children with arthritis.[131] The child is observed and timed performing common daily tasks (buttoning a shirt or blouse, putting on a shirt over the head, pulling on socks, cutting food with a knife and fork, getting in and out of bed, rising

to stand from sitting on the floor, picking up an object from the floor, walking 50 feet, and walking up a flight of steps). The child's time to complete each task is compared with a criterion standard based on a healthy control group. Items are scored 0 if the time is equal to or less than the criterion, 1 if the time is more than the criterion, and 2 if the child is unable to complete the task. Administration and scoring take 10 minutes and require minimal training and equipment. The scale and directions for administering the test are provided in the original paper.[132]

Quality of Life

Several measures have been developed to assess health status and QOL in children with arthritis. Three of the most frequently used are the Juvenile Arthritis Quality of Life Questionnaire (JAQQ),[133] Pediatric Quality of Life Inventory (PedsQL) Rheumatology Module 3.0,[134] and the Quality of My Life (QOML) questionnaire.[135] The QOML questionnaire consists of two separate VASs that measure overall QOL and HRQOL in children and adolescents. The QOL scale asks, "Overall, my life is," and the HRQOL scale asks, "Considering my health, my life is." The respondent (child or parent as proxy) records their response to each question on the 100-mm VAS for each question stem, scoring ranges from 0 ("the worst") to 100 ("the best"). Children and parents also complete a 5-point ordinal measure of change in QOL (much worse, somewhat worse, the same, somewhat better, much better) since the last visit. A study by Gong et al. reported the minimal clinically important difference (MCID) that indicates improvement was 7 mm for the overall QOL and 11 mm for the HRQOL scale. The MCID that indicated deterioration was −33 mm for QOL and −38 mm for HRQOL.[135]

Norm-Referenced Motor Assessments

Two norm-referenced assessments developed for all children to assess their motor function compared to peers that may be useful in JIA include the Peabody Developmental Motor Scales–2 (PDMS-2) and the Bruininks–Oseretsky Test of Motor Proficiency-2 (BOT-2). The School Function Assessment (SFA),[136] Validity and reliability of the school function assessment in elementary school students with disabilities and the informal school checklist shown in Appendix A can provide information on the child's function in school.

» Physical therapy examination and evaluation

Joint Examination

Display 17.5 shows the areas included in an physical therapy examination. In the presence of joint inflammation, the therapist may be able to assess joint swelling or effusion. Visual examination of the knee, ankle, wrist, or digits can often identify asymmetric joint swelling. Joint effusions can be detected by demonstrating fluctuation of synovial fluid

Components of the Physical Therapist Examination in Juvenile Idiopathic Arthritis

- Medical history
- Clinical observation
- Examination of the child's activities and participation in typical life settings (home, school, community) through standardized questionnaires, informal interview, or observation of child performing activities
- Examination of the child's gross motor skills for daily activities, play, and sports
- Systems review
  - Integumentary system
    - Examine skin for presence of rash, nodules.
    - Examine nails for pitting, onycholysis.
  - Musculoskeletal system
    - Joint status and integrity
    - Joint range of motion
    - Soft-tissue extensibility
    - Muscle bulk
    - Muscle strength and endurance
    - Postural alignment
  - Cardiopulmonary system
    - Resting and exercise HR
    - Aerobic capacity or performance on field test
  - Multiple systems
    - Pain
    - Gait pattern and parameters
    - Postural control

from one area of the joint to another; however, this type of physical examination has poor reliability. Joint swelling is best observed through imaging techniques especially for the hip, shoulder, spine, and SI joint. Joint tenderness may be assessed with firm pressure on the joint line, whereas enthesitis can be palpated at the tendinous insertion of the Achilles tendon, plantar fascia, or patellar tendon. A gentle squeeze to each individual MCP or MTP joint can identify metatarsalgia. Finally, the therapist can pass the back of their hand across the joint to identify subtle changes in temperature.[137]

Range of Motion

Examination of joint passive range of motion (PROM) provides valuable baseline information about pain, muscle guarding, muscle tightness, and joint contracture. Standard goniometric measurements should be recorded for all upper and lower extremity joints as a baseline. The large variability in ROM norms among children makes it difficult to monitor for changes in joint movement without an individual set of goniometric data points to compare. In the presence of muscle guarding, slow careful motion will often increase the available range over time. Hip rotation, especially internal rotation, is often limited in children with hip or SI joint inflammation. Hip flexion in a neutral plane of adduction and internal rotation is often limited with more severe disease.

With acute knee swelling, children will often demonstrate their best knee extension when lying prone compared to supine. In standing, they will tend to exhibit more flexion to reduce their pain. Children with ankle inflammation will have limitations in dorsiflexion and plantar flexion (PF). However, those with subtalar arthritis will be limited in hindfoot motion (inversion/eversion). Children with toe involvement may have limited great toe extension that can significantly impact the ability to move forward over the stance foot and achieve a push-off during gait. Arthritis in the shoulder girdle results in pain and restricted motion, especially with rotation. Elbow flexion contractures are common, occur early in the disease course, and are often accompanied by limited forearm supination. At the wrist, acute inflammation will limit flexion and/or extension. However, with chronic arthritis, there is often subluxation or a drift into ulnar deviation.

Goniometric measurements can help monitor the effects of medication on joint inflammation, because significant improvements can be made in a short period when limitations are related to inflammation and muscle guarding rather than to capsular tightness and contracture. Shortening of two joint muscles, the hamstring and gastrocnemius, leads to decreased flexibility in children with JIA. These muscles do not generally lengthen in response to medical treatment, and often require gentle stretching, positioning, or active movement to regain functional motion.

Children with chronic arthritis may present with limited ROM due to damage to the intra-articular structures. Crepitus, joint subluxation, and contracture are associated with chronic inflammation and more severe disease. The physical therapist should review the radiologist's report or view the child's radiographs if available. Knowledge of the extent of joint damage is important in developing an appropriate POC.

When evaluating ROM, it is also important to assess abnormal or asymmetric changes in skeletal structure, especially in younger children. Documentation of leg length, femoral anteversion/retroversion, genu varum/valgus, thigh–foot angle, and hindfoot varus/valgus provides the therapist with information regarding asymmetric joint involvement. These measurements will assist the therapist in determining the causal factors for observed postural and gait deviations. For example, in-toeing could be related to pain-induced forefoot supination, femoral anteversion, tibial torsion or hip weakness, and a good skeletal examination can help determine the origin of this deviation. Common patterns of joint impairments and subsequent activity restrictions in JIA are shown in Table 17.3

Muscle Strength

Muscle bulk, strength, and endurance should be assessed at the initial and follow-up visits. Measures of limb circumference (calf and thigh) document any asymmetries in muscle bulk and changes over time. MMTs can be used to measure

TABLE 17.3.	Common Patterns of Joint and Soft-Tissue Impairments in Juvenile Idiopathic Arthritis

Cervical Spine
- Most common in PoJIA and SoJIA
- Loss of extension, rotation
- Loss of normal lordosis
- May develop torticollis if asymmetric
- Chronic inflammation may lead to joint space narrowing with nerve root irritation.
- Fusion of zygapophyseal joints—often occurs first in C-2–C-3, but may progress to other levels
- Dysplasia of vertebral bodies
- Instability of C-1 to C-2 articulation may occur, but less common than in adult RA.

Temporomandibular Joints
- Most common in PoJIA; less common in oligoJIA
- Restriction in opening mouth; pain on chewing
- Greater functional loss if cervical spine extension is limited
- Mandibular asymmetry if unilateral involvement
- Undergrowth of the mandible (micrognathia)
- Malocclusion of the teeth
- May require orthodontic treatment

Shoulder Complex
- Most common in PoJIA
- Limited glenohumeral ABD and MR noted first; limited shoulder flexion
- Shortening of pectorals and scapular abductors
- Overgrowth of humeral head with irregular shape
- Shallow glenoid fossa with increased risk of subluxation
- Functional loss increases if elbow and wrist arthritis is present.

Thoracolumbar Spine
- Most common in ERA; sacroiliac arthritis common in JAS
- Motion may be limited by spasm of spinal extensors or short hip flexors.
- Scoliosis secondary to long-standing LLD
- Kyphosis in association with neck and shoulder arthritis
- Excessive lumbar lordosis secondary to hip flexion contracture
- Long-term systemic steroid therapy contributes to osteoporosis, wedging vertebral bodies, small compression fractures.

Hip
- Occurs in PoJIA and SoJIA; primary cause of disability
- Loss of extension, MR, and ABD
- Weakness of gluteus medius and deep hip LR; may cause Trendelenburg gait deviation
- Flexion contracture may be masked by increased lumbar lordosis.
- May have marked pain on weight bearing; pain may be referred to groin, buttocks, medial thigh, and knee.
- Femoral head overgrowth
- Osteoporosis
- Limited weight bearing in young child contributes to poorly developed hip joint with shallow acetabulum and trochanteric growth abnormalities.
- Lateral subluxation of femoral head, aggravated by short hip adductors
- Potential for protrusio acetabuli and AVN in persistent severe disease
- Potential for repair of articular cartilage with fibrocartilage during disease remission with improved weight bearing and mobility

Elbow
- Occurs in all types
- Involved early in disease course
- Loss of extension, forearm supination
- Overgrowth of radial head restricts ROM.
- Proximal radioulnar joint involved
- Ulnar nerve entrapment possible

Wrist
- Occurs in all types; occurs early in disease course
- Accelerated carpal maturation
- Undergrowth of ulna; ulna may migrate dorsally.
- Radial and intercarpal fusion
- Rapid loss of extension; shortening of wrist flexors; volar subluxation
- Wrist rests in flexion and ulnar deviation
- In older onset or RF-positive PoJIA, wrist may deviate radially.
- Distal radioulnar disease causes loss of forearm pronation and supination.
- Flexor tenosynovitis

Hand
- Involvement later in PoJIA and SoJIA than in oligoJIA; small joints of hand least commonly affected in JAS
- Premature epiphyseal fusion and growth abnormalities
- MCP and CMC subluxation
- Flexor tenosynovitis
- Loss of MCP flexion, terminal extension
- PIP contractures more common than DIP
- Marked decrease in grip strength
- Boutonniere less common than swan-neck deformities

Knee
- Most common joint involved early in all disease types
- Rapid weakness and atrophy of quadriceps, loss of patellar mobility
- Flexion contracture; may cause secondary hip flexion contracture
- Loss of hip flexion
- Overgrowth of distal femur contributes to LLD in unilateral disease.
- Knee valgus aggravated by short hamstrings, TFL, and ITB
- Posterior tibial subluxation secondary to prolonged arthritis or aggressive stretching of shortened hamstrings
- Risk of femoral fracture associated with osteoporosis

Ankle and Foot
- Occurs in all disease types
- Altered growth causes bony changes in the tarsals, with potential for fusion.
- Growth abnormalities due to early closure of epiphyses
- Early loss of ankle inversion, eversion; later loss of D-FL, PF, especially if standing and walking are limited
- Excessive hindfoot valgus or varus
- Excessive forefoot pronation or supination
- Loss of extension at MTP joints, with subsequent loss of push-off at terminal stance
- MTP subluxation
- Hallux valgus; hammertoes
- Overlapping of IPs
- Enthesitis at heel or knee is common in ERA.

ABD, abduction; AVN, avascular necrosis; CMC, carpometacarpal; D-FL, dorsiflexion; DIP, distal interphalangeal; ERA, enthesitis-related arthritis; IP, interphalangeal; ITB, iliotibial band; JAS, juvenile ankylosing spondylitis; LR, lateral rotation; MCP, metacarpophalangeal; MR, medial rotation; MTP, metatarsal phalangeal; oligoJIA, oligoarticular onset juvenile idiopathic arthritis; PIP, proximal interphalangeal; PF, plantar flexion; polyJIA, polyarticular onset juvenile idiopathic arthritis; RF-positive, rheumatoid factor positive; ROM, range of motion; sJIA, systemic onset juvenile idiopathic arthritis; TFL, tensor fascia latae.
Data in this table are summarized from Cassidy JT, Petty RE, eds. *Textbook of Pediatric Rheumatology*. 4th ed. W. B. Saunders; 2001. This listing is not inclusive, nor do all of the characteristics listed occur in every child with arthritis.

isometric strength in older children, but reliability is questionable. Care should be taken to assess that the child can move through their full ROM before applying resistance. Children with active inflammation may have difficulty with movement into their terminal range. This is often seen when testing a swollen knee for active extension. It is important to document the amount of muscle lag (motion lacking) as a measurement of future improvement. Resistance should be applied closer to the joint when there are concerns with active inflammation or joint instability. The therapist should gradually apply resistance while monitoring for discomfort.

Handheld or isokinetic dynamometers provide more objective and reliable measures of strength, especially for specific muscle groups, in children with arthritis.[138,139] Common patterns of weakness include hip extension and abduction, knee extension, ankle PF and dorsiflexion, shoulder flexion, abduction and rotation, elbow flexion and extension, wrist extension, and grip.

Children with JIA perform poorly on standardized measures of trunk flexor strength compared with age-, sex-, and size-matched healthy controls and age- and sex-based norms.[140,141] Lindehammar and Backman reported muscle weakness in knee extensors and elbow flexors regardless of the presence of active joint arthritis.[19] Weakness in the wrist flexors and ankle dorsiflexors (DFs) was increased with local joint inflammation. Brostrom et al., using an isokinetic dynamometer, found that girls with JIA had 40% less PF and 50% less DF strength compared with age- and sex-matched healthy controls.[142] The ratio of PF to DF strength was similar in both groups, suggesting that the disease affects both muscle groups equally. Weak ankle musculature negatively impacts gait in JIA.[23,141]

Two recent studies examined anaerobic capacity in JIA. Van Brussel et al. reported 94% of their sample ($N = 62$, ages 7–16 years) had significantly lower mean and peak anaerobic capacity (65% and 67%, respectively) compared with predicted values.[143] Deficits were larger in girls, and were found in children in clinical remission off medicines as well as in those with active disease. The largest impairments were in children with RF-positive polyJIA. Children with oligoJIA did not differ significantly from predicted values. Lelieveld et al. confirmed these findings in older adolescents. Strong negative correlations between anaerobic capacity, physical function, and overall well-being suggest that higher muscle fitness contributes to feeling better and being able to perform daily activities with less difficulty.[144]

Measures of functional strength using dynamic movements provide information about the child's daily activities. The 30-second chair-rise, timed floor-to-stand, and timed four-stair climb can provide objective measures that can be replicated in the clinic. In children without active arthritis or articular damage, a broad jump or hopping test can identify subtle muscle weakness. Special attention is given to antigravity muscles and those known to be weak in children with arthritis.

In very young children, strength is estimated by observing age-appropriate motor skills, such as squatting, rising up on toes, stair navigation, walking, running, or jumping. Toddlers should be able to complete a full squat and maintain the position for short periods of play. Children with either knee or ankle arthritis will often avoid squatting or shift their weight onto one leg while abducting the involved limb. Preschoolers with arthritis often have delayed development of an alternating pattern when walking up or down stairs. Instead, they choose to lead up with the uninvolved foot and lead down with the involved leg. Younger children may twist or turn sideways when coming downstairs to compensate for eccentric extensor weakness.

In older children, strength can be assessed using free weights to determine the maximum weight the child can lift through the available ROM for a specific muscle group (one maximal repetition [1 RM]). Other tests, such as a hand-grip dynamometer, vertical jump, or long jump have been found to correlate with 1 RM.[145] A 6 to 10 RM (maximum weight for 6 to 10 repetitions) is a sufficient measure of strength to establish a baseline, determine a training protocol, and evaluate progress.[146] Isometric testing performed at multiple joint angles provides an estimate of dynamic strength and may indicate weakness at specific points within the ROM. Muscle endurance is measured by having the child perform as many repetitions as possible, lifting a specified percentage, usually 60% to 80%, of the 6 or 10 RM. Tests of strength and endurance are performed on different days to avoid fatigue. A warm-up light activity typically precedes testing.

Postural Alignment

Height, weight, body composition, and posture should be included in the initial and follow-up physical therapy assessment to monitor the effects of the disease on growth and skeletal alignment.[147] A good postural examination should start at the top and document the head posture. Children with chronic disease may exhibit a forward head posture and micrognathia (retracted lower jaw). Torticollis may occur in children with asymmetric cervical spine arthritis. The child should be asked to demonstrate the ability to move their neck in all planes to their maximal ROM. School-aged children with JIA are at risk for a kyphotic thoracic spine and rounded shoulders with tight pectoral muscles. Scapular alignment may be asymmetric on the rib cage. An assessment of the spine may identify a scoliotic curve, kyphosis, or lordosis with anterior pelvic tilt.

Mobility of the lumbar spine should be examined in children with ERA using the modified Schober test (Fig. 17.11). With the child standing, with feet together and pointing forward, draw a line between the dimples of Venus (posterior superior iliac spine [PSIS]) to mark the lumbosacral junction. Place a mark on the spine 5 cm below and 10 cm above this line. Have the child lean forward with their knees slightly

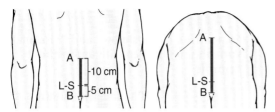

FIGURE 17.11. The modified Schober test of lumbar spine mobility. (Modified from Oatis CA. *Kinesiology: The Mechanics and Pathomechanics of Human Movement.* Lippincott Williams & Wilkins; 2004.)

bent and measure the distance between the two marks. This measurement should be greater than 21 cm. The increase in distance between the marks from baseline to a position of maximum forward flexion is used as an indicator of spinal mobility. An increase of less than 6 cm is considered abnormal.[148]

The horizontal symmetry of the dimples of Venus (PSIS) can also be used to quickly assess for leg length differences in the absence of a limb contracture. A radiograph is the most accurate method to obtain the true length of each limb segment. Leg length can also be examined in supine, measuring from the anterior superior iliac spine (ASIS) to the medial malleolus. The length of the femur and tibia should be measured separately if the child has a hip or knee flexion contracture. When differences are found, recheck spinal alignment after placing small lifts of known thickness under the shorter leg to level the pelvis.

In standing, make note of the base of support and whether the child is bearing weight equally on both legs. Young children often shift their weight off the affected lower limb to continue their motor play. Children with JIA may stand with excessive hip and knee flexion that can be asymmetric. Note the position of the knee in relation to the hip and the foot. Children may exhibit femoral anteversion or tibial torsion that may lead to a toe-out or toe-in pattern.

Therapists should perform a careful examination of the lower leg with an emphasis on the foot and ankle. Limited dorsiflexion often encourages a child to move into foot pronation to lower their heel to the floor. Pronation unlocks the child's midfoot, which may lead to a collapse of the longitudinal arch (pes planovalgus) that is often increased during the single-leg stance phase of gait.[149] Some children exhibit subtalar varus with a cavus forefoot. This is common in older children with enthesitis who subconsciously move into the position to avoid pain. Palpation under the longitudinal arch can identify plantar fascia tightness or fasciitis. Children with JIA are also at risk for toe deformities including hallux valgus, hammer toes, and claw toes. Using the Juvenile Arthritis Foot Disability Index (JAFI), 88% of participants reported some foot problems, 82% reported activity limitations, and 62% reported some restrictions in school and social participation related to foot impairments.[150]

Examination of sitting posture is also important to determine potential causes of muscle pain and fatigue during school and homework activities. Habitually sitting in a "slumped" posture characterized by a posterior pelvic tilt, thoracic kyphosis, and forward head position contributes to pectoral tightness and overlengthening of scapular stabilizers. Scapular weakness may result in difficulty or fatigue with overhead reaching activities.

Gait

Gait deviations in children with JIA are not uncommon, especially at the onset of the disease. Compared with healthy controls, children with JIA walk slower because of decreased cadence and step length, as well as a longer period of double support.[151–153] Gait mechanics were observed to return to normal in less severe cases and respond to treatment with intra-articular steroid injections.[151,154] Hendry et al. reported that mild-to-moderate walking disability continued in 25% of the subjects they followed up for 5 years despite a reduction in joint synovitis.[155]

Kinematic deficits include increased anterior pelvic tilt throughout the gait cycle, which may be a compensation for limited hip extension at terminal stance.[152,153] Limited terminal hip extension was observed in children whose walking speed was controlled on a treadmill.[153] Hartmann et al. speculated that limited hip extension may contribute to shortened step length and walking speed. Children with JIA also exhibit changes in knee kinematics during the gait cycle.[152] Kuntze et al. reported an alteration in knee motion as a compensatory mechanism to limit knee joint loading even in patients who denied joint pain.[153] During active knee arthritis, increased knee flexion during stance phase may be related to muscle guarding with hypertonia of the hamstrings and quadriceps femoris.[152]

Abnormal ankle kinematics is also observed in children with JIA and may be more responsive to treatment. Increased DF throughout the gait cycle with decreased PF at terminal stance has been reported. Data on ground reaction force during gait in JIA indicate lower heel-strike and push-off force.[152,156] Foot pain and deformities from long-standing arthritis negatively impact gait pattern and activities.[157] However, when medical treatment has been optimized, there is a significant reduction in foot deformity and functional disability.[156]

Gait deviations in children with JIA may also be related to LLDs. Changes in gait kinematics have been identified with a 5- to 10-mm leg length difference in typical teenagers.[158] Common gait changes due to limb length differences include an increased anterior pelvic tilt as well as a pelvic drop on the shorter side that is not necessarily accompanied by a thoracic trunk sway.[159] Teens also demonstrated increased hip, knee, and ankle flexion on the longer limb with increased knee extension and PF on the shorter limb. In typical teenagers, these gait deviations improved with the addition of a shoe lift.

Observational gait examination using a standardized recording form can provide useful information. A video of the child's gait provides a permanent record and is useful in monitoring change. By slowing or pausing the video recording, gait kinematics are more easily assessed. The child should be observed walking with and without shoes, although walking barefoot is often painful for some children. The gait symmetry, step and stride length, and alignment of the lower limb at heel strike, midstance, terminal stance, and swing are noted. Data from an instrumented gait mat provide a permanent record of the child's gait pattern. Velocity and cadence can be calculated by timing the walk. A full examination should include walking on level surfaces, inclines, stairs, curbs, and while running. Use of any assistive devices for mobility should be noted and also their influence on the child's gait pattern.

Motor Development and Functional Mobility

Standing, cruising, and walking should be encouraged at the expected age. Several studies report delayed motor development in young children with JIA.[160,161] One study by van der Net et al. examined motor development and functional skills in preschool and early school-age children with JIA, using standardized norm-referenced tests.[123] They found 45% of the preschool group, all with polyJIA, scored more than two standard deviations (SD) below the mean on the Bayley Scales of Infant Motor Development. Mean score for the early school-aged group on the Movement Assessment Battery for Children was within the normal range; however, 12% had severe delay and 20% were at risk for developmental delay. Functional skills assessed on the Pediatric Evaluation of Disability Inventory indicated that 70% of the early school-aged group scored greater than −2 SD on the mobility scale, suggesting that motor skill deficits become more evident as the demands for motor competence increase.[123]

Children with lower extremity arthritis may also exhibit difficulties with balance activities that require strength, ROM, and proprioception. Even in the presence of normal muscle strength, children with chronic arthritis may have deficits in proprioception due to chronic synovitis that may affect joint proprioceptors. Chronic muscle guarding may also limit the development of higher level balance and equilibrium responses. Balance can easily be screened by performing single-leg standing and hopping activities. Houghton and Guzman found that 40% of children with recent arthritis in a lower extremity joint were unable to maintain single-leg standing for 20 seconds, whereas all controls could complete at least one out of three trials.[162] Poor motor skills may limit a child's ability to participate in age-appropriate sports and contribute to a child's feelings of being less physically competent than that of their peers.

Aerobic Capacity and Performance

A large body of evidence shows that aerobic fitness is lower in children with JIA than that in healthy peers.[141,143,144]

DISPLAY 17.6 **Comparison of Physiologic and Performance Variables in Children with and without Arthritis**

Variable	Children with Arthritis Compared with Healthy Children
Peak VO₂	↓
Peak heart rate (HR$_{peak}$)	↓
Submaximal HR	↑
Peak workload	↓
Peak anaerobic power	↓
Performance-based fitness	↓
Muscle strength and bulk	↓

Impairments in aerobic capacity are greater in children with active disease than in those who are considered inactive; however, functioning is still diminished in both aerobic and metabolic functioning compared to that in healthy peers[163,164] (Display 17.6).

Van Brussel et al. measured peak oxygen uptake (VO$_{2peak}$) during a progressively graded exercise test on a cycle ergometer.[143] VO$_{2peak}$ was significantly reduced in 95% of their subjects with JIA. Several studies support an earlier meta-analysis demonstrating mean VO$_{2peak}$/kilogram body mass was 22% lower in children with JIA compared with age- and sex-matched healthy controls and reference values.[141] The largest deficits in VO$_{2peak}$ were found children with RF-positive polyJIA, while no impairment was found in children with oligoJIA.[143,144]

Giannini and Protas also reported that children with JIA had a lower peak workload and peak heart rate (HR) during exercise and shorter exercise time than did matched controls.[165] HR during submaximal exercise was also higher in children with JIA, suggesting that they work at a higher percentage of their peak exercise capacity than do healthy children. This may partly explain the fatigue frequently reported by children with JIA. Work by Helders et al. reported a significant and strong correlation ($r = 0.95$, $p < 0.001$) between peak workload (W$_{peak}$) and VO$_{2peak}$ in children with JIA during a progressive exercise test on a cycle ergometer.[166] This suggests that VO$_{2peak}$ can be predicted from W$_{peak}$, weight, and gender using the equation:

$$VO_{2peak} \text{ (L/min)} = (0.008 \times W_{peak} \text{ [Watts]}) + (0.005 \times \text{weight [kg]}) + (-0.138 \times \text{gender [1 = male, 2 = female]}) + 0.588$$

Field tests like the 1-mile or 9-minute walk/run test can provide an indication of the child's aerobic performance compared with published age- and sex-based health fitness criteria. Klepper et al. reported that children with polyJIA scored significantly lower on the 9-minute walk/run test than did healthy matched controls.[167] Unlike the controls, many children with JIA were unable to maintain a steady running pace. Test scores did not correlate significantly with active joint count or articular severity score, suggesting that performance may have been limited by other impairments, including low aerobic and muscular fitness, low motivation, or inexperience in distance or timed run tests.

The 6-minute walk test (6MWT) is another performance-related test developed to assess endurance in adults with cardiopulmonary disease, but is increasingly used to assess functional walking capacity in children with chronic health disorders. Standard guidelines for test administration have been published by the American Thoracic Society.[168] Reference values or prediction equations for the 6-minute walk distance (6MWD) in healthy children living in the United States have been published.[169] Paap et al. reported that children with JIA worked at 80% to 85% of their peak VO_2 and HR during the test, indicating that it is an intensive submaximal exercise test in children with JIA.[170] However, this test is not a good surrogate measure of VO_{2peak} in this population.[171] In the clinic, pre- and postwalk HR can be used to measure exercise intensity achieved during the test.

The cause of impaired aerobic fitness is multifactorial. Physiologic factors related to the disease process, including pain, mild anemia, and poor mechanical efficiency resulting from muscle atrophy, weakness, and joint stiffness, can impact the child's willingness and ability to be active. These impairments particularly impact children who develop JIA at a young age and those with persistent active disease. Several studies of school-age children found that neither active joint count nor articular severity scores were significantly correlated with aerobic fitness. Significant deficits were seen in children whose disease was in clinical remission off medications and also in those with active disease.[165,167,171] It appears that aerobic fitness in JIA does not improve without direct intervention despite improvement in disease status.

Pain

Pain is common despite improved medical management of the disease and has been reported in up to 86% of children with JIA.[172] Acute pain is associated with joint swelling at the onset of the disease, but it is reduced with intra-articular joint injections and medications. Chronic pain can evolve from acute pain and can be present even when the disease activity score is low. Rashid et al. followed up children with acute pain at the onset of their disease for 5 years.[173] Fifty percent of these children had "consistently low" pain that oscillated around the 1-cm mark on the VAS pain scale. One-third of the children experienced severe pain at initial diagnosis, with a rapid decline after 1 year followed by a 4-year plateau. A small cohort of children (17%) reported "consistently high" pain that trended along the 5-cm VAS score throughout the study. Children with enthesitis (30%) were more likely to report "consistently high" pain than did children with other JIA

subtypes. Pain at diagnosis was found to be one of the strongest predictors of chronic pain in children with JIA. Chronic pain is often associated with higher levels of stress, anxiety and depression, and sleep.[172,174]

Children with JIA appear to have a lower pain threshold and tolerance compared with healthy peers. One explanation may be prolonged activation of peripheral and central nociceptive systems, resulting in changes in pain processing and increased sensitivity to noxious stimuli.[175] Leegaard et al. found that changes in pain threshold do not actually correlate with disease duration.[176] Other factors that may contribute to a child's rating of pain include family pain histories, fluctuations in mood, stressful events, coping mechanisms, and overall health status.[172,175]

Pain examination should be frequent and comprehensive, including a pain history, self-report for children over the age of 4 years, parent report, and behavioral observations. In very young children, the therapist should be alert for pain behaviors validated in JIA, including bracing, muscle guarding, rubbing, rigidity, and flexing.[177] Display 17.7 lists self-report instruments that are useful in young children, including the Oucher, Wong-Baker Faces Pain Rating Scale, and the Poker Chip Tool.[178–180] The child can also indicate pain distribution and intensity on a body map using different colors to represent levels of pain intensity. Children at least 5 years old can report pain intensity on a numeric scale, a word graphic rating scale, or a VAS.

DISPLAY 17.7 Pediatric Pain Assessment Instruments Useful in Children with Juvenile Idiopathic Arthritis

Instrument (References)	Description
Oucher Scale[108]	• Ages 3–12 years • Measures pain intensity • Includes six faces and a scale from 0 to 100, from happy to very sad, scored as 0–5
Faces	• Suitable for children aged 3 years and older
Rating Scale[109]	• Scale includes six faces from happy to very sad, scored as 0–5; record face number child chooses • Child chooses face that best represents current feeling • Measures pain intensity and affect • Four red chips each representing a "piece of hurt"
Poker Chip Tool[110]	• Measures intensity from 1 piece to 4 pieces of hurt • Used for 3- to 4-year-olds • Correlates with Oucher

» Physical therapy intervention

A physical therapy POC should be developed on the basis of examination findings and child/family-centered goals. Treatment must be appropriate for the child's age and cognitive and psychosocial development. Physical activities and exercise must be graded on the basis of disease activity and severity. Developmentally based play can be useful to encourage young children to be active; however, joints with active disease or limited motion require direct attention (Display 17.8).

Pain Management and Comfort Measures

The first line of intervention to manage pain in JIA is adequate disease control using one or more of the systemic medications previously discussed. Children with chronic pain despite adequate disease control may benefit from nonpharmacologic treatments that provide temporary relief, while giving the child and parent some control over disease symptoms.[172] Reviews by Meng and Huang and Cameron and Chrubasik reported minimal evidence confirming the therapeutic effects of hot and cold modalities; however, they can be used per child preference with relatively little risk.[181,182] Using a heated blanket or taking a warm bath or shower can reduce morning stiffness. Exercising in a warm pool relieves pain and improves mobility. A home paraffin

unit may be used with adult supervision to provide prolonged warmth to arthritic hands. Locally applied cold may decrease intra-articular temperature and can be used to reduce joint pain and muscle spasm.[183] Cold along with rest, ice, compression, and elevation (RICE) applied immediately after an injury reduces inflammation, swelling, and pain. Placing a dry or damp warm towel between the cold source and skin allows the cold to penetrate slowly without stinging.

Balanced rest and exercise are necessary to manage pain and maintain joint mobility and function. A recent systematic review and meta-analysis by Kuntze et al. found that children with JIA who participated with land-based strengthening, Pilates, and aquatic exercise programs experienced a significant decrease in pain. In contrast, programs featuring repetitive jumping and high-impact tasks had high dropout rates secondary to pain.[153]

Restorative sleep is also essential for adequate pain management because poor sleep and fatigue negatively impact daytime function.[174,184,185] A systematic review completed in 2016 identified fatigue impacting 60% to 75% of all children with JIA. Pain was found to be the highest correlate with fatigue.[186] Simple measures to improve sleep and reduce morning stiffness include performing active ROM exercises before bed, using a sleeping bag to maintain body warmth during the night, and wearing resting splints to support joints in a functional position. Stretch gloves provide gentle compression and may relieve wrist and hand stiffness and pain. A cervical pillow helps reduce neck pain.

Education on pain and self-management has been shown to support other pain and comfort modalities well. This can be paired with biofeedback, which has also been shown through systematic reviews to be quite effective. Other methods of nonpharmaceutical pain management techniques include cognitive behavioral therapy (CBT), progressive relaxation therapy, and telephone consultation with a care provider. There is a paucity of evidence supporting the effectiveness of these interventions in children with JIA.[172] Distraction and imaginative play are useful in young children. Children with severe pain may require a multidisciplinary pain program. Connelly et al. found that adolescents experienced improvements in both pain and HRQOL through an online self-directed self-management training combined with online disease education.[187]

Therapeutic Exercise

Daily exercise has been widely recognized as beneficial to overall health through decreased risk for cardiovascular disease, decreased risk for type 2 diabetes, weight control, decreased risk for cancer, improved mental health and mood, and improved longevity. Exercise for children with JIA and other rheumatic diseases is likely no different; however, there is limited empirical evidence to support the extent of these benefits.[188,189] Nevertheless, it is essential that children with JIA and other rheumatic diseases are encouraged to meet the U.S. Center for Disease Control and Prevention (CDC)

DISPLAY 17.8 General Goals of Physical Therapist Intervention

Reduce Impairments in Body Structures and Functions
- Maintain/improve joint ROM
- Maintain/improve muscle bulk, strength, and endurance
- Maintain/improve health-related fitness
  - Reduce fatigue, improve stamina for physical activity
  - Reduce postural deviations/improve postural alignment

Maintain/Improve Child's Activities and Participation in the Home, School, and Community
- Basic and instrumental ADLs
- Functional mobility
- Gross motor skills for age-appropriate play, recreational activities, and sports
- Provide information and support to the child and caregivers.
- Provide information on the effects of arthritis on the body systems.
- Explain the benefits of daily exercise and provide clear instructions and illustration.
- Provide information to help the child manage pain and stiffness.
- Consult with school personnel to ensure child's full participation.
- Assist child and family to set achievable and meaningful goals.
- Encourage child and caregivers to actively participate in medical and therapy regimen.

and WHO recommendations for exercise to maintain joint health, remediate impairments, and achieve health-related physical fitness. Display 17.9 illustrates the components of a physical conditioning program that is graded to accommodate disease activity.

Range-of-Motion Exercise and Stretching

Techniques to preserve or increase joint mobility and soft-tissue extensibility include ROM exercise, positioning, and splinting. All joints with arthritis should be moved through the available range for three to five repetitions, preferably twice a day. Active range of motion (AROM) is optimal to preserve muscle function and joint mobility. Active assisted range of motion (AAROM) is used when the child is unable to perform full AROM. During active disease, care should be taken during PROM to prevent overstretching and tissue trauma. Games that elicit functional limb and trunk movement patterns are useful in very young children.

Gentle manual stretching to lengthen shortened soft tissues can begin once arthritis is under adequate control. Although there is little evidence for the effectiveness of any specific stretching regimen in JIA, research in other children indicates that dynamic stretching may be more beneficial than is static stretching.[190] Other studies have demonstrated that an intermittent stretching protocol of 30 seconds of stretch followed by 30 seconds of rest, repeated for a total stretch time of 90 seconds results in improved tissue range both short term and long term compared to static stretching alone.[190] This may lengthen tissues before placing the limb in a splint. Neuromuscular stretching techniques that promote autogenic or reciprocal inhibition of shortened muscle, including contract-relax, agonist contraction, and a combination of both, are useful in treating limited joint motion. The amount of resistance applied varies according to the child's tolerance.

Stretching techniques and ROM exercises must be graded according to disease status of individual joints. It is important to gain the child's cooperation to minimize pain and reflex muscle spasm. Aggressive passive stretching is avoided because of the risk of damage to epiphyseal areas at the tendon–bone interface. Using a long lever arm when stretching stiff hamstrings may cause posterior subluxation of the tibia. Stretching is always combined with active exercise

---

DISPLAY 17.9   Recommendations for Staging Physical Activity and Exercise in Juvenile Idiopathic Arthritis

Exercise Type	Disease State		
	Acute Disease	**Subacute and Chronic Disease**	**Inactive Disease/Clinical Remission On/Off Medications**
ROM/flexibility	Daily AROM or AAROM of all active joints and adjacent joints • 1–2 reps, 1–2 times/day	Daily AROM of all active joints and adjacent joints • 1–2 reps 1×/day • Active flexibility exercise • Modified yoga poses	Daily AROM of all active joints and adjacent joints
Aerobic activity	Balance rest for active joints with low-intensity, low-impact PA to maintain physical stamina, reduce load on inflamed joints • Exercise in warm pool • Tricycle or bicycle	Increase weight-bearing PA to promote bone health and lower limb muscle strength • Walking, low-impact dance • Use joint supports, splints, orthoses as recommended	Accumulate 60 min/d of moderate-to-vigorous PA • Aerobic dance, "step" aerobics, Tai chi, biking, swimming, jumping rope
Neuromuscular training • Minimize muscle atrophy Muscle strength • Muscle endurance • Muscle power • Neuromuscular control • Proprioception • Postural control • Coordination • Agility • Speed	One set of 1–6 reps of *submaximal* isometric muscle contractions performed at multiple points within the available pain-free ROM (performed several times/day) • One rep includes "ramp" up contraction for 2 s, hold for 6 s, "ramp" down for 2 s • 20 s rest between reps	Dynamic exercises • Must be able to perform 8–10 reps against gravity with good form and without pain before adding resistance • Use functional movements • To ⇑ muscle endurance, perform 15–20 reps with no added resistance • Use light weights, 0.5–2.5 kg (bottles filled with water or sand, handheld or cuff weights, elastic bands)	Resistance training • Determine starting weight based on a 6–10 RM or targeted number of reps • Include closed chain activities to promote bone health and improve proprioception Include coordination, speed, and agility drills to promote motor skills for safe age-appropriate physical play and sports

to encourage active use of the muscles in their new resting length and to actively use the joint throughout the new ROM.

Daily positioning in prone for at least 30 minutes allows a low-load prolonged stretch on hip and knee flexors. The child can lie prone on a bed or another firm surface with their pelvis level, legs extended, and feet hanging off the edge. A pillow placed under the chest or abdomen may improve comfort. Care should be taken for head position when there is cervical involvement. Although the evidence supporting the use of orthotics or splinting is inconsistent, commercial or custom-made resting splints can support inflamed joints, maintain proper joint alignment, and apply a gentle low-load stretch on the soft tissues (Fig. 17.12).[192,193] Figure 17.13 shows custom-made resting splints for the hands and knees. A posterior "shell" keeps the knee extended and maintains hamstring length during the night; this may reduce stiffness and allow the child to stand more easily upon arising.

Conservative approaches that provide a static progressive low-load stretch include serial splints or casts and dynamic splints. Custom-made serial splints are convenient because the therapist can mold and modify the splint as needed to accommodate the child's ROM. However, because these splints can be easily removed, their effectiveness depends on the child's adherence. In contrast, serial casts require a considerable amount of time and skill to apply and cannot be modified, but also cannot be removed by the child. Serial casting

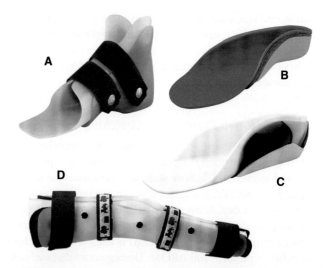

FIGURE 17.13. Sample of orthotics used for children with juvenile idiopathic arthritis (JIA) fabricated by Cascade DAFO in Ferndale WA. **A:** Supramalleolar orthotic-Fast Fit Leap Frog. **B:** Off-the-shelf Chipmunk shoe insert. **C:** Custom UCBL-DAFO 5.0. **D:** Banana peel circumferential knee extension splint. (DAFO® images courtesy of Cascade Dafo, Inc.)

is generally effective in reducing knee or elbow flexion contractures and improving wrist or ankle ROM. Protocols vary across clinics; however, typically the child wears the cast for 48 to 72 hours, after which it is removed. If the child still has limited joint mobility, a new cast is applied, and the process is repeated until full functional ROM is achieved. When the desired range is achieved, the final cast can be bivalved and made into a splint. During the next 1 to 2 weeks, the cast is worn for 18 to 24 hours a day as a splint, removing it only for exercise sessions or bathing to maintain the new range. For longer term range support, a custom-molded orthosis can be fabricated. Active exercise in a warm pool helps the child move the joint in its new ROM.[194]

Commercially available dynamic splints can be ordered to fit specific joints. This type of splint is not generally used on a joint with acute arthritis, instability, or bony erosion. Use of this type of splint can help wearers gain an average of 23.5 degrees of AROM through consistent use. The tension can be controlled by the physical therapist and set to the child's tolerance. Most children will tolerate a dynamic splint for 1-hour periods during the day; increased use shows significant linear increase in ROM gained.[195]

Exercise to Improve Muscular Performance

Strengthening activities are beneficial for all children with JIA. It is essential that muscles properly support arthritic joints during daily activity. The goal of the strengthening program is to allow children with JIA to return to age-appropriate recreational and fitness activities. The evidence supporting strength regimens for children with JIA is limited. The mode of exercise and the intensity and duration should be adjusted to the child's age, disease status, condition of individual

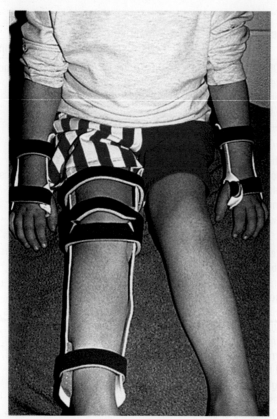

FIGURE 17.12. Aquaplast knee splints molded on child in prone.

joints, and current muscle function. The child's experience in strength training or sports should also be considered.[145]

During periods of active inflammation in the presence of pain and muscle guarding, the main goal of exercise is to maintain active ROM, muscle bulk, and muscle endurance. Isometric and active ROM exercises with gravity eliminated if necessary, should be performed at lower repetitions several times per day to tolerance. With lower extremity arthritis, exercises are generally performed in non–weight-bearing positions. Strength gains with isometric exercise are specific to the joint angle; therefore, isometric contractions should be performed in various positions including near the end ROMs. Five to ten repetitions daily may be sufficient to maintain muscle strength.[196] Aquatic activities are beneficial during this period because the child can move all joints through a large ROM with the weight of their limb supported. Cycling on level surfaces or the use of an upper extremity ergometer with minimal resistance can encourage multijoint movements. Electromyogram (EMG) biofeedback or ultrasound biofeedback may help the child isolate the muscle group and learn to regulate the intensity of the contraction.[197]

As the child's pain and inflammation decreases and they can move the limb against gravity for 8 to 10 repetitions without pain, a dynamic resistance program can be initiated.[196] Training includes concentric and eccentric contractions, achieving an appropriate balance between agonist and antagonist muscle groups across the joint. Young children and those with musculoskeletal impairments should begin with one to two sets of 8 to 12 repetitions of each exercise to build strength and muscle endurance.[145] The number of sets or repetitions can be increased, but should not exceed that which the child can perform without compensatory patterns that may compromise joint integrity. Proper technique and full ROM is critical.

External resistance can be added to progress the strengthening program. Weights or resistance bands should be placed close to and proximal to the joint. If elastic bands are used, lighter bands are used first, progressing to more resistive bands as strength increases, provided there is no joint pain or other signs of active disease. If using weights, begin at approximately 60% or less of 1 RM and progress to lesser than or equal to 80% 1 RM. Exercise intensity is based on the amount of weight the child can move through the ROM for 6 to 10 repetitions without discomfort, while maintaining proper exercise form.[145] Resistance training twice a week appears to be sufficient for healthy prepubertal children to achieve gains in muscle strength.[146] However, children with JIA may benefit from shorter sessions three times a week, with a day or two between sessions for recovery. Recent studies suggest that resistance-training programs lasting greater than 23 weeks are the most effective in attaining strength-related results.[145] To maximize proper form and technique, the prescription could include diagrams of all exercises to be performed.

Strengthening in weight-bearing positions can be included when children with active arthritis are able to maintain an appropriate weight-bearing posture and move without compensatory patterns. During active disease, care should be taken when using the weight of the body for resistance because eccentric muscle strength may still be inadequate for joint stability. In younger children, this would include the use of repetitive squatting and stair climbing if the child cannot be facilitated to complete the tasks using appropriate ergonomics.

Most children without joint deformity, who are being well managed with biologic or DMARD medications, can resume a more aggressive physical therapy program with the goal of returning to the sport and recreational activities they enjoy. The evidence suggests that children with medically controlled arthritis can improve muscle function through individualized progressive resistance training, with little to no exacerbation of disease symptoms.[198–201] The misconception that resistance training in children would impede skeletal growth has not been supported.[202] Strengthening exercises should target muscles supporting joints with arthritis and also muscles that may have become weak from disuse.

Strengthening programs should also incorporate activities to improve neuromotor control. A review by Kuntze et al. found that exercise protocols that featured strengthening exercises in conjunction with balance-proprioceptive changes had the biggest influence on functional activity capacity, such as 6-MWT, 10-stair climb, and functional reach tests.[200] Myer et al. described such a program in a single case study of a 10-year-old girl with quiescent oligoJIA who wished to return to competitive basketball.[203] The regimen included treadmill walking to improve symmetry in lower limb muscle function, progressive core and lower limb strengthening to improve postural control, and kinesthesia during jumping and landing. Resistance bands used during multidirectional movements simulated unanticipated challenges during games and practice sessions. Outcomes included improved control in single-limb stance, improved lower limb symmetry during gait and landing, and improved isokinetic strength ratio between lower limb flexors and extensors.

Once a child is exhibiting appropriate strength, ROM, balance, and coordination, they should be encouraged to participate in structured PA to maintain their strength and fitness. The Ottawa Panel Evidence-Based Practice Guidelines suggest that structured PA, such as Pilates, karate, and home and aquatic exercises, were all beneficial and well tolerated, with Pilates having the greatest influence on health outcomes.[204] Toddlers and young children may safely participate in dance, gymnastics, and soccer activities. However, as children get older and the demands of these sports increase, an individualized approach should be taken to determine whether the activity is still appropriate.

Children participating in strength training have improvements in motor skill performance, gains in speed and power, improved cardiovascular function and BMD, as well as a reduced risk of injury. Improvements in fatigue, energy, and well-being have also been reported on an anecdotal level.[202]

Exercise that Impacts Bone Density

Exercise that supports bone growth and strength in children has become a key component of PA recommendations for all children. In children with JIA, this is even more important because they are at higher risk for bone fragility. Children with JIA are commonly prescribed corticosteroids, which are well documented in their role of reducing bone density and increasing risk for fracture. A review by Huber and Ward identified that children with JIA tend to have lower BMD independent of corticosteroid exposure, and that subsequent risk for fracture may be higher with prolonged disease duration.[205] To evoke a change onto the bone, increased force is required. Typical exercises to promote BMD include jumping jacks, running, and weightlifting. Many of these "weight-loading" activities are more advanced and have higher impact and may not be tolerated by children with active disease. Fortunately, Sandstedt et al. found good tolerance and improved BMD in children who completed jump rope, core strengthening, and weighted arm and leg exercises for 12 weeks, indicating that many of the prescribed muscle-strengthening techniques described earlier will also positively influence bone health.[206]

Aerobic Conditioning

A 2008 Cochrane review found only three published RCTs that investigated the effects of aerobic training in JIA.[207] These studies compared land-based physical therapy with combined water- and land-based exercise, aquatic training versus standard medical care, and high-intensity land-based exercise to qigong, a form of gentle relaxation program similar to Tai chi.[184,208,209] All three studies reported that there were no adverse effects from exercise, but none found significant improvement in VO$_{2peak}$ following aerobic training. Possible reasons cited by the authors included low exercise frequency, insufficient intensity, poor adherence to center-based sessions, or failure to perform home exercise.

In a non-RCT to investigate the benefits of an 8-week aquatic exercise, pre- and postexercise capacity were measured using a cycle ergometer test. Anaerobic exercise capacity was found to improve following the aquatic program. However, there were no improvements in aerobic exercise capacity in the exercise group.[210]

Several non-randomized studies found significant improvements in other indicators of aerobic function, including higher distance run scores (land-based exercise), lower submaximal VO$_2$, increased exercise time (water, combined water, and land exercise), and decreased time to HR recovery (water). Most studies also report decreased disease signs and symptoms following training. Several review papers that provide an overview of exercise studies and recommendations for children with rheumatic diseases may be useful to clinicians in planning an exercise program for this population.[211–214] According to the literature, the recommendation for children with JIA who have impaired aerobic fitness is to train at least twice a week at an intensity of 60% to 85% of HR$_{max}$ for 45 to 60 minutes per session for at least 6 to 12 weeks.[211] Children who cannot tolerate a 30-minute session can begin with frequent short bouts of activity, increasing duration as their endurance improves. The child can monitor exercise intensity by counting pulse rate for 6 to 10 seconds, using a portable HR monitor, or estimating the exercise intensity on a rating of perceived exertion (RPE) scale.

As with any new exercise program, delayed-onset muscle soreness may occur early in the program, but should resolve with time. Teaching the child proper exercise form at the beginning of a training program and frequent monitoring are essential to prevent injury or increased pain. Pain reported by the child should be carefully assessed for a specific cause. Mild increase in joint pain may occur but should resolve within a few hours. Overuse injuries accompanied by joint swelling and pain should be treated with cold, elevation, and rest, and the exercise program should be modified to reduce potential injuries.

Surgery and Postoperative Physical Therapy

Surgical intervention in the JIA population is becoming less common with the shift in care to early and more aggressive medication. Well-timed selective surgical procedures can relieve pain and restore joint health and function in young children when conservative measures have failed.[215,216] Older children with joint damage may require reconstructive surgery to relieve pain and restore function. The decision to perform surgery is made by an interdisciplinary team based on an analysis of the risks and benefits. The physical therapist is involved in the preoperative examination and planning, as well as in the postoperative rehabilitation. Postoperative care and protocols can vary between different surgeons, between children, and even between sides. Always communicate with the surgical team to confirm precautions if you are working with someone postoperatively.

Preoperative physical therapy includes a conditioning program to improve strength, ROM and general stamina, and gait training with crutches or a walker. The child and parent also receive instruction in postoperative precautions to protect the surgical site during daily activities. Postoperative care is influenced by the surgical approach and type of implant or hardware used. As with any postoperative POC, communication with the surgeon regarding weight bearing or ROM precautions is essential.

Common Surgical Procedures

Soft-tissue releases (STRs) are performed to manage joint contractures that are unresponsive to conservative measures. This procedure involves making surgical cuts within the tight tissues to create length and relaxation. Reduced intra-arterial (IA) pressure and increased joint mobility improve joint nutrition and healing of the articular cartilage by fibrocartilage. Postoperative care is aimed at preserving muscle length and joint motion through splinting and ROM exercise.[217]

Supracondylar osteotomy may be performed in conjunction with STRs for a severe flexion contracture at the knee or when there is a valgus deformity and evidence of joint damage. This procedure involves cutting and repositioning the femur bone.

Synovectomy, or cutting of the joint capsule lining, is rarely performed in JIA because of the risk of postoperative pain and spasm and poor long-term results. However, the procedure may be done in combination with STRs to treat hip flexion contractures. It may also be done arthroscopically for acute synovitis of the knee, when effusion and overgrowth of inflamed synovium stimulate the adjacent epiphysis, resulting in lengthening of the limb. Tenosynovectomy may be indicated in a child with severe hand arthritis to prevent tendon rupture or reduce nerve entrapment from synovial proliferation.

Arthrodesis, or joint fusion, may be considered when a child has disabling pain and a high risk of natural joint ankylosis, for example, in advanced arthritis of the wrist, interphalangeal joints, ankle, or subtalar joints. Postoperative care includes immobilization in a cast, exercise, and positioning of adjacent joints to maintain mobility. Epiphysiodesis, or temporary surgical arrest of the growth plate, may be useful in some children with bony overgrowth leading to LLD.[215]

Children with irreversible joint damage may be candidates for total joint arthroplasty (TJA). Several factors are considered in the decision to perform TJA in a child with JIA, including the child's age, skeletal maturity, physical status, upper limb function, and the potential ability of the child and family to complete the lengthy and intensive postoperative rehabilitation. Ideally, surgery is delayed until the epiphyses have fused or there is little chance of further growth of the limb, although TJA may be necessary in younger children who have severe joint damage, disabling pain, and loss of function.[215] Custom-designed hip prostheses that are porous are typically used to accommodate the smaller bones in children with JIA and allow for biologic fixation, because cemented prostheses are more susceptible to loosening after several years. Timing of procedures is extremely important in a child who requires multiple joint replacements. In children with severe upper limb arthritis, fusion of a damaged or painful wrist may be necessary first to allow the child to use crutches after hip or knee surgery. When hips and knees must be replaced, the hip joints are usually done first. Both hips may be replaced at the same time if there is severe bilateral hip damage.[218]

Modifications to Activities and Participation

Children with uncontrolled disease or advanced joint deterioration may require modifications to their lifestyle to maintain optimal function. Modifications may be needed temporarily, such as during a disease flare, or long term for older children with advanced joint degeneration.

Joint Protection

During periods of active disease, parents and children need information on joint protection to reduce pain and limit potentially deforming mechanical forces on vulnerable joints. Children should use larger joints to perform tasks when possible, because they tolerate stress better than do smaller joints. For example, the child can carry large objects resting on the forearms rather than grasping them with their hands. They may use a backpack positioned close to the body's center of gravity or a rolling backpack to hold school books. Diagrams, demonstration, and practice of joint protection techniques may improve adherence.[219] Functional wrist and hand splints may decrease pain with grasping, gripping, or manipulative activities. Splints or adapted devices may also be useful in minimizing deforming mechanical forces during hand use.

Orthotics and Durable Medical Equipment

Children should be encouraged to walk within their home, school, and community to their joint tolerance. Ambulation encourages the maintenance of muscle strength, bone density, and aerobic fitness. All children should be encouraged to wear shoes that fit well and provide cushioning and support to the joints of the foot. High heels, platforms, and wedges are discouraged because they place added stress on the ankles as well as on the metatarsals. If worn frequently, they encourage Achilles tendon tightness, which is already a risk factor in JIA. Sneakers with a flexible sole, good arch support, and deep heel cup are often a good choice for most children to wear for walking and play activities. A shoe with a wide, deep toe box may be needed for children with hallux valgus, hammer toes, or claw toes. Examination of the child's shoes, both inside and out as well as the sole of the foot, helps identify pressure points from weight bearing or improper alignment.

Some children may require additional modification to the inside of their shoes. Children with metatarsalgia often benefit from a pad placed just proximal to the metatarsophalangeal joints to reduce pressure on these joints during gait. Children with mild metatarsalgia or hammer toes may also have increased comfort when using gel insoles inside their shoes. In children with pain and enthesitis at the calcaneal insertion of the Achilles tendon or plantar fascia, the addition of a gel heel cup or heel lift can reduce pain and improve gait. The heel lift should be removed once the pain is better managed with medication to discourage tightness of the plantar flexors.

The most common modification to the outside of the shoe is a full-length unilateral lift to correct an LLD. The evaluation for lift height needs to consider the age, growth potential, and standing posture of the child. In younger children, it is often beneficial to add a lift half to three-fourth the height of the discrepancy to encourage the shorter limb to grow. However, if the child has a knee flexion contracture on the longer involved limb, then a full-height lift would be appropriate to encourage increased active knee extension during standing and gait. Shoe lift recommendations should be re-assessed frequently. A quarter-inch lift may be added inside the shoe with the use of a dense noncollapsible foam. When a full-lift greater than quarter-inch is required, it should be added to the outside of the shoe by an orthotist, allowing for an adequate toe rocker. Finally, a child with a rigid great toe or ankle may benefit from a metatarsal bar added to the sole of the shoe to create a mechanical means of rolling over the foot during gait.

Often, shoes or shoe modifications are not enough to support the ankle or subtalar joint during weight-bearing activities. The child should then be fit with an orthotic that either supports their flexible foot deformity in a more neutral position or accommodates a more rigid deformity.[220] Often, a higher medial or calcaneal border is required to fully support the calcaneus in a more neutral position. A University of California Berkeley Laboratories (UCBL)-style orthotic has a higher trim line while still allowing full ankle motion. Children with JIA may have talar or metatarsal growth disturbances that require additional posting, especially if using an off-the-shelf product. It is important to assess whether forefoot posting is needed to maintain the calcaneus in a neutral position. It is important to encourage ankle motion during gait; however, there are times when a supramalleolar trim line may be needed to provide extra support during a flare when the child exhibits significant pain and muscle guarding. Rarely is there a need for ankle–foot orthotics unless there is severe arthritis with joint deformity.

Few children with JIA require an assistive device for ambulation; however, when changes in gait pattern are observed, or the child refuses to walk, the cause should be determined and addressed immediately. A child with pain or weakness in one leg can use a cane on the opposite side to unload the involved limb. A walker may be necessary for a child who has significant bilateral lower limb impairments. Platform attachments can be added for the child who also has limited upper limb motion.

Some children will need to use wheeled mobility for long distances in school or in the community to preserve energy. Tricycles or bicycles with training wheels are good options for young children. Older children can use a lightweight sports wheelchair or powered scooter to move around their school, college campus, or community. The child should be encouraged to get out of the wheelchair to stand and walk as tolerated to preserve muscular function and prevent contractures. Powered wheelchairs are generally reserved for children with severe disability.

Self-Care Activities

A primary goal for the child with JIA is to achieve independence in age-appropriate activities in all environments. The emphasis in young children is on basic ADLs and motor skills for play. Independence for an adolescent or young adult may revolve around the ability to drive, live independently in a college dormitory, and acquire a job.

The role of the therapist is to (1) assess the child's functional abilities using one of the standardized assessments described previously; (2) provide education and direct training in self-care activities, mobility, and motor skills; (3) suggest appropriate assistive devices, environmental modifications, and adaptive equipment, and train the child in their use; and (4) consult with school personnel to modify the environment to support independence. A child with minimal physical limitations may only need advice about the most efficient method of performing tasks, whereas a child with severe limitations may need instruction in the use of adaptive equipment or environmental modifications to promote independence. Dressing and hygiene aids that may be useful include Velcro closures on clothing and shoes, elastic shoelaces, a dressing stick, a buttonhook, a long-handled shoehorn, and a bath brush. Built-up handles on grooming items, eating utensils, and drawing and writing implements allow the child to be independent in these activities with less pain. The child with limited neck extension may need to use a straw to drink from a glass.

Home Modifications

Simple modifications in the home can increase a child's independence. These include replacing traditional doorknobs and faucets with levers, using a raised toilet seat, and installing safety bars in the bathtub or shower and additional handrails in stairways. The child should have easy and safe access to the bathtub, toilet, and sink. More substantial modifications may be needed if a child uses a wheelchair within the home, including widening doorways and adding a ramp or wheelchair lift at the entrance to the house.

Maintaining an Active Lifestyle: Recreation and Sports

Multiple studies report that children and adolescents with JIA engage in less vigorous PA and fewer organized sports than do their healthy peers.[221–223] Significant associations between PA level and VO_{2peak}, but not with disease activity, suggest a possible cause–effect relationship that provides direction for intervention.[223,224] The CDC recommends 60 minutes of daily moderate-to-vigorous PA for all children to achieve and maintain optimal health.[225] These recommendations apply to children with JIA as well, although the type and intensity of activity may need to be modified depending on the child's disease status and physical abilities. The use of a wearable activity tracker may encourage older children and adolescents to increase their activity throughout the day.[226]

Low-impact activities such as swimming, walking, dance, modified yoga, Tai chi, and cycling are the most appropriate choices when a child has active arthritis in weight-bearing joints. Bicycles can be adapted to lessen the stress to lower limb joints by setting the seat height so that the knee is at an angle of 30 degrees of flexion when the child's foot is at the apex of the downstroke.[227] Exercise in a heated (88° to

92°F) pool is recommended for children who have limited or painful mobility on land. Cooler pool temperatures (82° and 86°F) are more suitable for aerobic exercise, when joint stiffness is not a consideration.

School-age children should be encouraged to participate in physical education (PE) class. In 2018, Risum et al. found that most children with JIA are able to participate; however, 25% do require modifications. The physical therapist can consult with the instructor to adapt activities for the child. Somersaults and headstands should be avoided to prevent injury to the cervical spine. Children with wrist and hand arthritis should avoid weight bearing through their palms.[222]

Sports become more important as children reach school age. Safe and successful participation depends on the child's motor competence as well as physical stamina. Children with mild-to-moderate arthritis can participate in sports without disease exacerbation; however, high-impact loading should be avoided.[200] Sports with a high potential for collision, including football, hockey, and boxing, should be discouraged. A physical therapist can help children and families determine whether the child's preferred sport or recreational activity is a good "fit" for his or her physical abilities and motor skills. The activity should be analyzed to determine its collision or contact potential, demands for aerobic and muscular work, ROM, and neuromuscular skill. An exercise program designed to remediate specific problems may decrease the child's risk for injury. If the child chooses to play on a sports team, coaches should be made aware of the child's diagnosis and safety considerations, and children should be allowed occasional breaks from play during practice and games. The physical therapist can develop a preseason and in-season conditioning regimen if none exists.

School Participation

A child's ability to succeed in the school environment may be impacted by JIA. Chomistek et al. looked at self-reported barriers at school reported by children with JIA and identified physical barriers in 43.1% of subjects.[160] Participation in PE and sports may be limited or inconsistent owing to disease flares. Frequent disruptions to the child's school day as a result of medical appointments or visits to the nurse for medications can negatively impact the child's education.[161] However, only 23% of children utilized accommodations, and communication with both teachers and peers regarding their disease was low.

Children with JIA often require only a few modifications to their school program to be successful. Accommodations might include a second set of books for home, adapted writing tools, laptop computer for taking notes, and an easel-top desk for a child with cervical spine arthritis. Modifications in the child's schedule may be necessary to include visits to the nurse for medications, extra time to transition classrooms, and rest periods during the day. Children may benefit from standing and moving periodically to prevent stiffness or using

an elevator for transitions between floors. Families may need to modify lunch containers to make it easier for the child to access their meal independently. The school checklist (Appendix A) can be used to identify school-based problems.

Some schools provide program modifications and assistance voluntarily, but a formal evaluation by the school staff is often required to formalize the plan. Children with limited disease are often served under a 504 plan (Section 504 of the Vocational Rehabilitation Act), which outlines classroom accommodations. Children with more severe disease that significantly limits their ability to participate in school activities may benefit from an IEP (Individualized Education Plan). Under the Individuals with Disability Education Act (IDEA), children may qualify to receive specialized services including school therapies. Educational and vocational counseling is beneficial for adolescents and may begin as early as 14 years to prepare for the transition to postsecondary education or work.[228] The physical therapist can provide information to school personnel about the potential impact of JIA on school performance and suggest adaptations to the educational program.

Child and Family Education and Support

The demands placed on the family when a child is ill can be overwhelming. Successful management of JIA depends to a great extent on the ability of the child and caregivers to manage the medical and therapeutic regimen. Parents' attitudes regarding their child's pain was found to greatly impact the child's own adherence to treatment.[229] The therapist plays an important role in helping parents and the child to understand the effects of the disease and the benefits of medication, exercise, and other therapeutic procedures.

The effectiveness of treatment is highly dependent on adherence to the plan by the child and caregivers. Studies indicate that adherence to medications is higher than it is for exercise and is associated with lower disease activity. Moderate-to-high adherence to exercise is associated with better physical function, lower pain, and parental perception of global improvement. Parental adherence to exercise appears to be higher for younger children. Lack of time and failure to see the benefits of the prescribed activities contribute to lower adherence to exercise in older children and adolescents.[230–232] Active participation in managing the child's health care may be enhanced when both parent and child understand the effects of the disease and benefits of medication, exercise, and other therapeutic procedures.

Educational materials for families should be culturally appropriate and in the parent's preferred language. Materials for children should be appropriate to the child's cognitive and emotional development. Display 17.10 shows resources for children with arthritis, their families, and health professionals who care for them. Home exercise programs (HEPs) should be individualized to target the child's needs and limited to no more than seven simple exercises, requiring 20 to 30 minutes.

Organizations

Arthritis Foundation

1330 West Peachtree Street
Atlanta, GA 30309
1-800-238-7800
www.arthritis.org

Juvenile Arthritis Alliance

This virtual community of parents, volunteers, health professionals, and anyone affected by juvenile arthritis (JA) is connected through the Arthritis Foundation (AF) website and provides resources and opportunities for members to connect and share with others. An annual national conference brings together families and health professionals for education and recreation.
http://www.arthritis.org/juvenile-arthritis.php

American College of Rheumatology/Association of Rheumatology Health Professionals

The Association of Rheumatology Health Professionals (ARHP) is a multidisciplinary section of the ACR that provides education and resources to all health professionals caring for individuals with rheumatic diseases. Educational products and programs include the slide collection, online rehabilitation case studies, and training programs. The Annual Scientific Meeting brings together international researchers, clinicians, and educators with the purpose of sharing the latest research and clinical information related to the care of children and adults with rheumatic disease. The Pediatric Rheumatology Symposium (PRSYM) occurs every 3 years, and is dedicated exclusively to the needs of pediatric rheumatology clinicians and researchers.
www.rheumatology.org

Childhood Arthritis and Rheumatology Research Alliance

A network of rheumatologists and researchers working closely with families and patients to collaborate and find the best methods to treat and ultimately prevent or cure all pediatric RA community founded by families of children with JM who work together to educated, raise awareness, and support research toward better treatments and a cure for JM.
https://www.curejm.org/

Lupus Foundation of America

An organization with a mission to improve the QOL for all people affected by lupus through education, support, and advocacy.
https://www.lupus.org/resources/lupus-and-children

Pediatric Arthritis & Lupus Foundation (PAL Foundation)

A group of pediatric rheumatologists, researchers, and families working hand in hand to support research and treatments for children with arthritis and lupus.
https://pal-foundation.org/

Chronic Recurrent Multifocal Osteomyelitis Awareness

A website created by pediatric rheumatologists to provide information and resources.
http://crmoawareness.org/

Chronic Recurrent Multifocal Osteomyelitis Foundation

A nonprofit organization developed to support research, access to resources, and education to improve the health and well-being of individuals with CRMO and their families.
https://crmofoundation.org/

Camps

Several state AF chapters sponsor summer residential camps for children with arthritis or other rheumatic diseases. Contact your local AF chapter for information.

CureJM has hosted camps for children with JM and their siblings aged 3 to 12 called *Kids' Fun Camp*

The Painted Turtle camp has hosted medical condition-specific camp weekends for children and their families free of charge since 2004. https://www.thepaintedturtle.org/

Camp Sunshine hosts children and their families free of charge year round. They offer illness-specific sessions and include medical care and bereavement programming. https://www.campsunshine.org/

Exercise Programs for Young Children

Exercise Right Home exercise videos and resources. https://exerciseright.com.au/homeworkouts/

Arthritis Foundation Exercise Program (land-based)

Aquatic Exercise Program—warm water exercise program
Take Control with Exercise—Thera-Band Combo
Tai Chi (DVD)

303 Kid-Approved Exercises and Active Games (SmartFun Activity Books)
Authors: Wechsler K, Sleva M, McLaughlin DS. Alameda: Hunter House Inc., Publishers, 2013

Publications for Parents and Children
Raising a Child with Arthritis: From Infancy to Young Adulthood
Author: Charlotte Huff. Edited by: Richard Vehe MD. Arthritis Foundation, 2008

Kids Get Arthritis Too Newsletter
Arthritis Foundation periodic publication

Your Child with Arthritis—A Family Guide for Caregiving
Authors: Tucker Lori B, DeNardo Bethany A, Stebulis Judith A, Schaller Jane G. Baltimore: John's Hopkins University Press, 1996

It's Not Just Growing Pains
Author: Thomas JA Lehman, MD: Oxford University Press, 2004

The Official Patient's Sourcebook on Juvenile Rheumatoid Arthritis
A Revised and Updated Directory for the Internet Age
Editors: James N Parker, MD
Philip M Parker, PhD
ICON Health Publications, 2002
ICON Group International, Inc.
4370 La Jolla Village Drive, 4th Floor
San Diego, CA 02122

Myositis and You: A Guide to Juvenile Dermatomyositis for Patients, Families, and Health Care Providers
Authors: Rider LG, Pachman LM, Miller FW, Bollar H. Cure JM Foundation, 2007.

Publications for Clinicians
Kutcha G, Davidson I. *Occupational and Physical Therapy for Children with Rheumatic Diseases: A Clinical Handbook.* New York: Radcliffe Publishing; 2008
http://www.radcliffehealth.com/shop/occupational-and-physical-therapy-children-rheumatic-diseases-clinical-handbook.

The book *Raising a Child with Arthritis: A Parent's Guide* provides illustrations and instructions for ROM and postural exercises.[233] Exercises can be incorporated into daily activities for young children. Older children should be encouraged to express their personal goals and participate in developing the exercise program. Periodic reexamination and progression of the exercise prescription provide encouraging feedback to the child and parent.

Transition to Adult Health Care

Effective self-management of health care needs becomes especially important in late adolescence because estimates indicate that 50% to 60% of adolescents with JIA enter adulthood with mild disease activity. More individuals may continue to report pain and activity limitations as a result of their JIA.[234] Hilderson et al. followed up 44 subjects with JIA who were older than 16 years of age, had left pediatric care, and did not participate in a structured program of transitional care (PTC).[235] The majority of subjects (56.8%) who had persistent disease and associated activity limitations were still in specialized rheumatology care, 13.6% were followed up by a general practitioner, and 29.6% were no longer in medical follow-up. Of this latter group, 16.7% had disabilities and 42% reported persistent pain. The authors stress the need for interdisciplinary care programs throughout follow-up of children with JIA and structured transition from pediatric to adult health care.[235] A multicenter study by McDonagh et al. supports the use of an individualized PTC designed to reflect the developmental stages of adolescence.[236] They found significant improvement in adolescent and parent ratings of HRQOL, arthritis-related knowledge, and satisfaction with rheumatology care. Although not statistically significant, improvements were also found for independent health behaviors (managing medications and independent medical consultations) in the 12-month assessment.[236]

Older children and adolescents who participate in setting goals and making decisions about their own health care feel a greater sense of control. A study by Stinson and colleagues described how adolescents developed effective self-management skills through a dual process that included "letting go" by adults who manage their health care and "gaining control" of managing their own illness.[237] Common subthemes expressed by participants included "knowledge and awareness about the disease, listening to and challenging care providers, communicating with the doctor, managing pain, and managing emotions."[237]

Adolescents universally agreed on the need for more information and believed that web-based interventions could improve accessibility to this information. A study by Lelieveld et al. supports this belief. They found that an Internet-based program directed at children with JIA, aged 8 to 12 years, who had low daily PA, was safe, feasible, and effective in improving PA levels, endurance, and adherence to PA recommendations.[238]

Summary

This chapter presents information on the heterogeneous disorders included under the umbrella term JIA and a brief introduction to other rheumatic conditions one may encounter throughout their practice as a physical therapist. Although the exact etiology of many of these autoinflammatory and autoimmune diseases is not entirely understood, great strides continue to be made. Most children do well with early diagnosis and appropriate medical treatment to manage the inflammatory process. However, some with severe and persistent disease experience significant impairments, including joint pain and swelling, limited ROM, and muscle atrophy and weakness. Secondary impairments in aerobic fitness and exercise tolerance are common and may contribute to activity limitations and participation restrictions. The long-term prognosis depends on the child's age at disease onset, disease type and course, and the quality and consistency of health care. The goal of management is for the child to lead as normal a life as possible. Physical therapists play an important role on the multidisciplinary team to help the child and family achieve this goal.

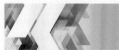

CASE STUDY

SARA

Sara is a 13-year-old girl with RF-negative polyJIA of 8 years' duration. After several years of mild disease activity, Sara presents with swelling in multiple joints, most notably both knees and the right ankle. She complains of pain and morning stiffness lasting 30 to 60 minutes and neck pain during the day. She lives with her parents, an older brother, and sister; and is in the eighth grade at a local public school.

Medical History

Sara was diagnosed with polyarticular JIA at 5 years of age. Her parents stated signs of the disease, including stiffness and irritability upon awakening, "bumps" on her elbows and shins, and altered gait pattern, were evident for at least a year before the diagnosis. At her first visit to the pediatric rheumatologist, she had active disease in most extremity joints and the cervical spine. Rheumatoid nodules were found on the extensor surface of the ulna and tibial crest bilaterally. She was originally treated with naproxen; however, after 6 months, during which she continued to have active disease, MTX given orally once a week was initiated. Signs of systemic disease were not evident at this time.

During the next several years, Sara continued to have disease flares in both knees, both hips, and the right ankle that were managed by IA steroid injections. Following each injection, she reported significant pain relief and was able to return to her normal activities. At the age of 11 years, Sara's JIA was determined to be in clinical remission on medication. However, her disease flared 6 months ago, with increased joint pain, morning stiffness, and fatigue that affected her school attendance and participation in PE and sports.

Current Complaints

Sara is being seen in clinic today to review her medications and HEP. She takes her MTX, but misses at least 30% of the prescribed dose of naproxen each week. She admits to poor adherence to the HEP, stating it doesn't help. According to Sara's mother, she has missed school or been late at least once a week for several months owing to disease symptoms. She does not meet the school's PE or sports requirement because of her JIA. She receives physical therapy and occupational therapy once a week in school and several accommodations under a 504 plan. These include lockers at either end of the school, a set of books for home, laptop computer for class notes, extra time for written examinations, and excuse from PE when she is unable to participate. Sara is also not bound by the school's attendance policy.

The rheumatologist confirmed that Sara has active arthritis in both of her wrists, knees, and right ankle. AROM and PROM are limited in the cervical spine, wrists, hips, right knee, and ankle; she has deformities of the toes in both feet. He added ETN once a week to Sara's medication regimen, continuing the once/weekly MTX and naproxen twice/day. IA steroid injections were scheduled for her next visit in 1 week, and she was referred to a physical therapist for an evaluation and review of her HEP, and to an occupational therapist (OT) for revision of her wrist splints and suggestions for adaptive equipment to improve her hand function. Sara was also referred to the child life specialist for assistance in managing her own health care needs.

Sara's Goals

Sara expressed two major concerns: (1) She would always have this disease and never be able to do the same activities as her friends; (2) she would not be able to keep up physically with the demands of high school. She stated her goals were to be like other kids, play on a sport team such as basketball or soccer, and hike and ski with her family.

Physical Therapist Examination
Questions Guiding the Examination
1. Are there specific activity limitations that negatively impact Sara's participation and overall QOL and prevent her from achieving her current goals?
2. Are there specific impairments that contribute to these problems?

Activity and Participation Findings

To answer the first question, several standardized assessments validated for children with JIA were used. The QOML questionnaire includes two 100-mm VAS that measure overall QOL and HRQOL; higher scores indicate better QOL.[73] Sara rated both her overall QOL and HRQOL as 40/100 mm. Using the 5-point categorical scale (much better to much worse), Sara rated her life as "much worse" than at her last clinic visit 3 months ago, indicating her JIA has a negative impact on her QOL.

Sara also completed the CAT$_{CHAQ38}$; the DI, calculated as the mean score for all 38 items, has a range of 0 to 3 where higher scores indicate greater disability.[69] Her DI was 1.50, suggesting moderate disability. She scored the following tasks as "unable to do" during the previous week: "play team sports with others in my class," "run a race," and "perform activities for a long time without getting tired." Pain during the previous week was scored as 60/100 mm on a VAS (higher scores indicate greater pain).

To answer the second question, several measures were performed, including a systems review, observational gait analysis, and two composites of the BOT-2, Body Coordination (Balance and Bilateral Coordination) and Strength and Agility (Running Speed and Agility and Strength). The tables given show Sara's scores on the BOT-2.

Composite Score Profile (Normative Mean on Standard Score = 50, SD = 10)

Composite	Standard Score	90% CI	Compared with Normative Values	Descriptive Category
Body coordination	36	32–40	≥1 SD	Below average
Strength and agility	37	33–41	≥1 SD	Below average

Subtest Profile (Normative Mean on Scale Score = 15; SD = 5)

Subtest	Scale Score	90% CI	Compared with Normative Values	Descriptive Category
Bilateral coordination	14	12–16	21 SD	Average
Balance	3	0–5	>22 SD	Well below average
Running speed and agility	8	6–10	>21 SD	Below average
Strength	8	5–11	>2SD	Below average

Body Structures and Function Findings

1. Signs of active joint disease
   - Both wrists, knees, and ankles had effusions with loss of joint contours; swelling was also noted around the right Achilles tendon.
   - Tenderness to palpation and mild withdrawal were noted at the abovementioned joints and at the right Achilles tendon.

2. ROM: All joints showed PROM within normal limits (WNL), with these exceptions:
   - Cervical spine rotation and lateral flexion to either side: limited by 50%
   - Right shoulder flexion: -20 degrees (0-160)
   - Elbow extension: -20 degrees (R), -30 degrees (L)
   - Wrist DF: (R) -25 degrees (0 to 45 degrees); (L) -25 degrees (0 to 55 degrees)
     - Resting position of R wrist/hand: ulnar deviation, MCP, and PIP flexion (alignment corrected with passive motion)
   - Pelvis in anterior tilted position; lumbar spine in excessive lordosis
   - Hip extension (modified Thomas test): -10 degrees (R) and (L)
   - Ober test: short tensor fascia lata (R)
   - Knee extension, measured in prone: -10 degrees (R), -5 degrees (L)
     - Hamstring length test (supine): -45 degrees (R), -35 degrees (L)
     - Prudential FITNESSGRAM sit-and-reach score: 8", below the minimum health fitness standard (HFS) of 10" for her age and gender[178]
   - Feet and ankles
     - (R) ankle PF: 0 degrees to 30 degrees; (R) ankle DF with the knee extended: 0 degrees
     - Hindfoot eversion: 0 degrees (R) and (L); inversion WNL
     - Pes cavus (R) and (L)

3. Muscle strength
   - Gross strength (MMT): lower limb = 4/5; upper limb = 3+/5
   - Functional ankle PF muscle endurance: able to perform eight bilateral heel rises
   - Grip strength measured with a modified blood pressure cuff: 60/20 mm Hg (R) and 80/20 mm Hg (L). According to Smythe and Helewa,[74] a rise of 20 mm Hg from the baseline of 20 mm Hg is equal to approximately 5 lb (2.27 kg) of force; Sara's grip strength, measured in pounds, was 10 lb (R) and 15 lb (L), considerably below the reported range of values for healthy, typically developing 13-year-old females: (39 to 79 lb [R], 25 to 76 lb [L]).[168]
   - PF curl-up test (abdominal strength and endurance) score: 8, below the minimum HFS of 18; PF-modified pull-up test (upper body strength and endurance) score: 1, below the minimum HFS of 4.[169]

4. Aerobic performance/exercise tolerance
   - 6MWD: 550 m, less than mean distance of 663 ± 50.8 m (95% CI: 651.0 to 675.0) reported for 12- to 15-year-old females[170]
     - Postwalk HR (170 bpm) was approximately 82% of age-related HR$_{max}$ and indicates a good effort and provides a target HR for exercise training.
   - Self-rated fatigue during the previous week: 50 on a 100-mm VAS

5. Body composition: Body mass index and skinfold thickness measures WNL for her age

6. Gait pattern: Footprint analysis with video
   - Decreased walking velocity: 75 cm/sec compared with 138.8 ± 4.7 cm/sec reported for a 12.6-year-old, males and females combined[171]

- Shortened right step length compared with left
- Majority of weight borne on lateral side of foot throughout stance phase
- Lack of push-off at terminal stance: decreased active ankle PF ROM and decreased hip extension

Evaluation and Diagnosis

Guiding Questions

1. Which impairments contribute to Sara's current activity and participation problems?
2. Which impairments must be addressed to prevent or minimize secondary problems?
3. What strengths and resources does Sara have that could support her overall QOL?

Participation Restrictions	Activity Limitations	Impairments
- Frequent school absence and tardiness - Inconsistent participation in PE - Unable to participate in sports with friends or family	- Difficulty transitioning between sitting on floor and standing - Difficulty negotiating steps - Difficulty with reach, grasp, and manipulation activities - Difficulty performing activities (complex motor skills) for PE and sports	*Musculoskeletal* - Active arthritis (joint swelling and pain) - Limited joint ROM / ↓ soft-tissue extensibility - Muscle weakness (hand grip, core trunk, and lower limb muscles) *Cardiopulmonary* - Impaired aerobic fitness - Impaired anaerobic fitness (speed/power) *Neuromuscular/ Multisystem* - Gait deviations: Slow walking speed, uneven step, stride length • Lower limb and foot pain when walking • Poor postural control (steady state on narrow base of support; anticipatory) • Poor bilateral coordination/movement speed

The first two columns in the given table list the priority activity and participation problems identified by Sara and her parents on the basis of information from the CHAQ, JAQQ, and interview. Column three lists the impairments believed to contribute to these problems.

- Active arthritis contributes to pain, tenderness, and limited AROM and PROM.
- Limited joint motion and soft-tissue shortening contribute to impaired movement patterns, fatigue, and pain during physical activities.
- Muscle weakness, fatigue, and poor power contribute to gross motor deficits.
- Impaired joint mobility and muscle performance contribute to gait deviations.
- Impaired proprioception, coordination, and speed may contribute to poor muscular control and postural stability during challenging physical activities.

- Poor adherence to prescribed medications and HEP and Sara's limited participation in her health care contribute to poor disease control and functional outcome.

Strengths and Resources

Although Sara's adherence to her medical and therapy regimen has been inadequate, she now appears more interested in managing her disease and improving her health status and functional capacity. Her parents are very supportive, and the school appears to be willing to accommodate her needs by making requested modifications to her educational program.

Prognosis

Guiding Questions

1. What would improve Sara's active participation in her health care?
2. What is the best POC with regard to medications and rehabilitation?

Question 1: The rheumatology team believed that inadequate disease control and poor adherence to her therapy regimen contributed to Sara's current problems. They thought adherence would improve if Sara were more involved in her own health care. Sara stated she wanted to participate in PE and sports with her family and friends. She is also concerned about adjusting to the physical and work challenges of high school next year. The child life specialist helped her understand how she might achieve her goals if her JIA was under better control by regular use of medication and adherence to her exercise regimen.

Question 2: The team believed that Sara's arthritis and functional status would improve following IA injections, the addition of ETN (Enbrel™), and improved adherence to the NSAID prescription and daily exercise regimen.[31] Sara agreed to a 6-month contract, listing her goals, therapy objectives, and a POC aimed at achieving these. An interim reevaluation was scheduled for 3 months. The contract included (1) following her full medication regimen, (2) performing home ROM and strengthening exercises, and (3) participating in an aerobic conditioning program designed by the physical therapist. She also agreed to wear resting hand splints each night while sleeping. Sara and her parents agreed to a 3-month trial of direct physical therapist and occupational therapist (OT) twice a week, with goals of improving ROM and strength, and her parents signed permission for the clinic physical therapist and OT to consult with the school PE instructor to discuss activity modifications so Sara could safely participate in PE.

Expected Outcomes (Goals to be achieved in 6 months with progress toward the goals observed at the 3-month follow-up visit):

- Improved adherence to medication should result in improved disease control, reduced joint pain, improved physical function, and HRQOL.[162-164]
  - Goal: Sara will show at least a 75% improvement in adherence to her medication schedule based on a daily log, with entries verified by one parent.
  - Goal: Sara will demonstrate improved capability to perform necessary and desired activities based on a reduction of greater than or equal to 0.13 on her self-reported CAT$_{CHAQ38}$ DI.[67]

- Goal: Sara's self-reported HRQOL score will show improvement based on an increase of greater than or equal to 11 mm in her score on the QOML VAS.[72]
- Sara's gait pattern will improve following joint injections and supportive therapy.
  - Goal: Sara will demonstrate increased walking speed and symmetry in step and stride length based on observational gait analysis and footprint recording.
- Available evidence suggests that Sara can improve her performance-related physical fitness through a physical conditioning regimen performed twice a week.[23,172]
  - Goal: Sara's 6MWD will increase by at least 48 m, the minimal detectable change (MDC) reported for healthy children on the 6MWT.[96]
  - Goal: Sara will demonstrate decreased fatigue with PA based on self-report using a 100-mm VAS, where higher values equal greater fatigue.
- Daily ROM and flexibility exercises should improve joint ROM and soft-tissue extensibility, resulting in decreased stiffness and pain.
  - Goal: Sara will demonstrate improved passive joint ROM based on goniometric measurement of the shoulders, hips, knees, and ankles.
- Improved physical status should allow Sara to increase her participation in physical activities with her family and friends. Sara will record progress using a daily diary.
  - Goal: Sara will actively participate in at least 75% of all PE activities each week, with or without modifications.
  - Goal: Sara will participate in at least one recreational PA with family or friends each week for at least 1 hour.

Intervention Plan

Following IA injections to the knees, right wrist, and right ankle, Sara was on non–weight bearing for 1 day. After 1 week of modified PA, she resumed all typical activities.

Coordination, Communication, and Documentation

The rheumatology team worked with Sara and her parents to determine techniques that would improve her adherence to the treatment plan. The nurse provided instruction to Sara and her parents to ensure correct administration of the weekly injections of ETN and reasons for following the exact prescription for taking the NSAID. The physical therapist provided written and oral instructions, demonstration, and illustrations of Sara's exercises. The OT made new resting wrist/hand splints and gave Sara assistive devices to improve her ability to perform ADLs. The child life specialist helped Sara establish a schedule for taking medications and develop a daily diary to keep a record of her medications, use of splints, HEP, PE, and recreational activities. Each section of the diary included space for Sara's comments. She was encouraged to contact the team with questions about her program or symptoms. The team, with the permission of Sara and her parents, sent a copy of the physical therapist and OT evaluations to the school and requested the PE instructor to consult with the clinic physical therapist to adjust activities so that Sara could increase her participation.

Patient Education

The clinic physical therapist discussed the findings of the physical examination with Sara and her parents. She discussed the impact of arthritis on joints and muscles, the potential sources of pain and stiffness, and secondary problems, including poor exercise tolerance and impaired motor skills. She explained that Sara's current functional problems were likely related to limited joint mobility and soft-tissue extensibility, pain, and poor aerobic and muscular fitness. She explained that intervention would be directed toward reducing these impairments. The therapy program would also include practice of the activities that were difficult for Sara.

Procedural Interventions

- Direct physical therapy 30 to 45 minutes twice a week and instruction in HEP

Interventions for Impaired Joint Mobility and Muscle Function

Direct therapy: Initial instruction in maintaining control of the trunk and lumbar spine by engaging abdominal muscles during all activities

1. AAROM for shoulder flexion, abduction in scapular plane, medial and lateral rotation, with attention to scapular position, movement, and scapulohumeral rhythm
2. Prone scapular progression exercises; progress to standing scapular exercises against a wall; progress to using light handheld weights when Sara can perform exercises without pain or compensatory movements
3. AAROM and AROM for serratus anterior; progress to exercise against resistance
4. Instruction in isometric exercise to improve neck stability
5. Stretching of shortened latissimus dorsi, lateral shoulder rotators and posterior capsule, hip flexors, hamstrings, and right gastrocnemius using autogenic and reciprocal inhibition
6. Stretching of right TFL
7. Strength training for hip extensors, deep external rotators, and abductors
   - Begin with AROM to teach correct technique for each muscle group.
   - Progress to graded resistance exercise using light weights or elastic bands.
   - Closed kinetic chain (CKC) exercise, including graded squats, lunges, and "step" training to improve strength, endurance, and control of lower extremity musculature
8. Gait training to improve lower limb weight bearing, step and stride length

Interventions to Address Impaired Motor Skills

1. Activities to improve proprioception, agility, and coordination once joint ROM and muscle strength improve and pain decreases
2. Gait training to increase walking velocity, using timed walks
3. Activity- or sport-specific training to ensure safe participation in physical activities and recreational sports

Home Exercise Program

1. Daily AROM exercises concentrating on cervical spine, shoulders, wrists, hips, knees, and ankles using illustrations from *Raising a Child with Arthritis*

2. Daily aerobic activity (Sara's choice), gradually increasing duration to at least 30 minutes a day and intensity to at least 75% of her age-based HR_{max}

Recommendations/Referrals

1. Referral to orthotist for custom insoles to accommodate pes cavus deformity and decrease pain under MTP joints
2. Recommendation for semirigid cervical collar when riding in school bus and car, and easel top for desk to decrease neck strain when reading

Reexamination

Sara was seen by the clinic physical therapist at her 3-month follow-up rheumatology appointment. She reported receiving physical therapy twice a week at school before classes begin and OT once a week during school time. She also attends all PE classes each week and participates in approximately 50% of the activities with some modifications. The school PE instructor and physical therapist are working together to improve Sara's gross motor skills and adapt difficult activities to allow her to participate with her classmates.

Findings of Reexamination
Activities and Participation

1. Sara's CAT_{CHAQ38} DI decreased from 1.50 to 1.30, exceeding the reported minimal clinically important improvement of greater than or equal to 0.13.
2. Her self-reported HRQOL improved from 40 to 70 mm, and she reported her life as somewhat better since her last clinic visit.

Body Structures and Functions

1. Signs of active joint disease
   - Mild swelling noted in the right knee, no tenderness or pain on passive motion
2. ROM, flexibility, and joint alignment
   - No change in cervical spine AROM, but no c/o PROM
   - (R) shoulder PROM: 0 to 170 degrees with stress pain at end range
   - Wrist DF: 0 to 60 degrees (R), 0 to 60 degrees (L)
   - Passive hip extension limitation: 5 degrees
   - Knee extension (examined prone): -5 (R); WNL (L)
   - (R) Ankle PROM: PF = 0 to 40 degrees; DF with knee extended = 0 to 5 degrees
   - Passive calcaneal eversion increased: 0 to 5 degrees
3. Standing posture
   - Sara continued to stand with an increased anterior pelvic tilt and lumbar lordosis, although she could correct this upon request by engaging her abdominal muscles.
   - Barefoot, Sara continued to stand with most of her weight over the lateral border of her foot; when wearing her custom-made in-shoe orthoses and sneakers, her weight was borne more evenly over the plantar surface of the foot.
4. Muscle strength and flexibility
   - Grip strength: 100/20 mm Hg (20 lb) (R); 140/20 mm Hg (30 lb) (L)
   - Score on the PF reported by Sara's school physical therapist improved.
   - Curl-up test: increased from 8 to 12 (HFS = 18)

- Modified pull-up test: increased from 1 to 5 (HFS ≥ 4)
- Sit-and-reach test: increased from 8″ to 9″ (HFS = 10″)

5. 6MWD increased from 550 to 610 m, exceeding the MDC of 48 m.
6. Gait velocity increased from 75 to 110 cm/sec. Gait pattern showed improved heel contact, weight more evenly distributed over the plantar surface of the foot during midstance, improved push-off on the medial side of the forefoot and hip extension at terminal stance, and increased step length.

Outcomes

1. A review of Sara's medication and activity diary indicated improved adherence to her medication regimen and HEP; this was supported by Sara's parents as well as by decreased signs of active arthritis and improved ROM in most joints.
2. Improvements in self-reported worst pain from 60 to 40 mm and worst fatigue from 50 to 20 mm over the previous week on the VASs reflect improved disease control.
3. Improvements in PF scores, walking speed, and 6MWD suggest increased stamina, as a result of improved adherence to her exercise program.
4. Clinically meaningful improvements in her physical function and QOL lend support to her improved health status and ability to manage her condition.

Plan

On the basis of Sara's improved physical status, the clinic therapist recommended continuing with direct physical therapy in school with an emphasis on increasing aerobic fitness, strength, and gross motor proficiency. She also suggested that the school physical therapist and the PE instructor work together with Sara on specific training for basketball to allow her to participate in an intramural league at school. Reevaluation was scheduled for her next clinic appointment in 3 months.

REFERENCES

1. Petty RE, Southwood TR, Manners P, et al. International League of Associations for Rheumatology classification of juvenile idiopathic arthritis: second revision, Edmonton 2001. *J Rheumatol.* 2004;31:390–392.
2. Martini A, Ravelli A, Avcin T, et al. Toward new classification criteria for juvenile idiopathic arthritis: first steps Pediatric Rheumatology International Trials Organization international consensus. *J Rheumatol.* 2019;46:190–197.
3. Thierry S, Fautrel B, Lemelle I, Guillemin F. Prevalence and incidence of juvenile idiopathic arthritis: a systemic review. *Joint Bone Spine.* 2014;81:112–117.
4. Ringold S, Angeles-Han ST, Beukelman T, et al. 2019 American College of Rheumatology/Arthritis Foundation guideline for the treatment of juvenile idiopathic arthritis: therapeutic approaches for non-systemic polyarthritis, sacroiliitis, and enthesitis. *Arthritis Care Res.* 2019;71:717–734.
5. Hersh AO, Prahalad S. Immunogenetics of juvenile idiopathic arthritis: a comprehensive review. *J Autoimmun.* 2015;64:113–124.
6. Fernando MM, Stevens CR, Walsh EC, et al. Defining the role of the MHC in autoimmunity: a review and pooled analysis. *PLoS Genet.* 2008;4:e1000024.

7. Hinks A, Marion MC, Cobb J, et al. The genetic profile of rheumatoid factor-positive polyarticular juvenile idiopathic arthritis resembles that of adult rheumatoid arthritis. *Arthritis Rheum.* 2018;70:957–962.

8. Ramsey LB, Moncrieffe H, Smith CN, et al. Association of SLCO1B1*14 allele with poor response to methotrexate in juvenile idiopathic arthritis patients. *ACR Open Rheumatol.* 2019;1:58–62.

9. Prahalad S, Zeft AS, Pimentel R, et al. Quantification of the familial contribution to juvenile idiopathic arthritis. *Arthritis Rheum.* 2010;62:2525–2529.

10. Clemens LE, Albert E, Ansell BM. Sibling pairs affected by chronic arthritis of childhood: evidence for a genetic predisposition. *J Rheumatol.* 1985;12:108–113.

11. Zeft A, Shear ES, Thompson SD, et al. Familial autoimmunity: maternal parent-of-origin effect in juvenile idiopathic arthritis. *Clin Rheumatol.* 2008;27:241–244.

12. Majumder S, Aggarwal A. Juvenile idiopathic arthritis and the gut microbiome: where are we now? *Best Pract Res Clin Rheumatol.* 2019;33:101496.

13. Lin YT, Wang CT, Gershwin ME, Chiang BL. The pathogenesis of oligoarticular/polyarticular vs systemic juvenile idiopathic arthritis. *Autoimmun Rev.* 2011;10:482–489.

14. Nigrovic PA. Autoinflammation and autoimmunity in systemic juvenile idiopathic arthritis. *Proc Natl Acad Sci USA.* 2015;112:15785–15786.

15. Seidman AJ, Limaiem F. Synovial fluid analysis. [Updated January 22, 2019]. In: *StatPearls [Internet].* Treasure Island, FL: StatPearls Publishing; January 2020. https://www.ncbi.nlm.nih.gov/books/NBK537114/

16. Burnham JM, Shults J, Dubner SE, et al. Bone density, structure, and strength in juvenile idiopathic arthritis: importance of disease severity and muscle deficits. *Arthritis Rheum.* 2008;58:2518–2527.

17. Simon S, Whiffen J, Shapiro F. Leg-length discrepancies in monoarticular and pauciarticular juvenile rheumatoid arthritis. *J Bone Joint Surg Am.* 1981;63:209–215.

18. Stoll ML, Kau CH, Waite PD, et al. Temporomandibular joint arthritis in juvenile idiopathic arthritis, now what? *Pediatr Rheumatol Online J.* 2018;16:32.

19. Lindehammar H, Backman E. Muscle function in juvenile chronic arthritis. *J Rheumatol.* 1995;22:1159–1165.

20. Rice DA, McNair PJ. Quadriceps arthrogenic muscle inhibition: neural mechanisms and treatment perspectives. *Semin Arthritis Rheum.* 2010;40:250–266.

21. Lindehammar H, Sandstedt P. Measurement of quadriceps muscle strength and bulk in juvenile chronic arthritis: a prospective, longitudinal, 2 year survey. *J Rheumatol.* 1998;25:2240–2248.

22. Lindehammar H, Lindvall B. Muscular involvement in juvenile idiopathic arthritis. *Rheumatology.* 2004;43:1546–1554.

23. Saarinen J, Lehtonen K, Malkia E, Lahdenne P. Lower extremity isometric strength in children with juvenile idiopathic arthritis. *Clin Exp Rheumatol.* 2008;26:947–953.

24. Bourdier P, Birat A, Rochette E, et al. Muscle function and architecture in children with juvenile idiopathic arthritis. *Acta Paediatr.* 2021;110(1):280–287

25. Singer NG, Ravelli A. Evaluation of musculoskeletal complaints in children: clinical evaluation. In: Hochberg MC, Smolen JS, Weisman MH, et al, eds. *Rheumatology.* 6th ed. Elsevier Ltd; 2015:815–819.

26. Herman MJ, Martinek M. The limping child. *Pediatr Rev.* 2015;36:184–195.

27. Swart JF, de Roock S, Prakken BJ. Understanding inflammation in juvenile idiopathic arthritis: how immune biomarkers guide clinical strategies in the systemic onset subtype. *Eur J Immunol.* 2016;46:2068–2077.

28. Mahmud SA, Binstadt BA. Autoantibodies in the pathogenesis, diagnosis, and prognosis of juvenile idiopathic arthritis. *Front Immunol.* 2019;9:3168.

29. Hemke R, Tzaribachev N, Barendregt AM, et al. Imaging of the knee in juvenile idiopathic arthritis. *Pediatr Radiol.* 2018;48:818–827.

30. Lanni S, Martini A, Malattia C. Heading toward a modern imaging approach in juvenile idiopathic arthritis. *Curr Rheumatol Rep.* 2014;16:416–425.

31. Shire NJ, Bardzinski BJ. Picture perfect: imaging techniques in juvenile idiopathic arthritis. *Imaging Med.* 2011;3:635–651.

32. Breton S, Jousse-Joulin S, Finel E, et al. Imaging approaches for evaluating peripheral joint abnormalities in juvenile idiopathic arthritis. *Semin Arthritis Rheum.* 2012;41:698–711.

33. Sudol-Szopinska I, Gietka P, Znajdek M, et al. Imaging of juvenile spondyloarthritis, part I: classifications and radiographs. *J Ultrason.* 2017;17:167–175.

34. Janow GL, Panghaal V, Frinh A, et al. Detection of active disease in juvenile idiopathic arthritis: sensitivity and specificity of the physical exam vs ultrasound. *J Rheumatol.* 2011;38:2671–2674.

35. Spannow AH, Pfeiffer-Jensen M, Andersen NT, et al. Ultrasonic measurements of joint cartilage thickness in healthy children: age- and sex-related standard reference values. *J Rheumatol.* 2010;37:2595–2601.

36. Consolaro A, Giancane G, Schiappapietra B, et al. Clinical outcome measures in juvenile idiopathic arthritis. *Pediatr Rheumatol Online J.* 2016;18:23.

37. Consolaro A, Ruperto N, Bazso A, et al. Development and validation of a composite disease activity score for juvenile idiopathic arthritis. *Arthritis Rheum.* 2009;61:658–666.

38. Nordal EB, Zak M, Aalto K, et al. Validity and predictive ability of the juvenile arthritis disease activity score based on CRP versus ESR in a Nordic population-based setting. *Ann Rheum Dis.* 2012;71:1122–1127.

39. Mcerlane F, Beresford MW, Baildam EM, et al. Validity of a three-variable juvenile arthritis disease activity score in children with new-onset juvenile idiopathic arthritis. *Ann Rheum Dis.* 2013;72:1983–1988.

40. Giannini EH, Ruperto N, Ravelli A, et al. Preliminary definition of improvement in juvenile arthritis. *Arthritis Rheum.* 1997;40:1202–1209.

41. Brunner HI, Lovell DJ, Finck BK, Giannini EH. Preliminary definition of disease flare in juvenile rheumatoid arthritis. *J Rheumatol.* 2002;29:1058–1064.

42. Weiss PF, Colbert RA, Xio R, et al. Development and retrospective validation of the juvenile spondyloarthritis disease activity (JSpADA) index. *Arthritis Care Res.* 2014;66:1775–1782.

43. Wallace CA, Ruperto N, Giannini EH. Preliminary criteria for clinical remission for select categories of juvenile idiopathic arthritis. *J Rheumatol.* 2004;31:2290–2294.

44. Wallace CA, Giannini EH, Huang B, et al. American College of Rheumatology provisional criteria for defining clinical inactive disease in select categories of juvenile idiopathic arthritis. *Arthritis Care Res.* 2011;63:929–936.

45. Consolaro A, Ruperto N, Pistorio A, et al. Development and initial validation of composite parent- and child-centered disease assessment indices for juvenile idiopathic arthritis. *Arthritis Care Res.* 2011;63:1262–1270.

46. Viola S, Felici E, Magni-Manzoni S, et al. Development and validation of a clinical index for assessment of long-term damage in juvenile idiopathic arthritis. *Arthritis Rheum.* 2005;52:2092–2102.

47. Singh YP, Aggarwal A. A modified juvenile arthritis damage index to improve articular damage assessment in juvenile idiopathic arthritis-enthesitis-related arthritis (JIA-ERA). *Clin Rheumatol.* 2012;31:767–774.

48. Sherry DD, Stein LD, Reed AM, et al. Prevention of leg length discrepancy in young children with pauciarticular juvenile rheumatoid arthritis by treatment with intraarticular steroids. *Arthritis Rheum.* 1999;42:2330–2334.

49. Zulian F, Martini G, Gobber D, et al. Comparison of intra-articular triamcinolone hexacetonide and triamcinolone acetonide in oligoarticular juvenile idiopathic arthritis. *Rheumatology.* 2003;42:1254–1259.

50. Gotte AC. Intra-articular corticosteroids in the treatment of juvenile idiopathic arthritis: safety, efficacy, and features affecting outcome.

A comprehensive review of the literature. *Open Access Rheumatol.* 2009;14:37–49.

51. Beukelman T, Patkar NM, Saag KG, et al. 2011 American College of Rheumatology recommendations for the treatment of juvenile idiopathic arthritis: initiation and safety monitoring of therapeutic agents for the treatment of arthritis and systemic features. *Arthritis Care Res.* 2011;63:465–482.

52. Stoll ML, Cron RQ. Treatment of juvenile idiopathic arthritis: a revolution in care. *Pediatr Rheumatol Online.* 2014;12:13.

53. Tukova J, Chladek J, Nemcova D, et al. Methotrexate bioavailability after oral and subcutaneous administration in children with juvenile idiopathic arthritis. *Clin Exp Rheumatol.* 2009;27:1047–1053.

54. Alsufyani K, Ortiz-Alvarez O, Cabral DA, et al. The role of subcutaneous administration of methotrexate in children with juvenile idiopathic arthritis who had failed oral methotrexate. *J. Rheumatol.* 2004;31:179–182.

55. Beresford MW. New insights into classification, measures of outcome, and pharmacotherapy. *Pediatr Drugs.* 2011;13:161–173.

56. Lovell DJ, Giannini EH, Reiff A, et al. Etanercept in children with polyarticular juvenile rheumatoid arthritis. Pediatric Rheumatology Collaborative Study Group. *N Engl J Med.* 2000;342:763–769.

57. Horneff G, De Bock F, Foeldvari I, et al. Safety and efficacy of combination of etanercept and methotrexate compared to treatment with etanercept only in patients with juvenile idiopathic arthritis (JIA): preliminary data from the German JIA registry. *Ann Rheum Dis.* 2009;68:519–525.

58. Emery P, Breedveld FC, Hall S, et al. Comparison of methotrexate monotherapy with a combination of methotrexate and etanercept in active, early, moderate to severe rheumatoid arthritis (COMET): a randomized, double-blind, parallel treatment trial. *Lancet.* 2008;372:375–382.

59. FDA approved drugs. Accessed September 1, 2020. https://www.accessdata.fda.gov/scripts/cder/daf/index.cfm?event=reportsSearch.process&rptName=1&reportSelectMonth=9&reportSelectYear=2020&nav

60. Lovell DJ, Ruperto N, Goodman S, et al. Adalimumab with or without methotrexate in juvenile rheumatoid arthritis. *N Engl J Med.* 2008;359:810–820.

61. Gerloni V, Pontikaki I, Gattinara M, et al. Efficacy of repeated intravenous infusions of an anti-tumor necrosis factor α monoclonal antibody, infliximab, in persistently active, refractory juvenile idiopathic arthritis. *Arthritis Rheum.* 2005;52:548–553.

62. Ruperto N, Lovell DJ, Quartier P, et al. Abatacept in children with juvenile idiopathic arthritis: a randomized, double-blind, placebo-controlled withdrawal trial. *Lancet.* 2008;372:383–391.

63. Brunner HE, Ruperto N, Zuber Z, et al. Efficacy and safety of tocilizumab in patients with polyarticular-course juvenile idiopathic arthritis: results from a phase 3, randomized, double-blind withdrawal trial. *Ann Rheum Dis.* 2015;74:1110–1117.

64. De Benedetti F, Brunner H, Ruperto N, et al. Catch-up growth during tocilizumab therapy for systemic juvenile idiopathic arthritis: results from a phase III trial. *Arthritis Rheumatol.* 2015;67:840–848.

65. Toplak N, Blazina S, Avcin T. The role of IL-1 inhibition in systemic juvenile idiopathic arthritis: current status and future perspectives. *Drug Des Devel Ther.* 2018;12:1633–1643.

66. Behrens EM, Beukelman T, Gallo L, et al. Evaluation of the presentation of systemic onset juvenile rheumatoid arthritis: data from the Pennsylvania systemic onset juvenile arthritis registry (PASOJAR). *J Rheumatol.* 2008;35:343–348.

67. Janow G, Schanberg LE, Setoguchi S, et al. The systemic juvenile idiopathic arthritis cohort of the childhood arthritis and rheumatology research alliance registry: 2010-2013. *J Rheumatol.* 2016;43:1755–1762.

68. Shimzu M, Nakagishi Y, Inoue N, et al. Interleukin-18 for predicting the development of macrophage activation syndrome in systemic juvenile idiopathic arthritis. *Clin Immunol.* 2015;160:277–281.

69. Ravelli A, Grom AA, Behrens EM, et al. Macrophage activation syndrome as part of systemic juvenile idiopathic arthritis: diagnosis, genetics, pathophysiology and treatment. *Genes Immun.* 2012;13:289–298.

70. Bennett TD, Fluchel M, Hersh AO, et al. Macrophage activation syndrome in children with systemic lupus erythematosus and children with juvenile idiopathic arthritis. *Arthritis Rheum.* 2012;64:4135–4142.

71. Singh-Grewal D, Schneider R, Bayer N, et al. Predictors of disease course and remission in systemic juvenile idiopathic arthritis. *Arthritis Rheum.* 2006;54:1595–1601.

72. Packham JC, Hall MA. Long-term follow-up of 246 adults with juvenile idiopathic arthritis: functional outcome. *Rheumatology.* 2002;41:1428–1435.

73. DeWitt EM, Kimura Y, Beukelman T, et al. Consensus treatment plans for new-onset systemic juvenile idiopathic arthritis. *Arthritis Care Res.* 2012;64:1001–1010.

74. Horneff G, Schulz AC, Klotsch J, et al. Experience with etanercept, tocilizumab and interleukin-1 inhibitors in systemic onset juvenile idiopathic arthritis patients from the BIKER registry. *Arthritis Res Ther.* 2017;19:256.

75. Nigrovic PA, Mannion M, Prince FH, et al. Anakinra as first-line disease-modifying therapy in systemic juvenile idiopathic arthritis. *Arthritis Rheum.* 2011;63:545–555.

76. Nigrovic PA. Is there a window of opportunity for treatment of systemic juvenile idiopathic arthritis? *Arthritis Rheum.* 2014;66:1405–1413.

77. Ringold S, Weiss PF, Beukelman T, et al. 2013 Update of the 2011 American College of Rheumatology recommendations for the treatment of juvenile idiopathic arthritis. *Arthritis Rheum.* 2013;65:2499–2512.

78. Guzman J, Orn K, Tucker LB, et al. The outcomes of juvenile idiopathic arthritis in children managed with contemporary treatments: results from the ReACCh-Out cohort. *Ann Rheum Dis.* 2015;74:1854–1860.

79. Ombrello MJ, Remmers EF, Tachmazidou I, et al. HLA-DRB1*11 and variants of the MHC class II locus are strong risk factors for systemic juvenile idiopathic arthritis. *Proc Natl Acad Sci USA.* 2015;112:15970–15975.

80. Al-Matar MJ, Petty RE, Tucker LB. The early pattern of joint involvement predicts disease progression in children with oligoarticular (pauciarticular) juvenile rheumatoid arthritis. *Arthritis Rheum.* 2002;46:2708–2715.

81. Ravelli A, Martini A. Juvenile idiopathic arthritis. *Lancet.* 2007;369:767–778.

82. Angeles-Han ST, Ringold S, Beukelman T, et al. 2019 American College of Rheumatology/Arthritis Foundation guideline for the screening, monitoring, and treatment of juvenile idiopathic arthritis-associated uveitis. *Arthritis Care Res.* 2019;71:703–716.

83. Ravelli A, Varnier GC, Oliveira S, et al. Antinuclear antibody-positive patients should be grouped as a separate category in the classification of juvenile idiopathic arthritis. *Arthritis Rheum.* 2011;63:267–275.

84. Nigrovic PA, Raychaudhuri S, Thompson SD. Genetics and the classification of arthritis in adults and children. *Arthritis Rheumatol.* 2018;70:7–17.

85. Ringold S, Weiss PF, Colbert RA, et al. Childhood arthritis and rheumatology research alliance consensus treatment plans for new-onset polyarticular juvenile idiopathic arthritis. *Arthritis Care Res.* 2014;66:1063–1072.

86. Selvang AM, Lien G, Sorskaar D, et al. Early disease course and predictors of disability in juvenile rheumatoid arthritis and juvenile spondyloarthropathy: a 3-year prospective study. *J Rheumatol.* 2005;32:1122–1130.

87. Weiss PF. Evaluation and treatment of enthesitis-related arthritis. *Curr Med Lit Rheumatol.* 2013;32:33–41.

88. Shih YJ, Yang YH, Lin CY, et al. Enthesitis-related arthritis is the most common category of juvenile arthritis in Taiwan and presents persistent active disease. *Pediatr Rheumatol Online J.* 2019;17:58.

89. Weiss PF, Klink AJ, Behrens EM. Enthesitis in an inception cohort of enthesitis-related arthritis. *Arthritis Care Res.* 2011;63:1307–1312.

90. Mistry RR, Patro P, Agarwal V, et al. Enthesitis-related arthritis: current perspectives. *Open Access Rheumatol.* 2019;11:19–31.

91. Stoll ML, Weiss PF, Weiss JE, et al. Age and fecal microbial strain-specific differences in patients with spondyloarthritis. *Arthritis Res Ther.* 2018;20:14.

92. Stoll ML, Nigrovic PA. Subpopulations within juvenile psoriatic arthritis: a review. *Clin Dev Immunol.* 2006;13:377–380.

93. Aviel YB, Tyrrell P, Schneider R. Juvenile Psoriatic Arthritis (JPsA): juvenile arthritis with psoriasis? *Pediatr Rheumatol Online J.* 2013;11:11.

94. Zisman D, Gladman DD, Stoll ML, et al. The juvenile psoriatic arthritis cohort in the CARRA registry: clinical characteristics, classification, and outcomes. *J Rheumatol.* 2017;44:342–351.

95. Huemer C, Malleson PN, Cabral DA, et al. Patterns of joint involvement at onset differentiate oligoarticular juvenile psoriatic arthritis from pauciarticular juvenile rheumatoid arthritis. *J Rheumatol.* 2002;29:1531–1535.

96. Mathiesen P, Orngreen M, Vissing J, et al. Aerobic fitness after JDM-a long-term follow-up study. *Rheumatol.* 2013;52:287–295.

97. Munters LA, Loell I, Ossipova E, et al. Endurance exercise improves molecular pathways of aerobic metabolism in patients with myositis. *Arthritis Rheum.* 2016;68:1738–1750.

98. Feldman BM, Rider LG, Reed AM, et al. Juvenile dermatomyositis and other idiopathic inflammatory myopathies of childhood. *Lancet.* 2008;371:2201–2212.

99. Philippi K, Hoeltzel M, Byun Robinson A, et al. Race, income and disease outcomes in juvenile dermatomyositis. *J Pediatr.* 2017;184:38–44.

100. Varnier GC, Pilkington CA, Wedderburn LR. Juvenile dermatomyositis: novel treatment approaches and outcomes. *Curr Opin Rheumatol.* 2018;30:650–654.

101. Rider LG, Koziol D, Giannini EH, et al. Validation of manual muscle test and a subset of eight muscles (MMT8) for adult and juvenile idiopathic inflammatories and myopathies. *Arthritis Care Res.* 2010;62:465–472.

102. Rennebohm RM, Jones K, Huber AM, et al. Normal scores for nine maneuvers of childhood myositis assessment scale. *Arthritis Rheum.* 2004;51:365–370.

103. Munters LA, Dastmalchi M, Andren V, et al. Improvement in health and possible reduction in disease activity using endurance exercise in patients with established polymyositis and dermatomyositis: a multicenter randomized controlled trial with a 1-year open extension follow-up. *Arthritis Care Res.* 2013;65:1959–1968.

104. Alexanderson H. Physical exercise as a treatment for adult and juvenile myositis. *J Intern Med.* 2016;280:75–96.

105. Alexanderson H, Munters LA, Dastmalchi M, et al. Resistive home exercise in patients with recent-onset polymyositis and dermatomyositis—a randomized controlled single-blinded study with a 2-year follow up. *J Rheumatol.* 2014;41:1124–1132.

106. Omori CH, Silva CA, Sallum AM, Rodrigues Pereira RM, et al. Exercise training in juvenile dermatomyositis. *Arthritis Care Res (Hoboken).* 2012;64(8):1186-94. doi: 10.1002/acr.21684. PMID: 22505288.

107. Zhao Y, Ferguson PJ. Chronic nonbacterial osteomyelitis and chronic recurrent multifocal osteomyelitis in children. *Pediatr Clin North Am.* 2018;65:783–800.

108. Roderick MR, Shah R, Roger V, et al. Chronic recurrent multifocal osteomyelitis (CRMO) advancing the diagnosis. *Pediatr Rheumatol Online J.* 2016;14:47.

109. Zhao Y, Wu EY, Oliver MS, et al. Consensus treatment plans for chronic nonbacterial osteomyelitis refractory to nonsteroidal anti-inflammatory drugs and/or with active spinal lesions. *Arthritis Care Res.* 2018;70:1228–1237.

110. Julia N, Katharina R, Hermann G, et al. Physical activity and health-related quality of life in chronic non-bacterial osteomyelitis. *Pediatr Rheumatol Online J.* 2019;17:45.

111. Levy DM, Kamphuis S. Systemic lupus erythematosus in children and adolescents. *Pediatr Clin North Am.* 2012;59:345–364.

112. Mayo Clinic: Lupus. February 5, 2021. https://www.mayoclinic.org/diseases-conditions/lupus/symptoms-causes/syc-20365789

113. Lambers WM, Westra J, Jonkman MR, et al. Incomplete systemic lupus erythematosus: what remains after application of American College of Rheumatology and systemic lupus international collaborating clinics criteria? *Arthritis Care Res.* 2020;72:607–614.

114. Smith EM, Lythgoe H, Midgley A, et al. Juvenile-onset systemic lupus erythematosus: update on clinical presentation, pathophysiology and treatment options. *Clin Immunol.* 2019;209:108274.

115. Margiotta DPE, Basta F, Dolcini G, et al. Physical activity and sedentary behavior in patients with Systemic Lupus Erythematosus. *PLoS ONE.* 2018;3:1–16.

116. Sule S, Fontaine K. Abnormal body composition, cardiovascular endurance, and muscle strength in pediatric SLE. *Pediatr Rheumatol Online J.* 2016;14:50.

117. Pinto AJ, Miyake CNH, Benatti FB, et al. Reduced aerobic capacity and quality of life in physically inactive patients with systemic lupus erythematosus with mild or inactive disease. *Arthritis Care Res.* 2016;68:1780–1786.

118. O'Dwyer T, Durcan L, Wilson F. Exercise and physical activity in systemic lupus erythematosus: a systematic review with meta-analysis. *Semin Arthritis Rheum.* 2017;47:204–215.

119. Pena-Romero A, Garcia-Romero MT. Diagnosis and management of linear scleroderma in children. *Curr Opin Pediatr.* 2019;31:483–490.

120. Florez-Pollack S, Kunzler E, Jacobe HT. Morphea: current concepts. *Clin Dermatol.* 2018;36:475–486.

121. Li, S. Scleroderma in children and adolescents: localized scleroderma and systemic sclerosis. *Pediatr Clin N Am.* 2018;65:757–781.

122. Christen-Zaech S, Hakim MD, Afsar S, et al. Pediatric morphea (localized scleroderma): review of 136 patients. *J Am Acad Dermatol.* 2008;59:385–96.

123. Van der Net J, van der Torre P, Engelbert R, et al. Motor performance and functional ability in preschool- and school-aged children with Juvenile Idiopathic Arthritis: a cross-sectional study. *Pediatr Rheumatol Online J.* 2008;6:2.

124. Ruperto N, Ravelli A, Pistorio A, et al. Cross-cultural adaption and psychometric evaluation of the Childhood Health Assessment Questionnaire (CHAQ) and the Child Health Questionnaire (CHQ) in 32 countries. Review of the general methodology. *Clin Exp Rheumatol.* 2001;19:S1–9.

125. Singh G, Athreya B, Fries J, et al. Measurement of health status in juvenile rheumatoid arthritis. *Arthritis Rheum.* 1994;37:1761–1769.

126. Norgaard M, Thastum M, Herlin T. The relevance of using the Childhood Health Assessment Questionnaire (CHAQ) in revised versions for the assessment of juvenile idiopathic arthritis. *Scand J Rheumatol.* 2013;42:457–464.

127. Sontichai W, Vilaiyuk S. The correlation between the Childhood Health Assessment Questionnaire and disease activity in juvenile idiopathic arthritis. *Musculoskeletal Care.* 2018;16:339–344.

128. Dempster H, Porpera M, Young N, et al. The clinical meaning of functional outcome scores in children with juvenile arthritis. *Arthritis Rheum.* 2001;44:1768–1774.

129. Brandon TG, Becker BD, Bevans KB, et al. Patient Reported Outcomes Measurement Information System (PROMIS) tools for collecting patient-reported outcomes in children with juvenile arthritis. *Arthritis Care Res.* 2017;69:393–402.

130. Morgan E, Mara CA, Huang B. Establishing clinical meaning and defining important differences for Patient Reported Outcomes Measurement Information System (PROMIS) measures in juvenile idiopathic arthritis using standard setting with patients, parents, and providers. *Qual Life Res.* 2017;26:565–586.

131. Klepper SE. Measures of pediatric function. *Arthritis Care Res.* 2011;63:S371–S382.

132. Lovell DJ, Howe S, Shear E. Development of a disability measurement tool for juvenile rheumatoid arthritis: the Juvenile Arthritis Functional Assessment Scale. *Arthritis Rheum*. 1989;32:1390–1395.

133. Degotardi P. Pediatric measure of quality of life. *Arthritis Rheum*. 2003;49:S105–S112.

134. Varni J, Seid M, Smith Knight T, et al. The PedsQL in pediatric rheumatology: reliability, validity, and responsiveness of the pediatric quality of life inventory generic core scales and rheumatology module. *Arthritis Rheum*. 2002;46:714–725.

135. Gong GUK, Young NI, Dempster H, et al. The quality of my life questionnaire: minimal clinically important difference for pediatric patients. *J Rheumatol*. 2007;34:581–587.

136. Davies PL, Pepper LS, Young M, et al. Validity and reliability of the school function assessment in elementary school students with disabilities. *Phys Occup Ther Pediatr*. 2004;24:23–43.

137. Smythe H, Helewa A. Assessment of joint disease. In Walker J, Helewa A, eds. *Physical Therapy in Arthritis*. W.B. Saunders; 1996.

138. Baschung Pfister P, de Bruin ED, Sterkele I, et al. Manual muscle testing and hand-held dynamometry in people with inflammatory myopathy: an intra-and interrater reliability and validity study. *PLoS ONE*. 2018;13:3.

139. Cuthbert S, Goodheart G Jr. On the reliability and validity of manual muscle testing: a literature review. *Chiropr Osteopat*. 2007;15:4.

140. Kwon HJ, Kim YL, Lee HS, et al. A study on the physical fitness of children with juvenile rheumatoid arthritis. *J Phys Ther Sci*. 2017;29:378–383.

141. Takken T, Hemel A, van der Net JJ, et al. Aerobic fitness in children with juvenile idiopathic arthritis. *J Rheumatol*. 2002; 29:2643–2647.

142. Brostrom E, Norlund MM, Cresswell AG. Plantar-and dorsiflexor strength in prepubertal girls with juvenile idiopathic arthritis. *Arch Phys Med Rehabil*. 2004;85:1224–1230.

143. Van Brussel M, Lelieveld OT, van der Net JJ, et al. Aerobic and anaerobic capacity in children with juvenile idiopathic arthritis. *Arthritis Care Res*. 2007;57:898–904.

144. Lelieveld OT, van Brussel M, Takken T, et al. Aerobic and anaerobic capacity in adolescents with juvenile idiopathic arthritis. *Arthritis Care Res*. 2007;57:898–904.

145. Stricker PR, Faigenbaum AD, McCambridge TM, et al. Resistance training for children and adolescents. *Pediatrics*. 2020;145(6): e20201011.

146. Faigenbaum AD, Milliken LA, Laud Rl, et al. Comparison of 1 and 2 days per week of strength training in children. *Res Q Exerc Sport*. 2002;73(4):416–424.

147. Bechtold S, Ripperger P, Dalla PR, Musculoskeletal and functional muscle-bone analysis in children with rheumatic disease using peripheral quantitative computed tomography. *Osteoporos Int*. 2005;16:757–763.

148. Houghton K. Review for the generalist: evaluation of low back pain in children and adolescents. *Pediatr Rheumatol*. 2010;8:20.

149. Merker J, Hartmann M, Kreuzpointer F, et al. Pathophysiology of juvenile idiopathic arthritis induced pes planovalgus in static and walking condition—a functional view using 3D gait analysis. *Pediatr Rheumatol Online J*. 2015;13:21.

150. Hendry G, Gardner-Medwin J, Watt GF, et al. A survey of foot problems in juvenile idiopathic arthritis. *Musculoskeletal Care*. 2008;6(4):221–232.

151. Brostrom E, Hagelberg S, Haglund-Akerlind Y. Effect of joint injections in children with juvenile idiopathic arthritis: evaluation of 3-D gait analysis. *Acta Paediatr*. 2004;93:906–910.

152. Hartmann M, Kreuzpointner F, Haefner R, et al. Effects of juvenile idiopathic arthritis on kinematics and kinetics of the lower extremities call of consequences in physical activities recommendations. *Int J Pediatr*. 2010;835984.

153. Kuntze G, Nesbitt C, Nettel-Aguirre A, et al. Gait adaptations in youth with juvenile idiopathic arthritis. *Arthritis Care Res*. 2020;72(7):917–924.

154. Montefiori E, Modenese L, DiMarco R, et al. Linking joint impairments and gait biomechanics in patients with juvenile idiopathic arthritis. *Ann Biomed Eng*. 2019;47:2155–2167.

155. Hendry GJ, Shoop-Worrall SJ, Riskowski JL, et al. Prevalence and course of lower limb disease activity and walking disability over the first 5 years of juvenile idiopathic arthritis: results from the childhood arthritis prospective study. *Rheumatol Adv Pract*. 2018;2:1–11.

156. Hendry GJ, Rafferty D, Barn R. Foot function is well preserved in children and adolescents with juvenile idiopathic arthritis who are optimally managed. *Gait Posture*. 2013;38:30–36.

157. Dekker M, Hoeksma AF, Dekker JHM, et al. Strong relationships between disease activity, foot-related impairments, activity limitations and participation restrictions in children with juvenile idiopathic arthritis. *Clin Exp Rheumatol*. 2010;28:905–911.

158. Khamis S, Carmeli E. The effect of simulated leg length discrepancy on lower limb biomechanics during gait. *Gait Posture*. 2018;61:73–80.

159. Bangerter C, Romkes J, Lorenzetti S. What are the biomechanical consequences of a structural leg length discrepancy on the adolescent spine during walking? *Gait Posture*. 2019;68:506–513.

160. Chomistek K, Johnson N, Stevenson R, et al. Patient-reported barriers at school for children with juvenile idiopathic arthritis. *ACH Open Rheumatol*. 2019;1:182–187.

161. Bouaddi I, Rostom S, Badri D, et al. Impact of juvenile idiopathic arthritis on school. *BMC Pediatr*. 2013;13:2.

162. Houghton KM, Guzman J. Evaluation of static and dynamic postural balance in children with juvenile idiopathic arthritis. *Pediatr Phys Ther*. 2013;25:150–157.

163. Rochette E, Bourdier P, Pereira B, et al. Impaired muscular fat metabolism in juvenile idiopathic arthritis in inactive disease. *Front Physiol*. 2019;10:528.

164. Van Pelt PA, Takken T, van Brussel M, et al. Aerobic capacity and disease activity in children, adolescents, and young adults with juvenile idiopathic arthritis (JIA). *Pediatr Rheumatol*. 2012;10:27.

165. Giannini MJ, Protas EJ. Aerobic capacity in juvenile rheumatoid arthritis patients and healthy children. *Arthritis Care Res*. 1992;4:131–135.

166. Helders PJ, Klepper SE, Takken T, et al. Juvenile idiopathic arthritis. In Campbell SK, Palisan RJ, Orlin MN, eds. *Physical Therapy for Children*. Elsevier Saunders; 2012:239–270.

167. Klepper S, Darbee J, Effgen S, et al. Physical fitness levels in children with polyarticular juvenile rheumatoid arthritis. *Arthritis Care Res*. 1992;5:93–100.

168. American Thoracic Society. ATS statement: guidelines for the six-minute walk test in children with juvenile idiopathic arthritis. *Arthritis Care Res*. 2005;53:351–356.

169. Klepper SE, Muir N. Reference values on the 6-minute walk test of children living in the United States. *Pediatr Phys Ther*. 2011;23:32–40.

170. Paap E, van der Net JJ, Helders PJ, et al. Physiologic response of the six-minute walk test in children with juvenile idiopathic arthritis. *Arthritis Care Res*. 2005;53:351–356.

171. Lelieveld OT, Takken T, van der Net JJ, et al. Validity of the 6-minute walking test in juvenile idiopathic arthritis. *Arthritis Care Res*. 2005;53:304–307.

172. Nijhof LE, Nap-van der Vlist MM, van de Putte EM, et al. Non-pharmacological options for managing chronic musculoskeletal pain in children with pediatric rheumatic disease: a systematic review. *Rheumatol Int*. 2018;38:2015–2025.

173. Rashid A, Cordingley L, Carrasco R, et al. Patterns of pain over time among children with juvenile idiopathic arthritis. *Arch Dis Child*. 2018;103:437–443.

174. Aviel YB, Stremler R, Bensler SM, et al. Sleep and fatigue and the relationship to pain, disease activity and quality of life in juvenile idiopathic arthritis and juvenile dermatomyositis. *Rheumatol*. 2011;50:2051–2060.

175. Munro J, Singh-Grewal D. Juvenile idiopathic arthritis and pain—more than simple nociception. *J Rheumatol.* 2013;40:7.

176. Leegaard A, Lomholt JJ, Thastum M, Herlin T. Decreased pain threshold in juvenile idiopathic arthritis: a cross-sectional study. *J Rheumatol.* 2013;40:1212–1217.

177. Jaworski TM, Bradley LA, Heck LW, et al. Development of an observational method for assessing pain behaviors in children with juvenile rheumatoid arthritis. *Arthritis Rheum.* 1995;38:1142–1151.

178. Beyer JE, Denyes MJ, Villarruel AM. The creation, validation, and continuing development of the Oucher: a measure of pain intensity in children. *J Pediatr Nurs.* 1992;7:335–346.

179. Wong DL, Baker CM. Pain in children: comparison of assessment scales. *Pediatr Nurs.* 1988;14:9–17.

180. Hester NO, Foster R, Kristensen K. Measurement of pain in children: generalizability and validity of the pain ladder and the poker-chip tool. In: Tyler DC, Kane EJ, eds. *Advances in Pain Research and Therapy.* Raven Press; 1990.

181. Meng Z, Huang R. Topical treatment of degenerative knee osteoarthritis. *Am J Med Sci.* 2018;355:6–12.

182. Cameron M, Chrubasik S. Topical herbal therapies for treating osteoarthritis. *Cochrane Database Syst Rev.* 2014;5:CD010538.

183. Oosterweld FG, Rasker JJ. Treating arthritis with locally applied heat and cold. *Semin Arthritis Rheum.* 1994;24:82–90.

184. Zamir G, Press J, Tal A, et al. Sleep fragmentation in children with juvenile rheumatoid arthritis. *J Rheumatol.* 1998;25:1191–1197.

185. Eyckmans L, Hilderson D, Westhovens R, et al. What does it mean to grow up with juvenile idiopathic arthritis? A qualitative study on the perspectives of patients. *Clin Rheumatol.* 2011;30:459–465.

186. Armbrust W, Siers NE, Lelieveld OT, et al. Fatigue in patients with juvenile idiopathic arthritis: a systematic review of the literature. *Semin Arthritis Rheum.* 2016;45:587–595.

187. Connelly M, Schanberg L, Ardoin S, et al. Multisite randomized clinical trial evaluating an online self-management program for adolescents with juvenile idiopathic arthritis. *J Pediat Psychol.* 2019;44:363–374.

188. Feldman BM. Exercise as medicine for children with arthritis. *J Rheumatol.* 2017;44:1103–1105.

189. Gualano B, Bonfa E, Pereira RMR, et al. Physical activity for paediatric rheumatic diseases: standing up against old paradigms. *Nat Rev Rheumatol.* 2017;13:368–379.

190. Chatzopoulos D, Doganis G, Lykesas G, et al. Effects of static and dynamic stretching on force sense, dynamic flexibility and reaction time of children. *Open Sports Sci J.* 2019;12:22–27.

191. Donti O, Papia K, Toubekis A, et al. Flexibility training in preadolescent female atheletes: acute and long-term effects of intermittent and continuous static stretching. *J Sports Sci.* 2018;36:1453–1460.

192. Brosseau L, Toupin-April K, Wells G, et al. Ottawa panel evidence-based clinical practice guidelines for foot care in the management of juvenile idiopathic arthritis. *Arch Phys Med Rehabil.* 2016;97:1163–1181.

193. Fellas A, Coda A, Hawke F. Physical and mechanical therapies for lower-limb problems in juvenile idiopathic arthritis. *J Am Podiatr Med Assoc.* 2017;107:399–412.

194. Melvin J, Wright FV. Procedure for serial casting of contractures from juvenile arthritis. In: Melvin J, Wright FV, eds. *Rheumatologic Rehabilitation: Pediatric Rheumatic Diseases.* AOTA; 2003.

195. Furia JP, Willis FB, Shanmugam R, et al. Systematic review of contracture reduction in the lower extremity with dynamic splinting. *Adv Ther.* 2013;30:763–770.

196. Minor MA, Westby MD. Rest and exercise. In: Robbins L, Burckhardt C, Hannan M, et al, eds. *Clinical Care in the Rheumatic Diseases.* 2nd ed. American College of Rheumatology; 2001.

197. Choi YL, Kim BK, Hwang YP, et al. Effects of isometric exercise using biofeedback on maximum voluntary isometric contraction, pain, and muscle thickness in patients with knee osteoarthritis. *J Phys Ther Sci.* 2015;27:149–153.

198. Catania H, Fortini V, Cimaz R. Physical exercise and physical activity for children and adolescents with juvenile idiopathic arthritis: a literature review. *Pediatr Phys Ther.* 2017;29:256–260.

199. Baydogan SN, Tarakci E, Kasapcopur O. Effect of strengthening versus balance-proprioceptive exercises on lower extremity function in patients with juvenile idiopathic arthritis. *Am J Phys Med Rehabil.* 2015;94:417–428.

200. Kuntze G, Nesbitt C, Whittaker J, et al. Exercise therapy in juvenile idiopathic arthritis: a systematic review and meta-analysis. *Arch Phys Med Rehabil.* 2018;99:178–193.

201. Emmanuelle R, Pascale D, Christophe H, et al. Single bout exercise in children with juvenile idiopathic arthritis: impact on inflammatory markers. *Mediators Inflamm.* 2018;2018:9365745. doi:10.1155/2018/9365745.

202. Sule SD, Fontaine KR. Slow speed resistance exercise training in children with polyarticular juvenile idiopathic arthritis. *Open Access Rheumatol Res Rev.* 2019;11:121–126.

203. Myer G, Brunner HI, Melson PG, et al. Specialized neuromuscular training to improve neuromuscular function and biomechanics in a patient with quiescent juvenile rheumatoid arthritis. *Phys Ther.* 2005;85:791–802.

204. Cavallo S, Brosseau L, Toupin-April K, et al. Ottawa panel evidence-based clinical practice guidelines for structured physical activity in the management of juvenile idiopathic arthritis. *Arch Phys Med Rehabil.* 2017;98:1018–1041.

205. Huber A, Ward L. The impact of underlying disease on fracture risk and bone mineral density in children with rheumatic disorders: a review of current literature. *Semin Arthritis Rheum.* 2016;46:49–63.

206. Sandstedt E, Fasth A, Fors H, et al. Bone health in children and adolescents with juvenile idiopathic arthritis and the influence of short-term physical exercise. *Pediatr Phys Ther.* 2012;155–162.

207. Takken T, Van Brussel M, Engelbert RH, et al. Exercise therapy in juvenile idiopathic arthritis: a Cochrane Review. *Eur J Phys Rehabil Med.* 2008;44:287–297.

208. Epps H, Ginnelly L, Utley M, et al. Is hydrotherapy cost-effective? A randomized controlled trial of combined hydrotherapy programmes compared with physiotherapy land techniques in children with juvenile idiopathic arthritis. *Health Technol Assess.* 2005;9:1–5.

209. Singh-Grewal D, Schneiderman-Walker J, Wright V, et al. The effects of vigorous exercise training on physical function in children with arthritis: a randomized controlled, single-blinded trial. *Arthritis Care Res.* 2007;57:1202–1210.

210. Bayraktar D, Savci S, Altug-Gucenmez O. The effects of 8-week water-running program on exercise capacity in children with juvenile idiopathic arthritis: a controlled trial. *Rheumatol Int.* 2019;39:59–65.

211. Klepper SE. Exercise in pediatric rheumatic diseases. *Curr Opin Rheumatol.* 2008;20:619–624.

212. Gualano B, Sa Pinto AL, Perondi B, et al. Evidence of prescribing exercise as treatment in pediatric rheumatic diseases. *Autoimmum Rev.* 2010;9:569–573.

213. Long AR, Rouster-Stevens KA. The role of exercise therapy in the management of juvenile idiopathic arthritis. *Curr Opin Rheumatol.* 2010;22:213–217.

214. Takken T, van der Net JJ, Kuis W, et al. Physical activity and health-related physical fitness in children with juvenile idiopathic arthritis. *Ann Rheum Dis.* 2003;62:885–889.

215. Bovid KM, Moore MD. Juvenile idiopathic arthritis for the pediatric orthopedic surgeon. *Orthop Clin North Am.* 2019;50:471–488.

216. Mitrogiannis L, Barbouti A, Theodorou E, et al. Surgical treatment of juvenile idiopathic arthritis: a review. *Bull Hosp Jt Dis.* 2019;77:99–114.

217. Arthritis Foundation: When Your Child with JIA Needs Surgery. February 5, 2021. https://www.arthritis.org/health-wellness/treatment/joint-surgery/preplanning/when-your-child-with-jia-needs-surgery

218. Emery HM, Bayer SL, Sisung CE. Rehabilitation of the child with a rheumatic disease. *Pediatr Clin North Am.* 1995;42:1263–1285.

219. Carmen D, Browne R. Joint protection education for children with arthritis: can handouts replace professional instruction? *Arthritis Rheum*. 1996;39:S1714.

220. Powell M, Seid M, Szer IS. Efficacy of custom foot orthotics in improving pain and functional status in children with juvenile idiopathic arthritis. *J Rheumatol*. 2005;32:943–950.

221. Norgaard M, Herlin T. Specific sports habits, leisure-time physical activity, and school-educational physical activity in children with juvenile idiopathic arthritis: patterns and barriers. *Arthritis Care Res*. 2019;71:271–280.

222. Risum K, Hansen BH, Selvaag AM, et al. Physical activity in patients with oligo- and polyarticular juvenile idiopathic arthritis diagnosed in the era of biologics: a controlled cross-sectional study. *Pediatr Rheumatol*. 2018;16:64.

223. Tarakci E, Yelden I, Mutlu EK, et al. The relationship between physical activity level, anxiety, depression, and functional ability in children and adolescents with juvenile idiopathic arthritis. *Clin Rheumatol*. 2011;30:1415–1420.

224. Lelieveld OT, Armbrust W, van Leeuwen MA, et al. Physical activity in adolescents with juvenile idiopathic arthritis. *Arthritis Care Res*. 2008;57:898–904.

225. Centers for Disease Control and Prevention. How much physical activity do children need? June 8, 2020. Accessed September 13, 2020. https://www.cdc.gov/physicalactivity/basics/children/index.htm

226. Heale LD, Dover S, Goh I. A wearable activity tracker intervention for promoting physical activity in adolescents with juvenile idiopathic arthritis: a pilot study. *Pediatr Rheumaol Online J*. 2018;16:66.

227. Wanich T, Hodgkins C, Columbier JA, et al. Cycling injuries of the lower extremity. *J Am Acad Orthop Surg*. 2007;15:748–756.

228. Farre A, Ryan S, McNiven A, et al. The impact of arthritis on the education and early work experiences of young people: a qualitative secondary analysis. *Int J Adolesc Med Health*. 2019:1–11.

229. Brandelli Y, Chambers CT, Tutelman PR, et al. Parent pain cognitions and treatment adherence in juvenile idiopathic arthritis. *J Pediatr Psychol*. 2019;44:1111–1119.

230. Feldman DE, deCivita M, Dobkin PL, e al. Effects of adherence to treatment on short-term outcomes in children with juvenile idiopathic arthritis. *Arthritis Rheum*. 2007;57(6):905–912.

231. Feldman DE, deCivita M, Dobkin PL, et al. Perceived adherence to prescribed treatment in juvenile idiopathic arthritis over a one year period. *Arthritis Care Res*. 2007;57:226–233.

232. April KT, Feldman DE, Zunzunequi MV, et al. Association between treatment adherence and health-related quality of life in children with juvenile idiopathic arthritis: perspectives of both child and parent. *Patient Prefer Adherence*. 2008;2(31):121–128.

233. Arthritis Foundation: Raising a Child with Arthritis. 2012. Accessed February 5, 2021. https://www.singlecare.com/blog/living-with-juvenile-idiopathic-arthritis/.

234. Vidqvist KL, Malin M, Varjolahti-Lehtinen T, et al. Disease activity of idiopathic juvenile arthritis continues through adolescence despite the use of biologic therapies. *Rheumatology*. 2013;52:1999–2003.

235. Hilderson D, Corstjens F, Moons P, et al. Adolescents with juvenile idiopathic arthritis: who care after age 16? *Clin Exp Rheumatol*. 2010;28:790–797.

236. McDonagh JE, Southwood TR, Saw KL, et al. The impact of a coordinated transitional care programme on adolescents with juvenile idiopathic arthritis. *Rheumatology (Oxford)*. 2007;46:161–168.

237. Stinson JN, Toomey PC, Stevens BJ, el al. Asking the experts: exploring the self-management needs of adolescents with arthritis. *Arthritis Care Res*. 2008;59:65–72.

238. Lelieveld OT, Armbrust W, Geertzen JH, et al. Promoting physical activity in children with juvenile idiopathic arthritis through an Internet-based program: results of a pilot randomized controlled trial. *Arthritis Care Res*. 2012;62:697–703.

School Activity and Participation Checklist

Children with arthritis or other musculoskeletal disorders may experience difficulty performing some necessary or desired activities in school. These activity limitations may negatively impact the child's participation in school programs. The given list includes many of the typical tasks performed in school. Please check any activity that is difficult for you/your child; please add any other activities that are difficult.

>> School attendance

_____ Getting to school on time is difficult for me because:

• I am stiff or hurt in the morning.
• I'm too tired to get ready for school.
• I need help getting dressed.

_____ I am often absent, late, or have to leave school early often because:

• I do not feel well.
• I have a doctor's appointment.
• I am tired.

>> Classroom activities

_____ I have trouble taking off/putting on my coat, hat, gloves, boots, etc.

_____ I have trouble using a pen, pencil, or crayons in school because:

• My arm or hands (fingers or wrist) hurt or get tired.
• The pen, pencil, crayon is too small to hold.

_____ I have trouble writing on the chalkboard.

_____ I have trouble raising my hand to ask or answer a question.

_____ I get stiff sitting in my chair for a long time.

_____ My teacher(s) will not let me stand up or walk around when I'm stiff.

_____ I get tired during the day and need to rest.

_____ I have trouble finishing my schoolwork on time.

_____ I have trouble writing fast when I take a test or class notes.

_____ My school doesn't have the things that help me do things at home (splints, easel for writing, chair cushion, other).

>> Physical education/recess

_____ I have trouble opening my gym locker.

_____ I have trouble changing clothes for gym.

_____ I have trouble taking a shower after gym class.

_____ I have trouble walking to the playground as fast as the other kids.

_____ I have trouble doing the same things in gym/on the playground as the other kids in my class.

_____ My gym teacher is afraid to let me do the same things as the other kids.

_____ My gym teacher doesn't understand that I can't do some of the things the other kids do. (List the things you have trouble doing.)

>> Getting around school

_____ I have trouble getting around the school (I am often late for the next activity) because:

• My classes are too far apart.
• The cafeteria or gym is too far away.

_____ I have trouble standing in lines for a long time, like in the cafeteria or during assemblies.

_____ I have trouble carrying my books, lunch tray, or other things while walking in school.

_____ I have trouble opening my milk carton, lunch box, or using a knife and fork during lunch.

_____ I have trouble opening heavy doors.

_____ I have trouble going up/down stairs.

_____ I have trouble using the bathroom at school.

_____ I have trouble during fire drills, earthquake drills, and other emergency drills.

_____ I often miss field trips because I have trouble walking long distances.

» Other problems

_____   My teacher(s) don't understand the problems I have because of my condition.

_____   My teacher(s) make a big deal of my condition, and it makes me feel different.

_____   Other kids make fun of me or say things that make me feel bad.

_____   I don't want anyone to know that I have arthritis (other condition).

_____   I have hand splints, but don't want to wear them in school.

_____   I sometimes forget to take my medicine because it is in the nurse's office.

Please add any other school-related problems you/ your child have because of their arthritis or other health condition.

_____

_____

_____

_____

Klepper S, Lopez R, Winn R, 2004

Rheumatology Transition Checklist for Teenagers

This checklist is to help you prepare to move on to adult care. You can achieve independence in matters of your health and future by actively participating in your care and planning transition to the next step: Care with an Adult Rheumatologist and Center.

	Plan to Start	Needs Practice	Can Do Independently Already	Comments and Contacts
Describe and understand your chronic condition				
Discuss concerns, any issues about transfer of care				
Participates in support group, camp, and teen programs. Interacts with teen, young adult "role models"				
Understands differences between pediatric and adult care, verbalizes expectations for moving on				
Prepares questions and speaks up at medical visit				
Participates in "Teen Visits"; partial visits without parent				
Takes medications, does exercises, treatment correctly				
Keeps "diary" information—medication, doses, provider names, phone numbers, and tracks relevant medical info				
Calls for prescription refilled, lab results, and schedules appointments; keeps contact numbers in cell phone				
Calls to report change in illness, new symptoms, concerns				
Knows insurance and has plans for continuous medical coverage after transfer				
Continues primary care visits—plans for primary care after transfer				
Understands and obtains reproductive health information and appointments				
Independent with self-care, chores, uses devices for ADLs if needed, volunteers, works part time				
Discusses how drugs, alcohol, cigarettes affect illness, pregnancy, and medication toxicities				
Contacts resources/agencies, i.e., Vocational Rehab, driving, college office for students with disabilities, financial aid, other:_____				
Discusses and plans for time to transfer care				
Chooses an adult physician—makes appointment				

Adult Rheumatologist:_____ Address:_____

Phone Number:_____ FAX #_____ First Appointment Date:_____

Comment:_____

Patricia A. Rettig, MSN, RN, CRNP, The Children's Hospital of Philadelphia, revised 10/1/10

» Healthcare transition resources

Visit the Health Care Transition Web site at:

http://hctransitions.ichp.edu/

This mailing list is a service of the Division of Policy and Program Affairs at the Institute for Child Health Policy (www.ichp.edu)

Arthritis Foundations
Atlanta, Georgia 30357-0669
(800) 283-7800
  a. Decision Making for Teenagers with Arthritis brochure
  b. JA Alliance/AF National and Regional Conferences for families and professionals

On TRAC – Taking Responsibility for Adolescent/Adult Care
British Columbia Children's Hospital
Room 2 D20 4480 Oak Street
Vancouver, B.C.
Canada 3V4
(604) 875-3472
  a. Annotated Bibliography
  b. Workshops, training, and consultation

RAP Journal for teens with JIA
Resource Handbook for Parents of Adolescent s with JIA
Janet McDonagh MD and Karen Shaw MD, Rheumatology
Institute of Child Health
Diana, Princess of Wales Children's Hospital
Steelhouse Lane
Birmingham, B4 6NH UK
Tel: 0121 333 8743

Parent Training and Information Center
PACER Center, Inc.
4826 Chicago Avenue South
Minneapolis, MN 55412
(612) 827-2966
  a. Speak Up for Health—handbook for parents
  b. Living Your Own Life—handbook for teenagers written by young people and adults with chronic illnesses or disabilities

» Additional resources

The Carra Group
  The Carra Group whose mission is to conduct collaborative research to prevent, treat, and cure pediatric rheumatic diseases.
    https://carragroup.org/
CreakyJoints
  CreakyJoints is a digital community for millions of patients with arthritis and their caregivers who are in search of education, support, advocacy, and patient-centered research.
    https://creakyjoints.org/

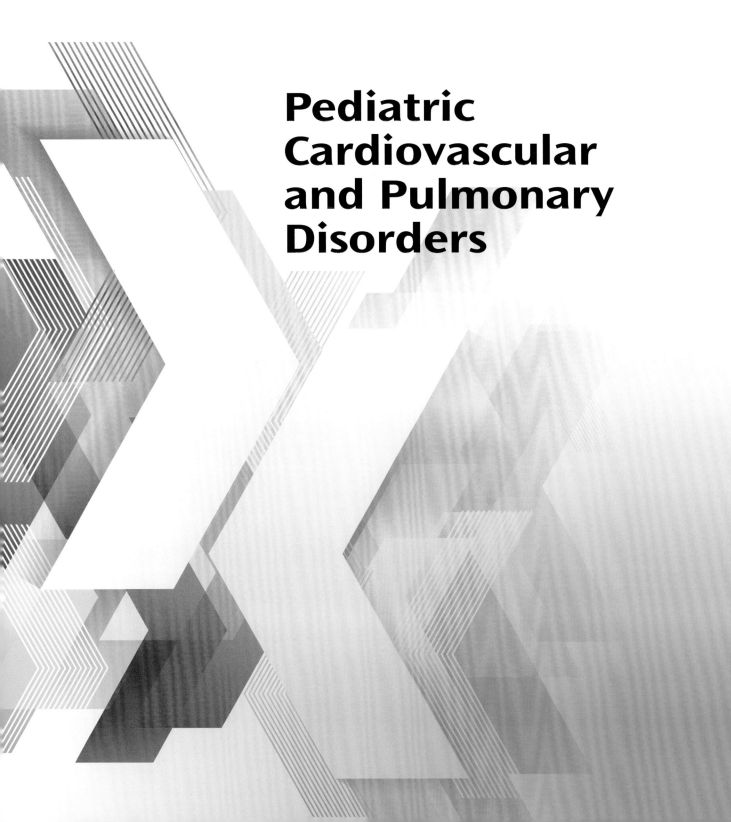

Pediatric Cardiovascular and Pulmonary Disorders

Cardiac Conditions

Heather Lever Brossman

≫ Introduction

Congenital heart disease (CHD) occurs in varying severities, ranging from mild to severe.[1] Moderate and severe CHD occurs in approximately 2.5 to 3 of every 1000 births, whereas mild CHD can occur up to 10 per 1000.[1] There are 25,000 babies born each year with CHD, and more than 1,000,000 individuals have reached adulthood and are living in the United States with a functionally significant CHD.[2] The mortality rates in infants with CHD have declined dramatically as a result of medical and surgical advances for their care, with up to 85% of infants born with CHD surviving to adulthood.[2] Because more children are surviving, more research is being done regarding neurodevelopmental outcomes for children with varying types of CHD, including cognition, language skills, gross and fine motor skills, and quality of life.[3–11] Pediatric physical therapists are likely to encounter infants, children, and adolescents with a cardiac disorder in every setting in which they practice. A physical therapist may see a child with CHD in the acute care setting preoperatively and/or postoperatively, in rehabilitation settings, in schools and home care, or in the outpatient setting. When treating the child with CHD, physical therapists should be familiar with the anatomy of the CHD, how it affects the child's cardiovascular system during exercise, and the secondary impairments of the CHD that are prevalent in this population. It is also important to note that CHD commonly accompanies other genetic disorders linked to developmental delays, for which they may see a physical therapist.[9]

Most congenital abnormalities of the heart can be detected between 8 and 12 weeks of gestation, when the heart is no larger than a peanut, although some may not be diagnosed until further along in gestation because of imaging techniques and growth.[12,13] In most CHD cases, it is speculated that genetic factors play a role in the acquisition of the defect, but the patterns of inheritance are not always clear, and are likely multifactorial.[9,14] There are several single-gene mutations identified in relation to genetic syndromes that include CHD (e.g., DiGeorge/22q11.2 microdeletion; CHARGE/CHD7 deletion/mutation).[9] Among the varying types of CHDs, each has its own incidence. Table 18.1 lists the more common congenital defects of the heart and their incidence in the general population.

To understand the various types of CHD, a clear understanding of normal cardiac development, anatomy, and physiology is important. It is beyond the scope of this text

TABLE 18.1. Incidence per Live Births of Congenital Heart Lesions	
Ventricular septal defects	1/1000
Patent ductus arteriosus (excluding preterm neonates)	1/2000
Coarctation of the aorta	1/2500
Atrial septal defects	1/3000
Tetralogy of Fallot	1/3500
Transposition of the great arteries	1/3500
Pulmonary stenosis	1/4000
Aortic valve stenosis	1/4500
Hypoplastic left heart syndrome	1/5500
Total anomalous pulmonary venous return	1/15,000
Tricuspid atresia	1/15,500
Truncus arteriosus	1/16,000
Pulmonary atresia	1/16,500

Wernovsky G, Gruber P. Common congenital heart disease: presentation, management and outcomes. In: Taeusch H, Ballard R, Gleason C, eds. *Avery's Diseases of the Newborn*. 8th ed. Philadelphia, PA: Elsevier Saunders; 2004:827–872.

to review cardiopulmonary physiology in detail; there are numerous excellent cardiopulmonary texts that can be referenced to understand structure and function.[15,16]

» Cardiac system development

The heart begins to form with four main components: (1) primary cardiac tube, (2) secondary, anterior heart field, (3) tertiary field cells, and (4) cardiac neural crest cells.[12] These four components combine in a modular manner to eventually develop into the basic four ventricles in the fetus. The primary cardiac tube forms the majority of the left ventricle, the secondary anterior field cells develop into the right ventricle and outflow tract, the tertiary field cells contribute to the atrial chambers and to portions of each ventricle. The cardiac neural crest cells contribute to the aortic arch and

coronaries. The component cells balloon and divide to connect to form the heart. Initially, there is a single ventricle leading into a large single vessel called the truncus arteriosus, and eventually the components bend and loop around to form two ventricles that separate as the septum grows vertically, and the truncus arteriosus separates into the aorta and pulmonary artery. The aortic and pulmonary valves develop, and the pulmonary artery loops around to lie in front of the aorta and attaches to the right ventricle. The foramen ovale remains open to allow blood to pass between the two atria, and the ductus arteriosus (DA) allows a connection between the aorta and the pulmonary artery. The four-ventricle heart is completely formed by 8 weeks of gestation, at which point the atria come to lie near the embryo's head and the ventricle toward the feet.[12] By 12 weeks, the heart is positioned normally in the fetal chest and is approximately 8 mm in length.[12] Development is primarily complete between the 10th and 12th weeks of gestation; thus, these first weeks are the critical period of cardiac development. Between 12 and 17 weeks, the heart doubles in size, and by 21 weeks of gestation triples in size.[12] During life in the womb, the right ventricle is dominant, with most of the fetal blood bypassing the lungs and reaching the left ventricle through the foramen ovale or the DA[17] (Fig. 18.1).

Normal Fetal Circulation

The fetal heart does not depend on the lungs for respiration, owing to high pulmonary resistance.[17] Rather, the fetus uses the low-resistance circulatory pathway of the placenta to obtain oxygen and to get rid of carbon dioxide (Fig. 18.2). In the fetus, the right and left ventricles exist in a parallel circuit. Blood travels through the umbilical vein through the ductus venosus to the fetal heart via the inferior vena cava to the right atrium, and through the foramen ovale to the left atrium. The superior vena cava leads to the right atrium, to the right ventricle, to the pulmonary artery, to the lungs or

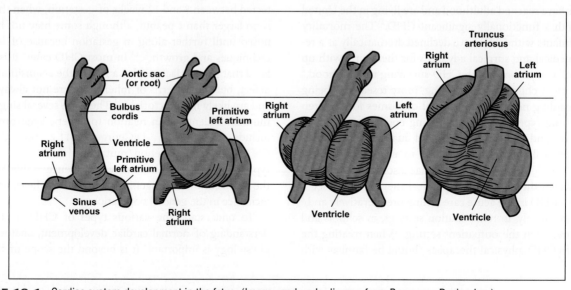

FIGURE 18.1. Cardiac system development in the fetus. (Image used under license from Brossman Design Inc.)

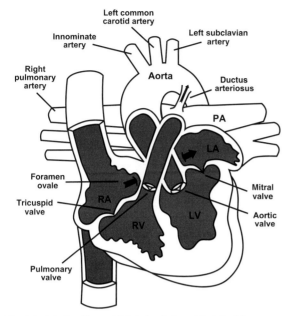

FIGURE 18.2. Normal fetal circulation. LA, left atrium; LV, left ventricle; PA, pulmonary artery; RA, right atrium; RV, right ventricle. (Image used under license from Brossman Design Inc.)

DA, bypassing the lungs, into the descending aorta to perfuse the bilateral lower extremities and body, then travels back to the placenta via the umbilical arteries.[17] The blood traveling through the left ventricle to the aorta perfuses the brain and upper extremities.[17] All of the blood flowing through the various chambers of the heart, and also through the arteries and veins, are rich in oxygen. In the fetus, the vessels of the pulmonary circulation are vasoconstricted, leading to high pulmonary vascular resistance.[17] Any blood traveling to the lungs, all of which is oxygen rich, will be utilized to develop

and nourish lung tissue. This blood flow through the heart and lungs also contributes to the size, shape, and function of the chambers of the heart and lung buds.

Changes Associated with Birth

At birth, several changes occur within the circulatory system. Figure 18.3 shows normal cardiac anatomy before and after birth. At birth as the first breath is taken, the lungs expand with air, and lung pressure falls; this allows blood to flow more easily into the lungs.[17] After reaching the lungs, the blood returns to the left atrium, which causes pressure to be higher on the left side of the atrial septum than on the right. This pressure differential and the increase in oxygen levels causes the foramen ovale, DA, and ductus venosus to functionally close shortly after birth.[17] The foramen ovale closes anatomically by 9 to 30 months, the DA by 2 to 3 months, and the ductus venosus by 7 to 14 days of life.[17] The body now relies on the lungs for obtaining oxygen and expelling carbon dioxide, and maintains separation of oxygenated and deoxygenated blood.

Normal Circulation after Birth

The heart is now essentially two pumps working in unison to propel blood through the blood vessels to the body. The right side of the heart receives deoxygenated blood from the body and pumps it through the pulmonary artery to the lungs. The left side receives oxygenated blood from the lungs and pumps it through the aorta to the body. Blood enters the right atrium via the inferior vena cava and superior vena cava, travels through the tricuspid valve to the right ventricle, and then through the pulmonary valve. The pulmonary

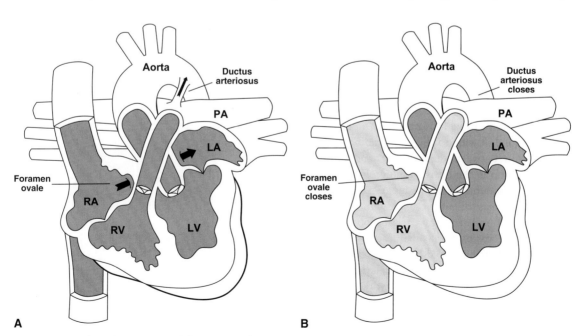

FIGURE 18.3. Normal cardiac structures **(A)** before and **(B)** after birth. LA, left atrium; LV, left ventricle; PA, pulmonary artery; RA, right atrium; RV, right ventricle. (Image used under license from Brossman Design Inc.)

valve, consisting of three semilunar cusps, prevents blood from returning to the right ventricle from the lungs. The blood then travels through the pulmonary artery to the lung and back through four pulmonary veins, which enter the posterior wall of the left atrium with no valves at the openings. The left atrioventricular valve, or the mitral valve, sits between the left atrium and ventricle, and it allows oxygenated blood from the left atrium to pass into the left ventricle. The left ventricle pumps the blood through the aortic valve, which also has three semilunar cusps leading to the aorta. The aortic valve is similar to the pulmonary valve except that its cusps are thicker and placed slightly differently. The left ventricle has a greater amount of pressure than does the right ventricle on account of higher systemic pressure of the body versus the lungs. Figure 18.3B depicts normal cardiac anatomy.

» Congenital heart defects

At any point in the development of the cardiac system, problems can arise leading to a CHD. It may be a persistent fetal pathway or a problem during development of the heart. Congenital heart defects are traditionally classified by the direction of altered blood flow (left-to-right shunting, duct-dependent systemic flow, duct-dependent pulmonary flow, or other,[14] according to level of severity (mild, moderate, or severe defects,[1] or according to whether the oxygenation process is affected. When the lesion causes oxygen saturations in the blood to be decreased, it is considered a cyanotic lesion; when blood oxygen saturation is not affected, it is an acyanotic lesion. Acyanotic lesions can block the flow of blood to the heart chambers (pressure issue) or alter the volume of blood traveling through the heart (volume issue).

Acyanotic Congenital Heart Defects

Volume-related acyanotic lesions include patent ductus arteriosus (PDA), atrial septal defects (ASDs), ventricular septal defects (VSDs), and atrioventricular septal defects (AVSDs). Both ASD and VSD are pictured in Figure 18.4. An increase in the volume of blood flowing to the lungs can be caused by a communication between the systemic and pulmonary sides of circulation in the heart, resulting in shunting of fully oxygenated blood back into the lungs. This type of blood flow is referred to as *left-to-right shunt*, with too much blood to the lungs and no change in arterial blood oxygen saturations. The symptoms of defects that lead to increased pulmonary blood flow include rapid breathing, even when asleep, as a consequence of congested lungs; delayed growth, as the extra calories are used by the increased work of breathing; sweating; heart failure; and severe difficulty in feeding.[14] Pressure-related acyanotic lesions include coarctation of the aorta, aortic stenosis, and pulmonary stenosis, and lead to increased pressure as blood leaves either ventricle. These lesions are demonstrated in Figure 18.5A–C.

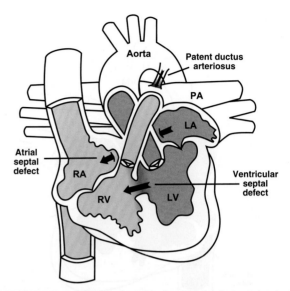

FIGURE 18.4. Atrial and ventricular septal defects and patent ductus arteriosus (PDA). LA, left atrium; LV, left ventricle; PA, pulmonary artery; RA, right atrium; RV, right ventricle. (Image used under license from Brossman Design Inc.)

Patent Ductus Arteriosus

PDA is associated with maternal rubella and prematurity. It occurs when the fetal communication between the aorta and the pulmonary artery (the DA described earlier) remains open after birth and allows blood flow between the two vessels. When the shunt does not close as it should, this is a PDA, and the pressure differential between the left and right sides of the heart causes too much blood to go to the lungs. The symptoms depend on the size of the opening and the degree of prematurity. A large opening can cause pulmonary

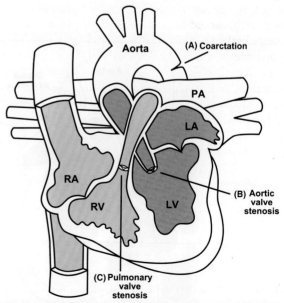

FIGURE 18.5. Several common congenital heart defects. **(A)** Coarctation of the aorta. **(B)** Pulmonary valve stenosis. **(C)** Aortic valve stenosis. LA, left atrium; LV, left ventricle; PA, pulmonary artery; RA, right atrium; RV, right ventricle. (Image used under license from Brossman Design Inc.)

congestion, congestive heart failure (CHF), and edema. Indomethacin may be given to decrease prostaglandin production to close the PDA in premature infants. In a full-term baby, surgery may be required if prostaglandins are unable to close the DA (see Fig. 18.4).

Atrial Septal Defects

An ASD is a hole in the wall separating the atria. This is most often caused by a patent foramen ovale, where the oval-shaped hole in the atrial wall that should close soon after birth does not close. Many ASDs will close spontaneously in the first few years of life. If it does not close, over many years, an ASD causes low pressure at the atrium and, consequently, results in gradual enlargement of the right atrium and ventricle. Symptoms include a heart murmur, an overactive right ventricle, and a large pulmonary artery. Surgery is usually performed if the ASD does not close by 2 to 3 years of age.[14] Surgery generally includes placing a Dacron patch or inserting a clamshell device via a catheter. Some surgeons will anticoagulate up to 6 months postoperatively to prevent clotting.

Ventricular Septal Defects

The ventricular septum consists of three distinct areas that fuse together to form the singular solid muscle wall of the ventricles. A VSD occurs when there is a failure of this fusion. With a VSD, some of the oxygen-rich blood in the left ventricle that should be pumped through the aorta is ejected directly to the right ventricle through a hole in the ventricular wall. Up to 50% of small VSDs close spontaneously and never become symptomatic.[14] With a large defect, excess blood goes to the lung and causes pulmonary congestion, which leads to shortness of breath. A large volume of blood returns from the lungs to the left heart, which, over time, becomes overburdened and enlarged. Heart failure may occur causing a backup of fluid in the lungs and other body tissues. For individuals with a large VSD, the signs and symptoms include dyspnea, feeding difficulties, poor growth, profuse perspiration, recurrent pulmonary infections, cardiac failure in early infancy, respiratory distress, and growth failure. If a VSD becomes symptomatic, it will require surgery, which is similar to that with the ASD with a Dacron patch to close the defect in the ventricle wall.

Atrioventricular Septal Defects

A complete AVSD involves the portion of the heart where the atrial septum meets the ventricular septum and the mitral and tricuspid valves. The result is a large hole spanning the septum and the presence of one large valve on both sides. If the defect includes the entire septum, it is considered a complete common atrioventricular canal (CAVC). Blood flow shunts left to right because of the greater force generated by the left myocardium. Signs and symptoms include lung congestion, pulmonary hypertension, increased work of breathing, and feeding intolerance. AVSDs are associated with Down syndrome: 70% of infants with CAVC have Down syndrome.[14] This defect will require surgery in the first few months of life.

Coarctation of Aorta

In coarctation of the aorta, the aorta is pinched or narrowed after it leaves the heart. This defect increases pressure in the arteries closest to the heart, the head, and the arms, causing upper body hypertension, with reduced circulation and diminished pulses in the lower extremities. Coarctation in newborns is not evident until the DA closes and the obstruction of blood flow from the left ventricle results in heart failure and shock, requiring respiratory support and prostaglandin E_1 to reopen the ductus.[14] The problem occurs after DA closure because as the ductus closes, it shortens into a thin cord, and like a noose, this cord pinches off the aorta, making it narrower where the DA was located. The left ventricle then has to pump blood directly through the constriction, often resulting in left ventricular failure and symptoms including increased work of breathing, sweating, and wheezing. Symptoms in older children may include headache, leg cramps, and a pale appearance. Blood pressure differs between the upper extremities (high) and lower extremities (low). Most children require surgery to remove the constriction and reconnect the aorta.[14] In 10% to 15% of children, re-coarctation occurs, requiring further intervention, often with balloon dilation via angioplasty.[14]

Aortic Stenosis

Aortic stenosis occurs when there is a fusion, thickening, or narrowing of the aortic valve. This valve defect leads to obstruction of flow from the left ventricle to the aorta, increasing the work of the left ventricle to pump to the body. Aortic stenosis is often identified at birth when an infant is critically ill with left ventricular failure and shock.[14] Aortic atresia occurs if the aortic valve fails to form during gestation, or is blocked. It can be identified in utero. If found later, signs and symptoms may include fatigue, murmur, chest pain, fainting, or arrhythmia. Surgical intervention options include using balloon dilation via catheterization, performing valvuloplasty to separate fused leaflets of the valve or artificial valve replacement.

Pulmonary Stenosis

Pulmonary stenosis occurs with a thickening of the area below or above the valve. This stenosis leads to pulmonary valve obstruction, causing increased work of the right ventricle to pump to the lungs. Signs and symptoms may include respiratory distress, fatigue, murmur, or chest pain. Just as with aortic stenosis, surgical intervention options include using balloon dilation via catheterization, performing valvuloplasty to separate fused leaflets of the valve, or using a homograft to replace the stenotic valve or artery. Pulmonary atresia occurs when the pulmonary valve does not form during gestation, or is blocked and can be diagnosed in utero. The treatment is for the DA to remain open until surgery can be completed.[14]

Cyanotic Heart Defects

A cyanotic heart defect causes a decrease in oxygen saturation, which causes the lips, toes, toenail beds, and fingernails to appear blue (*cyanosis* is Greek for blue). The resulting chronic arterial oxygen desaturation stimulates erythropoiesis, an increased red blood cell formation that results in polycythemia, an overabundance of red blood cells. This condition increases blood viscosity, which increases the risk of cerebrovascular accidents and microvascular problems.[14] The cyanotic heart defects include tetralogy of Fallot (TOF), double-outlet right ventricle (DORV), transposition of the great arteries (TGA), and hypoplastic left heart syndrome (HLHS) as shown in Figures 18.6 to 18.9.

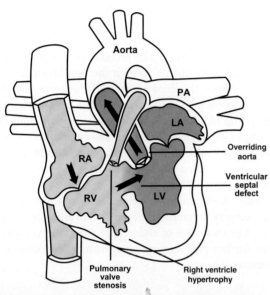

FIGURE 18.6. Tetralogy of Fallot. LA, left atrium; LV, left ventricle; PA, pulmonary artery; RA, right atrium; RV, right ventricle. (Image used under license from Brossman Design Inc.)

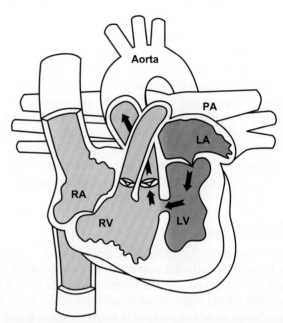

FIGURE 18.8. Double-outlet right ventricle. LA, left atrium; LV, left ventricle; PA, pulmonary artery; RA, right atrium; RV, right ventricle. (Image used under license from Brossman Design Inc.)

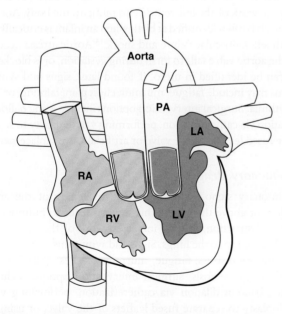

FIGURE 18.7. Transposition of the great arteries. LA, left atrium; LV, left ventricle; PA, pulmonary artery; RA, right atrium; RV, right ventricle. (Image used under license from Brossman Design Inc.)

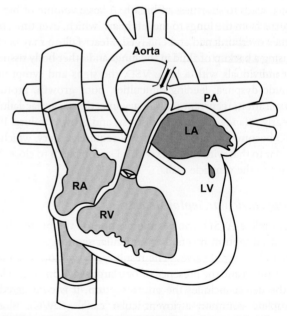

FIGURE 18.9. Hypoplastic left heart syndrome. LA, left atrium; LV, left ventricle; PA, pulmonary artery; RA, right atrium; RV, right ventricle. (Image used under license from Brossman Design Inc.)

Tetralogy of Fallot

TOF is the most common cyanotic congenital heart defect and has four components.[14] The first basic component is a large VSD with blood mixing freely between the ventricles. The second component is pulmonary stenosis, which causes a right ventricular outflow tract obstruction. The third component is an aorta positioned above the VSD (overriding aorta). Finally, hypertrophy of the right ventricle is caused by increased pressure owing to the right ventricular outflow obstruction. Blood flow to the pulmonary artery is obstructed, so oxygen-poor blood finds it easier to enter the aorta than the pulmonary artery. The resulting decreased oxygen levels in the arteries and tissues of the body cause cyanosis, with symptoms of tiring easily, fainting, and shock.[14] Surgical correction to optimize outcomes is typically performed as early in a child's life as possible.[14] Figure 18.6 depicts TOF.

Transposition of the Great Arteries and Double-Outlet Right Ventricle

TGA (see Fig. 18.7) occurs when the aortic artery arises from the right ventricle and the pulmonary artery from the left ventricle.[14] These errors cause deoxygenated blood to circulate around the body, and the already oxygenated blood returns to the lungs. In DORV (see Fig. 18.8), the aorta and the pulmonary artery arise from the right ventricle. The only outlet from the left ventricle is via a VSD, which shunts blood into the right ventricle and causes mixing of oxygenated and deoxygenated blood leaving the heart.[14] Signs and symptoms include cyanosis, poor feeding, poor weight gain, decreased appetite, and increased respiratory rate. One-third of children with TGA require urgent intervention within hours of birth to create an ASD to allow mixing of blood. All children with TGA require an arterial switch operation to repair the defect a few days after birth.[14]

Hypoplastic Left Heart Syndrome

HLHS is the most serious of the congenital malformations with the poorest prognosis (see Fig. 18.9). In HLHS, the left ventricle is underdeveloped or absent, and the mitral valve and/or aortic valve are absent (atresia) or too small. The presence of a PDA keeps the child alive by allowing flow from the left atrium back to the right heart. Signs and symptoms include cyanosis, poor feeding, poor weight gain, increased work of breathing, lethargy, and, ultimately, shock and multiorgan failure. Symptoms are usually minimal until the DA closes. Keeping the DA open with prostaglandin E$_1$ until surgery can be performed keeps the child alive. Children with HLHS typically undergo a three-stage repair.[18] In the first stage, surgery may include a Blalock–Taussig shunt or Norwood procedure, the right ventricle becomes the primary pumping chamber, and a shunt is placed between arterial and pulmonary blood supplies to increase blood flow to the lungs. This typically occurs in the first few days or weeks of life. The second stage, the bidirectional Glenn procedure, occurs around 4 to 6 months of age. In this operation, the shunt is taken down, and the superior vena cava is connected to the pulmonary artery, allowing more venous blood to be oxygenated. The final stage, the Fontan procedure, is typically done between 3 and 6 years of age.[18,19] The inferior vena cava is attached directly to the pulmonary artery, and an opening or fenestration is made to allow extra blood to go back to the right atrium. Following the Fontan surgery, all venous blood goes to the lungs. This staged repair is a palliative surgery and may have late complications.[18,19] If the palliation fails, heart transplantation may be suggested as an option.[18]

» Heart transplantation

Heart transplantation may be recommended for children with less than 2 years of predicted survival due to heart failure or cardiomyopathy associated with CHD. CHF is a syndrome with many pathophysiologic and compensatory mechanisms in the body's attempt to maintain the normal ventricular ejection of blood from the heart to the vital organs. Right heart failure presents with hepatomegaly, peripheral edema, and cyanosis. Left heart failure presents with pulmonary edema and poor perfusion. The clinical presentations of CHF are listed in Table 18.2. Heart failure occurs in some children with CHD owing to the nature of their artificial circulatory systems. For example, the use of the right ventricle as the main systemic circulation ventricle may cause the right ventricle to fail, because it is not intended to pump against systemic pressures.[19]

Heart transplantation is generally considered for children with end-stage heart disease that is unresponsive to medical management or when conventional surgical intervention is not a realistic or viable option.[20,21] Transplantation is truly

TABLE 18.2.	Clinical Presentation of Congestive Heart Failure
Onset of rapid breathing	Change in behavior
Edema	Irritability
Fatigue	Excessive sweating
Poor feeding	Vomiting
Oliguria	Tachycardia
Pulmonary/systemic vein	Peripheral vasoconstriction
Engorgement	Wheezing
Tachypnea	Nasal flaring
Chest retractions	
Failure to thrive	

the exchanging of a set of undesirable lethal circumstances for another set of circumstances. Transplantation presents a lifelong risk of graft loss (acute and chronic rejection), graft coronary disease, nonspecific graft failure, death from infection, oncogenesis, and other organ failure.[21] Complex CHD and cardiomyopathy account for 90% of pediatric heart transplantations; however, two-thirds of *infant* heart transplants are due to CHD, whereas two-thirds of *adolescent* heart transplants are due to cardiomyopathy.[21,22] In 2009 (latest report), nearly 550 heart transplants were performed, with the distribution evenly spread between three age groups (infants, children aged 1 to 10, and adolescents).[22] In the first year of life, children with a single ventricle, such as HLHS and DORV, have the greatest risk of requiring transplantation.[21]

A heart transplant operation involves excising the original heart, inserting the donor heart, and then performing a reanastomosis of atria and great arteries to the donor heart. The vagus nerve is removed, and the sympathetic cardiac nerves are severed. This means that a transplanted heart is denervated. Without the vagus nerve, there is loss of sympathetic control of the heart, which causes an altered heart rate response, higher resting heart rate, and lower heart rate increase with exercise.[20,23]

Survival data continue to improve each year as techniques and postoperative management are refined.[21] The overall 5-year survival rate for pediatric cardiac transplant is about 70%. The median survival (the age at which 50% of recipients are still alive) for children receiving transplants is 18.4 years in infancy, 16.4 years during childhood, and 12.0 years during adolescence.[22]

Heart transplantation has its own set of circumstances, of which the physical therapist must be aware. Immediately after heart transplantation due to denervation, children have a higher resting heart rate, lower exercise heart rate, and a lower heart rate recovery.[23] Physical therapists mainly need to be aware of the denervation of the heart posttransplantation, as well as signs and symptoms of rejection, infection, and graft versus host disease. One longitudinal study showed that each year following transplant, children's resting heart rate drops, and exercise heart rate and heart rate recovery increase, suggesting that pediatric heart transplant recipients may have the ability for long-term reinnervation.[23] For the physical therapist, this means that warm-ups and cooldowns are vital for exercise, which we discuss in more detail later in the chapter.

» Physical therapy examination

History

A physical therapy examination should begin with a thorough history, including demographic information, medical/surgical history, family and social history, developmental history, and chief complaint. Demographics of the child and family include age, date of birth, primary language, and race. It is important to recognize that families come from all over the world to centers that perform CHD operations and cardiopulmonary transplantation. The family should be an integral part of physical therapy intervention. Understanding family structure, culture, and history will assist in involving the family in all aspects of the care of their child.[24]

Next, gather medical and surgical history, which may be very complex in children with CHD, including multiple surgeries, medical complications, or comorbidities. It is important to obtain a thorough and accurate history, because this provides a picture of the child's medical course. Medications the child is taking should be documented, including blood thinners (e.g., Lovenox/enoxaparin, Coumadin/warfarin), anti-arrhythmics, and immunosuppressives. These medications have side effects such as longer bleeding times, which should be noted for physical therapy treatment. Birth history should be obtained, including whether the child was born full term or prematurely and whether the CHD diagnosis was made prenatally or after birth. Social history should be gathered. Social history should include the living situation, including house setup (stairs, etc.), family members who live in the home, who will be involved in the care of the child, and other environments for the child including school or day care. This information can help determine who will be involved in the child's care, and also discharge recommendations or education/training needs. Family history is also important information to gather, including birth order, siblings or relatives with CHD, or other medical history. It may be important to discuss with the family that a child with a CHD is very different from, for example, an uncle who died from atherosclerosis. Developmental history includes gathering information about developmental skill achievement and the age at which the child achieved various developmental milestones. Is the child or siblings receiving early intervention services or have they ever received other therapies? A developmental history should also include questions regarding daily schedules, sleep patterns, prior level of function, and ability to perform activities of daily living (ADLs).

A final component of history gathering is the child and family's chief complaint. The chief complaints for infants with CHD are generally poor feeding, failure to thrive, or delayed milestones. Chief complaints for adolescents are often lethargy, fatigue, general malaise, and exercise intolerance. It is important to understand what the family believes is the main reason for a hospitalization, episode of outpatient therapy, or early intervention services. A thorough history of current signs and symptoms will assist the physical therapist in determining appropriate examination techniques.

Laboratory Values

Numerous laboratory values are important to the physical therapist. The most basic of these is a complete blood count (CBC). A CBC gives information about hemoglobin levels, white blood cells, and other basic functions. Along with a CBC, some children may have international normalized ratio (INR) or anti-Xa levels that indicate how much the blood is thinned or thickened. A higher value indicates that the blood is thinner and represents a higher risk of bleeding, whereas a lower number represents a greater risk of clotting. If the child had a recent cardiac catheterization, the values from that procedure identify the central pressures and oxygen saturations. These values provide a baseline for how much mixing between oxygenated and deoxygenated blood occurs, and the degree to which central pressures are altered. As oxygen saturations decrease, there may be increasing complaints of fatigue, dizziness, lethargy, and general malaise. Figure 18.10 shows normal heart catheterization values for the various chambers of the heart. The values in the circles are the oxygen saturations, and the other values are the normal pressures for the various chambers and vessels of the heart.

A cardiac catheterization is an invasive examination where catheters are inserted into a vein in the groin and threaded into the heart under fluoroscopic guidance. The catheter enters the systemic venous and arterial systems to measure hemodynamic pressures and oxygen saturations. Radiographic material may be injected through the catheters to take cine radiographs of the heart and its structures. The right ventricle and pulmonary artery pressures are usually about one-fifth that of the left ventricle and aorta because of the high systemic pressure the left side of the heart must overcome to pump blood out of the aorta. The right heart is the deoxygenated side and generally has oxygen saturations in the 60s; the left side is the oxygenated side with the oxygen saturations in the high 90s (98% to 100%).

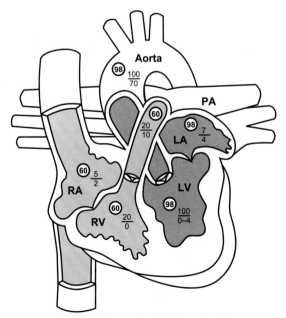

FIGURE 18.10. Cardiac catheterization values in a normal heart. LA, left atrium; LV, left ventricle; PA, pulmonary artery; RA, right atrium; RV, right ventricle. (Image used under license from Brossman Design Inc.)

Age-Appropriate Arterial Blood Gas Values

Arterial blood is the most reliable way to measure O_2 transport (Table 18.3). Hypoventilation causes a shift to the right on the normal oxyhemoglobin dissociation curve with an increase in CO_2 and a decrease in pH, causing a respiratory acidosis. Hyperventilation causes a shift to the left with a decrease in CO_2 and an increase in pH, causing a respiratory alkalosis. A PaO_2 of 60 to 80 mm Hg corresponds with a SaO_2 of 90% to 95%, which is mild hypoxia. A PaO_2 of 40 to 60 mm Hg corresponds with a SaO_2 of 60% to 90%, or moderate hypoxia. A PaO_2 of less than 40 mm Hg corresponds with a SaO_2 of less than 60% and is considered severe hypoxia.

Vital Signs

Arterial blood gas determination often requires an invasive line, and is not always indicated. Pulse oximeters may provide a proxy for saturations. Other vital signs to consider are heart rate, blood pressure, and respiratory rate. Consider these values for children at rest, and observe how they change with position changes and activity to give an indication of the child's cardiovascular response to activity. The trends of the vital signs are very important. If possible, a resting cardiac rhythm strip should be examined for arrhythmia, and documented. A sinus tachycardia is commonly found in response to low cardiac output. Be aware of other conditions, such as transplantation, that may impact heart rate or rhythms, as noted earlier. Vital signs should be monitored as strength, functional mobility, and exercise tolerance is examined.

General Appearance

During any physical examination, there should be a discussion with the parents about the best way to approach the child. One can watch monitors to document vital signs before entering the room. For young children, beginning with play or playing with the caregiver will help the child gain comfort in the presence of a therapist. Letting them explore equipment, including stethoscopes or blood pressure cuffs is helpful. For adolescents, explain the purpose of being there, and explain to them and their caregiver what will be done. Utilizing age and cognitively appropriate descriptions of the activities that will be performed is appropriate. This explanation should precede the actual examination. While introducing the therapist and their role, the child's state of consciousness

TABLE 18.3.	Age-Appropriate Arterial Blood Gases		
	pH	PCO₂	PO₂
Preterm infant at 1–5 hr	7.29–7.37	39–56	52–67
Term infant at 5 hr	7.31–7.37	32–39	62–86
Preterm and term infant at 5 d	7.34–7.42	32–41	62–92
Children, adolescents, adults	7.35–7.45	35–45	80–100

can be observed. Some children with CHD may be very ill at initial examination. Some children may be on musculoskeletal blockade, due to the inability of their cardiovascular system to tolerate any movement or excitement, whereas others may be lightly sedated or fully engaged. The state of consciousness will dictate the level to which the child can cooperate with simple commands appropriate for age. The use or discontinuation of any supportive equipment, lines, or devices should be documented. The documentation of the presence of or change in medical interventions provided will give an idea of the child's current or past health status, and the considerations for positioning and scar management. These devices and lines will vary by setting and acuity, and are discussed in more detail later in the chapter. The child should be monitored for edema or ascites, which may result from retained fluid or abdominal fluid overload when the heart becomes unable to maintain adequate cardiac output. The general coloring should be noted—anemia causes paleness, polycythemia causes plethora, and oxygen desaturation causes cyanosis. The individual's body type as cachectic, obese, or appropriate for age should be noted.

Pain

Pain should be well documented with age-appropriate pain scales. For children who can verbalize and rate their own pain, a self-report of pain is preferred using a visual analog scale (VAS) or the Wong–Baker FACES scale.[25,26] An observational/behavioral pain scale may be used. These include the face, legs, activity, cry, and consolability (FLACC) and the COMFORT scales, which have been validated for infants and young children,[27] in postoperative cardiac care,[28] and for critically ill children in intensive-care settings.[29,30]

A simple rating scale or VAS has the child rate their pain on a scale from 0 to 10 or to mark along a 10-cm line, with 0 being no pain and 10 the worst pain.[26] The Wong–Baker FACES is for children with a cognitive age of 3 to 7 years and uses a VAS from no hurt to hurts worst.[25] The FLACC assessment scale is a behavioral scale that has the rater observe five categories: face, legs, activity, cry, and consolability. Each category is scored from 0 to 2: 0 is a relaxed and calm behavior, 1 is an increase in pain behaviors noted, and 2 is the most pain in each category. Therefore, a total score of 10 means the worst pain, and the range of scores is 0 to 10.[27] The COMFORT scale, another behavioral scale, has the observer examine and rate seven areas: alertness, calmness, respiratory response, cry, physical movement, muscle tone, and facial tension. Each area is rated 1 through 5, with 1 being the least pain and 5 the most pain, the highest score is 35.[29] The management of pain is very important, because it impacts both movement and respiratory function. Therapists will be better able to provide interventions if there is good pain control. This may mean requesting a directed time for pain medication and scheduling therapy around pain medications.

Equipment and Devices

Most children with CHD in the inpatient setting will have cardiorespiratory monitors and pulse oximetry continuously monitoring their vital signs. Many children will have a peripheral intravenous line, arterial line, or central line. An arterial line is placed directly into the artery and can be used to continuously monitor blood pressure and blood gases. A central line, such as a Broviac catheter or port, is inserted into central circulation and used to administer medications or fluids, or for drawing blood. A peripherally inserted central catheter is also a central line that is placed more distally to the heart, generally in an arm. Those who are postsurgical may have chest tubes in place to help drain fluid. Some children may have supplemental oxygen delivered by oxygen masks, nasal cannulas, or oxygen hoods. Those requiring supplemental nutrition may have nasogastric or gastrostomy tubes.

Because children require more support, other equipment or devices may be introduced, including pacer wires, mechanical ventilation, extracorporeal membrane oxygenation (ECMO), or ventricular assist devices (VADs). Pacer wires are centrally placed on the heart for emergent needs for electrical intervention for the heart and are usually removed within 7 days postoperatively. These lines must be treated with respect and care, and children with pacer wires in place may not be stable for out-of-bed activity.

ECMO is similar to a heart–lung machine, supplying an artificial heart and lung outside the body. The machine adds oxygen into the blood and removes carbon dioxide, giving the child's heart and lungs time to rest and heal. ECMO does not cure the disease; it just gives the child physiologic support as he or she heals. Indications for ECMO include acute transplant rejection and respiratory failure. ECMO is generally used for short-term treatment, and is considered a bridge to transplant or recovery.[31] In Figure 18.11, a child is receiving ECMO. During ECMO, a physical therapist will provide a positioning program to maintain midline orientation of the limbs, especially positioning of the lower extremities to prevent contractures. It is important not to

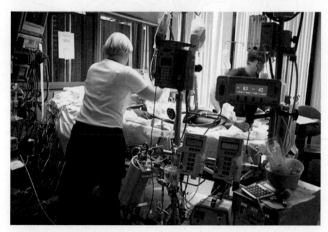

FIGURE 18.11. A child receiving extracorporeal membrane oxygenation (ECMO).

kink the blood flow circuit; therefore, passive range of motion of some joints may be contraindicated. There are many sequelae of ECMO including thrombosis that can lead to stroke and necrosis of the extremities (especially distally). It is important to be aware of these sequelae as a child is being removed from ECMO, and their function can be reexamined.

A VAD is an external device that assists the right or left ventricle to pump blood. A left ventricular assist device (LVAD) will assist pumping to systemic circulation, whereas a right ventricular assist device (RVAD) will assist pumping to pulmonary circulation. Adults have been using VADs for many years, and these include internal device options. In the past few years, internal VAD options have been utilized as a bridge to transplantation, and, occasionally, to destination therapy, in children (mean age 11 years) with 1-year survival rates greater than 80%.[31] Adverse effects that include device malfunction, adverse neurologic sequelae, bleeding, and infection.[31]

VADs can be utilized over a long period, often as a bridge to transplantation, and they allow for exercise conditioning and training while awaiting transplantation.[32] The VAD monitors heart rate, stroke volume, and cardiac output; but blood pressure and oxygen saturation are monitored manually. It is important to consider subjective reports of exertion, pain, and dyspnea.[32] The literature suggests that children should participate in early mobilization as soon as medically stable following VAD placement.[32] Exercise training should progress as tolerated while a VAD remains in place. A child with an external LVAD can be seen ambulating in Figure 18.12. It may be helpful to have those with a VAD use an abdominal binder for upright activities.

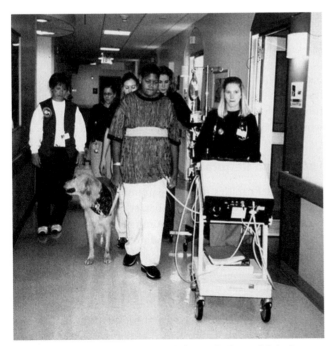

FIGURE 18.12. A child with a left ventricular assist device ambulating with a physical therapist.

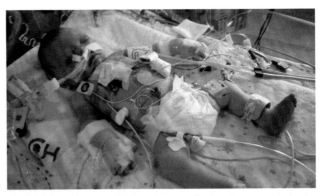

FIGURE 18.13. An infant postoperatively with a nasotracheal tube.

Mechanical ventilation is utilized both pre- and postoperatively for children with CHD. Preoperatively, the ventilator is used to assist with breathing during respiratory distress. Postoperatively, it is used while returning to breathing independently. The ventilator may be connected to an endotracheal tube or tracheostomy tube. An endotracheal tube may be placed in the nose or mouth to assist with breathing. Figure 18.13 shows a postoperative infant with a nasotracheal tube. Airway suctioning to keep the child clear of secretions is of the utmost value when a child is intubated. Always be sure to clear the ventilator tubing of water before listening to breath sounds because the water may distort the actual sounds. If physical therapists do not perform suction in the venue, a person who is able to suction the child should be aware of the interventions, should suctioning become necessary during treatment. Without a clear airway it is unlikely that gross motor skills will be optimal. Providing midline orientation, especially to prevent a head preference, is very important. Some children will pull away from the ventilator and will have a head preference facing away from the ventilator, whereas some will hold still facing the ventilator, afraid to move and pull the tubing. Less invasive modes of ventilation may include continuous positive airway pressure (CPAP), bilevel positive airway pressure (BiPAP), nitric oxide ventilation, or oxygen via nasal cannula. Children may require these modes of ventilation continuously or intermittently while sleeping or with activity. It is important to communicate with the medical team to understand the reasons for ventilation, and also to monitor vital signs while working with children who are using a ventilator.

Integument

The state of the integumentary system should be examined, beginning with the general appearance of the skin. Does it look glossy, turgid, loose, bruised, or broken down? Anticoagulation can lead to bruising and skin breakdown, and fluid retention can lead to glossy or turgid skin. Surgical sites and incisions should be examined, including clamshell, median sternotomy, thoracotomy, and small incisions for chest tubes, central lines, or other tubes. These sites may be sutured or stapled closed, but occasionally may be left open with a surgical dressing. Scar mobility should be examined in all directions. Documentation should occur as to whether scars move well or are bound down to the tissue underneath, and also whether scars are painful. A typical chest of a child following heart surgery is seen in Figure 18.14.

The extremities should be examined, and digital clubbing documented, as a sign of prolonged hypoxia, where the tip of the distal phalanx becomes bulbous and the nail of the digit exits at an increased angle. Clubbing is common in patients with cyanotic CHD or chronic lung disease leading to hypoxia. An example of clubbing is presented in Figure 18.15. Capillary refill in the extremities should be examined. This is done by pushing down on the nail bed, which should blanch and rebound 1 to 2 seconds after pressure is relieved. Capillary refill ideally should be examined by compression of the big toe. Children with CHD are at risk for wounds after their surgical procedures because of long operative times with positioning on hard surgical tables at awkward angles to access the necessary organs. Children should be examined after each surgical procedure to view their skin over bony prominences.

Edema should also be evaluated. The most common method of measuring edema is to apply pressure with one or two fingers to the affected area for several seconds, then observe how deep the area depresses and how long it takes to return to normal. The result is graded on a 1+ to 4+ scale,

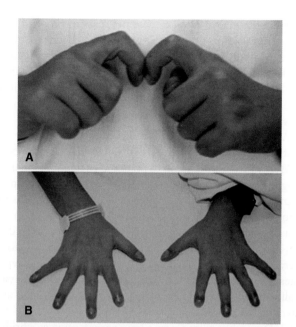

FIGURE 18.15. (**A**) No space present between forefingers signifies digital clubbing. (**B**) A child with digital clubbing and cyanosis in his extremities.

where 1+ is the least and 4+ is the worst. Edema may also be measured using circumferential measurements of the affected area. This method may be helpful to compare changes in the amount of edema over time. Peripheral and central edema may be evident with children with CHD. Peripheral edema is due to the inability of the heart to maintain adequate cardiac output. The autonomic nervous system is attempting to increase cardiac output by retaining fluid from the kidneys. This makes the heart work even harder, and the fluid accumulates in the periphery in the dependent extremities. Central edema or jugular venous distension results from fluid overload because the fluid is retained centrally owing to the heart's ability to pump being compromised and fluid backs up into the lungs and venous system of the body. Adolescents with Fontan circulation are at risk for lymphatic dysfunction due to increased pulmonary lymphatic pressures, which can result in peripheral or central edema.[19]

Thorax and Respiratory Examination

Thoracic deformities should be examined, including pectus excavatum, pectus carinatum, barrel chest, rib flaring, and mid-trunk folds. Pectus excavatum is where the chest caves inward, resulting in the tightening of the upper chest musculature. Pectus carinatum is where the chest bows outward, resulting in a deformity of the sternum. Both pectus excavatum and carinatum may be due to surgical procedures or altered chest pressures due to respiratory status.[33] Barrel chest deformities can be due to the overinflation of the lung tissue, rib flaring is due to an imbalance of the abdominal muscles with the diaphragm, and a mid-trunk fold is due to muscle imbalance of the chest wall to counteract the diaphragm.

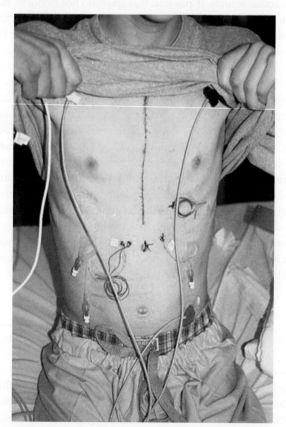

FIGURE 18.14. A adolescent following transplantation, with numerous lines and surgical incisions.

Examination of the rib angles and intercostal spaces for age appropriateness and mobility is important.[33–35]

To evaluate the thoracic cage of a child with CHD, the therapist must have knowledge of age-appropriate thoracic cage structure. Newborns have narrow rib spaces, horizontal ribs, a triangular shape to the chest wall, minimal neck space, and chest separate from the abdomen.[35] Three- to six-month-old children will have a normal pectus, more rectangular shape, and horizontal ribs. They will be normal upper chest breathers with only anterior expansion possible. Six- to 12-month-old children will have an even more pronounced rectangular shape, and lateral expansion will be added to their respiratory repertoire, giving them rib space opening as well as increasing the length of the neck. This is a significant stage in the respiratory development of the thorax.[35] There will be a more barrel-shaped appearance of the chest. The rib cage is beginning to be pulled downward owing to a more upright posture and the more continuous effects of gravity on the thorax. This change provides the child a better length–tension relationship for the diaphragm and the intercostal muscles. In this stage, the diaphragm and all the accessory musculature patterns of breathing are available. This trend in the development of the thorax continues for several more years as the rib cage gradually rotates downward and the intercostal spaces widen.[35] Figure 18.16A–C shows a newborn, a 3-month-old, and an 8-month-old with normally configured chest walls. An infant with CHD may have respiratory compromise, which may alter typical muscular function of the chest and, if not addressed, may lead to chest wall deformities.

Examining thoracic cage mobility means ascertaining movement of the ribs. Can the child flex laterally? Do the ribs move with respiration? How is abdominal and upper chest movement? Muscular development should be symmetric, without hypertrophy of accessory muscles of respiration. Chest wall movement can be examined by palpation and measurement. By placing hands over the upper lobe of the lungs with the heel of the hand at the fourth rib, fingertips at the upper trapezii, and thumb at the sternal angle, symmetry, extent of movement, and general movement may be examined. Measure the thoracic circumference with a tape measure at three levels: axilla/third rib, xiphoid, and half way from xiphoid to umbilicus. Wrap a tape measure around the thorax until it overlaps, then measure the change in circumference during normal inhalation and exhalation. Adult data suggest that during quiet breathing, the chest wall should move approximately 2 to 3 mm at the upper chest, 3 to 4 mm at the lower chest, and 6 to 7 mm at the abdomen; during deep inhalation, it should move 19 to 18 mm at the upper chest, 16 to 20 mm at the lower chest, and 17 to 25 mm at the abdomen.[36] These values vary slightly by gender. No published data exist for pediatric values.

Children with CHD may present with respiratory issues as their primary complaint, given the integral relationship between the heart and lungs. Including respiratory examination as detailed in Chapter 19 will assist in examination of the child's status.

Musculoskeletal Examination

An examination of range of motion, postural alignment, and sensation is also necessary. Scoliosis, kyphosis, or a syndromic deviation of the musculoskeletal system may be present and can impact the child's posture, respiration, and pain before, during, or after surgery for CHD. Figure 18.17 shows common postural deviations in a child with CHD. Flexibility can be examined by functional range of motion, a sit-and-reach test, and lateral flexion measurements. Measure from the axilla to the base of the ribs and then the base of the ribs to the pelvis; there should be a 1:2 ratio. Nerve palsies and signs of thrombosis are also important to screen for as they can happen postsurgically, during prolonged positioning, or with anticoagulation medication.

Strength

Measurement of strength must consider children who are at risk for myopathy, osteopenia, and osteoporosis secondary to steroids preoperatively or following transplantation. Manual muscle testing and dynamometry should be considered. Manual muscle testing may not offer an accurate measure of the child's strength, whereas dynamometry can provide

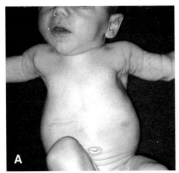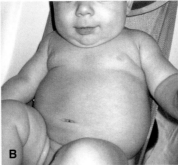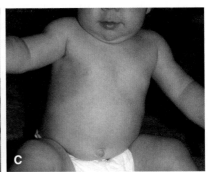

FIGURE 18.16. **(A)** A newborn and a normal chest wall shape. **(B)** A normal 3-month-old's chest wall shape. **(C)** An 8-month-old child with a normal chest wall.

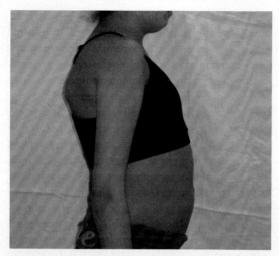

FIGURE 18.17. A child with common postural deviations associated with congenital heart disease (CHD).

TABLE 18.4.	Dyspnea Index	
		Score
Breathlessness barely noticeable		1
Breathlessness moderately bothersome		2
Breathlessness severe, very uncomfortable		3
Most severe breathlessness ever experienced		4

an alternative, objective means to specifically measure strength. Breathing techniques should be taught, breathing out on the exertion, while measuring strength to avoid Valsalva maneuver (breath holding) during exertion. An eight-repetition maximum to fatigue should be considered, rather than a one-repetition maximum so as to determine initial level of muscular endurance.

Functional Mobility

Functional mobility examination includes bed mobility, transfers, balance, gait, and stairs, as well as developmentally appropriate activities. Most activities can be evaluated on the first day postoperatively, and more as medical status improves and as children move from acute care to outpatient and early intervention settings. Functional activities, such as transfers, ambulation over a specified distance, or stair climbing, can be timed and provides useful test–retest data by which to measure progress. Developmental motor skills should be evaluated as able and standardized assessment tools utilized to provide an objective examination of gross motor skills.

Aerobic Capacity and Endurance

Aerobic capacity can be examined using formal exercise testing or timed walk tests. The 6-minute walk test is a self-paced walking test designed to measure the submaximal level of functional exercise, and is endorsed by the American Thoracic Society as the gold standard for evaluation of functional exercise capacity.[37] It has been validated in children[38] and for children with CHD,[39] with normative values available for healthy children as young as 3 years old.[40,41] During a 6-minute walk test, the child is given specific and age-appropriate directions to walk as fast as possible, without running, for a total of 6 minutes. Children are instructed to walk at their own pace, but to try to walk as far as they can to cover the greatest distance possible in the allotted time. Rest breaks

are allowed, but the time keeps going. Children should be instructed to inform the evaluation if they have chest discomfort, dizziness, severe shortness of breath, unsteadiness, or blurred vision. The distance walked, rate of perceived exertion (RPE), dyspnea index (DI), and vital signs before, during, and after the testing should be recorded. The 6-minute walk distance correlates with oxygen uptake at maximal exercise (VO_{2max}),[38,39] which has been shown in children with CHD to be correlated with increased risk of heart failure, hospitalization, and death when below 50% of predicted values.[42–44] Thus, the 6-minute walk test can give the physical therapist an idea of functional capacity when compared with peers and prognostic information, and assist in goal setting.

While examining aerobic capacity, shortness of breath and level of exertion should be observed. Breathlessness can be evaluated using the DI (Table 18.4). Children rate how breathless they feel with certain activities, and they respond with a number from a chart that is shown to them. Breathlessness can also be examined by counting how many syllables they are able to speak per breath (8 to 10 syllables per breath is normal) or how long they can maintain a vowel sound without taking a breath (10 to 15 seconds is normal). These measures provide a baseline value to reexamine over time to determine whether ratings, syllables, or time change. Perceived exertion can be monitored using the Borg RPE scale (Table 18.5).

TABLE 18.5.	Borg Rate of Perceived Exertion Scale	
6		
7	Very, very light	
8		
9	Very light	
10		
11	Fairly light	
12		
13	Somewhat hard	
14		
15	Hard	
16		
17	Very hard	
18		
19	Very, very hard	
20		

The child should be asked, "How hard do you feel you are working?" This is meant to include overall work, breathing, muscle exertion, and fatigue. The child should integrate information from the peripheral working muscles and joints, the cardiovascular and pulmonary systems, and the central nervous system. A rating of 6 is analogous to no work at all, whereas a rating of 20 is the hardest work ever done. A newer Borg scale from 0 to 10 points is also commonly used.

» Physical therapy evaluation, diagnosis, and prognosis

Following the physical therapy examination, the therapist must integrate the examination findings and clinical expertise to synthesize the complete evaluation and determine the individual's physical therapy diagnosis and prognosis. This process helps determine the plan of care and the outcomes expected. The goals of a physical therapy plan of care are directly related to examination findings and may include improving the individual's endurance, strength, range of motion/flexibility, balance, functional mobility or gross motor skills, posture, respiratory/ventilatory status, scar and chest wall mobility, chest expansion, airway clearance, and providing child and family education (Table 18.6). The plan of care should specify the anticipated frequency and duration of physical therapy intervention, as well as the areas to be addressed. Frequency and duration will vary according to individual needs, and the setting (e.g., acute care, outpatient, or community settings).

Coordination, Communication, and Documentation

Physical therapists should collaborate with other services, including cardiology, genetics, neurology, otolaryngology, orthopedics, social work, feeding specialists, occupational therapy, or speech therapy, and recommend consults as needed for specialists not involved. It is important to advocate for the child to access the services he or she deserves. In the inpatient setting, participating in rounds with the medical team will allow collaboration. In the outpatient or community settings, establishing a relationship with the child's care team will help determine important medical information or change in status. Several tertiary hospital centers have initiated team-based neurodevelopmental follow-up programs for children with CHD to enable collaboration and regular follow-up on issues across disciplines. Referrals to early intervention (0 to 3 years) and school-based services (3 to 21 years) are also encouraged on the basis of the child's age.

» Physical therapy intervention

Child- and Family-Related Instruction

Family and caregiver education should focus on the family unit as a whole, including the specific needs of the child. It is important to emphasize the difference between CHD and adult coronary artery disease. The child should be able to explore and play within boundaries based on his or her specific CHD, not based on fear of participation as may happen in

TABLE 18.6.	Physical Therapy Goal Areas and Sample Goals

Endurance
Patient will have improved endurance as evidenced by increased 6-min walk distance to at least 450 m to keep up with peers.

Strength
Patient will have improved strength by at least 5 lb on dynamometry in bilateral gluteus maximus and quadriceps to climb stairs independently.

Respiratory/ventilatory status
Patient will have improved respiratory coordination during functional mobility as evidenced by ability to coordinate inhale and exhale with sit-to-stand transfer while maintaining saturation >90%.

Balance
Patient will have increased balance as evidenced by increased score on the Pediatric Balance Scale to 56/56 to maintain safe functional mobility without falls.

Functional mobility or gross motor skills
Patient will have improved gross motor skills to at least 37th percentile on standardized gross motor testing to age-appropriately interact with environment.

Posture
Patient will have improved posture with ability to maintain scapular retraction, chin tuck, and shoulders back for at least 5 min while sitting without verbal cues.

Range of motion/flexibility
Patient will have improved hip flexor flexibility with Thomas test to neutral to maintain upright posture for standing and walking.

Scar and chest wall mobility
Patient will have increased sternal scar mobility as evidenced by Vancouver Scar Scale score decrease by at least 3 points to allow full trunk rotation without pain.

Chest expansion
Patient will have improved chest wall expansion while seated as evidenced by increased circumferential excursion by at least 0.5 cm at diaphragm level to improve oxygenation.

Airway clearance
Patient will be independent with use of home airway clearance device with proper technique demonstrated on 3/3 trials without verbal cues.

Patient and family education
Patient's family will be independent with home positioning program as evidenced by 100% return demonstration without cues.

adults. Child and family education should include discussion about sternal precautions, optimal positioning options for different ages, therapy outcomes and role of early intervention, importance of physical activity, and understanding self-limitation. Children and families should start to understand that exercise should be a lifelong habit. Health, wellness, and fitness programs including cardiac rehabilitation programs and YMCA programs are an important component of lifelong health habits. In addition, literature has shown that long-term cardiac outcomes, mortality, self-esteem, and emotional state are all improved with increasing exercise tolerance and motor skills.[42–46]

Procedural Interventions

Positioning

Providing and promoting varied positions will enable the physical therapist to begin to achieve goals related to preventing musculoskeletal abnormalities, improving pulmonary parameters, and promoting age-appropriate skills. Proper positioning can help provide midline orientation, prevent contractures, promote development, and improve pulmonary status. Positioning may include turning schedules, special devices or equipment, or recommendations for postures and positions. While a child is an inpatient and has had a neuromuscular blockade or sedation, decreased mobility, and in-dwelling lines and tubes, rotation schedules can reduce the possibility of skin pressure and breakdown. The therapist must coordinate changes in the infant's position with other nursing procedures to avoid unnecessary stimulation. Positioning devices such as Multi-Podus boots help control plantar flexion contractures, enhance hip rotation, and protect the heel from pressure. Molded foot and ankle orthoses, towel rolls, and gel pillows will help prevent secondary integument issues for children with CHD who are not mobile. Scar massage can help prevent binding down of scars after skin healing, enhance skin movement to reduce range-of-motion limitations, and limit deformities from surgical scars. Scar massage can begin 6 weeks after a sternal incision to allow time for bone healing of the sternum.

Positioning can also enhance oxygen transport and pulmonary function. Infants, even those with endotracheal tubes, have increased oxygenation while in prone versus other positions, especially supine.[47] A mismatch of ventilation and perfusion is a common cause of arterial hypoxemia. Small children have better ventilation to the uppermost lung. Larger children have better ventilation to the dependent lung, similar to that of the adult pattern. Specific body positioning can allow matching of ventilation and perfusion to a specific lobe of the lung.[48] Atelectasis versus hyperinflation in the lung should be considered. A chart similar to the one shown in Table 18.7 to place the child in different positions and see where the best ventilation–perfusion matching may be so as to raise SpO_2 and decrease heart rate, blood pressure, and respiratory rate should be considered. Prone positioning in infants with CHD can assist with maintaining hip extension range of motion, chest expansion, trunk and head strength, and attainment of gross motor skills.[49,50] Positioning should also play a role in the outpatient or early intervention plan of care to promote optimal lung function, developmental skills, and to allow engagement with the environment. These positions may include prone (as described earlier) and side-lying to encourage reaching in a gravity-eliminated position. Other positioning should be specific to the child's needs.

Postural Education and Awareness

Most therapeutic exercises and activities can begin with postural training and education. This may mean using elastic wrap or other tools for tactile cues during upright posture to minimize thoracic kyphosis and rounded shoulders. Other techniques include exercises to improve postural control, strengthen postural muscles, and hands-on interventions for postural education.

Flexibility

Flexibility exercises should also begin early and, depending on the child's presentation, commonly include stretches for muscles, including pectoralis major, Achilles/gastrocnemius/soleus group, hip flexors, hamstrings, and upper extremities, and chest expansion for thoracic cage mobility. Bolsters, balls, and towel rolls for thoracic cage stretching may assist in making stretching tolerable. Stretches may need to be held for long periods and may be completed as part of a home program while a child watches television or reads. All flexibility activities should consider sternal precautions that are present for 6 weeks postoperatively.

TABLE 18.7.	**Vital Sign Trends**									
Breathing Patterns/Vital Sign Trends			RR		SpO₂%		HR		BP	
Position	Sequence	1 min	3 min	1 min	3 min	1 min	3 min	1 min	3 min
Supine									
Side-lying									
Sitting/upright									
Prone									

BP, blood pressure; HR, heart rate; RR, respiratory rate.

Breathing Exercises

Breathing activities should be incorporated into intervention to foster deep breathing, help maintain ventilation, assist with pain control, and promote coordinated breathing patterns. Breathing games such as blowing bubbles, air hockey, blowing a windmill, and sniffing stickers are an excellent start to improve the child's respiratory status. Diaphragmatic breathing training, inspiratory muscle trainers, incentive spirometers, and deep-breathing techniques can be utilized in children as young as 18 months. Finding a strategy that works with the developmental level of the child and one that the child finds "fun" is the goal. More extensive information about breathing exercises can be found in Chapter 19.

Aerobic and Endurance Training

Aerobic exercise prescription should be individualized on the basis of the previous testing during the physical therapy examination. An exercise regimen should include principles of mode, frequency, duration, and intensity,[51] and identified precautions. Mode may be a bicycle, treadmill, elliptical, upper body ergometer (UBE), or may be overground exercise such as walking. The frequency should be a minimum of three times a week and up to seven times a week. When a child is very ill, the duration may be as little as short bouts of 2 to 5 minutes, with rest breaks between bouts. Lower intensity stretching may be tolerated during rest breaks. Duration should progress to 30 to 45 minutes as the child improves or transitions to the outpatient or early intervention setting. Intensity can be determined from a stress or functional exercise test performed before training. Generally, intensity should begin at 60% to 65% of the maximal level of work. Intensity can also be prescribed on the basis of RPE with the Borg scale, which should fall between 11 and 15 on the 20-point scale. Very deconditioned children may need to start with lower intensity activities or alternate short-duration and higher intensity activities with lower intensity activities. During activity, the therapist should monitor the vital signs, including heart rate, blood pressure, RPE, DI, respiratory rate, and SpO_2. Some children may benefit from electrocardiogram (ECG) monitoring during aerobic activity. During training, the therapist can instruct some children to take their own heart rate, respiratory rate, RPE, and DI. Identifying their own vital signs will foster the independence necessary to continue exercise independently once they are ready to move to autonomous activity. It is important to remember that following heart transplant, there is not a normal exercise response due to loss of the vagus nerve, and therefore requires warm-up to increase the heart rate to have an effect from the circulating catecholamines in the blood, followed by a cooldown.

Strength Training

Strength training is an important component of physical therapy for children of an appropriate age. Following cardiac surgery, children generally have sternal precautions in

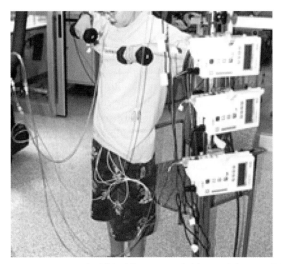

FIGURE 18.18. A child with a congenital heart defect participating in strength training.

place for 6 to 8 weeks, which may include lifting precautions for greater than 10 lb. With this caveat, strength training is a valuable tool in the treatment of children with CHD both pre- and postoperatively. Children should always be taught proper breathing techniques with lifting to prevent a Valsalva maneuver and an unnecessary rise in blood pressure. Figure 18.18 shows a child participating in strength training.

Airway Clearance Techniques

These topics are covered in detail in Chapter 19. Positioning, as discussed earlier, and postural drainage should be utilized immediately postoperatively. Mechanical airway clearance techniques such as percussion, vibration, shaking, and the high-frequency chest wall oscillation may require a short wait postoperatively, but other airway clearance techniques, such as Acapella or autogenic drainage, can be utilized as appropriate.

Functional Mobility

Transfer training, gait training, balance training, and stair climbing are functional tasks that should be included as necessary in physical therapy intervention. Transfer training should include ways to move that decrease discomfort and improve independence. This may mean teaching log rolling postoperatively while using deep-breathing techniques, or giving a child a "hug pillow" to hold over surgical sites. For small children, this may mean teaching family members how to pick up and hold their child in such a way as to pose as little discomfort as possible. Gait training, balance training, and stair climbing should be initiated as soon as they are able and medically stable. This may involve coordinating care with nursing staff, respiratory staff, or medical team members to allow safe completion. Once children are discharged to outpatient or early intervention programs, gait training, balance training, or stair training may need to continue to improve speed, stability, or technique.

Developmental Activity

Play is the means by which young children explore their world. A child with CHD who is awaiting surgery or is very ill and hospitalized has little exposure to physical exploration. Age-appropriate gross and fine motor play is very important for this population. Although there may be many tubes and wires to manage in the acute care setting, an infant should be exposed to all positions, including prone. Parent education and involvement of early intervention personnel in the home should also promote position changes, prone position, and progression of motor skills as tolerated. This effort may start with getting the infant accustomed to prone by starting with semi-prone positioning over a towel roll or prone on the shoulder of the caregiver. Prone positioning is the forerunner of many early developmental skills, including creeping, crawling, and upper extremity weight bearing and will assist in promoting infant development.[49,50] This position is important for children with poor feeding, reflux, and respiratory issues. Families should be encouraged to promote prone positioning during awake, alert, and calm periods during the day to help the infant gain head control and feel comfortable in prone. It is unusual for a child to have difficulty in prone after practice. Prone is seldom a contraindicated position, with the exception of a thoracic wound that is not closed or for the first 2 weeks following a sternal incision. Figure 18.19 shows an infant with a nasotracheal tube being placed in prone, and an infant following two cardiac surgeries working on prone skills in the home setting. Crawling should be encouraged in children with CHD because it improves all the muscle groups that are impacted by the surgical procedures done to correct or palliate CHD. Ambulatory children should be encouraged to ambulate postoperatively as soon as they are medically stable. Children receiving mechanical ventilation can ambulate with a team effort to maintain their ventilatory support and the safety of their airway. Children with chest tubes can also ambulate with little limitation, and ambulation may help hasten chest tube removal. Higher level motor skills may be delayed in children with CHD and should be promoted during therapy sessions.[3–6,10]

Home Programming

Recommendations should be made for home exercise programs, according to the child's needs and age. Any of the above activities can be transitioned to home program activities because he or she is safe and stable to complete them without supervision. Parents should be encouraged to participate in sessions, and to assist with carryover of home activities.

» Neurodevelopmental outcomes of congenital heart disease

Children with CHD are at high risk for a myriad of neurodevelopmental challenges, the causes of which are multifactorial and not yet fully understood. Early developmental milestones, including cognition, language, and motor skills, are often delayed. One report found that 54% of infants with any type of single ventricle defect were receiving early intervention for a developmental domain by 6 months, 62% by 12 months, and 67% by 2 years, whereas 45% of infants with two ventricle defects were receiving developmental intervention by 6 months, 43% at 12 months, and 52% at 2 years.[6] Another study reported an overall rate of developmental delay of 25% for children following Fontan completion.[10] Uzark et al. demonstrated that 46% of children status post–heart transplantation present with language delay and 63% with visual motor deficits.[52] They also found a decrease in intelligence quotient (IQ), with the lowest IQs being in children with CHD as the primary reason for transplant.[52] Seventy-four percent of children with single ventricle defects and 29% of children with two ventricle defects scored below the 5th percentile on specific gross motor testing at 6 months.[6] Up to 50% of children with TGA present with decreased psychomotor skills at 1 year of age,[3] up to 40% present with motor or gait abnormalities at 4 years of age,[5] and, by 8 years of age, 54% present with gait abnormalities and 63% with motor abnormalities.[4]

Although the factors causing neurodevelopmental challenges are not fully known, they likely involve an interaction

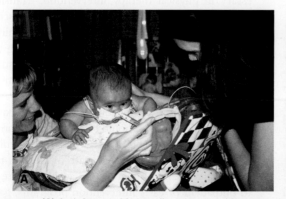
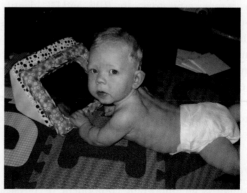

FIGURE 18.19. **(A)** An infant awaiting cardiac surgery, with nasotracheal intubation, working on prone skills in physical therapy with physical therapist and mother. **(B)** An infant with congenital heart defect following two surgeries working on prone skills in the home setting.

of the preoperative, intraoperative, and postoperative events. Oxygenation levels following the first stage of single ventricle repair have been found to be associated with composite developmental score.[53] Whether a child undergoes circulatory arrest or low-flow cardiopulmonary bypass during surgery may also impact outcomes, because children with TGA who underwent circulatory arrest have been shown to have up to 30% more delays at 1, 4, and 8 years of age.[3–5] In addition, several studies have found that length of stay following surgical intervention can impact neurodevelopmental outcome, such that each increased day of length of stay was shown to lead to a 1.4-point decrease in full-scale IQ and a 1.6-point decrease in math IQ.[54,55] Increased length of stay has been shown to be the greatest predictor of decreased motor skills at 1 year for children with HLHS.[7]

Concern regarding the neurodevelopmental implications in children with CHD has become a significant focus of cardiac management for these children. A recent scientific statement from the American Heart Association recommends regular surveillance for neurodevelopmental delays in children with CHD with referral for full evaluation and intervention when there is concern for delay.[9] Although initial surveillance may often occur in the cardiology or pediatrician visits, physical therapists should be involved for evaluation and monitoring of motor skills in early intervention, outpatient, and hospital-based settings for children with CHD.

Summary

Physical therapy is an integral component of the care of a child with CHD in the inpatient, outpatient, and community-based settings. Physical therapists are a vital component of the care of all children with cardiac disorders to improve posture, mobility, development, and, ultimately, the ability to keep up with peers and participate and thrive in their family, school, and community environments.

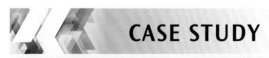

CASE STUDY

TODDLER WITH HYPOPLASTIC LEFT HEART SYNDROME FOLLOWING TWO CARDIAC SURGERIES

History of Present Illness and Chief Complaint
Baby X is a 13-month-old male with HLHS who presents for developmental assessment in a multidisciplinary outpatient clinic setting. Baby X has a history of gross motor delay, and his parents are concerned that he does not put his feet down to stand.

Birth and Medical History
Baby X was diagnosed prenatally with HLHS and was born full term in the Special Delivery Unit at a children's hospital and

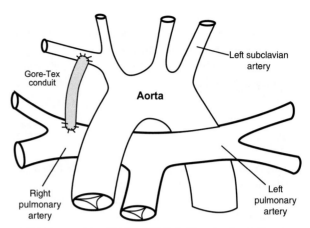

FIGURE 18.20. Modified Blalock–Taussig shunt. (Image used under license from Brossman Design Inc.)

transferred immediately to the Cardiac Intensive Care Unit for stabilization.

Surgical History
Baby X underwent a stage one repair with Blalock–Taussig shunt on day 3 of life (Fig. 18.20), which was complicated by left vocal cord paralysis and venous sinus thrombus. He had a bidirectional Glenn procedure at 4.5 months.

Current Medications
Lasix 0.8 mg 1 per day; Lovenox 0.7 mg 1 per day; Benefiber 1 tsp per day.

Social History
Baby X's parents are very involved in his care, and his mother stays home with him. He has been receiving early intervention physical therapy weekly since 8 months of age.

Physical Therapy Examination
General appearance/lines/tubes: Baby X presents with mild cyanosis and has no external supportive devices or lines.
State of consciousness: He is awake, alert, and oriented and interactive with parents in the examination room.
Pain: FLACC score of 0 out of 10.
Vital signs at rest: Heart rate = 130, SpO_2 = 87%, blood pressure in the right upper extremity = 92/59, respiratory rate = 30.
Integument/skin integrity: Median sternotomy scar well healed with good scar mobility. Capillary refill: <3 seconds.

Thoracic Cage and Respiratory Examination
Baby X presents in no obvious distress, with a respiratory rate of 30 breaths per minute. He uses primarily upper chest breathing, although he has some diaphragmatic excursion. When working hard, he demonstrates increased cyanosis and mild intercostal retractions. He clears his lungs using cough and sneeze independently. Baby X has a mild pectus carinatum with age-appropriate rib spacing and good chest wall mobility. He does not tolerate chest wall circumferential measurements due to age.

Musculoskeletal Examination
Baby X presents with full passive range of motion in bilateral upper and lower extremities, and with mild hypotonia in bilateral

lower extremities. Formal manual muscle test not performed because of age, but presents with decreased lower extremity strength evidenced by decreased standing skills detailed later. Functional skills are detailed under developmental assessment.

Developmental Examination

Supine: brings feet to mouth, reaches across midline, and tracks bilaterally

Prone: pushes up onto palms, reaches with either upper extremity in prone, starting to move onto all fours

Rolling: rolls bilaterally supine to prone, leading with hips

Pull to sit: with + chin tuck

Sitting: sits independently, reaches out of base of support, manipulates toys in sitting

Transitions: per report, transitions sit to prone, but not supine or prone to sit

Standing: does not stand or place feet on ground, very resistant to lower extremity weight bearing

The Peabody Developmental Motor Scales, 2nd edition, was administered with scores at the 16th, 2nd, and 37th percentile for stationary/balance skills, locomotor skills, and object manipulation skills, respectively. Gross motor quotient is 79 (8th percentile).

Physical Therapy Evaluation and Diagnosis

Baby X is a 13-month-old male with HLHS status post (s/p) stage two repair. He presents to physical therapy with decreased leg strength and decreased weight bearing, impacting his standing and walking skills, leading to delayed gross motor skills. He presents with overall gross motor skills at the 8th percentile on the Peabody Developmental Motor Scales, 2nd edition, with performance at the 16th, 2nd, and 37th percentile for stationary/balance skills, locomotor skills, and object manipulation skills, respectively. This corresponds to the 7- to 12-month level. His delayed motor skills impact his ability to age-appropriately interact with his environment.

Plan of Care

Early intervention physical therapy once per week, with a focus on standing skills. Parent education for standing skills and shoe wear.

Goals (for 12 weeks)

1. Baby X will stand at a support surface when placed for 5 minutes without loss of balance.
2. Baby X will pull to stand at support surface independently.
3. Baby X will cruise laterally for 5 feet each direction.
4. Baby X will take steps for 10 feet forward with one hand held.

Procedural Interventions

Parent education: Role of shoe wear, ways to encourage standing and walking, continue scar massage

Developmental skills: Play activities to encourage standing; transfers to standing, cruising, and walking

Strengthening: Via standing and walking repetition activities

REFERENCES

1. Hoffman JI, Kaplan S. The incidence of congenital heart disease. *J Am Coll Cardiol.* 2002;39(12):1890–1900.
2. Green A. Outcomes of congenital heart disease: a review. *Pediatr Nurs.* 2004;30(4):280–284.
3. Bellinger DC, Jonas RA, Rappaport LA, et al. Developmental and neurologic status of children after heart surgery with hypothermic circulatory arrest or low-flow cardiopulmonary bypass. *N Engl J Med.* 1995;332(9):549–555.
4. Bellinger DC, Wypij D, duPlessis AJ, et al. Neurodevelopmental status at eight years in children with dextro-transposition of the great arteries: the Boston circulatory arrest trial. *J Thorac Cardiovasc Surg.* 2003;126(5):1385–1396.
5. Bellinger DC, Wypij D, Kuban KC, et al. Developmental and neurological status of children at 4 years of age after heart surgery with hypothermic circulatory arrest or low-flow cardiopulmonary bypass. *Circulation.* 1999;100(5):526–532.
6. Hoskoppal A, Roberts H, Kugler J, et al. Neurodevelopmental outcomes in infants after surgery for congenital heart disease: a comparison of single-ventricle vs. two-ventricle physiology. *Congenit Heart Dis.* 2010;5(2):90–95.
7. Knirsch W, Liamlahi R, Hug MI, et al. Mortality and neurodevelopmental outcome at 1 year of age comparing hybrid and Norwood procedures. *Eur J Cardiothorac Surg.* 2012;42(1):33–39.
8. Majnemer A, Limperopoulos C, Shevell M, et al. Long-term neuromotor outcome at school entry of infants with congenital heart defects requiring open-heart surgery. *J Pediatr.* 2006;148(1):72–77.
9. Marino BS, Lipkin PH, Newburger JW, et al. Neurodevelopmental outcomes in children with congenital heart disease: evaluation and management: a scientific statement from the American Heart Association. *Circulation.* 2012;126(9):1143–1172.
10. McCrindle BW, Williams RV, Mitchell PD, et al. Relationship of patient and medical characteristics to health status in children and adolescents after the Fontan procedure. *Circulation.* 2006;113(8):1123–1129.
11. Newburger JW, Sleeper LA, Bellinger DC, et al. Early developmental outcome in children with hypoplastic left heart syndrome and related anomalies: the single ventricle reconstruction trial. *Circulation.* 2012;125(17):2081–2091.
12. Cook AC, Yates RW, Anderson RH. Normal and abnormal fetal cardiac anatomy. *Prenat Diagn.* 2004;24(13):1032–1048.
13. Godfrey ME, Messing B, Cohen SM, et al. Functional assessment of the fetal heart: a review. *Ultrasound Obstet Gynecol.* 2012;39(2):131–144.
14. Wernovsky G, Gruber P. Common congenital heart disease: presentation, management and outcomes. In: Taeusch H, Ballard R, Gleason C, eds. *Avery's Diseases of the Newborn.* 8th ed. Elsevier Saunders; 2004:827–872.
15. Frownfelter D, Dean E, eds. *Cardiovascular and Pulmonary Physical Therapy: Evidence and Practice.* 5th ed. Elsevier Mosby; 2005.
16. Hillegass E, ed. *Essentials of Cardiopulmonary Physical Therapy.* Saunders; 2011.
17. Blackburn S. Placental, fetal, and transitional circulation revisited. *J Perinat Neonatal Nurs.* 2006;20(4):290–294.
18. Feinstein JA, Benson DW, Dubin AM, et al. Hypoplastic left heart syndrome: current considerations and expectations. *J Am Coll Cardiol.* 2012;59(1 Suppl):S1–S42.
19. Fredenburg TB, Johnson TR, Cohen MD. The Fontan procedure: anatomy, complications, and manifestations of failure. *Radiographics.* 2011;31(2):453–463.
20. Mendeloff EN. The history of pediatric heart and lung transplantation. *Pediatr Transplant.* 2002;6(4):270–279.

21. Webber SA, McCurry K, Zeevi A. Heart and lung transplantation in children. *Lancet.* 2006;368(9529):53–69.

22. Kirk R, Edwards LB, Kucheryavaya AY, et al. The registry of the International Society for Heart and Lung Transplantation: fourteenth pediatric heart transplantation report—2011. *J Heart Lung Transplant.* 2011;30(10):1095–1103.

23. Singh TP, Gauvreau K, Rhodes J, et al. Longitudinal changes in heart rate recovery after maximal exercise in pediatric heart transplant recipients: evidence of autonomic re-innervation? *J Heart Lung Transplant.* 2007;26(12):1306–1312.

24. Kuhlthau KA, Bloom S, VanCleave J, et al. Evidence for family-centered care for children with special health care needs: a systematic review. *Acad Pediatr.* 2011;11(2):136–143.

25. Garra G, Singer AJ, Taira BR, et al. Validation of the Wong-Baker FACES Pain Rating Scale in pediatric emergency department patients. *Acad Emerg Med.* 2010;17(1):50–54.

26. Howard R, Carter B, Curry J, et al. Pain assessment. *Paediatr Anaesth.* 2008;18(suppl 1):14–18.

27. Merkel S, Voepel-Lewis T, Malviya S. Pain assessment in infants and young children: the FLACC scale. *Am J Nurs.* 2002;102(10):55–58.

28. Bai J, Hsu L, Tang Y, et al. Validation of the COMFORT Behavior scale and the FLACC scale for pain assessment in Chinese children after cardiac surgery. *Pain Manag Nurs.* 2012;13(1):18–26.

29. Johansson M, Kokinsky E. The COMFORT behavioural scale and the modified FLACC scale in paediatric intensive care. *Nurs Crit Care.* 2009;14(3):122–130.

30. Voepel-Lewis T, Zanotti J, Dammeyer JA, et al. Reliability and validity of the face, legs, activity, cry, consolability behavioral tool in assessing acute pain in critically ill patients. *Am J Crit Care.* 2010;19(1):55–61; quiz 62.

31. Potapov EV, Stiller B, Hetzer R. Ventricular assist devices in children: current achievements and future perspectives. *Pediatr Transplant.* 2007;11(3):241–255.

32. Corra U, Pistono M, Mezzani A, et al. Cardiovascular prevention and rehabilitation for patients with ventricular assist device from exercise therapy to long-term therapy. Part I: exercise therapy. *Monaldi Arch Chest Dis.* 2011;76(1):27–32.

33. Massery M. Musculoskeletal and neuromuscular interventions: a physical approach to cystic fibrosis. *J R Soc Med.* 2005;98(suppl 45):55–66.

34. Massery M. The Linda Crane Memorial Lecture: the patient puzzle: piecing it together. *Cardiopulm Phys Ther J.* 2009;20(2):19–27.

35. Massery M. Chest development as a component of normal motor development: implications for pediatric physical therapists. *Pediatr Phys Ther.* 1991:3–8.

36. Ragnarsdottir M, Kristinsdottir EK. Breathing movements and breathing patterns among healthy men and women 20-69 years of age. Reference values. *Respiration.* 2006;73(1):48–54.

37. ATS Committee on Proficiency Standards for Clinical Pulmonary Function Laboratories. ATS statement: guidelines for the six-minute walk test. *Am J Respir Crit Care Med.* 2002;166(1):111–117.

38. Li AM, Yin J, Yu CC, et al. The six-minute walk test in healthy children: reliability and validity. *Eur Respir J.* 2005;25(6):1057–1060.

39. Moalla W, Gauthier R, Maingourd Y, et al. Six-minute walking test to assess exercise tolerance and cardiorespiratory responses during training program in children with congenital heart disease. *Int J Sports Med.* 2005;26(9):756–762.

40. Geiger R, Strasak A, Treml B, et al. Six-minute walk test in children and adolescents. *J Pediatr.* 2007;150(4):395–399, e391–e392.

41. Li AM, Yin J, Au JT, et al. Standard reference for the six-minute-walk test in healthy children aged 7 to 16 years. *Am J Respir Crit Care Med.* 2007;176(2):174–180.

42. Diller GP, Dimopoulos K, Okonko D, et al. Exercise intolerance in adult congenital heart disease: comparative severity, correlates, and prognostic implication. *Circulation.* 2005;112(6):828–835.

43. Fredriksen PM, Therrien J, Veldtman G, et al. Lung function and aerobic capacity in adult patients following modified Fontan procedure. *Heart.* 2001;85(3):295–299.

44. Inuzuka R, Diller GP, Borgia F, et al. Comprehensive use of cardiopulmonary exercise testing identifies adults with congenital heart disease at increased mortality risk in the medium term. *Circulation.* 2012;125(2):250–259.

45. Fredriksen PM, Kahrs N, Blaasvaer S, et al. Effect of physical training in children and adolescents with congenital heart disease. *Cardiol Young.* 2000;10(2):107–114.

46. Rhodes J, Curran TJ, Camil L, et al. Sustained effects of cardiac rehabilitation in children with serious congenital heart disease. *Pediatrics.* 2006;118(3):e586–e593.

47. Balachandran R, Nair SG, Sivadasan PC, et al. Prone ventilation in the management of infants with acute respiratory distress syndrome after complex cardiac surgery. *J Cardiothorac Vasc Anesth.* 2012;26(3):471–475.

48. Bhuyan U, Peters AM, Gordon I, et al. Effects of posture on the distribution of pulmonary ventilation and perfusion in children and adults. *Thorax.* 1989;44(6):480–484.

49. Kennedy E, Majnemer A, Farmer JP, et al. Motor development of infants with positional plagiocephaly. *Phys Occup Ther Pediatr.* 2009;29(3):222–235.

50. Kuo YL, Liao HF, Chen PC, et al. The influence of wakeful prone positioning on motor development during the early life. *J Dev Behav Pediatr.* 2008;29(5):367–376.

51. American College of Sports Medicine. *ACSM's Guidelines for Exercise Testing and Prescription.* 6th ed. Lippincott, Williams & Wilkins; 2000.

52. Uzark K, Spicer R, Beebe DW. Neurodevelopmental outcomes in pediatric heart transplant recipients. *J Heart Lung Transplant.* 2009;28(12):1306–1311.

53. Hoffman GM, Mussatto KA, Brosig CL, et al. Systemic venous oxygen saturation after the Norwood procedure and childhood neurodevelopmental outcome. *J Thorac Cardiovasc Surg.* 2005;130(4):1094–1100.

54. Mahle WT, Visconti KJ, Freier MC, et al. Relationship of surgical approach to neurodevelopmental outcomes in hypoplastic left heart syndrome. *Pediatrics.* 2006;117(1):e90–e97.

55. Newburger JW, Wypij D, Bellinger DC, et al. Length of stay after infant heart surgery is related to cognitive outcome at age 8 years. *J Pediatr.* 2003;143(1):67–73.

Pulmonary and Respiratory Conditions

Heather Lever Brossman

>> Introduction

Pulmonary diseases and respiratory disorders continue to be major causes of both mortality and morbidity for children in the United States and throughout the world. Respiratory viruses and bacteria continue to cause acute and sometimes fatal respiratory infections in infants and children. Vaccines against both bacterial and viral agents have decreased the incidence of certain acute respiratory infections, and are commonly employed for children at risk for respiratory disease.

In the United States, up to 20% or more of children younger than 18 years of age have been reported to have a chronic respiratory problem such as asthma, wheezing, bronchial hyperreactivity, cystic fibrosis (CF), and bronchopulmonary dysplasia.[1] Chronic lung disease in children has morbidity statistics that are staggering. An estimated 5.5 million children (7.5%) in the United States have been diagnosed with asthma,[2] which is responsible for 14 million missed days of school annually.[3] It is also important to note that childhood asthma is most prevalent among those of black and multiracial ethnicity. In addition, respiratory illness is the most common reason for hospitalization in children with severe neurologic impairment, and is the most common cause of death in these children.[4,5] These statistics may seem surprising, yet they are not to health care professionals who spend a great deal of time treating children with primary pulmonary diseases or respiratory problems secondary to other conditions.

The information in this chapter will enable readers to understand the fragility of the neonatal and pediatric respiratory system, the developmental process of the pulmonary system, and the need for aggressive treatment of disorders of the system. These introductory topics include growth and development of the respiratory tract and predisposition to acute respiratory failure in infants and children. Physical therapy examination and specific intervention for infants and children with pulmonary disorders follow. Medical information and a discussion of physical therapy for four major respiratory problems in children—atelectasis, respiratory muscle weakness, asthma, and CF—are presented, followed by questions for future research.

» Growth and development of the lungs

A brief review of the major periods of lung development is useful in discussing the interrelationship between lung and airway growth and specific childhood diseases. A description of lung development also provides insight into some unique aspects of the growth, particularly in number, of pulmonary alveoli.

Four specific periods of lung growth have been confirmed and include the embryonic, pseudoglandular, canalicular, and saccular periods from postconception weeks 0 to 6, 6 to 16, 16 to 24, and 24 to 40 (term), respectively.[6] Because alveolar growth continues after birth, a fifth period, alveolar, is also noted. The earliest sign of lung development occurs during the *embryonic period*, from 0 to 6 weeks' gestation. Endodermal tissue of the primitive foregut expands into an anterior lung pouch when the embryo is 4 mm long. During this period, in which there is a separation of the trachea and esophagus, aberrations in development may lead to one of several configurations of tracheoesophageal fistulae—abnormal communication between the two structures (Fig. 19.1). Four days later, the future trachea differentiates into right and left bronchial buds—the precursors of each lung. Mesenchymal cellular tissue surrounding the developing bronchial buds will later differentiate to become muscle, connective tissue, and cartilage within the bronchial walls. Also developing from the mesenchyme is vascular tissue that will soon connect the primitive pulmonary artery to the pulmonary veins. Noncellular tissue will provide the elastic and collagen fibers that support the lung structures.[7] Vascular development is congruent with bronchial buds and airway branching.[8]

The lung buds continue to grow and subdivide into smaller airways during the 5th to 16th week of gestation, termed the *pseudoglandular period* because the lung tissue looks similar to glandular cells. During this period, many of the early cells differentiate into specific types of airway cells. Tall bronchial epithelium lines the primitive airways, and there is a burst of growth between the 10th and 14th weeks. Mucous-secreting glands and supportive cartilage appear late in the pseudoglandular period and continue their

growth through the canalicular period. Branching and subdivision produces 8 to 32 bronchial generations, with the greatest number of divisions occurring in those lung areas that are most distant from the hilum, or the root of the lungs. The bronchial tree is complete from the glottis to the terminal bronchioles by the end of the pseudoglandular period, and the diaphragm is beginning to form. Similar development of the pulmonary vascular system occurs concurrently.[8]

The major events that mark the 16th to 26th week, the canalicular period, are thinning and flattening of the epithelium that will become the type I pneumocytes or alveolar cells. Type II cells also begin to appear at this time and are the lamellar cells that ultimately produce surfactant. In addition, a critical occurrence is the appearance of pulmonary capillaries. The capillaries, which protrude into the epithelium, provide close proximity of the blood supply to the airways. Thinning of the epithelium and capillary development provide the apparatus—the air–blood interface—for respiration. Gas exchange can take place by the end of the canalicular period.[8]

At approximately 26 weeks, the energy of the developing lung begins to form outpouchings of the terminal bronchioles called saccules. This "terminal sac" or "saccular" period continues until about birth when the alveolar period begins, at which time the saccules have begun to branch into many alveolar pockets or ducts. These ducts are in continued proximity to the tiny capillaries formed during the canalicular period. Once sufficient numbers of alveolar/capillary units are present, life may be sustained, provided that the biochemical substance surfactant is present within the alveoli.

Surfactant, as noted, is a phospholipid material secreted by type II cells that line the pulmonary alveoli. Surfactant reduces surface tension within the alveolus, thus allowing inflation of the alveolus with smaller pressures and less work by the infant than would be needed to inflate a surfactant-deficient alveolus. Surfactant appears at its mature chemical level at approximately 34 weeks of gestation and indicates maturity of the lung by allowing the maintenance of continuous respiration.[9]

The postnatal period is characterized initially by an 18- to 24-month period of rapid growth of both surface area and volume of lung tissue for gas exchange through continued subdivision of the alveolar ducts to form alveolar sacs (i.e., the true alveoli). The current consensus is that alveolar number is largely completed by 6 months of age, although some development may continue through 24 months.[8] Of note is that the vasculature grows to an even greater degree than do the air spaces in this earlier of the postnatal phases. In the second of the postnatal phases, there is more parallel growth in the alveoli and capillaries. From the 25 million alveoli present at birth, there is a 12-fold increase by 8 to 10 years, at which time the adult number of approximately 300 million is achieved. Destructive processes within the period of alveolar multiplication may limit the potential for achieving the adult number of pulmonary alveoli.[10]

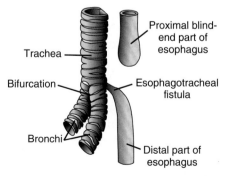

FIGURE 19.1. Tracheoesophageal fistula. (From Sadler TW. *Langman's Medical Embryology*. 9th ed. Lippincott Williams & Wilkins; 2002.)

» Predisposition to respiratory failure

The following information is presented to describe more fully several mechanisms of acute respiratory failure and its rapid development in children and infants. Although acute respiratory failure is not a disease, it is often the final common pathway for many diseases that affect the developing respiratory system.

Several structural and metabolic factors in the pediatric population, although entirely normal, predispose them to acute respiratory failure. Respiratory failure can be defined as a condition in which impairment of gas exchange within the lungs poses an immediate threat to life. Downes and associates were among the first to state that clinical signs and arterial blood gas determinations should be used to monitor infants and children for the development of acute respiratory failure.[11] The arterial blood gas levels compatible with respiratory failure are 75 mm Hg of carbon dioxide and 100 mm Hg of oxygen when the child is receiving an inspired oxygen concentration of 100%. Respiratory failure exists when either of these arterial levels is reached in the presence of any of the following clinical signs—decreased or absent inspiratory breaths sounds, severe inspiratory retractions with accessory muscle use, cyanosis with inspiration of 40% oxygen, depressed consciousness and response to pain, and poor skeletal muscle tone.

The most important general factor predisposing infants and children to acute respiratory failure is their high incidence of respiratory tract infections. During the first several years of life, when immunologic defenses are developing, the child is at risk for infections. This risk increases as the environment of the toddler expands, particularly with early enrollment in day care, preschool, and other similar exposures to various infectious agents transmitted by classmates, teachers, and other personnel. As the number of children in day care programs has increased in recent decades, the concurrent increase in the incidence of respiratory infections has been predictable. Indeed, recent research has focused on the economic impact of these infectious episodes and the economic benefits to developing and instituting infection control programs.[12]

Two major structural factors—airway size and poor mechanical advantage for the respiratory muscles—contribute to respiratory failure in a young child. According to calculations applied to the work of Effmann, the diameter of the tracheal lumen in children younger than 1 year of age is smaller than is the diameter of a lead pencil.[13] A large percentage of the young child's peripheral bronchioles are smaller than 1 mm in diameter. A small amount of mucus, bronchospasm, or edema can effectively not only occlude the peripheral airways but may also obstruct the larger, more proximal bronchi. With sufficient airway blockage, respiratory failure may quickly ensue.

Additional major structural issues that predispose infants and children to respiratory failure involve several items that cumulatively cause poor mechanical advantage to the respiratory bellows of the child's thorax:

1. Type I fatigue-resistant muscle fibers are not present in adult proportions in the diaphragm or other ventilatory muscles of the infant until 8 months of age.[14] This lack of fatigue-resistant fibers allows the infant's respiratory muscles to tire quickly, causing alveolar hypoventilation that may lead to respiratory failure.
2. There is a greater work of breathing cost that may reach 10% of basal metabolic rate when the preterm infant must use the diaphragm to distort its ribcage in times of stressful breathing. Should the infant have lung disease as well, the increased metabolic demands of the diaphragm may predispose preterm infants to fatigue and may contribute to respiratory failure.[15]
3. Poor development of the ability to cough either spontaneously or with direct laryngeal stimulation renders the infant's airways susceptible to obstruction by mucus.[16]
4. Horizontal alignment of the infant's rib cage and the round (rather than oval) configuration of the chest provide poor mechanical advantage to the intercostal and accessory muscles of respiration. These muscles lift the ribs and sternum to increase thoracic diameter and lung volume.
5. Increased chest wall compliance during infancy can result in sternal retractions associated with increased inspiratory effort during times of illness. The relative lack of stiffness in the infant thorax can simulate a flail chest. Intense inspiratory efforts may paradoxically decrease thoracic volume at a time when just the opposite response is necessary, and ventilation is further compromised with the potential for hypoventilation. Developmental changes in the chest wall during the second year of life result in chest wall compliance similar to that of adults.[17]
6. The baby's position may affect diaphragmatic excursion. The infant who is in a supine position works harder to ventilate because the abdominal viscera may impede the full descent of the diaphragm.

A third important issue for the physical therapist is respiratory metabolism. The high metabolic rate of the child causes increased consumption of oxygen, increased heat loss, and increased water loss secondary to a faster respiratory rate. The range of normal respiratory rates for children is shown in Figure 19.2.

In addition to having muscle fibers that are susceptible to early fatigue, as noted earlier, the young child or infant has a relatively poor muscle fuel supply. Glycogen supply in the muscle tissue is small in the infant, and is depleted quickly when muscular activity is increased, which occurs during respiratory distress.[18]

The factors described—general, structural, and metabolic factors—although developmentally and chronologically normal and appropriate, may combine to render the young respiratory tract fragile and prone to failure during periods of stress, which are commonly seen in respiratory diseases.

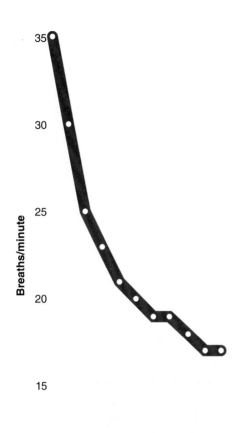

FIGURE 19.2. Respiratory Rates in Children.
This graph shows normal respiratory rates in children, which are higher than the normal rates in adults. Accordingly, bradypnea and tachypnea in a child are defined by the child's age.

» Physical therapy examination of children with respiratory disorders

Careful examination of the infant or child with respiratory distress can offer useful information. The younger the child, the more the therapist may need to rely on careful observation, because the infant or young child cannot participate actively in a chest examination. An age-appropriate description of the activities that the therapist will be performing should precede the actual physical examination. The following organization of the examination is based on the Guide to Physical Therapist Practice.[19]

History

A complete medical chart review should be the first aspect of the physical therapy examination of a child. The review should provide information regarding the child's medical history—the clinical course of the child's current illness, including signs and symptoms and their precipitating factors;

any previous treatment for the illness; and reasons for the referral to physical therapy. In addition to the information in the chart, members of the child's health care team can provide invaluable and immediate information regarding the child's current state. Chest radiographs and other forms of imaging are useful in identifying specific areas of the lung or thorax that may be affected by the illness. A complete radiographic interpretation is beyond the scope of physical therapy practice.

Given here are specific questions the physical therapist should ask the child and family while completing their history.

Living Environment

Does the home or other discharge destination provide the space and resources needed for respiratory items such as oxygen, ventilator, and suction device?

General Health Status

Has the infant or child displayed a normal developmental history? Have motor milestones been reached at appropriate times? Is there a history of ongoing or recurrent medical problems?

Medical/Surgical History

Have there been recent hospitalizations, illnesses, or surgical interventions of note? Does the child or parent report comorbidities or past illnesses that may affect the current condition? Is there knowledge of genetic diseases within the family?

Current Condition/Chief Complaint

What is the recent concern leading to the request for physical therapy? Is this a recurrence of a previous problem? Is the child receiving physical therapy, including airway clearance (AC), at home? What are the child/family expectations for this episode of care?

Functional Status/Activity Level

Has the child been functioning at an age-appropriate level?

Medications

What medications is the child taking, and is there any potential impact on the physical therapy regimen? (Aerosol medications such as bronchodilators, mucolytics, and hypertonic saline often precede AC.)

Other Clinical Tests

Review all laboratory values, including pulmonary function tests, arterial blood gas values, and pulse oximetry, all imaging information, exercise tests, and any other potentially informative studies.

Review of Systems

The systems review is a brief and gross examination, a "quick check," used to gather additional information and to detect other health problems that should be considered in the diagnosis, prognosis, and plan of care.

Cardiovascular/Pulmonary Systems

This brief review of the child should include blood pressure determination, measurement of pulse and respiratory rate, and documentation of any gross indications of edema.

Integument

Are the color and integrity of the skin normal? Are any old or new scars apparent? Are current wounds healing properly?

Musculoskeletal System

Measure and record the child's height and weight. Identify any obvious physical asymmetries. Examine gross muscle strength and range of motion (ROM) to the degree possible, depending on the age of the child and the ability to cooperate.

Neuromuscular System

Determine whether grossly coordinated and age-appropriate movement or movement patterns are seen.

Tests and Measures

Ventilation and Respiration/Gas Exchange

Of all the tests and measures administered to the child with pulmonary disease, none is more important than those assessing ventilation and respiration. Many signs and symptoms associated with ventilation and gas exchange have a direct bearing on the interventions that the therapist will choose. A traditional chest examination includes the four classic approaches of inspection, auscultation, palpation, and mediate percussion.

The physical therapist has several objectives related to the chest examination:

Identify the pulmonary problems and symptoms noted.
Examine coexisting signs of pulmonary disease.
Determine the need for additional tests and measures such as
    exercise testing when appropriate.
Formulate a prognosis and a plan of care.
Identify treatment goals.

Inspection

The inspection phase of the chest examination documents clinical characteristics of the presenting symptoms, which may indicate what other components of the examination are necessary.

Inspection includes the following:

Examining the child's general appearance
Inspecting the head and neck
Observing the chest
Considering the child's breath, speech, cough, and sputum

GENERAL APPEARANCE First, the therapist should note the state of consciousness of the child and the level to which the child can cooperate with simple commands. Is the child's body habitus normal, obese, or cachectic? Are there obvious postural issues such as kyphosis, scoliosis, or unusual postures? Children who are dyspneic often assume a forward bent position.

During the extremity examination, the therapist notes digital clubbing, painful swollen joints, tremor, and edema. Clubbing of the fingers or toes is associated with CF, as shown in Figure 19.3A and B.[20] Painful swollen joints may indicate pseudohypertrophic pulmonary osteoarthropathy[21] rather than the osteoarthritis or rheumatoid arthritis more familiar to physical therapists. Bilateral pedal edema may indicate cor pulmonale or right heart failure in those with long-standing CF and chronic lung disease with hypoxemia.[22]

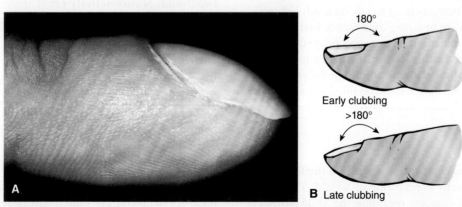

FIGURE 19.3. A: Clubbing of the fingers is seen in patients with cystic fibrosis and other respiratory and cardiovascular disease. **B:** In clubbing, the angle between the nail plate and the proximal nail fold increases to 180 degrees or more.

The therapist also notes all equipment and monitoring devices used in managing the child and the impact of those devices on planned interventions (e.g., mechanical ventilator, oxygen hood or mask, and intravenous or arterial lines).

INSPECTION OF THE HEAD AND NECK The child's face often shows signs of respiratory distress and oxygen deficit. Of these signs, *flaring of the alae nasi* and *cyanosis* of the mucous membranes are commonly seen in those with acute respiratory distress. *Head bobbing* that coincides with the respiratory cycle may be the result of attempts to use the accessory muscles of inspiration by an infant who has inadequate strength to stabilize the head and neck. *Audible expiratory grunting* is thought to be an effort by the infant and young child to maintain airway patency and prevent airway collapse during expiration. Grunting is most commonly heard during lower respiratory tract disorders.

EXAMINATION OF THE STRUCTURES OF THE THORACIC CAGE In this portion of the physical examination, the shape and symmetry of the thorax are noted, as are any unusual characteristics of the skin, including rashes, scars, and incisions. The thorax of the infant is more rounded in configuration than is the adult thorax, and the ribs attach to the vertebrae almost at 90 degrees, which makes further elevation almost impossible.[23] The anteroposterior diameter of the thorax in the infant is likely to be equal to its transverse diameter, whereas in the adult's thorax, there is usually a much greater transverse diameter. As infants develop, from the third to the sixth month, they begin to reach out to their environment, developing the agonistic and antagonistic upper extremity muscle relationships. The shape of the thoracic cage becomes more rectangular in the anterior plane, although the ribs are still horizontal. From the sixth month and up to a year, children assume upright postures against gravity, and ventilation is no longer inhibited by contact with a support surface. The child's movement into and out of gravity's resistance develops a balance of trunk flexion and extension. For children meeting developmental milestones, head control is well developed, and the head is able to move independent of the trunk. Among the more common abnormalities of the thorax are congenital defects, including pectus excavatum (or funnel chest) and pectus carinatum (or pigeon breast); barrel chest, usually associated with hyperinflation of the lungs, in which the anterior-to-posterior measurement of the thorax is greater than is the lateral measurement; and the several thoracic deformities associated with scoliosis. Muscle development of the thorax should also be examined for symmetry and for the presence of hypertrophy of the accessory muscles of inspiration, which suggests chronic dyspnea.

EXAMINATION OF MOVEMENT OF THE THORACIC CAGE Respiratory rate is the first item measured when examining the moving chest. Counting respirations should be done inconspicuously and is often done when counting the pulse rate.

For children and infants on cardiorespiratory monitoring, noting values before engaging with the individual may be helpful. As previously noted, in Figure 19.2, the younger the child, the greater the normal resting respiratory rate. Tachypnea refers to an abnormally high respiratory rate and bradypnea refers to a low respiratory rate, while keeping in mind the normal variation in infant and childhood respiratory rates.

The pattern and regularity of breathing should also be evaluated, particularly in neonates and in children with neuromuscular disorders. Short periods of apnea are not particularly unusual and may be referred to as *periodic breathing* in neonates. True apnea exists when apneic periods exceed 20 seconds. Apnea can be associated with respiratory distress, sepsis, and central nervous system (CNS) hemorrhage. In addition to the rate and regularity, the ratio of inspiration to expiration (I:E) should be determined. This I:E ratio is usually approximately 1:2. Infants and children with obstructive airway disease, such as asthma and bronchiolitis, may have a marked increase in expiratory time; as a result, their I:E ratio may become 1:4 or 1:5. Synchronous motion of the abdomen and thorax should be observed. On inspiration, both thoracic expansion and abdominal bulging should be noted. When this synchrony is lost, a "seesaw" motion of thoracic expansion with abdominal indrawing occurs on inspiration, with the opposite movements being noted on expiration. The presence of chest wall retractions should be noted. Retractions, or indrawing, may occur in suprasternal, substernal, subcostal, or intercostal areas. Retractions, seen more frequently in pediatrics, occur as a result of the compliant thorax of the infant and young child and an increased respiratory effort. During respiratory distress, the muscles of either inspiration or expiration, or both, place sufficient pull on the as yet largely cartilaginous thorax to cause indrawing in several areas. When retractions are severe, they may reduce effective inspiration.

Audible sounds during breathing can be heard and may be notable. *Stridor,* a crowing sound during inspiration, suggests upper airway obstruction or possible laryngospasm. During expiration, one may also hear grunting sounds, particularly in infants with respiratory distress. Expiratory *grunting* may represent a physiologic attempt to prevent premature airway collapse. *Gurgling* sounds heard during both ventilatory phases commonly indicate copious secretions in the larger airways.

EVALUATION OF COUGHING AND SNEEZING Infants probably use sneezing more than coughing as both a protective and a clearance mechanism for the airway. Older infants and children must be able to cough effectively to clear secretions or other debris from their airway. It is important to determine the ability to cough in a child with neuromuscular disease. With neuromuscular disease and associated abdominal muscle weakness, the child may be at risk for secretion retention and aspiration of feedings, which may require some mechanical assistance for secretion removal.

Auscultation

Auscultation—listening to the lungs with a stethoscope—is a useful method of examination. The stethoscope used for auscultation of the infant and young child is a smaller version of that used for adults. The therapist should warm the stethoscope before using it, and, depending on the age of the child, the therapist may show how it is used by demonstrating on a child's doll or on a puppet. Because of the proximity to the thoracic surface of the child's airways, and to the thin chest wall in the young child and infant, sounds are easily transmitted, and anatomic specificity may be reduced. A particular sound, therefore, although heard in one area of the thorax, may not correspond to the lung segment directly below the area in which the sound is heard. As a result, auscultation, particularly in the neonate or premature neonate, may not be as precise as in the older child or adult. Nonetheless, the therapist should attempt to ascertain the presence of normal and abnormal breath sounds throughout the lung fields. The therapist should also try to identify adventitious sounds, such as wheezes, crackles, rubs, and crunches.

Wheezes are musical sounds thought to be produced by airflow through narrowed airways. They may be inspiratory or expiratory and may be monophonic or polyphonic. Expiratory wheezes are probably more common and represent airway obstruction from bronchospasm or secretions.

Crackles (sometimes called *rales*) are nonmusical sounds that may be heard during inspiration or expiration. They may represent previously deflated airways opening suddenly. Expiratory crackles often denote fluid in the larger airways.

Rubs are coarse, grating leathery sounds that often indicate inflammatory tissues rubbing against one another.

Crunches are crackling sounds often heard over the mediastinum when air has leaked into that area.

The audible sounds of stridor and expiratory grunting were mentioned earlier. Because of the ease of transmission of sound through the infant's thorax, the therapist should attempt to correlate auscultatory findings with roentgenographic changes and other physical findings during the examination and treatment planning portion of the encounter.

Palpation

Palpation of the thoracic cage in the infant or child can help identify the following circumstances:

Position of the mediastinum via palpation of the trachea
Palpation for rhonchal fremitus (the feeling of turbulent airflow around secretions) is also a useful means to localize secretion in the larger airways.

Palpation for local areas of rib cage motion and the symmetry of that motion as the chest expands is also useful in older children.[24] Thoracic cage movement can be measured, but has not been highly researched as of this writing, and no normative values have been published. Ventilation may be highly individual, and changes within a person may be

meaningful. "Best Practice" numbers from courses of experts in the field of pediatric chest wall excursion[24] recommend using for children older than a year.

Measurement Location	Children Older Than a Year	Children Older Than Age 3
Third rib	One-eighth of an inch	Two-eighth of an inch
Xiphoid	Two-eighth of an inch	Three-eighth of an inch
Halfway between xiphoid and umbilicus	Three-eighth of an inch	Four-eighth of an inch

The recruitment pattern should be larger as you move superior to inferior. In the teenage years, children obtain the adult shape, with the ribcage occupying greater than half of the trunk cavity with a rectangular frontal plane and elliptical anterior posterior plane shape. The apex of the upper chest is wide and convex, and the lower chest is fully integrated with the abdominals. The intercostal spaces should be wide, allowing for the ribs to move individually. Side bending examination should reveal separation between each rib, and between the rib and pelvis. The ribs should have no flat lines, with nice curved lines through the entire rib cage. The activity of the muscles of inspiration can also be determined via their direct palpation. Palpation can also be employed to help identify and localize areas of chest pain in the child.

Mediate Percussion

This last of the four skills in a traditional respiratory examination enables the therapist to identify areas of abnormal lung density, and evaluate the extent of diaphragmatic motion. The technique requires tapping the finger of one hand against the nail of a finger placed firmly in a rib interspace. The actual sound or percussion note can denote air-filled versus non–air-filled lung tissue. The more hollow/resonant the sound, the greater is the likelihood of an air-filled lung. The more dull or flat the sound, the more likely the lung is poorly aerated in that specific area.

In addition, percussion can also identify diaphragmatic motion. The percussion note changes from resonant (air-filled) to dull (airless) at the base of the lungs, where the diaphragm is located. The therapist percusses the rib interspaces from lung apex to base. When dullness is encountered, the therapist has the child exhale fully, causing the diaphragm to ascend. The therapist percusses to mark the highest level of ascent. Next, the child inspires completely, and percussion tracks the descending diaphragm until the limit of descent is identified. Diaphragmatic excursion is the distance traveled between maximum ascent and maximum descent.

Aerobic Capacity and Endurance

Aerobic capacity and endurance are commonly defined by the term *maximal oxygen uptake*. This measurement is an indication of (1) the ability of the cardiovascular system to provide oxygen to working muscles and (2) the ability of those muscles to extract oxygen for energy generation. Such testing can provide much useful information about the patient such as the following:

Identify the baseline ability.
Determine aerobic capacity during functional activities.
Predict the response to physiologic demands during periods of increased or stressful activity.

Recognize limitations in the face of an increased workload.

Many modes of testing that range from observation of symptomatic responses during a standard exercise challenge to instrumented, technically sophisticated invasive aerobic testing in an exercise laboratory are used. Exercise testing in a laboratory typically involves progressive and incremental increases in exercise intensity while the child is walking on a treadmill or riding a bicycle ergometer. Exercise testing sites should have the capacity for continuous electrocardiographic monitoring, periodic heart rate and blood pressure measurement, cutaneous oximetry and arterial blood gas determination, and expired gas analysis; they should also have an oxygen source. In addition, a cardiac defibrillator, other emergency equipment and supplies, and proper personnel for their use must be immediately available in case of cardiopulmonary emergency. Maximal and submaximal testing may be performed.

When a formal laboratory is not available or not practical, a 6- or 12-minute timed walking test,[25,26] a shuttle walking test,[27] or a step test[28] are simple and well-studied alternatives, and these are discussed later in the chapter.

Anthropometric Characteristics

Measurement of height and weight percentiles, body mass index, and peripheral edema are all important measures of anthropometric characteristics for children with pulmonary disorders. Height and weight along with body mass index values are important in determining physical growth, stature, and nutrition in the child. Nutritional status has a significant impact on lung function and, hence, on exercise capacity in children.[29] Monitoring of cor pulmonale—congestive right heart failure—is an important reason for measuring edema in the child with chronic lung disease, particularly those with CF and severe asthma. Cor pulmonale often results from long-standing arterial hypoxemia, hypercapnia, and respiratory acidosis, all of which add to right ventricle afterload, leading to right ventricular hypertrophy.[30] Right ventricular failure is associated peripheral edema, likely manifested as pedal and ankle edema. The physical therapist may use simple girth measurements, volumetric displacement, and figure-of-eight girth measurements to monitor the early development of peripheral edema and its progression.[31] In addition, sudden gross weight gain may indicate a rapid onset of cor pulmonale; therefore, periodic weight measurement is useful.

Arousal and Cognition

The child should be oriented to time and space and should be able to respond both to questions of a cognitive nature and to varied environmental stimuli given the limitations of developmental age. The therapist should determine the general state of consciousness and ability to respond to questions and requests.

Assistive and Adaptive Devices

Assistive and adaptive devices such as crutches, walkers, wheelchairs, splints, raised toilet seats, and environmental control systems are not inherent needs for most children who have acute or chronic pulmonary problems. Some pulmonary-related devices that children might use include nebulizers, supplemental oxygen by nasal cannula or mask, mechanical ventilator, tracheotomy tube, and, in some cases, a port for provision of supplemental nutrition. A major exception to this pattern concerns children whose respiratory impairment is secondary to a musculoskeletal or neuromuscular disease for which such devices as walkers, wheelchairs, and others would be appropriate.

Environmental, Home, and Work (Job/School/Play) Barriers

Major environmental barriers of importance for the child with pulmonary disease involve the physical demands of attending school and playing in various environments. In addition, the therapist should enquire about the presence or absence within the home or school environment of dust, vapors, and known or possible allergens or other inhalation hazards. These can be evaluated through interviews of the child and parent or caretaker regarding the home, school, and play environments.

Integumentary Integrity

The review of systems mentioned will have been useful to the clinician in identifying any existing or potential skin impairments. Major findings are likely to involve pallor or cyanosis in individuals who are hypoxemic. Children with CF are also likely to exhibit digital clubbing.[20]

Muscle Performance

Gross muscle performance should be documented in the review of systems. However, because increasing evidence indicates that peripheral muscle dysfunction exists independent of ventilation limitations in persons with CF, the physical therapist must be particularly careful to document and follow up on strength measures. Studies indicate that chronic lung disease results in muscle weakness, placing voluntary maximal strength measures at about 80% of that of similar persons without chronic lung disease. Mechanisms leading to this strength deficit have been identified as inactivity that leads to muscle deconditioning, malnutrition, and a myopathic process. Regardless of their cause, it is clear that peripheral muscle strength deficits lead to exercise limitation and intolerance.[32,33] More recently, a great deal of attention has focused on physical rehabilitation of children in intensive care and the development of intensive care unit–acquired weakness.[34,35] Although this recent work refers to adult care, it is likely that children suffer from similar deficits following long periods of intensive care.

Muscle performance can be measured in many different ways, including manual muscle testing, dynamometry using handheld devices or more sophisticated technology-assisted systems, and functional muscle testing. Functional muscle testing often employs timed walking tests, a shuttle walking test, or a step test.[25-28] Although these several approaches examine more than discrete muscle function, they offer a more practical examination of muscle performance because it occurs during a child's daily activities.

Other Important Tests and Measures

Although this chapter deals with disorders of the pulmonary system, the therapist must consider all systems when examining a child. A functional combination of several systems can be examined by considering exertion and dyspnea.

EXERTION AND DYSPNEA Perceived exertion, commonly quantified with the revised 10-point Borg scale, and quantification of dyspnea are two important indicators of potential problems with cardiopulmonary function not previously noted in this chapter. The Borg scale of perceived exertion was originally designed as a scale with a range of scores from 6 to 20. The scale was later revised to a 10-point scale ranging from 0 to 10, with 0 equating to no exertion at all and 10 identifying very strong exertion. The Borg scale correlates well with physiologic measures of maximal oxygen uptake and heart rate in adults. However, recent work has demonstrated that the Borg scale is best understood by children older than 7 years of age, because younger children do not yet have the capacity to understand exercise intensity descriptors typically associated with adult-perceived exertion scales.[36] Pictorial scales have therefore been developed specifically for children, but research on their use has largely been for typical children. The Dalhousie Dyspnea and Perceived Exertion Scales,[37] the Pictorial Children's Effort Rating Table (P-Cert), and OMNI walking scales are pictorial perceived exertion scales that have been developed specifically for children.[38,39] Another test of dyspnea is the 15-count dyspnea test in which the child simply inhales deeply and counts aloud to 15 during the exhale. It is easy to explain and perform, and can be used by any child capable of counting fluently to 15 in any language. It is best used in conjunction with a subjective score, and either the Borg scale or a visual analog score is appropriate.[40-42]

A group of visual dyspnea scales for children was published by McGrath et al. in 2005. The descriptive drawings demonstrated and measured throat closing, chest tightness,

and effort in a group of 79 children, including those with asthma, CF, and no lung disease. The authors stated that the measures appeared to measure the three constructs built into the visual aids.[43]

Neuromotor development and sensory integration testing is often necessary for a child who has experienced periodic or chronic episodes of hypoxemia that often occur with pulmonary disorders. Inadequate oxygenation for a period of time may cause minor or major CNS deficit, resulting in a developmental delay.

Examination of pain—both its source and perceived level—is an important part of the examination. Identification of painful areas of the thorax is often accomplished via palpation and questioning the child or parent. If a painful site is identified, it is appropriate for the clinician to use some pain scale or pain diary to determine the child's level of pain, its attributes, and its effect on daily activity, as well as methods of reducing or modifying the painful stimulus. This issue of an age and developmentally appropriate rating scale for pain in children has been addressed in the past two decades. The Faces Pain Scale, developed by Bieri, was an early and significant attempt to use a scale that was suitable for children, but suffered from having seven faces on the scale and was difficult to correlate with the more commonly employed 5- or 10-point analog pain scales.[44] More recently, Hicks and colleagues revised the scale by Bieri in a manner that made it more easily comparable with either a 5- or 10-point analog pain scale. The revised Face Pain Scale was not significantly different from either of the analog scales previously noted.[45] Figure 19.4 shows the Faces Pain Scale.

Postural abnormalities can result from *or* can cause respiratory disorders. Scoliosis with a primary curvature of greater than 60 degrees often results in thoracic restriction and a decrease in lung volumes, as will severe pectus excavatum.[46] Some chronic lung diseases, such as severe recurring asthma and CF, lead to a hyperinflated, barreled chest with abducted and protracted scapulae. These possibilities must be considered in the examination of the child with pulmonary disorders.

Finally, an evaluation of the family's knowledge and ability to participate in the child's care is important when planning discharge from the hospital. Many pediatric pulmonary disorders are chronic, and will require continuing and

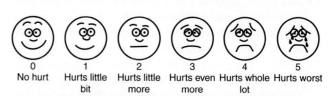

FIGURE 19.4. The Wong-Baker FACES Pain Rating Scale. (Reprinted with permission from Wong-Baker FACES Foundation. Wong-Baker FACES® Pain Rating Scale. 2020. Retrieved March 15, 2021, with permission from http://www.WongBakerFACES.org)

effective care at home. The physical therapist is an important family educator and troubleshooter and must participate in formal and informal teaching.

» Physical therapy for children with pulmonary disease and respiratory disorders

Physical therapy for the infant or child with pulmonary disease or respiratory disorder can be categorized into three general areas that often overlap:

1. AC for removal of secretions, either by traditional postural drainage with percussion and vibration (PDPV) or with more contemporary techniques that are discussed at some length
2. Breathing exercises and retraining
3. Physical reconditioning including aerobic exercise, strength training, and other types of exercise for the thorax

Of course, the degree to which these three areas are used and the specific interventions employed will depend not only on the disease process but also on the age and level of ability and cooperation of the child. Neonates and infants will be treated almost exclusively with traditional AC procedures, including positioning to alter ventilation and perfusion. Simple breathing games and activities can be incorporated into the regimen as needed when the child becomes a toddler. As the child grows older, exercises for breathing retraining, physical reconditioning, and postural exercises become possible. Also, measures for AC that depend on breathing control, such as autogenic drainage (AD), active cycle of breathing, and positive expiratory pressure (PEP) devices become more applicable as the older child can coordinate the necessary breathing maneuvers. The next section of the chapter presents the more classic studies that helped establish the efficacy of the numerous types of intervention.

Airway Clearance

Removal of secretions from the child's airway is the main goal of AC. Of all types of physical therapy treatment for children with respiratory problems, AC in its many formats and approaches has been the most extensively studied. Despite limited compelling evidence based on controlled studies, AC is widely accepted and used universally. Perhaps the universal use of AC suggests that "lack of evidence does not mean lack of effectiveness." AC includes both traditional methods—positioning for gravity-assisted drainage of the airways, manual techniques for loosening secretions, and removal of secretions by coughing and suctioning of the airway. AC has also come to include active cycle of breathing techniques (ACBT), PEP devices, oscillating PEP (Flutter® and Acapella®), high-frequency

chest wall oscillation (HFWCO), and intrapulmonary percussive ventilation (IPV). Each of these techniques is described here.

Postural Drainage with Percussion and Vibration

POSITIONING FOR GRAVITY-ASSISTED DRAINAGE Using a working knowledge of bronchopulmonary segment anatomy, the therapist can position the infant or child to drain areas of the lung in which secretions are found during the chest examination. The positions place the segment or lobe of lung to be drained uppermost, with the bronchus supplying that lung area in as close to an inverted position as possible. In adults and older children, specific positioning for segmental drainage often involves the use of treatment tables or tilting beds. In infants and young children, the therapist's lap and shoulder serve as the "treatment table." The infant or toddler can be held and comforted while in each of the drainage positions (Fig. 19.5A and B). When the child reaches 3 or 4 years of age, the transition may be made from lap to treatment table, but many therapists and parents will continue to use the lap for children up to 4 or 5 years of age. The older child or teen can use an exercise table or pillows for proper positioning.

One point of caution must be raised regarding tipping infants into traditional head-down positions. In a series of well-designed studies over a period of 8 years, Button et al. clearly demonstrated that infants with CF had significant gastroesophageal reflux and resulting decreased long-term lung function associated with head-down positioning during PDPV.[47,48] With this clear evidence, the use of head-down positions for PDPV has become contraindicated in CF centers around the world.

MANUAL TECHNIQUES OF PERCUSSION AND VIBRATIONS The manual techniques of percussion and vibration are used to loosen or dislodge secretions from the bronchial wall, thus allowing easier removal when the child coughs, sneezes, or undergoes airway aspiration with a suction catheter. Although some obvious differences exist, the techniques used are quite similar to those performed on adults. One of the major differences is the amount of force used for either percussion or vibration. Common sense should dictate that minimal amounts of force should be used on the thorax of a premature infant who weighs 1 to 2 kg or less. Increased amounts of percussion and vibration force can be safely applied as the infant grows and as the bones and muscles of the thorax become stronger.

As with adults, the percussion and vibration should be applied to the area of the thorax that corresponds to the lung and airways in which secretions are present. Another difference in the pediatric group is that a therapist's percussing or vibrating hand often covers the entire thorax of an infant or a toddler. As a result, other implements have been suggested for percussion and vibration in the infant. Several items

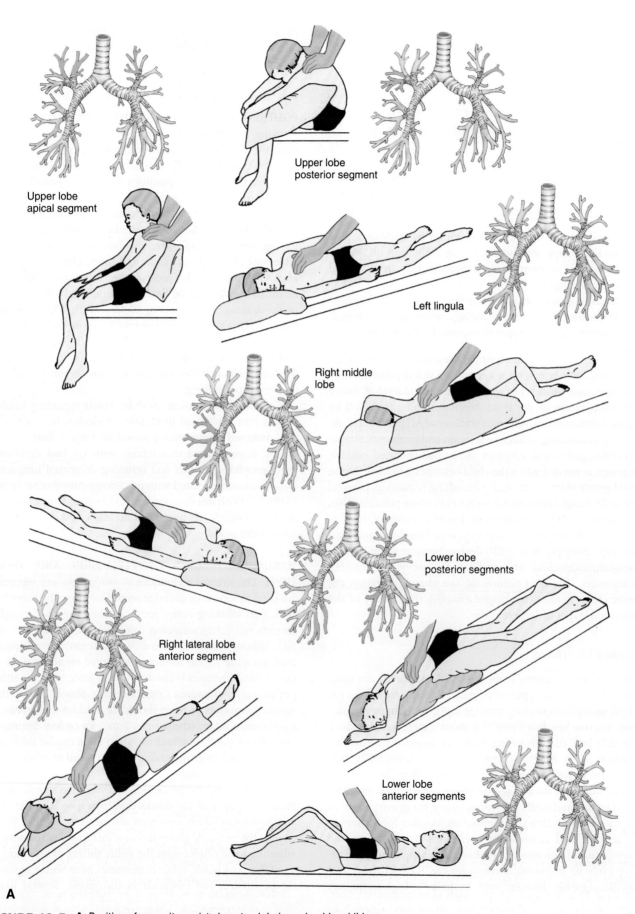

Upper lobe
apical segment

Upper lobe
posterior segment

Left lingula

Right middle
lobe

Right lateral lobe
anterior segment

Lower lobe
posterior segments

Lower lobe
anterior segments

A

FIGURE 19.5. A: Positions for gravity-assisted postural drainage in older children.

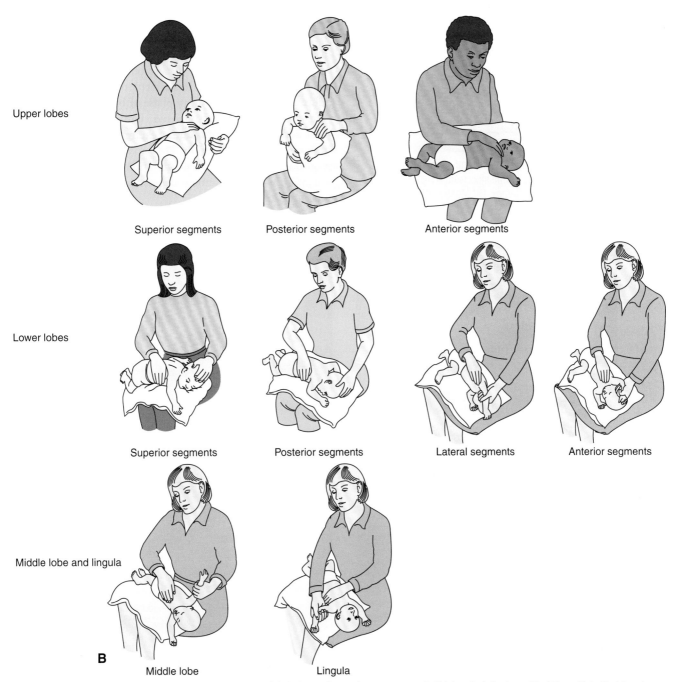

Upper lobes

Superior segments   Posterior segments   Anterior segments

Lower lobes

Superior segments   Posterior segments   Lateral segments   Anterior segments

Middle lobe and lingula

B

Middle lobe   Lingula

FIGURE 19.5. (*Continued*) **B:** Positions for bronchial drainage for major segments of all lobes in infants and toddlers. Note that head-down positions may be contraindicated in children with gastroesophageal reflux. This procedure is most readily performed with the infant on your lap, with your hand on the chest over the area to be cupped or vibrated. (From Pillitteri A. *Maternal and Child Nursing.* 4th ed. Lippincott, Williams & Wilkins; 2003.)

used for percussion are shown in Figure 19.6, and different hand configurations for percussion of the infant are shown in Figure 19.7A–E. Contraindications for chest percussion in the neonate commonly include a significant drop in transcutaneous (or arterial) oxygen level during percussion; rib fracture or other thoracic trauma; and hemoptysis.[49] There are also various conditions under which percussion for a

child should be used carefully: poor condition of the infant's skin; coagulopathy; osteoporosis or rickets; cardiac arrhythmias; apnea and bradycardia; increased irritability during treatment; subcutaneous emphysema; and subependymal or intraventricular hemorrhage.[50] Vibration, which may be used in addition to or in place of percussion, is less vigorous than is percussion. There are few true contraindications

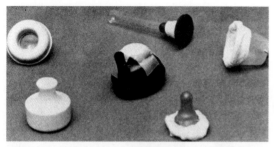

FIGURE 19.6. Commercially available and adaptable devices for percussion. (Reproduced by permission from Irwin S, Tecklin JS. *Cardiopulmonary Physical Therapy.* CV Mosby; 1985.)

to vibration, with the exception of hemoptysis and reduced oxygenation during treatment. Because vibration is usually done during the expiratory phase of breathing, and because the infant with respiratory disease often has a rate of 40 or more breaths per minute, it is difficult to coordinate manual vibration with the expiratory phase of breathing. Some persons use various battery-powered vibrators that can be held against the infant's thorax during expiration and then quickly removed during inspiration. The modifications and precautions for both percussion and vibration become fewer as the infant grows, and treatment begins to parallel more closely that used for an adult.

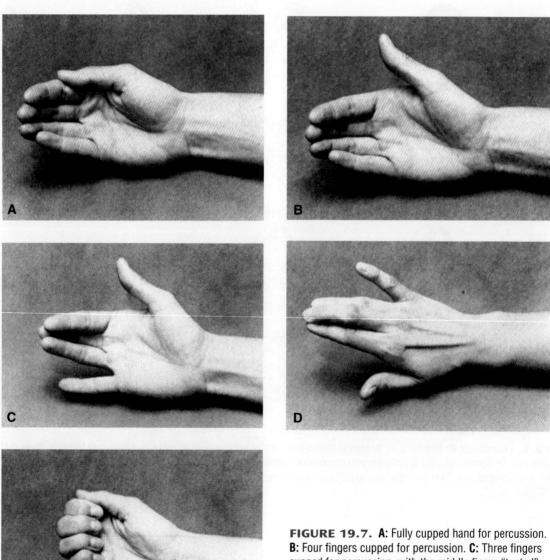

FIGURE 19.7. **A:** Fully cupped hand for percussion. **B:** Four fingers cupped for percussion. **C:** Three fingers cupped for percussion, with the middle finger "tented" (anterior view). **D:** Three fingers cupped for percussion, with the middle finger "tented" (posterior view). **E:** Thenar and hypothenar surfaces for percussion. (Reproduced by permission from Irwin S, Tecklin JS. *Cardiopulmonary Physical Therapy.* CV Mosby; 1985.)

COUGHING AND SUCTIONING Infants and young children will seldom cough on request. Toddlers and school-aged children have the language skills to understand the request for coughing, but will often choose not to cough. Imaginative means, including storytelling, coloring games, and nursery rhymes have been suggested to entice young children to cooperate.[51] In addition, the author has found that by prompting these young children either to laugh or cry (preferably the former), a useful and productive cough can often be elicited. External stimulation of the trachea ("tracheal tickling") using a circular or vibratory motion of the fingers against the trachea as it courses behind the sternal notch may be another useful technique for removing loosened secretions (Fig. 19.8). However, given the relatively small size and fragility of the structures involved with this technique, great care must be employed to avoid injury. Coughing is particularly difficult for the child who has undergone thoracic surgery. Splinting the incision with the hands or with a doll or stuffed animal pressed close to the child's chest promotes the development of an effective cough (Fig. 19.9).

Airway aspiration by suctioning is often needed, particularly in the neonate, to remove secretions. Suctioning must always be done carefully because it has significant risks, even when performed under the best circumstances. Despite the

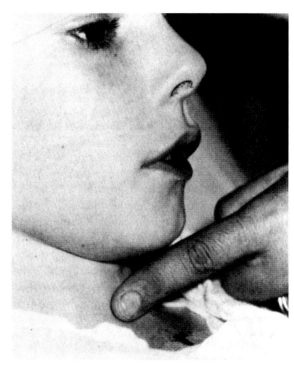

FIGURE 19.8. Placement of the finger for the tracheal "tickle" maneuver. (Reproduced by permission from Irwin S, Tecklin JS. *Cardiopulmonary Physical Therapy.* CV Mosby; 1985.)

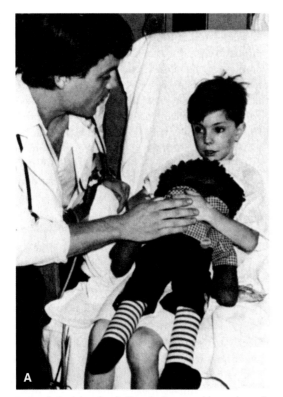

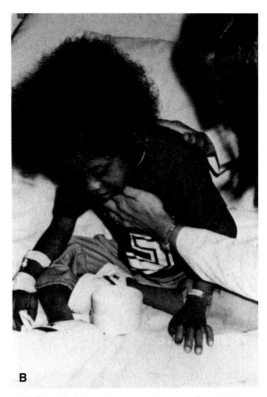

FIGURE 19.9. A: Incisional splinting during coughing using a favorite stuffed toy. **B:** Manual compression over the midsternum to facilitate expectoration of sputum. (Reproduced by permission from Irwin S, Tecklin JS. *Cardiopulmonary Physical Therapy.* CV Mosby; 1985.)

many protocols available, endotracheal suctioning is always a potential hazard, particularly in the pediatric and neonatal populations.[52]

Contemporary Approaches to Airway Clearance

During the past two or three decades, several new approaches to AC were developed. The earlier of the new approaches included breathing maneuvers used to loosen and transport mucus as the common feature. In addition, the techniques were designed to eliminate the need for an individual other than the child to perform necessary AC. These approaches were developed primarily for children and young adults with CF, although they are appropriate for all individuals with chronic lung disease that produces copious sputum. The 1990s saw the development of several new AC techniques that employed various modes of oscillation to either the chest wall or the airway. These include oscillatory PEP (Flutter® and Acapella®), IPV, and HFWCO (the Vest® and SmartVest®). Each of these AC techniques is discussed.

AUTOGENIC DRAINAGE This approach was introduced by Chevalier and described by Dab and Alexander:

1. The child sits in an upright or sitting position.
2. The child takes deep breaths at a "normal or relatively slow" rhythm.
3. Secretions move upward as a result of the breathing.
4. When secretions reach the trachea, they are expelled with either a gentle cough or slightly forced expiration.

The authors recommend that slightly forced expiration be used because of their belief that the high transmural pressures that develop during coughing effectively cause airway collapse, thereby rendering the coughing effort ineffective.[53,54]

Current use of AD recommends tidal breathing at differing lung volumes rather than deep breathing. That is, the child will breathe at a normal volume, but will begin this controlled breathing with most of the resting lung volume previously expelled. After several breaths at low lung volume, the child moves the tidal breathing to a midlung volume and then, following several additional breaths, to a higher lung volume. The movement of air through the smaller to the larger airways is thought to loosen secretions in the smaller, more peripheral airways and move them proximally. The child should be taught to suppress active coughing until huff coughing (controlled coughing with an open glottis) can clear the secretions from the respiratory system. Although controlled research is minimal, at least two studies have shown AD to be effective and equivalent to other accepted AC techniques.[50,55] In addition, evidence exists to support AD as a well-accepted method of AC.[55] The author has worked with many children in whom this technique has been successful in clearing the airways, particularly with copious thick secretions. A notion has circulated that AD is a difficult

technique to teach and learn. This may be highly overstated and an essentially incorrect idea. AD is most commonly used for children who are highly motivated and old enough to control their breathing well.

FORCED EXPIRATORY TECHNIQUE The forced expiratory technique (FET) was developed in New Zealand, but was popularized in the late 1970s and into the 1980s by Pryor, Webber, Hodson, and Batten, all from Brompton Hospital in London.[56] As with AD, the primary benefit derived from FET is that it can be performed without an assistant. Because the Brompton group expressed great concern about what they believed to be misinterpretations of their original description, their description of FET is provided here in a direct quotation from the original article.

> The forced expiratory technique (FET) consists of one or two huffs (forced expirations), from mid-lung volume to low lung volume, followed by a period of relaxed, controlled diaphragmatic breathing. Bronchial secretions mobilized to the upper airways are then expectorated and the process is repeated until minimal bronchial clearance is obtained. The children can reinforce the forced expiration by self compression of the chest wall using a brisk adduction movement of the upper arm.[56]

In a subsequent article that attempts to clarify the various components of FET, the authors place particular emphasis on huffing to low lung volumes in an effort to clear peripheral secretions. In addition, the phrase "from midlung volume" has been clarified to mean taking a medium-sized breath before initiating the huffing. The authors recommend that children use FET while in gravity-assisted positions, and further suggest that pauses for breathing control and periods of relaxation are part of the overall technique.[57]

Owing to continuing differences in interpretation of the FET, it was reconstituted by the Brompton group into a series of activities called *active cycle of breathing technique* (ACBT). The ACBT employs a number of individual skills, including controlled breathing, FET, huff coughing, and thoracic expansion exercises. As was the case with the FET, there have been no attempts at controlled research for the ACBT by the individuals who developed the technique, but some data exist to support ACBT.[56,57]

POSITIVE EXPIRATORY PRESSURE BREATHING PEP breathing was developed in Denmark in an attempt to maintain airway patency and employ channels of collateral ventilation to provide airflow distal to accumulated secretions. Airflow in the distal portions of the airway is presumed to dislodge and move secretions proximally toward larger airways. In addition, PEP provides expiratory resistance that appears to stabilize smaller airways, thereby preventing their early collapse during expiration and huff coughing. PEP is thought to be effective in both reducing air trapping and enhancing secretion removal. The original technique relied on breathing through an anesthesia face mask, but more recent devices use mouthpieces.

When using PEP, the therapist attempts to have child breathe with a level of expiratory pressure of approximately 15 cm H_2O. Devices to provide PEP usually offer varied resistance and have some type of indicator to identify when the 15 cm of pressure has been achieved. The child attempts to maintain that level of pressure throughout the expiratory phase of breathing for 10 to 15 breaths followed by ACBT with huff coughing to clear the secretions. Some recommend using PEP breathing while the child assumes each of the several bronchial drainage positions.[58] Figure 19.10

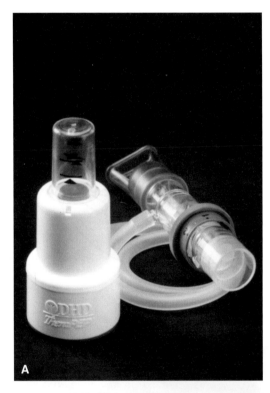

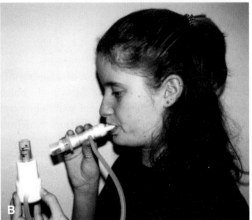

FIGURE 19.10. A: An example of a positive expiratory pressure device (TheraPEP, DHD Healthcare, Canastota, NY). **B:** Thera-PEP device in use (compliments of A. Tecklin).

shows a commercially available PEP device (Smith's Medical, St. Paul, MN).

FLUTTER® The Flutter is a small, handheld pipelike device that produces an oscillating resistance during expiration. The oscillations are created by a small ball within the device that is moved out of its seat during expiration, but then rapidly moves back into its seat through the effects of gravity. The ball is then moved out of the seat again by the continuing force of the expiratory airflow. This repeated movement of the ball rapidly opens and occludes the orifice of the device that results in the rapid oscillations or vibrations transmitted into the airway. These rapid oscillations are thought to loosen the secretions for ease of removal. As with PEP breathing, airway collapse is reduced by the PEP generated by the device. Use of the Flutter is followed by attempts to clear secretions by ACBT or huff coughing. Figure 19.11A–E shows the Flutter device (Vario Raw SA; distributed by Scandipharm, Inc., Birmingham, AL). Research has shown Flutter to be an effective AC treatment when compared with PDPV for hospitalized children with CF.[59]

ACAPELLA® This is another small handheld device capable of providing both PEP and oral oscillation. Unlike Flutter, Acapella generates oscillation using a special valve. A benefit of the Acapella is that it is capable of providing oscillation in any position, thereby being less technique dependent than is the Flutter. There are two versions of the device. I recommend the Acapella Choice® because that model can be disassembled for more complete disinfection and cleaning. Figure 19.12 shows the Acapella Choice (Smith Medical, St. Paul, MN).

HIGH-FREQUENCY CHEST WALL OSCILLATION HFCWO is a newer means of AC that employs an air pulse generator and a garment—a vest—that has inflatable bladders attached to the compressor by large, flexible tubing. The air pulse generator provides pulses at varying frequencies (5 to 20 Hz) and at varying pressures into the inflatable bladders. The air pulses entering the bladder produce oscillations that are transmitted to the chest wall. King's work on dogs suggested that the bursts of air produced a shearing force on secretions within the airways and actually increased airflow into and out of the airways.[60] At least one researcher has referred to this air movement as a "staccato cough."[61] These rapidly recurring bursts of air, or staccato coughs, provide a shear force that cleaves the secretions from the walls of the airways. In addition to the shear forces, the air bursts reduce the viscosity of the secretions[62] and move the secretions upward where they can be coughed or suctioned out.[63] All lobes of the lungs are treated at the same time and the child may sit upright throughout the entire treatment without having to assume the 10 to 12 different positions required for PDPV. Figure 19.13 is the MedPulse Smart Vest® (Electromed-USA, New Prague, MN)

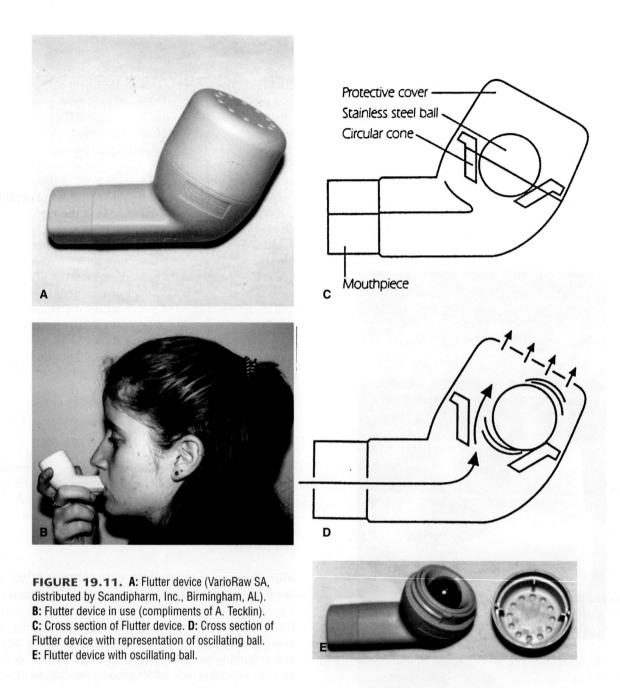

FIGURE 19.11. A: Flutter device (VarioRaw SA, distributed by Scandipharm, Inc., Birmingham, AL). **B:** Flutter device in use (compliments of A. Tecklin). **C:** Cross section of Flutter device. **D:** Cross section of Flutter device with representation of oscillating ball. **E:** Flutter device with oscillating ball.

Breathing Exercises and Retraining

Because many of the commonly used breathing exercises require voluntary participation by the child, the classic methods for teaching improved diaphragmatic descent, increased thoracic expansion, and pursed-lip breathing may not be useful in the infant or young child. Some therapists employ neurophysiologic techniques, such as applying a quick stretch to the thorax to facilitate contraction of the diaphragm and intercostal muscles, to increase inspiration for the baby or young child.

The toddler can participate in games that require deep breathing and control of breathing. Asking the child to breathe in time to music or to the beat of a metronome can present the skill of paced breathing. Blowing bubbles from a bubble wand or blowing a pinwheel will help emphasize increased control and prolonged expiration, which may be useful for the child with obstructive disease. Numerous types of incentive spirometers are also useful for enhancing deep inspiration after either medical or surgical diseases. Incentive spirometry has been studied extensively and is generally considered to be a useful adjunct to postoperative pulmonary care and a means of strengthening respiratory muscles. Improving ventilation to the lower lobes using diaphragmatic breathing and lateral costal expansion may help reduce postoperative pulmonary complications, but as with other

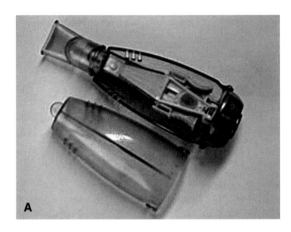

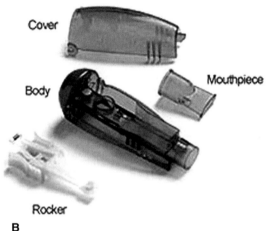

Cover

Mouthpiece

Body

Rocker

B

FIGURE 19.12. A: Acapella Choice airway clearance device. **B:** Acapella Choice disassembled for cleaning. (Smith's Medical, Watford, UK.)

breathing techniques, evidence for efficacy is lacking in both adult and pediatric care.

Participation in and cooperation with breathing exercises usually improves as the child grows older. When appropriate, the therapist may use manual contact to teach diaphragmatic breathing, lateral costal expansion, and segmental expansion. Depending on the findings from the examination of the moving chest, the therapist will choose one or more of these types of breathing exercises. The older child with severe, perennial asthma and the child or adolescent with advanced CF will often exhibit many of the same characteristics as adults with chronic obstructive pulmonary disease (COPD). Paced diaphragmatic breathing may be very useful for these children and young adults. Reduced energy expenditure of breathing is often considered a benefit of diaphragmatic breathing. Because exercise intolerance becomes a problem for children with asthma and CF, paced diaphragmatic breathing may improve the child's ability to walk, climb stairs, and perform other vigorous physical activities. Pursed-lip breathing may also be useful for breath control in the child with chronic lung disease. Relaxation exercise for the child with asthma is often suggested as a means of

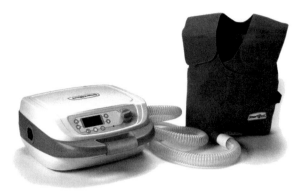

FIGURE 19.13. The MedPulse SmartVest Airway Clearance System (Electromed, New Prague, MN).

reducing breathlessness. Although there is little or no scientific evidence of any change in the pulmonary function of these children with relaxation exercise, there is strong anecdotal evidence of a reduction in the anxiety associated with dyspnea.

Physical Development

Activities to improve physical function in the infant or child with a pulmonary disorder may begin in the neonatal nursery. When physiologic conditions permit, physical therapy interventions should be done with the infant removed from the isolette or warming bed. The handling and tactile stimulation provided by the AC session may be helpful adjuncts to the sensorimotor development of the infant, who may spend great amounts of time in a supine position. Of course, this type of movement is not always possible, particularly for the critically ill baby. As the pulmonary condition improves, the infant should begin to receive, in addition to respiratory physical therapy, appropriate intervention to evaluate and, if necessary, to treat delays in motor development.

Physical Training

Children with asthma and CF and those with respiratory disease secondary to neuromuscular or musculoskeletal problems represent two distinct groups for whom physical training is important. A case example of each group follows in this chapter. Programs of physical training usually include exercises to improve strength and ROM, posture, and cardiovascular endurance.

Strength training is helpful in both groups of children. Children with severe asthma and moderately advanced CF are often limited in strength owing to inactivity and chronic or periodic hypoxemia. In addition, evidence in the past decade has shown that children with CF have weakness in their peripheral muscles associated with diminished maximal workload, even without diminished pulmonary or nutritional status.[33] Darbee and Cerny advocated a strengthening program involving isotonic resistive exercise performed at a high number of repetitions rather than high levels of resistance. They also recommended that exercise should stress the shoulder girdle and thoracic musculature as a means of facilitating the respiratory pump.[64] Orenstein et al. demonstrated increased upper body strength and physical work capacity over a 1-year training program for children with CF.[65]

Decreased ROM is more commonly a problem for those with neuromuscular/musculoskeletal problems than for those with asthma and CF. Nonetheless, children with asthma and CF have been found to have reduced thoracic motion associated with chronic hyperinflation, and may be at risk for both loss of shoulder motion and development of kyphoscoliosis. Exercises for deep breathing, thoracic expansion, segmental expansion, and upper extremity function can help either prevent loss of motion or regain motion that has been lost.

Just as other skeletal muscles respond to training for both endurance and strength, the muscles of inspiration and expiration will respond similarly. Studies of children with chronic lung disease and groups with specific respiratory muscle weakness have shown that significant improvement in respiratory muscle function accompanies breathing activities aimed at either endurance or strength, or both. Inspiratory muscle endurance training and strengthening have resulted in improvement in numerous physiologic indices and have also shown functional and psychosocial benefits.[66,67] Expiratory muscle strengthening may benefit exercise tolerance and surely should enhance the force of expiratory maneuvers, including coughing.[68] These exercises are described later in this chapter.

The child with chronic lung disease will benefit from a program of cardiovascular training or conditioning. Because running precipitates exercise-induced bronchospasm in children with asthma, this group of young children seems to respond much better to swimming programs.[69] Children and young adults with CF participate throughout the United States in organized walking or jogging groups. The popularity of these groups can be traced to Orenstein and colleagues, who first popularized jogging for children with CF and who then studied the benefits for those children.[70]

Regardless of the specific exercise or physical reconditioning program, and regardless of the pediatric pulmonary problem, there is a major role for the physical therapist in treating children with lung disease.

The next section of this chapter describes four common disorders of the respiratory tract in children and their physical therapy evaluation and treatment.

» Atelectasis

Atelectasis, or incomplete expansion of a lung or a portion thereof, was first described by Laennec in 1819.[71] Primary atelectasis occurs in the neonate as a result of pulmonary immaturity, and at any age as a result of inadequate respiratory effort. Secondary atelectasis occurs when gas in a lung segment is reabsorbed without subsequent refilling of that segment. Common causes of secondary atelectasis in children

include external compression of lung tissue, obstruction of the bronchial or bronchiolar lumen, and respiratory compromise secondary to musculoskeletal or neuromuscular disorders.[72]

Primary atelectasis in small areas of the newborn lung is a common finding during the first few days of life. The sick neonate with poor respiratory effort and generalized weakness may not fully expand all areas of the lung for several weeks. Major areas of secondary atelectasis may be the result of abnormal thoracic content such as an enlarged heart or great vessels, congenital or acquired lung cysts, diaphragmatic hernia, and congenital lobar emphysema, each of which compresses lung tissue or the airways. Atelectasis seen by the physical therapist is caused frequently by airway obstruction secondary to accumulation of mucus or other debris, including meconium, amniotic content, foreign bodies, and aspirated gastrointestinal contents. Multiple AC techniques as part of preoperative preparation along with mobility has been shown to be an important feature in treating atelectasis—an important issue for those who are acutely ill and unable to move or change position.[73]

Medical Information

Signs and symptoms of atelectasis depend on the degree of involvement of the lungs. Small areas may be asymptomatic, but common findings in larger areas of atelectasis include decreased chest wall excursion of the affected hemithorax, tachypnea, inspiratory retractions, and cyanosis if the atelectasis is large. The trachea, which can be palpated, will deviate toward the involved lung because of volume loss, and a dull percussion note, which indicates an airless lung, will be present. By auscultation, breath sounds will be reduced or absent. The radiograph will often demonstrate a sharply demarcated area of consolidation, although patchy areas of atelectasis are not uncommon in acute respiratory tract infection.

Medical management

Medical management of obstructive atelectasis is directed toward removal of the obstructing material or condition. When atelectasis is associated with an acute infection, therapy to treat the infection will often eradicate the atelectasis. Good hydration may decrease the viscosity of the mucus, thereby aiding in its removal. A bronchodilator may widen the bronchus, thus allowing air past the obstruction to enhance AC techniques, including PDPV, PEP, and various forms of oscillation—internal and chest wall, and AD. Finally, early mobilization while in bed is an important consideration.[73]

When an obstruction is caused by a neoplasm or another structure that occludes the airway or exerts pressure over the lung parenchyma, surgical removal of the item may be indicated. Endobronchial aspiration using a suction catheter may help remove airway debris, and repositioning of a poorly placed endotracheal tube may correct atelectasis. If none of these more conservative measures is successful, particularly in an acute scenario, bronchoscopy, using either a rigid or a flexible bronchoscope with administration of general or local anesthesia, is indicated to remove the intraluminal mucus or debris.[74]

Prognosis is usually good if the underlying disease process is not life-threatening and if the duration of the atelectasis has not been prolonged. Permanent damage to the bronchial architecture and lung parenchyma can occur with delayed or incomplete resolution of atelectasis and related postoperative pulmonary complication.

Physical Therapy Examination

A thorough review of the child's chart is necessary to fully understand the pathophysiology of the condition and to identify the type and etiology of atelectasis (primary or secondary). The treatment for each type will include similar efforts to increase respiratory effort, but only secondary atelectasis requires AC.

Review of the radiographic findings will identify the location of the atelectasis. The therapist should use the roentgenogram as a clinical tool when treating a child with atelectasis. Lateral and posteroanterior exposures provide a three-dimensional view of the lung fields to more accurately locate the area of atelectasis. Figure 19.14 shows two radiographs with different types of atelectasis. The child's chest configuration and breathing pattern should be noted. A large atelectasis narrows the rib interspaces and decreases excursion of the involved hemithorax. The muscular pattern of respiration should be noted—diaphragmatic versus accessory—and the child's respiratory rate should be determined. Palpation may indicate a shift of the trachea toward the atelectasis owing to volume loss in the involved lung, as noted in the figure. The airless lung area has a dull percussion note that helps the therapist locate the atelectasis. Auscultatory findings will vary. The most frequent change is a diminution of breath sounds in the involved area. Complete obstruction of a large or main bronchus associated with the atelectasis may result in complete absence of breath sounds. With patchy or incomplete atelectasis, crackles may be heard for the first of several deep breaths; however, with subsequent deep breaths, the alveoli may open and the crackles may decrease.

Other considerations in evaluating the child include the following:

1. Mobility—has the child been on bed rest for a long period?
2. Pain—can the child take a deep breath and cough despite the level of pain?
3. Cough—can the child cough, or is there insufficient strength or neurologic competence for an effective cough?

Physical Therapy Procedural Interventions

Several studies support physical therapy interventions for the *prevention* of postoperative atelectasis in adults and children who have had surgery. Therapeutic methods used in these studies included bronchial drainage, percussion, vibration, deep breathing[73,75,76] maximal inspiratory efforts,[77] and electrical stimulation of the thorax with direct current.[78] The success of each treatment regimen was unequivocal.

Finer and associates found a significant decrease in the incidence of postextubation atelectasis in infants who were treated with bronchial drainage, vibration, and oral suctioning when compared with a similar control group treated only with bronchial drainage.[75] A more recent Cochrane review by Flenady and Gray found that AC techniques reduced post extubation atelectasis in a small group of infants who were being extubated.[76] A methodologically sound study by Wong compared traditional chest physical therapy techniques with a lung squeezing approach. There was clear evidence of decreased nonresolution of atelectasis following lung squeezing than with traditional treatment.[77] Atelectasis after extubation occurs commonly in infants, and is presumably caused by excessive bronchial secretions. These studies have

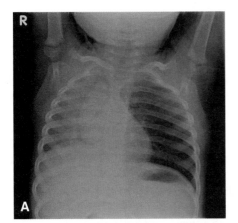
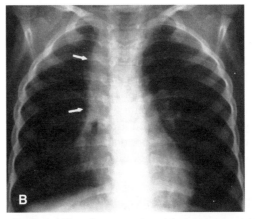

FIGURE 19.14. A: The chest film shows tracheal deviation and mediastinal shift, and compression atelectasis of the right lung due to hyperinflation of the left lung, which compresses the lung on the right side. **B:** Sublobar atelectasis. Asthmatic child with acute asthma attack. Note area of apparent consolidation in the right paratracheal region (*arrows*). This represents collapse of one portion of the right upper lobe.

not evaluated the treatment of atelectasis; however, they have evaluated its prevention, which is the best treatment.

Postoperative atelectasis is often a combination of primary and secondary atelectasis. Secretions are more abundant owing to irritation of the airway by the anesthetic gases and tube manipulations. With incisional pain, and with the generalized weakness that accompanies thoracic or abdominal surgery, the child has a less effective cough and the volume of inspirations is decreased. Deep breathing to achieve maximal inspiration will often be sufficient to resolve small areas of atelectasis. These efforts should be initiated early in the postoperative period—in the recovery room if possible—to prevent atelectasis. Coaching the child to breathe deeply, splinting the incision to reduce pain, and using proprioceptive techniques to facilitate the inspiratory musculature can help the child increase the depth of respiration. Positioning the child to drain the major lung fields and percussion/vibration followed by attempts to cough will aid in the prevention of pulmonary complications. Incentive spirometers, used as a breathing game, will stimulate deeper inhalations. Percussion and coughing become critical components of the treatment if the child develops atelectasis despite preventive measures. Aggressive percussion of the chest over the atelectasis and splinted coughing will work to mechanically dislodge and clear the obstructing mucus. Should percussion prove too aggressive and result in increased pain, vibration of the chest is a good alternative intervention.[79] Endotracheal suctioning to remove accumulated mucus and to further stimulate coughing is often employed for postoperative atelectasis. Early mobilization of the child after surgery and the resultant need for increased ventilation may help mobilize secretions by causing the child to breathe deeply.

Children with medical chest conditions develop atelectasis as a result of retained secretions, and one of the many types of AC may be employed. These children without incisional pain can often tolerate liberal and more aggressive use of manual techniques. Bronchial drainage with localized percussion will often dislodge the obstructing secretions, and coughing will clear the airway. Other techniques such as ACBT, PEP, intra-airway oscillation, and HFCWO are also likely to be effective in loosening the obstructing debris. Many physicians also suggest nebulized mucolytics and bronchodilators as well as bland aerosols to thin and moisten the secretions and to deliver a bronchodilator. The rationale for these procedures of inhalation is that thinned, moist secretions will drain more easily from a bronchus that is maximally dilated. Primary atelectasis caused by respiratory muscle weakness can be resolved by deep breathing and strengthening of the respiratory muscles and change in position to afford better aeration to the poorly ventilated lung areas.

» Respiratory muscle weakness

Respiratory muscle weakness in children, as in adults, may result from any disorder affecting a link in the chain of neuromuscular events that produce contraction of the respiratory muscles. Weakness or paresis of the respiratory muscles may be either mild and transient or severe and irreversible. The underlying pathologic process is the primary determinant of the duration and severity of the weakness. The physical therapist should develop a therapeutic regimen to treat the muscle weakness and to prevent or treat the resultant pulmonary symptoms within the limitations imposed by the disorder.

In the past two decades, a growing population of community-living, ventilator-dependent children has arisen as a result of improved technology and care for chronic ventilatory failure.[80,81] A major improvement in the ability of families and caregivers to maintain these children at home has been due to the acceptance and *relative* ease of care through noninvasive ventilation and improved secretion control.[82,83] Many of these children require physical therapy for deficits and impairments associated with respiratory pump failure and for the delay in motor skill development caused by reliance on the mechanical ventilator, be it invasive or noninvasive ventilation provided in a hospital, residential facility, or home.

Medical Information

Diffuse pathology of the CNS (e.g., viral encephalitis or barbiturate intoxication) may lead to respiratory failure by paralyzing portions of the respiratory muscle pump. Abnormal neural control mechanisms and reflexes may ablate or reduce the physiologic response to chemical and mechanical stimuli. These stimuli may occur within the lungs, the brain stem, the blood, and cerebrospinal fluid (CSF). Examples of childhood disorders that result in a reduced response to respiratory stimuli are familial dysautonomia, sleep apnea, and obesity-hypoventilation syndrome. Focal lesions may affect many nervous system sites such as the medullary centers that generate the inspiratory drive and may cause marked changes in ventilatory patterns.

Spinal cord lesions in the high cervical region may result in total ventilatory paralysis. Because the phrenic nerve, which innervates the diaphragm, leaves the spinal cord at the C3 to C5 level, a lesion at or above that level will likely affect many muscles of respiration. Injury to the high-thoracic or low-cervical cord often results in decreased lung volume and reduced chest wall compliance due to impairment of thoracic musculature. Coughing, which is critically important for removing debris from the airways, will be inadequate if the abdominal muscles are paralyzed. These factors may cause respiratory insufficiency that may progress to respiratory failure, which may be an early sign of neuromuscular disease.[84] Acute respiratory care and long-term rehabilitation are essential components of a treatment plan for the child with a spinal cord lesion or injury.

Diseases of the neuromuscular system are not uncommon in children. Respiratory deficits can result from acute inflammatory polyneuritis (Guillain–Barré syndrome). Because recovery from Guillain–Barré syndrome is often complete, the respiratory weakness must be treated aggressively, and rehabilitation should include acute and long-term measures. The progressive loss of anterior horn cells seen in the spinal muscular atrophies (SMAs) may reduce respiratory muscle function, leading to paralysis and death secondary to respiratory failure. Degenerative diseases of the muscle (e.g., Duchenne myopathy) are characterized by progressive deterioration of pulmonary function later in the course of the disease. Adequate arterial oxygen and carbon dioxide values are maintained only through active efforts. Death is often the direct result of respiratory failure, which often follows the development of pneumonia. When these syndromes are fatal, it is usually attributable to respiratory failure.

The thoracic cage normally provides for adequate function of the respiratory musculature. Abnormalities of the thorax, such as idiopathic scoliosis, scoliosis secondary to neuromuscular disease, and other specific congenital abnormalities, may result in a loss of mechanical advantage of the respiratory muscles. In addition to specific abnormalities, chest wall compliance in individuals with chronic neuromuscular disease appears to decrease through the lifespan, which results in increased work of breathing.[85,86]

Medical Management

The examples just mentioned can cause respiratory muscle weakness or mechanical disadvantage, which may also lead to the requirement for long-term management by mechanical ventilation, as noted earlier. Mallory and Stilwell identify the physical therapist as a member of the typical team of caregivers for these technology-dependent children.[87] In addition, of the seven rehabilitation goals they have identified for the ventilator-dependent child, six are directly related to physical therapy knowledge, skills, and scope of practice. These seven goals are as follows:

1. Increase in muscle strength
2. Increase in attention and cognition
3. Decrease in spasticity
4. Increase in chest wall movement
5. Accessory muscle breathing while upright
6. Diaphragmatic breathing
7. Assisted cough

All goals, with the possible exception of the second one, are direct benefits derived from physical therapy.[86,87]

Physical Therapy Examination

The physical therapy examination for a child with respiratory muscle weakness should follow the recommended sequence

TABLE 19.1.	Recommendations for Varied Types of Exercise in Cystic Fibrosis	
	General Exercise and Training Recommendations	
	Patients with Mild to Moderate CF Lung Disease	Patients with Severe CF Lung Disease
Recommended activities	Cycling, walking, hiking, aerobics, running, rowing, tennis, swimming, strength training, climbing, roller-skating, (trampolining)	Ergometric cycling, walking, strengthening exercise, gymnastics, and day-to-day activities
Method	Intermittent and steady state	Intermittent
Frequency	Three to five times per week	five times per week
Duration	30–45 min	20–30 min
Intensity	70%–85% HR_{max}; 60%–80% peak VO_2; LT; GET	60%–80% HR_{max}; 50%–70% peak VO_2; LT; GET
Oxygen supplementation	Indicated, if SaO_2 drops below 90% during exercise	Indicated, if SaO_2 drops below 90% during exercise (cave: resting hypoxia)
Activities to avoid	Bungee jumping, high diving, and scuba diving	Bungee jumping, high diving, scuba diving, and hiking in high altitude
Potential risks associated with exercise, and training	Dehydration Hypoxemia Bronchoconstriction Pneumothorax Hypoglycemia[*] Hemoptysis Oesophageal bleedings Cardiac arrhythmias Rupture of liver and spleen Spontaneous fractures[†]	

HR_{max}: maximum heart rate; peak VO_2: peak oxygen consumption; LT: lactate threshold; GET: gas exchange threshold; SaO_2: oxygen saturation.
[*]Depending on the existence of an impaired glucose tolerance.
[†]Depending on the existence of untreated CF-related bone disease.
From Williams CA, Benden C, Stevens D, et al. Exercise training in children and adolescents with cystic fibrosis: theory into practice. *Int J Pediatr.* 2010;2010:670640.

presented earlier.[23] Specific attention should be paid to breathing pattern, respiratory muscle strength, chest and shoulder mobility, and AC (see Case Study, H. E., and Table 19.1).

Determining breathing pattern is a major part of the examination. Minute ventilation—the product of the respiratory rate and the tidal volume—determines the arterial $PaCO_2$. The respiratory rate can be counted for 30 seconds or 1 minute, remembering that the child's normal respiratory rate at rest varies with age (a younger child will have a higher rate). Figure 19.2 presents respiratory rates in children. Tidal volume can be easily measured with a mechanical or electronic handheld spirometer used at the bedside. Figure 19.15 shows a child using a spirometer. As with respiratory rate, tidal volume varies depending on the child's height. A taller child has a larger predicted tidal volume. The pattern and symmetry of muscular effort should be identified. Is the child using primarily the diaphragm, intercostal muscles, accessory muscles, or glossopharyngeal muscles? Is the muscular pattern similar for each hemithorax?

The therapist has several methods available for evaluating respiratory muscle strength. The measurement of maximal static inspiratory and expiratory pressures is simple and inexpensive, but requires the child's full cooperation. These pressures can be measured with appropriate pressure manometers, and measurements can be repeated as often as necessary. Reference values for maximal static respiratory pressures in children and adolescents were established by Domenech-Clar et al. In their conclusion, they state that both maximum inspiratory and expiratory pressures increase with age and are consistently higher in males.[88] Infants have also been studied. Airway pressures during crying have been an index of respiratory muscle function in infants

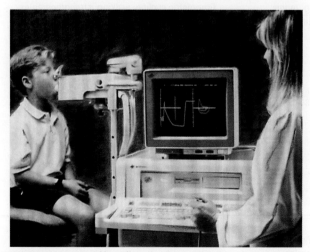

FIGURE 19.15. Use of a spirometer to evaluate lung function. Person being tested takes in a full breath, seals the lips over the mouthpiece of the spirometer, and then blows out as hard and as fast as possible for at least 6 seconds. Nose clips may be applied to ensure that no air escapes through the nose. (Nath JL. *Programmed Learning Approach to Medical Terminology*, 3rd ed. Philadelphia: Wolters Kluwer, 2019.)

for many years, with differences in normal infants clearly distinguished from that in infants with neuromuscular disorders.[89,90]

Evaluation of chest wall mobility includes determining expansion of the chest wall in the anteroposterior, transverse, and vertical directions during inspiration. Thoracic dimensions should be measured with a tape measure or chest calipers during inspiration and expiration to document chest motion. Active ROM in the spine and the shoulder girdle should be examined, including glenohumeral, acromioclavicular, and sternoclavicular joints. Decreased motion at any one of these joints may result in reduced thoracic expansion.

Auscultation of the lungs of a child with respiratory weakness will serve several functions. Decreased breath sounds will help identify areas that are poorly ventilated. Lung areas with decreased or absent sounds may correlate with decreased chest motion or muscular effort. Breath sounds are the most reliable clinical tool for ensuring good ventilation. Breath sounds can help the therapist evaluate the need for AC. If crackles and wheezes are heard, AC and removal of secretions are probably necessary. Breath sounds may indicate the resolution or progression of pulmonary complications, such as pneumonia or atelectasis, and the therapist may choose to modify treatment accordingly.

The therapist should evaluate the child's cough. Integral components of a cough include several distinct phases. Stimulation or triggering of a cough is related to some irritant in the tracheobronchial system, which activates a deep inspiration. Normally, the increased inspiratory volume flows into small airways behind secretions or debris. Coordinated glottis closure is followed by sudden contraction of the expiratory muscles to markedly increase intrathoracic pressure, which can reach 300 mm Hg pressure. The glottis opens, pressure is released, and secretions and other debris are sheared from the airway walls and moved proximally in the tracheobronchial tree. With neuromuscular dysfunction, the child may lack any or all cough-related function. Evaluation of inspiratory effort and volume, and abdominal muscle strength is important in examining coughing and can be objectively done with maximal inspiratory and expiratory pressure measurements. The child must also coordinate the three components—inspiratory, glottis closure, and expiratory effort—into an effective, sputum-producing skill.[91]

Cough effectiveness can be determined by cough peak flow measurements. The child attempts to produce a cough after a maximal inspiration. The cough force is measured via a peak flow meter attached to the child by a mouthpiece or mask. Cough peak flows of less than 160 L/min during respiratory exacerbation are considered inadequate to protect against secretion retention and respiratory failure.[92]

Overall strength, mobility, and coordination, as well as the developmental level of the child, must be evaluated to plan a realistic rehabilitation program. A child who can actively locomote in some manner is less likely to suffer pulmonary complications, and may improve pulmonary function as a by-product of the rehabilitative effort. An aggressive therapeutic regimen is necessary, both to provide early mobility and to strengthen the respiratory musculature, thus improving ventilatory function.

Evaluation of oral motor function—swallowing and feeding—is beyond the realm of physical therapy and often requires an interdisciplinary effort by physicians, physical therapists, occupational therapists, speech pathologists, other therapists, and nurses. Swallowing should be evaluated for two reasons: Eating is the best way for a child to thrive nutritionally, and aspiration of feedings is a major cause of respiratory problems in developmentally delayed and neurologically impaired children.[93] It is clear that as muscle weakness progresses, swallowing dysfunction and aspiration of saliva and food can be problematic.[94]

Physical Therapy Interventions

Physical rehabilitation for the child with neurologic impairment should include an exercise program to improve or maintain respiratory function. The exercises should strengthen inspiratory and expiratory muscles, especially the abdominal muscles that are necessary for effective coughing. In addition, exercise, AC, and related techniques are among the recommendations of the British Thoracic Society guideline for respiratory management of children with neuromuscular weakness.[95]

A traditional method of "strengthening" the diaphragm using abdominal weights has not withstood rigorous scientific evaluation.[96] More physiologically appropriate methods of improving inspiratory muscle strength and endurance are currently used. Resistive breathing for improving inspiratory and expiratory strength will improve maximal respiratory pressures. Endurance studies have similarly shown the benefit of repetitive inspiratory and expiratory exercise with increasing periods of time and increasing resistive loads. Respiratory muscle training is a recognized approach to reduce the progressive decline in respiratory function in children with Duchenne myopathy and SMA. Studies have shown continuing improvement over a period of up to 6 months of training, with much of the improvement sustained at a point as long as 6 months following the cessation of the formal exercise regimen.[93] Training effects are dose dependent, but appear most effective in children who have more slowly progressive neuromuscular disease.[97] Despite numerous studies showing at least short-term benefit to respiratory muscle strength and endurance, there is little evidence of the functional benefit of this exercise in the long term.

Active and resistive exercises for the neck will strengthen the accessory muscles of inspiration (i.e., the sternocleidomastoid and scalene muscles). Although accessory muscle use increases the energy cost of breathing, the accessory muscles may provide increased inspiratory volume to prevent respiratory insufficiency in the child with neuromuscular disease. Active and resistive exercises for strengthening of the abdomen, which may help develop a strong, effective cough, are well known by physical therapists.

Improving the pattern of breathing of a child with neuromuscular disease may provide two benefits. First, an improved ratio of alveolar ventilation to dead space ventilation occurs when a slower, deeper pattern of breathing replaces a fast and shallow mode. The therapist may have the child attempt a slower and deeper pattern of breathing using various clinical cues, including counting, a metronome, or a spirogram. Avoiding inefficient or counterproductive muscular effort is the second possible benefit of changing the pattern of breathing. A child with respiratory distress may appropriately use the accessory muscles to aid inspiration and may use the abdominal muscles to enhance full expiration. This muscular pattern, however, can become habitual. If the diaphragm provides adequate ventilation, unnecessary muscular effort is exerted if the child continues to use the accessory muscles. Various training methods have been suggested, including relaxation exercises and neurosensory techniques, but no scientific data support these endeavors, nor do they suggest that short-term changes in muscular patterns during the therapeutic session have a residual effect or replace the inefficient patterns.

Although the importance of maintaining or improving the mobility of the thorax in children has been identified and related treatment plans have been outlined, no controlled studies of the techniques have been conducted. Active breathing exercises to improve thoracic mobility have been suggested for localized areas or for the entire chest. Manual stretching of the chest wall has been advocated, but has not been tested. Active or passive exercise to improve shoulder girdle mobility in children with paralysis may also improve thoracic excursion. Clinical studies must be undertaken to justify the time-consuming procedures used in the name of respiratory exercises. This notion of little evidence has been supported by a recent Cochrane Review[98] and an independent systematic review of breathing exercises.[99] The authors of the Cochrane Review stated:

The results of this systematic review cannot inform clinical practice as no suitable trials were identified for inclusion. Therefore, it is currently unknown whether these interventions offer any added value in this group or whether specific types of breathing exercise demonstrate superiority over others.[98]

AC is an important therapeutic regimen for hospital, residential, and home treatment programs because many children with respiratory weakness and general inactivity accumulate secretions. If the parent suspects an increase in secretions as a result of a respiratory tract infection, the AC techniques described may prevent the development of pneumonia or atelectasis. If the child cannot cough well and if secretions are problematic, oral or nasal suctioning may be necessary to maintain a clear airway. Parents should be trained in aspiration techniques, and should have proper suctioning equipment in the home. Two additional approaches may help evacuate secretions when a child with neuromuscular weakness is unable to cough effectively. Manually assisted cough is achieved by helping the child inhale to maximal capacity by performing an "air-stacking" maneuver, being insufflated via a bag and mask effort, or with a breath provided by a mechanical ventilator. The caregiver then performs an abdominal thrust or thoracic squeeze as the child relaxes the glottis. The sudden expulsive thrust or squeeze attempts to mimic a cough by promoting a higher expiratory flow than is possible by the weakened musculature. The second approach uses mechanical insufflation/exsufflation (MIE). This mechanical device, originally described during the polio epidemics of the early 1950s, can produce positive pressure that will insufflate the lungs followed by pressure reversal to an expiratory pressure that simulates a cough.[100] MIE has been shown useful in children with neuromuscular disease and impaired cough in numerous studies including children with Duchenne muscular dystrophy (DMD), and SMA.[93,101,102] Despite many articles and textbooks that describe detailed physical therapy programs for children with neuromuscular weakness of the chest, there is a dearth of well-substantiated clinical research to support many of the suggested treatment procedures.

» Asthma

The following description of asthma is a direct quotation from an official American Thoracic Society/European Respiratory Society Statement.[103]

Asthma is a heterogeneous condition. Its natural history includes acute episodic deterioration (exacerbations) against a background of chronic persistent inflammation and/or structural changes that may be associated with persistent symptoms and reduced lung function. Trigger factor exposure combines with the underlying phenotype, the degree of hyperresponsiveness and of airflow obstruction, and the severity of airway inflammation to cause wide variability in the manifestations of asthma in individuals.

Medical Information

Asthma is among the most prevalent chronic childhood conditions in the United States affecting approximately 7 million children, which accounts for 9.6% of children. Asthma is more prevalent in non-Hispanic black children, with the percentage for this group at 16%.[104] There is enormous morbidity associated with the condition, including days lost from school, emergency room (ER) visits, hospitalizations, and health care costs. There are approximately 2 million yearly visits to the ER in the United States related to acute asthma among all ages.[105] Further, from 6% to 13% of those with asthma exacerbations require hospital admission.[13,14,104]

Asthma in children is characterized by several factors. Boys seem to predominate over girls by as much as a 2:1 ratio. Exercise-induced bronchoconstriction is common in most children with asthma, and may be a specific phenotype for some children, with a reported incidence of up to 90%.[106] Children with asthma are often allergic, with the inhaled

or ingested allergen triggering a type 1 immunoglobulin E (IgE)–mediated response. Symptoms may also be provoked by viral infections and by dry, cold air in some. Finally, the increasing mortality and continuing high morbidity associated with childhood asthma are attributable, in part, to an increasing incidence of asthma in the inner-city population.[105]

The physiologic changes responsible for the signs and symptoms of asthma are thought to be initiated when IgE in the sensitized child binds with receptor sites on mast cells. The IgE binding causes the release of histamine and tryptase from mast cells in the airways. Histamine provokes bronchoconstriction, vasodilation within the bronchial walls, and mucous secretion. Tryptase has similar effects, but it also generates bradykinin, a very powerful bronchoconstrictor. The activated mast cells begin to manufacture numerous inflammatory mediators, including prostaglandins and leukotriene. These inflammatory mediators—histamine, prostaglandin D_2, leukotriene C_4, and others—stimulate a response that increases bronchial smooth muscle contraction, causes mucous secretions from the airways, and causes bronchial edema.[107] The result of these three processes is often an obstruction of the airways. As airway obstruction progresses, expiratory airflow decreases, lung volumes and airway resistance increase, airway conductance decreases, and ventilation/perfusion inequality leads to arterial hypoxemia. The various pathophysiologic aspects of asthma appear to have a major hereditary component. However, asthma seems to have a complex genetic model without any clear pattern of inheritance.

A fascinating aspect of asthma in children is the exercise-induced component. With strenuous exercise for a period, usually 5 to 10 minutes, a child can develop many manifestations of asthma (e.g., dyspnea, wheezing, and airway obstruction) that may reverse spontaneously or with treatment.[108] This exercise component is important to the physical therapist developing a conditioning program to increase exercise tolerance in the child with asthma. The response can be managed by having the child premedicate using appropriate oral or inhalation medications before the exercise session to counteract the likely asthmatic response.

Medical Management

Medical management of the child with asthma has two major phases—treatment of the acute attack and control of chronic asthma.

Treatment goals for the acute attack in the ER include reversal of hypoxemia, if present; reduction in airway obstruction; and treatment of airway inflammation. β2-agonists, which can be administered in several modes—including inhalation, subcutaneously, and intravenously—relax bronchial smooth muscle. Short-acting β2-agonists are the recommended first-line therapy for the acute asthma exacerbation. Albuterol sulfate is the most commonly used β2-agonist for acute asthma.[109] Anticholinergic medications, most commonly ipratropium bromide, produce bronchodilation by blocking the effects of acetylcholine on the parasympathetic autonomic nervous system in the airways. The parasympathetic response includes bronchial smooth muscle constriction. β2-Agonists are often used with anticholinergics in multiple doses for best effects.[109] Systemic corticosteroids in the ER are recommended for individuals with moderate or severe asthma to help reduce the inflammatory changes within the airways. A study of almost 900 subjects found a reduction in hospital admission rates when corticosteroids were given within 1 hour of ER presentation.[110] Supplemental oxygen is used to maintain an O_2 saturation of approximately 95%.

The long-term medical management for control of chronic asthma has several components: pharmacologic, environmental, and immunologic. The pharmacologic agents used may include β2 sympathomimetic agents delivered orally or by aerosol; oral preparations of theophylline; anti-inflammatory agents including inhaled and oral corticosteroids; and cromolyn sodium delivered by inhalation. Two newer groups of medication for long-term treatment of asthma include leukotriene receptor antagonists (LTRA) and long-acting β2-agonists (LABA). LTRA reduces the ability of certain leukotrienes—inflammatory mediators—to produce bronchial constriction by interfering with their attachment to receptor sites. LABAs have been in use for almost two decades, but their safety and efficacy are still unsure. A recent Cochrane review states: "The current systematic review seriously questions the benefit of LABAs in children, although it also demonstrates that they appear safe when combined with inhaled corticosteroids."[111]

Control of environmental factors plays a major role in asthma therapy. A dust-free environment is imperative for the child, and special air-filtration units may be required for the child's room. Several multifaceted, randomized controlled trials have shown that reducing multiple early allergen exposures with environmental controls is associated with a decreased risk of asthma.[112] Among the several major allergens noted for removal from the child's environment are dust mites, pets, cockroach, mouse, mold, tobacco smoke, endotoxin, and air pollution. If the youngster chooses to be active in athletics, care must be taken either to avoid levels of activity that may provoke bronchospasm or to use appropriate medication before engaging in asthma-inducing levels of physical exertion.

Immunotherapy (allergy shots) is another method of long-term therapy for allergic asthma. Once allergens are identified by skin testing, extracts of these allergens are given in gradually increasing strengths via periodic subcutaneous injections. The rationale is that the child's immunologic system will respond to the small doses of allergen by producing circulating antibodies. Once sufficient levels of antibodies are developed, environmental exposure to the allergen will result in no symptoms of asthma because the acquired antibodies will alleviate the allergic response of the child. A recent review has established the efficacy of both subcutaneous immunotherapy and sublingual immunotherapy.[113]

Physical Therapy Examination

As with medical care, physical therapy examination and management of children with asthma is largely based on the clinical situation at the time (i.e., whether the child is in an acute, subacute, or chronic stage of the disease). The hospitalized child with status asthmaticus (intractable acute asthma) will not tolerate either AC or physical training. A notable exception for AC is when the child is intubated and mechanically ventilated and control of airway secretions is part of care.

The physical therapist's examination of a child receiving mechanical ventilation should include lung auscultation to identify the location of bronchial secretions and to ascertain whether areas of the lungs are poorly ventilated. The pattern of ventilation and use of accessory muscles should be noted. Measurements of the thorax, including thoracic index, should be made during inspiration and expiration to determine chest mobility. Several or all of these evaluated items will be abnormal. The therapist must reevaluate these items with each treatment until the thoracic index, breath sounds, and pattern of breathing have improved.

A long-term rehabilitation plan for the child with asthma must also examine exercise tolerance, strength, and posture. Exercise tolerance may be evaluated by several well-studied and easily performed tests. These commonly include the 6-minute walk test,[114] the step test,[115] and the 20-minute shuttle run test.[116] Quantitative strength measurement of major muscle groups can be made with equipment that is readily available in the physical therapy department. Posture can be evaluated using a grid system.

Physical Therapy Interventions

As noted earlier under Physical Therapy Examination, there is little, if any, rationale for physical therapy for the child with status asthmaticus.[117] Status asthmaticus renders a child too dyspneic, anxious, scared, and physically unable to cooperate with the therapist for AC, breathing activity, posture and ROM evaluation, or any rehabilitative endeavors. When the severe bronchospasm begins to reverse, accumulated secretions are often encountered in the previously narrowed airways. Aggressive AC is imperative during this subacute stage, but must be administered within tolerance. Secretions retained in the airways predispose the child to atelectasis and bronchial infection. AC at this time is indicated within the limits of the youngster's tolerance and endurance. Secretion volume, color, consistency, and the child's vital signs including pulse oximetry before, during, and after treatment should be recorded.

In the long-term care of asthmatic children, intermittent AC treatments may be useful when secretions are present, but treatments are not used routinely as in other conditions, such as CF. Parents should use AC techniques at the first sign of a respiratory infection or increased mucus production and should know the drainage positions and manual techniques and the techniques of use of newer AC modalities to treat the child at home. One of the only reported controlled studies of the effects of AC via bronchial drainage and percussion in children with asthma involved 21 outpatients. These children, who had mild to moderate asthma, were divided into a treatment group and a control group. The mean forced expiratory volume (FEV_1) for the treatment group increased by 10.5% 30 minutes after therapy. The control group had a slight decrease in mean FEV_1 during the same period. The difference in mean FEV_1 values was significant at the 0.05 level.[118]

In previous editions of this chapter, various traditional breathing exercises for children with asthma were discussed. They are omitted in this edition owing to a complete lack of supporting evidence for their efficacy.

Relaxation techniques have also been advocated to reduce the anxiety and physical stress associated with an episode of asthma. Many anecdotal and verbal reports lend support to the benefits of relaxation techniques in children with asthma, but controlled studies are lacking. Two systematic reviews have been published—one regarding relaxation exercises for asthma and the second, more recent, review on psychological interventions for children with asthma. Huntley et al. found some evidence for muscular relaxation exercises improving lung function, but no other benefits were noted owing to poor methodology and inherent difficulties with this type of study.[119]

The second systematic review found some data to suggest relaxation therapy was beneficial, but, in general, studies showed widely varied approaches and lack of sufficient data.[120]

Physical rehabilitation to improve aerobic endurance, work capacity, and strength are major goals in the long-term management of asthmatic children. Children with chronic asthma are often less physically active than are their unaffected peers. Exercise-induced bronchospasm may restrict a child with asthma from participating in vigorous exercise, and the child may, therefore, be unable to respond to physical demands in daily life. Appropriate medication before vigorous exercise may attenuate the bronchospastic response, and the child can derive the enjoyment, social interaction, and physiologic benefits of exercise.[121,122] A formal physical training program should be preceded by quantitative evaluation of the child's response to strenuous exercise. The initial evaluation determines the level of exercise needed to improve strength and endurance, and is a baseline against which the results of subsequent studies can be compared to determine improvement or deterioration. Among the more commonly used methods of physical training are free running, treadmill running, bicycle ergometry, and swimming.

There is conclusive evidence supporting physical training and exercise for individuals with asthma. Most significant is that physical training/activity does not exacerbate asthma symptoms or disease control.[123,124] Mancuso et al. recently demonstrated an improved quality of life following a 1-year program of increased physical activity. Asthma quality-of-life quotient improved during the year of activity from 5.0 to 5.9,

a clinically important difference. Although not specifically for children, there were children 12 years of age and older who participated in the program.[125] A Cochrane Review of physical exercise in asthma found that many modes of exercise—running, walking, cycling, swimming, and others—were well tolerated without detrimental effects on symptoms. Cardiopulmonary and aerobic fitness levels improved along with quality-of-life measures. However, as is also found in adults with COPD, physical training had no significant effect on resting lung function.[126]

In addition to traditional land-based exercise showing promise for improving physical status and quality of life in individuals with asthma, swimming as a training mode has been shown to have beneficial effects in children with asthma. Sly and associates studied the effects of swimming by assigning children to either a treatment group or a control group. The treatment group participated in a swimming program for 2 hours three times a week for 13 weeks. Although no changes were recorded in pulmonary function or basic personality traits, a marked decrease in wheezing days was noted in the treatment group, as was also seen with land-based exercise studies cited earlier. The mean number of days of wheezing for the treatment group was 31.3 during the 13 weeks before the training program; this figure declined to 5.7 days of wheezing during the swimming program. A similar control group of asthmatic children had a mean of 10.1 and 13.2 days' wheezing, respectively, before and during the 3-week control period.[127]

Fitch and associates published the results of a 5-month swimming program in 46 asthmatic children compared with a control group of 10 nonasthmatic children. Outcome measures included asthma score (based on wheeze, cough, and sputum), physical work capacity at a heart rate of 170, drug score (based on the amount of medication), FEV_1 values, and response to an exercise challenge on a treadmill. A marked improvement in asthma score, drug score, and physical work capacity followed the training period. A concomitant improvement in posture was noted. No change was reported in FEV_1 or the severity of exercise-induced asthma. The authors concluded that swimming is an effective method of physical training in asthmatic children.[128]

More recent studies include a 2009 report by Wang and Hung, who followed up 30 children with asthma randomly assigned to a swimming group or usual care during a 6-week period. There was a significant improvement in peak expiratory flow rate in the experimental group compared with that in the control group (330 L/min, 95% confidence interval [CI]: 309 to 351 vs. 252 L/min, 95% CI: 235 to 269) after the swimming intervention. There was also a significant decrease in the severity of asthma in the experimental group compared with that in the control group. The authors suggested that swimming may be an effective nonpharmacologic intervention for the child or adolescent with asthma.[129] A 2011 study using a prospective longitudinal examination of data on 5,738 children sought to find information on recreational swimming pool attendance and asthma and allergy at 7 and 10 years of age. The results showed that by 7 years of age, more than 50% of the children swam once a week or more. Children with high cumulative totals of swimming had a decreased likelihood of developing asthma at both 7 and 10 years of age, and also showed a significant improvement in forced mid-expiratory flow of 0.2 standard deviations. As seen with land-based physical training, swimming provided clinical and physiologic benefits to a large cohort of children as regards development of asthma.[130] A recent systematic review supported swimming as a safe and effective means of physical training for children with asthma. The authors stated that swimming is "well-tolerated in children and adolescents with stable asthma, and increases lung function (moderate strength evidence) and cardiopulmonary fitness (high strength evidence)."[131]

It is very clear that children with asthma will benefit from physical training using the more traditional modes of treadmill, bicycle, and running or jogging as well as swimming.

» Cystic fibrosis

Medical Information

CF is the most common life-limiting genetic disorder affecting, primarily, Caucasians. The disease is inherited in an autosomal recessive pattern. It is estimated to occur in 1 of every 3,500 births in the United States, and has a carrier rate of approximately 1 in 29 persons. When two carriers have a child, there is a 25% chance that the child will have CF, a 50% chance that the child is a carrier of the gene, and a 25% chance that the child will be completely free from the CF gene. Accurate genetic testing is currently available when CF is suspected or when there is a high risk of inheritance owing to family history of the disorder. CF is a generalized disorder of the exocrine glands, which, in its fully manifested state, produces elevated sweat electrolyte concentrations, pancreatic enzyme deficiency, and chronic inflammatory and suppurative pulmonary disease. The clinical presentation of CF varies, but usually includes combinations of productive cough, abnormally frequent and large stools, failure to thrive, recurrent pneumonias, rectal prolapse, nasal polyposis, and clubbing of the digits. Because of its variable presentation, CF is often misdiagnosed as asthma, allergy, celiac disease, and chronic diarrhea. The well-informed health professional should consider CF when any of these symptoms are encountered.

The gene for CF, the *cystic fibrosis transmembrane conductance regulator (CFTR)*, was identified in 1989 on the long arm of chromosome 7.[132] Although one mutation is responsible for approximately 85% of all cases of CF—F508del—more than 1,000 mutations of the *CFTR* gene are recognized. The major hypothesis of CFTR dysfunction states that the absence of CFTR is responsible for a decrease in chloride and water secretion and transport by airway epithelial and submucosal cells, thereby resulting in thick and dehydrated mucus.[133] However, the diversity of organ system involvement

in CF suggests that other mechanisms are also associated with the CFTR. Regardless of the specific mechanisms, it is agreed that all exocrine glands are impaired to some degree and the variable dysfunction results in a wide spectrum of symptoms and complications in CF.

The incidence in the United States has been mentioned. CF is much less common in the black population, occurring in 1 of about 17,000 births among African Americans. CF is considered uncommon in the Asian population. The course of the disease, similar to its presentation, is variable. Although severe lung and gastrointestinal disease can be fatal for children with CF, survival rates have improved steadily over the past several decades, with an increasing percentage of individuals living beyond 40 years in developed countries.[134]

The pulmonary disease associated with CF causes the greatest mortality. Pulmonary involvement in CF begins with the production and retention of thick, viscous, poorly hydrated secretions within the airways. These secretions provide a medium in which bacterial pathogens flourish. The resultant infections produce inflammation, more secretions, and additional obstruction; and a vicious cycle is begun. The earliest pathologic changes may be reversed with aggressive treatment. With continued reinfection, bronchiolitis and bronchitis progress to bronchiolectasis and bronchiectasis. The latter two processes, which are irreversible, destroy elements within the walls of the airways.

In addition to these destructive processes, hyperplasia of mucous-secreting glands and cells occurs within the lungs. Large quantities of thick, purulent mucus are produced, causing the airway obstruction that is common in CF. If the obstruction is partial, a ball-valve process may result in which airways that widen on inspiration allow air into the lungs. When those same airways narrow with expiration, the air becomes trapped, thereby producing hyperaeration of the lung distal to the obstruction. Complete airway obstruction results in absorption atelectasis distal to the obstruction. Small areas of hyperaeration and atelectasis often exist in adjacent areas, and present a honeycomb pattern on a chest roentgenogram. The rapidity of pulmonary progression and success of treatment play major roles in determining the survival of a child with CF.

Pulmonary complications often include massive hemoptysis, pneumothorax, lobar atelectasis, and pulmonary hypertension with cor pulmonale. These problems have been discussed at length by others.[135-138]

Medical Management

Management of CF is directed toward decreasing pulmonary infection and airway obstruction, replacing pancreatic enzymes to help reverse the nutritional deficiency, and providing appropriate psychosocial and emotional support to the child and family. Control of pulmonary infection is the major therapeutic objective. Sputum culture and sensitivity tests to identify pathogens and determine appropriate antimicrobial drugs enable the physician to plan a rational course of medications. The most common bacteria-causing infections in children with CF vary with age. *Staphylococcus aureus, Pseudomonas aeruginosa*, and *Haemophilus influenzae* are the most frequently identified pathogens in the early years of life. *H. influenzae* infection decreases as the child ages. Antimicrobial agents are used aggressively, and may be given orally, parenterally, and by inhalation. In the past two decades, the bacterium *Burkholderia cepacia* has become recognized as contributing to infection in people with CF. *B. cepacia* is largely antibiotic resistant and may be transmitted in an epidemic-like manner. Some strains of *B. cepacia* are associated with a syndrome of rapid progression of lung disease, ending in death within several months. It must be noted, however, that not all *B. cepacia* infections react in this manner. The Cystic Fibrosis Foundation (CFF), in 2013, recommended isolating individuals with CF at CFF events to prevent or reduce the likelihood of cross-infection.[139]

Reduction of airway obstruction is the most time-consuming aspect of comprehensive treatment of CF. Reduction of sputum viscosity by aerosolized or oral medications is thought to enhance physical efforts to loosen and drain mucus from the airways. Physical therapy is a major part of the care and is detailed later.

Replacement of pancreatic enzymes is essential for the 85% of children with pancreatic dysfunction. Traditionally, the recommended diet for those with CF has included high-protein, high-carbohydrate, and low-fat foods. With more effective pancreatic preparations, many children have liberalized their intake of fat. Despite apparent control of pancreatic insufficiency with enzymes, children with CF may need up to 50% more calories than their age- and weight-matched peers. Continually underweight children, or those who experience weight loss with a progression of disease, may benefit from commercial dietary supplements. Supplements must be chosen carefully and added to the diet, and a nutritionist's counseling is necessary.

Psychosocial and emotional support for children with CF and their families is the responsibility of all professionals who work with this population. Issues that must be confronted include chronic life-shortening illness, genetic disease, cost of drugs and care, time-consuming treatments, and death of a child, denial, and guilt. Other issues emerge as children reach adulthood: marriage, occupations, and dependence on others for treatment. A counselor or social worker plays a major role on the CF team. A large body of literature is available regarding psychosocial aspects of the children with CF and their families.

Two newer approaches to pulmonary treatment include lung transplantation and gene therapy. Lung transplantation for those with end-stage disease has been successful. Unfortunately, there are major problems with transplantation, including an uncertain waiting time for donor organs and the development of obliterative bronchiolitis following transplantation. A study published in 2007 in the *New England Journal of Medicine* and a related editorial provide varied perspectives on this extraordinarily difficult treatment.[140,141] More recent work by Thabut et al. shows a significant survival benefit after lung transplant, with approximately 68% of subjects surviving at 3 years following transplantation.[142] Lung transplantation for CF will continue to develop as a major treatment option for advanced lung disease in CF.

Gene therapy trials followed the identification of the *CFTR* in 1989. Researchers attempted to introduce normal versions of the CFTR into the airways, but successes were limited. One of the biggest issues in gene therapy has been finding a way to introduce the normal genes into the airways of patients. The most commonly tried approach was using a viral vector as a gene transfer agent to carry the genes into the lungs. To date, results have been limited owing to many different factors and lack of an effective gene transfer agent.

A nationwide network of centers is dedicated to the treatment of CF. These centers are sponsored by the CFF, and can reach almost every population center in the United States. The CFF sponsors research projects, fellowships, conferences, fund raising, and other activities in its mandated task of providing the best care for children and adults with CF (see CFF.org). As a result of the CFF Drug Development Pipeline, a medication developed by Vertex Pharmaceuticals was approved by the U.S. Food and Drug Administration for use in individuals with one specific mutation of the *CFTR* gene—G551D—which represents approximately 4% of the population with CF. The medication, called *Kalydeco®* (ivacaftor), helps improve the function of the specific CFTR in this group and improves pulmonary function values and reduces sweat chloride values.[143] This medication is considered a proof-of-concept breakthrough with work on Kalydeco and similar possible medications continuing.

Physical Therapy Examination

Physical therapy examination for the child with CF is similar to the process described early in this chapter based on the Guide to Physical Therapist Practice.[19] Emphasis in CF must be placed on the bronchial secretions that cause the numerous pulmonary problems and complications.

Auscultation for secretions must be done with the expectation of finding many areas with sonorous wheezes, harsh breath sounds, and crackles (all abnormal breath sounds), which are associated with secretions. Of course, the findings will vary depending on the degree of lung impairment in the child. The sounds may not change for several days in a patient with advanced disease, and auscultation on an intermittent, rather than daily, basis may be helpful.

A determination of the child's ability to cough and raise secretions is very important. An acutely ill child with CF who cannot cough effectively risks further deterioration in airway function. The chest radiograph and other imaging are useful in identifying specific anatomic areas of lung disease and infection. Many believe that the three-dimensional view of the lungs afforded by posteroanterior and lateral chest films provides specific information to help direct treatment.

Also, the child's physical capabilities, including strength and aerobic fitness, should be a focus of the examination. Children with CF participate in less physical activity than do their healthy non-CF peers despite those with CF having good lung function.[144] Therefore, strength testing and cardiopulmonary exercise testing should be performed when appropriate to develop an exercise reconditioning program appropriate to the child's tolerance.

The most valid and accurate manner for formal exercise testing includes laboratory maximal exercise testing by treadmill for measurement of peak oxygen consumption (peak VO_2), which is considered the best index of cardiopulmonary function.[145] Orenstein developed a group of runners with CF in the late 1970s. He reported safe and beneficial results of a 3-month cardiopulmonary fitness program, which heralded more and more importance ascribed to cardiopulmonary or aerobic "fitness" in the population with CF.[65] In addition to enhancing exercise, fitness, and quality of life, the concept of exercise capacity has been shown to have prognostic features for survival in CF.[146,147] Owing to limitations of time, space, and financial concerns related to laboratory exercise testing, several widely used "clinical tests" of exercise among physical therapists working with children with CF have been popularized and included in exercise evaluation. The following are three commonly used clinical tests for exercise evaluation in CF.

1. The 6-minute walk test is well known by physical therapists. The child is asked to walk as far as possible in a 6-minute period, with the distance walked being the primary outcome. Other values can be measured, but should not interfere with the time or distance. The child walks alone at a self-paced speed on a straight, flat course of no less than 30 m with small traffic cones at each end of the course for a turnaround point. If the child is receiving supplemental oxygen, it should be used.[148]

2. Subjects performing a step test are instructed to step up and down on a step at a height of 15 cm. The step frequency is kept constant at a pace controlled by a metronome. The duration of the test is 3 minutes, with the subject maintaining a rate of 30 steps per minute for 3 minutes by stopwatch. The child is encouraged to switch the leading leg during the 3-minute test period. If the test is aborted early, owing to muscle fatigue or dyspnea, the number of steps taken must be counted.[149]

3. The modified shuttle walking test may be performed in either 12- or 15-level formats. Children must move around two markers over a 10-m course in cadence with "beeps" from a prerecorded tape. Work at each level—12 or 15—continues for 1 minute, and the speed of the increases by 0.61 km/h each minute. There are a maximum of 15 levels. The test ends when subjects have completed the required work, state that they are unable to continue, or fail to achieve the course marker on two consecutive beeps. Selvadurai et al. validated the 10-m modified shuttle walk test in children with CF.[150]

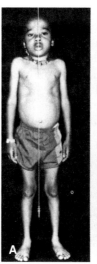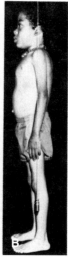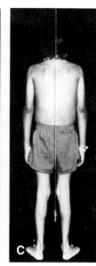

FIGURE 19.16. Postural abnormalities in a child with cystic fibrosis. **A:** Anterior view. Notice that the shoulders are held high, especially on the right. This posture appears to offer better mechanical advantage to the accessory muscles for breathing. The lower ribs are flared, and the thorax appears barreled and elongated because of the hyperinflation of the lungs. A full postural evaluation might reveal other, less obvious abnormalities. **B:** Lateral view. The thoracic kyphosis and barreled chest seen here are common findings in children with obstructive pulmonary disease and hyperinflation of the lungs. **C:** Posterior view. The shoulders appear high, with a protraction of the scapulae. Notice the enlargement of the thorax in relation to the rest of this patient's body. Pronated feet are also noticeable. (Reproduced by permission from Irwin S, Tecklin JS. *Cardiopulmonary Physical Therapy.* CV Mosby; 1985.)

Evaluation of the child's posture, including mobility of the chest wall, should be determined for several reasons. Children with CF often have hyperinflated lungs, so the chest wall may appear barreled and fixed, very similar to adults with COPD. Figure 19.16 shows a young child with CF and thoracic changes due to advanced pulmonary disease. A noncompliant thorax increases the work of breathing. If chest wall changes occur, the child may have difficulty developing the necessary inspiratory and expiratory pressures and flow rates to cough effectively and to increase ventilation during physical stress. Thoracic index, thoracic girth, and rib motion should be determined during full inspiration and full expiration.

The barrel-shaped configuration of the hyperinflated thorax will likely increase the normal thoracic kyphosis. Scapular protraction also becomes evident. With the anatomic changes in the upper thorax that accompany hyperaeration, ROM of the shoulder girdle must be measured too. A comprehensive examination should include those postural items that may affect both function and cosmesis.

Physical Therapy Management

Physical therapy for infants and children with CF begins invariably with AC techniques taught to the parents of newly diagnosed children. This usually includes positioning for gravity drainage, and manual techniques of percussion and vibration, keeping in mind the concern previously noted regarding head-down drainage positions. As the child ages, other AC techniques can begin at age-appropriate times. Exercise for both aerobic fitness and strengthening will begin at differing times in a child's life, depending on the specific progression of lung disease and activity levels of the individual.

Airway Clearance

A major role of physical therapy for the child with CF is in the aggressive use of AC—including bronchial drainage, chest percussion, vibration, and suctioning (if necessary), and the many newer and effective techniques developed and popularized in the past three decades. Treatment should be generalized as needed because mucus is produced in all areas of the lungs; but if the examination identifies specific lobes or segments with advanced disease or that appear to have increased production of mucus, emphasis for treatment should center on these segments. Early studies of conventional bronchial drainage, percussion, and vibration in CF during the 1960s and 1970s helped document their efficacy. Lorin and Denning, for instance, demonstrated that twice the amount of sputum per cough and per treatment was obtained when a combined treatment regimen of gravity drainage, percussion, and vibration was compared with cough alone.[151] Tecklin and Holsclaw found improvement in forced vital capacity and peak expiratory flow rate after bronchial drainage, percussion, and vibration in 26 children with CF.[152] Feldman and associates have demonstrated remarkable improvement in flow rates at low lung volumes 45 minutes after treatment in nine subjects with CF.[153] In Feldman's study, the isovolume flow rate near 25% of forced vital capacity increased from baseline by 70% 45 minutes after treatment.[154] These changes in small airway flow rates are consistent with the results of Motoyama.[155]

Desmond and coworkers employed a crossover design to determine whether pulmonary function decreased over a 3-week period during which physical therapy was withheld. There was a statistically significant decrease in flow rates reflective of small airway function, forced expiratory flow (FEF 25% to 75%) and V_{max60} (total lung capacity [TLC]), each of which declined by 20% after 3 weeks of no therapy. These values returned to their prior levels shortly after resumption of physical therapy.[156]

Current Airway Clearance Techniques

As individuals with CF have grown older to the point where the median age of survival approaches 40 years, the importance of independent treatment is now paramount. The contemporary techniques are used extensively throughout the world because they provide independence

in self-care without the need for an assistant to provide the manual techniques.

AUTOGENIC DRAINAGE AD, described previously, improves pulmonary function and secretion removal when compared with several other AC techniques.[157-160] AD is most commonly used by teenagers and adults with CF owing to the need for good breathing control and personal motivation required. One of the drawbacks with AD is that it requires individual training by the physical therapist, and some individuals have difficulty learning and performing the technique. Those who are able to participate report good acceptance and use of the procedure and independence in its use.

POSITIVE EXPIRATORY PRESSURE MASK The PEP mask, described earlier in the chapter, may hold the greatest promise in terms of independent removal of excess secretions in children with CF and is used throughout the world. Two long-term studies of PEP breathing have been reported. McIlwaine et al., long-time supporters of PEP, recently compared two groups of subjects with CF who were assigned randomly to a PEP group or a HFCWO group. At the end of 12 months, the PEP group had a lower frequency of pulmonary exacerbations, but there were no differences in lung function, health-related quality of life scores, or personal satisfaction with treatments.[161] Darbee et al. found notable improvements in pulmonary function following low-PEP or high-PEP treatment in individuals with CF. In addition to increased lung function, including oxygen saturation, those using PEP had increased sputum expectoration with high PEP. Darbee also discussed the physiologic rationale for PEP.[162]

FLUTTER AND ACAPELLA The Flutter® was developed to offer a measure of independence to young adults with CF and included an oscillatory aspect to PEP. Several studies of the Flutter found no difference between the device and other modalities of AC. It appears that the Flutter is well accepted by many children and is equivalent to the effects on sputum clearance and pulmonary function of other types of AC.[163] A negative aspect of the Flutter is its dependence on gravity for proper use. The Acapella is a device with a specific valve that enables oscillation without regard to position, and for this reason may be easier to use than is the Flutter. As with many AC devices, the Acapella provides AC effects similar to most other techniques.[163]

HIGH-FREQUENCY CHEST WALL OSCILLATION HFCWO has gained acceptance throughout many CF centers in the United States and internationally largely because of its ease of application. Warwick and Hansen examined the efficacy of high-frequency chest compression (HFCC) in a long-term but uncontrolled study of 16 subjects with CF. All but one of those subjects showed improvement in their respiratory impairment during the trial.[154] Subsequent evaluations of HFCWO demonstrated that the technique was at least as beneficial to subjects with CF as conventional physical therapy and PEP breathing both in short-term and in long-term studies.[164,165] The "vest," as HFCWO is called by children, has provided a useful, independent means for both children and adults with CF to perform daily AC without an assistant to provide manual techniques. The only drawback to the vest is its high cost, but many insurance carriers will provide excellent levels of support for this device.

In summary, gravity-assisted bronchial drainage with manual techniques as the "gold standard" for children with CF is no longer the case because numerous other interventions have been determined to be equally efficacious. When working with children and adults with CF, the therapist must consider many alternatives for AC and secretion removal. Despite the publication and presentation of several hundred comparisons of the many AC techniques, comments made by Jennifer Pryor and Eleanor Main hold true. Pryor stated in 1999:

If objective differences are small, individual preferences and cultural influences may be significant in increasing adherence to treatment and in the selection of an appropriate regimen or regimens for an individual.[166]

Main, in 2013, reflected on the lack of conclusive evidence regarding AC in CF despite numerous Cochrane Reviews and several unsuccessful recent attempts at long-term comparative studies:

Strong patient preference, lack of blinding and the requirement for effortful and demanding participation over long intervals will continue to derail efforts to find the best AC technique for CF, unless they are addressed in future clinical trials.[167]

Given the current evidence, this author believes that the choice of procedures should be based on age, disease severity, caregiver availability, need for independence, and child/family preference. The decision falls largely on the child and family members who are ultimately responsible for this daily procedure.

MODIFICATIONS OF AIRWAY CLEARANCE PROCEDURES

Modifications of usual treatment procedures are often necessary for acutely ill children or for those with certain complications. There is little or no evidence to support one technique versus another. In a child with major hemoptysis, chest percussion and vibration should be discontinued temporarily because the physical maneuvers may dislodge a blood clot and prolong the bleeding. AC techniques that employ breathing—PEP, AD, Flutter, and Acapella—may be useful in an attempt to remove accumulated blood from the airways.

Pneumothorax is a complication of CF, and is commonly treated with an intrapleural chest tube with suction. Gravity drainage is appropriate, although percussion and vibration at the site of tube insertion are contraindicated. PEP and other breathing approaches to AC may enable continued treatment of excessive secretion. With advanced lung disease, the child may benefit from any of the techniques that they are able to use and find tolerable and acceptable.

Physical Exercise

There is little question about the benefits of exercise and physical conditioning for children with CF. More than 30 years ago, Cropp and associates showed that children with CF, excepting those with advanced lung disease, had a normal *cardiovascular* response to exercise. Children with advanced disease were likely to have arterial oxygen desaturation during exercise due to ventilator limitations.[168] Marcus and colleagues demonstrated that children with advanced CF who exercised with a fraction of inspired oxygen (FiO_2) of 30% worked longer, had higher maximal oxygen consumption, and experienced less oxygen desaturation than they did while exercising at room air. This suggested that children with advanced disease were also able to improve their exercise tolerance with supplemental oxygen during training.[169] Muscle fatigue as a limiting factor in physical exercise was identified by Moorcraft et al. on the basis of 78 of 104 subjects with CF who reported needing to stop exercise owing to muscular fatigue.[170]

Treadmill walking or running, cycle ergometer training, free running or walking, and strengthening exercises are useful methods of increasing cardiovascular fitness, endurance, and general muscular strength. See Table 19.1.[171]

The relevance of these findings is that physical training and reconditioning, in a formal or informal program, is safe and beneficial in all children except those with severe lung disease. Even those with severe disease have been shown to benefit from an exercise program if supplemental oxygen is provided.

Summary

This chapter has attempted to provide a summary of unique characteristics of lung disease in children, growth and development of the respiratory system, and the reasons why children and infants are predisposed to acute respiratory failure. Examination of the child with pulmonary disease and treatments aimed at reducing the severity of pulmonary disease in infants and children have been reviewed. Four major respiratory disorders have been described, along with a discussion of appropriate physical therapy examination and management. Published evidence for the physical therapy methods has been reviewed. Physical therapy for children with lung disease has been shown to be efficacious, depending on the treatment employed and the problems addressed.

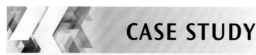

CASE STUDY

H.E., a 14-year-old Caucasian boy with a history of DMD diagnosed at 4 years of age, was referred for pulmonary physical therapy evaluation. This case study focuses on the cardiovascular/pulmonary needs of this patient.

Examination
History
H.E. was a full-term infant who appeared to be developing normally until approximately 3 years of age, when his parents noted that he had difficulty rising easily from the floor and could not easily ascend stairs. Upon stating their concerns to the pediatrician, H.E. was sent for laboratory testing and a muscle biopsy. The testing indicated abnormally high serum creatinine kinase, and a muscle biopsy was performed. The resulting diagnosis of DMD was made. He was referred to a large children's hospital for follow-up and continuing care. As the years progressed, H.E.'s weakness became more pronounced, and he developed some of the classic physical characteristics including increasingly severe lumbar lordosis, several contractures including plantar flexion, and hip and knee flexion contractures. He was still ambulatory, although he and his mother reported that the distance was steadily decreasing and the speed was getting slower.

Review of Systems
Integument
There were no obvious or stated problems in this area.

Musculoskeletal
Numerous contractures in the lower extremities were obvious along with severe lumbar lordosis. Elbow contractures were also noted, although not as severe as those of the lower extremities. There was obvious weakness, particularly in the shoulders and hip musculature.

Neuromuscular
Ambulation, balance, and transfers were all significantly abnormal and limited. H.E. currently functions from a power wheelchair.

Cardiovascular/Pulmonary
Heart rate, respiratory rate, and blood pressure were all within normal limits.

Communication, affect, cognition, language, and learning style appeared unimpaired.

Tests and Measurements
General Summary of Function
At the time of his referral, an examination of overall physical function revealed that H.E. could ambulate 25 feet in 20 seconds, roll from a prone to a supine position and back to a prone position, and had adequate sitting balance. He was unable to run, ascend or descend stairs, rise from the floor or from a chair, sit up from a supine position, or assume a posture on all fours. A modified manual muscle examination indicated strength that was graded from "poor" to "absent" for all isolated muscle groups, with the exception of wrist extensors, which were graded as

"fair" to "good." H.E. could function from an electric wheelchair, and he could ambulate slowly using a walker with supervision.

Ventilation, Respiration/Gas Exchange
H.E.'s breathing pattern was examined, and was found to be a diaphragmatic pattern with appropriate intercostal muscle use while at rest and during exertion; his accessory respiratory muscles became active during inspiration and expiration. His respiratory muscle strength was measured using maximum static inspiratory pressure (MSIP), inspiratory capacity (IC), and slow inspiratory vital capacity (IVC). The MSIP was 60% of predicted values; the IC was 45% of predicted values; and the IVC was 45% of predicted values. His maximal static expiratory pressure, a measure of expiratory muscle strength, was 35% of predicted values.

Chest wall expansion was determined with a tape measure, and found to be approximately 2.5 cm at maximal inspiratory effort. Passive motion was adequate at the glenohumeral joints. Coughing was evaluated as being weak and questionably functional. As previously noted, his limited IC and reduced expiratory pressures were largely responsible for the impaired cough.

Evaluation, Diagnosis, and Prognosis
On the basis of the data gathered specific to his current pulmonary issues, H.E. would receive a classification at cardiovascular/pulmonary pattern 6E ventilatory pump dysfunction or failure. This would be a pattern specific to his respiratory muscle impairment for which he was referred. His prognosis would be 8 to 10 weeks of care with episodes of physical therapy two times per week for the first several weeks, and reduced to weekly thereafter.

Interventions
Coordination, communication, and documentation would focus on interaction with the muscular dystrophy center at the children's hospital where H.E. is followed up. Patient instruction would focus on instruction of H.E. and his parents and other caregivers regarding a home exercise program to improve his respiratory muscle strength, enhance his coughing, and provide for AC as needed. In addition, they would be trained in proper AC and assisted cough techniques, including various devices to support AC.

Procedural Interventions
Therapeutic Exercise
Active cycle of breathing to enhance diaphragmatic excursion, maximal inspiration, and FET to aid in improving ventilation to the lower lobes, maintain/improve chest expansion, and aid in secretion removal

Continuing with ongoing strength training and ROM exercise with emphasis on thorax and shoulder girdle to maintain thoracic compliance

Inspiratory and expiratory muscle strengthening using simple handheld devices to maintain/increase respiratory muscle strength

AC as needed using HFCWO with SmartVest or airway oscillation with either Acapella or Flutter device; should secretion removal become problematic, equipment for airway aspiration or insufflation–exsufflation recommended.

REFERENCES

1. Yeatts K, Davis KJ, Sotir M, et al. Who gets diagnosed with asthma? Frequent wheeze among adolescents with and without a diagnosis of asthma. *Pediatrics.* 2003;111(5, pt 1):1046-1054.
2. Centers for Disease Control and Prevention. National Health Interview Survey (NHIS) Data: 2018. Lifetime and Current Asthma. US Department of Health and Human Services. 2016-2018. https://www.cdc.gov/asthma/most_recent_national_asthma_data.htm. Accessed August 13, 2020.
3. Nurmagambetov T, Kuwahara R, Garbe P. The economic burden of asthma in the United States, 2008-2013. *Ann Am Thorac Soc.* 2018;15(3):348-356.
4. American Lung Association. (2012). Trends in asthma morbidity and mortality. https://www.lung.org/research/trends-in-lung-disease/asthma-trends-brief
5. Westbom K, Bergstrand K, Wagner P, et al. Survival at 19 years of age in a total population of children and young people with cerebral palsy. *Dev Med Child Neurol.* 2011;53:808-814.
6. Boyden E. Development and growth of the airways. In: Hodson AW, ed. *Development of the Lung.* Marcel Dekker Inc; 1977:3-35.
7. Haddad GG, Fontan JJP. Development of the respiratory system. In: Berman RE, Kliegman RM, Jensen HB, eds. *Nelson's Textbook of Pediatrics.* 17th ed. Saunders; 2004:1357-1359.
8. Smith LJ, McKay KO, van Asperen PP, et al. Normal development of the lung and premature birth. *Pediatr Respir Rev.* 2010;11:135-142.
9. Avery ME. Hyaline membrane disease. *Am Rev Respir Dis.* 1975;111:657-688.
10. Polgar G, Weng TR. The functional development of the respiratory system. *Am Rev Respir Dis.* 1979;120:625-695.
11. Downes JJ, Fulgencio T, Raphaely RC. Acute respiratory failure in infants and children. *Pediatr Clin North Am.* 1972;19:423-445.
12. Ackerman SJ, Duff SB, Dennehy PH, et al. Economic impact of an infection control education program in a specialized preschool setting. *Pediatrics.* 2001;108(6):E102.
13. Effmann EL, Fram EK, Vock P, et al. Tracheal cross-sectional area in children: CT determination. *Radiology.* 1983;149(1):137-140.
14. Siren PMA, Siren MJ. Critical diaphragm failure in sudden infant death syndrome. *Ups J Med Sci.* 2011;116(2):115-123.
15. Guslits BG, Gaston SE, Bryan MH, et al. Diaphragmatic work of breathing in premature human infants. *J Appl Physiol.* 1987;62(4):1410-1415.
16. Leith DE. The development of cough. *Am Rev Respir Dis.* 1985;131(5):S39-S42.
17. Papastamelos C, Panitch HB, England SE, et al. Developmental changes in chest wall compliance in infancy and early childhood. *J Appl Physiol.* 1995;78:179-184.
18. Pagliara AS, Karl IE, Haymond M, et al. Hypoglycemia in infancy and childhood. *J Pediatr.* 1973;82:365-379.
19. Guide to Physical Therapist Practice 3.0. Alexandria, VA: American Physical Therapy Association; 2014. Available at http://guidetoptpractice.apta.org/
20. Nakamura CT, Ng GY, Paton JY, et al. Correlation between digital clubbing and pulmonary function in cystic fibrosis. *Pediatr Pulmonol.* 2002;33(5):332-338.
21. Nathanson I, Riddlesberger MM Jr. Pulmonary hypertrophic osteoarthropathy in cystic fibrosis. *Radiology.* 1980;135(3):649-651.
22. Boat TA. Cystic fibrosis. In: Berman RE, Kliegman RM, Jensen HB, eds. *Nelson's Textbook of Pediatrics.* 17th ed. Saunders; 2004:1447.
23. Gaultier C. Respiratory muscle function in infants. *Eur Respir J.* 1995;8:150-153.
24. Massery M. Chest development as a component of normal motor development: implications for pediatric physical therapists. *Pediatr Phys Ther.* 1991;3(1):3-8. doi:10.1097/00001577-199100310-00002
25. Li AM, Yin J, Yu CC, et al. The six-minute walk test in healthy children: reliability and validity. *Eur Respir J.* 2005;25(6):1057-1060.
26. Gulmans VA, van Veldhoven NH, de Meer K, et al. The six-minute walking test in children with cystic fibrosis: reliability and validity. *Pediatr Pulmonol.* 1996;22(2):85-89.
27. Tomkinson GR, Leger LA, Olds TS, et al. Secular trends in the performance of children and adolescents (1980-2000): an analysis of 55 studies of the 20m shuttle run test in 11 countries. *Sports Med.* 2003;33(4):285-300.
28. Holland AE, Rasekaba T, Wilson JW, et al. Desaturation during the 3-minute step test predicts impaired 12-month outcomes in adult patients with cystic fibrosis. *Respir Care.* 2011;56(8):1137-1142.
29. Steinkamp G, Wiedemann B. Relationship between nutritional status and lung function in cystic fibrosis: cross sectional and longitudinal analyses from the German CF quality assurance (CFQA) project. *Thorax.* 2002;57(7):596-601.
30. Palevsky HI, Fishman AP. Chronic cor pulmonale. Etiology and management. *JAMA.* 1990;263:2347.
31. Mawdsley RH, Hoy DK, Erwin MP. Criterion-related validity of the figure-of-eight method of measuring ankle edema. *J Orthop Sports Phys Ther.* 2000;30:149.
32. de Meer K, Jeneson JA, Gulmans VA, et al. Efficiency of oxidative work performance of skeletal muscle in patients with cystic fibrosis. *Thorax.* 1995;50:980-983.
33. de Meer K, Gulmans VA, van Der Laag J. Peripheral muscle weakness and exercise capacity in children with cystic fibrosis. *Am J Respir Crit Care Med.* 1999;159(3):748-754.
34. Engel HJ, Tatebe S, Alonzo PB, et al. Physical therapist–established intensive care unit early mobilization program: quality improvement project for critical care at the University of California San Francisco Medical Center. *Phys Ther.* 2013;93:975-985.
35. Nordon-Craft A, Moss M, Quan D, et al. Physical rehabilitation of patients in the intensive care unit requiring extracorporeal membrane oxygenation: a small case series. *Phys Ther.* 2012;92:1494-1506.
36. Marinov B, Mandadjieva S, Kostianev S. Pictorial and verbal category-ratio scales for effort estimation in children. *Child Care Health Dev.* 2008;34:35-43.
37. Pianosi H. Dalhousie pictorial scales measuring dyspnea and perceived exertion during exercise for children and adolescents. *Ann Am Thor Soc.* 2015;12(5):718-726. doi:10.1513/AnnalsATS.201410-477OC
38. Yelling L. Validity of a pictorial perceived exertion scale for effort estimation and effort production during stepping exercise in adolescent children. *Eur Phys Educ Rev.* 2002;8(2):157-175. doi:10.1177/1356336X020082007
39. Roemmich B. Validity of PCERT and OMNI walk/run ratings of perceived exertion. *Med Sci Sports Exerc.* 2006;38(5):1014-1019. doi:10.1249/01.mss.0000218123.81079
40. Prasad R. Fifteen-count breathlessness score: an objective measure for children. *Pediatr Pulmonol.* 2000;30(1):56-62. doi:10.1002/1099-0496(200007)30:1<56::AID-PPUL9>3.0.CO;2-R
41. Chen MJ, Fan X, Moe ST. Criterion-related validity of the Borg ratings of perceived exertion scale in healthy individuals: a meta-analysis. *J Sports Sci.* 2002;20(11):873-899.
42. Pfeiffer KA, Pivarnik JM, Womack CJ, et al. Reliability and validity of the Borg and OMNI rating of perceived exertion scales in adolescent girls. *Med Sci Sports Exerc.* 2002;34(12):2057-2061.
43. McGrath PJ, Pianosi PT, Unruh AM, et al. Dalhousie dyspnea scales: construct and content validity of pictorial scales for measuring dyspnea. *BMC Pediatr.* 2005;5:33.
44. Bieri D, Reeve R, Champion G, et al. The Faces Pain Scale for the self-assessment of the severity of pain experienced by children: development, initial validation and preliminary investigation for ratio scale properties. *Pain.* 1990;41:139-150.
45. Hicks CL, von Baeyer CL, Spafford PA, et al. The Faces Pain Scale-Revised: toward a common metric in pediatric pain measurement. *Pain.* 2001;93(2):173-183.
46. Koumbourlis AC, Stolar CJ. Lung growth and function in children and adolescents with idiopathic pectus excavatum. *Pediatr Pulmonol.* 2004;38(4):339-343.

47. Button BM, Heine RG, Catto-Smith AG, et al. Postural drainage in cystic fibrosis: is there a link with gastro-oesophageal reflux? *J Paediatr Child Health*. 1998;34(4):330-334.

48. Button BM, Heine RG, Catto-Smith AG, et al. Chest physiotherapy in infants with cystic fibrosis: to tip or not? A five-year study. *Pediatr Pulmonol*. 2003;35(3):208-213.

49. Crane L. Physical therapy for the neonate with respiratory disease. In: Irwin S, Tecklin JS, eds. *Cardiopulmonary Physical Therapy*. 3rd ed. CV Mosby; 1995.

50. Savci S, Ince DI, Arikan H. A comparison of autogenic drainage and the active cycle of breathing techniques in patients with chronic obstructive pulmonary diseases. *J Cardiopulm Rehabil*. 2000;20(1):37-43.

51. DeCesare J. Physical therapy for the child with respiratory dysfunction. In: Irwin S, Tecklin JS, eds. *Cardiopulmonary Physical Therapy*. 3rd ed. CV Mosby; 1995.

52. Morrow BM, Futter MJ, Argent AC. Endotracheal suctioning: from principles to practice. *Intensive Care Med*. 2004;30(6):1167-1174.

53. Dab I, Alexander F. Evaluation of a particular bronchial drainage procedure called autogenic drainage. In: Baran K, Van Bogaert K, eds. *Chest Physical Therapy in Cystic Fibrosis and Chronic Obstructive Pulmonary Disease*. European Press; 1977:185-187.

54. Dab I, Alexander F. The mechanism of autogenic drainage studied with flow volume curves. *Monogr Paediat*. 1979;10:50-53.

55. Miller S, Hall DO, Clayton CB, et al. Chest physiotherapy in cystic fibrosis: a comparative study of autogenic drainage and the active cycle of breathing techniques with postural drainage. *Thorax*. 1995;50(2):165-169.

56. Pryor JA, Webber BA, Hodson ME, et al. Evaluation of the forced expiratory technique as an adjunct to postural drainage in treatment of cystic fibrosis. *Br Med J*. 1979;2:417-418.

57. Partridge C, Pryor J, Webber B. Characteristics of the forced expiratory technique. *Physiotherapy*. 1989;75:193-194.

58. Hofmyer JL, Webber BA, Hodson ME. Evaluation of positive expiratory pressure as an adjunct to chest physiotherapy in the treatment of cystic fibrosis. *Thorax*. 1986;41:951-954.

59. Gondor M, Nixon PA, Mutich R, et al. Comparison of Flutter device and chest physical therapy in the treatment of cystic fibrosis pulmonary exacerbation. *Pediatr Pulmonol*. 1999;28(4):255-260.

60. King M, Zidulka A, Phillips DM, et al. Tracheal mucus clearance in high-frequency oscillation: effect of peak flow bias. *Eur Respir J*. 1990;3:6.

61. Warwick W. High frequency chest compression moves mucus by means of sustained staccato coughs. *Pediatr Pulmonol*. 1991;(suppl 6):283, A219.

62. Tomkiewicz RP, Biviji A, King M. Effects of oscillating air flow on the rheological properties and clearability of mucous gel simulants. *Biorheology*. 1994;31(5):511-520.

63. King M, Phillips DM, Zidulka A, et al. Tracheal mucus clearance in high-frequency oscillation. II: chest wall versus mouth oscillation. *Am Rev Respir Dis*. 1984;130(5):703-706.

64. Darbee J, Cerny F. Exercise testing and exercise conditioning for children with lung dysfunction. In: Irwin S, Tecklin JS, eds. *Cardiopulmonary Physical Therapy*. 3rd ed. CV Mosby; 1990:570.

65. Orenstein DM, Hovell MF, Mulvihill M, et al. Strength vs aerobic training in children with cystic fibrosis: a randomized controlled trial. *Chest*. 2004;126(4):1204-1214.

66. Keens TG, Krastins IRB, Wannamaker EM, et al. Ventilatory muscle endurance training in normal subjects and patients with cystic fibrosis. *Am Rev Respir Dis*. 1977;116:853-860.

67. Enright S, Chatham K, Ionescu AA, et al. Inspiratory muscle training improves lung function and exercise capacity in adults with cystic fibrosis. *Chest*. 2004;126(2):405-411.

68. Weiner P, Magadle R, Beckerman M, et al. Comparison of specific expiratory, inspiratory, and combined muscle training programs in COPD. *Chest*. 2003;124(4):1357-1364.

69. Weisgerber MC, Guill M, Weisgerber JM, et al. Benefits of swimming in asthma: effect of a session of swimming lessons on symptoms and PFTs with review of the literature. *J Asthma*. 2003;40(5):453-464.

70. Orenstein D, Franklin BA, Doershuk CF, et al. Exercise conditioning and cardiopulmonary fitness in cystic fibrosis. *Chest*. 1981;80:392.

71. Laennec RTH, Forbes J, trans. *Diseases of the Chest*. 4th ed. Thomas Cowperthwaite and Co.; 1819.

72. Sharma A. Respiratory Distress. In: Kliegman RM, Toth H, Bordini BJ, Basel D, eds. *Nelson Pediatric Symptom Based Diagnosis*. 1st ed. Elsevier; 2018:39-60.

73. Felcar JM, Guitti JCS, Marson AC, et al. Preoperative physiotherapy in prevention of pulmonary complications in pediatric cardiac surgery. *Rev Bras Cir Cardiovasc*. 2008:383-388.

74. Ferreyra G, Long Y, Ranieri VM. Respiratory complications after major surgery. *Curr Opin Crit Care*. 2009;15(4):342-348.

75. Thoren L. Postoperative pulmonary complications: observations on their prevention by means of physiotherapy. *Acta Chir Scand*. 1954;107:193-205.

76. Stein M, Cassara EL. Preoperative pulmonary evaluation and therapy for surgery patients. *JAMA*. 1970;211:787-790.

77. Bartlett RH, Gazzinga AB, Graghty JR. Respiratory maneuvers to prevent postoperative complications. *JAMA*. 1973;224:1017-1021.

78. Hymes AC, Yonehiro EG, Raab DE, et al. Electrical surface stimulation for treatment and prevention of ileus and atelectasis. *Surg Forum*. 1974;25:222-224.

79. Finer MN, Moriartey RR, Boyd J, et al. Postextubation atelectasis. A retrospective review and a prospective controlled study. *J Pediatr*. 1979;94:110-113.

80. Flenady VJ, Gray PH. Chest physiotherapy for preventing morbidity in babies being extubated from mechanical ventilation. *Cochrane Database Syst Rev*. 2002;(2):CD000283.

81. Wong I, Fok TF. Randomized comparison of two physiotherapy regimens for correcting atelectasis in ventilated pre-term neonates. *Hong Kong Physiother J*. 2003;21:43-50.

82. Chen YC, Wu LF, Mu PF, et al. Using chest vibration nursing intervention to improve expectoration of airway secretions and prevent lung collapse in ventilated ICU patients: a randomized controlled trial. *J Chin Med Assoc*. 2009;72(6):316-322.

83. Graham RJ, Fleegler EW, Robinson WM. Chronic ventilator need in the community: a 2005 pediatric census of Massachusetts. *Pediatrics*. 2007;119:e1280-e1287.

84. Kennedy JD, Martin AJ. Chronic respiratory failure and neuromuscular disease. *Pediatr Clin North Am*. 2009;56:261-273.

85. Wolfe LF, Joyce NC, McDonald CM, et al. Management of pulmonary complications in neuromuscular disease. *Phys Med Rehabil Clin N Am*. 2012;23(4):829-853.

86. Yang ML, Finkel RS. Overview of paediatric neuromuscular disorders and related pulmonary issues: diagnostic and therapeutic considerations. *Paediatr Respir Rev*. 2010;11(1):9-17.

87. Mallory GB, Stillwell PC. The ventilator-dependent child: issues in diagnosis and management. *Arch Phys Med Rehabil*. 1991;72:43-55.

88. Domènech-Clar R, López-Andreu JA, Compte-Torrero L, et al. Maximal static respiratory pressures in children and adolescents. *Pediatr Pulmonol*. 2003;35(2):126-132.

89. Shardonofsky FR, Perez-Chada D, Carmuega E, et al. Airway pressures during crying in healthy infants. *Pediatr Pulmonol*. 1989;6:14-18.

90. Shardonofsky FR, Perez-Chada D, Milic-Emili J. Airway pressures during crying: an index of respiratory muscle strength in infants with neuromuscular disease. *Pediatr Pulmonol*. 1991;10:172-177.

91. Finder JD. Airway clearance modalities in neuromuscular disease. *Paediatr Respir Rev*. 2010;11:31-34.

92. Gauld LM, Boynton A. Relationship between peak cough flow and spirometry in Duchenne muscular dystrophy. *Pediatr Pulmonol*. 2005;39:457-460.

93. Wanke T, Toifl K, Formanek D, et al. Inspiratory muscle training in patients with Duchenne muscular dystrophy. *Chest*. 1994;105:475-482.

94. Aloysius A, Born P, Kinali M, et al. Swallowing difficulties in Duchenne muscular dystrophy: indications for feeding assessment and outcome of videoflurooscopic swallow studies. *Eur J Paediatr Neurol*. 2008;12:239-245.

95. Hull J, Aniapravan R, Chan E, et al. British Thoracic Society guideline for respiratory management of children with neuromuscular weakness. *Thorax*. 2012;67(suppl 1):i1-i40. doi:10.1136/thoraxjnl-2012-201964

96. Merrick J, Axen K. Inspiratory muscle function following abdominal weight exercises in healthy subject. *Phys Ther*. 1981;61:651-656.

97. Winkler G, Zifko U, Nader A, et al. Dose-dependent effects of inspiratory muscle training in neuromuscular disorders. *Muscle Nerve*. 2000;23(8):1257-1260.

98. Barker NJ, Jones M, O'Connell NE, et al. Breathing exercises for dysfunctional breathing/hyperventilation syndrome in children. *Cochrane Database Syst Rev*. 2013;12:CD010376. doi:10.1002/14651858.CD010376.pub2

99. Cup EH, Pieterse AJ, ten Broek-Pastoor JM, et al. Exercise therapy and other types of physical therapy for patients with neuromuscular diseases: a systematic review. *Arch Phys Med Rehabil*. 2007;88:1452-1461.

100. Miske L, Hickey E, Kolb S, et al. Use of the mechanical in exsufflator in pediatric patients with neuromuscular disease and impaired cough. *Chest*. 2004;125:1406-1412.

101. Barach AL, Beck GL, Bickerman HA, et al. Physical methods simulating mechanisms of the human cough. *J Appl Physiol*. 1952;5:85-90.

102. Bach JR. Amyotrophic lateral sclerosis: prolongation of life by noninvasive respiratory aids. *Chest*. 2002;122:92-98.

103. Reddel HK, Taylor DR, Bateman ED, et al. Asthma control and exacerbations. *Am J Respir Crit Care Med*. 2009;180:59-99.

104. Adams PF, Kirzinger WK, Martinez ME. Summary health statistics for the U.S. population: National Health Interview Survey, 2011. National Center for Health Statistics. *Vital Health Stat*. 2012;10(255).1-110

105. Moorman JE, Rudd RA, Johnson CA. National surveillance for asthma–United States, 1980-2004. *MMWR Surveill Summ*. 2007;56:1-54.

106. Rowe BH, Bota G, Clark S. Comparison of Canadian versus American emergency department visits for acute asthma. *Can Respir J*. 2007;14:331-337.

107. Haslett C. Asthma: cellular and humoral mechanisms. In Seaton D, Leitch AG, Seaton D, eds. *Crofton and Douglas's Respiratory Diseases*. Wiley Publishers; 2008:916-917.

108. National Asthma Education and Prevention Program. *Expert Panel Report III: Guidelines for the Diagnosis and Management of Asthma*. National Heart, Lung, and Blood Institute; 2007 (NIH publication no. 08-4051).

109. Craven D, Kercsmar CM, Myers TR, et al. Ipratropium bromide plus nebulized albuterol for the treatment of hospitalized children with acute asthma. *J Pediatr*. 2001;138(1):51-58.

110. Rowe BH, Spooner CH, Ducharme FM, et al. Early emergency department treatment of acute asthma with systemic corticosteroids. *Cochrane Database Syst Rev*. 2001;1:CD002178.

111. Ni Chroinin M, Lasserson TJ, Greenstone I, et al. Addition of long-acting beta-agonists to inhaled corticosteroids for chronic asthma in children. *Cochrane Database Syst Rev*. 2009;3:CD007949.

112. Rao D, Phipatanakul W. Impact of environmental controls on childhood asthma. *Curr Allergy Asthma Rep*. 2011;11(5):414-420.

113. Kim JM, Lin SY, Suarez-Cuervo C, et al. Allergen-specific immunotherapy for pediatric asthma and rhinoconjunctivitis: a systematic review. *Pediatrics*. 2013;131(6):1155-1167.

114. Andrade LB, Silva DA, Salgado TL, et al. Comparison of six-minute walk test in children with moderate/severe asthma with reference values for healthy children. *J Pediatr (Rio J)*. 2014;90(3):250-257. doi:10.1016/j.jped.2013.08.006

115. Jinzhou Y, Fu Y, Zhang R, et al. The reliability and sensitivity of indices related to cardiovascular fitness evaluation. *Kinesiology*. 2008;40(2):139-146.

116. Liu L, Plowman S, Looney M. The reliability and validity of the 20-metre shuttle test in American students 12-15 years old. *Res Q Exerc Sport*. 1992;63:360-365.

117. Schechter MS. Airway clearance applications in infants and children. *Respir Care*. 2007;52(10):1382-1390; discussion 1390-1391.

118. Huber AL, Eggleston PA, Morgan J. Effect of chest physiotherapy on asthmatic children (abstract). *J Allergy Clin Immunol*. 1974;53:2.

119. Huntley A, White A, Ernst E. Relaxation therapies for asthma: a systematic review. *Thorax*. 2002;57(2):127-131.

120. Yorke J, Fleming SL, Shuldham C. A systematic review of psychological interventions for children with asthma. *Pediatr Pulmonol*. 2007;42(2):114-124.

121. Milgrom H, Taussig LM. Keeping children with exercise-induced asthma active. *Pediatrics*. 1999;104:e38.

122. Bonini M, Di Mambro C, Calderon MA, et al. Beta2-agonists for exercise-induced asthma. *Cochrane Database Syst Rev*. 2013;10:CD003564.

123. Mendes F, Cukier A, Stelmach R, et al. Which asthmatic patients benefits most from aerobic training program? Paper presented at: European Respiratory Society Annual Congress; September 18-22, 2010; Barcelona, Spain. http://www.incor.usp.br/sites/incor2013/docs/imprensa/congresso-euro-respiratory/set-2010/Which-Asthmatic-Patients-Benefits.pdf

124. Moreira A, Delgado L, Haahtela T, et al. Physical training does not increase allergic inflammation in asthmatic children. *Eur Respir J*. 2008;32(6):1570-1575.

125. Mancuso CA, Choi TN, Westermann H, et al. Improvement in asthma quality of life in patients enrolled in a prospective study to increase lifestyle physical activity. *J Asthma*. 2013;50(1):103-107.

126. Carson KV, Chandratilleke MG, Picot J, et al. Physical training for asthma. *Cochrane Database Syst Rev*. 2013;9:CD001116.

127. Sly RM, Harper RT, Rosselot I. The effect of physical conditioning upon asthmatic children. *Ann Allerg*. 1972;30:86-94.

128. Fitch KD, Morton AR, Blanksby BA. Effects of swimming training on children with asthma. *Arch Dis Child*. 1976;51(3):190-194.

129. Wang JS, Hung WP. The effects of a swimming intervention for children with asthma. *Respirology*. 2009;14(6):838-842.

130. Font-Ribera L, Villanueva CM, Nieuwenhuijsen MJ, et al. Swimming pool attendance, asthma, allergies, and lung function in the Avon Longitudinal Study of Parents and Children cohort. *Am J Respir Crit Care Med*. 2011;183(5):582-588.

131. Beggs S, Foong YC, Le HC, et al. Swimming training for asthma in children and adolescents aged 18 years and under. *Cochrane Database Syst Rev*. 2013;(4):CD009607.

132. Rommens JM, Iannuzzi MC, Kerem B, et al. Identification of the cystic fibrosis gene: chromosome walking and jumping. *Science*. 1989;245:1059-1065.

133. Pilewski JM, Frizzell RA. Role of CFTR in airway disease. *Physiol Rev*. 1999;79(1)(suppl):S215-S255.

134. Simonds NJ. Ageing in cystic fibrosis and long-term survival. *Paediatr Respir Rev*. 2013;14(suppl 1):6.

135. Flume PA, Yankaskas JR, Ebeling M, et al. Massive hemoptysis in cystic fibrosis. *Chest*. 2005;128:729-738.

136. Flume PA, Strange C, Ye X, et al. Pneumothorax in cystic fibrosis. *Chest*. 2005;128:720-728.

137. Slattery DM, Waltz DA, Denham B, et al. Bronchoscopically administered human DNase for lobar atelectasis in cystic fibrosis. *Pediatr Pulmonol*. 2001;31:383-388.

138. Bright-Thomas RJ, Webb AK. The heart in cystic fibrosis. *J R Soc Med*. 2002;95(suppl 41):2-10.

139. Cystic Fibrosis Foundation. Infection prevention and control policy. https://www.cff.org/Care/Clinical-Care-Guidelines/Infection-Prevention-and-Control-Care-Guidelines/ accessed 2/4/2021

140. Liou TG, Adler FR, Cox DR, et al. Transplantation and survival in children with cystic fibrosis. *N Engl J Med*. 2007;357:2143-2152.

141. Allen J, Visner G. Lung transplantation in cystic fibrosis—primum non nocere? *N Engl J Med*. 2007;357:2186-2188.

142. Thabut G, Christie JD, Mal H, et al. Survival benefit of lung transplant for cystic fibrosis since lung allocation score implementation. *Am J Respir Crit Care Med*. 2013;187(12):1335-1340.

143. Ramsey BW, Davies J, McElvaney NG, et al. A CFTR potentiator in patients with cystic fibrosis and the G551D mutation. *N Engl J Med*. 2011;365:1663-1672.

144. Nixon PA, Orenstein DM, Kelsey SF. Habitual physical activity in children and adolescents with cystic fibrosis. *Med Sci Sports Exerc.* 2001;33(1):30-35.

145. Radtke T, Stevens D, Benden C, et al. Clinical exercise testing in children and adolescents with cystic fibrosis. *Pediatr Phys Ther.* 2009;21(3):275-281.

146. Nixon PA, Orenstein DM, Kelsey SF, et al. The prognostic value of exercise testing in patients with cystic fibrosis. *N Engl J Med.* 1992;327:1785-1788.

147. Moorcroft AJ, Dodd ME, Webb AK. Exercise testing and prognosis in adult cystic fibrosis. *Thorax.* 1997;52:291-293.

148. ATS Committee on Proficiency Standards for Clinical Pulmonary Function Laboratories. ATS Statement: guidelines for the six-minute walk test. *Am J Respir Crit Care Med.* 2002;166:111-117.

149. Narang I, Pike S, Rosenthal M, et al. Three-minute step test to assess exercise capacity in children with cystic fibrosis with mild lung disease. *Pediatr Pulmonol.* 2003;35:108-113.

150. Selvadurai HC, Cooper PJ, Meyers N, et al. Validation of shuttle tests in children with cystic fibrosis. *Pediatr Pulmonol.* 2003;35(2):133-138.

151. Lorin MI, Denning CR. Evaluation of postural drainage by measurement of sputum volume and consistency. *Am J Phys Med.* 1971;50:215-219.

152. Tecklin JS, Holsclaw DS. Evaluation of bronchial drainage in patients with cystic fibrosis. *Phys Ther.* 1975;55:1081-1084.

153. Feldman J, Traver GA, Taussig LM. Maximal expiratory flows after postural drainage. *Am Rev Respir Dis.* 1979;119:239-245.

154. Warwick WJ, Hansen LG. The long-term effect of high frequency chest compression therapy on pulmonary complications of cystic fibrosis. *Pediatr Pulmonol.* 1991;11:265-271.

155. Motoyama EK. Lower airway obstruction. In: Mangos JA, Talamo RD, eds. *Fundamental Problems of Cystic Fibrosis and Related Diseases.* Intercontinental Medical Book Corp; 1973.

156. Desmond KF, Schwenk F, Thomas E, et al. Immediate and long-term effects of chest physiotherapy in patients with cystic fibrosis. *J Pediatr.* 1983;103:538-542.

157. McIlwaine PM, Davidson AGF. Cystic fibrosis, basic and clinical research. Comparison of expiratory pressure and autogenic drainage with conventional percussion and drainage therapy in the treatment of cystic fibrosis. In: *Proceedings of the 17th European Cystic Fibrosis Conference, Copenhagen, Denmark.* Amsterdam, Netherlands: Elsevier Science BV; 1991:54.

158. Pfleger A, Theissl B, Oberwalder B, et al. Self-administered chest physiotherapy in cystic fibrosis: a comparative study of high-pressure PEP and autogenic drainage. *Lung.* 1992;170:323-330.

159. Miller S, Hall D, Clayton CB, et al. Chest physiotherapy in cystic fibrosis: a comparative study of autogenic drainage and active cycle of breathing technique (formerly called FET). *Pediatr Pulmonol.* 1993;(suppl 9):267.

160. Butler-Simon N, McCool P, Giles D, et al. Efficacy and desirability of autogenic drainage vs. conventional postural drainage and percussion. *Pediatr Pulmonol.* 1995;(suppl 253):179.

161. McIlwaine MP, Alarie N, Davidson GF, et al. Long-term multicentre randomized controlled study of high frequency chest wall oscillation versus positive expiratory pressure mask in cystic fibrosis. *Thorax.* 2013;68(8):746-751.

162. Darbee JC, Ohtake PJ, Grant BJ, et al. Physiologic evidence for the efficacy of positive expiratory pressure as an airway clearance technique in patients with cystic fibrosis. *Phys Ther.* 2004;84(6):524-537.

163. West K, Wallen M, Follett J. Acapella vs. PEP mask therapy: a randomised trial in children with cystic fibrosis during respiratory exacerbation. *Physiother Theory Pract.* 2010;26(3):143-149.

164. Arens R, Gozal D, Omlin KJ, et al. Comparison of high frequency chest compression and conventional chest physiotherapy in hospitalized patients with cystic fibrosis. *Am J Respir Crit Care Med.* 1994;150(4):1154-1157.

165. Tecklin JS, Clayton RG, Scanlin TF. High frequency chest wall oscillation vs. traditional chest physical therapy in CF- a large, one-year, controlled study. *Pediatr Pulmonol.* 2000;459(Suppl. 20).

166. Pryor JA. Physiotherapy for airway clearance in adults. *Eur Respir J.* 1999;14:1418-1424.

167. Main E. What is the best airway clearance technique in cystic fibrosis? *Pediatr Respir Rev.* 2013;14(suppl 1):10-12.

168. Cropp GJA, Pullano TP, Cerny FJ, et al. Adaptation to exercise in cystic fibrosis. *CF Club Abstr.* 1979;20:32.

169. Marcus CL, Bader D, Stabile MW, et al. Supplemental oxygen and exercise performance in patients with cystic fibrosis with severe pulmonary disease. *Chest.* 1992;101:52-57.

170. Moorcraft AJ, Dodd ME, Howarth C, et al. Muscular fatigue, ventilation, and perception of limitation at peak exercise in adults with cystic fibrosis. *Pediatr Pulmonol.* 1996;(suppl 13):306.

171. Williams CA, Benden C, Stevens D, et al. Exercise training in children and adolescents with cystic fibrosis: theory into practice. *Int J Pediatr.* 2010;2010:670640.

Fitness and Prevention

Kathleen Coultes

» Children with obesity

Pediatric physical therapists (PTs) can be found in a variety of practice settings. Whether working in early intervention, acute care, educational arenas, or within community and outpatient settings, the epidemic of pediatric obesity can be readily appreciated. In 2018, the American Physical Therapy Association (APTA) established a mission statement that reads, "Building a community that advances the profession of physical therapy to improve the health of society."[1] Because childhood obesity has clearly become a health crisis, this chapter is dedicated to increasing the knowledge base of pediatric PTs in the definitions, prevalence, trends, and health impacts, as well as suggesting clinical paths that might be taken to begin halting this epidemic, thus offering tools by which the mission of the APTA and the vision of "transforming society by optimizing movement to improve the human experience" may be met.[1] Because obesity was formally established as a diagnosis by the American Medical Association (AMA) in June, 2013, the International Classification of Functioning, Disability and Health (ICF) framework as well as the APTA Guide to Physical Therapist Practice are considered in the call to action for pediatric PTs to become primary service providers in health promotion and wellness.[2,3]

» Scope of the issue

Despite the comprehensive efforts from health policymakers, industry, and media to bring to light the major health consequences related to obesity, research indicates that it remains an issue of epidemic proportion. The American College of Sports Medicine (ACSM) has defined obesity as "percent fat at which disease risk increases."[4] The U.S. Centers for Disease Control and Prevention (CDC) reports that findings from the National Health and Nutrition Examination Survey (NHANES) 2015 to 2016 continue to suggest alarming statistics regarding obesity in the United States. In the country, 39.6% of adults and 18.5% of children and adolescents were found to be obese. Overall, the prevalence of obesity among adolescents (12 to 19 years) at 20.6% and school-aged children (6 to 11 years) at 18.4% was higher than that among preschool-aged children (2 to 5 years) at 13.9%. School-aged boys (20.4%) had a higher prevalence of obesity than did preschool-aged boys (14.3%). Adolescent girls (20.9%) had a higher prevalence of obesity than did preschool-aged girls (13.5%) (Fig. 20.1).[5]

Another area of concern for health care providers is the rise in the number of young children, between 3 and 5 years of age, who are now being identified as obese. Estimates in 2005 to 2006 were that 10.7% of these young children were obese, as compared to 2015 to 2016 where the percentage rose to 13.9%.[5-7] As integral members of the early intervention team, PTs are often in homes providing care for children at this age. Knowledge translation of this information to parents should be part of the plan of care for these children.

Although this survey did suggest that the rapid increases seen in childhood obesity in the 1980s and 1990s have not continued, current estimates by the AMA have suggested that rates of childhood obesity have increased more than three-fold in the past 30 years.[6] Table 20.1 shows the increase in childhood obesity as described by the NHANES.[8] These numbers represent just a moment in time, because prevalence figures are constantly changing for this health crisis.

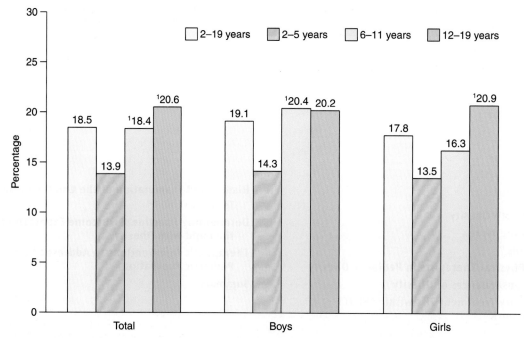

FIGURE 20.1. Prevalence of obesity among youth aged 2 to 19 years, by sex and age in the United States, 2015–2016[5]. [1]Significantly different from those aged 2 to 5 years. NCHS, National Health and Nutrition Examination Survey, 2015–2016.

In addition to the prevalence information available regarding age variations in obesity, it is important that health care providers recognize racial, ethnic, and socioeconomic disparities in obesity prevalence rates. Again, referring to the NHANES 2015 to 2016, it has been found that obesity rates are highest among non-Hispanic black and Hispanic children than among non-Hispanic white and non-Hispanic Asian children.[9]

Table 20.2 further defines the disparity. This information can provide PTs with a profile for those clients of at-risk populations when seen for developmental, orthopedic, or other diagnosis that may decrease the child's overall activity level.

TABLE 20.1.	Prevalence of Overweight, Obesity, and Severe Obesity among Children and Adolescents Aged 2–19 Years, by Sex: United States, 1971–1974 through 2015–2016

		Percentage (Standard Error)																		
		All*						Boys						Girls*						
Survey Period	Sample (*n*)	Overweight		Obesity		Severe Obesity		Overweight		Obesity		Severe Obesity		Overweight		Obesity		Severe Obesity	
1971–1974	7,041	10.2	(0.6)	5.2	(0.3)	1.0	(0.1)	10.3	(0.8)	5.3	(0.5)	1.0	(0.2)	10.1	(0.8)	5.1	(0.4)	1.0	(0.2)
1976–1980	7,351	9.2	(0.4)	5.5	(0.4)	1.3	(0.2)	9.4	(0.6)	5.4	(0.4)	1.2	(0.3)	9.0	(0.5)	5.6	(0.6)	1.3	(0.3)
1988–1994	10,777	13.0	(0.7)	10.0	(0.5)	2.6	(0.4)	12.6	(0.9)	10.2	(0.7)	2.7	(0.5)	13.4	(0.9)	9.8	(0.8)	2.6	(0.4)
1999–2000	4,039	14.2	(0.9)	13.9	(0.9)	3.6	(0.5)	15.0	(1.9)	14.0	(1.2)	3.7	(0.7)	13.4	(0.8)	13.8	(1.1)	3.6	(0.6)
2001–2002	4,261	14.6	(0.6)	15.4	(0.9)	5.2	(0.5)	14.2	(0.7)	16.4	(1.0)	6.1	(0.8)	15.0	(0.9)	14.3	(1.3)	4.2	(0.6)
2003–2004	3,961	16.5	(0.8)	17.1	(1.3)	5.1	(0.6)	16.6	(1.0)	18.2	(1.5)	5.4	(0.8)	16.3	(0.9)	16.0	(1.4)	4.7	(0.7)
2005–2006	4,207	14.6	(0.9)	15.4	(1.4)	4.7	(0.6)	14.7	(1.2)	15.9	(1.5)	4.9	(0.8)	14.6	(1.0)	14.9	(1.6)	4.5	(0.7)
2007–2008	3,249	14.8	(0.7)	16.8	(1.3)	4.9	(0.6)	14.3	(0.7)	17.7	(1.4)	5.5	(0.8)	15.4	(1.5)	15.9	(1.5)	4.3	(0.8)
2009–2010	3,408	14.9	(0.8)	16.9	(0.7)	5.6	(0.6)	14.4	(1.0)	18.6	(1.1)	6.4	(1.0)	15.4	(0.9)	15.0	(0.8)	4.7	(0.6)
2011–2012	3,355	14.9	(0.9)	16.9	(1.0)	5.6	(0.7)	15.4	(1.3)	16.7	(1.4)	5.7	(0.9)	14.5	(1.4)	17.2	(1.2)	5.5	(0.8)
2013–2014	3,523	16.2	(0.6)	17.2	(1.1)	6.0	(0.6)	16.4	(0.8)	17.2	(1.3)	5.6	(0.6)	16.0	(1.0)	17.1	(1.6)	6.3	(0.9)
2015–2016	3,340	16.6	(0.8)	18.5	(1.3)	5.6	(0.8)	15.7	(1.0)	19.1	(1.7)	6.3	(1.0)	17.6	(1.2)	17.8	(1.2)	4.9	(0.9)

Overweight is body mass index (BMI) at or above the 85th percentile and below than the 95th percentile from the sex-specific BMI-for-age 2000 CDC Growth Charts. Obesity is BMI at or above the 95th percentile. Severe obesity is BMI at or above 120% of the 95th percentile.
* Excludes pregnant females.
NCHS, National Health and Nutrition Examination Survey.
From Centers for Disease Control and Prevention. *NCHS Health E – Stat.* Accessed October, 2019. www.cdc.gov/NCHS/data/hestat/obesity_Child_15_16/obesity_child_15_16.htm

TABLE 20.2. Obesity among Children and Adolescents Aged 2 to 19 Years				
Race and Hispanic† Origin and Percentage of poverty Level	1988–1994	2003–2006	2009–2012	2013–2016
Both sexes‡	10.0	16.3	16.9	17.8
Not Hispanic or Latino				
White only	9.2	14.7	14.0	14.7
Black or African American only	12.5	20.7	22.1	20.4
Asian only	—	—	—	9.8
Hispanic or Latino	—	—	21.8	23.6
Mexican origin	14.3	20.9	21.9	24.2
Percent of poverty level§:				
Below 100%	12.6	18.9	20.9	21.0
100%–199%	10.2	17.4	18.5	20.7
200%–399%	9.4	17.1	15.9	16.9
400% or more	4.7*	11.0	11.5	12.2

* Estimates are considered unreliable.
† Persons of Hispanic and Mexican origin may be of any race. Starting with 1999 data, race-specific estimates are tabulated according to the 1997 Revisions to the Standards for the Classification of Federal Data on Race and Ethnicity and are not strictly comparable with estimates for earlier years. The non-Hispanic race categories shown in the table conform to the 1997 Standards. Starting with 1999 data, race-specific estimates are for persons who reported only one racial group. Before data year 1999, estimates were tabulated according to the 1977 Standards. Estimates for single-race categories before 1999 included persons who reported one race; or if they reported more than one race, identified one race as best representing their race. See Appendix II, Hispanic origin; Race.
‡ Includes persons of all races and Hispanic origins, not just those shown separately.
§ Percentage of poverty level was calculated by dividing family income by the U.S. Department of Health and Human Services' poverty guideline specific to family size, as well as the appropriate year and state. Persons with unknown percentage of poverty level are excluded (6% in 2013–2016). See Appendix II, Family income; Poverty.
—, Data not available.
Excel version (with more data years and standard errors when available): https://www.cdc.gov/nchs/hus/contents2018.htm.Table_027.[9]

In the adult population, obesity rates were found to be inversely associated with income and educational levels in women, with increased body mass index (BMI) found in those adults with less income and education. However, the relationship between income and obesity in children is less consistent, with some indication of the opposite relationship being true.[10] This led to the recommendation by the White House Task Force on Childhood Obesity in 2010 that "efforts to reeducate ethnic disparities in obesity must target factors other than income and education, such as environmental, social, and cultural factors."[10]

Beyond racial, ethnic, and socioeconomic disparities, there exist regional disparities within the United States. Although the NHANES reports data from actual physical examination data, the Behavioral Risk Factor Surveillance System (BRFSS) is a national survey of self-reported health information. See Figure 20.2 for the BRFSS trends.[11]

Because it has been clearly identified as a national health crisis, obesity in both children and adults has taken a huge financial toll on the health care system. Although specific health impairments are addressed later in the chapter, it is important to point out here that obesity has been estimated to cause 112,000 deaths per year in the United States.[10] The White House Task Force on Childhood Obesity Report to the President in 2010 documents the financial burden to the health care system, with an estimated $1,429 more in medical expenses incurred annually by adults with obesity

as compared to normal-weight peers. Estimates on medical spending on adults attributed to obesity topped $40 billion in 1998, with an increased estimate to $147 billion in 2008. Direct medical costs were estimated at $3 billion per year for children due to excess body weight. It also reported alarming statistics on how overweight and obese children are more likely to become obese adults. A study that suggests obese 6- to 8-year-olds were approximately ten times more likely to become obese adults than were those with lower BMIs was revealed. It goes on to say that the association may be stronger for obese adolescents than for younger children.[10]

Presence of developmental disabilities has also been clearly associated with increased prevalence of childhood obesity. Table 20.3 shows the impact on prevalence for various conditions that are seen regularly with children already receiving physical therapy in early intervention, school-age services, or outpatient settings.

In 2000, the APTA House of Delegates adopted its official vision statement for the future of physical therapy entitled Vision 2020. The following excerpt relates to how this obesity epidemic is within the scope of practice for physical therapists: "By 2020, physical therapy will be provided by physical therapists who are doctors of physical therapy, recognized by consumers and other health care professionals as the practitioners of choice to whom consumers have direct access for the diagnosis of, interventions for, and prevention of impairments, activity limitations, participation restrictions, and

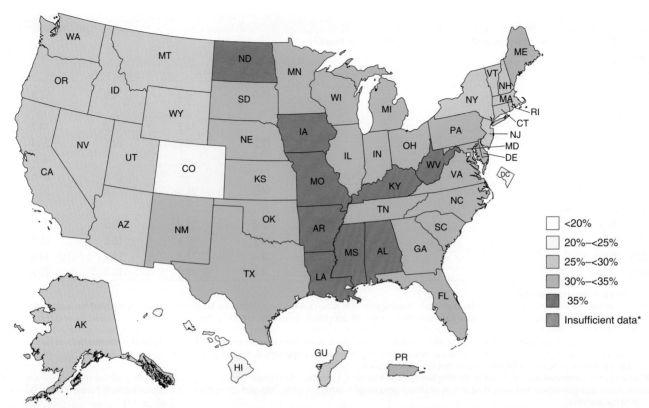

FIGURE 20.2. Map: Overall obesity. [†]Prevalence of Self-Reported Obesity Among U.S. Adults by State and Territory, BRFSS, 2018. Prevalence estimates reflect Behavioral Risk Factor Surveillance System (BRFSS) methodologic changes started in 2011. These estimates should not be compared to prevalence estimates before 2011. *Sample size <50 or the relative standard error (dividing the standard error by the prevalence) ≥ 30%.

TABLE 20.3. Developmental Disabilities and Obesity Prevalence	
With attention deficit hyperactivity disorder	17.6%
With intellectual disability	19.8%
With learning disorder/other developmental disability	20.3%
With any learning behavioral developmental disability	20.4%
With autism	31.8%
With Down syndrome	47.8%

From Phillips KL, Schieve LA, Visser S, et al. Prevalence and impact of unhealthy weight in a national sample of US adolescents with autism and other learning and behavioral disabilities. *Matern Child Health J.* 2014;18:1964-1975; Basil JS, Santoro SL, Martin LJ, et al. Retrospective study of obesity in children with downs syndrome. *J Pediatr.* 2016;173:143-148.

environmental barriers related to movement, function, and health." Of importance to the discussion of the role of physical therapists in the treatment of pediatric obesity is the commitment to prevention and health promotion. The vision statement went on to say: "Physical therapy, by 2020, will be provided by physical therapists who are doctors of physical therapy and who may be board-certified specialists. Consumers will have direct access to physical therapists in all environments for client management, prevention, and wellness services. Physical therapists will be practitioners of

choice in clients' health networks and will hold all privileges of autonomous practice. Physical therapists may be assisted by physical therapist assistants who are educated and licensed to provide physical therapist directed and supervised components of interventions. Guided by integrity, lifelong learning, and a commitment to comprehensive and accessible health programs for all people, physical therapists and physical therapist assistants will render evidence-based services throughout the continuum of care and improve quality of life for society. They will provide culturally sensitive care distinguished by trust, respect, and an appreciation for individual differences. While fully availing themselves of new technologies, as well as basic and clinical research, physical therapists will continue to provide high level direct care. They will maintain active responsibility for the growth of the physical therapy profession and the health of the people it serves."[12] It is into the arena of health and wellness that PTs must traverse to become the practitioners of choice to maximize the *prevention of impairments, activity limitations, participation restrictions, and environmental barriers related to movement, function, and health* of children with obesity and who are overweight. Furthermore, proponents have defined "integration of prevention and wellness strategies into the physical therapy intervention" as a critical role in the practice of physical therapy[2] (Guide to Physical Therapist Practice).

» Definitions

The classification of childhood obesity is distinct from that of adult obesity, because it is dependent not only on height and weight but also on age and sex, because of the variations in a maturing body. The BMI, typically utilized as the measure of adult obesity, is defined by the CDC as a number calculated from the measure of a person's height and weight. BMI expresses this relationship as a ratio of weight (in kilograms) divided by height squared (meters). It is considered to be a reliable measure of body fatness, as a relatively easy and inexpensive screening tool to look at weight categories that may be used as health indicators. It also has been found to identify the fattest individuals correctly, with "acceptable accuracy at the upper end of the distribution."[13] In children and adolescents, BMI is calculated and compared to that of others of the same age to determine the percentile for age. The advantage of utilizing the body mass index–for-age (BMI-for-age) value as the indicator for determining the nutritional status in children is that it provides a guideline based on weight and height taking into consideration that interpretation depends on age, because normal body fat differs in boys and girls as they mature. As of April 2012, the CDC defined overweight children between the ages of 2 and 18 years, to have a BMI at or above the 85th percentile and lower than the 95th percentile for children of the same age and sex. Childhood obesity was defined as a BMI at or above the 95th percentile for children of the same age and sex using the CDC growth chart (see Figs. 20.3 and 20.4).[14] In 2013, a new weight status category was identified to describe children who were at or above 120% of the 95th percentile of BMI for age.[15] This category has grown out of the need to further categorize the extreme values of BMI for age. It should be noted that the CDC growth charts do not reflect the severe obesity weight status categories.[16]

To truly be practitioners of choice for wellness, PTs must learn to integrate prevention and wellness strategies into interventions. It is also necessary for PTs to have a working knowledge of the various aspects of health-related fitness and wellness terminology to increase the impact they might have working with the pediatric client with obesity. The ACSM clearly defines physical fitness as "a multidimensional concept" consisting of "a set of attributes that people possess or achieve that relates to the ability to perform physical activity, and is comprised of skill-related, health-related, and physiologic components."[4] PTs are often involved in return to the skill-related component of fitness, such as rehabilitation following a sports injury. Agility, balance, coordination, and speed are just a few of the functional skills often addressed in the treatment. Health-related fitness measures include the ability of an individual to perform activities of daily life with stamina. It precludes the effects of inactivity, such as an overall state of deconditioning. This type of fitness may be the most impacted in children with obesity, because they are not able to perform many of the activities that would be enjoyed by same-aged peers. Understanding that health-related fitness is inclusive of body composition, muscular strength, and endurance, cardiovascular endurance, as well as flexibility, should be considered in designing long- and short-term goals. Other components of obesity and measurement must be understood for PTs to attain a role in promoting fitness, health, and wellness for the pediatric population. To review, *body composition* refers to the relative amount of fat versus fat-free body mass. It has been found that healthier body composition in youth is associated with an improved cardiovascular profile later in life and a decreased morbidity. A balance of caloric intake and energy expenditure determines body composition. Recent studies have examined the question of whether calories are weighted differently, with the consumption of certain types of foods being better for burning calories and maintaining weight loss than are others[17] (see Display 20.1 for more information). Waist *circumference measurements* have also been used as a health indicator, along with BMI for age. It has been found that central adiposity, which is measured by circumferential measurement, is associated with hyperlipidemia, cardiovascular disease risk factors, and type 2 diabetes. Studies have suggested that an increased measure of central adiposity at age 8 years could increase the risk of cardiovascular disease in adolescence by four times over that of children with smaller waist circumferential measurements.[18] Muscular *strength and endurance* are often measured by standardized youth fitness tests, such as those used in physical education curriculum. Examples of such tests might include curl-up or push-up tests, as well as more comprehensive tests such as the FITNESSGRAM.[19] Pediatric PTs routinely measure strength as part of the subtests of gross motor tests such as the Peabody Developmental Motor Scales–2nd edition or the Bruininks–Oseretsky Test of Motor Proficiency 2nd edition, although these test items do use jumping that requires the children to overcome body weight to complete the task. In "typical" scenarios such as this, PTs must use their judgment to determine whether the risk of injury of testing a young child who is obese balances the benefits of the standardized testing results. *Cardiorespiratory endurance* is the ability of the body to deliver oxygen to tissues at levels appropriate to the activity. Children who are physically active have been found to have more high-density lipoproteins, lower triglycerides, less low-density lipoproteins, lower BMI, improved insulin sensitivity, and lower systolic blood pressure.[18] Flexibility is another aspect of fitness that is often tested in children to help determine their overall fitness level. The ACSM defines flexibility as the ability of a joint to move through the full range of motion. There are many factors that influence the flexibility of a joint, including extensibility of muscle, tendons, ligaments, and the joint capsule.[4] Education of the PT routinely includes measurements of flexibility, such as use of a goniometer or tape measure. In the fitness arena, field tests include sit and reach tests and the v-sit and reach. Both tests measure flexibility across multiple joints, and therefore offer more information to a more general state of the flexibility of the individual than the more joint-specific goniometric tests.

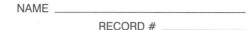

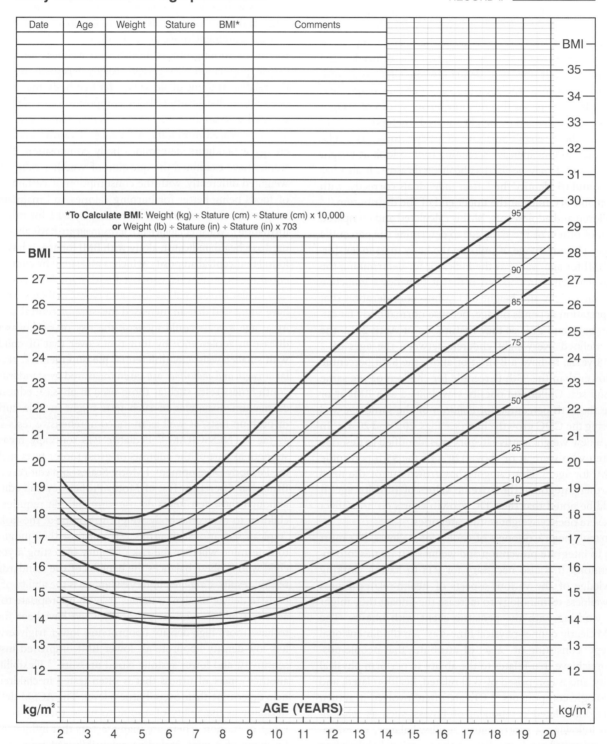

2 to 20 years: Boys
Body mass index-for-age percentiles

NAME _____

RECORD # _____

Date	Age	Weight	Stature	BMI*	Comments

*To Calculate BMI: Weight (kg) ÷ Stature (cm) ÷ Stature (cm) x 10,000
or Weight (lb) ÷ Stature (in) ÷ Stature (in) x 703

Published May 30, 2000 (modified 10/16/00).

SOURCE: Developed by the National Center for Health Statistics in collaboration with
the National Center for Chronic Disease Prevention and Health Promotion (2000).
http://www.cdc.gov/growthcharts

SAFER·HEALTHIER·PEOPLE™

FIGURE 20.3. U.S. Centers for Disease Control Growth Chart for body mass index (BMI) for age for boys, 2 to 20 years of age. The BMI-for-age growth charts are available at https://www.cdc.gov/growthcharts/clinical_charts.htm.

2 to 20 years: Girls
Body mass index-for-age percentiles

NAME _____

RECORD # _____

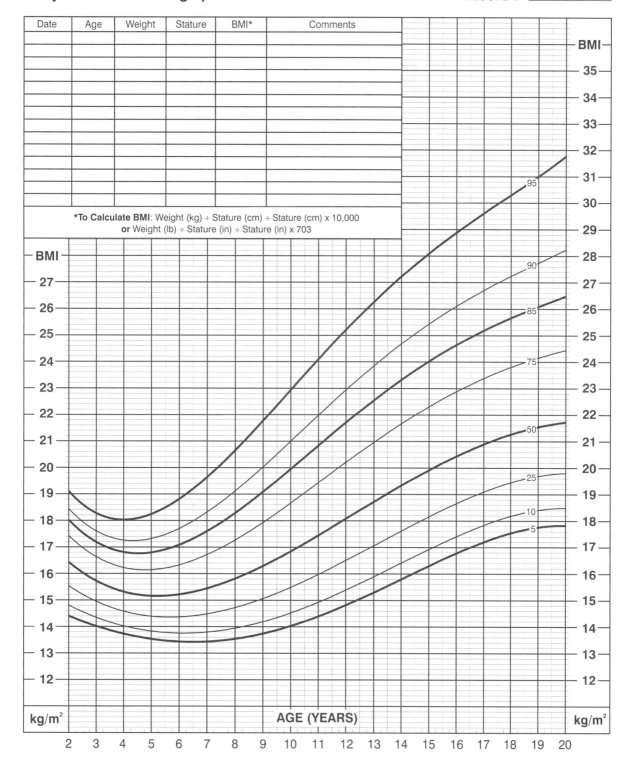

*To Calculate BMI: Weight (kg) ÷ Stature (cm) ÷ Stature (cm) x 10,000
or Weight (lb) ÷ Stature (in) ÷ Stature (in) x 703

Published May 30, 2000 (modified 10/16/00).
SOURCE: Developed by the National Center for Health Statistics in collaboration with
the National Center for Chronic Disease Prevention and Health Promotion (2000).
http://www.cdc.gov/growthcharts

SAFER·HEALTHIER·PEOPLE™

FIGURE 20.4. U.S. Centers for Disease Control Growth Chart for body mass index (BMI) for age for girls, 2 to 20 years of age. The BMI-for-age growth charts are available at https://www.cdc.gov/growthcharts/clinical_charts.htm.

Although pediatric PTs are not experts in the area of nutrition, some basic information is valuable in being an integral part of an interdisciplinary team working together to combat childhood obesity.

Recent evidence has been found disproving the theory of energy in equals energy out.[17,20,21] Although it is still an undeniable truth that calories taken in through food must be burned through physical activity and basal metabolic functioning to avoid being stored in the body, just how this occurs is being called into question. Robert Lustig, MD has done significant research in this area, and is now suggesting the theory that the quality of the calorie determines how much is burned and how much is stored. Breaking it down further, he describes four examples of calorie categories:

Fiber—delays absorption of calories; uses example of eating 160 calories in almonds leads to absorption of only 130. It is suggested that the bacteria in the intestine use some of the calories, thereby delaying the absorption of the remaining calories into the bloodstream.

Protein—owing to the thermic effect of food, one must put two times the amount of energy into metabolizing proteins as with carbohydrates. This leads to proteins using more energy and therefore calorie burn, in its processing. It is also stated that proteins reduce hunger better than do carbs by reducing hunger hormones.

Fat—It is noted that fats release 9 calories per gram when burned. However, although some are considered "bad" fats, like trans fats, which clog arteries, others are considered "healthy" fats such as Omega-3 fats, which are considered heart healthy.

Sugars—consists of two chemicals—fructose and glucose. Every cell in the body uses glucose for energy, whereas fructose is metabolized in the liver as fat and not used for energy as glucose is. Fructose is the key ingredient in soda, candy, and processed foods.

In keeping abreast of nutrition evidence and research, PTs may be able to dispel myths that children and their families may hold in developing a healthier diet.

Furthermore, the field tests have normative data to compare the children with their peers.[18]

The ACSM describes elements of physiologic fitness as distinct from health-related fitness components "in that it includes nonperformance components that relate to biological systems influenced by habitual activity."[4] Metabolic fitness, morphologic fitness, and bone integrity may be included in this category. In looking at the APTA vision statement including health promotion and wellness as integral to practice, it is in this physiologic fitness arena that growth is necessary in the treatment of youth with obesity. Tests and measures in the physical therapy evaluation will help identify goals to maximize all fitness measures in those children with obesity, even if that is not the primary diagnosis being treated. PTs are now an integral part in maximizing fitness within the rehabilitation process. Applying the multifactorial concepts of

fitness within the treatment program of children with obesity and continuing to center on evidence-based research in the design of such programs will help establish the role of PTs within the multidisciplinary team focused on the goal of decreasing the incidence of pediatric obesity.

» Role of physical therapists in pediatric obesity

PTs have been defined by the APTA as "health care practitioners who maintain, restore, and improve movement, activity, and health enabling individuals of all ages to have optimal functioning and quality of life" and who "are involved in promoting health, wellness, and fitness through risk factor identification and the implementation of services to reduce risk, slow the progression of or prevent functional decline and disability." Within this definition, the role of a PT within pediatric obesity is defined. The battle to combat the growing incidence of childhood obesity begins with the concepts of active living and healthy lifestyle. Considering the definition of "active living" as a way of life incorporating physical activity into daily routine, there is a unique opportunity to promote this healthy living as pediatric PTs, whether in the educational setting, community, or in a medically based facility. Because PTs are experts in the musculoskeletal system and gross motor development, and are practitioners who assist in health promotion and prevention of impairment, their role is clear in the treatment of pediatric obesity. Because maximizing independent movement potential and quality of life are staples of the role of PTs in the pediatric population, their function within the treatment of those children with obesity is multifactorial. Beyond the interventions for physical impairments, a PT should be part of the multidisciplinary team working with the families in the education and prevention of comorbid impairments in the medical arena, the community, and in educational settings. In 2008, the U.S. Department of Health and Human Services established the guidelines for physical activity in children and adolescents as 60 minutes or more each day of moderate to vigorous physical activity to maximize healthy growth and development. Incorporating the concepts of health-related fitness, it is further suggested that the hour of physical activity includes the components of aerobic, muscle strengthening, and bone strengthening. The guidelines further delineate aerobic recommendations to include at least moderate- to vigorous-level activity most days and vigorous level 3 days a week. Muscle and bone strengthening activities are also recommended at least 3 days a week.[22] These are guidelines that should be considered in developing a comprehensive home exercise program for all children and adolescents, but especially those with increased weight status. Moderate physical activity is described as a perceived level of exertion of 5 or 6 and vigorous as 7 or 8. It is important to use objective measures such as the modified Borg Scale or any other visual scale appropriate to the age of the child.[3]

Physical activity refers to a movement of the body by the skeletal muscles that result in energy expenditure. To differentiate, *exercise* is physical activity that is planned, structured, and repetitive and has the purpose of improvement or maintenance of one or more components of physical fitness.[4,18] Although PTs may be considered experts in therapeutic exercise as a key component of the rehabilitative treatment procedure, a research report published in 2011 by Schlessman et al. suggests only one in three PTs "were thinking of or preparing to incorporate wellness promotion into practice and only 54% were incorporating wellness into practice."[23] Because there has been an increase in the attention given to the role of health prevention in post–baccalaureate degree programs, the perception of PTs as a lead in this area is growing.[23]

The general public has not yet realized the role of PTs as leaders in health promotion and wellness. Studies of parents of preschoolers indicate that they did not recognize weight concerns in their children, nor did they know what action to take when presented with the issue. This suggests a lack of public knowledge of the role PTs play in pediatric health promotion and a need to explore the opportunity for PTs to get more involved in this area. As integral members of the early intervention team, PTs are charged with increasing the gross motor skill acquisition of the children and families they service. As Nervik et al. suggested in 2011, gross motor development in children aged 3 to 5 may be impacted by higher BMIs.[8] It has been suggested that between the ages of 3 and 7, the development of fat tissue makes this a critical time for obesity prevention. This is the time in which a child's BMI typically reaches its lowest point, to then begin rising through adolescence. Because preschool years have been found to be a critical time for obesity prevention because of the timing of the development of fat tissue, PTs can begin the education of both parents and early education professionals at preschool and daycares on the importance of physical activity for this young population.[8,24] Barriers do exist in putting wellness promotion into practice. The lack of resources, time, and funding as well as difficulty with keeping the families and children engaged in programs are among these barriers.[23] As PTs are often introduced to the children and their families in the course of rehabilitation for the comorbidities of obesity, a unique opportunity does exist to be on the frontlines of promoting a healthy lifestyle choice and educating families in health-related fitness guidelines for children.

» Health consequences of obesity

Just as the sheer numbers of children who are overweight and obese have increased at an alarming rate, so too have the long- and short-term health consequences being seen at hospitals and clinics throughout the country in this population. The impact of obesity exists not only in the medical arena but also can be seen throughout the educational system. It is well documented that associated with primary childhood obesity are increases in high blood pressure, type 2 diabetes, breathing disorders, sleep disorders, chronic low-grade systemic inflammation, orthopedic musculoskeletal issues, and psychosocial impacts. As already noted, studies have suggested that children with obesity may have difficulty with developmental motor skill acquisition.[8] There is an increased risk of long-term consequences such as increased incidence of adult obesity, with over 50% of overweight adolescents now meeting the criteria for the metabolic syndrome (insulin resistance, hypertension, hyperlipidemia, and abdominal obesity), adverse socioeconomic impact, cardiovascular disease, and premature morbidity.[25] It has been estimated that up to one-third of the population of the United States will develop type 2 diabetes during their lifetime. With a two-fold increase in the mortality risk as early as the fourth decade of life for those adolescents who are obese, this epidemic has been reported to threaten to reverse the gains in life expectancy occurring through improvements in clinical treatments of hypertension, hyperlipidemia, and smoking. That being said, data suggest that this generation of children will be the first to not outlive their parents.[10,25] Furthermore, a study released by the National Institutes of Health in 2014 suggested that severe obesity in adults could have a dramatic impact on life expectancy, with a decrease up to 14 years reported.[26]

Although many of the secondary impairments of pediatric obesity are beyond the scope of PT practice, the areas of orthopedic and musculoskeletal dysfunction are often examined and treated by PTs. Blount's disease, slipped capital femoral epiphysis, spinal dysfunction, and fractures are just a few of the diagnoses that may be directly related to the child being overweight or obese. Research suggests that being overweight can impact the body's response to weight-bearing activities that are a part of physical activity. Gait changes, including changes in velocity, cadence, energy usage, and biomechanical changes leading to abnormal knee loading and foot discomfort have also been linked to children who are overweight or obese.[27]

In addition to comorbidities related to obesity, pediatric PTs must also be aware of those children most frequently seen in therapy, and the impact the primary dysfunction may have on their ability to be physically active. According to the CDC, only 47% of adolescents without a disability were meeting the suggested guideline of 60 minutes of physical activity 5 days a week in a survey performed in 2017.[28]

Although the positive effects of physical activity have been well documented to have a benefit to overall health and well-being, it has been found that for people with a disability, an active lifestyle is even more beneficial.[29] Because those individuals with childhood-onset physical disabilities such as cerebral palsy (CP), myelomeningocele (MMC), or brain injury are now living longer, health care is shifting focus toward health promotion and wellness to help prevent secondary conditions and improve quality of life into adulthood.[29] Buffart et al. found that the overall health-related physical fitness was poor in youth with MMC. This is of particular concern when considering life expectancy of persons with MMC has increased and lifestyle-related diseases such as cardiovascular disease and diabetes will be of increasing concern.[30] Pan and Frey published a study outlining the paucity of information surrounding the physical activity level of children with autism spectrum disorder (ASD). They found that youth with ASD might have less opportunity for physical activity owing to social and behavioral deficits as well as difficulty with peer interaction. Although they found no consistent pattern in physical activity of youth with ASD, findings suggested that increasing opportunities were needed to address extracurricular physical activity, particularly during adolescence.[31] In a more recent study conducted by McCoy et al., adolescents with ASD were found to be 72% more likely to be obese than were typically developing peers. They were reportedly 60% less likely to engage in regular physical activity 3 or more days a week than were their peers without autism.[32] This presents another opportunity for PTs in the educational setting to provide assistance and adaptations to improve participation in physical activity opportunities for the students they service. Surrounding youth with CP, it has been suggested that these children live the most sedentary lifestyles among those with pediatric disabilities.[33] In a study examining self-reported levels of activity in adolescents with CP, it was found that physical activity participation was related to level of gross motor function and that physical activity decreased with increasing age. The inverse relationship between physical activity level and age is consistent with data on the physical activity of nondisabled peers. What was notable was the decrease in variation and intensity level of the physical activity employed by those with CP when contrasted with their same-aged peers.[34] Focusing treatment approach, home exercise programs, and discharge planning in physical therapy to a strategy of lifelong fitness and physical activity is imperative to maximizing the potential of those children with CP. Encouraging increased physical activity is important for health promotion and is suggested to improve the overall functional independence, social integration, and life satisfaction for all children, both with and without childhood-onset physical disabilities.

It is widely reported that a significant barrier to all children achieving healthy weight and activity levels is time spent sedentary while using technology such as smart phones and screens. In a survey of 1,600 youth, between the ages of 8 and 18, teens self-reported spending an average of 7 hours and 22 minutes on smartphones. Youth between the ages of 8 and 12 reported usage times averaging 4 hours and 44 minutes. Time spent on the phone was reported to watch videos and television, play games, and access social media.[35] There are new arenas that PTs can help promote, including active video gaming, as a viable option for increasing activity levels in kids of all levels of ability.[36]

A qualitative study was performed looking at personal and environmental barriers to engage in physical activity in young adults with childhood-onset physical disabilities. As is comparable to the general population, barriers related to attitude and motivation existed—in conjunction with fatigue,

---

DISPLAY 20.2 **A Model for Inclusion: Special Olympics**

Existing since 1968, the Special Olympics has strived to include all people, specifically those with intellectual disability, into an arena of competition to promote inclusion and camaraderie within the context of competition in sports and physical activities.

The mission of Special Olympics is "to provide year-round sports training and athletic competition in a variety of Olympic-type sports for children and adults with intellectual disabilities, giving them continuing opportunities to develop physical fitness, demonstrate courage, experience joy and participate in a sharing of gifts, skills and friendship with their families, other Special Olympics athletes and the community."

It is through involvement in programs such as these that physical therapists continue to increase public awareness of the role they play in health promotion and wellness in all arenas.

Special Olympics, Inc. Our mission. Accessed October 10, 2013. www.specialolympics.org/mission.aspx

---

having injuries related to the condition, and lack of information and professional support—were perceived as barriers to physical activity.[28] Those children with autism also can have barriers related to social skills, frustration tolerance, and behavior-limiting participation in physical activities with peers.[37] Barriers that are not just unique to children with autism, including deficits in motor skill level compared to peers, sequencing issues, as well as difficulty with sequencing, can all lead to decreased participation in play throughout childhood. This suggests yet another role PTs might have as health care providers to work with coaches and staff that can promote physical activity for all children. By helping to alleviate barriers, educating clients and families as to the recommendations by the CDC of physical activity, and helping to determine the correct balance between activity and rest to reduce fatigue, PTs can begin to bridge the gap in activity levels for children with physical impairments. It is noted that although studies have been reported documenting improved levels of physical activity of those with acquired short- and long-term physical disability, future studies are warranted to determine efficacy of rehabilitation professionals to provide counseling and advice on physical activity and whether such intervention would impact physical activity levels in youth with childhood-onset physical disabilities.[29] (See Display 20.2 for an example of increasing opportunities for physical activity for those with special needs.)

» How obesity treatment fits within the ICF framework

The World Health Organization (WHO)'s ICF framework can be utilized as a guide to develop clinical pathways and critical thinking in the treatment of impairments related to pediatric obesity (Fig. 20.5).[38] In contrast to the Guide

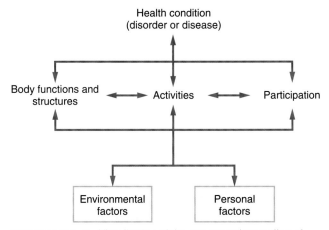

FIGURE 20.5. Visualization of the current understanding of interaction of various components of the International Classification of Functioning, Disability and Health (ICF).[27]

to Physical Therapist Practice 3, the ICF offers a model of health and functioning as opposed to a disability model. This classification system describes human functioning within the daily lives of individuals with a health condition. It is generally agreed upon that those individuals with obesity experience disability in terms of their ability to participate in activities within both daily and community functioning. In a pediatric population, these activities could include mobility in and around an educational setting, recreational activities, or even their ability to progress with self-care activities. Tolerance for physical activity could impede social development and lead to further issues. Looking only at the presence of obesity, whether as a primary or secondary diagnosis, does not offer a clinician enough information on how the child's participation in daily activities may be affected. The ICF can be used to evaluate the dynamic impact obesity can have on the function, activities, and participation by looking at two distinct components. First, the impairments that might be present with the disability of obesity on the body structures and functioning and the impact this might have on performance and participation in activities are evaluated. Secondly, the contextual component of obesity is examined in the psychosocial views of health and well-being, and includes personal and environmental factors. This dynamic interaction between health conditions and environmental and personal factors moves away from the disablement models emphasizing the individual as being handicapped by the diagnosis (Fig. 20.6). The APTA has been clear in identifying the ICF as a means of using language of function and health, understood by those both in and out of the health care arena, which might be utilized to enhance communication between health care provider and patient, policy makers, and payers.

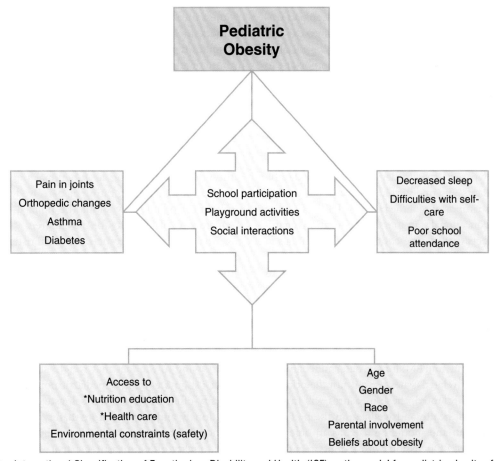

FIGURE 20.6. International Classification of Functioning, Disability and Health (ICF) as the model for pediatric obesity effects on health and functioning of a pediatric patient.

By using this language, communication within the health care community might be enhanced, leading to a clearer picture of the role physical therapists might play in the broader concept of rehabilitation of those children with obesity. Furthermore, conversations might be stimulated regarding interdisciplinary collaboration in research, resulting in overall improved clinical care.[38–40]

» History and examination of the child with obesity

In the case of pediatric obesity, it is very important to recognize that the child may *not* be seeking physical therapy for diagnosis and treatment of obesity; rather, it may exist as a comorbidity of a more physical impairment, such as back or knee pain. It is imperative to be comprehensive in the history and physical aspects of the examination to include consideration of the whole body structure and function that may be related to the functional limitations of the presenting diagnosis. Particular attention must be paid to risk factors, including ethnicity, cultural beliefs, family/caregiver resources, education, social interaction, activities, and support systems. General health status questions will lead to information regarding physical functioning, psychological functioning, level of physical fitness, and general health perception. Physical functioning would include perceived mobility issues or sleep patterns or issues. Psychological functioning might look into existing conditions such as depression, anxiety, memory, or social issues related to weight status. It would also be important to assess the family because it might relate to overall home environment and health-related fitness. Intake information about medications currently being used by the child for comorbidities may also offer vital information regarding weight status in the child. Knowledge of the potential for weight gain as a side effect of some antipsychotic drugs used in some cases to treat attention deficit hyperactivity disorder or autism, mood stabilizers, antidepressants, and oral steroids such as those used to treat asthma is also important for the pediatric PT.[41,42] In some cases, parents or educational staff may need education regarding these side effects that may be contributing to changes in the weight status of a child.

Within a systems review, attention should be paid to cardiopulmonary-related measures, as indicated earlier in the discussion of health-related fitness measures. Blood pressure, resting heart rate, and respiratory rate are important factors to monitor when proposing an exercise plan for a child with obesity. Anthropometric measurements must be recorded, including height, weight, and BMI for age determined in children who have weight-related issues, even if not the primary diagnosis. As previously noted, these measures will impact the return to maximal health and wellness in the pediatric client. BMI for age can and should be used as an objective measure for health risk. Discussion with parents regarding the weight status category can open a dialogue to provide education regarding the potential health risks of obesity.

A comprehensive review of the musculoskeletal and neuromuscular systems must be performed, because impairments may result in developing joints related to a child's elevated weight status. Because it relates to both primary diagnosis and overall health-related fitness level, it is important to measure muscle performance as well, through manual muscle testing and other measurements outlined earlier. Weight status can also impact posture and alignment, and must be measured on examination. For the obese population, ventilation and respiration measures may also need to be examined, to ensure safety with aerobic and strengthening activities within the treatment plan. As previously noted, gross motor skills and coordinated movements may also be impacted if a child is obese. The child and family's motivation for change and expectations for results must be measured as well to determine goal attainment strategies.

Tests and Measures

Although the PT may use a variety of specific tests and measures in the examination of a pediatric client for a specific diagnosis, it is important to address those measures that quantify the effect weight status may have on overall prognosis and outcomes. As previously noted, there are a variety of tests to look specifically at both health- and skill-related fitness measures that may be useful in some populations. For others, looking at the Guide to Physical Therapist Practice supplies a framework with which to specifically measure those children with obesity. In the area of aerobic capacity and endurance, standardized testing protocols can be utilized such as arm, cycle, or wheelchair ergometer tests, step tests (such as the Harvard step test), or walk/run testing such as the 6-minute walk test. All of these measures offer standards with which to compare results. Timed up and go, timed floor to stand, and the 30-second walk tests can be easily used in the educational setting as functional measures of performance. Modified Borg rating of perceived exertion or other self-report of intensity should be utilized to determine adequate level of intensity for the children.

Measuring anthropometric characteristics, including body composition and dimensions, have already been discussed. In the area of arousal, attention, and cognition, it may be beneficial to evaluate motivation and expectation level as well as overall quality-of-life ratings using a self-assessment tool such as the ***Child Health Questionnaire***.[43] This type of assessment may be necessary, because it has been documented that severely obese children report lower health-related quality of life. Owing to the fact that weight status can be associated with a stigma within the pediatric population, the child with obesity often displays lower self-esteem, and reports feeling sad, lonely, and nervous more than typical weight peers do.[10] Although not always included in a physical therapy examination, quality-of-life measures, particularly in the overweight youth, may offer another outcome area to improve overall wellness.

In examining the circulatory system, measures should include the standard blood pressure, heart rate, and respiratory rate with the addition of electrocardiogram (ECG) if the child has severe obesity and may need further medical clearance to participate in endurance activities. Pulse oximetry, respiratory rate, rhythm and pattern, the Borg rating of perceived exertion scale, and dyspnea visual analog scale are means by which a PT can document baseline cardiorespiratory status and document improvement throughout the course of physical therapy.

As discussed in health-related fitness testing, muscle performance testing can occur in a variety of ways. Beyond manual muscle testing, other functional tests might be utilized such as sit to stand tests, sit up tests, or squat testing, for example. Also noted is the strength portion of standardized tests such as the Bruininks–Oseretsky Test of Motor Proficiency–2 subtest.

In the examination of the child with obesity, particular attention should be paid to posture and alignment to determine further risk factors related to weight status, such as increased genu valgus at the knees, or issues at the subtalar joint resulting in pain with activity. An examination of self-care issues may also be necessary with the population in the highest weight percentiles for children to help with problem solving for the family in the area of home management when the child cannot be safely lifted because of weight.

» Determining functional outcome expectations for the child with obesity

The PT should focus interventions for children with obesity and increased weight status on decreasing the risk of cardiovascular, pulmonary, and musculoskeletal disorders. Therapeutic exercise, aerobic conditioning, functional training, education and training of children and their families, and overall lifestyle modifications will all be strategies used to attain the overarching goal of improved health status and well-being. Anticipated functional outcomes affecting participation aspects of activity could include the following:

- Improved ability to perform physical actions such as jumping activities is well documented.
- Awareness and use of community resources is improved.
- Behaviors that foster healthy habits, wellness, and prevention strategies are acquired and documented through self-assessments.
- Decision making is enhanced regarding health and use of health care resources by the child and family both at home and in school.
- Child and family knowledge of personal and environmental factors and barriers associated with weight status and obesity is increased.
- Performance levels in self-care, school, play, community, or leisure activities are improved by self-reported measures.
- Attendance at school is improved.

More outcomes related to body structure and function related to obesity might include the following:

- Increased muscle performance, strength and joint range of motion
- Improved aerobic capacity and endurance
- Improved tolerance of positions and activities both at home, in school and within the community
- Improved sense of well-being, as documented through questionnaires or surveys
- Improved measures of skill-related fitness
- Decrease in risk factors

Other secondary outcomes that are broader in spectrum would include decreasing utilization and cost of health care services and optimizing use of physical therapy services. This utilization of PT to include attention to weight status in children who present with other primary impairments results in a more efficient use of health care dollars.

» Therapeutic interventions to address obesity in the pediatric population

Whether the child with obesity is receiving physical therapy in a medical setting or in the educational environment, particular attention must be paid to structuring therapeutic interventions in a safe, effective manner to meet goals. Increased monitoring of perceived level of exertion, respiratory rates, and blood pressure and heart rates may be indicated in this population to maintain a safe working zone. Child and family education is necessary on monitoring heart rate. Because of the variation in resting heart rate in children, target heart rate for children younger than 18 is not as reliable a measure as in adults. Rating perceived exertion is a safe way to monitor intensity.[44] There are options beyond the Borg for rating exertion in children. The Pictorial Children's Effort Rating Table (PCERT) and OMNI child scales are two other self-rating scales for children that offer a PT the ability to grade the exercise intensity for the pediatric population.[45,46] In terms of health-related fitness, aerobic capacity and endurance conditioning are areas of need that will require specific attention. Interventions to improve cardiovascular endurance may include aquatics, walking or wheelchair propulsion programs, gait training on treadmills, cycle ergometers, and elliptical training activities.

In the area of flexibility, beyond the typical interventions such as both manual and self-stretching, group activities such as yoga have become available to children both in the educational setting and in the community. Strength and endurance for more skill-related fitness is also to be considered in the interventions for children with obesity. Beyond active assisted, active, and resistive exercises, more comprehensive exercise approaches have been used such as Pilates or Power Yoga.

20.3   Recommendations to Motivate Children and Families to Exercise

Encourage	Discourage
Fitness education for family members	Comparing child with physically active peers
Having fun with activities	
Begin with lower intensity exercises	Participation more important than winning
Include child/family in goal identification	Gradual progression of exercise program
Develop achievable goals that enhance quality of life	Maintain appropriate level of reinforcement
	Do not be demanding, exercise should be its own reward
Give positive reinforcement as appropriate	

Adapted from McWhorter JW, Wallmann HW, Alpert PT. The obese child: motivation as a tool for exercise. *J Pediatr Health Care.* 2003;17:11-17.

Motivation is another key aspect of therapeutic intervention that must be understood by the PT working with a child with obesity. To encourage optimal effort in exercises and interventions, it becomes necessary to properly motivate these youth who may already have a negative view of physical activity. Display 20.3 offers guidelines for increasing participation in therapeutic exercise in children.[47]

There are various approaches taken by PTs who treat children with obesity. As with many children, it is clear that interventions need to be individualized for each client. Furthermore, because this has become a health problem of epidemic proportions, it is clear that an interdisciplinary approach to treating these children provides a comprehensive means to achieving the goal of reducing the incidence of obesity in general. Health care providers, such as primary care physicians and PTs, must partner with the community through the educational team, and those with an "environmental" stake in the effort such as local and state governments and health insurers who are in a position to extend the reach of strategies to promote a healthy lifestyle. Display 20.4 describes part of a Commonwealth of Pennsylvania growth screening program related to body weight determination. Taking advantage of unique opportunities to be part of a larger wellness community may be available to PTs as primary interventionists in the treatment of pediatric obesity. Being a part of a school wellness committee or assisting with performing a School Health Index are examples of school-based health initiatives in which PTs could be an integral part of improving the wellness of the community. Display 20.5 shows a report about a PT-led project to partner with a local school district. The PT is this chapter's author.

20.4   Pennsylvania's Growth Screening Program

In response to the growing obesity epidemic, some states developed school health initiatives to begin to gain control over the issue. In 2003, PA Department of Health initiated the Nutrition and Physical Activity Plan to Prevent Obesity and Related Chronic Diseases. Parental awareness of the BMI-for-age measure as a tool to measure growth was set as one of the goals of the program. Over the course of three school years, the program was mandated for all students in the kindergarten through 12th grade to have BMI for age documented with notifications being offered to parents should the measure fall outside the norms for age. The procedure set forth by the state includes annual screening of height and weight, with attention given to the average growth velocity as a measure of normal growth, and use of the CDC growth charts to determine BMI-for-age statistics for each student in the district. Interpretation of the findings fall into one of three categories:

Weight within acceptable range—Even when findings are within a normal range for testing, parent notification of results are recommended to decrease possibility of a student being singled out for being overweight.

Weight less than 5th percentile—Includes both BMI for age <5th percentile and stature for age <5th percentile; recommendations include sending parent/guardian notification home in a timely manner with additional recommendation for follow-up by primary care provider for nutritional concerns and information on community-based food supplementation programs.

Weight equal to or greater than 85th percentile—Includes BMI for age greater than or equal to 85th percentile; recommendations include parental notification, encouraging healthy eating and regular physical activity, and recommendation for follow-up with primary care provider for blood pressure, total cholesterol, family history, assess exogenous causes of overweight, and for type 2 diabetes screening.

Furthermore, the PA Department of Health (DOH) requests each school district to submit the data each school year. On the website, the DOH offers a variety of handouts and resources accessible to both the districts and the families to increase the knowledge base of healthy nutrition and living an active lifestyle.[48]

Department of Health. Procedures for the growth screening program for Pennsylvania's school-aged population. https://www.health.pa.gov/topics/school/Pages/Growth-Screen.aspx

20.5   Toward a Larger Wellness Community: A Physical Therapist Collaborates with a Community Elementary School in Securing a Federal Grant

Through the Carol M. White Physical Education Program (PEP), the U.S. Department of Education provides grants "to LEAs [local educational agencies] and community-based organizations (CBOs) to initiate, expand, or enhance physical education programs, including after-school programs, for students in kindergarten through 12th grade. Grant recipients must implement programs that help students make progress toward meeting state standards."[49] In 2007, a physical therapist partnered with a community elementary school nurse and physical education department to procure a 2-year grant in the amount of 175,000 dollars. The physical therapist served as the project director and chief investigator for the grant, which opens up a new role in the wellness arena. The following is an excerpt from the grant report: "The purpose of **The Healthy Kids/Healthy Community Program** is to ensure students in a high risk population are healthier and therefore better able to learn and that the staff at Penrose Elementary will be properly trained and supported to promote a healthy school environment. This has been a collaborative effort between (school) and (health system) with other community partners, focusing on the needs of this underserved population, with particular attention to ensure specific needs are being met for those children already at risk for adult obesity. Specifically, three areas were identified as focal points for this project.

1. Students will receive nutrition education both as a classroom based curriculum and as a component of after-school wellness programs
2. Children identified as overweight or at risk of overweight as per the established CDC guidelines of a BMI-for-age at or above the 85th percentile, will be eligible and encouraged to participate in after-school programming which will focus on teaching these children how to live an active, healthy lifestyle. For those children who have special needs, a separate program will focus on increasing their activity levels by adapting current PE/fitness programming or by establishing individualized fitness plans. Use of components of the Fitnessgram will be used to assess fitness changes as related to activity levels in random group of students.
3. Promote comprehensive increases in moderate to vigorous activity throughout the school day by increasing the number of playground activities available to all students, and improving the organization of the recess yard. Fitnessgram measures as part of the PE program will be used to assess the overall fitness changes with increasing activity options at lunch recess. Furthermore, professional development of the staff, towards creating a healthy school environment will be available. As a final component in achieving an inclusive program, parents will be invited to participate in fitness nights to further their knowledge and experience of wellness.

Using a collaborative approach, exploring available resources from the (school district), an after-school program, nutrition education professionals, and utilizing and training the current staff on available low/no cost programs (such as professional student capital) has enabled (health system), a community-based health system with strong ties to the community, to assist (elementary school) to utilize its expertise in health and wellness to meet the current standards for Health, Safety and Physical Education. The overarching goal of the PEP program this year is to increase the activity levels of students in Kindergarten to 5th Grade to 150 minutes a week and those students in 6th through 8th Grade to 225 minutes a week."

Summary

As PTs strive to achieve the designation of health care professionals who are experts in health promotion and wellness, it is imperative that clinicians achieve a level of knowledge regarding assessment and intervention for children and adolescents who are obese. The role of a PT within the larger interdisciplinary team allocated to begin the process of reversing the epidemic of childhood obesity continues to be defined. As experts in the area of gross motor development, and as part of a larger response to optimize function and enhance movement in children with obesity, PTs have an opportunity to enhance overall quality of life for these children. There is an additional case to be made for PTs to be educators for families and the larger community in addressing pediatric health promotion and wellness.

REFERENCES

1. American Physical Therapy Association. APTA Mission statement adopted. 2018. Accessed September 2019. www.apta.org/mission
2. American Physical Therapy Association. APTA guide to physical therapist practice 3.0. Accessed November 19, 2020. guidetoptpractice.apta.org
3. AMA adopts new policies on second day of voting at annual meeting. Released June 18, 2013. Accessed September 2013. www.ama-assn.org/AMA/pub/news/news/2013/2013-06-18-new-AMA-policies-annual-meeting.page
4. American College of Sports Medicine. *ACSM's Guidelines for Exercise Testing and Exercise Prescription.* Williams and Wilkins; 1995.
5. Centers for Disease Control and Prevention. National Health and Nutrition Examination Survey, 2015-2016. Accessed October 2019. www.cdc.gov/nchs/products/databriefs/db288.htm
6. Ogden CL, Carroll MD, Kit BK, et al. Prevalence of obesity and trends in BMI among US children and adolescents, 1999–2010. *JAMA.* 2012;307(5):483-490.
7. Nervik D, Martin K, Rundquist P, et al. The relationship between body mass index and gross motor development in children aged 3 to 5 years. *Pediatr Phys Ther.* 2011;23:144-148.
8. Centers for Disease Control and Prevention. NCHS Health E – Stat. Accessed October 2019. www.cdc.gov/NCHS/data/hestat/obesity_Child_15_16/obesity_child_15_16.htm
9. Centers for Disease Control and Prevention. Obesity among children and adolescents aged 2–19 years, by selected characteristics: United States, selected years 1988–1994 through 2013–2016. Accessed October 2019. www.cdc.gov/nchs/data/hus/2018/027.pdf
10. White House Task Force on childhood obesity report to the president: solving the problem of childhood obesity within a generation. May 2010. Accessed March 2013. www.letsmove.goc/sites/letsmove.gov/files/TaskForce_on_Childhood_Obesity_May2010_FullReport.pdf
11. Centers for Disease Control and Prevention. Prevalence of self-reported obesity among U.S. adults. BRFSS, 2018 State Obesity Map. Accessed November 2019. http://www.cdc.gov/obesity/data/prevalence-maps.html
12. American Physical Therapy Association. Vision 2020. Accessed March 2019. http://www.apta.org/vision2020/
13. Krebs NF, Himes JH, Jacobson D, et al. Assessment of child and adolescent overweight and obesity. *Pediatrics.* 2007;120(4):S193-S228.
14. Centers for Disease Control and Prevention. Overweight and obesity. Accessed January 20, 2021. https://www.cdc.gov/obesity/childhood/index.html
15. Gulati AK, Kaplan DW, Daniels SR. Clinical tracking of severely obese children: a new growth chart. *Pediatrics.* 2012;130(6):1136-1140.

16. Centers for Disease Control and Prevention. Clinical growth charts. Accessed October 2019. http://www.cdc.gov/growthcharts/clinical_charts.htm#set2

17. Ebbeling CB, Swain JF, Feldman HA, et al. Effects of dietary composition on energy expenditure during weight-loss maintenance. *JAMA.* 2012;307(24):2627-2634.

18. Ganley KJ, Paterno MV, Miles C, et al. Health related fitness in children and adolescents. *Pediatr Phys Ther.* 2011;23:208-220.

19. FITNESSGRAM. Accessed January 20, 2021. https://fitnessgram.net/

20. Lustig RH. Still believe "A Calorie is Just a Calorie"?. Huffington Post Healthy Living. Accessed October 2013. www.huffingtonpost.com/rober-lustig-md/sugar-toxic_b_2759564.html

21. Gelman L. 3 Reasons a calorie is not a calorie. *Reader's Digest.* July 26, 2013.

22. U.S. Department of Health and Human Services. Physical activity guidelines for Americans. Accessed November 2019. www.health.gov/paguidelines/pdf/paguide.pdf

23. Schlessman AM, Martin K, Ritzline PD, et al. The role of physical therapists in pediatric health promotion and obesity prevention: comparison of attitudes. *Pediatr Phys Ther.* 2011;23:79-86.

24. Whitaker RC, Pepe MS, Wright JA, et al. Early adiposity rebound and the risk of adult obesity. *Pediatrics.* 1998;101(3):e5. Accessed October 2013. http://pediatrics.aappublications.org/content/101/3/e5.full

25. Lynn CH, Miller JL. Bariatric surgery for obese adolescents: should surgery be used to treat the childhood obesity epidemic? *Pediatr Health.* 2009;3(1):33-40.

26. National Institutes of Health. NIH study finds extreme obesity may shorten life expectancy up to 14 years. Accessed November 2019. https://www.nih.gov/news-events/news-releases/nih-study-finds-extreme-obesity-may-shorten-life-expectancy-14-years

27. Pathare N, Haskvitz EM, Selleck M. Comparison of measures of physical performance among young children who are healthy weight, overweight, or obese. *Pediatr Phys Ther.* 2013;25:291-296.

28. Centers for Disease Control and Prevention. Youth risk behavior surveillance—United States, 2017. *Morbidity and Mortality Weekly Report.* 2018;67(8). 1-114

29. Buffart LM, Westendorp T, van den Berg-Emons H, et al. Perceived barriers and facilitators of physical activity in young adults with childhood-onset physical disabilities. *J Rehabil Med.* 2009;41:881-885.

30. Buffart LM, van den Berg-Emons RJG, van Wijlen-Hempel MS, et al. Health related physical fitness of adolescents and young adults with myelomeningocele. *Eur J Appl Physiol.* 2008;103:181-188.

31. Pan CY, Frey GC. Physical activity patterns in youth with autism spectrum disorders. *J Autism Dev Disord.* 2006;36:597-606.

32. McCoy SM, Jakicic JM, Gibbs BB. Comparison of obesity, physical activity, and sedentary behaviors between adolescents with autism spectrum disorders and without. *J Autism Dev Disord.* 2016;46:2317-2326.

33. Longmuir PE, Bar-Or O. Factors influencing the physical activity levels of youths with physical and sensory disabilities. *Adapt Phys Activ Q.* 2000;17:40-53.

34. Maher C, Williams MT, Olds T, et al. Physical and sedentary activity in adolescents with cerebral palsy. *Dev Med Child Neurol.* 2007;49(6):450-457.

35. Rideout V, Robb MB. *The Common Sense Census: Media Use by Tweens and Teens.* Common Sense Media; 2019. Accessed October 2019. www.commonsensemedia.org/sites/default/files/uploads/research/2019-census-8-to-18-full-report-updated.pdf

36. Rowland JL, Malone LA, Fidopiastis CM, et al. Perspectives on active video gaming as a new frontier in accessible physical activity for youth with physical disabilities. *Phys Ther.* 2016;96:521-532.

37. Srinivasan SM, Pescatello LS, Bhat AN. Current perspectives on physical activities and exercise recommendations for children and adolescents with autism spectrum disorders. *Phys Ther.* 2014;94:875-889.

38. Winstein C, Pate P, Ge T, et al. The Physical Therapy Clinical Research Network (PTClinResNef), methods, efficacy, and benefits of a rehabilitation research network. *Am J Phys Med Rehabil.* 2008;87:937-950.

39. World Health Organization. *International Classification of Functioning, Disability, and Health.* World Health Organization; 2001.

40. Forhan M. An analysis of disability models and the application of the ICF to obesity. *Disabil Rehabil.* 2009;31(16):1382-1388.

41. American Academy of Child and Adolescent Psychiatry. Weight Gain from Medication: Prevention and Management. Accessed January 20, 2021. www.aacap.org/AACAP/Families_and_Youth/Facts_for_Families/FFF-Guide/Preventing-and-Managing-Medication-Related-Weight-094.aspx

42. UCLA Department of Medicine. When Your Weight Gain Is Caused by Medicine. Accessed January 20, 2021. https://healthinfo.uclahealth.org/Library/Wellness/WeightControl/56,DM300

43. CHQ. Child Health Questionnaire TM. Accessed October 2013. www.healthactchq.com/chq.php

44. Kasai D, Parfitt G, Tarca B, et al. The Use of Ratings of Perceived Exertion in Children and Adolescents: A Scoping Review. *Sports Med.* 2021;51:33–50.

45. Lagally KM. Using rating of perceived exertion in physical education. *J Phys Educ Recreat Dance.* 2013;84(5):35-39.

46. Roemmich JN, Barkley JE, Epstein LH, et al. Validity of PCERT and OMNI walk/run ratings of perceived exertion. *Med Sci Sports Exerc.* 2006;38(5):1014-1019.

47. McWhorter JW, Wallmann HW, Alpert PT. The obese child: motivation as a tool for exercise. *J Pediatr Health Care.* 2003;17:11-17.

48. Procedures for the growth screening program for Pennsylvania's school-aged population. https://www.health.pa.gov/topics/school/Pages/Growth-Screen.aspx

49. Carol M. White physical education program. Accessed September 2013. www2.ed.gov/programs/whitephysed/index.html

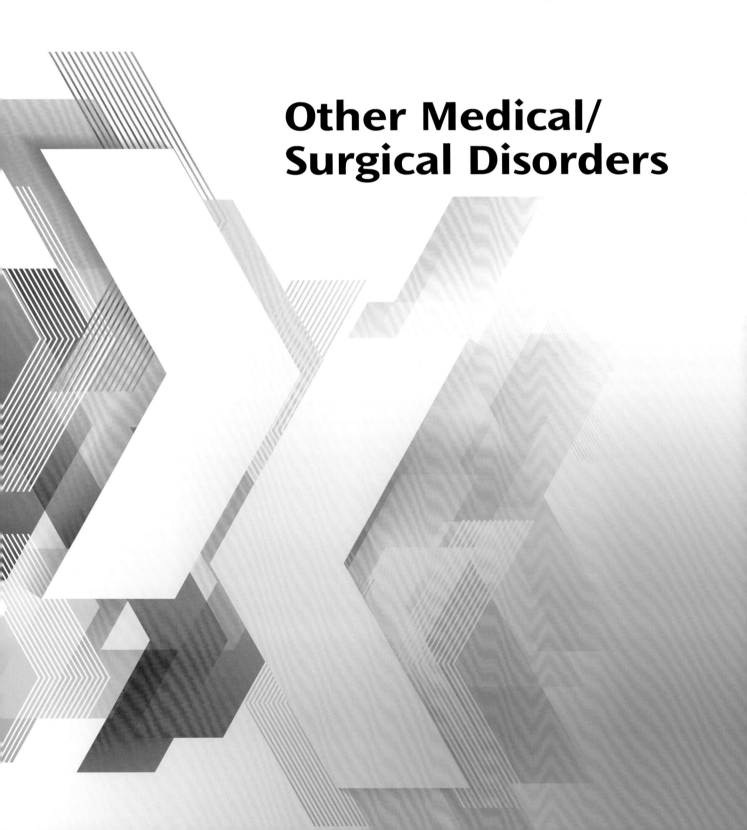

PART

VI

Other Medical/ Surgical Disorders

Oncologic Disorders

Stacey DiBiaso Caviston, Megan Ryninger, and Lauren B. Ward

» Introduction

Each year more than 11,000 children and adolescents in the United States are diagnosed with cancer.[1] As a result of improved diagnostic testing and medical interventions, survival rates for young adults who had cancer in childhood is 84%,[1] and it is estimated that 429,000 survivors of childhood cancer are living in the United States.[2] Therefore, more young adults than ever before are now living with the short- and long-term effects of cancer and the medical interventions used to save their lives. As the number of children with cancer and the number of survivors increase, so does the need for physical therapists (PTs) to learn more about early detection, treatment interventions for common types of pediatric cancer, and the short- and long-term side effects arising from the cancer and its treatment. PTs have a responsibility to understand the continuum of care for these children. This includes from the time of the diagnosis of cancer, to appropriate types of physical therapy interventions throughout the treatment, to educating children and families about the short- and long-term complications that they may experience as they relate to the scope of physical therapy practice primarily in the areas of the musculoskeletal, neuromuscular, integumentary, and cardiopulmonary systems.

PTs are in a unique position to assist children with their cancer care and advance the body of research, considering their education and training in those functional areas most adversely impacted by the disease and its treatment. These areas include disease prevention, education, and intervention, with a focus on a variety of impairments including range of motion (ROM), strength, motor planning, balance and coordination, fatigue, assistive devices, prosthetics and orthotics, and functional mobility. The ultimate goal of physical therapy for children with cancer is to improve their quality of life (QOL) and ability to participate in family and community activities.

Cancer is the uncontrolled growth of cells that do not function properly. As these cells increase in number, they tend to crowd out normal healthy cells or develop into a solid mass, causing signs and symptoms of disease to appear. Typically, the cancer develops at a primary site, but it may *metastasize* or spread to other areas of the body. The term *cancer* is often used to refer to various types of cancer. In children, leukemia, brain tumors, lymphomas, Wilms tumor, neuroblastoma, retinoblastoma, rhabdomyosarcoma, osteosarcoma, and Ewing sarcoma family of tumors are the most common types.[3] In contrast, adults most frequently develop prostate, breast, lung, colon, and rectal cancer.[1]

» Common types of pediatric cancer

Leukemia

Leukemia is the most prevalent type of pediatric cancer, accounting for 28% of all cancer cases in children younger than 15 years of age.[1] The disease takes its name from *leukocyte* (white blood cell) and the Greek word ending *emia,* which indicates a condition of the blood. Normal leukocytes are essential in helping the body remove foreign substances such as viruses, bacteria, and fungi. Leukemia, a malignant disorder of the blood and the blood-forming tissues of the bone marrow, is characterized by an overproduction of abnormal leukocytes. There are several different types of leukemia, and they are typically classified by the type of cell that gives rise to the cancerous cells (lymphoid or myeloid) and by the speed at which the cells replicate, quickly (acute) or slowly (chronic). In contrast to acute leukemias, chronic leukemias are less common in children, accounting for less than 5% of the cases of all pediatric leukemia.[4]

The most common pediatric leukemia is acute lymphoblastic leukemia (ALL), also known as acute lymphocytic leukemia or acute lymphoid leukemia. ALL accounts for 75% of all leukemia cases in children younger than 15 years of age.[3] It is most common in children 2 and 3 years of age. ALL is considered acute because immature lymphocytes proliferate rapidly and because the disease is fatal without treatment. However, with appropriate medical intervention, survival rates for children with ALL are now above 90%.[3]

The second most common pediatric leukemia is acute myeloid leukemia (AML), also referred to as myelocytic, myelogenous, or nonlymphoblastic leukemia. It accounts for 15% to 20% of all leukemia cases in children younger than 15 years of age.[5] AML is the rapid proliferation of immature myeloid cells. The survival rate for children with AML is less favorable than that for children with ALL; however, recent survival rates have risen to 65% to 70%.[3]

Genetic factors are assumed to play a role in causing acute leukemia. For example, children with Down syndrome, Klinefelter syndrome, Li–Fraumeni syndrome, and neurofibromatosis are more likely to develop leukemia than are children without these conditions.[1] Another possible factor in the development of acute leukemia is exposure to ionizing radiation and certain toxic chemicals.[3]

The signs and symptoms of leukemia are caused by an overproduction of a specific cell type that crowds out normal healthy cells, causing anemia, thrombocytopenia, and neutropenia and producing the identifiable side effects of leukemia such as fatigue, bruising, bleeding, infection, bone pain, fever, and enlarged lymph nodes and spleen.[1]

Medical intervention for children with leukemia includes multiagent chemotherapy, which can be given for 2 to 3 years, depending on the type of leukemia and the protocol. It is typically only when ALL relapses, that is, when the cancer cells return, that children will receive a stem cell transplant. Children with AML undergo chemotherapy as well, but the treatment is typically more intense and shorter in duration. At some cancer centers, children with AML receive stem cell transplantation (if a donor is available) soon after their cancer is under remission. Other centers hold this option as a means of treatment should the cancer return.[3]

Central Nervous System Tumors

Central nervous system (CNS) tumors are the second most commonly diagnosed pediatric cancer and the most commonly diagnosed solid tumor in children (Table 21.1).[6] These tumors account for 26% of childhood malignancies, and most frequently occur in children during the first decade of

TABLE 21.1.	Common Pediatric CNS Tumors[1,6,7,10,17,36]				
Type of Tumor	**Histology**	**Location**	**CNS Occurrences (%)**	**Peak Age of Incidence**
Astrocytoma Low-grade I, II (i.e., juvenile pilocytic astrocytoma, diffuse astrocytomas, optic gliomas) High-grade III, IV (i.e., anaplastic astrocytoma, glioblastomas)	Astrocytes (glial cells)	Cerebellum, cerebrum, thalamus, or hypothalamus	52	5
Embryonal tumors (medulloblastoma, atypical teratoid/rhabdoid tumor [ATRT])	Neuroepithelial	Cerebrum, cerebellum	10–20	1–10
Brainstem gliomas (diffuse midline glioma, diffuse intrinsic pontine glioma [DIPG])	Glial cells	Midbrain/pons/medulla	10–20	5–10
Ependymoma	Ependymal	Fourth ventricle	5–6	<5

CNS, central nervous system.

life.[6] The most common location of pediatric tumors is in the posterior fossa, accounting for 60% of all tumors in the brain (CHOP.edu). Common tumor types found in this location include medulloblastoma, juvenile pilocytic astrocytoma (JPA), diffuse intrinsic pontine glioma (DIPG), and atypical teratoid/rhabdoid tumor (ATRT). The remaining 40% of pediatric brain tumors are located in the cerebral hemispheres (CHOP.edu). The most common type of tumors found in this area of the brain are astrocytomas, gangliomas, and craniopharyngiomas. Signs and symptoms of brain tumors in children vary widely according to the size and location of the tumor. They may include headaches; seizures; drowsiness; changes in speech, vision, or hearing; behavioral changes; nausea or vomiting; poor coordination; weakness; and impaired balance.[7]

Medical intervention for children with brain tumors depends on the type and location of the tumor and may include surgery, radiation therapy, and chemotherapy.[6] Survival rates for children with CNS tumors vary depending on the type of tumor, size, and location. Children and adolescents with a CNS cancer have an overall survival rate of 74%.[6]

Lymphoma

The third most common type of cancer in children is lymphoma, including Hodgkin disease and non-Hodgkin lymphoma (NHL). Lymphomas account for 8% of all pediatric cancers.[1,3] These malignancies arise in the lymphoid cells and have their own biologic subtypes.[3] Hodgkin disease is more common in older children and adolescents, whereas NHL is more prevalent in younger children.[3] The signs and symptoms of Hodgkin disease include painless supraclavicular or cervical adenopathy, nonproductive cough, fatigue, anorexia, slight weight loss, night sweats, and pruritus.[8] NHL is typically classified into four subcategories[8]:

1. Burkitt and Burkitt-like lymphoma (small noncleaved cell lymphoma)
2. Lymphoblastic lymphoma (T-cell lymphoma)
3. Diffuse large B-cell lymphoma
4. Anaplastic large cell lymphoma

The clinical signs and symptoms of NHL may include changes in bowel habits; nausea; vomiting; swelling of the abdomen, face, neck, or upper limbs; dysphagia; and dyspnea.[8] The survival rate for children and adolescents with Hodgkin disease is 98%, and for those with NHL is 91%. (cancer facts and figures). Medical treatment of lymphoma typically includes chemotherapy and radiation therapy.[8]

Neuroblastic Tumors

The neuroblastic tumors include neuroblastoma, ganglioneuroblastoma, and ganglioneuroma.[9] These tumors are the most common extracranial solid tumors occurring in children, with the median age being 16 months. These tumors develop from primordial neural crest cells, with the most common sites of origin including the adrenal region (48%), extra-adrenal retroperitoneum (25%), and chest (16%).[10] Neuroblastoma is the most common cancer in infants younger than 1 year old. It accounts for 6% of all childhood cancers, about 800 new cases each year in the United States. Nearly 90% of cases are diagnosed by age 5, with the average age at diagnosis being 1 to 2 years of age.[1] Neuroblastomas commonly develop in the adrenal glands, sympathetic nervous system, ganglia of the abdomen, and sympathetic ganglia of the chest or neck.[3,9] The signs and symptoms of neuroblastoma depend largely on the location of the tumor. These include a palpable fixed hard mass in the neck or abdomen area and pain and paralysis if the tumor involves the spinal cord or peripheral nerves.[9] It most often spreads to the lymph nodes, bones, bone marrow, liver, and skin in infants and children, and often (in two-thirds of the cases) before it is diagnosed.[3]

A biopsy is performed to diagnose neuroblastoma. A computed tomography (CT) scan and magnetic resonance imaging (MRI) can reveal where the tumors are located in the body. An metaiodobenzylguanidine (MIBG) scan is used to detect spread to other parts of the child's body by injecting a radioactive substance into the body. Certain factors affect prognosis and treatment options as well as chance of recovery. The stage and risk group provide important information about the treatment and anticipated response to treatment. The International Neuroblastoma Staging System (INSS) and the International Neuroblastoma Risk Group Staging System (INRGSS) are used to determine the stage of neuroblastoma. These staging systems use results from surgery or imaging tests, respectively, to determine the stage of neuroblastoma.[3] The Children's Oncology Group (COG) places children in risk groups (low, intermediate, high) based on the stage of the tumor and prognostic factors including age and tumor histology and biology. Treatment is based on risk groups. Surgery, chemotherapy, radiation therapy, stem cell transplant, and immunotherapy are used to medically manage cases of neuroblastoma.[3]

The survival rate for children with neuroblastoma depends on the age at diagnosis, disease stage, and tumor histology.[2,9] The younger the child is at diagnosis, the greater the chances of survival. The 5-year survival rate for children in the low-risk group is higher than 95%. Children in the intermediate risk group have a 5-year survival rate of 90% to 95%. Children in the high-risk group have a 5-year survival rate around 40% to 50%.[1]

Sarcoma

The word *sarcoma* means a malignant tumor arising from cells of mesenchymal origin. These cells typically mature into skeletal muscle, smooth muscle, fat, fibrous tissue, bone, and cartilage.[11] The medical intervention for sarcoma may include neoadjuvant (preoperative chemotherapy) and adjuvant (after surgery) chemotherapy, surgery, and/or radiation therapy. The primary goal of medical treatment is to improve survival of the child and to preserve as much function of the affected extremity as possible. Factors used to determine the type of medical intervention include the tumor's size, location, and response to presurgical chemotherapy and containment of the disease to the primary site.[12]

Osteosarcoma

Osteosarcoma is the most common bone tumor in adolescents, with the most prevalent age of diagnosis between the ages of 10 and 30.[3,13] Teens are the most affected.[3] The tumor occurs most commonly in the long bones, primarily in the metaphyseal area of the distal femur, proximal tibia, or proximal humerus.[13] The primary symptom of osteosarcoma is pain in the involved site, specifically pain that progresses over time and may wake a child from sleep. A palpable mass may be present in the affected limb. Other symptoms may include decreased ROM or gait abnormalities. Some children may present with pathologic fracture at or near the tumor site.[10,13] Standard medical interventions for osteosarcoma include neoadjuvant chemotherapy, local control, and then adjuvant chemotherapy. Local control surgery options include amputation and limb-sparing procedures. Both are discussed later in this chapter. Factors used to determine the form of surgery include the tumor's size, location, and response to presurgical chemotherapy. The medical team also takes the child's age and skeletal maturity, as well as their overall prognosis into consideration when offering surgical options to a child/family. Survival rates for children with metastatic osteosarcoma (30%) are not as favorable as are those for children whose disease is localized (75%).[10]

Ewing Sarcoma

Ewing sarcoma is the second most common type of bone malignancy in children and adolescents, with a mean age of 15 years old at diagnosis.[14] Ewing sarcoma is a small, round, blue cell tumor that arises from bones or surrounding soft tissue. Common sites for Ewing sarcoma are the lower extremity long bones (41%), pelvis (26%), chest wall (16%), spine (6%), hand/foot (3%), and the skull (2%). Signs and symptoms include pain and/or swelling at the tumor location.[14] A palpable mass may also present at the site.[14] Medical intervention for children with Ewing sarcoma include neoadjuvant chemotherapy, local control of the tumor site, and then adjuvant chemotherapy. Local control options for Ewing sarcoma include surgery and/or radiation therapy. The plan for local control is based on tumor location, size, and the risks of morbidity or decreased functional outcome with surgical resection. The prognosis for Ewing sarcoma in children varies widely, depending on the tumor location. The overall 5-year survival rate for children with localized Ewing sarcoma is approximately 70%.[3] The survival rate is lower for those children who develop metastatic disease (15% to 30%).[3]

Rhabdomyosarcoma

The most common soft-tissue sarcoma in neonates to children 14 years of age, rhabdomyosarcoma is the sixth most common cancer in children and adolescents.[3,11] The most prevalent sites for a rhabdomyosarcoma are the head and neck, followed by the urinary and reproductive organs, extremities, and trunk.[10,11] Signs and symptoms of rhabdomyosarcoma include the appearance of a mass or the disturbance in a normal body function such as a tumor in the nasopharynx that causes an obstruction and discharge.[11] Medical treatment for children with rhabdomyosarcoma includes surgical removal of the tumor, chemotherapy, and radiation therapy.[11] As was the case with the other sarcomas, the survival rate for children with rhabdomyosarcoma depends on the tumor size, location, and cellular composition, how successful surgical removal was, and whether the tumor is contained to one site. Children younger than 15 years at diagnosis have a 5-year survival rate of 65% in contrast to those 15 to 19 years of age, who have a 47% survival rate.[2,3]

Retinoblastoma

Retinoblastoma, the most common childhood eye cancer, is a malignancy of the retina that originates from multipotent precursor cells. It accounts for only 2% of all childhood cancers. In the United States, 200 to 300 children are diagnosed with retinoblastoma each year. It is most common in infants and very young children, rarely occurring in children older than 6 years of age.[3] The disease may be hereditary or nonhereditary; the hereditary form presents primarily in infants.[15] The nonhereditary form occurs when the gene spontaneously develops a new mutation, and it is more prevalent in children than in infants.[15] The median age of retinoblastoma is 2 years of age.[3] Three out of four children will have unilateral involvement, whereas one out of four will have bilateral involvement.[3] The two most common signs and symptoms of retinoblastoma are leukocoria (lack of the normal red reflex of the eye) and strabismus (eyes cross).[15] Medical intervention for children with retinoblastoma is very multifaceted and may include external beam radiotherapy, intensity-modulated radiation therapy (IMRT) and proton radiation laser photocoagulation, cryotherapy, thermotherapy, systemic chemotherapy (~6 months to shrink the tumor), intra-arterial chemotherapy (chemotherapy given in the artery that feeds the eye), and/or intravitreal chemotherapy (chemotherapy injected into the eye).[15] If these treatments fail, enucleation (removal of the eye) is performed. Stem cell transplants in conjunction with high-dose chemotherapy can be used in children with retinoblastoma that has spread outside the eye.[3] Overall, nine out of ten children in the United States with retinoblastoma are cured unless cancer has spread outside of the eye. The 5-year survival rate for infants and children with retinoblastoma now exceeds 95%.[3,10]

Wilms Tumor

Wilms tumor, also called nephroblastoma, is the most common malignancy of the kidney in children.[16] About 5% of all childhood cancers are Wilms tumor, with 500 to 600 new cases diagnosed each year in the United States.[3] It mostly occurs in young children, with average age of diagnosis between 3 and 4 years of age.[3,16] The primary signs and symptoms of Wilms tumor are abdominal swelling or mass, fever, anemia, and hypertension.[16] The majority of children have disease in only one kidney, and only 5% to 10% of cases are bilateral. About nine out of ten Wilms tumors have a favorable histology with a good chance of a cure. The COG staging system is most often used to describe the extent of spread of Wilms tumors. The system divides the tumors into five stages.

The COG staging system[16]:

- Stage I: Contained in kidney and was removed by surgery
- Stage II: Grown beyond kidney, either into nearby fatty tissue or blood vessels, but was removed completely by surgery
- Stage III: Not fully removed by surgery, and cancer remains in abdomen
- Stage IV: Spread by blood to organs away from the kidney, such as lungs, liver, brain, bones, or other lymph nodes
- Stage V: Tumor found in both kidneys at time of diagnosis

Medical intervention for Wilms tumor consists of surgical resection, chemotherapy, and radiation therapy.[16] The type of intervention depends on the stage. The goal is to remove the primary tumor with surgery. Sometimes chemotherapy and radiation can be used to shrink the tumor before surgery. Radiation may also be needed after surgery to eliminate the remaining tumor cells. Chemotherapy drugs most often used include vincristine, actinomycin D, doxorubicin, cyclophosphamide, etoposide, irinotecan, and carboplatin. The 4-year survival rate for children with Wilms tumor is 95% to 100% in stages I to III and V, and 85% to 90% with stage IV.[3]

» Disease and medical intervention factors that influence physical therapy practice

When a child presents with signs and symptoms suggestive of cancer, a physician orders specific diagnostic tests. A complete blood count test is very frequently performed to evaluate the function of the bone marrow. The normal blood values listed in Table 21.2 are only a general range because these values vary slightly according to the child's gender and age.[25] Children undergoing treatment for cancer typically have lower blood counts. Therapists working with this population should have a strong working knowledge of these norms and also the signs and symptoms of altered values. The newest literature demonstrates no adverse effects when PTs working with children undergoing cancer treatment evaluate and treat them depending on their symptoms versus previously accepted guidelines.[21]

A bone marrow aspiration or bone marrow biopsy is performed by direct insertion of a needle into the bone, typically the iliac crest bone. The sample is then examined microscopically to detect the presence of cancer cells. A lumbar puncture is performed by insertion of a needle into the lumbar vertebrae area; cerebrospinal fluid is withdrawn to determine whether the cancer involves the cerebrospinal fluid. PTs must understand that a child who has undergone either a bone marrow aspiration or a lumbar puncture may experience discomfort with movement or feel sore in these areas for a few days and take this into consideration when performing the physical therapy examination and planning for that session's intervention program. For example, if a child has difficulty transitioning from a sitting position to standing, it may not be due to lower extremity weakness but instead to the discomfort in the hip or low back area, and the problem will resolve in a few days.

If a child presents with pain or swelling in an extremity, radiography, ultrasound, CT, or MRI is performed. Examination of the imaging results is helpful in identifying the

TABLE 21.2. Blood Counts and Symptoms[7]				
	Red Blood Cells (Erythrocytes)	Platelets (Thrombocytes)	Hemoglobin	White Blood Cells (Leukocytes)
Function	CO_2 and O_2 transport	Clotting of blood	CO_2 and O_2 transport	Defense against infection
Normal values	Male: $4.7-5.5 \times 10^6/\mu L$ Female: $4.1-4.9 \times 10^6/\mu L$	$150,000-350,000/\mu L$	$10-13$ g/100 mL	$4,500-11,000/mm^3$
Name of low value	Anemia	Thrombocytopenia	Anemia	Bacterial, viral, and/or fungal infection
Symptoms of low values	Pallor Fatigue	Bruising Petechiae	Pallor Fatigue	Infection

tumor's location. Further testing, for example, of a needle biopsy sample, is required to determine the type of tumor on the basis of the cell's morphologic characteristics. The location of the tumor may have an impact on the surrounding tissues such as causing joint contractures or changing the child's lower extremity weight-bearing status, thus limiting ambulation and functional mobility.

Before prescribing a course of medical treatment, the oncologist will determine the tumor's grade and stage by identifying the specific type of cancer on a cellular level, its exact location, and whether the cancer has spread to other areas of the body. The tumor's grade, which indicates its degree of malignancy, is determined on the basis of the microscopic appearance of the tumor cells, the tendency of the tumor to spread, and its growth rate. A system frequently used in the determination of cancer grade is that of the World Health Organization (WHO).[17] The system starts with grade I (a tumor that grows slowly and has a slightly abnormal appearance) and ends with grade IV (a tumor that reproduces most rapidly and has the undifferentiated cells).[17] Staging classifications are used to describe whether the disease is contained to the primary site, and, if not, the extent of its spread. Although the exact cause of the cancer is often unknown, genetic and environmental factors have been linked to many of the common pediatric cancers. It is important for the oncologist to understand these genetic factors because they may also affect the type of intervention chosen for the child. The PT must also understand the grading and staging systems to tailor the physical therapy intervention program and plan of care around the child's specific needs. For example, if a child has a lower extremity osteosarcoma and the therapist is working on gait training and the child is becoming short of breath with increased work of breathing, the therapist will want to know if the child has lung metastases and modify the session accordingly.

Pediatric cancers are typically treated with multiple modalities such as surgery, chemotherapy, radiation therapy, or stem cell transplantation. Medical intervention is based on the type of cancer and the extent of disease. There are different phases of treatment: induction, consolidation, and maintenance. During the induction phase, the child receives high doses of chemotherapy and, possibly, other modalities such as radiation therapy, with the goal of achieving remission as quickly as possible (no cancer cells present). To eliminate any remaining cancer cells, children continue to receive high doses of chemotherapy during the consolidation phase. During the maintenance phase, children receive lower doses of chemotherapy with the goal of preventing disease relapse.

Immunotherapy is a newer type of cancer treatment being successfully used in the pediatric population. This type of treatment genetically alters the body's own immune cells to train white blood cells to seek out and kill cancer cells. "Chimeric antigen receptor (CAR) T-cell therapy for B-Cell ALL was the first-ever cell therapy to receive FDA approval,"[7] and is now an available treatment option for relapsed or refractory disease at many cancer centers (Fig. 21.1). A possible serious side effect is cytokine release syndrome (CRS) that can be life-threatening. Children receiving CAR T-cell therapy are monitored closely for this side effect by the medical team. Monoclonal antibodies are another form of immunotherapy in which man-made antibodies are used to target-specific cancer cells in the body and destroy them. Examples of these include bevacizumab and cetuximab. They are given intravenously and usually have fewer side effects than does chemotherapy.[1] New immunotherapy treatments are currently being researched and approved for treatment of pediatric cancers.

Chemotherapy

Chemotherapeutic agents are chemicals used to interfere with rapidly dividing cancer cells, thus resulting in cell death. Multiagent chemotherapy is used to prevent resistance to one drug and allows administration of higher doses. Chemotherapy is the primary intervention for many types of cancers such as leukemia and lymphoma. It is often combined with other treatment modalities such as surgery and radiation therapy. For example, children with osteosarcoma or Ewing sarcoma often receive neoadjuvant chemotherapy for approximately 10 to 12 weeks before surgery to help shrink the tumor.[18,19] They also receive adjuvant chemotherapy to aid in elimination of any cancer cells that have spread to other areas of the body.

Chemotherapeutic agents are administered in a variety of ways, including intravenous, oral, and intramuscular routes. Most agents do not readily cross the blood–brain barrier. To target disease in the CNS, these agents are injected directly into the cerebrospinal fluid, typically through a catheter inserted in the lumbar area or in the brain.[20] This mode of administration, which is called intrathecal, is commonly used for administration of methotrexate.

Chemotherapeutic agents cause secondary side effects (Table 21.3). Not all agents cause the same side effects, nor do they occur within the same period of time. Certain classes of drugs or specific agents can cause harmful effects such as neurotoxicity, cardiotoxicity, or pulmonary complications. Please refer to Table 21.3 for the list of common side effects. One common side effect of chemotherapy is chemotherapy-induced peripheral neuropathy (CIPN). CIPN occurs secondary to the neurotoxic effects of frequently used chemotherapy agents including vinca alkaloids (most common vincristine) and platinum agents (most common cisplatin). CIPN occurs in children receiving treatment for both CNS and non-CNS cancers, occurring in 20% to 85% of children with non-CNS cancers.[21,22] CIPN can lead to sensory, motor, and/or autonomic nerve dysfunction. Impairments primarily affect the peripheral extremities, hands and feet, within weeks of administration.[22] The earliest and most common clinical sign related to CIPN is a decreased Achilles tendon reflex, which can occur within a month of chemotherapy. The primary indication of peripheral neuropathy is weakness and or sensory changes in the distal extremities. The most common impairment in the lower extremities is

CAR T-cell Therapy

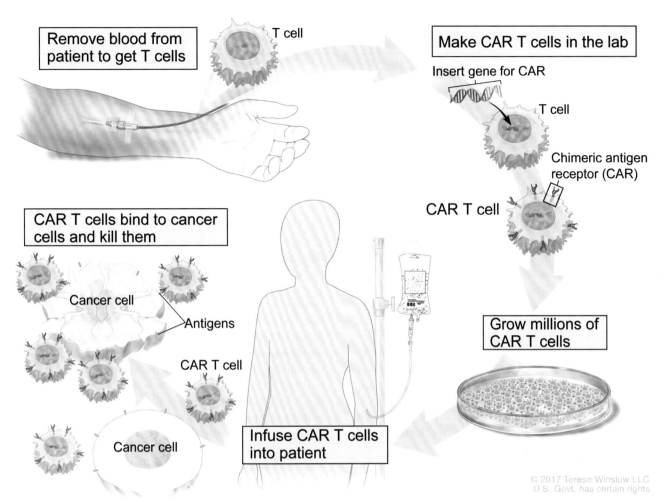

FIGURE 21.1. Diagram depicting treatment with chimeric antigen receptor (CAR) T-cell therapy. (From National Cancer Institute at the National Institutes of Health, https://www.cancer.gov/publications/dictionaries/cancer-terms/def/car-t-cell-therapy. Accessed December 2018. © 2017 Terese Winslow LLC, U.S. Govt. has certain rights.)

TABLE 21.3.	Specific Chemotherapeutic Agents and Common Side Effects Pertinent to Physical Therapy[3,21-25]		
	Common Side Effects		
Chemotherapeutic Agents	**Short Term**	**Long Term**	**Common Types of Cancer**
Vincristine	Hypertension, motor difficulties, CNS depression, peripheral neuropathy, alopecia, constipation, anorexia, jaw pain, leg pain, weakness, paresthesia, numbness, myalgia, cramping	Peripheral neuropathy, decreased gross and fine motor skills	Leukemia, Hodgkin disease, neuroblastoma, lymphomas, Wilms tumor, and rhabdomyosarcoma
Cisplatin	Bradycardia, nausea, vomiting, bone marrow suppression, ototoxicity, peripheral neuropathy	Ototoxicity, nephrotoxicity	Osteosarcoma, Hodgkin disease and non-Hodgkin lymphoma, brain tumors
Methotrexate	Malaise, fatigue, dizziness, alopecia, photosensitivity, nausea, vomiting, diarrhea, anorexia, mucositis, glossitis, myelosuppression, arthralgia, osteopenia	Osteoporosis, bone fracture, infertility, renal toxicity, hepatotoxicity, neuropsychological-cognitive deficits	Leukemia, osteosarcoma, non-Hodgkin lymphoma

(continued)

TABLE 21.3.	Specific Chemotherapeutic Agents and Common Side Effects Pertinent to Physical Therapy[3,21-25] (continued)		
	Common Side Effects		
Chemotherapeutic Agents	Short Term	Long Term	Common Types of Cancer
Dexamethasone	Hypertension, increased susceptibility to infection, myopathy, increased appetite, mental changes	Growth suppression, bone demineralization, osteonecrosis	Leukemia, brain tumors, and other types of malignancy
Ifosfamide	Somnolence, dizziness, polyneuropathy, alopecia, dermatitis, nausea, vomiting, anorexia, diarrhea, constipation, myelosuppression	Cardiotoxicity, nephrotoxicity	Hodgkin disease and non-Hodgkin lymphoma, acute and chronic lymphocytic leukemia, sarcoma
Doxorubicin	Alopecia, nausea, vomiting, mucositis, diarrhea, bone marrow suppression	Cardiotoxicity, myocarditis	Lymphoma, leukemia, soft-tissue sarcoma, neuroblastoma, osteosarcoma

foot drop, decreased ankle dorsiflexion (DF) strength and active DF ROM, and neuropathic pain or sensory loss.[22] The order in which the clinical presentation occurs may vary; the PT may observe weakness in a child's intrinsic muscle of the hands and feet followed by weakness of the anterior tibialis, or the child may experience neuropathic pain without any signs of muscle weakness. Generally, with a reduction in the dose of the chemotherapy agent or when administration of the drug is stopped, the symptoms of neurotoxicity decrease. However, newer research suggests some residual deficits in ankle strength, ROM, gait, and gross motor skills may persist. Research data show 30% of children experiencing CIPN have resulting deficits later in life.[21,22]

Drugs such as methotrexate can cause myelosuppression within a week of their administration. Myelosuppression is a process in which bone marrow activity is decreased, resulting in low production of platelets, red blood cells, and white blood cells and a corresponding increase in the risk of bleeding, fatigue, and infection. Methotrexate can also cause long-term neuropsychological problems with memory deficits and visual-spatial and motor coordination impairments.[3,23-25] Steroids such as dexamethasone can cause proximal weakness, hypertension, emotional lability, increased appetite, and immunosuppression. Long-term effects can include growth suppression, bone demineralization osteonecrosis, and avascular necrosis (AVN).[3]

The neurotoxic effects of the drugs are particularly a concern for the developing nervous system of young children. Given the young age at diagnosis, significant developmental concerns arise because children receive neurotoxic drugs while still growing. This can have profound effects on motor, cognitive, social, and psychosocial effects on development.[3,26-27]

Radiation Therapy

Radiation therapy is the use of ionizing radiation to disrupt the structure of the tumor cells' DNA, which limits the cells' ability to further reproduce. Unlike chemotherapy, radiation does not cause cell damage throughout the body; it only damages cells in the area of the body where it is given (COG).

Radiation therapy is delivered by an external radiation beam (most common), or internal placement of radiation material near the tumor. Radiation therapy can be used alone or, more frequently, is used in combination with other treatments such as surgery and chemotherapy.[28,29] Radiation therapy delivered before surgical removal of a tumor can shrink the tumor mass, thus decreasing the amount of damage to the surrounding healthy tissues. Radiation is used after surgery to destroy any cells that may have spread from the primary site.[30] Total body irradiation is also used with chemotherapy to destroy the child's bone marrow in preparation for receiving a stem cell transplant.

Radiation therapy may cause numerous short- and long-term side effects (Table 21.4), which are mainly related to the area and the surrounding tissues that received the radiation.[28-35] Some of the side effects of radiation include fatigue/somnolence syndrome, effects on skin, and slowed bone growth. Scoliosis can be a late effect from chest wall radiation. Side effects from radiation are particularly severe in infants and children who are still growing. Radiation therapy significantly impacts the neuropsychological and musculoskeletal systems of children. Cranial radiation leads to fibrosis of the brain; therefore, radiation to the brain is avoided in children younger than 3 years old because of the severity of neurocognitive effects on the developing brain.[1,3]

Surgery

Surgical procedures typically performed for the children patient with cancer include tumor biopsy, central line and shunt placement, and tumor resection, with or without extensive surgical reconstruction.

Tumor Biopsy

Typically, before any medical intervention takes place, a biopsy of a portion of the tumor or a bone marrow aspiration is obtained to determine the cell type and stage of cancer. These procedures are performed under general anesthesia, conscious sedation, or local anesthesia. Unfortunately, with some brain tumors, primarily those of the brainstem,

TABLE 21.4.	Short- and Long-term Side Effects of Radiation[28-35]	
Short Term	**Long Term**	**Implication for Physical Therapists**
Skin	Fibrosis	Pain
Redness	Pathologic fracture	Decreased ROM
Blistering	Bone growth abnormalities	Decreased strength
Hair loss	Osteonecrosis/avascular necrosis	Decreased endurance
Fibrosis	Osteoporosis	Decreased functional mobility
Fatigue	Cardiac complications	Decreased balance
Cognitive deficits	Hypertension	Decreased neuropsychological function
	Thyroid dysfunction	Motor accuracy, sensory integration, memory, concentration
		Decreased quality of life and participation in community and family activities

ROM, range of motion.

a biopsy cannot be performed because of the high risk of damage to surrounding tissue.

Central Line and Shunt Placement

Because most children receive intravenous chemotherapy agents over an extended period of time, a surgically placed indwelling catheter that leads directly into a major blood vessel near the heart may be required. These lines are often called a central line, or Broviac or Hickman catheter. The Broviac catheter is an external catheter that leads into a major vessel such as the external or internal jugular. An internal catheter (port) is placed into the same major vessel, but it remains under the skin and is accessed with a needle each time the child needs to receive medication or to have blood drawn. A central line being pulled out accidentally constitutes a medical emergency owing to the risk of infection and bleeding. Therefore, special precautions must be taken to keep the area around the catheter clean, dry, and protected from injury.

Surgical placement of a ventriculoperitoneal shunt is often required when a brain tumor results in increased intracranial pressure. It is important for PTs to know the following signs and symptoms of increased cranial pressure owing to a brain tumor or a shunt malfunction. These include headaches, vomiting, diplopia, depressed mental status, papilledema, and changes in motor function.[36]

Surgical Resection

Most solid tumors will require surgical resection. However, some are too large to be resected, or are located where surgical resection would be risky. Examples include brainstem glioma or neuroblastoma that extends into the spinal cord. However, for malignant tumors, surgical resection is typically the optimal choice. To increase the chance that the tumor does not return or spread to other areas of the body, the surgeon will make every effort to completely resect the tumor with a clean margin of tissue with no cancer cells. Because it is not always known whether any cells have spread beyond the primary tumor site, chemotherapy and radiation

therapy may also be given to the child to make every effort to rid the body of all cancerous cells.

Other Surgical Procedures

For children with an upper or lower extremity bone or soft-tissue tumor, surgical options such as amputation, rotationplasty, and limb-sparing procedures are available.[37-39] Each surgical option has risks and benefits. Children and families are encouraged to consult with a multidisciplinary team including orthopedics, PTs and occupational therapists (OTs), oncologists, radiologists, and social workers to determine which option is best suited for each individual child.

LIMB-SPARING SURGERIES Limb-sparing surgeries fall into two categories: endoprosthetic reconstruction and biologic reconstruction. Endoprosthetic reconstruction entails surgical removal of the tumor with clear margins and reconstruction of the limb with a custom endoprosthetic device. Benefits of this option include immediate weight bearing postoperatively, allowing for early rehabilitation and return to functional activities. For children who have not reached skeletal maturity, the lower extremity can be reconstructed using an expandable endoprosthesis or contralateral epiphysiodesis.[12] After the expandable prosthesis is implanted, the surgeon can lengthen the child's leg without opening the surgical site. Use of this noninvasive procedure decreases the risk of infection and the time required for healing. Potential complications of endoprosthetic reconstruction can include the need for multiple surgical revisions due to loosening of the hardware, growth, fracture, or infection. Decreased ROM around the surgical joint is also common, impacting a child's ability to complete functional activities. Other complications include leg length discrepancies or the need for conversion to amputation.[12,37,40-42] Thus, it is important for PTs to plan for these types of complications and provide preventive measures if possible, such as exercises to prevent contractures and activity recommendations to decrease the wear and tear on the prosthesis.

BIOLOGIC RECONSTRUCTION Biologic reconstruction surgeries may use a bone allograft or an autograft to aid in rebuilding the removed portion of bone. Vascularized autografts are frequently harvested from the fibula or iliac crest. There are multiple options for surgical approaches in this category and considerations such as age, tumor size, and location are taken into account. A child's physical activity level and long-term goals for return to activity and sport should also be considered. Short-term limitations of these surgeries include delayed bone healing because of ongoing chemotherapy, which leads to a prolonged period of non–weight bearing. In some cases, a child may need to remain non–weight bearing for close to a year following surgery. However, long-term benefits can include decreased future surgical procedures and ability to participate in higher level activities such as sports, running, and jumping without risk of hardware failure.

AMPUTATION This surgical procedure results in removal of a portion of an extremity. The extent of the amount of limb removed depends on the tumor's location, type, and size. Amputation is typically performed when it is not possible to make a wide-enough excision to achieve clean margins, or when surgery is so extensive that the extremity is no longer functional.[40] After deciding that a child needs an amputation, the surgeon makes every effort to provide the child with a residual limb that is conducive to the functional use of a prosthetic device. The short-term complications of

an amputation may include psychological distress related to a drastic change in body image, slow healing of the surgical site if the child is receiving chemotherapy, inadequate wound coverage, neuropathic pain, phantom limb sensation, and increased energy expenditure for functional activities.[40] Long-term complications include psychological distress related to a drastic change in body image; skin blisters, redness, or bruising on the residual limb due to growth or weight changes; phantom limb pain and sensation; musculoskeletal pain; and increased energy expenditure for activities of daily living (ADLs).[40] In children, the need for different sized prostheses as a child grows or a heavier, expandable prostheses is also a consideration.

ROTATIONPLASTY This surgical procedure is sometimes performed in lieu of an amputation; however, it is still considered a form of amputation.[40] Rotationplasty is not the standard of care at many of the children's hospitals in the United States. Rotationplasty removes a femoral tumor while preserving the neurovascular bundle and the distal portion of the lower leg and foot (Fig. 21.2). The lower leg is turned 180 degrees and attached to the proximal femur in such a way that the foot can serve as the functional knee joint and as a weight-bearing surface for a prosthesis. The resultant residual limb does not require multiple surgical revisions and it is longer than if a below-knee amputation had been performed.[12] This longer limb provides the child with the chance for higher functional abilities.[43]

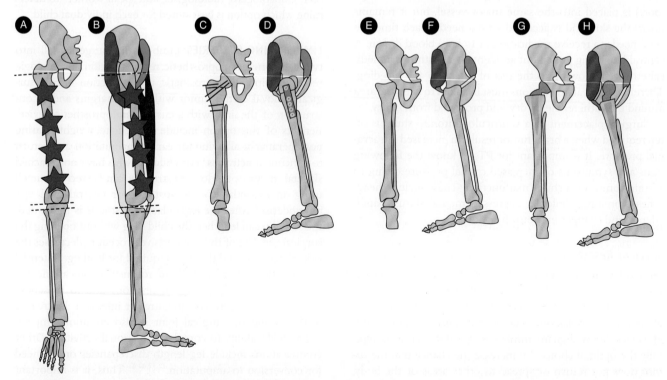

FIGURE 21.2. Rotationplasty. (Bernthal NM, Monument MJ, Randall RL, et al. Rotationplasty: beauty is in the eye of the beholder. *Oper Tech Orthop.* 2014;24(2):103-110. doi:10.1053/j.oto.2013.11.001)

Furthermore, children who have undergone rotationplasty can participate in recreational activities and sports, as can those who have had an amputation.[44,45] In the short term, the wound heals poorly; and in both the short and long term, the extremity has poor cosmesis compared to other surgical options. Researchers have studied QOL in children who have undergone a rotationplasty and determined that they do not show reduction in psychosocial adaptation compared with the healthy population.[46,47]

Bone Marrow Transplantation and Peripheral Stem Cell Transplantation

Bone marrow transplantation (BMT) or peripheral blood stem cell transplantation (PSCT) is performed in children with leukemia (relapsed ALL or chronic myelogenous leukemia) or other hematologic diseases (e.g., aplastic anemia, severe combined immunodeficiency [SCID], and sickle cell disease) that involve the bone marrow. The purpose is to replace the child's bone marrow with his or her own marrow or donor bone marrow capable of producing healthy cells. Bone marrow is typically harvested by the repeated insertion of a large needle into the donor's bone (e.g., the iliac crest) and withdrawal of the marrow. The stem cells, the most immature cell that further differentiates into mature cells, are obtained by taking blood from the donor via a process called *apheresis*. There are three common forms of BMT or PSCT:

1. Allogeneic transplants from a histocompatible donor
2. Autologous transplants from the child's own cells
3. Syngeneic transplants from an identical twin

The protocol being used and the policies of the institution where the transplantation takes place will determine whether the child receives a BMT or PSCT. The more common procedure currently performed is the PSCT. Some institutions are also now performing umbilical cord blood transplants.

Children who receive a BMT or a PSCT first receive combination chemotherapy to achieve a state of remission (no identifiable cancer cells in the body). The child is then admitted to the hospital for the conditioning phase. For approximately 1 week, the child receives chemotherapeutic agents (e.g., thiotepa) and total body irradiation, depending on his or her age and the treatment protocol. The goal of the conditioning phase is to provide complete bone marrow suppression. Because the child's white blood cell, red blood cell, and platelet counts drop, the child requires special care during this period to prevent infection and hemorrhaging. On the day of transplant, the child then receives an infusion of bone marrow or peripheral stem cells. For approximately 6 weeks, the child stays in an isolated room equipped with a positive pressure and an air filtration system to help prevent infection. Engraftment, the process by which donor marrow begins to produce healthy cells, typically takes 10 to 17 days.[48] Until the body produces its own cells, the child will require antibiotics to prevent infection and transfusions of red blood cells and platelets. Children may require red blood cell and platelet transfusions for up to 6 months and may not have adequate white blood cells to fight infection for 6 to 12 months.[48] Thus, PTs must be knowledgeable of the child's blood count levels to plan for the physical therapy session.

Transplant recipients do not produce healthy bone marrow cells for a period. Therefore, the recipient has an increased risk of infection, bleeding, and severe fatigue. Children who receive allogeneic transplants are at risk for developing some form of graft-versus-host disease (GVHD), a process by which the transplanted marrow (graft) starts to attack the child's (host) organs. There are two types of GVHD: acute and chronic. Acute GVHD can begin as early as the first month after the transplantation, when the engraftment process is taking place. Acute GVHD most commonly affects the skin, the gut, and the liver. These symptoms include a rash, itchy skin, skin discoloration, dry mouth, mouth ulcers, diarrhea, and weight loss. Chronic GVHD occurs months after the child receives the transplant and affects the skin and gastrointestinal system. Specific complications may include changes in the skin pigmentation and texture; possible development of joint contractures; dry mouth and ulcer formations; difficulty in swallowing and malabsorption, which may cause the child to lose weight; chronic liver disease; and problems with the eyes such as dryness, pain, and sensitivity to light.[49] The drugs prednisone, cyclosporine, and methotrexate are commonly given to child to prevent GVHD or to decrease the severity of the reaction.[49] Long-term complications include those that were previously listed under chemotherapy and radiation therapy. PTs should evaluate and provide intervention for children with GVHD to assist in the prevention of the development of joint contractures, decreased strength, and functional mobility.

Stem cell rescue is a process by which the child's own stem cells are extracted and stored. The child is then able to receive very high doses of chemotherapeutic agents, after which he or she receives a transfusion of his or her own cells. This procedure allows children with cancers such as medulloblastoma and neuroblastoma to receive multiple rounds of very high doses of chemotherapy.

» Physical therapy examination and evaluation

Medical and Social History

Obtaining a thorough medical and social history is one of the key components of any physical therapy examination. This process helps the PT select the types of questions to ask the child, directs the specific types of tests and measurements that are chosen, and ultimately guides the plan of care.

If the child's chart is available, it is ideal to obtain the following information before meeting the child:

1. Diagnoses, including pertinent past medical history
2. Disease grade and stage
3. Medical history, including child's growth and development
4. Current medical treatment, including the types of chemotherapeutic agents the child is receiving and other medical treatments
5. Current blood values, that is, hemoglobin concentrations, white and red blood cell counts, and platelet counts
6. Recent imaging results
7. Precautions/restrictions in the community

After obtaining the required medical information, it is important for the therapist to build a rapport with the child and the family. This is when the therapist asks about the child's social history. With whom does the child live? Does he or she have any siblings? What is the household setup? What grade has he or she completed in school? What sports or other leisure activities does the child enjoy? What is their daily routine like? What was their previous level of function? Have they previously had rehabilitation therapies? The therapist will use the answers to these questions as a basis for discussing areas with which the child is having difficulty at home, at school, or in the hospital. Often, it isn't until the therapist begins the examination that the child and family realize how much trouble the child is really having with specific tasks performed during their daily routines.

Systems Review

Specific impairments from different types of cancer can develop because of the cancer itself or the medical interventions required to treat the cancer. These impairments can have a profound effect on the child's physical mobility, cognitive, psychological and social function, communication, self-care, and participation level in their daily routines.[26,27] It is therefore important that the therapist identify areas of concern immediately and focus the examination on those target areas. The systems review is a helpful way to guide the physical therapy examination. As soon as the therapist sees the child, whether this occurs in his or her hospital room, the clinic, the child's classroom, or home, the therapist can identify the current key issues. Keeping a list of the essentials in mind helps with efficiency and thoroughness:

1. Musculoskeletal: weakness, ROM limitations, joint contractures, foot drop
2. Neuromuscular: signs of pain such as antalgic gait pattern, facial grimacing, guarding an area, sensory neuropathy; increased or decreased muscle tone, facial paralysis, difficulty hearing, seeing, and/or communicating, impaired balance; neurocognitive deficits that will limit the child's ability to follow directions
3. Cardiovascular and pulmonary: nasal flaring, increased work of breathing or respiratory rate

4. Integumentary: scars from previous surgeries; facial skin color that demonstrates possible low hemoglobin or liver function problems, for example, bruising that signals a low platelet count; skin changes from radiation

Tests and Measurements

To perform a thorough and comprehensive examination, the therapist can use a framework such as the WHO's International Classification of Functioning, Disability, and Health (ICF) including body functions/structures, activity, and participation. According to the WHO, the term *body function and structure* refers to the physiologic functions of body systems, including the body's psychological functions and anatomic parts, such as organs and limbs and their components. Activity refers to the execution of a task or action by an individual and participation refers to involvement in a life situation.[50] The WHO model takes into account the interactions between all three components of the model and the child's individual environmental and personal factors. Each child will require an individualized examination based on the specific diagnoses and common side effects of the medical intervention the child has received or is receiving.

The International Classification of Functioning, Disability, and Health-Childhood Cancer (ICF-CC) model was recently published, and focuses on identifying the body impairments, activity limitations, and participation restrictions among children and adolescents with cancer to assist in "defining rehabilitation goals and interventions" of this population.[21] Figure 21.3 shows this model filled out for the health condition of childhood and adolescent cancer.[21] Table 21.5, also by Tanner et al.,[21] outlines the key areas of focus in each category and the recommended clinical assessments to objectively measure them. For individual children, some areas will be more applicable and will require further testing.

Body Function and Structure (Impairments)

Musculoskeletal

The musculoskeletal component of the examination is important for children with cancer because they often have problems with ROM, strength, and postural alignment. Deficits in these areas are common in children who have experienced side effects of chemotherapy or radiation therapy, surgical alterations of the skeletal system, or weakness from prolonged inactivity. When assessing ROM, the therapist should give particular attention to the joints above and below any area where a surgical procedure has recently been performed. Children will often guard the area around the surgical site because of pain or fear. For example, immediately after a brain tumor resection, a child may have decreased cervical spine ROM or may tilt his or her head laterally to compensate for visual deficits. For a few days after a central line placement, a child may not want to perform full-shoulder flexion or trunk ROM because the chest area is sore. After an aggressive distal femur or proximal tibia limb-sparing procedure, a child's hip,

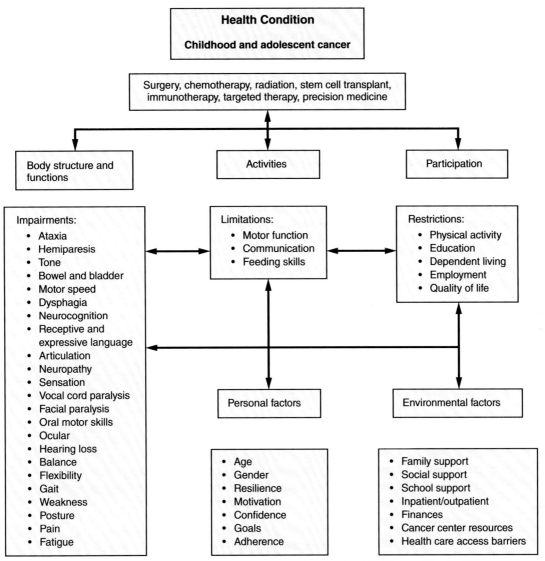

FIGURE 21.3. World Health Organization's International Classification of Functioning, Disability, and Health (ICF).

TABLE 21.5.	Recommended Clinical Assessments for Functional Impairments, Activity Limitations, and Participation Restrictions in Children, Adolescents, and Young Adults with Cancer[21]
Impairments	**Clinical Assessment**
Ataxia	• Box and Block Test (BBT)[97] • International Cooperative Assessment of Ataxia Rating Scale (ICARS)[98] • Scale for the Assessment and Rating of Ataxia (SARA)[99]
Muscle tone	• Hypertonia Assessment Tool (HAT)[100] • Modified Ashworth Scale (MAS)[101]
Dysarthria	• Dysarthria Examination Battery (DEB)[102] • Frenchay Dysarthria Assessment-2nd ed. (FDA-2)[103] • Speech sample
Apraxia	• Apraxia Profile[104] • Kaufman Speech Praxis Test for Children (KSPT)[105] • Speech sample

(continued)

TABLE 21.5.	Recommended Clinical Assessments for Functional Impairments, Activity Limitations, and Participation Restrictions in Children, Adolescents, and Young Adults with Cancer[21] (continued)
Impairments	**Clinical Assessment**
Dysphagia	• Clinical bedside swallow evaluation • Flexible endoscopic evaluation of swallowing (FEES) • Marshalla Oral Sensorimotor Test (MOST)[106] • Videofluoroscopic Swallow Study (VFSS or modified barium swallow [MBS])
Neurocognition	• Beery–Buktenica Developmental Test of Visual-Motor Integration-6th ed. (Beery VMI)[107] • Behavior Rating Inventory of Executive Functioning-2nd ed. (BRIEF-2)[108] • Children's Kitchen Task Assessment (CKTA)[109] • Children's Orientation and Amnesia Test (COAT)[110] • Cognitive-Linguistic Quick Test (CLQT)[111] • Digit Span Test, Verbal Fluency Test, Grooved Pegboard Test, Trail Making Test[112-114] • Miller Function and Participation Scales-VMI Scale[115] • National Institutes of Health Toolbox cognition[116] • The Pediatric Test of Brain Injury (PTBI)[117] • Scales of Cognitive Ability for Traumatic Brain Injury (SCATBI)[118] • Test of Visual Perceptual Skills (TVPS)[119] • The Test of Memory and Learning-2nd ed. (TOMAL-2)[120] • Test of Reading Comprehension-4th ed. (TORC-4)[121] • Weekly Calendar Planning Activity (WCPA)[122]
Receptive and/or expressive language impairment	• Ages and Stages Questionnaires (ASQ-3)[123] • Clinical Evaluation of Language Fundamentals-Preschool-2nd ed. (CELF-P2)[124] • Clinical Evaluation of Language Fundamentals-5th ed. (CELF-5)[125] • Comprehensive Assessment of Spoken Language-2nd ed. (CASL-2)[126] • Expressive One-Word Picture Vocabulary Test-4th ed. (EOWPVT-4)[127] • Oral and Written Language Scales-2nd ed. (OWLS-2)[128] • Peabody Picture Vocabulary Test-5th ed. (PPVT-5)[129] • Preschool Language Scale-5th ed. (PLS-5)[130] • Receptive-Expressive Emerging Language Test-3rd ed. (REEL-3)[131] • Receptive One-Word Picture Vocabulary Test-4th ed. (ROWPVT-4)[132] • The Rossetti Infant-Toddler Language Scale[133] • Test of Adolescent and Adult Word Finding (TAWF)[134] • Test of Integrated Language and Literacy Skills (TILLS)[135] • Test of Language Development-4th ed. (TOLD-4)[136] • Test of Word Finding-3rd ed. (TWF-3)[137]
Articulation	• Clinical Assessment of Articulation and Phonology-2nd ed. (CAAP-2)[138] • Goldman–Fristoe Test of Articulation-3rd ed. (GFTA-3)[139] • Structured Photographic Articulation Test-3rd ed. (SPAT-D III)[140]
Peripheral muscle weakness	• Dynamometry • Manual muscle test (MMT) • Pediatric-modified Total Neuropathy Score (Ped-mTNS)[141] • Total Neuropathy Score-Pediatric Vincristine (TNS-PV)[142]
Sensation impairment	• Ped-mTNS[141] • TNS-PV[142] • Monofilament testing • Point/dull testing • Vibration testing
Vocal cord paralysis	• Endoscopy/laryngoscopy
Facial paralysis	• House–Brackmann Scale[143] • Oral Motor Examination
Oral motor skills for feeding and speech	• Oral Motor Examination
Ocular impairment	• Observation of functional skills (e.g., reading, handwriting, environmental navigation) • Screening of visual acuity (LEA Symbols or age-appropriate eye chart)[144] • Screening of visual fields and ocular motility • The Oregon Project for Visually Impaired and Blind Preschool Children[145]

TABLE 21.5. Recommended Clinical Assessments for Functional Impairments, Activity Limitations, and Participation Restrictions in Children, Adolescents, and Young Adults With Cancer[21] (*continued*)

Impairments	Clinical Assessment
Hearing loss	• Audiometry • Auditory Brainstem Response (ABR) • Otoacoustic Emissions (OAEs)
Balance	• Pediatric Balance Scale (PBS)[146] • Bruininks–Oseretsky Test of Motor Performance-2nd ed. Balance scale (BOT-2)[147] • Modified Clinical Test of Sensory Integration in Balance (mCTSIB)[148]
Contractures	• Active and passive range of motion (ROM)
Fibrosis	• Active and passive ROM
Gait	• Edinburgh Visual Gait Scale (EVGS)[149] • Computerized gait analysis • 30-second Walk Test (30sWT)[150]
Weakness	• Dynamometry[151] • Manual muscle test (MMT)[152] • Functional strength tests[153] • BOT-2 Strength subtest[147]
Posture	• Adam's Forward Bend Test[154] • Foot Posture Index (FPI-6)[155]
Pain	• CRIES Scale[156] • Faces Pain Scale-Revised (FPS-R)[157] • Numerical Rating Scale (NRS)[158] • revised Face Legs Activity Cry and Consolability (FLACCr)[159] • Visual Analog Scale (VAS)[160]
Fatigue	• Adolescent Fatigue Scale (FS-A)[161] • Childhood Fatigue Scale (FS-C)[162] • Parent Fatigue Scale (FS-P)[162] • Patient-Reported Outcomes Measurement Information System (PROMIS) fatigue item banks[163]
Activity limitations	
Gross and fine motor skills	• Ages and Stages Questionnaire (ASQ-3)[123] • Battelle Developmental Inventory[164] • Bayley Scales of Infant and Toddler Development-4th ed. (Bayley-4)[165] • Bruininks–Oseretsky Test of Motor Proficiency-2nd ed. (BOT-2)[166] • Miller Function and Participation Scales • 9-Hole Peg Test[167] • Peabody Developmental Motor Scales-2nd ed. (PDMS-II)[168] • Print Tool[169] • Purdue Pegboard Test[170] • Test of Handwriting Skills-Revised (THS-R)[171] • Timed up and go (TUG)[172] • Timed up and down stairs (TUDS)[173]
Communication	• See receptive and/or expressive language impairment • Language sample • Observation of communication interactions
Feeding	• Oral motor feeding evaluation
Participation restrictions	
Dependent living	• Unable to recommend
Education	• School Function Assessment[174]
Employment	• Unable to recommend
Physical activity level	• 6-minute Walk Test (6MWT)[175] • FitnessGram PACER Test[176]
Quality of life	• Children's Assessment of Participation and Enjoyment (CAPE)[177] • Preferences for Activities of Children (PAC)[177] • The Pediatric Quality of Life Inventory (PedsQL) Generic Core Scales,[178] Multidimensional Fatigue Scale,[178] Cancer Module,[178] or Brain Tumor Module[179] • PROMIS[180]

knee, and ankle ROM may be limited. GVHD after a BMT can cause limited ROM at joints; therefore, it is important to maintain frequent and accurate ROM measurements in this population. Another important factor to consider when testing a child's ROM and strength is the type of chemotherapy the child is receiving or has received. As previously discussed, some neurotoxic agents, specifically vincristine, can cause CIPN, resulting in a decrease in distal strength and active range of motion (AROM). Therefore, the therapist will want to focus on the ankle and hand strength in children receiving vincristine or other chemotherapy agents causing CIPN using manual muscle testing (MMT) or dynamometry, as well as functional measurements of strength. It is important to frequently reassess strength and ROM while a child is actively undergoing chemotherapy treatment. Steroids can cause steroid myopathy, resulting in proximal weakness; therefore, assessing core strength is important as well.[21,22]

Postural alignment should be examined in this population as well. Looking for asymmetries that could be the result of surgery, hemiparesis, and scoliosis is important especially in examining later effects of cancer. Examining foot posture is important if CIPN is present because of weakening of the foot intrinsic musculature leading to pes planus or calcaneal valgus.[21]

When performing the strength component of the examination, the therapist must consider the child's blood count levels and ability to comprehend directions for MMT. The therapist should also observe the child's functional strength abilities safely while performing activities such as walking, climbing stairs, and performing transitional movements such as sit-to-stand.

Neuromuscular

When examining a child's neuromuscular system (i.e., conducting tests of pain, muscle tone, balance, motor control, vision, sensation, and sensory integration), it is important for the therapist to consider the complex interplay of the neuromuscular system with all the other systems in the body, the environment, and the task. If a child with a brainstem glioma presents with increased or decreased muscle tone or stiffness in the right lower and upper extremity, the therapist must consider how this impairment affects the child's active and passive ROM, isolated muscle strength, proprioception, functional abilities, and ADL, while also taking into account the child's cognitive abilities, age, family support, and motivation.

Sensory changes are common with CIPN. Frequent examinations of the sensory system along with strength and function are important to determine the degree of CIPN. The pediatric modified total neuropathy scale (ped m-TNS) can be used to measure CIPN, which assesses light touch, sharp–dull discrimination, vibratory sensation, distal strength, and reflexes, as well as taking into account subjective measures of pain and function.[22] The ped m-TNS should be performed frequently throughout a child's course of treatment.

Balance and coordination deficits are common in children who have had CNS or peripheral nervous system tumors or who have experienced side effects of chemotherapy or radiation therapy, surgery, and/or weakness from prolonged inactivity. As previously stated, therapists must consider other systems (e.g., vision, hearing, sensation, muscle tone, and cognition) and environmental factors when examining a child's balance and coordination abilities. A few common tests used to examine balance and coordination in children (Table 21.6) include eyes open or closed, single-limb stance, timed up and down stairs, timed up and go, dual-task activities, and tandem walking.[51,52] The vestibular system can also be affected with certain types of brain tumors and with chemotherapy agents such as the platinum agents. A vestibular screen is therefore warranted in the case of a balance impairment.[53]

It is important that the PT determine whether a child is experiencing pain, and, if so, to identify the location, intensity, quality, onset/duration, and aggravating and alleviating factors. Pain is measurable in all individuals regardless of age. Depending on the child's age and cognitive abilities, a variety of tools are available: (1) the FLACC (face, legs, activity, cry, and consolability) scale for infants to children 5 years of age; (2) the FACES scale for children 5 to 13 years of age; and (3) self-reporting numeric scales (0 to 10) or a visual analog scale for children older than 13 years. A child may experience nociceptive pain and/or neuropathic pain. Nociceptive pain, commonly described as aching or throbbing pain, is typically caused by bone, joint, muscle, skin, or connective tissue damage from the disease itself, from medications such as steroids, or from surgery. In contrast, neuropathic pain is typically described as burning, tingling, or piercing, and it is caused by injury to a nerve, either from surgery, chemotherapeutic agents, or radiation therapy.[54-56] Neuropathic pain is common when receiving chemotherapy agents such as vincristine that cause CIPN. Studies show that 49% to 62% of children report pain during treatment.[21]

Integumentary

Examination of the integumentary system tells the therapist a great deal about a child. The color and texture of the skin alone may offer the therapist some information that will lead to further examination. For example, pallor suggests anemia; jaundice, liver dysfunction; dry and itchy skin, GVHD; cold skin, poor circulation; hot skin, infection; drainage with a foul odor, infection; blisters, poorly fitted brace; red/blistered skin, radiation burns; and ulcers, pressure sores. PTs will want to examine the mobility of a scar and note any scar adhesions. PTs play a critical role in the identification and management of the integumentary issues that children with cancer may experience. The PT must take the time to examine the integumentary system thoroughly, document the findings, and communicate and coordinate the plan of care with the physician.

TABLE 21.6. Possible Physical Therapy Diagnoses Based on Medical Diagnosis

Medical Diagnosis	Physical Therapy Diagnosis	Possible Causes
Leukemia/lymphoma	Pain	Peripheral neuropathy, bone pain from buildup of blast cells in the bone marrow, joint, and bone mainly due to osteonecrosis
	Decreased sensation	Peripheral neuropathy, nerve root compression
	Decreased strength	Peripheral neuropathy, steroids, inactivity
	Decreased ROM	Peripheral neuropathy, osteonecrosis
	Decreased endurance and fatigue	Inactivity, chemotherapy, radiation therapy, stem cell transplant
	Decreased functional mobility	Decreased strength, endurance, pain
	Decreased participation in community activities	Self-confidence, fear, other social concerns such as friendships and previously listed impairments, limited handicapped-accessible accommodations
CNS and peripheral nervous system tumor	Pain	Tumor impingement (spinal cord or peripheral nerve root impingement), peripheral neuropathy, or surgical pain
	Decreased sensation	Peripheral neuropathy, CNS damage
	Decreased strength	Tumor impingement, surgical pain, fear, immobility, inactivity
	Decreased ROM	Surgical incision site, decreased motor control, abnormal muscle tone
	Decreased balance and coordination	Poor motor control, ataxia, paralysis/paresis, decreased vision, vestibular dysfunction
	Decreased functional mobility	Visual deficits, decreased strength, endurance
	Decreased participation in community activities	Previously listed impairments and limited handicapped-accessible accommodations
Bone and soft-tissue tumors	Pain	Tumor impingement, surgical pain, neuropathic pain, chemotherapy, osteoporosis
	Decreased sensation	Surgical nerve damage, chemotherapy
	Decreased strength	Immobility, nerve damage, CNS metastases
	Decreased ROM	Immobility, nerve damage, scar adhesions
	Open wound	Failure of incision site to close, infection

CNS, central nervous system; ROM, range of motion.

Cardiopulmonary

Children with cancer may experience cardiopulmonary complications due to the effects of chemotherapy, radiation, prolonged bed rest, generalized fatigue, or skeletal abnormalities caused by a tumor, surgery, or radiation therapy. Certain chemotherapy agents can cause cardiopulmonary side effects; for example, doxorubicin can have cardiotoxic effects, and cyclophosphamide can lead to pulmonary complications. The PT must perform a comprehensive respiratory, skeletal (rib cage), and endurance examination. A good starting point is observation of the child, which will reveal increased work of breathing, nasal flaring, respiratory rate, and skeletal asymmetries that affect the cardiorespiratory system. More detailed measures will include using a pulse oximeter to obtain a child's resting heart rate before he or she performs an endurance examination and the therapist calculates his or her target heart rate range.

The child's age and abilities will guide the type of endurance tests the therapist chooses. For infants and toddlers, endurance testing may include observation of skin color, vital signs, and breathing patterns while the child is playing. For testing of the older child and adolescent, more structured methods are available such as a treadmill test at a variety of levels, step tests, and run/walk tests, including the 2-, 6-, and 9-minute tests.[75,76] While the child is performing the endurance tests, the therapist can monitor the child's heart and respiratory rates. Tools are available to examine the energy required to perform specific tasks. The physiologic cost index is an objective way to calculate a child's energy expenditure. The rating of perceived exertions scale is a subjective scale of how hard the child reports that he or she is working.[57-62]

Activity (Activity Limitations)

Motor Function

Children with cancer may experience difficulty with motor function, including gross and fine motor skills. Treatment- and disease-related effects impact the development of motor function and can have a profound effect on participation in daily activities, socialization, and QOL. Studies show limitations in gross motor and fine motor skills across cancer diagnoses during cancer treatment and into survivorship. Survivors with ALL score lower on gross motor and fine motor assessments by 5% to 54%.[21] Examinations of gross motor skills can be performed using standardized assessments (Table 21.5). Scores can be compared to the general population or be used to show change over time with an individual. Interventions to improve motor function include impairment-based physical therapy and individual- or group-based exercise training programs. Physical therapy has been shown to improve motor function if initiated early on, and rehabilitation has shown improvement in children with ALL, CNS, and bone tumors.[21,63-65]

Ambulation/Locomotion

Children with cancer may experience difficulty with ambulation and locomotion as a result of the disease and treatment effects. These deficits may occur because of the effects of drugs such as vincristine that cause foot drop, weakness due to nerve root impingement, bone pain from the buildup of blast cells in the bone marrow, or structural changes from a limb-sparing or amputation procedure. The therapist will first identify the child's primary means of mobility, whether it is walking, crawling, or using a wheelchair. Second, the therapist will identify the amount of assistance or the type of assistive device required for the child to perform the task. Third, the therapist will examine the quality of the gait pattern or other means of mobility. Foot orthotics and bracing such as supramalleolar orthoses (SMOs) and ankle–foot orthoses (AFOs) are often used in improving alignment and/or the gait pattern of the individual with a gait impairment due to foot drop caused by CIPN or a hemiparesis from a brain tumor.

Participation (Participation Restrictions)

A critical component of the examination is identification of how the child's body structure/function and activity limitations are affecting the child and the family at home, work, school, or play. It is important to discuss with the child and caregiver the child's level of involvement in activities such as eating at the dinner table with the family, bathing, participating in leisure activities or play with friends, going to school, and participating in sports. This can be achieved using oral communication, observation, and structured questionnaires or self-reported outcome measures. Some commonly used pediatric-specific questionnaires are the PedsQL, Short Form 36, PROMIS Fatigue and PROMIS Physical Function and Mobility.[85,86] Identifying these participation restrictions are critical to the QOL of the child, adolescent, and survivor of pediatric cancer as they participate in major life events throughout their lifetime including play, engagement at home with family, school, work, and transitioning into adulthood.

Level of physical activity is a major component of participation in daily activities. Questions related to fatigue and energy level should be asked. The PROMIS Fatigue is an effective self-reported outcome measure used to determine an individual's level of fatigue. Fatigue is the symptom of greatest distress for children and adolescents with cancer, with 50% to 76% experiencing fatigue.[21] This includes physical, emotional, cognitive tiredness, or exhaustion related to cancer or cancer treatments.[21] Evidence shows a significant reduction in fatigue with physical activity across cancer types. Clinical guidelines recommend physical activity, relaxation, and mindfulness as primary fatigue interventions in children with cancer. The physical activity recommendation for children is 60 minutes a day; barriers should be discussed and addressed if this is unable to be met.[21] Physical activity recommendation should be tailored to the specific needs of the individual.

» Diagnosis, prognosis, and plan of care

The physical therapy diagnosis and prognosis for pediatric cancer will vary depending on the specific type of cancer (including grade, stage, and overall medical prognosis), medical intervention, and family dynamics. The following physical therapy diagnoses are common for children with cancer: pain (neuropathic/nociceptive), fatigue, decreased ROM, decreased strength, decreased balance and coordination, decreased endurance, developmental delays, poor wound closure, decreased functional mobility, and decreased participation in community activities (Table 21.6). For each child, the plan of care and goals will require individual consideration depending on the child's unique circumstances. The PT's role is to assist children with cancer in the prevention of secondary complications of the cancer and medical interventions; to promote health, wellness, fitness, and normal development; to limit the degree of disability; to promote rehabilitation; and to restore function in children with chronic and irreversible disease.[66] To fulfill this role, the PT should provide physical therapy intervention for children with cancer with an equal emphasis on body structure/function impairments, activity limitations, and participation restrictions.[67] The timeline for physical therapy intervention and the child and caregiver's goals will depend on the individual child and the medical diagnosis and prognosis.

Physical Therapy Intervention

There is an increasing amount of evidence to support the need for physical therapy services for children with cancer. Pediatric cancer happens during a critical period of development as the child's systems are growing and changing. The neurotoxic effects of cancer treatment can have a profound effect on the child's developing systems; therefore, it is crucial to intervene early. Physical therapy intervention for children with cancer is beneficial on all levels of care from body function/structure limitations to activity limitations to participation limitations. Physical therapy can help prevent loss of function, restore function, compensate for loss, or be adaptive if recovery is not possible. Literature supports the following benefits of exercise for adults with cancer: improved hemoglobin concentrations, reduced duration of neutropenia and thrombocytopenia, reduced severity of diarrhea and pain, reduced duration of hospitalization, reduced reports of nausea, decreased emotional distress, increased lean body weight, improved physical performance, improved functional capacity, improved QOL index, improved flexibility, decreased fatigue, improved concentration, and increased skeletal mass.[68-79] Studies have shown that rehabilitation services may reduce the loss of function and/or developmental delay in children and adolescents with cancer. Early rehabilitation has been recommended to reduce long-term complications of childhood cancers. A recent National Initiative in Cancer Rehabilitation expert group recommended that integrating rehabilitation into oncology care can help maximize the functional capabilities of cancer survivors. This National Institutes of Health (NIH) initiative requires specialists in multiple disciplines to provide services to children with cancer from diagnosis, throughout their course of treatment and into survivorship to optimize overall function and QOL.[21,80]

Promoting a culture of mobility that includes physical activity early on during diagnosis, throughout treatment, and into survivorship has been shown to help address disease- and treatment-related complications in the cancer population.[81] Studies specifically related to physical therapy intervention for children with cancer have been focused primarily on children with leukemia, with growing evidence in the solid tumor and CNS tumor population. Children receiving medical intervention for ALL demonstrate significant improvements in lower extremity strength and ankle DF ROM when they participate in a physical therapy program.[65,82,83] Systemic review of PT interventions show improvement in gross motor function as well as strength in the ALL population. Inpatient rehabilitation has been shown to improve mobility and ADLs in children with CNS tumors.[84] Studies are starting to reveal anticancer effects of physical activity, with overall lower relapse rates and mortality in adult cancers, and lower relapse mortality rate in childhood cancer survivors.[85,86] Overall, rehabilitation interventions that treat physical and cognitive deficits have led to improved QOL, improving participation in life roles and activities in those with cancer.[21] There is a great need for additional research in the area of pediatric cancer rehabilitation interventions, its impact on cancer, treatments, and long-term survivorship.

There are different ways of delivering rehabilitation service, proactive versus reactive approaches. The Prospective Surveillance Model (PSM) is based on surveillance of common impairments and limitations, early detection of these, education to prevent adverse events, rehabilitation when impairments are identified, and encouragement of physical activity throughout treatment and thereafter. The symptom-based model relies on frequent screens from health care providers to identify impairments and refer to rehabilitation when needed. Both should include episodic physical therapy care, defined periods of physical therapy to meet certain specified goals with breaks in between when a plateau is reached or goals are met, followed by time frames for reexamination.[64,65,80]

Coordination, Communication, and Documentation

Because of the rapidly changing needs of children with cancer, it is important that the PT take the time to appropriately coordinate, communicate, and document all aspects of the physical therapy care. Physical therapy coordination, communication, and documentation require different approaches, depending on the location of services such as inpatient, outpatient, and school-based services. Regardless of the location of services, it is oftentimes challenging to coordinate appointment times around the child's sleep schedule, a procedure that requires sedation, and other medical appointments; to identify the child's blood counts before physical therapy; and to talk with the physician or nurse if changes are observed. To maximize the physical therapy session, it is imperative that the PT take responsibility in all three of these areas. Multidisciplinary collaboration is important for the effective management of children with cancer. The multidisciplinary team can include medical doctors (MDs), registered nurses (RNs), OTs, speech pathologists, psychologists, neuropsychologists, social workers, case managers, child life specialists, and orthotists/prosthetists. Communication among the health care providers, family, and child is critical for the continuous assessment and the most effective treatment of the child with cancer. For example, a PT may notice a significant change in ankle strength in a child receiving vincristine affecting his gait pattern and functional mobility. Reporting this immediately to the oncology provider may result in a dose reduction of the chemotherapy agent, preventing further weakness and decline in motor function.

Child/Family Education

A primary role of the PT is to provide information, to educate, to motivate and inspire, and to instruct children, caregivers, and siblings. Fulfillment of this role is essential in optimizing the benefits of physical therapy services. Therefore, a responsibility of the PT is to empower the child and family to take an active role in improving the child's health and well-being. The PT must discuss which activities are of interest to the child and family and offer positive encouragement for the activities the child can do.

It is important to educate the family and child early on, preferably at diagnosis or in the first month of treatment regarding the role of physical therapy, the importance of physical activity and performing a home exercise program, the signs and symptoms to expect during medical treatment, and when to notify the physical therapy or medical team of adverse effects or difficulty with mobility.

Physical therapy interventions must be age appropriate and, most importantly, meaningful to the child and the caregiver. Physical therapy instruction for a child with cancer may consist of showing a child how to get out of bed for the first time after surgery; helping him or her learn how to properly use an assistive device, orthosis, or prosthesis; or helping him or her perform specific therapeutic exercises. The PT may deliver the instructions orally or by manual guidance, visual demonstration, or written handouts. Through child, family, and therapist collaboration, ideas are generated on how the child and family can participate in activities together, with the goal of enhancing the child's performance, functioning, and, ultimately, QOL.

Procedural Intervention

Each intervention session between the therapist and a child with cancer is unique because of the complexity of the disease, the medical intervention, and the individual needs of the child and family. A physical therapy session may require modifications because the child has a low blood count, fever, pain, headache, vomiting, diarrhea, generalized fatigue, or drainage from a wound, or because the child has a specific request. Therefore, the PT should be prepared to modify the intervention session on the basis of the child's needs at that moment, keeping in mind the short- and long-term goals of the therapy. Physical therapy interventions (Table 21.7) may include nonpharmacologic pain management, therapeutic exercise, aerobic exercise, gait training, or a fitting for an assistive device, wheelchair, orthosis, or prosthesis. Most importantly, the pediatric PTs must be creative and engage the child.

» Survivorship

There are an estimated 420,000 survivors of childhood cancer in the United States, and 15,000 children and adolescents diagnosed each year. Overall, childhood cancer survival has improved markedly over the past 40 years largely because of significant improvements in the medical management of these cancers.[2,87,88] The 5-year relative survival rate for all childhood cancers combined is now 84%, although rates vary considerably depending on cancer type and stage, patient age, and other characteristics.[88] Deficits and resolution of deficits can occur any time during cancer treatment and even years after treatment. With the increase in life expectancy, late effects are commonly experienced by adult survivors of childhood cancer.[3] Late effects are the complications or adverse events that occur months or years following the completion of treatment and can impact any organ system in the body. "The Childhood Cancer Survivor Study (CCSS), funded by the National Cancer Institute and other organizations, was started in 1994 to better understand these late effects, increase survival and minimize harmful health effects."[2] Survivors often develop mild to severe long-term impairments of the musculoskeletal (muscle weakness, osteonecrosis, osteoporosis, leg length discrepancy),

TABLE 21.7.	Suggested Physical Therapy Interventions	
Area of Focus	**Intervention**	**Frequency**
Pain	Modalities	As needed
	Ice, heat, massage	
	Positioning	
	Assistive device	
	Neuropathic pain	
	Compression stocking	
	Deep pressure	
	Physician-prescribed medications	
Strengthening	Therapeutic exercises	3–5 days a week
	Functional activities	
	Stair climbing	
	Squats	
Stretching	CPM machine	Five times a week to daily
	Splinting, bracing, orthotic	
	Manual stretching, self-stretching	
Aerobic/endurance	Walking	5 days a week
	Treadmill	
	Bike	
	Stair stepper	
	Swimming	
	Dancing	
Manual techniques	Manual guidance	As needed
	Neurodevelopmental treatment	
	Self-directed	
Motor learning principles	Knowledge of performance	As needed
	Knowledge of results	
	Blocked practice	
	Random practice	

CPM, continuous passive motion.

neuromuscular (peripheral neuropathy, pain, poor motor control), cardiopulmonary (cardiomyopathy, pulmonary fibrosis, fatigue, decreased exercise tolerance, obesity), and integumentary systems (fibrosis, radiation dermatitis), as well as neurocognitive dysfunction (memory and processing delays).[89,90] Of the childhood cancer survivors, 60% to 90% will experience one or more chronic health conditions, and 20% to 80% will experience life-threatening complications during adulthood.[2] Early recognition of late effects offers the best opportunity to provide appropriate treatment, thus minimizing the impairments associated with late effects that can significantly impact employment, life participation, and QOL.[21,26,27,91]

Long-term follow-up by a multidisciplinary team is essential in providing the care required to optimize the health and QOL of childhood cancer survivors. Unfortunately, long-term follow-up care is often not provided or accessed by these survivors. Physicians and PTs should routinely monitor these survivors to identify the onset of adverse late effects and initiate appropriate therapeutic interventions. It is important for PTs to obtain a detailed medical history from the child, family, or primary medical contact regarding the diagnosis, treatments, and medications received during cancer-related care so as to most appropriately evaluate and treat any identified late effects.

The COG has developed guidelines that provide the PT advice on appropriately screening and managing this growing population of childhood cancer survivors in an effort to provide them with consistent care and reduce the long-term health risks they face. These guidelines, as well as "Health Links" (patient education on guideline-specific topics), are available at www.survivorshipguidelines.org.[92] Research has demonstrated the effectiveness of early intervention, and education and has demonstrated the ability of exercise and physical therapy interventions to moderate many of the late effects reported by survivors.[91,93-96] Rehabilitation intervention in this population has been shown to reduce the impact of cancer and its treatment, improve QOL, optimize function, and play a role in reducing morbidity and mortality.[21,26,27] In summary, childhood cancer survivors and their families can benefit from physical therapy interventions as they transition from diagnosis through active treatment and to survivorship. More research is still needed, however, on the effects of rehabilitation in this special population.

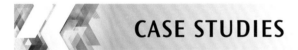

CASE STUDIES

ACUTE LYMPHOBLASTIC LEUKEMIA

History

Three-year-old Emily presented to her pediatrician with excessive bruising, accompanied by reports of wanting her parents to carry her rather than having to walk. She had no significant past medical history and was performing all age-appropriate skills until 3 weeks ago. Her white blood cell count was high. Analysis of bone marrow aspirate and cerebrospinal fluid from a lumbar puncture showed an overproduction of blast cells and CNS involvement.

Emily was diagnosed as having ALL and was referred to a hospital approximately 60 minutes from her hometown to receive treatment. She was enrolled on a standard risk protocol to receive combination chemotherapy (prednisone, dexamethasone, vincristine, daunorubicin, doxorubicin, L-asparaginase, methotrexate, cyclophosphamide, and cytarabine). Chemotherapy will last approximately 2.5 years and will be administered in phases: induction, consolidation, interim maintenance, intensification, and maintenance therapy.[7]

Emily lives at home with her mother, father, and two older brothers. She enjoys playing with her dolls, riding her bike, and going to the playground. Before diagnosis, Emily attended pre-school half days, 3 days a week. Emily's parents both typically work out of home. They are currently alternating working from home to take care of her, and she has not been to preschool since her diagnosis.

Emily was referred to physical therapy by the oncology team during her hospital admission at diagnosis due to her decrease in walking. Her initial PT goals focused on patient and family education as well as on increasing functional mobility.

Physical Therapy Systems Review

Upon initial greeting, Emily was bright and was very comfortable talking with the PT when her father was holding her. She appeared fearful of movement. Her muscle tone appeared within normal limits (WNL) to mildly low. Vision, hearing, and sensation appeared intact. She didn't appear to be in any pain while her father was holding her. She was mildly pale, with a few healing bruises. Her respiratory rate and breathing pattern appeared normal at rest.

Physical Therapy Tests and Measures

Emily presented with full AROM in her neck, trunk, upper extremities, and lower extremities. Her strength was examined while she was playing with toys and was grossly 4/5 (0 to 5 scale). Emily tracked toys right/left/up/down and responded to all auditory stimuli in the room.

Upon further testing, Emily's sensation was WNL as measured by light touch, and her muscle tone was also WNL. She had no pain, as measured by the FLACC scale, when she was sitting and playing; however, when she was in a standing position, her FLACC pain score was 5. Emily pointed to her lower extremities when in standing. As reported, Emily's skin color was mildly pale and she presented with three large bruised areas, which were healing. Emily's skin around her central line was clean and dry. She presented with decreased endurance, as indicated by her increased work of breathing and increased heart and respiratory rates while she performed functional tasks such as transitioning from sitting to standing and ambulating.

With encouragement from the PT and her dad, Emily ambulated independently for 2 feet, slowly with a short step length, and then began to cry. When engaged in play, Emily was able to stand independently with her hand on a bench and cruise right and left for 3 feet. Emily transitioned from sitting on a bench to standing with moderate assistance, and from standing to sitting on the floor by half-kneeling with her hand on her knees and then on the floor, with minimal assistance for balance. She crawled on her hands and knees for a distance of 4 feet independently. She would not attempt to ascend a step.

Physical Therapy Diagnosis

- Nociceptive pain caused by increased blast cell production in the bone marrow and arthralgia from high-dose methotrexate and intrathecal cytarabine

- Decreased overall strength—differential of side effect of steroids during induction therapy and/or decreased activity since diagnosis
- Decreased endurance—differential of side effect of medications and/or recent decrease in activity
- Decreased functional mobility due to pain, limited strength, decreased endurance, and nausea
- Decreased participation in play and nonattendance at school

Physical Therapy Prognosis

Emily is expected to return to full, independent mobility. After she receives chemotherapy for a few more weeks, her bone pain from initial disease should resolve. Over the next 3 months, Emily will undergo additional rounds of chemotherapy and steroids as well as other medical interventions to stage and treat her cancer (spinal taps, etc.). It is anticipated that she will return to independent mobility during this time, but also have periods where she demonstrates intermittent weakness, fatigue, pain, and decreased functional mobility.

Goals as Determined with Emily and Her Family

- At 1 week, Emily will perform floor to stand with one upper extremity on a stable surface, independently during play activities and will ambulate 100 feet with one hand held.
- At 4 weeks, Emily will ambulate independently without assistance, transition from ring sitting to standing independently and without upper extremity assist, and ascend and descend three steps with one hand on a rail and age-appropriate supervision.
- At 6 weeks, Emily will ascend and descend three steps independently without use of a railing, jump up independently with both feet leaving the floor 1 inch, and participate in play at home with siblings for 20 minutes at a time without a sitting rest.
- Ongoing goals include Emily's family independently assisting her with the exercise program provided by her inpatient PT and encouraging active play when she feels well.

Plan of Care

Emily will receive physical therapy three times a week as an inpatient to address her mobility and child/parent education goals. If Emily continues to demonstrate the need for weekly skilled physical therapy at the time of discharge from the hospital, she will be referred to outpatient physical therapy in her local community or at her cancer center. If Emily demonstrates improvements in her mobility and age-appropriate gross motor skills by discharge from the hospital, she will be referred to PT follow-up in the oncology clinic on a consultative basis, in conjunction with medical visits in clinic to monitor for signs of peripheral neuropathy, steroid myopathy, decreased mobility and/or gross motor skills, and so on. The plan for physical therapy services with Emily will involve educating Emily and her family in the following areas: activities to regain function, normal development, resuming activities that are important to

Emily and her family such as going to the park and riding their bikes together as a family, and future concerns such as the development of peripheral neuropathy or osteonecrosis. The PT may find that Emily could benefit from a referral to occupational therapy to assist with fine motor skills or ADLs with a focus on age-appropriate developmental skills.

Physical Therapy Patient-Related Instruction

Activity: Ankle DF active/passive ROM and family instruction on signs and symptoms of peripheral neuropathy due to vincristine (foot drop, tripping, poor grip strength)—Frequency: five times a week. Intensity: mild heel cord stretch. Duration: Hold for 30 seconds with three repetitions. Active ankle DF throughout the day.

Activity: Strengthening exercises—Frequency: five times a week. Intensity: fun, functional, strengthening activities such as squatting to pick up a toy off the ground; tossing a ball overhead, from the mid-chest region, and underhand; painting a picture while standing at the kitchen table, squatting to pick up a different color marker; and doing ankle pumps while listening to music. Duration: Throughout the day, because she will not tolerate long periods of exercise at one time; therefore, three sets of ten repetitions are recommended.

Activity: Ambulation—Frequency: throughout the day, when she needs to transition from one activity to another. Intensity/duration: short distances to start with and build up over time.

Activity: Aerobic exercise, tricycle riding—Frequency: 7 days a week. Intensity: slow and controlled. Duration: 5 minutes to start with and build up to 10 minutes. She should be wearing a helmet (Fig. 21.4).

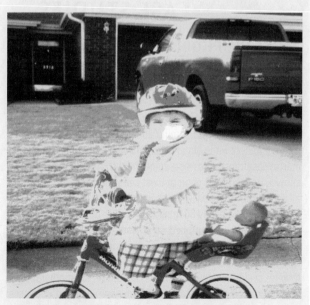

FIGURE 21.4. Emily playing outside on her bike.

Physical Therapy Procedural Intervention

The PT will help Emily and her parents perform active ankle DF exercise and ankle DF stretching and review procedures with the parents for ensuring proper alignment. The therapist will encourage Emily to play a game such as basketball that requires her to transition from standing to squatting to pick up the ball, walking over to the basket, and tossing the ball into the basket. This activity will assist Emily with her upper and lower extremity strength and ambulation skills. While Emily rides a tricycle, the therapist will monitor her heart rate with a pulse oximeter and visually observe her respiratory rate, skin color, and breathing pattern. During the physical therapy session, the therapist will be able to determine Emily's improvements in ROM, strength, endurance, and functional mobility, and then make recommended suggestions to Emily and her family on how to modify her home or inpatient exercise program. In skilled follow-up sessions, the therapist will assess gait pattern, foot posture, and active ankle ROM to monitor for CIPN.

Episode of Care

Three months after Emily received the initial diagnosis of ALL, she met all her previously set goals and was actively participating in family activities such as bike rides and time on the playground. She was scheduled for PT follow-up in the clinic every 2 to 3 months.

At her next PT examination, during the intensification phase of treatment, Emily developed peripheral neuropathy, as indicated by frequent tripping while she was walking and running. The physical therapy examination in the clinic indicated that Emily had weak intrinsic musculature in her feet and hands and decreased active ankle DF strength. Emily's oncology team decreased her dose of vincristine to reduce the effects of the peripheral neuropathy, the PT in conjunction with an orthotist provided Emily with bilateral solid AFOs to help prevent falls and to protect the alignment of her ankle structure, and Emily was referred to OT for an examination of her fine motor abilities. Emily continued to perform her ankle DF stretching and strengthening exercises as previously recommended and was followed up weekly by the PT in the oncology clinic for 6 weeks to provide gait training with the new braces, strength measurements and updates to her home program, and child and family education as needed. After this episode of care, Emily was then followed up by the PT in the oncology clinic every 1 to 2 months, and over time demonstrated resolution of her CIPN symptoms. Emily was eventually able to wean out of her AFOs.

When Emily completed her medical intervention for cancer about a year later, she no longer needed to use an AFO and was walking independently without any gait deviations. She was able to keep up with peers in active play settings at school and on the playground. Throughout her life, Emily will be followed up by an interdisciplinary team, including a PT, through the survivorship clinic at her cancer center because of her increased risks of musculoskeletal, cardiopulmonary, integumentary, and neurocognitive side effects from her cancer and the treatment for it.

OSTEOSARCOMA

Medical History

John, a 12-year-old boy with no significant medical history, presented to a local orthopedic physician with a history of intermittent but progressive pain of his left distal thigh. Diagnostic X-ray revealed a distal femoral lesion. John was then referred to the cancer center at a local pediatric hospital and an MRI was ordered. The MRI showed a destructive bone lesion with extension into the lateral soft tissues and into the bone epiphysis. Bone biopsy revealed cells consistent with osteosarcoma. Positron emission tomography (PET) scan results were negative for metastasis outside of the primary lesion.

A family meeting was held with John, his family, and members of the interdisciplinary team of the cancer center. The oncology team recommended port placement and for neoadjuvant chemotherapy to begin within a week. They also recommended a G tube for anticipated nutritional needs. The orthopedic team recommended that John ambulate with toe touch weight bearing (TTWB) because of the tumor compromising the integrity of the bone.

John received physical therapy during his admission at diagnosis, where the main focus was on mobility with axillary crutches while maintaining TTWB and child and family education on the importance of maintaining TTWB, safety with mobility with crutches, and instruction and completion of a home program for overall strengthening, balance, and endurance. Upon discharge from the hospital, the PT recommended that John begin an episode of outpatient physical therapy to coincide with his continued neoadjuvant chemotherapy in preparation for his future surgery for local control of the tumor.

After 14 weeks of chemotherapy, John was reevaluated by his orthopedic surgeon and oncologist and admitted for his local control procedure. John, his family, and the doctors agreed that John would receive a resection of his left distal femur osteosarcoma and reconstruction with a femoral expandable prosthesis and hinged knee replacement. John had no major complications and started using a continuous passive motion (CPM) device hours after surgery with knee flexion parameters of −10 to 30 degrees of flexion. John started physical therapy on postoperative day 1 with a focus on functional mobility training, left knee AROM and passive ROM, therapeutic exercises, and family education.

Social History

John lives at home with his mother and two younger brothers. He is in the eighth grade and enjoys playing soccer and basketball and motorcycle riding. John's mother has a full-time job outside the home, and he sees his father only once every few months.

Physical Therapy Systems Review

When the PT arrived in John's hospital room, he was in bed with a Foley catheter, central venous line, and pain pump in place. He was receiving an analgesic through an epidural catheter in his lumbar spinal area to assist with lower extremity pain management. His mom and both brothers were present. John was alert and oriented, but reluctant to begin physical therapy because of concerns about falling and pain.

Physical Therapy Tests and Measures

John presented with full AROM in his neck, upper extremities, and right lower extremity. John's CPM had been set at −10 to 30 degrees of motion per surgeon orders, and mom and RN reported that John used the device overnight per recommendations. The therapist removed John's left leg from the CPM device and performed gentle passive ROM exercises; the left hip and ankle demonstrated a full ROM and 40 degrees of left knee flexion. He had decreased trunk mobility owing to the placement of his epidural catheter. His strength was 5/5 as measured by MMT in the bilateral upper extremities and right lower extremity. John's strength in the left lower extremity (LLE) was limited because of pain and fear of movement. His hamstring strength was 2/5 and his ankle DF was 3/5.

John followed directions spoken at a normal voice level. He had lost sensation to light touch in his bilateral lower extremities owing to the effects of the epidural. John reported pain in his LLE as a 3 on the 0 to 10 self-report scale. His incision was covered with a surgical dressing that was scheduled to be changed later in the day with the orthopedics team.

John required minimal assistance to protect the epidural while transferring from a supine to a sitting position in his bed. He required maximum assistance for support of his LLE to scoot to the edge of the bed. The PT placed a hinged knee brace, which was locked in extension, on John's LLE before he got out of bed. With the brace locked in full-knee extension, John then transferred from sitting on the edge of the bed to standing using his crutches and moderate assistance of one person. John ambulated 5 feet to a chair in his room and transferred from standing to sitting with moderate assistance of one person.

Physical Therapy Diagnosis

- Nociceptive pain from the surgical site
- Decreased strength from change in alignment of the muscle pull
- Increased energy expenditure with functional activities such as walking
- Decreased functional mobility due to pain, limited strength and balance, and nausea from the anesthesia
- Decreased participation in school, sports, and socialization with friends

Physical Therapy Prognosis

John's strength and functional mobility are expected to improve. He may continue to lack full-knee extension secondary to the changes in the biomechanical alignment of his knee structure.

Goals as Determined with John and His Family—timeframe of this inpatient admission, about 1 week.

- John will transfer from a supine position to sitting edge of bed independently.

- John will transfer from a sitting to a standing position with crutches, weight bearing as tolerated, and supervised assistance of mom.
- John and his mother will be able to independently use the CPM device and don and doff John's lower extremity brace.
- John will independently ambulate 50 feet with crutches, weight bearing as tolerated on LLE.
- John will ascend and descend 12 steps with one hand on the rail and one hand on a crutch, weight bearing as tolerated on LLE, and with contact guard assistance from mom for safety.

Plan of Care

John will receive physical therapy daily while on the inpatient unit. After he is transferred home, he will return for outpatient physical therapy two times a week for 1 month, and then be followed up once a week to make modifications to his home exercise program.

Physical Therapy Client-related Instruction

The PT will provide John and his mother with instruction on the use of his equipment, exercises, and safety.

Activity: Instruction on use of the CPM device and how to increase the ROM by 10 degrees each day per surgeon orders
Activity: Instruction on donning and doffing the lower extremity brace, which John is to wear when getting out of bed and during ambulation
Activity: Instruction on active LLE ROM exercises
Activity: Transfer training
Activity: Gait training weight bearing as tolerated on LLE

Physical Therapy Procedural Intervention

The PT will provide John with manual guidance, tactile cues, and oral instruction to achieve his goals.

Episode of Care

John was discharged from the hospital on postoperative day 5. He began outpatient physical therapy 2 days after his discharge from the hospital and continued to attend two times a week as recommended. John resumed chemotherapy per the oncology team 3 weeks after surgery to allow his surgical incision time to heal.

After 6 weeks of outpatient physical therapy that included strengthening and stretching exercises, John achieved 100 degrees of passive left knee flexion and 92 degrees of active left knee flexion. He had a knee extension lag of approximately 20 degrees. John's full AROM in his left knee was 20 to 92 degrees of knee flexion. His LLE strength was hip flexion/extension and abduction/adduction 5/5, hip internal rotation 4−/5, hip external rotation 4/5, knee extension 3+/5, knee flexion 4−/5, and ankle DF/plantar flexion/inversion/eversion 5/5.

John used the CPM device for 6 weeks at night only. When he was not performing his exercises during the day, he wore his knee brace unlocked to continue to work on increasing his knee flexion ROM. After he completed the use of the CPM device, John wore his knee brace at night locked in full extension to assist him in preventing the development of a knee flexion contracture because he still did not have full active knee extension ROM.

After 2 months of physical therapy two times a week, John's sessions were decreased to once a week because he was independent in his exercise program and was showing signs of progress. He had seen the orthopedics team for a follow-up visit during this time, and was cleared for full weight bearing without an assistive device. John had achieved active knee flexion to 110 degrees and continued to lack 10 degrees of active knee extension to achieve full extension. He ambulated with a mild lateral trunk deviation to the left; however, with oral cues, he could ambulate with his trunk in the midline position. He could ascend and descend 12 stairs, alternating feet to step slowly with his hand on the rail for minimal support. John now wore the lower extremity brace only to sleep in at night, and he wore a small knee brace during the day to provide tactile cues and comfort to his LLE.

Eight months after John's surgery, he completed his chemotherapy. John and the PT noticed he had increased trunk flexion to the left. John had grown over the past 8 months, and, as a result, his right leg was longer than his left causing a lateral lean as a compensatory measure. John was referred back to the orthopedic surgeon for evaluation to determine whether his prosthesis needed to be lengthened. The surgeon was in agreement with the findings of John and his PT and scheduled a procedure to lengthen John's endoprosthetic. After the lengthening procedure, John's LLE was sore and he required gentle knee ROM exercises and the use of crutches for 2 days. He then returned to his normal prelengthening functioning.

Twelve months after John's surgery, he came to the PT once every 3 months for checkup visits including full strength, ROM, and gait evaluation, as well as updates to his home program as needed. John returned to school full time and was planning to swim on his high-school swim team the following winter.

REFERENCES

1. American Cancer Society. *Cancer Facts & Figures 2020*. American Cancer Society; 2020.
2. National Cancer Institute. www.cancer.gov. Accessed 2020.
3. American Cancer Society. www.cancer.org. Accessed 2020.
4. Altman AJ, Fu C. Chronic leukemias of childhood. In: Pizzo PA, Poplack DG, eds. *Principles and Practices of Pediatric Oncology*. 6th ed. Lippincott Williams & Wilkins; 2011:611-637.
5. Cooper TM, Hasle H, Smith FO. Acute myelogenous leukemia, myeloproliferative and myelodysplastic disorders. In: Pizzo PA, Poplack DG, eds. *Principles and Practices of Pediatric Oncology*. 6th ed. Lippincott Williams & Wilkins; 2011:566-610.
6. Blaney SM, Haas-Kogan D, Pussaint TY, et al. Tumors of the central nervous system. In: Pizzo PA, Poplack DG, eds. *Principles and Practices of Pediatric Oncology*. 6th ed. Lippincott Williams & Wilkins; 2011:717-808.
7. Children's Hospital of Philadelphia. www.chop.edu. Accessed October 2020.
8. Leukemia & Lymphoma Society. www.lls.org. Accessed 2020.
9. Brodeur BM, Hogarty MD, Mosse YP, et al. Neuroblastoma. In: Pizzo PA, Poplack DG, eds. *Principles and Practices of Pediatric Oncology*. 6th ed. Lippincott Williams & Wilkins; 2011:886-922.
10. St. Jude Children's Research Hospital. www.stjude.org. Accessed October 2020.
11. Wexler LH, Meyer WH, Helman LJ. Rhabdomyosarcoma. In: Pizzo PA, Poplack DG, eds. *Principles and Practices of Pediatric Oncology*. 6th ed. Lippincott Williams & Wilkins; 2011:923-953.
12. Hosalkar HS, Dormans JP. Limb sparing for pediatric musculoskeletal tumors. *Pediatr Blood Cancer*. 2004;42:295-310.
13. Gorlick R, Bielack S, Teot L, et al. Osteosarcoma: biology, diagnosis, treatment and remaining challenges. In: Pizzo PA, Poplack DG, eds. *Principles and Practices of Pediatric Oncology*. 6th ed. Lippincott Williams & Wilkins; 2011:1015-1044.
14. Hawkins DS, Bolling T, Dubois S, et al. Ewing's sarcoma. In: Pizzo PA, Poplack DG, eds. *Principles and Practices of Pediatric Oncology*. 6th ed. Lippincott Williams & Wilkins; 2011:987-1014.
15. Margolin JF, Rabin KR, Seuber CP, et al. Retinoblastoma. In: Pizzo PA, Poplack DG, eds. *Principles and Practices of Pediatric Oncology*. 6th ed. Lippincott Williams & Wilkins; 2011:809-837.
16. Fernandez C, Geller JI, Ehrlich PDF, et al. Renal tumors. In: Pizzo PA, Poplack DG, eds. *Principles and Practices of Pediatric Oncology*. 6th ed. Lippincott Williams & Wilkins; 2011:861-885.
17. American Brain Tumor Association. www.abta.org. Accessed February 2020.
18. Meyers PA, Schwartz CL, Krailo M, et al. Osteosarcoma: a randomized, prospective trial of the addition of ifosfamide and/or muramyl tripeptide to cisplatin, doxorubicin, and high-dose methotrexate. *J Clin Oncol*. 2005;23(9):2004-2011.
19. Womer RB, West DC, Krailo MD, et al. Randomized controlled trial of interval-compressed chemotherapy for the treatment of ewing sarcoma: a report from the Children's Oncology Group. *J Clin Oncol*. 2012;30(33):4148-4154.
20. Adamson PC, Bagatell R, Balis FM, et al. General principles of chemotherapy. In: Pizzo PA, Poplack DG, eds. *Principles and Practices of Pediatric Oncology*. 6th ed. Lippincott Williams & Wilkins; 2011:279-355.
21. Tanner L, Keppner K, Lesmeister D, et al. Cancer rehabilitation in the pediatric and adolescent/young adult population. *Semin Oncol Nurs*. 2020;36:150984.
22. Gilchrist LS, Tanner L. The pediatric-modified total neuropathy score: a reliable and valid measure of chemotherapy induced peripheral neuropathy in children with non-CNS cancers. *Support Care Cancer*. 2013;21:847-856.
23. Wheeler DL, Vander Griend RA, Wronski TJ, et al. The short- and long-term effects of methotrexate on the skeleton. *Bone*. 1995;16:215-221.
24. Harten G, Stephani U, Henze G, et al. Slight impairment of psychomotor skills in children after treatment of acute lymphoblastic leukemia. *Eur J Pediatr*. 1984;142:189-197.
25. Mattano L. The skeletal remains: porosis and necrosis of bone in the marrow transplantation setting. *Pediatr Transplant*. 2003;7:71-75.
26. Ness KK, Mertens AC, Hudson MM, et al. Limitations on physical performance and daily activities among long term survivors of childhood cancer. *Ann Intern Med*. 2005;143:639-647.
27. Ness KK, Hudson MM, Scrimm S, et al. Neuromuscular impairments in adult survivors of childhood acute lymphoblastic leukemia; associations with physical performance and chemotherapy doses. *Cancer*. 2012;118:828-838.
28. Krasin MJ, Rodriguez-Galindo C, Billups CA, et al. Definitive irradiation in multidisciplinary management of localized Ewing's sarcoma family of tumors in pediatric patients: outcome and prognostic factors. *Int J Radiat Oncol Biol Phys*. 2004;60:830-838.
29. Oberlin O, Rey A, Anderson J, et al. Treatment of orbital rhabdomyosarcoma: survival and late effects of treatment—results of an international workshop. *J Clin Oncol*. 2001;19:197-204.
30. Davis AM, O'Sullivan B, Turcotte BR, et al. Function and health status outcomes in a randomized trial comparing preoperative and postoperative radiotherapy in extremity soft tissue sarcoma. *J Clin Oncol*. 2002;20:4472-4477.
31. Grossi M. Management and long-term complications of pediatric cancer. *Pediatr Clin N Am*. 1998;45:1637-1651.

32. Cooper JS, Fu K, Marks J, et al. Late effects of radiation therapy in the head and neck region. *Int J Radiat Oncol Biol Phys.* 1995;31:1141.

33. Jentzsch K, Ginder H, Cramer H, et al. Leg function after radiotherapy for Ewing's sarcoma. *Cancer.* 1981;47:1267-1278.

34. Williams KY, Cox RS, Donaldson SS. Radiation induced height impairment in pediatric Hodgkin's disease. *Int J Radiat Oncol Biol Phys.* 1993;28:85-92.

35. Nysom K, Holm K, Michaelsen KF, et al. Bone mass after allogeneic BMT for childhood leukaemia or lymphoma. *Bone Marrow Transplant.* 2000;25:191-196.

36. Thapar K, Taylor MD, Laws ER, et al. Brain edema, increased intracranial pressure, and vascular effects of human brain tumors. In: Kaye AH, Laws ER, eds. *Brain Tumors: An Encyclopedic Approach.* Churchill Livingston; 2001:189-215.

37. Neel MD, Wilkins RM, Rao BN, et al. Early multicenter experience with a noninvasive expandable prosthesis. *Clin Orthop Relat Res.* 2003;415:72-81.

38. Rougraff BT, Simon MA, Kneisl JS, et al. Limb salvage compared with amputation for osteosarcoma of the distal end of the femur. A long-term oncological, functional, and quality-of-life study. *J Bone Joint Surg Am.* 1994;76:649-656.

39. Tunn PU, Schmidt-Peter P, Pomrenke D, et al. Osteosarcoma in children. *Clin Orthop Relat Res.* 2004;421:212-217.

40. Nagarajan R, Neglia JP, Clohisy DR, et al. Limb salvage and amputation in survivors of pediatric lower-extremity bone tumors: what are the long-term implications? *J Clin Oncol.* 2002;20:4493-4501.

41. Renard AJ, Veth RP, Schreuder HWB, et al. Function and complications after ablative and limb-salvage therapy in lower extremity sarcoma of bone. *J Surg Oncol.* 2000;73:198-205.

42. Jeys LM, Grimer RJ, Carter SR, et al. Risk of amputation following limb salvage surgery with endoprosthetic replacement, in a consecutive series of 1261 patients. *Int Orthop.* 2003;27:160-163.

43. McClenaghan BA, Krajbich JI, Prone AM, et al. Comparative assessment of gait after limb-salvage procedure. *J Bone Joint Surg Am.* 1989;71:1178-1182.

44. Fuchs B, Sims FH. Rotationplasty about the knee: surgical technique and anatomical considerations. *Clin Anat.* 2004;17:345-353.

45. Fuchs B, Kotajarvi BR, Kaufman KR, et al. Functional outcome of patients with rotationplasty about the knee. *Clin Orthop Relat Res.* 2003;415:52-58.

46. Veenstra KM, Sprangers MAG, Van Der Eyken JW, et al. Quality of life in survivors with Van Ness-Borggreve rotationplasty after bone tumour resection. *J Surg Oncol.* 2000;73:192-197.

47. Hillman A, Hoffman C, Gosheger G, et al. Malignant tumor of the distal part of the femur or the proximal part of the tibia: endoprosthetic replacement or rotationplasty: functional outcome and quality-of-life measurements. *J Bone Joint Surg.* 1999;81:462-468.

48. Horwitz EM. Bone marrow transplantation. In: Steen G, Mirro J, eds. *Childhood Cancer: A Handbook from St. Jude Children's Research Hospital.* Perseus Publishing; 2000:155-165.

49. Bain LJ. *A Parent's Guide to Childhood Cancer (The Children's Hospital of Philadelphia).* Dell Publishing; 1995:89-100.

50. World Health Organization. International classification of functioning, disability, and health. http://www.who.int/classifications/icf/en/. Accessed January 2005.

51. Habib Z, Westcott S. Assessment of anthropometric factors on balance tests in children. *Pediatr Phys Ther.* 1998;10:101-108.

52. Zaino CA, Gocha Marchese V, Westcott SL. Timed up and down stairs test: preliminary reliability and validity of a new measure of functional mobility. *Pediatr Phys Ther.* 2004;16:90-98.

53. Prayuenyong P, Taylor JA, Pearson SE, et al. Vestibulotoxicity associated with platinum-based chemotherapy in survivors of cancer: a scoping review. *Front Oncol.* 2018;25(8):363.

54. Schechter NL, Berde CB, Yaster M. *Pain in Infants, Children, and Adolescents.* 2nd ed. Lippincott Williams & Wilkins; 2003.

55. Jensen MP, Karoly P, Braver S. The measurement of clinical pain intensity: a comparison of six methods. *Pain.* 1986;27:117-126.

56. Wong DL, Hockenberry-Eaton M, Wilson D, et al. *Wong's Essentials of Pediatric Nursing.* 6th ed. Mosby; 2001.

57. The American Alliance for Health, Physical Education, Recreation and Dance. *Health Related Physical Fitness: Test Manual.* 1980.

58. Butler P, Engelbrecht M, Major RE, et al. Physiological cost index of walking for normal children and its use as an indicator of physical handicap. *Dev Med Child Neurol.* 1984;26:607-612.

59. Nene A. Physiological cost index of walking in able-bodied adolescents and adults. *Clinical Rehabilitation.* 1993;7(4):319-326.

60. Chin T, Sawamura S, Fujita H, et al. The efficacy of physiological cost index (PCI) measurement of a subject walking with an Intelligent Prosthesis. *Prosthet Orthot Int.* 1999;23:45-49.

61. Marchese VG, Ogle S, Womer RB, et al. An examination of outcome measures to assess functional mobility in childhood survivors of osteosarcoma. *Pediatr Blood Cancer.* 2004;42:41-45.

62. Grant S, Aitchison T, Henderson E, et al. A comparison of the reproducibility and the sensitivity to change of visual analogue scales, Borg scales, and Likert scales in normal subjects during submaximal exercise. *Chest.* 1999;116:1208-1217.

63. Tanner LR, Hooke MC. Improving body function and minimizing activity limitations in pediatric leukemia survivors; the lasting impact of the Stoplight Program. *Pediatr Blood Cancer.* 2019;66:e27596.

64. Tanner LR, Hooke MC. The Stoplight Program; a proactive physical therapy intervention for children with acute lymphoblastic leukemia. *J Pediatr Oncol Nurs.* 2017:34-347-357.

65. Marchese VG, Chiarello LA, Lange BJ. Effects of physical therapy intervention for children with acute lymphoblastic leukemia. *Pediatr Blood Cancer.* 2004;42:127-133.

66. American Physical Therapy Association. Guide to physical therapist practice. 2nd ed. *Phys Ther.* 2001;81:9-746.

67. Marchese VG, Chiarello LA. Relationships between specific measures of body function, activity, and participation in children with acute lymphoblastic leukemia. *Rehabil Oncol.* 2004;22:5-9.

68. Dimeo FC, Tilmann MHM, Bertz H, et al. Aerobic exercise in the rehabilitation of cancer patients after high dose chemotherapy and autologous peripheral stem cell transplantation. *Cancer.* 1997;79:1717-1722.

69. Dimeo FC, Stieglitz RD, Novelli-Fischer U, et al. Effects of physical activity on the fatigue and psychological status of cancer patients during chemotherapy. *Cancer.* 1999;85:2273-2277.

70. Dimeo FC, Fetscher S, Lange W, et al. Effects of aerobic exercise on the physical performance and incidence of treatment-related complication after high-dose chemotherapy. *Blood.* 1997;90:3390-3394.

71. Winningham ML, MacVicar MG, Bondoc M, et al. Effects of aerobic exercise on body weight and composition in patients with breast cancer on adjuvant chemotherapy. *Oncol Nurs Forum.* 1989;16:683-689.

72. MacVicar MG, Winningham ML, Nickel JL. Effects of aerobic interval training on cancer patients' functional capacity. *Nurs Res.* 1989;38:348-351.

73. Young-McCaughan S, Sexton D. A retrospective investigation of the relationship between aerobic exercise and quality of life in women with breast cancer. *Oncol Nurs Forum.* 1991;18:751-757.

74. Courneya KS, Keats MR, Turner AR. Physical exercise and quality of life in cancer patients following high dose chemotherapy and autologous bone marrow transplantation. *Psychooncology.* 2000;9:127-136.

75. Courneya KS, Friedenreich CM, Sela RA, et al. The group psychotherapy and home-based physical exercise (group-hope) trial in cancer survivors: physical fitness and quality of life outcomes. *Psychooncology.* 2003;12:357-374.

76. Hayes S, Davies PSW, Parker T, et al. Quality of life changes following peripheral blood stem cell transplantation and participation in a mixed-type, moderate-intensity, exercise program. *Bone Marrow Transplant.* 2004;33:553-558.

77. Hayes S, Davies PSW, Parker T, et al. Total energy expenditure and body composition changes following peripheral blood stem cell

transplantation and participation in an exercise program. *Bone Marrow Transplant.* 2003;31:331-338.

78. Mock V, Burke MB, Sheehan P, et al. A nursing rehabilitation program for women with breast cancer receiving adjuvant chemotherapy. *Oncol Nurs Forum.* 1994;21:899-907.

79. Courneya KS, Friedenreich CM. Relationships between exercise during treatment and current quality of life among survivors of breast cancer. *J Psychosoc Oncol.* 1997;15:35-56.

80. Stout NL, Silver JK, Alfano CM, et al. Long term survivorship care after cancer treatment: a new emphasis on the role of rehabilitation services. *Phys Ther.* 2019;99:10-13.

81. Spina NM, Augustine L. Creating a culture of mobility: hospital based pediatric oncology considerations. *Rehabil Oncol.* 2017;35(1):48-50.

82. Wright MJ, Hanna SE, Halton JM, et al. Maintenance of ankle range of motion in children treated for acute lymphoblastic leukemia. *Pediatr Phys Ther.* 2003;15:146-152.

83. Wright MJ, Halton JM, Barr RD. Limitation of ankle range of motion in survivors of acute lymphoblastic leukemia in childhood: a cross-sectional study. *Med Pediatr Oncol.* 1999;32:279-282.

84. Wacker K, Tanner L, Ovans J, et al. Improving functional mobility in children and adolescents undergoing treatment for non-central nervous system cancers: a systemic review. *PM R.* 2017;9(9S2):S385-S397.

85. Cormie P, Zopf EM, Zhang X, et al. The impact of exercise on cancer mortality, recurrence, and treatment related adverse effects. *Epidemiol Rev.* 2017;39(1):71-92.

86. Scott JM, Li N, Liu Q, et al Association of exercise with mortality in adult survivors of childhood cancer. *JAMA Oncol.* 2018;4(10):1352-1358.

87. Siegel RI, Miller KD, Jemal A. Cancer statistics 2018. *Cancer J Clin.* 2018;68:7-30.

88. The National Cancer Institute. The childhood cancer survivor study: an overview. http://www.cancer.gov/cancertopics/coping/ccss. Accessed February 2013.

89. Marchese VG, Miller M, Niethamer L, et al. Factors affecting childhood cancer survivors' choice to attend a specific college: a pilot study. *Rehabil Oncol.* 2012;30(1):3-11.

90. Landier W, Bhatia S. Cancer survivorship: a pediatric perspective. *Oncologist.* 2008;13(11):1181-1192.

91. Ness KK, Morris EB, Nolan VG, et al. Physical performance limitations among adult survivors of childhood brain tumors. *Cancer.* 2010;116(12):3034-3044.

92. Children's Oncology Group. Long-term follow-up guidelines for survivors of childhood, adolescent, and young adult cancers. www.survivorshipguidelines.org. Accessed February 2013.

93. Ness KK, Leisenring WM, Huang S, et al. Predictors of inactive lifestyle among adult survivors of childhood cancer: a report from the childhood cancer survivor study. *Cancer.* 2009;115(9):1984-1994.

94. Wampler MA, Galantino ML, Huang S, et al. Physical activity among adult survivors of childhood lower-extremity sarcoma: a report from the Childhood Cancer Survivor Study. *J Cancer Surviv.* 2012;6:45-53.

95. Järvelä L, Niinikoski H, Lähteenmäki P, et al. Physical activity and fitness in adolescent and young adult long-term survivors of childhood acute lymphoblastic leukemia. *J Cancer Surviv.* 2010;4(4):339-345.

96. Mulrooney DA, Dover DC, Li S, et al. Twenty years of follow-up among survivors of childhood and young adult myeloid leukemia: a report from the Childhood Cancer Survivor Study. *Cancer.* 2008;112(9):2071-2079.

97. Mathiowetz V, Federman S, Wiemer D. Box and block test of manual dexterity: norms for 6-19 year olds. *Can J Occup Ther.* 1985;52:241-245.

98. Storey E, Tuck K, Hester R, et al. Inter-rater reliability of the International Cooperative Ataxia Rating Scale (ICARS). *Mov Disord.* 2004;19:190-192.

99. Weyer A, Abele M, Schmitz-Hubsch T, et al. Reliability and validity of the scale for the assessment and rating of ataxia: a study in 64 ataxia patients. *Mov Disord.* 2007;22:1633-1637.

100. Knights S, Datoo N, Kawamura A, et al. Further evaluation of the scoring, reliability, and validity of the Hypertonia Assessment Tool (HAT). *J Child Neurol.* 2014;29:500-504.

101. Bohannon RW, Smith MB. Interrater reliability of a modified Ashworth scale of muscle spasticity. *Phys Ther.* 1987;67:206-207.

102. Drummond S. *Dysarthria Examination Battery.* Pearson Assessments; 2003.

103. Enderby P, Palmer R. *Frenchay Dysarthria Assessment.* 2nd ed. Pro-Ed; 2008.

104. Hickman L. *Apraxia Profile.* Communication Skills Builders; 1997.

105. Kaufman N. *Kaufman Speech Praxis Test for Children.* Northern Speech Services; 1995.

106. Marshalla P. *Marshalla Oral Sensorimotor Test.* Super Duper Publications; 2007.

107. Beery KE, Beery NA. *The Beery-Buktenica Developmental Test of Visual-Motor Integration (Manual).* 6th ed. Pearson Assessments; 2010.

108. Sherman E, Strauss E, Spreen O. *Behavior Rating Inventory of Executive Function (BRIEF): A Compendium of Neuropsychological Tests, Administration, Norms, and Commentary.* 3rd ed. Oxford University Press; 2006.

109. Rocke K, Hays P, Edwards D, et al. Development of a performance assessment of executive function: the Children's Kitchen Task Assessment. *Am J Occup Ther.* 2008;62:528-537.

110. Ewing-Cobbs L, Levin HS, Fletcher JM, et al. The Children's Orientation and Amnesia Test: relationship to severity of acute head injury and to recovery of memory. *Neurosurgery.* 1990;27:683-691;discussion 691.

111. Helm-Estabrooks N. *Cognitive-Linguistic Quick Test.* Psychological Corp; 2001.

112. Wechsler D. *WISC–III: Wechsler Intelligence Scale for Children: Manual.* 3rd ed. Psychological Corporation; 1991.

113. Benton AL, Hamsher KD, Sivan A. *Multilingual Aphasia Examination.* In: Lutz FL, ed. 3rd ed. Psychological Assessment Resources, Inc.; 1994.

114. Trites RL. *Neuropsychological Test Manual.* Royal Ottawa Hospital; 1977.

115. Miller LJ. *Miller Function and Participation Scales: Examiner's Manual.* Pearson; 2006.

116. Weintraub S, Dikmen SS, Heaton RK, et al. Cognition assessment using the NIH Toolbox. *Neurology.* 2013;80(suppl 3):S54-S64.

117. Hotz G, Helm-Estabrooks N, Nelson N, et al. *Pediatric Test of Brain Injury.* Brookes Publishing; 2010.

118. Adamovich B, Henderson J. *Scales of Cognitive Ability for Traumatic Brain Injury (SCATBI).* Riverside Publishing; 1992.

119. Martin NA. *Test of Visual Perceptual Skills.* 4th ed. Academic Therapy Publications; 2017.

120. Reynolds CR, Voress JK. *Test of Memory and Learning.* 2nd ed. Pro-Ed; 2007.

121. Brown VL, Wiederfolt JL, Hammill DD. *Testing of Reading Comprehension.* 4th ed. Pro-Ed; 2009.

122. Toglia J. *Weekly Calendar Planning Activity: A Performance Test of Executive Function.* AOTA Press; 2015.

123. Squires J, Bricker D, Twombly E, et al. *Ages and Stages Questionnaires.* 3rd ed. Brookes Publishing; 2009.

124. Semel E, Wiig EH, Secord WA. *Clinical Evaluation of Language Fundamentals-Preschool.* 2nd ed. Psychological Corp; 2004.

125. Wiig EH, Semel E, Secord WA. *Clinical Evaluation of Language Fundamentals.* 5th ed. NCS Pearson, Inc.; 2013.

126. Carrow-Woolfolk E. *Comprehensive Assessment of Spoken Language.* 2nd ed. Western Psychological Services; 2017.

127. Martin NA, Brownell AR. *Expressive One-Word Picture Vocabulary Test.* 4th ed. Pro-Ed; 2010.

128. Carrow-Woolfolk E. *Oral and Written Language Scales.* 2nd ed. Western Psychological Services; 2011.

129. Dunn DM. *Peabody Picture Vocabulary Test.* 5th ed. NCS Pearson, Inc.; 2018.

130. Zimmerman IL, Steiner VG, Pond RE. *Preschool Language Scale*. 5th ed. NCS Pearson, Inc.; 2011.

131. Bzoch KR, League R, Brown VL. *Receptive-Expressive Emerging Language Test*. 3rd ed. Pro-Ed; 2003.

132. Martin NA, Brownell AR. *Receptive One-Word Picture Vocabulary Test*. 4th ed. Pro-Ed; 2011.

133. Rossetti L. *The Rossetti Infant-Toddler Language Scale*. LinguiSystems; 2006.

134. German DJ. *Test of Adolescent and Adult Word Finding*. 2nd ed. Pro-Ed; 2016.

135. Nelson N, Plante E, Helm-Estabrooks N, et al. *Test of Integrated Language and Literacy Skills (TILLS)*. Brookes Publishing; 2016.

136. Hammill DD, Newcomer PL. *Test of Language Development*. 4th ed. Western Psychological Services; 2008.

137. German DJ. *Test of Word Finding*. 3rd ed. Pro-Ed; 2015.

138. Secord WA, Donahue JS. *Clinical Assessment of Articulation and Phonology*. 2nd ed. Super Duper Publications; 2014.

139. Goldman R, Fristoe M. *Goldman Fristoe Test of Articulation*. 3rd ed. NCS Pearson, Inc.; 2015.

140. Dawson J, Tattersall P. *Structured Photographic Articulation Test*. 2nd ed. Janelle Publications; 2016.

141. Gilchrist LS, Tanner L. The pediatric-modified total neuropathy score: a reliable and valid measure of chemotherapy-induced peripheral neuropathy in children with non-CNS cancers. *Support Care Cancer*. 2013;21:847-856.

142. Smith EM, Li L, Hutchinson RJ, et al. Measuring vincristine-induced peripheral neuropathy in children with acute lymphoblastic leukemia. *Cancer Nurs*. 2013;36:E49-E60.

143. House JW, Brackmann DE. Facial nerve grading system. *Otolaryngol Head Neck Surg*. 1985;93:146-147.

144. Hyvärinen L, Näsänen R, Laurinen P. New visual acuity test for preschool children. *Acta Ophthalmol*. 1980;58:507-511.

145. Anderson S, Boigon S, Davis K, et al. *The Oregon Project for Visually Impaired and Blind Preschool Children*. 6th ed. Southern Oregon Education Service District; 2007.

146. Franjoine MR, Gunther JS, Taylor MJ. Pediatric balance scale: a modified version of the Berg Balance Scale for the school-age child with mild to moderate motor impairment. *Pediatr Phys Ther*. 2003;15:114-128.

147. Dietz JC, Kartin D, Kopp K. Review of the Bruininks-Oseretsky test of motor proficiency, second edition (BOT-2). *Phys Occup Ther Pediatr*. 2007;27:87-102.

148. Cohen H, Blatchly CA, Gombash LL. A study of the clinical test of sensory interaction and balance. *Phys Ther*. 1993;73:346-351.

149. Wright M, Twose D, Gorter JW. Multidimensional outcome measurement of children and youth with neuropathy following treatment of leukemia: cross-sectional descriptive report. *Rehabil Oncol*. 2019;37:160-166.

150. van Brussel M, Helders PJ. The 30-second walk test (30sWT) norms for children. *Pediatr Phys Ther*. 2009;21:244.

151. Beenakker E, Van der Hoeven J, Fock J, et al. Reference values of maximum isometric muscle force obtained in 270 children aged 4-16 years by hand-held dynamometry. *Neuromuscul Disord*. 2001;11:441-446.

152. Cuthbert SC, Goodheart GJ Jr. On the reliability and validity of manual muscle testing: a literature review. *Chiropr Man Therap*. 2007;15:4.

153. Secomb JL, Nimphius S, Farley OR, et al. Relationships between lower-body muscle structure and, lower-body strength, explosiveness and eccentric leg stiffness in adolescent athletes. *J Sports Sci Med*. 2015;14:691-697.

154. Côté P, Kreitz BG, Cassidy JD, et al. A study of the diagnostic accuracy and reliability of the scoliometer and Adam's forward bend test. *Spine (PhilaPa 1976)*. 1998;23:796-802; discussion 803.

155. Redmond AC, Crosbie J, Ouvrier RA. Development and validation of a novel rating system for scoring standing foot posture: the Foot Posture Index. *Clin Biomech*. 2006;21:89-98.

156. Krechel SW, Bildner J. CRIES: a new neonatal postoperative pain measurement score. Initial testing of validity and reliability. *Paediatr Anaesth*. 1995;5:53-61.

157. Hicks CL, von Baeyer CL, Spafford PA, et al. The Faces pain scale_revised: toward a common metric in pediatric pain measurement. *Pain*. 2001;93:173-183.

158. Tsze DS, von Baeyer CL, Pahalyants V, et al. Validity and reliability of the verbal numerical rating scale for children aged 4 to 17 years with acute pain. *Ann Emerg Med*. 2018;71:691-702. e693.

159. Malviya S, Voepel–Lewis T, Burke C, et al. The revised FLACC observational pain tool: improved reliability and validity for pain assessment in children with cognitive impairment. *Paediatr Anaesth*. 2006;16:258-265.

160. Bailey B, Gravel J, Daoust R. Reliability of the visual analog scale in children with acute pain in the emergency department. *Pain*. 2012;153:839-842.

161. Mandrell BN, Yang J, Hooke MC, et al. Psychometric and clinical assessment of the 13-item reduced version of the Fatigue Scale–Adolescent instrument. *J Pediatr Oncol Nurs*. 2011;28:287-294.

162. Hinds PS, Yang J, Gattuso JS, et al. Psychometric and clinical assessment of the 10-item reduced version of the Fatigue Scale-Child instrument. *J Pain Symptom Manage*. 2010;39:572-578.

163. Lai JS, Stucky BD, Thissen D, et al. Development and psychometric properties of the PROMIS® pediatric fatigue item banks. *Qual Life Res*. 2013;22:2417-2427.

164. Newborg J. *Battelle Developmental Inventory*. 2nd ed. Riverside Publishing; 2008.

165. Bayley N, Aylward GP. *Bayley Scales of Infant and Toddler Development*. 4th ed. NCS Pearson, Inc.; 2019.

166. Bruininks RH. *Bruininks–Oseretsky Test of Motor Proficiency*. AGS Publishing; 2005.

167. Smith YA, Hong E, Presson C. Normative and validation studies of the Nine-hole Peg Test with children. *Percept Mot Skills*. 2000;90:823-843.

168. Folio MR, Fewell RR. *Peabody Developmental Motor Scales*. 2nd ed. Pro-ed; 2000.

169. Olsen JZ, Knapton EF. *The Print Tool*. Handwritingwithout Tears; 2008.

170. Buddenberg LA, Davis C. Test-retest reliability of the Purdue Pegboard Test. *Am J Occup Ther*. 2000;54:555-558.

171. Gardner MF. *Test of Handwriting Skills*. Western Psychological Services; 1998.

172. Katz-Leurer M, Rotem H, Lewitus H, et al. Functional balance tests for children with traumatic brain injury: within-session reliability. *Pediatr Phys Ther*. 2008;20:254-258.

173. Zaino CA, Marchese VG, Westcott SL. Timed up and down stairs test: preliminary reliability and validity of a new measure of functional mobility. *Pediatr Phys Ther*. 2004;16:90-98.

174. Coster W, Coster W, Deeney TA, et al. *School Function Assessment*. Psychological Corporation; 1998.

175. ATS Committee on Proficiency Standards for Clinical Pulmonary Function Laboratories. ATS Statement: guidelines for the six-minute walk test. *Am J Respir Crit Care Med*. 2002;166:111-117.

176. Chun DM, Corbin CB, Pangrazi RP. Validation of criterion-referenced standards for the mile run and progressive aerobic cardiovascular endurance tests. *Res Q Exerc Sport*. 2000;71:125-134.

177. King GA, Law M, King S, et al. Measuring children's participation in recreation and leisure activities: construct validation of the CAPE and PAC. *Child Care Health Dev*. 2007;33:28-39.

178. Varni JW, Burwinkle TM, Katz ER, et al. The PedsQL in pediatric cancer: reliability and validity of the Pediatric Quality of Life Inventory Generic Core Scales, Multidimensional Fatigue Scale, and Cancer Module. *Cancer*. 2002;94:2090-2106.

179. Palmer SN, Meeske KA, Katz ER, et al. The PedsQL Brain Tumor Module: initial reliability and validity. *Pediatr Blood Cancer*. 2007;49:287-293.

180. DeWalt DA, Gross HE, Gipson DS, et al. PROMIS® pediatric self-report scales distinguish subgroups of children within and across six common pediatric chronic health conditions. *Qual Life Res*. 2015;24:2195-2208.

Burn Injuries

Alison Hayward and Joseph Ableman

>> Introduction

Every day, over 300 children (0 to 19 years of age) in the United States are treated in an emergency room for burn-related injuries, and two of them will die because of those injuries.[1] Younger children are more likely to sustain a burn injury from hot liquids or steam, whereas older children are more likely to sustain a burn injury from direct contact with fire (e.g., fireworks).[1] Burn injury, as part of the category of unintentional injuries (drowning, motor vehicle accidents, and suffocation, etc.), is a common cause of death in children under the age of 4 years and the third leading cause of death for all those younger than 19 years.[2]

This type of injury to the integumentary system may require the involvement of a multidisciplinary team of health professionals to stabilize the body's response to such an injury and to promote the restoration of health and functioning. Understanding the physical impact of such an injury to the largest organ of the human body requires an understanding of that organ and its response to injury as well as patient management during the acute and postacute phases of recovery. Collaborating with the multidisciplinary team members and understanding the use of invasive and noninvasive interventions to repair and restore the skin and body movement will support care that promotes healing to allow the child that has sustained this type of injury to function optimally and participate in society.

>> Etiology

Burns have numerous causes, including thermal injuries attributable to residential fires, automobile accidents, playing with matches, improper handling of firecrackers and scalds caused by kitchen or bathroom accidents. Chemical burns occur because of contact, ingestion, inhalation, or injection of acids, alkalis, or vesicants. Electrical burns happen when there is contact with faulty electrical wiring, electrical cords, or high-voltage power lines.[3]

The mechanism of thermal injury is closely correlated with the child's age. For example, toddlers often sustain a scald burn from pulling hot liquids off surfaces (e.g., boiling water off a stove, hot tea off a table); they also sustain unintentional scald burns from bathtub accidents, where the home's water heater temperature is set too high. Hot tap water is a common cause of scald burns among children and correlates with more deaths and hospitalizations than any other hot liquid burns.[4,5] Tap water can cause a full-thickness burn in under 5 seconds at 140° F. Hot liquids such as coffee, tea, soup, or cocoa can reach temperatures hot enough to cause a scald burn.[4] Toddlers are also at risk for electrical burns caused by putting objects into uncovered electrical outlets or by chewing on wires leading to electrical products. Flame burns from playing with matches and contact burns caused by touching hot objects (e.g., iron, oven door, stove top, curling irons, door on a working fireplace) happen with the school-age group. As children grow and become more adventurous, the mechanism of burn injury correlates with the risks these children and adolescents take.

Male children are at higher risk for burn-related deaths and injuries than their female counterparts. Children under the age of 4 years and those with disabilities are at higher risk for burns. The mortality rates from burn injuries for Native Americans and African Americans are two to three times higher than those for Caucasian children.[5]

Lorch et al., in 2011, studied the etiology of burn injuries in infants brought to the emergency department for medical attention. They found that males outnumbered females (55% and 45%, respectively) and that African Americans comprise 47% of the those seen. Most burns seen in this study occurred in the home, and most commonly in the kitchen. Scald burns were the most common (hot liquids either in the bath or in the kitchen), followed by contact burns from touching a hot appliance such as the stove top, iron, or heater.[6]

Shah et al., in 2011, studied the epidemiology and profile data of children with burn injuries from the national burn registry. They too found scalds to be the most common mechanism of injury resulting from hot liquids, cooking oils, or bath water. As a single food item, they found hot noodles (microwaved) were responsible for most of the burns reviewed. They also found that gasoline burns, electrical burns, and burns caused by motor vehicle accidents were more likely in children older than 10 years. Nonaccidental or child abuse accounted for 6.7% of all the burns reviewed.[7]

Child Abuse and Neglect

According to the Department of Health and Human Resources, in 2018, over 678,000 children were confirmed to be victims of child abuse in the United States.[8] Child abuse crosses all socioeconomic classes; educational levels; and religious, ethnic, and cultural groups.[8] It is the cause of death for almost five children every day, the most likely perpetrator being one or both parents and the victim most likely to be an infant, 1 year old or younger. Most such children are victims of neglect, and 46% suffer some type of physical abuse. Shah et al. revealed that children under the age of 1 year were more likely to be burned by nonaccidental causes, attributable to the demands of a newborn on new or single parents.[7]

Up to 8% of infants and children admitted to the hospital for burns are victims of abuse. Suspicion of abuse arises when the injuries are non–splash related, have linear demarcations (e.g., glove/stocking distribution or dip patterns), or burns to the buttocks and no other area of the body. Contact burns with symmetric shapes may also signify intentional burns (e.g., circular lines consistent with a stovetop burner). Children with inflicted burns are more likely to have burns on both hands, feet, and legs, and a higher total body surface area (TBSA) may be involved.[9] To try to distinguish between an accidental and an intentional burn, documentation should include the pattern, location, and depth of the burn. Certain burn patterns will raise suspicions, for instance, scald burns to the perineum, buttocks, and lower extremities, especially those with sharply defined lines between burned and unburned skin.[10] In the hospital setting, suspicion of abuse or neglect is investigated by an interdisciplinary team including physicians, nurses, social workers, psychologists, and physical therapists. The following are some of the factors in a child's case that may indicate abuse or neglect:

- Child is brought for treatment by an unrelated adult
- An unexplained delay of 12 or more hours in seeking treatment
- Inappropriate parental affect: Parents appear inattentive to child; lack empathy; may appear to be under the influence of alcohol or drugs
- Attribution of guilt for injury to the child's sibling or to him/her
- An injury inconsistent with its description
- History of injury inconsistent with the developmental capacity of the child
- History of accidental or nonaccidental injury to the patient or siblings
- History of failure to thrive
- Historical accounts of the injury that differ with each interview
- Injury localized to genitalia, perineum, and buttocks (because of frequency with which injury occurs related to toilet training)
- "Mirror image" injury of extremities (Fig. 22.1)
- Inappropriate affect of child; child appears withdrawn with flattened affect
- Evidence of unrelated injuries, for example, scars, bruises, welts, fractures

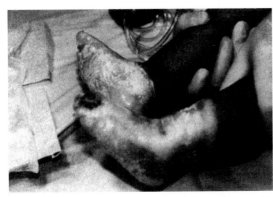

FIGURE 22.1. "Mirror image" burns to bilateral feet and lower legs, a pattern consistent with abuse via dunking in hot water.

It is mandatory under state law for professionals, including physical therapists, to report *suspected* cases of child abuse. Through a thorough examination of the child, including visualization of the skin, especially on the buttock and back, the physical therapist can examine for signs and symptoms of abuse and document the reported mechanism of injury, and the location, size, and depth of the injury, to aid in the determination of the current health and safety of the child and to decide whether a referral to a protective service is warranted.

» Prevention

Because of the high incidence and common pattern of distribution of types of burn injuries among children of various age groups, prevention efforts have been directed toward educating parents, children, and others about how these injuries occur and how they can be prevented. The National SAFE KIDS Campaign was the first national organization dedicated to prevention of childhood injuries. It was founded in 1988 and has over 600 SAFE KIDS coalitions and chapters across the United States. Injury prevention efforts in the area of thermal injuries include distribution of smoke alarms and assistance in amending plumbing codes to include "antiscald" technology and a maximum water heater temperature of 120° F. Other prevention tips include using the back burner of the stove and turning pot handles inward so as to avoid young children pulling down on the handles. For older children, cooking safety is imperative, including the proper and safe use of the microwave oven. Safety training by parents may include not allowing children to use the microwave oven until they are tall enough to reach the items, using oven mitts to remove the item, and slowly opening the container after removing it from the oven. For other household areas, parents should consider using a sturdy screen around a fireplace or outdoor fire pit, keeping candles away from anything that can burn, and placing matches and flammable liquids out of the reach of children.[11]

Injury prevention is commonly called the three E's: education, engineering (including environmental change), and law enforcement. Such prevention initiatives led to changes in the laws for children's sleepwear, smoke detector use, and setting water heaters to less than 120° F.[12]

Several suggestions for preventing childhood burn injuries include the following:

- Lowering water heater temperature settings to 120° F or lower
- Keeping cords to coffee pots and cups with hot liquids out of reach of young children
- Keeping young children in a safe place during food preparation and serving
- Turning pot handles toward the back of the stove and cooking on rear burners when possible
- Supervising children in the bathtub and testing bath water with a thermometer before placing the child in the tub
- Keeping young children in a safe place when using appliances such as a clothes iron or curling iron, and allowing these items to cool while out of the reach of children
- Discouraging the use of infant walkers
- Placing safety caps on electrical outlets
- Teaching children that matches are tools, not toys
- Teaching older children and adolescents about (1) the dangers of high-voltage wires and (2) the dangers of and safe use of gasoline and other flammable liquids
- Teaching children about the dangers of fireworks
- Creating and practicing a family fire escape plan
- Installing and maintaining smoke detectors and alarms in the house

Additionally, other prevention efforts have focused on federal regulations mandating the use of flame-retardant fabrics and materials in such articles as children's sleepwear and mattresses to help decrease the number and severity of burns resulting from the ignition of these items. In April 1996, the Consumer Product Safety Commission relaxed the standard for children's sleepwear flammability, which became effective on January 1, 1997. However, as of June 2000, all manufactured or imported sleepwear must be flame resistant or snug fitting, and a warning label must be attached to each item.[13]

» Structures and functions of the skin

The skin, like the heart and lungs, is a vital organ of the body and, in fact, is the largest organ, varying in thickness from 0.5 mm in the eyelids to 4 mm in the palms and soles.[14] The skin is composed of the more superficial and thinner (20 to 400 µm) layer, the epidermis, and the deeper and thicker (440 to 2500 µm) layer, the dermis.[14] The dermis can be divided into two layers: the more superficial papillary dermis and the deeper reticular dermis. In the basal layer of the epidermis are granules of melanin that give skin its color. The dermis is vascular, and the epidermis, although avascular, has its deeper layers nourished by fluid from the dermis (Fig. 22.2). Sweat glands, hair follicles, and sebaceous glands are contained in the skin, and nails are found on the fingers and toes. Sensory nerves and sympathetic fibers to vessels, to arrector pili

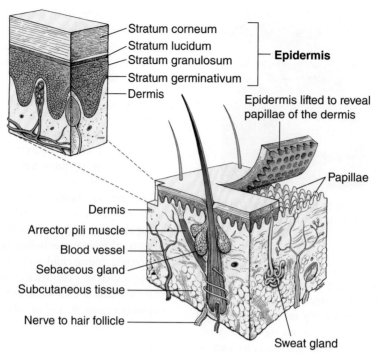

FIGURE 22.2. Structure of the skin.

muscles, and to sweat glands abound in the skin.[14] The skin helps regulate body temperature, preserves body fluids, protects against infection (by serving as a barrier and also by having certain bactericidal abilities), protects against radiation, and acts as a barrier to help protect vital organs and other body structures against external objects and fluids. Because of nerve endings that sense touch, pain, and temperature, the skin aids in both protective and discriminatory sensation. It also assists in vitamin D production. The skin, along with its appendages, can help reveal an individual's race, age, sex, and health. Ridges in the skin on the fingertips give each person a unique set of fingerprints. The skin on the face, with fluctuations in blood flow (e.g., blushing) and with the action of the underlying muscles, can express an individual's emotions. Whenever the skin is significantly damaged or destroyed, these functions may become impaired. Because it is an organ, its damage or destruction produces both local and systemic effects.[14]

>> Classification of burns

Burns can be classified by depth of tissue involvement and by size via the percentage of TBSA and by mechanism of injury. For purposes of initial triage, burns are also classified as minor, moderate, or major.

Burn Depth

Burns can be classified according to the depth of skin damaged or destroyed (Fig. 22.3). Superficial burns (formerly referred to as first-degree burns) are most commonly sunburn.

They will heal without scar formation or pigment changes. Deeper burns are classified as partial-thickness burns (formerly known as second-degree burns) or as full-thickness burns (previously referred to as third-degree burns). Partial-thickness burns can be either superficial or deep. Superficial partial-thickness burns involve the epidermis and the papillary dermis. Nails, hair, oil and sweat glands, and nerves are spared. They are painful, appear red, and frequently present with blisters. Superficial partial-thickness burns will heal in about 2 weeks or less without scarring.[15]

Deep partial-thickness burns injure structures deep into the reticular dermis. Structures affected include nails, hair follicles, and the function of sebaceous glands. These burns are waxy white in appearance and are pliable. Such burns may be insensitive to light touch but painful to deep pressure. If they become infected, dry out, or have impaired circulation, deep partial-thickness burns can convert to full-thickness wounds. Deep partial-thickness burns will heal spontaneously by epithelial cells from remaining dermal appendages, but the time required for healing may be 3 to 6 weeks or longer, and such burns heal with scar tissue that can hypertrophy and contract. Although deep partial-thickness burns will heal spontaneously without skin grafting, many surgeons elect to excise and apply skin grafts to these wounds when possible and indicated because of the prolonged healing times and frequently poor functional and cosmetic outcomes.

Full-thickness burns, by definition, destroy the full thickness of the skin. Such burns can appear as cherry red, white, or brown and leathery, and thrombosed veins may be visible. Hairs can be easily extracted owing to the death of hair follicles.[15] Full-thickness burns are less painful than

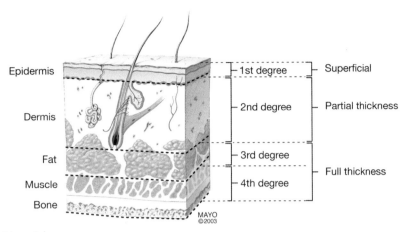

FIGURE 22.3. Depth of burn injury.

partial-thickness burns owing to the destruction of the peripheral nerves. However, this does not mean that there is no pain associated with full-thickness burns. Activation of the nerves around the periphery of the burn, exposure of the wound to air by removal of dead tissue, or manipulation of the wound can cause extreme pain. Full-thickness burns will not heal without skin grafting. Even with skin grafting, such burns may result in scar contraction and hypertrophy. Figure 22.4 demonstrates both deep partial- and full-thickness burns to the shoulder and chest.

The actual depth of injury may not be accurately or easily determined on the first day, even by the most experienced clinician. Burn injuries frequently present with varying depths of involvement and are usually not uniform in depth; such factors as how the injury occurred, the thickness of body skin in the area of the burn, and whether or not the individual was wearing clothes have a bearing on the depth of injury. The skin of infants and young children is thinner than that of adults, so, for example, a hot liquid that would cause a superficial, partial-thickness burn in an adult may cause a deeper injury in an infant or toddler. Knowing the depth of the burn is important in determining the immediate needs

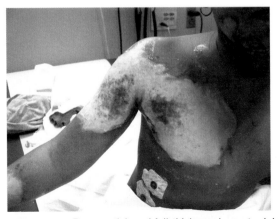

FIGURE 22.4. Deep partial- and full-thickness burns to right upper extremity and trunk. Darkened areas with no capillary refill and no pain sensation are signs of a full-thickness injury.

the child's resuscitation and stabilization, acute medical care, wound care, and burn closure options, as well as providing a prognosis and reasonable outcomes.

Burn Size

Burn injuries are also classified according to size or TBSA burned. The TBSA is counted as a percentage up to 100%, 100% indicating involvement of the entire body without sparing. There are several accepted methods of estimating the extent of the body surface area involved. The first is the palmar method, where the palm of an individual's hand is estimated to be about 1% of the TBSA. A second method, more traditionally utilized in the triage of adults, is the "Rule of Nines." According to this rule, in an adult, the head represents 9% of the TBSA, each upper extremity counts as 9%, the trunk represents 36%, each lower extremity represents 18%, and the genitalia are assigned 1%. However, a child's head (especially that of a baby) is larger in proportion to the body than an adult's head, and a child's lower extremities are smaller in proportion to the body than an adult's lower extremities are. For example, the head of a baby younger than 1 year is counted as 18%, whereas each lower extremity represents 13.5%. Because of such differences, modified versions of the "Rule of Nines" are used to calculate the TBSA burned in children. The most accurate measurement across the age groups and one that has been modified for the pediatric population is the Lund and Browder chart.[15] This chart assigns different percentages to body parts, according to the child's age. Use of a body diagram and the appropriate age-matched percentage will allow for more accurate triage and initial emergency care.[16] The examination form in Figure 22.5 shows the body diagrams and surface area percentages associated with the Lund and Browder chart. These two-dimensional measuring methods do not take into consideration individual body shape, sex, age, body mass, or the irregular shape of the injury. Computer-aided methods are being developed and utilized to aid in the accuracy of the initial burn examination.[17]

BURN ASSESSMENT

(PATIENT PLATE IMPRINT)

CAUSE OF BURN: _____

DATE OF BURN: _____ TIME OF BURN: _____

WEIGHT: _____

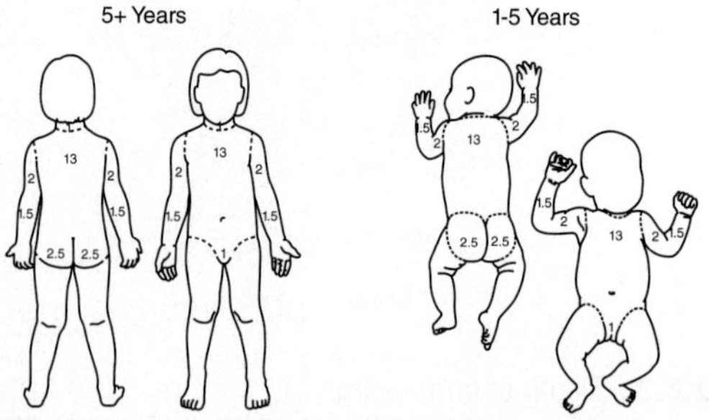

5+ Years   1-5 Years

Lund & Browder Chart

Area: *For all body parts except trunk, buttocks, and genitalia, the number in the table represents only the anterior or posterior surface of the body. Need to double number if both anterior and posterior are burned.	Age/Years					% of Body Surface Area Burned: _____		
	0-1	1-4	5-9	10-15	ADULT	PARTIAL THICKNESS	FULL THICKNESS	TOTAL
*Head	9.5%	8.5%	6.5%	5%	3.5%			
*Neck	1%	1%	1%	1%	1%			
Anterior Trunk	13%	13%	13%	13%	13%			
Posterior Trunk	13%	13%	13%	13%	13%			
Right Buttock	2.5%	2.5%	2.5%	2.5%	2.5%			
Left Buttock	2.5%	2.5%	2.5%	2.5%	2.5%			
Genitalia	1%	1%	1%	1%	1%			
*Right Upper Arm	2%	2%	2%	2%	2%			
*Left Upper Arm	2%	2%	2%	2%	2%			
*Right Lower Arm	1.5%	1.5%	1.5%	1.5%	1.5%			
*Left Lower Arm	1.5%	1.5%	1.5%	1.5%	1.5%			
*Right Hand	1.25%	1.25%	1.25%	1.25%	1.25%			
*Left Hand	1.25%	1.25%	1.25%	1.25%	1.25%			
*Right Thigh	2.25%	3.25%	4.25%	4.25%	4.75%			
*Left Thigh	2.25%	3.25%	4.25%	4.25%	4.75%			
*Right Leg	2.5%	2.5%	2.75%	3%	3.5%			
*Left Leg	2.5%	2.5%	2.75%	3%	3.5%			
*Right Foot	1.75%	1.75%	1.75%	1.75%	1.75%			
*Left Foot	1.75%	1.75%	1.75%	1.75%	1.75%			
Signature: _____					TOTAL			
Date: _____								

FIGURE 22.5. Lund and Browder chart for burn size estimation.

The importance of accuracy with burn size estimation has implications for referral to a burn center, proper fluid resuscitation in the acute medical treatment, and overall morbidity and mortality resulting from the large inflammatory and hypermetabolic response. Attention to the changing body proportion size of a growing child must be taken into account.[18]

Mechanism of Injury

Burns are also classified according to the mechanism of injury: scald, contact, flash, flame, chemical, radiation, or electrical. Knowing the causative agent or method is important in determining appropriate treatment. For example, if an individual sustains a chemical burn, knowing which chemical caused the burn is necessary in order to apply the correct antidote and in determining the need for copious water lavage, which would not necessarily be done for an electrical burn or a flame burn. In electrical burns, there is typically a wound at the points of entry and exit, which would not be found in scald burns. Recognizing the mechanism of injury and correlating the presentation of the burn will aid in developing a plan of care and in ruling out child abuse.

Indications for Referral to a Burn Center

Burns can be classified as minor, moderate, or major according to guidelines established by the American Burn Association (ABA) for purposes of triage. For example, a minor burn for an adult would be a partial-thickness burn involving less than 10% of the TBSA; this case could be treated as an outpatient. A minor burn for a child would be a partial-thickness burn involving less than 5% of the TBSA. A moderate burn involves a TBSA of less than 20% in an adult and less than 10% in a child, or a 5% full-thickness burn, which requires hospitalization. A major burn involves a TBSA greater than 20% in an adult and greater than 10% in a child and would justify referral to a burn center. The ABA recommends that an individual with the following injuries be referred to a burn center:

- Partial-thickness burns greater than 10% TBSA
- Burns of the face, hands, feet, genitalia, perineum, or major joints
- Full-thickness burns in any age group
- Electrical burns
- Chemical burns
- Burns with inhalation injuries
- Burn injury in children with preexisting medical disorders that could complicate management
- Burns in children at a hospital without qualified personnel or equipment
- Burn injury in children that will require special social, emotional, or rehabilitative intervention.[19]

» Pathophysiology

Dimensions of Injury

Regardless of the mechanism of injury, each burn wound consists of three zones that are identified concentrically around the center portion of the injury. The most central area of the burn is the zone of coagulation, which had the most contact with the heat source. The cells in this zone have been permanently damaged. Extending outwardly is the zone of stasis, where the cells have decreased blood flow and respond to resuscitation to save viable tissue. The outermost zone of burn injury is the zone of hyperemia. These cells have sustained the least damage and should recover within 10 days.[15]

Burn Wound Healing

Destruction of the skin impairs this organ from performing its basic functions to protect underlying tissues and organs, regulate body temperature and body fluid levels, and protect the body from infections. Once an injury has occurred, the body responds with a chain of events at both the local and the systemic levels. Burn wound healing can be categorized into three phases: inflammation, proliferation, and maturation/remodeling.

Inflammatory Phase

Once an injury has occurred, the disruption of epidermal and dermal structures signals the healing process to occur. Platelets come in contact with the injured tissue, fibrin is deposited, more platelets are trapped, and a thrombus is formed. A local vasoconstriction also occurs and, in combination with the thrombus, blocks the injured tissue from systemic circulation, thus achieving hemostasis at the site of injury. The major goals of the inflammatory phase are to provide for this hemostasis and the breakdown and removal of cellular, extracellular, and pathogen debris, which will in turn signal the repair process to start. Cytokines and growth factors attract responder cells and help regulate the repair process.[20]

Proliferative Phase

The proliferative phase, which is dominated by fibroblast activity, follows the inflammatory phase. The goals of the proliferative phase are to assist wound healing and restore skin integrity. The main processes involved in this second stage are angiogenesis, collagen synthesis, and wound contraction. Collagen is deposited at the wound site as early as 48 hours after a burn. Type I collagen is seen by days 4 to 7 after injury. Granulation tissue forms as endothelial cells migrate to the wound and will continue until the wound is completely reepithelialized. The cells migrate from the periphery toward the center of the wound (i.e., the wound will heal from the outside toward the middle).[20] Reepithelialization is more rapid when the stratum granulosum layer of the epidermis is intact, as with superficial partial-thickness burns. The burn wound will remain in this phase until epithelialization is complete or until the wound is surgically treated (e.g., covered with a skin graft).

Maturation/Remodeling Phase

The maturation or remodeling phase is the final phase of wound healing. This phase actually began as granulation tissue formed in the earlier proliferative phase. During the remodeling phase of burn wound healing, collagen synthesis and lysis occurs, thus creating scar tissue. During the remodeling phase, the collagen is reorganized into a more compact area. An imbalance in collagen synthesis will result in a hypertrophic or keloid-type scar.[20]

» Scar hypertrophy and contraction

There are two common, though potentially avoidable, sequelae of deep partial-thickness and full-thickness burns: scar hypertrophy and scar contraction. Scar hypertrophy and scar contraction can impede both physical and psychological functioning. Scar hypertrophy is a raised, thick, usually hard, often knotty appearing area of scar tissue (Fig. 22.6) that results from an imbalance of collagen synthesis and collagen lysis. A hypertrophic scar is raised, but does not exceed the original boundaries of the wound. A keloid scar is raised and extends beyond the boundaries of the original wound (Fig. 22.7). Factors that may predict scar formation include a genetic tendency, depth of the wound, extended healing time, wounds in individuals with more skin pigment, and young people who tend to scar more than the elderly.[21,22]

Hunt[23] stated that increased tension, which promotes collagen deposition and lessens collagen lysis, may contribute to the formation of hypertrophic scars, evidenced by the appearance of hypertrophic scars in areas of motion, such as the joints.

Chan et al., in 2012, examined the correlation of the time to skin grafting and hypertrophic scarring. They acknowledged that in addition to the age of the child and the mechanism of the burn injury, factors that played a role in hypertrophic scar formation included race, genetic predisposition, site, and depth of the burn. Other complications such as a prolonged inflammatory phase, or wound colonization, also increased the scarring process. They performed split thickness skin grafting in porcine models and concluded that early grafting of deep dermal burns had better histology and clinical scar outcomes. They noted that contemporary surgical practice was to delay grafting until 14 to 21 days post injury, but their study advocated for earlier grafting as the best scar outcomes were observed in skin grafts performed within 14 days of the injury.[24]

Scar contraction is the pulling or shortening of scar tissue, which can result in the loss of joint motion or skin

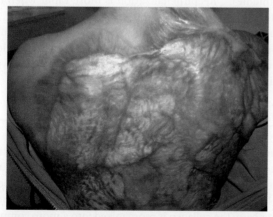

FIGURE 22.6. Hypertrophic scarring along patient's back following split-thickness skin grafts.

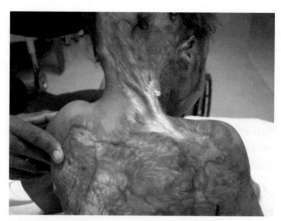

FIGURE 22.7. Note the keloid scar at right side of neck. Notice the band-like formation.

mobility, and disfigurement, especially when located on the face. Scar contracture is a fixed shortening of the scar tissue that may be amenable only to surgery. Contraction may be attributed to myofibroblasts, cells with contractile properties, found in the healing burn wound.[22] Scar contraction over a joint can lead to loss of joint range of motion (ROM) or postural and gait deviations. Because of the contracting force of scar tissue, which results in loss of skin mobility, loss of joint ROM can also result from contracting scar tissue adjacent to, although not covering, a joint.[22] In 2009, Richard et al. developed the concept of the cutaneous functional unit (CFU). CFUs are fields of skin that move when a joint moves. Skin movement was found to be positively correlated with joint ROM.[25] It was suggested that skin required for joint movement extends past the skin in joint creases. What is initially a loss of motion from a contracting scar can, if left uncorrected, lead to a gradual shortening of the joint capsule, surrounding muscles, tendons, and ligaments.

The processes of scar contraction and hypertrophy begin almost as soon as the burn wound begins healing, although initially may not be readily visible. Collagen formation begins within 24 hours of the burn injury. There is a high rate of collagen synthesis in the wound,[26] and such activity returns to a normal rate by 6 to 12 months.[27] The scar is initially red because of an increased blood supply, but it usually fades over time. When the scar is no longer actively hypertrophying and contracting, it is said to be mature. The period of scar maturation for most children is approximately 12 to 18 months. For adults, this period may be shorter. While the scar is active, particularly during the first 6 months, the processes of hypertrophy and contraction can be controlled or corrected by nonsurgical approaches, such as pressure, splinting, and ROM exercises. As scar maturation progresses, these treatments become less effective in altering the scar. After the scar is mature, most nonsurgical treatments are no longer effective, and surgery, if indicated, may afford the only treatment alternative.

» Burn center

In 1999, the ABA published guidelines for the development and operation of burn centers and updated the guidelines for verification for burn centers in 2006. These verification criteria continue to be reviewed by a committee each spring, and changes, if any, take effect the following first of January. To achieve verification as a burn center, the center has to meet rigorous standards, and participate in onsite and ongoing review by the ABA. Several criteria pertain specifically to the presence and provision of physical therapy services, including ongoing pediatric specific education and being able to provide age-appropriate therapeutic equipment. As of 2020, there were 62 verified burn centers in the United States.[28]

» Burn team

In its guidelines for burn centers, the ABA specifies whose personnel should staff the burn center, as well as which specialists and personnel should be on call or available for consultation. (The criteria state that "both physical and occupational therapy should be represented in the burn center staff.") Within the ABA guidelines, each burn center establishes its own burn team. Personnel who comprise the burn team and their specific roles may vary from institution to institution or according to the individual needs of a given child or the particular phase of healing, although there is generally a core team.[29] The pediatric burn team frequently includes a surgeon, a nurse, an occupational therapist, a physical therapist, a social worker, a respiratory therapist, a dietitian, a child life therapist, a hospital chaplain, a discharge planner, various specialists (e.g., pediatrician, pulmonologist, psychiatrist, plastic surgeon, infection control specialist, pharmacist, speech language pathologist, school teacher), and, most importantly, the child and family. Because many children do not have a traditional nuclear family, it is often necessary to determine who, in the child's view, comprises the family.

» Burn therapist certification

In 2011, the Burn Rehabilitation Therapist Competency Tool (BRTCT) was developed by the American Burn Association Rehabilitation Committee to define core knowledge and skill sets required of physical and occupational therapists working with children who have sustained a burn, during acute hospitalization and initial rehabilitation.[30] This was later updated and expanded in 2017 to define competencies for burn rehabilitation therapists treating children during long-term rehabilitation and outpatient phases of care to reflect the involvement of these disciplines across the continuum of care.[31] To recognize this specialized knowledge, skill, and experience relevant to working in this environment, the ABA created a specialty certification for burn therapists, the Burn

Therapist Certified (BT-C) program. The certification includes requirements for applicants to have worked for at least 2 years in burn care, 4,000 hours in direct patient care with the burn population in the 5 years prior to application, and the demonstration via portfolio that the applicant has met defined standards and objectives for at least four domains of burn rehabilitation practice as outlined in the development of the BRTCT.[32]

» Initial treatment and medical management

The initial treatment and medical management of the child with a burn depends, in part, on the depth, size, and location of the burn; the presence of other concomitant injuries, such as smoke inhalation; the age of the child; and the premorbid health of the child. The injury itself will trigger physiologic responses that, in turn, will affect treatment requirements.

» Systems review

Pulmonary System

Establishing and maintaining an adequate airway and breathing are the first concerns when treating a thermally injured child. If the child has inhaled steam or noxious gases, intubation may be necessary owing to bronchospasm and the development of upper airway edema,[33] possibly resulting in airway obstruction within hours. Oxygen is administered if the child has inhaled high levels of carbon monoxide. The endotracheal tube may be removed once the edema has subsided, which usually occurs within a few days.[33] Children with more extensive airway or lung injuries will require sustained or more involved treatment.

Cardiovascular System

The circulatory changes that occur following a burn injury have been discussed earlier. These changes are termed *burn shock*. The loss of fluid, increased capillary permeability, and vasodilation that occur all cause decreases in the circulatory volume and reduced cardiac output. Proper fluid resuscitation is key to recovering normal cardiac output. Inadequate fluid replacement can lead to poor tissue perfusion, organ dysfunction, and death.[15]

Fluid Resuscitation

Because of the inflammatory process and increased capillary permeability in children with deep partial-thickness or full-thickness burns, fluid leaves the blood and is dispersed into the interstitial spaces. Children with burns of less than 10% to 20% of their TBSA, depending on other considerations, may be able to compensate for this fluid shift physiologically through such measures as vasoconstriction and urine retention.[33] Thus, smaller burns tend to cause edema only in the burn wound and immediately surrounding tissues. Large TBSA burns (>20%) cause a systemic or total body inflammatory response. Children with burns involving a greater percentage of TBSA will develop hypovolemic shock and can die if not treated. Replacement of the circulating fluid loss is termed *fluid resuscitation*. Fluids cannot be administered orally to children with larger area burns because of ileus (obstruction of the bowel), which occurs secondary to shock. Fluids, with electrolytes similar to serum, and colloid are given intravenously. Children with smaller burns may be able to take fluids orally. However, children, in particular, may be unwilling to drink and may therefore require intravenous fluids. In a few days, with adequate fluid replacement, the fluid in the interstitial spaces returns to the intravascular spaces, and the children will have a diuresis, signaling successful fluid resuscitation.[33] After fluid resuscitation, the children may still require replacement of fluids because fluid is also lost through the burn wound and because the child may be unwilling or unable to take sufficient fluids orally.

A urinary catheter is placed in children with large burns to monitor urine output during resuscitation. Children with perineal burns may also require catheterization to keep bandages dry or to protect newly placed skin grafts during the skin graft phase.

Renal System

As a result of loss of fluid from intravascular spaces, renal vasoconstriction can occur and may cause renal failure because of decreased renal blood flow and decreased glomerular filtration. Electrical burn injuries may cause extensive damage to tissue, resulting in the release of myoglobin, which may occlude the kidneys' filtration system, thus leading to renal failure.

Circulatory System

Full-thickness burned skin is inelastic. Because of the body's response to injury and fluid resuscitation, the child will become edematous. In children with greater than 20% TBSA burns, this is a systemic response that also occurs in the unburned parts of the body. In the case of circumferential burns of the extremities, the combination of inelastic skin and increasing edema can cause a tourniquet effect, resulting in compromised circulation to the distal extremities. If treatment is not initiated, ischemia and tissue damage or necrosis can occur. Signs of compromised circulation include pallor, decreased skin temperature, delayed capillary refill, numbness/tingling, loss of a distal pulse via Doppler, and decreased chest wall excursion in the case of trunk burns. Compartment pressures of greater than 30 mm Hg also indicate the need for surgical intervention. The surgeon will attempt to relieve the pressure by performing an escharotomy, which is a surgical incision through the burned tissue.

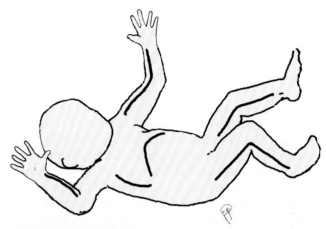

FIGURE 22.8. This diagram shows where surgical incisions (escharotomy) are performed in children who have compromised blood flow caused by circumferential full-thickness burns. The incisions are made laterally and/or medially with the child in the true anatomic position, as shown.

These incisions are usually along the lateral and medial sides of the affected extremity. In the chest, longitudinal incisions are made along the anterior axillary lines and a transverse incision at the costal level.[15] Figure 22.8 shows common sites for an escharotomy.

In 2009, Orgill and Piccolo released practice guidelines for burn care clinicians regarding escharotomy and decompressive therapies. Their review of the burn care literature supports the implementation of decompressive techniques following a burn injury to alleviate further tissue necrosis and preserve nerve function. If pressure is still not relieved by an escharotomy, these incisions may need to be extended, and the fascia released via a fasciotomy.[34]

Musculoskeletal System

Owing to the association between fire and traumatic injuries, it is not uncommon to have a burn injury and concomitant bone fracture. Examination of the musculoskeletal injury will often be delayed while the potential life-threatening injuries are addressed and stabilized. Children who are unresponsive or unable to report specific pain may be at risk for having fractures or other musculoskeletal injuries unnoticed on primary or secondary surveys. The therapist may be the first clinician to discover an undiagnosed musculoskeletal injury. Children likely to have musculoskeletal injuries are those involved in an automobile accident with a resulting fire or those who jumped from a burning building. Both burns and fractures can cause soft tissue swelling, thus requiring an escharotomy in the case where circulation is compromised. Nonoperative management of fractures includes using a splint or traction. Use of a circumferential cast is discouraged because of swelling and the inability to examine the wounds properly. Internal fixation is also beneficial because it increases the rate of fracture healing. Surgery for internal fixation should occur within 48 hours after injury; otherwise, bacterial colonization is presumed. Surgical fixation of the fracture will allow for a reduction in pain at the fracture site and for physical therapy interventions.[35]

» Nutrition

In response to the burn injury, the child will be in a hypermetabolic state, and caloric and nutritional requirements are greatly increased. The hypermetabolic and inflammatory response caused by a burn is demonstrated by an increase in protein, proinflammatory cytokine, and catabolic hormone levels. These findings increase energy requirements, which can result in muscle wasting because of a catabolic state. If this posttraumatic response is prolonged, it can lead to multiple organ dysfunction and death. Raising of room temperatures and nutritional supplementation have been efficient in modulating the hypermetabolic responses.[36] Adequate nutrition is necessary to prevent wasting and to promote proper wound healing. The child with a burn may be unwilling to eat because of the injury and a strange environment. The severity or location of the burns may make it difficult or impossible to eat. A child with a larger burn may find it hard to consume the volume of food necessary to obtain sufficient calories. Additionally, the child will be prohibited from eating on days when a surgical procedure is scheduled. Because of such factors, the child may receive a large portion of nutrition through enteral tube feedings or through peripheral vein infusions. Enteral nutrition is the preferred route of nutritional support because it offers maintenance of the gastrointestinal (GI) mucosal integrity by delivering nutrients into the GI tract. An additional benefit of enteral tube feedings is that they may continue during a surgical procedure so long as the child is not in a prone position.[37]

A nutritional evaluation should be done on admission following a thermal injury. This will include review of medical, nutritional, and medication histories, and laboratory data, and an examination. The clinician will evaluate plasma protein levels, more specifically, albumin and prealbumin. The normal range for serum albumin is 3.5 to 5 g/dL. Low levels of albumin may signify a poor potential to heal. Prealbumin is a transport protein for thyroid hormone. Normal serum prealbumin levels range from 16 to 40 mg/dL, with values less than 16 mg/dL associated with malnutrition. The half-life of prealbumin is 2 to 3 days, thus making it a good predictor of nutritional status.[38]

» Pain management

Burn-associated pain is one of the most relevant complaints in children with burn injuries. Burn pain intensity can vary because of the inflammatory response and the changes in levels of inflammatory mediators. In partial-thickness burns, nerve endings are still viable and cause significant pain, whereas full-thickness burns are less painful owing to the

damage to the nerve endings. Medical and therapeutic interventions such as dressing changes, wound cleansing, and physical therapy can cause pain. Tengvall et al., in 2010, did a retrospective study on subjects' memories of pain after their burn injury. They found that they remember pain throughout the recovery from the initial injury, to care within the hospital or burn center, and through transition to home and with any new physical limitations.[39]

In 2003, Martin-Herz et al. investigated pediatric pain control practices in North American Burn Centers. Their study results were compared with a study, completed in 1982, that revealed that 17% of burn units recommended using no opioid analgesics and 8% did not use any analgesics during pediatric wound care.[40] The newer survey revealed significant changes in the use of opioids during pediatric burn dressing changes. Morphine appeared to be the "gold standard" for medicating the child before, during, and after a painful procedure.[41] Twenty-five percent of the responders in the survey utilized psychotropic medications in combination with opioids. Background pain control and breakthrough pain control was also best controlled by IV morphine. Only 8% of centers responding stated that they routinely utilized an anesthesia-based pain service for helping with pain management.[42]

In 2010, Bayat et al. studied analgesia and sedation for children undergoing burn wound care. They identified the different types of burn pain experienced by children. These included background pain, which was relatively constant from the time of injury through the initial healing period. Next was procedural pain, which was described as burning or stinging during wound cleansing and dressing changes, and often included significant anxiety and distress. Next was breakthrough pain, which was worsening of background pain because of a decrease in blood levels of analgesia and which may require additional medication or use of a self-controlled analgesia (PCA) pump. The last type of pain they looked at was postsurgical pain, which was longer lasting but less severe than procedural pain.[43] Medications used for procedural analgesia or sedation should have a rapid onset, limited side effects, and allow for resumption of activities and oral intake following the procedure. Common medications might include nonsteroidal anti-inflammatory drugs (NSAIDs), opiates (morphine, oxycodone, fentanyl), benzodiazepines (for sedation and anxiety), nitrous oxide, and ketamine (for sedation and amnesia/analgesia).[43,44]

When addressing procedural pain, the services of child life specialists and/or music therapists may be of benefit with a nonpharmacologic approach. In addition, these team members may help to prepare the child for the procedure itself. The child's pain and anxiety must be considered and treated appropriately throughout all phases of healing. Age-specific distraction techniques can be seen in Table 22.1.

Medication for pruritus should also be considered, because itching can be a source of discomfort and pain and may limit child tolerance for interventions. Antihistamines are a commonly prescribed medication for pruritus. Opioids

TABLE 22.1.	Nonpharmacologic Pain Management
Age Range	Participation Motivators/Distraction Techniques
Under 2 yr	Use parents to help; rattles, bubble blowing, singing, videos
2–7 yr	Singing, looking at a book, videos, magic wand
7–11 yr	Allow them to participate as indicated; headphones for music, videos, sticker chart
11 yr and over	Give precise information regarding the intervention; music, videos, video games, reward chart

themselves can cause itching, so careful documentation of the occurrence of itching and whether or not it is related to burn wound healing or medication is important.[42]

Besides specific medications and pain management techniques, the facility and each professional should have a treatment approach that has a goal of caring for the burn child in a way that causes the least amount of pain.

» Burn wound management

The primary goals of wound management are to provide an optimal environment for wound healing, to provide a healthy tissue bed to receive a skin graft, and to protect healing tissue or a recently placed graft. Such goals are accomplished mainly through adequate nutrition, removing dead tissue, keeping the wound clean and minimizing bacterial invasion, preventing the wound or new skin graft from drying out, and protecting newly healing tissue or recent skin graft(s) from disruptive mechanical abrasion. There are nonsurgical and surgical interventions that comprise overall burn wound management. Prior to any wound cleansing or dressing changes, the child should be premedicated.

Nonsurgical Interventions

Wound Cleansing

HYDROTHERAPY Hydrotherapy is used in some burn centers as a part of wound management. Showering, immersion (bathing), or a spray table can be used. The purpose of hydrotherapy is to help remove the old topical antimicrobial agent, to clean the wound, to help superficially debride the wound, to increase circulation to promote wound healing, and to provide an environment for participation in age-appropriate self-care activities and exercises. Conventional hydrotherapy such as use of a Hubbard tank or whirlpool in burn care is mostly outdated. The drawbacks of it are that it can spread infection, increase the length of time required for a dressing change, increase cost (because of the additional personnel required to perform the procedure and clean the equipment),

and increase edema (especially if a limb is placed in a dependent position). Furthermore, many children, may find it traumatic to be in a tub of water. Because of the drawbacks of hydrotherapy, some burn centers limit its use to specific wounds or to certain phases of wound healing or use handheld shower heads to help clean the wound.

In 2010, Davison et al. reviewed hydrotherapy in North American Burn Centers. The results of their study showed a decrease in the use of hydrotherapy from a high of 95% of the burn centers using it in 1990 to 83% at the time of the study. The trend toward early excision of dead tissue and the increase in nosocomial infections led to a decrease in the use of immersion hydrotherapy from 81% to 45%, in favor of showering methods.[45]

Dressing Changes

Most children with burns will undergo bandage (also called dressing) changes from daily to every few days, depending on the dressings used. Considerations before beginning a dressing change include appropriate premedication for the activity, having the dressing change take place in an environment outside of the child's hospital room to maintain his or her room as a safe space, and involving team members such as child life services to prepare the child for what to expect and how to participate with nonpharmacologic interventions to assist with pain management. Even very young children can participate in removing their dressings, which may help minimize pain and offer some sense of control and independence in a situation in which they might otherwise feel helpless. Because some of the pain experienced during a dressing change is caused by exposure of the wound to air, such exposure time should be limited. Limiting the exposure time to air will help prevent the tissue from drying out and will also limit exposure to bacteria. To minimize the time required for a dressing change, bandages should be prepared ahead of time so that they may be quickly applied. Health care professionals who wish to observe the child's wound should be present at the time of the dressing change so that he/she is not waiting with an undressed wound for them to arrive. If the parent desires, and if appropriate, the parent's presence during the dressing change can be beneficial for both the parent and the child. In some cases, however, children may cry more in the presence of a parent because they expect the parent to rescue them from the dressing change.

In some burn centers, therapists are responsible for, or may assist with, daily wound care for both inpatients and outpatients. (It may also be the case that the therapist, before or during performance of outpatient therapy, will need to change the child's bandage.) During a dressing change, the old bandage is removed and the wound may be superficially debrided (nonviable tissue removed). While the wound is being cleaned and examined, ROM is measured without the dressings in place to establish how much ROM the child should work toward for the remainder of the therapy day.

Topical Agents

In a burn injury, the protective barrier of the skin is lost, and the burn wound becomes a host for bacteria. Topical antimicrobial agents play a vital role in helping minimize bacterial colonization of the wound, decrease vapor loss, prevent desiccation, and control pain.[46] Several topical antimicrobial agents may be employed depending on the specific wound and the organisms to be controlled. New products are released on the market regularly that contribute to the ever changing practice of burn wound care. Today's highest quality wound care includes choosing the right product for the right child with the right wound burden, which can include standard products as well as new high-tech ones. The following examples are among the many options available for providing excellent wound care.

Silver sulfadiazine (Silvadene) is the most commonly used topical agent.[3] Silvadene is a white, opaque cream that is painless on application, has fair eschar penetration, and has a broad antibacterial spectrum.[46] Silvadene can't be used by patients with sulfa allergies.[3] Silvadene has also been shown to cause neutropenia when applied on large surface area burns.[46] Mafenide acetate (Sulfamylon) is another topical agent available in liquid or cream form, is painful on application, has excellent eschar penetration, and has a broad antibacterial spectrum. Mafenide acetate is utilized on burns of the external ear to reduce suppurative chondritis.[46] Sulfamylon can be used on partial-thickness burns that are resistant to Silvadene and to increase eschar penetration/separation. Sulfamylon is contraindicated for use in children with metabolic acidosis.[3] Other topical agents used in burn wound management include silver nitrate, which has broad antibacterial coverage and is applied as a solution on burn wounds or graft sites. Petroleum-based products such as gentamicin and bacitracin are used on superficial burns or on areas where the skin is very thin (e.g., eyelids, scrotum).[46]

Acticoat dressing is another alternative to topical antimicrobial creams. It has been shown to be more effective than Silvadene and silver nitrate against gram-negative and gram-positive organisms. Acticoat is a three-ply gauze with an absorbent rayon and polyester core. The coating to Acticoat is nonadherent to the wound and is flexible. The child would need to undergo debridement prior to Acticoat placement. A bulky layer of wet gauze is wrapped around the Acticoat and then covered with dry gauze. Daily dressing changes include removing the gauze dressings, inspecting the Acticoat for slippage from the wound bed, and reapplying wet gauze and dry gauze. Once adhered, the Acticoat is left in place until reepithelialization occurs. This process will decrease the risk of infection (from daily wound cleansing) and discomfort associated with dressing changes.[47]

AQUACEL Ag Hydrofiber is a moisture-retentive topical dressing used in the acute management of burns. It consists entirely of carboxymethylcellulose, which forms into a gel on contact with burn exudate. This gel promotes a moist wound healing environment while still managing moderate amounts of burn exudate.[48] This hydrofiber, with 1.2% ionic silver, releases silver within the dressing for up to 2 weeks. It can be applied on an acute burn and left in place until healing occurs, thus decreasing pain and length of hospitalization.[49] Caruso et al. performed a randomized clinical study comparing AQUACEL Ag and silver sulfadiazine for the management of partial-thickness burns. Compared with silver sulfadiazine, AQUACEL Ag was associated with less pain and anxiety during dressing changes. Children using the traditional silver sulfadiazine dressing had more flexibility and ease of movement during use in comparison with those using AQUACEL Ag. Overall, in this study the AQUACEL Ag group demonstrated greater benefits with fewer dressing changes, less nursing time, and fewer preprocedural opiate medications.[50] These benefits clearly support implementation of AQUACEL use in the pediatric setting where pain reduction and decreased length of hospitalization are overall goals. Al-Ahdab and Al-Omawi reported the use of AQUACEL Ag in a newborn with scald burns. Their choice of AQUACEL Ag was based on the dressing being shown to be less painful because it required fewer dressing changes. The effectiveness of the dressing was noted by the rapid healing of the partial-thickness burns in their neonatal case study and absence of wound infection.[41]

Functional Dressings

Dressings should not excessively inhibit motion. The thumb, for example, should not be wrapped into the palm, nor should bandages restrict chest expansion. However, bandages can be used to help position the child. For example, bulky bandages can be used in place of splints to support the fingers and wrists in infants and toddlers.

Additionally, applying the topical antimicrobial agent to the gauze and then applying the gauze to the wound (instead of applying the topical agent directly to the wound and then applying the gauze) will also help minimize pain during the dressing change. A nonadherent gauze such as Exu-Dry, Adaptic, or Xeroform will decrease the pain associated with dressing removal. A bulky bandage is used to secure the topical agent and nonadherent dressing in place. Tubular netting is then placed over the bulky bandage to secure it in place. The tubular netting can be cut/fabricated into many styles (e.g., sleeve, shirt, stocking) for the specific body part. Figure 22.9 shows a functional dressing for the hand, which gives the child more freedom of use while playing or engaging in activities of daily living (ADLs).

Positioning with dressing application should be followed. Burns across joints or at the hands or feet require special attention with dressing application. Positioning is utilized to protect the burn wounds, decrease edema, and counteract wound and scar contraction by putting the tissue in an elongated position. For example, burns across the antecubital fossa should be wrapped and splinted into extension. Burns on the plantar/dorsal surface of the foot and calf should be wrapped and splinted into neutral dorsiflexion.[40]

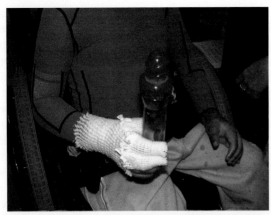

FIGURE 22.9. Functional wrapping of a hand burn. Individual finger dressings allow for easier movement and performance of activities of daily living.

Biologic and Synthetic Dressings

Advances in burn wound management surround the invention and improvements made in the area of biologic or synthetic dressings. Biobrane is a synthetic dressing that can be used on superficial partial-thickness burns, over autografts, on donor sites, and in the treatment of toxic epidermal necrolysis (TEN). It is a nylon fabric that is combined with a silicone film, where collagen is incorporated. The nylon fabric comes into contact with the burn wound and adheres until reepithelialization occurs. It is placed on the burn wounds in the operating room and secured with staples or sutures, and once it has adhered to the wound, no other dressing is necessary.[51]

Some of the more common biologic dressings are allografts and xenografts. An allograft is a graft of skin from a cadaver, which has been harvested within 24 hours of death and preserved via cryopreservation (at a skin bank). A xenograft is skin harvested from a species that is different from the recipient. Quite often referred to only as xenograft, porcine xenograft comes from a pig and can help protect and facilitate healing of partial-thickness burns as well as debriding exudative wounds. Work in Brazil has been conducted exploring the use of tilapia skin, a resource more readily available in the area, as another xenograft for use in the treatment of children with superficial partial-thickness burn wounds. In a pilot study by Júnior et al., tilapia skin showed similar time to healing compared with standard treatments with a benefit of fewer dressing changes.[52] Xenografts used for superficial partial-thickness burns function like an artificial scab, promote healing, and slough off when the wound is healed underneath. Both xenografts and allografts are pretreated biologic dressings that can be applied to excised tissue. Underneath, healing can begin, and the wound bed becomes sufficiently vascularized to prepare for autografting.

Surgical Management

Once burn size and depth estimations have been made and the initial burn wound management has commenced, further wound management may include surgery.

Because a superficial partial-thickness burn will heal in approximately 2 weeks with normal skin, the goals of the surgeon in such cases are to keep the wound free of infection, to provide adequate nutrition and fluids, and to manage pain until the wound is healed. Depending on the size and location of the superficial partial-thickness burn, the age of the child, and the ability of the parent, many of these burns can be treated on an outpatient basis and without surgery.

A deep partial-thickness burn can heal without surgical intervention if adequate medical treatment and wound management are provided. The progression of deep partial-thickness burns will usually take one of two pathways. The first includes the filmy eschar separating from the wound edges, allowing epithelial buds to resurface the wound. In the second pathway, following separation of the eschar, the wound heals by granulation tissue. The presence of granulation tissue will increase the risk of hypertrophic scarring. This situation, along with large TBSA of deep partial-thickness burns, makes surgical intervention via grafting more probable. The surgeon may elect to graft the deep partial-thickness burn in a procedure called tangential excision and grafting.[3] Such excision and grafting can be done within the first week of the burn injury and is ideally performed 2 to 5 days after the burn injury (termed *early excision and grafting*). Early excision and grafting may also apply to other wounds, particularly full-thickness wounds, which may be excised to fascia. Tangential excision and grafting of deep partial-thickness wounds during the first week shortens the hospital stay, lessens pain, decreases the incidence of infection, and improves cosmetic and functional outcome by minimizing the amount of hypertrophic scar tissue development and scar contraction.[53]

There are drawbacks associated with early tangential excision and grafting of deep partial-thickness wounds, however, and not all children are candidates for this procedure. Early excision and grafting of deep partial-thickness burns usually involves significant intraoperative blood loss that may require substantial transfusion; this may not be recommended for those who are medically unstable or those with inhalation injury.[54] When a burn involves a significant percentage of TBSA, and particularly when the burn area consists of both deep partial-thickness and full-thickness burns with a limited number of donor sites for skin grafts, excision and grafting of deep partial-thickness burns can be delayed in hopes of healing under skilled wound care. When this does not occur, skin grafting surgeries are often staged to allow for healing of donor sites which can be reharvested multiple times.

Skin Graft and Donor Site

There are several different types of grafts, depending on the source of the skin. An autograft is skin that is surgically shaved from an unburned part of the child's body (called the donor site) and placed on the burned area. Removal of the skin to be used for grafting is called harvesting. In cases where infection is present or TBSA is large, autografting may not be possible and alternative grafts, including xenografts and allografts, can be used as a temporary biologic dressing. These are often used in preparation for autografting to test the receptivity of the wound bed for an autograft.[55] Ultimately, unless significant extenuating circumstances are present, all allografts and xenografts are removed from the child, and autografts are used as the final surgical intervention to allow wound closure.

With an autograft, either a full thickness or partial thickness of skin can be harvested. If a full-thickness piece of skin from the unburned donor site was taken and placed on the burned area, the burn would heal, but a wound of similar dimensions to the burn would remain at the donor site. Full-thickness skin grafts (FTSGs) (0.025 to 0.030 inches thick) are used mostly in reconstructive surgery, over pressure points, or wherever extra skin thickness is needed. More commonly, only a partial- or split-thickness (approximately 0.008-inch thick) portion of skin is taken (STSG). Some areas of the body are preferred donor sites because of the thickness, texture, or color of the skin; because they are areas that will heal well; because they are in areas that are easy to harvest during surgery; and because they are in a region not usually visible. Common preferred donor sites include the lateral thighs and buttocks. However, when these areas are burned, or occur among extensive burns, almost any skin on the body can be used. A split-thickness donor site is similar to a superficial partial-thickness burn, with healing occurring within 14 days via reepithelialization. After the child has been anesthetized, the skin is shaved from the donor site with an electric knife—known as a dermatome—with settings to adjust the thickness of skin excised. The procedure is called a sheet graft when the skin is placed "as is" on the excised burned area (also known as the recipient or graft site) (Fig. 22.10). Alternatively, the skin may be placed in a skin mesher before its application to the recipient site. The mesher cuts small slits in the graft, after which the graft may be stretched or expanded before placement on the recipient site. Such a graft is known

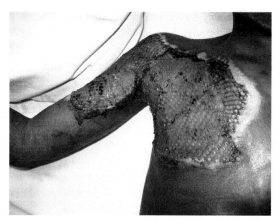

FIGURE 22.11. Meshed split-thickness skin graft.

as an expanded mesh graft (Fig. 22.11). The main purpose of meshing is to allow a skin graft to cover a larger area than could otherwise be covered using a sheet graft. The amount of graft expansion achieved is expressed as a ratio of the expanded to the unexpanded size. For example, an expanded mesh graft that covers one and a half times its original or unmeshed size would be referred to as a 1.5:1 mesh graft. One advantage of a mesh graft over a sheet graft is that there is less likelihood that hematomas or serous fluid will collect under the graft, causing the graft to be nonadherent. A disadvantage of a mesh graft, particularly a large-ratio mesh graft, is scarring that occurs within the interstices, or holes, which can hypertrophy and contract. The permanent meshed pattern of the graft may also be cosmetically unattractive.[56] Because sheet grafts provide a better cosmetic outcome with less contraction and hypertrophy, they are the graft of choice in burns involving less than 30% of TBSA that are not excessively colonized by bacteria and other microbes. Sheet grafts should also be used on the face, neck, and hands and are often preferred for other functional areas of the body, such as the feet and the axillae. The surgeon may secure the graft with surgical staples, stitches, a fibrin sealant, Steri-strips, or a combination of these techniques.[57] The graft usually takes 3 to 7 days to become adherent or to "take." The grafted area is protected during this period by bulky dressings. If the graft site is over a joint, the joint is usually immobilized with a splint during this initial period, and exercise of the joint is discontinued for that same period. Movement or shearing forces can result in graft loss. Infection, inadequate nutrition, the development of a hematoma, a poor graft bed, and inadequate debridement are other factors that can contribute to graft loss or less than optimal graft take.

Once healed, donor sites can be reharvested, up to three or four times in the case of a large TBSA burn. Harvesting of the skin over irregular surfaces can be achieved by injecting saline to contour such areas.[58]

Before the skin graft can be placed, the burned, necrotic skin, called *eschar*, must be removed. This is usually accomplished surgically, but enzymatic debrider may also be used on partial-thickness wounds. Surgical excision usually extends down to a level of viable tissue. Excision

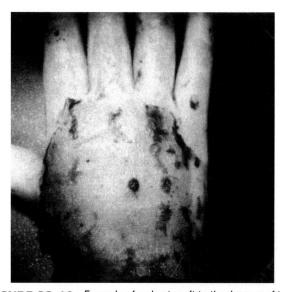

FIGURE 22.10. Example of a sheet graft to the dorsum of the hand.

of eschar may occur immediately before placing the skin graft, or, depending on the depth and extent of the wound, it may be done earlier, in a separate operation. If an excised full-thickness wound is not grafted during the same procedure, it is frequently covered with a dermal substitute or biologic dressing to allow the wound bed to develop vasculature in preparation for a skin graft at the site.

In the case of a burn involving a large percentage of TBSA, even when multiple donor sites are available, the surgeon may elect not to graft the entire burn at once because of the stress of surgery to the child, particularly if the child is already medically compromised or unstable. If the grafts do not take, not only is there still a large TBSA burn, but the donor sites are now additional wounds that must be healed, and the donor sites cannot be reused for about 10 days.

Cultured Autografts and Dermal Substitutes

Advances in wound healing and surgical techniques have improved the outcome and increased survival of those with burns. Among these advances are two that increase survival in massively burned individuals who lack sufficient donor sites: cultured autografts and dermal substitutes.

In the 1980s, cultured epithelial autografts (CEAs) or keratinocytes were the newest advancement in wound closure of the severely burned individual. In the case of CEAs, a small piece of unburned skin measuring approximately 1 square inch is harvested from the child and grown in a laboratory. Within several weeks or less, there is enough skin to cover an entire body, and this skin can be grafted onto the child from whom the original sample was taken. However, there are drawbacks and problems with cultured autografted skin. Wound closure must be delayed until the skin is grown, and the rate of graft adherence varies from 15% to 80% depending on the occurrence of graft site infection.[59] Standard physical therapy regimens, in particular those involving ROM and mobilization, must be altered or their implementation delayed in many cases. Sood et al., in 2009, performed a retrospective study of children with congenital nevi and burns who required CEA for wound coverage. They studied 29 children over an 18-year period, with all participants surviving, and those with burns averaging over 50% TBSA. The final CEA "take" success rate was over 75%, with a 99-day mean length of hospitalization. Contractures were the major long-term complication in most of the children. The CEA proved to be a durable wound coverage option in large TBSA burns.[59]

Several dermal substitutes or dermal analogs are now available. One such substitute, Integra (Integra LifeSciences Corp., Plainsboro, NJ), is an artificial dermis composed of two layers: a dermal replacement layer of bovine tendon collagen and a substitute epidermal layer of silicone.[40] Integra is placed on the excised wound. The porous dermal replacement layer serves as a matrix for the infiltration of elements from the wound bed that construct a neodermis. While the child's own neodermis is being constructed, the bovine collagen dissolves. During the period of neodermis construction, about 2 weeks, the silicone epidermal layer acts to control moisture loss from the wound. After neodermis construction is complete, the surgeon removes the silicone layer and replaces it with very thin autografts from the child. One major benefit of Integra is lack of scar formation associated with its use. Other benefits are

- its immediate availability for use,
- provision for immediate postexcisional wound coverage,
- early ambulation and rehabilitation,
- delayed autografting of the neodermis, if necessary,
- more rapid healing and better cosmetic outcome of donor sites because of ultrathin autograft use, and
- ability to save certain donor sites for use on cosmetically sensitive areas.[60]

Some disadvantages of Integra are that it lacks hair follicles and sweat glands. However, sensory function returns at the same level and time course as with normal STSG autografting.[61] Integra is expensive but may be justifiable if its use can decrease morbidity and mortality and improve outcome. Also, the high cost of the product may be offset by the lower costs associated with wound closure interventions and decrease the rehabilitation and future reconstructive needs of the child.

An additional dermal substitute is Novosorb BTM (Polynovo Biomaterials Pty, Ltd). It is a 2-layer synthetic matrix that is applied to a wound after excision. When placed in the wound bed, its outer layer acts as a barrier by preventing moisture loss.[62] The thicker matrix layer provides a scaffolding for cell and vascular regeneration.[63] Once mature, typically in 2 to 3 weeks, the upper layer is removed and a skin graft can be applied.[64] This product is less expensive than Integra yet still associated with improved cosmetic outcomes.

Other new technology such as the ReCell Spray on Skin™ system is currently indicated for children with acute burns who are 18 years or older.[65]

AlloDerm (LifeCell Corp., The Woodlands, TX) is another dermal replacement product, which is applied once the antigenic epidermis and antigenic cells from the dermis are removed from human cadaver skin through a patented process. AlloDerm leaves a dermal matrix that will accept an ultrathin STSG. Less scarring and contraction result with AlloDerm and an ultrathin STSG than with an STSG alone, and the combination of ultrathin grafts with AlloDerm results in quicker healing and less scarring of donor sites.[40] The color of the combined AlloDerm and STSG closely resembles the surrounding skin. As is the case with Integra, the high cost of AlloDerm may be offset by the lower costs of decreased length of stay and fewer rehabilitation needs or future reconstructive surgeries.

» Physical therapy examination

The physical therapist plays a crucial role in the rehabilitation of the child with a burn. The therapist's goals for the child who has been burned are

- to assist with burn wound management,
- to maintain or increase active and passive ROM,
- to manage soft tissue contours,
- to maintain and increase strength and endurance,
- to promote normal development and function,
- to inhibit loss of motion, deformity, hypertrophic scarring, and contractures,
- to minimize pain with activity and promote use of age-appropriate management strategies,
- to promote a return to meaningful participation in social roles such as playing with peers or participation in school.

The physical therapist is involved in the continuum of care for children with thermal injuries from the acute through the rehabilitative and reconstructive phases. The therapist is a member of the burn team and consults with other team members, including the child and parents, when providing interventions and assisting with the plan of care.

Examination/Evaluation

Depending on the setting in which the physical therapist is working, the burn injury will be in a different phase of healing (e.g., inflammation, proliferation, and maturation). You may be examining a new burn, one that has undergone excision and grafting, one that is healing following a graft, or one that has begun to demonstrate scarring months after the original injury.

History

Whether reviewing the child's chart or conducting a detailed child/parent interview, key pieces of information are needed. These include the date of injury, the mechanism of injury, what the child was wearing, what was done immediately at the scene prior to the arrival of emergency services, and what medical or surgical interventions the child has received. The circumstances of the injury and the pattern of the burn will assist the team in ruling out child abuse. Knowing what the child was wearing may give a better idea of the appearance of the burn. For example, knowing whether a child had clothing on that wasn't fire retardant or had a diaper on that spared the groin area will assist the therapist in a full evaluation. If there was clothing on, was it removed? Because there are still many home remedies for burns, it is important to ask the family members what first aid was provided at the scene. Was water poured on the area? Was any ointment or other substance applied to the burn? Many people still put ice, oils, ointments, or even butter on burns because these remedies have been passed down through generations; however, these can affect the healing process and influence the examination of the burn. A social and environmental history should be obtained. What type of structure the child lives in, who lives in the home, what school the child attends and at which grade level, and what mode of transportation the child uses, are all questions to ask to assist with early discharge planning. If the child was burned in a house fire, is the home inhabitable, were other family members injured, and does the family need assistance to secure safe housing prior to discharge? For the child in the rehabilitation setting, return to and reintegration into the school setting need early planning to assist teachers and students in what to expect on their return. Past medical history, educational history, and developmental history that may influence the child's recovery or physical therapy interventions are also important to document.

Review of Systems

CARDIOVASCULAR PULMONARY The circulatory changes following a thermal injury are called burn shock. Cardiac output is decreased owing to fluid losses, vasodilation, and decreased circulating volume. Fluid resuscitation is key to regaining normal resting values of cardiac output.[15] Children with singed hair on the face or hairline, oral edema and blisters, hoarseness, and carbonaceous sputum have signs and symptoms of inhalation injury and need close monitoring of their respiratory status. They often require 100% oxygen or even intubation to protect their airway and provide adequate respiratory support.[15] The physical therapist in the acute care setting must be aware of normal vital signs, oxygen saturation, and the effects of interventions on these parameters. Severe thermal injuries will result in decreased pulmonary function, which can last several years. The initial obstructive respiratory phase often develops into a restrictive pattern as seen on pulmonary function tests.[66] Other factors that could influence pulmonary function include chest wall burns and the need for a tracheotomy. Suman et al.[66] reported increased pulmonary function in children who underwent exercise tolerance interventions, recommending them to be a component of a comprehensive outpatient intervention program for children following thermal injuries.

NEUROMUSCULAR Depending on the burn depth, circulatory compromise can result from edema formation. The child is at risk for compartment syndrome, which can affect nerves and muscle viability.[15] The child is also at risk for peripheral nerve compression caused by immobility and improper positioning (e.g., peroneal nerve compression associated with externally rotated lower extremities).

MUSCULOSKELETAL If the child was involved in a motor vehicle accident with vehicle fire or jumped from a burning home, there is a bone fracture risk. The fractures may not be found initially if the child is unresponsive and the initial trauma survey is concentrated on the thermal injury. With a deep hand burn, flexor or extensor tendons may be exposed, requiring careful attention to prevent tendon rupture.

Heterotopic ossification is a complication that often occurs most often at the elbow in children following a thermal injury. Other joints affected by immobility may be the hip and shoulder, even if not directly affected by the thermal injury. In the acute phase, a ramification of heterotopic ossification is pain, whereas further into the child's recovery, function is limited. Surgical intervention is often required to improve ROM and ADLs such as feeding and self-care.[67]

Children with severe burns are at risk for development of critical illness myopathy (CIM) and critical illness polyneuropathy (CIP). This may be attributable to the high incidence of multiorgan dysfunction in children with severe burns and prolonged ICU- and ventilator-dependent days. Banwell et al. suggested that CIM/CIP occurs at an incidence of 1.7% in pediatric ICUs.[68] Children with burns are likely underrepresented in this population because some hospitals care for children with burns in the pediatric ICU, whereas others care for them in a specialized burn ICU. Kukreti et al. noted that it is difficult to differentiate between the two diagnoses of CIM and CIP. They reported there were no proven therapies that prevent or reverse these diagnoses.[69] As with any critically ill child, the physical therapist should be attentive to daily changes in the child and report their findings to the team so that timely and appropriate interventions can be provided.

INTEGUMENTARY Examination of the integumentary system should include an estimation of burn depth and TBSA involved. The physical therapist can utilize a body diagram to make notations on the areas that are burned, as well as graft sites or scars that are present. The Lund and Browder chart could be utilized to determine TBSA. Identifying structures of the skin as well as tissue type, capillary refill, and mechanism of injury will aid in determining burn depth.

For a child who underwent skin grafting, on removal of the postoperative dressings, examination of graft adherence can be described in percentage of graft "take." For example, for an STSG that has completely adhered and with no signs of open wound, the graft has 100% take.

Scar-rating tools may be helpful in a more comprehensive examination/evaluation of burn scars. Both subjective and objective tools exist. The Vancouver Scar Scale (VSS) is a widely used subjective scar rating tool (Fig. 22.12). This visual examination tool rates the scar according to its pigmentation, vascularity, pliability, and height, assigning a score for each. The scores can then be compared over time.[70] Multiple studies have found the VSS or the mVSS to lack acceptable intra-rater reliability.[71,72] Although multiple objective scar examining tools exist, no single tool has been identified by the ABA as a gold standard. Objective tools do not address common scar-associated problems such as pain and pruritus.[73] In addition to such tools, the child's perception of the scar should be taken into consideration.[74]

Examination of the nonburned skin is another component of the integumentary review. The acutely burned child may be immobile because of medical instability, and careful inspection of nonburned skin on a daily basis is imperative, as the immobile child is at risk for pressure ulcers. Contributing factors for pressure ulcers, in addition to immobility, are decreased nutrition, altered consciousness, and altered sensory perception, in the case of compartment syndrome. Areas at risk for pressure ulcers include bony protuberance such as the occiput, sacrum, or heels. Splints are used to maintain joint position and preservation. Splints can also cause pressure ulcers owing to improper fit or application and volume shifts from edema. Daily inspection of the skin and proper fit of splints is part of the acute care therapist's examination and subsequent interventions. The Braden Q scale is a skin risk assessment scale utilized in the pediatric population. It was adapted from the Braden scale, which was established for determining adults at risk for pressure sores. This scale is often done by the bedside nurse but can be implemented by any member of the health care team.[75]

Photography is another important component of the integumentary examination. In addition to the body diagrams, a photo may allow for further evaluation, once the burn has been covered by dressings. A photograph will also allow another clinician, who missed the dressing change, to view the wound. This approach avoids subjecting the child to an unnecessary dressing change. Advantages of digital photography (over 35-mm film) include image verification, immediate printing, and ease of collecting a series of photographs to document change. Many of the current systems used for creating electronic records for children allow for the storage of digital pictures, which makes it convenient for a team of providers to view how wounds are changing as the child progresses along the continuum of care. Photography can also be utilized as a communication tool between therapists and nurses in the case of specific dressing or splint application.[76]

Tests and Measures

PAIN The child's pain management should be a priority. Following an acute burn, children experience pain not only from the original injury, but also from daily procedures, including dressing changes and therapy. These procedures stimulate the nociceptive afferent fibers on a daily basis during their recovery.[42] Before physically examining the child (or during interventions), pain must be evaluated. Pain scales for children are readily available and are valid measures. The Wong–Baker FACES scale is a self-reporting scale from which the child can pick from six different faces (no hurt to hurts as much as you can imagine) with a resultant score of 0 to 10.[77] For children older than 7 years, a self-reporting numeric scale of 0 to 10 can be used. For unresponsive children or those unable to use the self-reporting scales, a behavioral scale should be used. The Pain Observation Scale for Young Children (POCIS) and the COMFORT Behaviour Scale (COMFORT-B) are two pain behavior observation tools that have shown good reliability and construct validity for use with young children with burns for the measurement of procedural and background pain.[78-80] Scored as either a 0 or 1 for the presence or absence of each item between two labeled categories, the

VANCOUVER GENERAL HOSPITAL
OCCUPATIONAL THERAPY DEPARTMENT

BURN SCAR ASSESSMENT
PATIENT NAME:

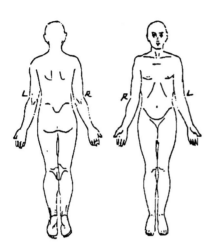

PIGMENTATION (M)
0   normal—color that closely resembles
    the color over the rest of one's body
1   hypopigmentation
2   hyperpigmentation

VASCULARITY (V)
0   normal—color that closely resembles
    the color over the rest of one's body
1   pink
2   red
3   purple

PLIABILITY (P)
0   normal
1   supple—flexible with minimal resistanc
2   yielding—giving way to pressure
3   firm-inflexible, not easily moved,
    resistant to manual pressure
4   banding—rope-like tissue that
    blanches with extension of scar
5   contracture—permanent shortening of
    scar producing deformity or distortion

HEIGHT
0   normal—flat
1   < 2 mm
2   < 5 mm   Scale in mm
3   > 5 mm

Date	Scar #	Pigmentation	Vascularity	Pliability	Height	Total	OT init

FIGURE 22.12. Vancouver Scar Assessment Scale.

POCIS contains seven behavioral items with possible scores ranging from 0 to 7, 0 indicating no pain and 7 severe pain. Comprising six behavioral items with five specific defined answer categories for each item with increasing scores from 1 to 5, the COMFORT-B total score can range from 6 to 30, 6 representing no pain and 30 the most severe pain. Each tool has its strengths and weaknesses, the POCIS being quicker and easier to use, whereas the COMFORT-B allowing for more degrees of severity within a measured behavioral category.[78] Documentation of the pain score is done daily by the therapist before, during, and after the interventions as well as periodically by nursing in the acute care setting.

SENSATION Sensory testing is part of the examination of an acute burn. The child's ability to detect touch or pain at the burn site indicates the depth of the burn. Insensate areas, which are not painful despite the burn, may indicate a full-thickness injury. Edema in the acute phase of a burn formation may be rapid and extensive. Edema formation can be severe enough to compromise blood flow to the extremities and lead to compartment syndrome and altered sensation. Careful examination of skin color, temperature, and the presence of numbness/tingling are necessary.[15] Children with increased lower extremity or groin edema may assume a position of lower extremity external rotation. This position can compress the peroneal nerve, causing numbness and tingling and leading to foot drop during gait. For children in later stages of healing, or in the scar maturation phase, careful examination of sensation will aid in planning interventions. Children with foot burns, who lack normal sensation owing to the depth of the burn or following a graft on the plantar surface, should be instructed in safety concerns of going barefoot. Children and their parents must be aware of the dangers of walking barefoot and need to carefully inspect the skin for any cuts, punctures, or infections.

RANGE OF MOTION On initial examination of the acute burn, ROM of all joints, both affected and unaffected, should be carefully measured. If the child can participate, active-assistive ROM is beneficial to give the child some form of control while also giving you an idea of the ROM limits. Passive range of motion (PROM) can be performed with caution in the acute phase, especially in an unresponsive child. Aggressive PROM is contraindicated over exposed tendons/joints owing to the risk of rupture. Care must also be taken at the shoulder joint to avoid joint or brachial plexus injury.

During the remodeling phase of healing, daily examination of ROM with the bandages removed is important. Observing and measuring the ROM without the dressings allows the therapist to view healing structures and to examine any scar tissue for blanching. Blanching tissue signifies the end of the ROM prior to tearing the skin.[40] Once blanching is noted, the clinician has a clear idea of what ROM to expect from the child for the rest of the day during all therapies. Pushing the child past the point of blanching can lead to a tearing of the skin. This auto release of scar tissue along a line of stress mimics what would be done surgically. It can be considered as sparing a child from an expensive surgical release. However, it is also painful and creates a new open wound that needs to be dressed and managed.

For children well into the scar maturation phase, ROM determination of scarred joints needs to be done in multiple planes of movement to fully measure the ROM and scar blanching. For example, a child with a scar on the anterior shoulder area may not show limitations in straight plane movements but may be limited with overhead activities such as throwing a ball. Taking the shoulder joint and subsequent scars through multiplanar motions provides a more thorough examination.

MOBILITY/GAIT If the child is allowed to be mobile, examination of the level of independence with transfers in and out of bed and a chair, and with ambulating should occur. With lower extremity burns, the child may have an antalgic gait and may need an assistive device. Following grafts, the child may have pain/limitations at the donor sites, which are frequently on the thigh, thus impacting mobility and gait. During the scar maturation phase, truncal and leg scars may inhibit normal walking or running patterns.

ACTIVITIES OF DAILY LIVING A thorough examination includes the child's ability to participate in ADLs. Depending on the child's age, the level of baseline participation will be different. For example, the toddler may be able to remove clothes/shoes, but will need assistance with donning them. The child's ability to participate in ADLs may also include dressing changes in the acute phase, as well as scar management and donning compression garments during the scar maturation phase. The adolescent is expected to be independent with all ADLs. Appropriate standardized testing, such as the WeeFIM for a child 6 to 16 years of age, may be appropriate to evaluate changes in function over time.[81]

» Interventions

Pain Management

Prior to any interventions for the child with a thermal injury, pain should be evaluated using a standardized and age-appropriate system of measurement. There can be different types and causes of pain, including those associated with the injury itself, wound care techniques, debridement, grafting, and therapeutic interventions. Depending on the type and timing of the intervention, pain evaluation could determine the use of a pharmacologic approach, nonpharmacologic approach, or a combination of the two.[82] Intervention strategies include providing medications to the child prior to a painful or anxiety-provoking procedure. Medications may include nonsteroidal anti-inflammatory agents, which reduce pain and modify the systemic inflammatory response. Opiates have been proven useful in alleviating burn pain. Benzodiazepines are effective for anxiety control. Ketamine, a dissociative anesthetic, is also widely used to provide comfort and has an amnesic effect, so the child does not have memory of the painful procedure.[82]

Nonpharmacologic interventions include cognitive-behavioral therapy; relaxation training; hypnosis and guided imagery; biofeedback; distraction; art, music, and play therapies; and the use of virtual reality and augmented reality devices.[82-84] In 2011, Miller et al. studied the differences in pain experiences in children who used standard distraction techniques (TV, video games, stories, toys, and caregiver support) and those who used a multimodal distraction device (MMD). The MMD is a customized handheld device (console and content) that is interactive via movement, touch screen, and multisensory feedback. There are two components to the device, one for procedural preparation and the other for distraction. The MMD group demonstrated a reduction in pain experiences during burn care procedures and decreased treatment length.[85]

A child life specialist could also be included in either preparing the child for the procedure or aiding in distraction during the procedure. If a child life specialist or music therapist is not available, the provider should be prepared, prior to providing interventions, with age-appropriate distraction activities. These may include bubbles, books, and magic wands for younger patients and portable radio/compact disc players, video games, or DVDs for older patients.

Wound Care

Acute Management

Depending on the institution, the mode of wound cleansing and dressing application will already be established. The physical therapist may play a primary role in wound care or an adjunctive role if nursing has the lead role in cleaning the wounds and applying dressings. Daily or twice-daily dressing changes may be ordered in the early stages of burn wound management.

Preparation for wound cleansing and dressing change includes providing timely medications prior to the intervention to the child, coordinating staff who need to examine the child, and preparing the room and supplies. The room temperature should be at least 86° F to minimize heat loss and lower the metabolic rate of the child.[15] Wounds should be gently cleansed to remove old topical agents and devitalized tissue and to decrease pain.[86] Wound beds should not be scrubbed to the point of bleeding, although bleeding may occur in the healing epithelium. Removal of intact blisters is controversial. Some believe that the area under the blister is sterile and can remain intact, unless it becomes very tense or erythematous. Others believe that remaining blisters may interfere with an ongoing examination process. Guidance from your trauma, plastic, or burn surgeon will dictate the institution's policies.

Once the wound is cleansed, timely application of the topical agents and dry dressings will aid in decreasing the child's pain when the wounds are left open to the air for prolonged periods.

Ideal burn dressings will serve multiple functions. They should be nonadherent to the healing wound; absorb exudates; provide a warm, moist environment for healing; protect the wounds from further damage; reduce pain; and allow for functional use of the affected area.[86] Functional wrapping of the affected areas is often best done by the physical or occupational therapist. The therapist can suggest positions for placement or positioning of the extremities or affected joints and have the bandage applied so as to maximize function. Examples of this approach include wrapping the elbow into extension when a burn covers the antecubital fossa; individually wrapping fingers and toes; and positioning the ankle in neutral dorsiflexion to avoid a plantar flexion contracture, thereby inhibiting movement.

There are several layers to a good burn dressing. The contact layer is just that—it comes in contact with the burn and is low to nonadherent. The topical agent (most commonly Silvadene) is typically embedded into large pieces of gauze that can be laid directly on the skin. For burns to the saddle/buttock area, a diaper covered with Silvadene can be used. Other examples of commercially available contact layer dressings include Exu-Dry, Conformant, Xeroform, and Adaptic. The next layer is the intermediate absorbent layer and is usually dry gauze or absorptive pads (Exu-Dry). The outermost layer serves to hold the other two layers in place and includes rolls of gauze or tubular elastic netting. The netting can be made into garments, thus securing the bandages from slipping and exposing the burns. Tape should be avoided because it makes removal of the dressing more difficult and can also migrate onto good or burned tissue, thus creating pain and anxiety at dressing removal.[86] Ongoing wound/skin management includes moisturizing cream, sunscreen, and occasionally dressings for an open wound.

Splinting and Positioning

The purpose of splinting and positioning during the acute phase of recovery is to help control edema, provide support for edematous extremities, provide joint protection, immobilize exposed tendons, immobilize joints in the postoperative period to improve graft take, and inhibit wound contraction and loss of motion. Splinting children during this phase of care is often unnecessary, except in the case of older children and adolescents and those who are extensively burned. Care must be taken to prevent pressure sores because these children are at high risk owing to increased moisture and decreased mobility. Pressure sores in the burn population can occur because of hypovolemia, decreased oxygenation, prolonged bed rest, or splints that are poorly fitting or have been improperly applied. Causes of pressure ulcers are attributed to shear, friction, and unrelieved pressure. The most common sites for pressure ulcers are the sacrum/coccyx and heels, and the ankle, buttocks, and occipital area are also vulnerable. The child who requires surgical intervention is also at risk because of prolonged immobilization during the operation if appropriate pressure-relieving devices are not used.[75]

For positioning in bed during the first few days of hospitalization, the child who is on bed rest must have appropriate devices in place. Heel and elbow protectors can be used as well as gel pillows for bony prominences. An interdisciplinary approach to proper positioning is key to managing this issue. Appropriate positioning programs and devices are effective only when implemented correctly. Education and communication between therapists and nurses will aid in this process. A whiteboard in the child's room is often used as a visual and written communication tool, as well as documentation in the child's chart and included in the child/family education and handouts.

When using splints, the therapist must consider the skin integrity, edema formation, and proper fit of the device. The zone of stasis lies immediately beneath the burn and has a compromised state of circulation; this area is sensitive to increased pressure. If splints or elastic bandages are applied too tightly, the zone of stasis could convert to a deeper wound. Care must also be taken when using devices on nonburned areas because they too could cause skin breakdown. Splints made to prevent contractures or protect structures during the early phase of wound healing must be monitored daily to ensure proper fit. They may need to be adjusted daily to accommodate for edema formation or changes in dressings. As edema increases, splints or elastic bandages holding the splints in place can cause increased compression, leading to a pressure sore. Meticulous skin inspection during dressing changes must occur during the edema formation stage and as the burn heals so as to ensure proper fit.[75]

Proper bed positioning must begin as soon as the child is admitted, either to an intensive care unit or a regular unit. For children on bed rest, care must be taken to avoid shear forces. The Agency for Healthcare Research and Quality has made recommendations to minimize shear, including avoiding elevating the head of the bed higher than 30 degrees for a prolonged period of time. The skin and fascia of the torso tend to remain static, whereas the deep fascia and skeleton slide toward the bottom of the bed when the head is raised. The skin on the scapula and buttocks is then put on traction, causing a shearing force. With sufficient traction, blood supply is compromised, and a pressure ulcer can develop. The physical therapist can advise the team on the best way to transfer a child. For example, if a child has burns or compromised skin to the buttocks and upper thighs, the therapist may recommend the use of a mechanical lift in place of transfers, using a sliding board to decrease the risk of shearing across already compromised skin.

Repositioning the child in bed should occur at least every 1 to 2 hours, if he/she is medically stable. Adhering to the lower limits of this time frame will be helpful as different tissues have different tolerances to ischemia from pressure.[75]

There is an axiom that states that the position of comfort—flexion—is the position of contracture for children who have been burned. Children are therefore splinted or positioned to counteract contracting forces. The neck should be positioned in a neutral position or slight extension. Pillows under the head are prohibited because they promote cervical flexion. The shoulders should be positioned in approximately 90 degrees of abduction and in slight protraction. Elbows should be placed in extension and supination (Fig. 22.13). Wrist/hands should be positioned in slight wrist extension, slight metacarpophalangeal (MCP) joint flexion, proximal interphalangeal/distal interphalangeal extension, and thumb abduction, as shown in Figure 22.14. Hips are placed in neutral extension and slight abduction, neutral rotation. Knees are placed in full extension and ankles in neutral dorsiflexion (no plantar flexion). Figure 22.15 shows recommended anticontracture positioning. All of these anticontracture positions can be attained either with towel rolls, splints, or other positioning devices that are commercially available.[40]

Splints are fabricated over a uniform layer of dressings to ensure proper day-to-day fit and are monitored closely owing to the edema issues.

Specialized splints can be fabricated for specific body parts. Airplane splints are made for axillary burns. Microstomia prevention appliances (MPAs) are special devices to assist in mouth/lip stretching. A multiring collar is a flexible neck orthosis that allows circumferential pressure to the neck to

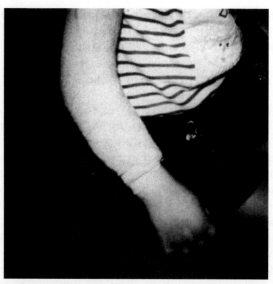

FIGURE 22.13. Elbow extension splint to prevent or correct elbow flexion contracture.

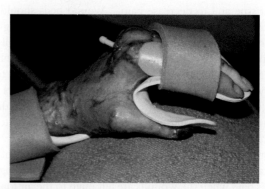

FIGURE 22.14. Example of a hand splint to prevent contractures.

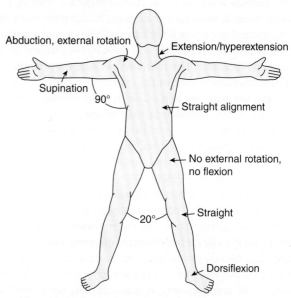

FIGURE 22.15. Positioning for contracture avoidance.

assist increasing ROM and is easier to fabricate than traditional thermoplastic splints.[87]

Casting

Casting may be used during both the acute and rehabilitation phases to maintain a specific position in children when a splinted position is difficult to sustain. For example, it may be preferable to immobilize the MCP joints in flexion while allowing active use of the distal joints. Serial casting is effective in correcting contractures in both pediatric and adult burn children in whom other methods of regaining motion have failed, in noncompliant children,[88] in children whose splints easily slip or are removed, or in those for whom other methods, such as dynamic splinting, cannot be used. Once motion is regained through serial casting, it must be maintained through continued casting or splinting and ROM exercise. Depending on the cast material used, a cast can be bivalved, padded as necessary, and used for splinting purposes. Depending on the child and the phase of healing, casts made of either plaster or synthetic materials may be used. Synthetic casting material can be particularly useful when working with children because the material may set more quickly and may be removed by unwrapping or cutting with scissors instead of using a cast saw, which has the potential to frighten the child or cause skin disruption owing to vibration over fragile skin.

Range of Motion

Active ROM (AROM) exercises during the emergent phase help control edema and initiate early motion. Muscle contraction serves as a pumping mechanism to aid venous and lymphatic return.[89] ROM exercises should be performed during dressing changes when the bandages do not restrict motion, the therapist can see the limitations in motion resulting from edema, the wound can be viewed, and the child has received pain medication.

Active ROM exercises should commence on admission and continue throughout the rehabilitative and scar management phases. Active exercise will help decrease edema as well as preserve muscle, tendon, and joint function.[89] Development of rapport with the child and family is important, especially prior to attempting challenging exercises. Choosing activities that are an interest of the child will motivate the child to participate in active exercise. Such activities could include catching/throwing a ball overhead for upper extremity/shoulder burns, playing baseball (for trunk rotation), and riding a bike (for lower extremity burns). ADLs can also be implemented to gain active ROM. Stepping into/out of a bathtub requires increased hip/knee ROM; reaching up onto a counter or into a cabinet requires adequate shoulder ROM. Those children with true muscle weakness caused by deconditioning or nerve damage may require assistance with active ROM exercises. Both active and active-assisted exercises provide sensory feedback, increase circulation, maintain

muscle function, and allow for preserving fine and gross motor skills.[40]

PROM exercises are implemented for children who are unable to move on their own. Children who are critically ill or heavily sedated/medicated may not be able to participate in AROM exercises, and PROM exercises are then implemented. PROM exercises are an important part of a postburn therapy program because they maintain elasticity of joint structures, muscle, and tendons and help to minimize the formation of contractures.[89] Stretching exercises can be achieved either via traditional PROM by the therapist or by the child using a self-stretch premise. Self-stretching can be achieved by using overhead pulleys for shoulder ROM or a towel stretch for ankle dorsiflexion. Stretching, no matter when it is done, should be slow, gentle, and sustained. A good teaching point for parents or children of an appropriate age is to maintain a "low load with a long hold" when stretching. Remember that blanching of tissue/scar is the sign of the appropriate stretch. PROM could be performed in the operating room if the child is undergoing a surgical procedure. For a child who is resistant to all stretching, active ROM, or positioning, the opportunity to examine ROM under anesthesia is valuable. Caution must be taken, however, to protect joints from subluxation or dislocation during this exam.[40]

Massage

Massage of scar tissue and skin grafts helps maintain motion by freeing restrictive bands and increasing circulation.[90] Massage may also be helpful in decreasing itching. Initially, only gentle massage should be employed, because the newly healed tissue is often too fragile to tolerate much friction. Many children enjoy massage because it decreases itching, but other children find massage painful or may be able to cooperate with this intervention. Although all burns should have scar tissue and skin grafts lubricated by lotions—preferably two to three times each day—the therapist may select particular areas of concern for massage and may also instruct the parent in massage of these areas. Massage should be done before specific ROM exercises, especially passive ROM exercises.

Nedelec et al. studied the immediate and long-term effect of massage on adult hypertrophic scars.[91] Several things were identified that can be of benefit to the pediatric physical therapist. First, massage is a therapeutic touch and can temporarily reduce itching and pain, as well as increasing motion. Second, these effects do not persist long term. The study suggests that massage therapy does not provide added benefit over conventional treatment for increasing scar elasticity, reducing erythema, or reducing scar thickness when compared with conventional treatment alone.

Ambulation

Once cleared by the physician, mobility should commence as soon as possible in the acute postburn phase and/or after autografting. For children with acute burn injury or donor sites on their legs, premedication may reduce pain during mobility. For those with lower extremity burns or grafts, elastic bandage compression is necessary to give vascular support prior to ambulating. Following a lower extremity graft, the child, at the discretion of the surgeon, may be on bed rest for up to 3 to 7 days to permit graft adherence. The recent trend is to mobilize those with burns as early as possible to avoid joint stiffness and risks of immobility such as deep vein thrombosis and pulmonary embolism.[89] In 2012, Nedelec et al. published practice guidelines for early ambulation after lower extremity grafting following a review of relevant literature and a formal consensus exercise to identify gaps in the literature.[92] These guidelines include the following: (1) initiation of an early postoperative ambulation protocol immediately, or as soon as possible, after lower extremity grafting unless criteria of exclusion were encountered, (2) application of external compression before ambulation, and (3) continuous immobilization of the joint until the first dressing change if graft is placed across the joint. Optionally, the introduction of gradual weight bearing was recommended if full weight bearing was not immediately tolerated. The presence of fractures, a preinjury inability to walk, overriding social or psychiatric conditions, medical status prohibiting mobilization and graft on the plantar surface of the foot were all cited as criteria to defer early ambulation.

To begin mobility, the treating physical therapist should make it a priority to coordinate with the bedside nurse, child, and child's family to establish the plan for mobility, which includes premedication. Depending on the size of injury, injury location, or whether it is the acute phase of injury or postoperatively, it may be the case that the child has been mobile with assistance from the family or nursing staff. Reported tolerance to this activity should be noted by the therapist. Prior to initiating movement from the bed surface, compression should be applied distal to proximal over the area of wound. Any necessary bracing or splinting should be in place to immobilize joints with overlying autograft as appropriate. If the child has not been out of bed or positioned upright, the child should be evaluated for any evidence of orthostatic hypotension. If orthostatic hypotension is present and persistent, the use of a tilt table or bed features that gradually introduce the upright position may be utilized before progressing to sitting at the edge of the bed or standing.

When tolerated, the child should be assisted to the edge of the bed with care to avoid shearing over areas of autograft by bridging toward the edge of the bed, log rolling, and pushing up to a seated position, or, if the child is small enough, lifted and transferred to a seated position. At this time, use of a standing frame or Moveo XP (DJO Global, Lewisville, TX), a device that combines the ability to introduce graded weight bearing like a tilt table with active movement of lower extremities, may be appropriate to work toward standing unsupported for the child who has undergone a prolonged period of bed rest. An important consideration for transfers to standing is the surface height from which the child will be attempting a stand so that a safe return to sitting is possible if tolerance to standing is impaired. A parent's lap on the floor, a wheelchair after transfer via a lift, or a step stool at bedside are all good alternatives to a bed that may not be suited to the height of the child. After standing has been achieved, a progression from lateral weight shifting to stepping in place may occur to determine the child's ability to safely bear weight. It is at this time that an assistive device such as a walker or crutches may be introduced if the patient is poorly tolerant of weight bearing or demonstrates movement patterns that would make unsupported ambulation unsafe. In the early stages of ambulation after an acute burn injury or during early mobility in the postoperative period, the emphasis should be placed on the act of mobilizing. Work toward establishing a more normalized gait pattern should occur as pain and edema are resolving and restrictive dressings are minimized. After ambulation, the lower extremities should be elevated and temporary compression removed.

Exercises

Sakurai et al. studied the benefits of exercise in children with burns. They found increased physical functioning, muscle mass, strength, and cardiovascular endurance.[93] Exercise that incorporates repetitive movement of extremities and increased core body temperature, thus increasing blood flow, may alter scar elasticity and increase ROM. Celis et al.[94] found that a supervised exercise program produced beneficial outcomes in children with thermal injuries. They reported a decreased number of scar releases needed for functional improvement in comparison with their control group.[94]

Children with an inhalation injury as well as thermal injury are at risk for decreased exercise tolerance owing to decreased pulmonary function. Children may have an initial obstructive pattern of disease, which can last up to 2 years after the initial injury. This obstructive pattern then develops into a restrictive pattern for up to 8 years after burn. Suman et al.[66] examined the effects of an exercise program in severely burned children. The subjects did resistance and aerobic training 3 days per week, and increases in pulmonary function and subsequent improved exercise tolerance were noted.[66]

Cucuzzo et al. compared the efficacy and effects of an inpatient exercise program versus traditional outpatient therapy in children who sustained a burn injury.[95] The inpatient program included a general conditioning prescription for exercise. This program included moderate intensity, progressive resistance training with aerobic and general conditioning exercises for 1 hour three times per week. Strength training utilized free weights, and aerobic training included motorized treadmill, stationary bike, or independent walking. The results showed, on the basis of the gains in strength and functional outcomes recorded by their study group, that severely burned children could participate safely in this type of supervised exercise program.[95]

The advent of more sophisticated computer software has enabled video games to begin to play a role in burn rehabilitation. In 2012, Yohannon et al. looked at the adjunctive use of the Nintendo® Wii™ during sessions.[96] Children in this study received traditional PROM and exercises, and either designated Wii™ games or therapist-chosen interventions. Those in the Wii™ group showed less pain responses, decreased anxiety, and greater enjoyment.[96]

Scar Management

Following burn wound healing, or skin grafting, scar formation may occur. Skin and scar care progresses from the initial open wound phase into the scar maturation phase as the wounds heal. Once the wounds or grafts have healed, it is important to keep the skin well moisturized. Remember, burned skin has impaired ability to self-lubricate. Application of a moisturizer throughout the day will decrease the risk of skin cracks and decrease itching. Massaging in the lotion with enough pressure to create blanching may assist in releasing the scar tissue and increase ROM.[40] Putting too much pressure too soon on the scars can cause blisters to form and require massage to be discontinued and should therefore be avoided. Massage may help break up collagen fibers, which in turn will soften the scar.[97]

Compression has also been used to combat the formation of hypertrophic scarring. Early compression can begin once the wounds or grafts have healed. Compression can begin in the form of Ace wrapping, elastic cotton tubular stockings, or adhesive wraps (Figs. 22.16 and 22.17). Once edema has stabilized and the grafts or burns have completely healed, the child may be measured for a custom compression garment. Pressure garments have four main functions, namely, to restore function, relieve symptoms, prevent scar recurrence, and promote an aesthetic appearance. Pressure results in the

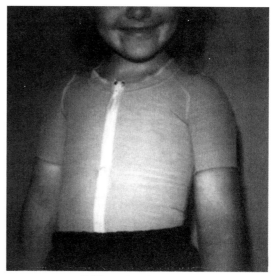

FIGURE 22.17. Child wearing the temporary compression vest from Figure 22.16.

reduction of intercollagen fibers, which helps to flatten the excessive collagen that is deposited during the proliferative phase of healing. Pressure levels for these garments should be 24 mm Hg or more, and applied for a minimum of 12 months. Pressure garments are worn for 23 hours a day, allowing removal for bathing/skin care. Pressures exceeding 24 mm Hg occlude vessels, leading to hypoxia and fibroblast degeneration and altered collagen synthesis. This process then helps flatten the scar.[97] Early application of pressure is necessary for optimal outcomes. Pressure is applied as soon as reepithelialization has occurred and continues through the maturation phase. Children are issued two sets of garments owing to the constant wear and the need for the garments to be washed. They will need to be evaluated for proper fitting periodically, typically every 3 months, unless outgrown sooner, because of wear from usage, growth, or surgical interventions.[98] Several commercially available options are made for children, with a wider variety of colors and appliqués to try to increase their use (Fig. 22.18).

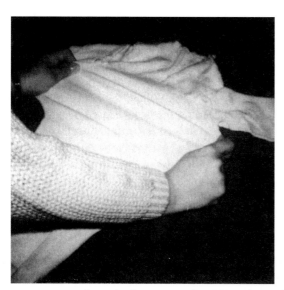

FIGURE 22.16. Example of a compression vest made out of tubular elastic netting.

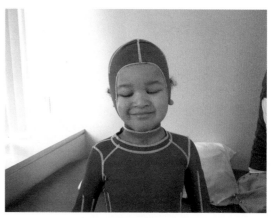

FIGURE 22.18. Example of custom compression mask and jacket.

To apply uniform pressure over convex or concave areas, foam, rubberized materials, or thermoplastic splinting material may be used as inserts under the garments. Areas often needing more custom pressure include finger web spaces, the palm, the interscapular area, and the central face.[40] Silicone linings and inserts have also been used as an adjunct to compression therapy. The mechanism of action by silicone is hydration and occlusion of the scar. Silicone elastomers (putty) were made to solve concavity problems, especially in web spaces. Benefits of using silicone sheets include comfort in application and little to no hindrance of movement. Disadvantages include frequent need to renew the sheets, loss of mobility when used over a joint, and excessive sweating.[99] Most manufacturers of compression garments offer some form of silicone lining that can be sewn directly into the garment over specified areas. Use of compression and silicone combined was studied in 2009 by Harte et al.[100] Their randomized controlled trial included subjects using compression garments with silicone sheeting or compression garments alone for burn scar management. There were no statistically significant changes in the VSS scores between the groups, but both groups showed a reduction in the scores with use of both types of garments.[100]

Facial burns require special attention, given the importance of cosmetic appearance following a burn. Children with facial burns will have the social stigma of looking different and may have to bear a long-term psychological impact of disfigurement. Compression therapy for the face can occur in three different ways. Custom compression garments are available for the face but usually cover the entire face and head, thus "hiding" the deformities. Clear plastic masks allow the clinician to see the pressure applied to the scars directly under the mask; however, the child's face and scars are fully visible. A third option is a silicone mask held in place with a facial pressure garment.[101]

The transparent plastic face mask was introduced in 1979 by Rivers et al. as an alternative to the elastic face mask to control facial scarring (Fig. 22.19).[102] As its name implies, the transparent face mask is a piece of hard, transparent plastic in the form of a custom-fitting face mask secured to the face by means of straps. The mask is constructed by forming heated plastic over a modified positive mold of the child's face. In the past, the mold would need to be made in the operating room with the child anesthetized owing to the use of plaster, which requires that the child not move. Digital scanning technology has made that procedure obsolete. The Total Contact Scanner, by Total Contact Inc (www.totalcontact.com), is a digital surface scanner that allows for noncontact scanning. The original system used a low-power helium-neon laser projected from the moving scanner head to the child's face. This required the child to sit still while unsupported on a chair or wheelchair. Newer, hand-held scanners, from Total Contact Inc, have come to market that allow for scanning to occur even if the child is not yet able to get out of bed. The scan is transmitted to a computer, which captures all the surface data. These data are then sent to the company, which produces a positive mold, over which a negative mold of the plastic/silicone face mask is made. The therapist can then adjust the fit of the mask by making the necessary changes to the positive mold and reheating the mask. Partnering with a local prosthetic and orthotic provider may be an alternative method of obtaining a full contact face mask, because many other scanner and computer technologies exist that would allow for such fabrication. This collaboration between burn therapist and orthotist/prosthetist typically includes fabrication by the orthotist/prosthetist and joint fitting of the mask. The time and resources saved by not having the child undergo anesthesia are quite beneficial.

The advantages of the transparent face mask versus the elastic face mask are as follows:

- The mask can be constructed and applied to the child within 72 hours, depending on how close the facility is to the fabricator of the mask and the type of adjustments that are required once fit.
- The therapist can see exactly where pressure is being adequately applied by observing blanching of the scar. The transparent mask can be adjusted accordingly by the therapist to increase or decrease pressure in specific areas.
- The child's face is visible to other people.
- The transparent mask usually does not require the construction and exact placement of inserts.
- The transparent face mask may cause fewer problems with head growth and malocclusion than the elastic mask.

There are also several disadvantages of the transparent face mask, including the following:

- Although both types of mask must be replaced as the child grows and the mask wears out, the cost of a new transparent mask is probably greater.
- The plastic used to construct the transparent mask is rigid, permits little movement of the facial muscles, and often limits mandible motion.

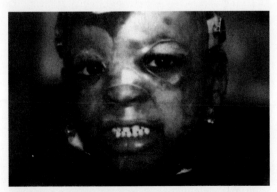

FIGURE 22.19. Transparent face mask for facial burn compression.

- The transparent mask may not cover as many areas on the head as the elastic mask. (However, the transparent mask can be used with a chin strap or alternated with an elastic mask.)
- Perspiration is increased underneath the transparent mask, and plastic may be more uncomfortable than elastic.

Although not a modality provided by physical therapists, laser therapy is now being used more commonly in the treatment of hypertrophic scarring after burn injury. There are two laser types most often used in the treatment of burn scar, pulsed dye laser (PDL) and ablative fractional CO_2 laser (AFCL). Each laser type targets different attributes of the scar, PDL reducing redness and pruritus and AFCL improving overall texture and thickness.[103-105] Zuccaro et al. performed a retrospective before-and-after study of children with hypertrophic burn scars treated with laser therapy, most of which underwent procedures with the use of PDL and AFCL in combination.[106] Outcome measures included the Vancouver Scar Scale (VSS) and Toronto Pediatric Itch Scale (TPIS), a tool validated to measure postburn pruritus in children under the age of 5.[107] A total of 125 subjects were treated over the duration of the study with greater than 50% under the age of 5 at first treatment, having mean age of 6.62 years (SD, 5.36). Of those treated, 51 had before-and-after scores for the VSS for at least one procedure on a total of 71 scarred areas. After a single treatment VSS total scores decreased from 7.37 (SD, 2.46) to 5.76 (SD, 2.29), $P < 0.005$. Additionally, the subset of subjects under 5 showed improvement in TPIS scores from 1.2 (SD, 0.70) before the first laser session to 0.35 (SD, 0.74) before the second laser session, $P < 0.005$.

Child and Family-Related Instructions

Throughout the continuum of care following a burn injury, the child and caregivers will need ongoing teaching. Initially, the parents may help with burn dressing changes, application of splints, and exercises. As the child returns to home and school, caregivers must assume all care, including skin and graft care, scar management, night splints, day splints, compression garments, massage, and, in many cases, being parents to other siblings. When possible, practicing interventions in a controlled setting may help parents be more comfortable than carrying out the intervention on their own child. This can occur in a classroom-type setting where parents can practice on mannequins or on each other, gain confidence, and then work with their own child. Children who are old enough to follow directions and a schedule are able to learn their self-care and often prefer to have control over parts of it. A written home program for exercises, splint application, and compression garment wearing schedules will aid in the caregiver's carryover.

» Outcomes on the quality of life

Children who sustain a burn injury, especially one of extensive TBSA, incur cosmetic and functional impairments that may never be completely corrected. Psychosocial implications for children include an altered body image and acceptance by their family, peers, and schoolmates, with potentially disfiguring and disabling effects from their original injury. A study by Sheridan et al. in 2000 showed that extensively burned children ($\geq$70% of the body surface) do not necessarily report a poor quality of life.[108] Even though they can't be returned to their preburn status, appearance, and function, their acute care team, support after discharge, and family support can produce satisfying long-term outcomes.[108]

The child who sustains a burn injury undergoes long-term hospitalization, painful procedures and rehabilitation, and lifelong disfigurement. Landolt et al. in 2002 looked at predictors of quality of life in pediatric burn survivors. Their results demonstrated an almost normal outcome concerning health-related quality of life. The family environment was one of the main predictors of quality-of-life outcome. The overall quality of life and psychological adjustment were best predicted by greater family cohesion, higher expressiveness, and fewer conflicts within the family. Age at injury was the second most important variable to predicting quality of life. Children who sustained a burn at a younger age had a better quality of life at follow-up. Younger children may more easily deal with their scars and integrate disfigurement into their developing body image, whereas older children may have more difficulties with body image as they develop through adolescents.[109] In a study by Murphy et al. in 2015, 50 people who sustained a burn injury (16 to 21.5 years of age and 2 to 12 years post injury) revealed a greater need for long-term psychosocial intervention for males, those with larger TBSA, those burned after school entry, and those transitioning into adulthood.[110]

The impact of a thermal injury on the family and siblings was reviewed by Mancuso et al. in 2003.[111] Sibling research has shown that relationships among themselves are among the most significant in preparing a child for adulthood. The studies revealed that siblings had fewer signs of internalizing problems and were less withdrawn and showed fewer depressive symptoms and fewer somatic problems than the control group. Compared with the control group, those siblings of children with moderate to severe injuries did have more difficulties with social competence. This finding corresponds with the severity of injury causing an increased duration of care, potentially more absence of parents, and more family attention to the injured sibling. The siblings appeared to do well at school, and the social competence piece may have been related to their ability to have friends at their home, in light of the disfigurement of their sibling. Even under stressful events, the well siblings are adjusting socially, emotionally, and behaviorally.[111]

» Social supports for children and families

When a child sustains a burn injury, it can impact the entire family, not only in the acute phase of recovery but for years afterward. In a study by Duke et al., children (<18 years old) who sustained an unintentional burn injury had significantly higher rates of hospital admissions, post burn event, because of mental health issues such as mood and anxiety disorders, psychotic disorders, or mental and behavioral conditions related to drug or alcohol abuse as compared with a matched uninjured group.[112] Understanding the various factors that impact the rehabilitation of the child is important to provide necessary and individualized support for the child and family. (Children who sustain intentional burn injuries will have additional factors that impact acute and long-term care.) Ongoing services to monitor and address any psychiatric, academic, psychological, or social issues that may arise is appropriate to optimize the child and family's functioning post injury and acute recovery. Linkage to appropriate psychological services and social groups, such as summer camps for children who have sustained a burn injury, or parent support groups, can be helpful and appropriate depending on the availability of the resources and the family's needs. Under Section 504 of the Rehabilitation Act, the student who has a condition that substantially limits a major life activity, such as his or her education, is entitled to an evaluation and, if determined appropriate, the development of a Section 504 Plan.[113] This Plan, which may include the provision of physical therapy services, is to provide reasonable accommodations that will enable the student to participate in the school's regular education curriculum.

Like many chronic or lifelong conditions in children, the physical therapist's "patient" often consists of more than the child and includes the parents or other significant caregivers in the child's life. Working with the multifaceted perspective can facilitate optimal recovery and appropriate support services for children who have sustained a burn injury and their families.

Summary

Physical therapists play a vital role in the interdisciplinary burn care team. They function in many different roles, from acute burn wound management to positioning, splinting, ROM, and functional mobility to scar management and return to home and school reintegration. Pediatric physical therapists, in any setting across the continuum of care, should be prepared to provide interventions for these children as well as to be advocates for their psychosocial needs on reentry into the community. Ongoing continuing education and mentorship will provide the best experience to gain clinical competence in the area of care for the child with thermal injuries.

CASE STUDIES

JADE

Jade is a 6-year-old girl who was admitted to her local hospital following an accident at home. She was leaning over a candle in her mom's bedroom, when her hair braids caught fire and set her shirt on fire. Her mom put out the flames with a blanket and removed Jade's shirt immediately, calling 911 in the process. Jade received emergency care within minutes and was transported to the hospital. She was referred to physical therapy on postburn day 1.

On initial examination, Jade appeared to have superficial partial-thickness burns to her face and deep partial-thickness burns to her arm and chest, with some questionable areas of deeper burns at her right upper chest and arm (Fig. 22.4). She received local wound care and ongoing burn depth estimation as structures evolved. On postburn day 2, the areas at the upper right chest and upper right arm appeared to have a brown coloration and no capillary refill and did not cause her pain on palpation. It was determined at that time that these areas were full-thickness injuries, and the plastic surgeon decided on skin grafting. On postburn day 6, she underwent excision of the eschar and split-thickness grafting with her right thigh as the donor site (Fig. 22.11). She was immobilized in the operating room with an airplane splint to protect the graft from shearing as well as to maintain preoperative ROM.

On postoperative day 5, the dressings were removed with 100% graft take (Fig. 22.20). She was allowed to mobilize on postoperative day 5, with pain limiting her right lower extremity ROM from the donor site. She required assistance with ambulation for short distances. She remained in the airplane splint until postoperative day 7, when she began gentle active-assisted ROM exercises. She was discharged on postoperative day 8 to home, with follow-up therapy for ROM and scar management. She was also seen by occupational therapy for ROM, splinting, and ADLs as well as compression garments.

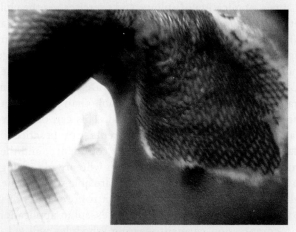

FIGURE 22.20. Healed meshed split-thickness skin graft (same child from Figure 22.4)

FRANKIE

Frankie is a 3-year-old boy who was involved in a house fire, sustaining 60% TBSA burns to his face, trunk, upper extremities, and lower extremities. He developed severe compartment syndrome, sepsis, and respiratory complications in addition to his massive burns. He was treated at a local burn center. During his acute hospitalization, Frankie developed decreased circulation to both feet and required bilateral below-knee amputations. He underwent local wound care and multiple grafting procedures to achieve wound closure. After a prolonged hospitalization, he was transferred to a rehabilitation hospital for further care.

Initially, Frankie had multiple open wounds that required daily dressing changes as well as graft care. He had significant loss of ROM at both knee joints (held in extension) as well as limited ROM in his upper extremities. He underwent serial casting of both knee joints, which was successful in achieving functional ROM. He required occupational therapy and physical therapy to regain the use of his hands, ADLs, bed mobility, and preparation for prosthetic training. He began prosthetic training but had a setback as he developed an open wound at the end of one residual limb and accentuated growth of his fibula faster than his tibia on the other residual limb. This impacted gait training for several months.

Once Frankie's open wounds had healed, new liners and sockets were developed to relieve pressure on both areas, and he was cleared to begin standing. He began a standing program both static at the edge of a mat and in a mobile prone standing frame. He had foreshortened prostheses, which he tolerated well, and began ambulation about 4 days after he began standing (Fig. 22.21). He progressed to platforms on his pylons and quickly to Solid Ankle Cushion Heel (SACH) feet. He progressed to ambulating 200 feet with a rolling walker and supervision (Fig. 22.22). His limitations in full knee joint flexion limit his ability to transition, as well as ascend and descend stairs. Owing to nerve damage to his left hand, he was unable to utilize Lofstrand crutches and worked toward independent ambulation without an assistive device. He continues to work on fine motor skills with occupational therapy (Fig. 22.23).

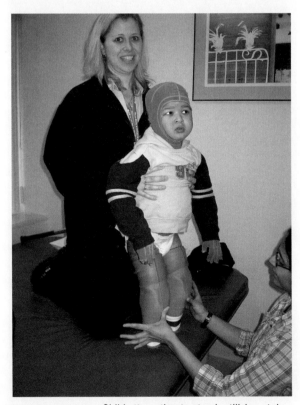

FIGURE 22.21. Child attempting to stand, utilizing stubbies as prostheses.

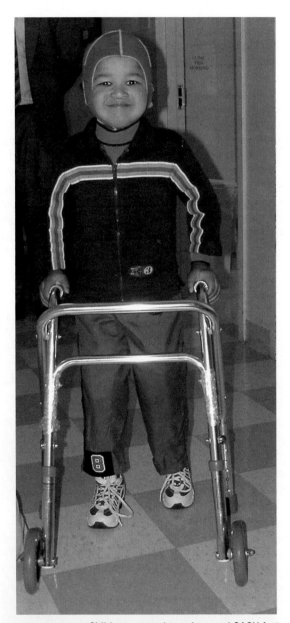

FIGURE 22.22. Child progressed to pylons and SACH feet and was able to ambulate with supervision with a rolling walker.

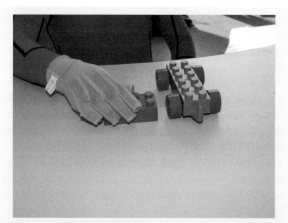

FIGURE 22.23. Child using play to increase hand function.

Frankie developed several sites of hypertrophic and keloid-type scarring at his face, neck, upper extremities, trunk, and lower extremities (Fig. 22.7). He is utilizing custom compression garments with a mask, jacket, and pants. His new prosthetic liners are actually custom fit and are providing excellent compression for his lower extremities while being worn. While out of the prostheses, he has a custom compression garment that he tolerates well (Fig. 22.18). He has undergone injections of steroids to his keloid scar on his neck and had a Z-plasty done to release the neck scar. He participated in the hospital's day rehabilitation program for 5 months and then transitioned to outpatient care. He required scar revision surgery for the back and side of his head/neck. For this, he underwent tissue expander placement (Fig. 22.24) at his scalp. This enabled the surgeon to have enough nonburn/scar tissue to cover the previous defect (Fig. 22.7). Once the tissue expanders were removed, the scarred tissue was excised and the nonscarred tissue moved into its place (Fig. 22.25).

Frankie is now able to ambulate independently in the community with new prostheses and Impulse feet by Ohio Willow Wood (Fig. 22.26). This energy-storing foot has allowed him to achieve better heel strike and push-off during the gait cycle. He can now ascend and descend a full flight of stairs

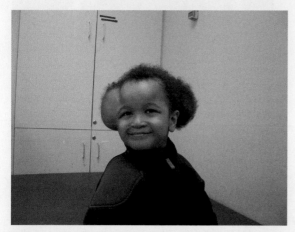

FIGURE 22.24. Child with tissue expanders in his scalp.

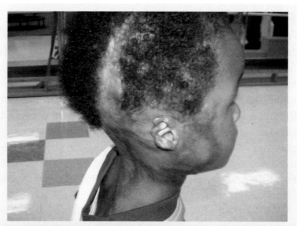

FIGURE 22.25. Patient status after tissue expander removal and corrective surgery.

and practice bus steps with supervision. He receives school-based physical therapy services as well as outpatient services to address his ongoing scar management, function, and prosthetic needs.

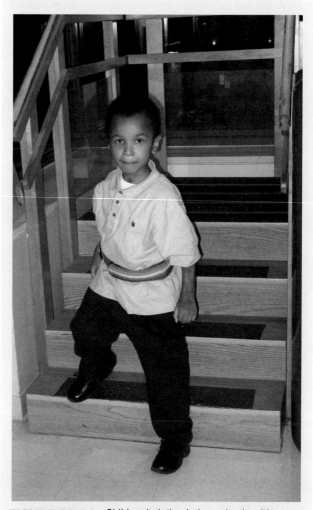

FIGURE 22.26. Child ambulating independently with bilateral prostheses.

REFERENCES

1. Centers for Disease Control and Prevention, National Center for Injury Prevention and Control. *Burn prevention. Child Safety and Injury Prevention.* 2019. Accessed July 27, 2020. https://www.cdc.gov/safechild/burns/index.html

2. Centers for Disease Control and Prevention, National Center for Injury Prevention and Control. *10 Leading causes of death, United States. All Races, Both Sexes.* 2018. Accessed July 27, 2020. https://www.cdc.gov/injury/wisqars/LeadingCauses.html

3. Johnson RM, Richard R. Partial thickness burns: identification and management. *Adv Skin Wound Care.* 2003;16(4):178-187.

4. Firefighters Burn Institute Youth Fire Setters Program. Scald Burn Facts and Figures. Firefighters Burn Institute. Accessed February 1, 2021. https://firesetter.org/scald-burn-facts-and-figures/

5. Fast Facts. Fire and Burn Injuries Among Children in 2018. *SafeKids Worldwide.* 2020. Accessed February 1, 2021. https://www.safekids.org/sites/default/files/documents/2020_fast_facts_fire_burn_v1.pdf

6. Lorch M, Goldberg J, Wright J, et al. Epidemiology and disposition of burn injuries among infants presenting to a tertiary-care pediatric emergency department. *Pediatr Emerg Care.* 2011;27(11):1022-1026.

7. Shah A, Suresh S, Thomas R, et al. Epidemiology and profile of pediatric burns in a large referral center. *Clin Pediatr.* 2011;50(5):391-395.

8. U.S. Department of Health and Human Services. *Administration for children and families. Child Maltreatment 2018.* Published January 2020. Accessed March 6, 2021. https://www.acf.hhs.gov/sites/default/files/documents/cb/cm2018.pdf

9. Zenel J, Goldstein B. Child abuse in the pediatric intensive care unit. *Crit Care Med.* 2002;30(11 Suppl):S515-S523.

10. Gornor G. Medical evaluation for child physical abuse: what the PNP needs to know. *J Pediatr Health Care.* 2012;26(3):163-170.

11. Safe Kids Worldwide. *Burn and scald prevention tips.* Accessed February 1, 2021. https://www.safekids.org/tip/burns-and-scalds-prevention-tips

12. Dowd MD, Keenan HT, Bratten SL. Epidemiology and prevention of childhood injuries. *Crit Care Med.* 2002;31(11 Suppl):S385-S392.

13. Consumer Product Safety Commission. Office of Compliance. *Children's Sleepwear Regulations.* 2001. Accessed February 1, 2021. https://www.cpsc.gov/s3fs-public/pdfs/blk_pdf_regsumsleepwear.pdf

14. Lockhard RD, Hamilton GF, Fyfe FW. *Anatomy of the Human Body.* JB Lippincott; 1969.

15. Merz J, Schrand C, Mertens D, et al. Wound care of the pediatric burn patient. *AACN Clin Issues.* 2003;14(4):429-441.

16. Lund CC, Browder NC. The estimation of areas of burns. *Surg Gynecol Obstet.* 1944;79:352.

17. Sheng WB, Zeng D, Wan Y, et al. BurnCalc assessment study of computer-aided individual three-dimensional burn area calculation. *J Transl Med.* 2014;12:242. doi:10.1186/s12967-014-0242-x

18. Chan Q, Barzi F, Cheney L, et al. Burn size estimation in children: still a problem. *Emerg Med Australas.* 2012;24:181-186.

19. *American Burn Association.* Burn center referral criteria. Accessed July 2020. http://ameriburn.org/wp-content/uploads/2017/05/burncenterreferralcriteria.pdf

20. Sussman C, Bates-Jensen B. Wound healing physiology: acute and chronic. In: Sussman C, Bates-Jensen B, eds. *Wound Care: A Collaborative Practice Manual.* Wolters Kluwer/Lippincott Williams & Wilkins; 2007:26-33.

21. Wallace HJ, Cadby G, Melton PE, et al. Genetic influence on scar height and pliability after burn injury in individuals of European ancestry: a prospective cohort study. *Burns.* 2019;45(3):567-578. doi:10.1016/j.burns.2018.10.027

22. Ward RS. Management of scar. In: Sussman C, Bates-Jensen B, eds. *Wound Care: A Collaborative Practice Manual.* Wolters Kluwer/Lippincott Williams & Wilkins; 2007:309-318.

23. Hunt TK. *Fundamentals of Wound Management in Surgery—Wound Healing: Disorders of Repair.* Chirurgecom; 1976.

24. Chan Q, Harvey J, Graf N, et al. The correlation between time to skin grafting and hypertrophic scarring following an acute contact burn in a porcine model. *J Burn Care Res.* 2012;33(2):e43-e48.

25. Richard RL, Lester ME, Miller SF, et al. Identification of cutaneous functional units related to burn scar contracture development. *J Burn Care Res.* 2009;30:625-631.

26. Diegelmann RF, Rothkop LC, Cohen LK. Measurement of collagen biosynthesis during wound healing. *J Surg Res.* 1975;19:239-243.

27. Barnes MK, Morton LF, Bennett RC, et al. Studies on collagen synthesis in the mature dermal scar in the guinea pig. *Biochem Soc Symp.* 1975;3:917-920.

28. American Burn Association. *Verification criteria.* Accessed February 1, 2021. http://ameriburn.org/quality-care/verification/

29. American Burn Association. *Rehabilitation. Resources.* 2020. Accessed February 2, 2021. http://ameriburn.org/quality-care/rehabilitation/

30. Parry I, Esselman PC; Rehabilitation Committee of the American Burn Association. Clinical competencies for burn rehabilitation therapists. *J Burn Care Res.* 2011;32(4):458-467.

31. Parry I, Forbes L, Lorello D, et al. Burn Rehabilitation Therapists Competency Tool—Version 2: an expansion to include long-term rehabilitation and outpatient care. *J Burn Care Res.* 2017;38(1):e261-e268.

32. *American Burn Association. Certification.* Accessed August 2020. http://ameriburn.org/quality-care/certification/

33. Kim L, Martin H, Holland A. Medical management of paediatric burn injuries: best practice. *J Paediatr Child Health.* 2012;48:290-295.

34. Orgill D, Piccolo N. Escharotomy and decompressive therapies in burns. *J Burn Care Res.* 2009;30(5):759-768.

35. Blasier RD. Treatment of fractures complicated by burn or head injuries in children. *J Bone Joint Surg.* 1999;81(A7):1038-1043.

36. Barret JP, Herndon DN. Modulation of inflammatory and catabolic responses in severely burned children by early burn wound excision in the first 24 hours. *Arch Surg.* 2003;138(2):127-132.

37. Jenkins ME, Gottschlich MM, Warden GD. Enteral feeding during operative procedures in thermal injuries. *J Burn Care Rehabil.* 1994;15(2):199-205. doi:10.1097/00004630-199403000-00019

38. Huckleberry Y. Nutritional support and the surgical patient. *Am J Health Syst Pharm.* 2004;61(7):671-684.

39. Tengvall O, Wickman M, Wengstrom Y. Memories of pain after burn injury-the patient's experience. *J Burn Care Res.* 2010;31(2):319-327.

40. Ward RS. Physical rehabilitation. In: Carrougher GJ, ed. *Burn Care and Therapy.* Mosby; 1998:293-327.

41. Al-Ahdab M, Al-Omawi M. Deep partial scald burn in a neonate: a case report of the first documented domestic neonatal burn. *J Burn Care Res.* 2011;32(1):e1-e6.

42. Martin-Herz SP, Patterson DR, Honari S, et al. Pediatric pain control practices of North American Burn Centers. *J Burn Care Rehabil.* 2003;24(1):26-36.

43. Bayat A, Ramaiah R, Bhananker S. Analgesia and sedation for children undergoing burn wound care. *Expert Rev Neurother.* 2010;10(11):1747-1759.

44. Luhmann JD, Kennedy RM, Porter FL, et al. A randomized clinical trial of continuous-flow nitrous oxide and midazolam for sedation of young children during laceration repair. *Ann Emerg Med.* 2001;37(1):20-27.

45. Davison PG, Loiselle F, Nickerson D. Survey on current hydrotherapy use among North American burn centers. *J Burn Care Res.* 2010;31(3):393-399.

46. Patel P, Vasquez S, Granick M, et al. Topical antimicrobials in pediatric burn wound management. *J Craniofac Surg.* 2008;19(4):913-922.

47. Tredget EE, Shankowsky HA, Groeneveld A, et al. A matched-pair, randomized study evaluating the efficacy and safety of Acticoat silver-coated dressing for the treatment of burn wounds. *J Burn Care Rehabil.* 1998;19(6):531-537.

48. AQUACEL® Ag. *The dual-purpose antimicrobial dressing: absorbency with the power of silver.* Accessed February 2, 2021. https://www.convatec.com/advanced-wound-care/aquacel-dressings/hydrofiber-technology/

49. Caruso DM, Foster KN, Hermans MH, et al. Aquacel® Ag in the management of partial-thickness burns: results of a clinical trial. *J Burn Care Rehabil.* 2004;25(1):89-97.

50. Caruso DM, Foster KN, Blome-Eberwein SA, et al. Randomized clinical study of hydrofiber dressing with silver or silver sulfadiazine in the management of partial-thickness burns. *J Burn Care Res*. 2006;27(3):298-309.

51. Barre JP, Dziewulski P, Ramzy PI, et al. Biobrane versus 1% silver sulfadiazine in second-degree pediatric burns. *Plast Reconstr Surg*. 2000;105:62-65.

52. Júnior EML, de Moraes Filho MO, Forte AJ, et al. Pediatric burn treatment using tilapia skin as a xenograft for superficial partial-thickness wounds: a pilot study. *J Burn Care Res*. 2020;41(2):241-247. doi:10.1093/jbcr/irz149

53. Xiao-Wu W, Herndon DN, Spies M, et al. Effects of delayed wound excision and grafting in severely burned children. *Arch Surg*. 2002;137(9):1049-1054.

54. Sheridan FL. Burns. *Crit Care Med*. 2002;30(11S):S500-S514.

55. Carrougher GJ. Burn wound assessment and topical treatment. In: Carrougher GJ, ed. *Burn Care and Therapy*. Mosby; 1998:133-165.

56. Parks DH, Wainwright DJ. The surgical management of burns. In: Carvajal HF, Parks DH, eds. *Burns in Children: Pediatric Burn Management*. Year Book Medical Publishers; 1988:158, 166.

57. Gibran N, Luterman A, Herndon D, et al. Comparison of fibrin sealant and staples for attaching split-thickness autologous sheet grafts in patients with deep partial-or full-thickness burn wounds: a phase 1/2 clinical study. *J Burn Care Res*. 2007;28(3):401-408.

58. Mozingo DW. Surgical management. In: Carrougher GJ, ed. *Burn Care and Therapy*. Mosby; 1998:233-248.

59. Sood R, Balledux J, Koumanis D, et al. Coverage of large pediatric wound with cultured epithelial autografts in congenital nevi and burns: results and technique. *J Burn Care Res*. 2009;30(4):576-583.

60. Integra LifeSciences Corp. *Medical economics of Integra artificial skin*. Accessed October 2013. www.integralife.com

61. Burk JF. Observations on the development and clinical use of artificial skin: an attempt to employ regeneration rather than scar formation in wound healing. *Jpn J Surg*. 1987;17:431-438.

62. Dearman BL, Li A, Greenwood JE. Optimization of a polyurethane dermal matrix and experience with a polymer-based cultured composite skin. *J Burn Care Res*. 2014;35(5):437-448.

63. NovoSorb BTM. *PolyNovo Limited*. 2020. Accessed August 21, 2020. https://usa.polynovo.com/product-btm/

64. Greenwood JE, Schmitt BJ, Wagstaff MJD. Experience with a synthetic bilayer Biodegradable Temporising Matrix in significant burn injury. *Burns Open*. 2018;2(1):17-34.

65. Kowal S, Kruger E, Bilir P, et al. Cost-Effectiveness of the Use of Autologous Cell Harvesting Device Compared to Standard of Care for Treatment of Severe Burns in the United States. *Adv Ther*. 2019;36:1715–1729. Accessed February 1, 2021. https://doi.org/10.1007/s12325-019-00961-2

66. Suman O, Mlcak RP, Herndon DN. Effect of exercise training on pulmonary function in children with thermal injury. *J Burn Care Rehabil*. 2002;23(4):288-293.

67. Gaur A, Sinclair M, Caruso E, et al. Heterotopic ossification around the elbow following burns in children: results after excision. *J Bone Joint Surg*. 2003;85(A8):1538-1543.

68. Banwell BL, Mildner RJ, Hassall AC, et al. Muscle weakness in critically ill children. *Neurology*. 2003;61:1779-1782

69. Kukreti V, Shamim M, Khilnani P. Intensive care unit acquired weakness in children: critical illness polyneuropathy and myopathy. *Indian J Crit Care Med*. 2014;18(2):95-101. doi:10.4103/0972-5229.126079

70. Baryza MJ, Baryza GA. The Vancouver Scar Scale: an administration tool and its inter-rater reliability. *J Burn Care Rehabil*. 1995;16:535-538.

71. Lee KC, Bamford A, Gardiner F, et al. Investigating the intra-and inter-rater reliability of a panel of subjective and objective burn scar measurement tools. *Burns*. 2019;45(6):1311-1324. doi:10.1016/j.burns.2019.02.002

72. Nedelec B, Correa JA, Rachelska G, et al. Quantitative measurement of hypertrophic scar: interrater reliability and concurrent

73. validity. *J Burn Care Res*. 2008;29(3):501-511. doi:10.1097/BCR.0b013e3181710881

73. Lee KC, Dretzke J, Grover L, et al. A systematic review of objective burn scar measurements. *Burns Trauma*. 2016;4:14. doi:10.1186/s41038-016-0036-x

74. Martin D, Umraw N, Gomez M, et al. Changes in subjective vs. objective burn scar assessment over time: does the patient agree with what we think. *J Burn Care Rehabil*. 2003;24(4):239-244.

75. Gordon M, Gottschlich MM, Helvig EI, et al. Review of evidence-based practice for the prevention of pressure sores in burn patients. *J Burn Care Rehabil*. 2004;25(5):388-410.

76. Van LB, Sicotte KM, Lassiter RR, et al. Digital photography: enhancing communication between burn therapists and nurses. *J Burn Care Rehabil*. 2004;25(1):54-60.

77. Wong D, Baker C. Pain in children: comparison of assessment scales. *Pediatr Nurs*. 1988;14(1):9-17.

78. de Jong A, Baartmans M, Bremer M, et al. Reliability, validity, and clinical utility of three types of pain behavioural observation scales for young children with burns aged 0 to 5 years. *Pain*. 2010;150:561-567.

79. de Jong AEE, Bremer M, Schouten M, et al. Reliability and validity of the pain observation scale for young children and the visual analogue scale in children with burns. *Burns*. 2005;31:198-204.

80. de Jong AEE, Tuinebreijer WE, Bremer M, et al. Construct validity of two pain behaviour observation measurement instruments for young children with burns by Rasch analysis. *Pain*. 2012;153:2260-2266.

81. Serghiou MH, Rose MW, Pidcock FS, et al. The WeeFIM [R] instrument—a paediatric measure of functional independence to predict longitudinal recovery of paediatric burn patients. *Dev Neurorehabil*. 2008;11(1):39-50. doi:10.1080/17518420701520644

82. Stoddard FJ, Sheridan RL, Saxe GN, et al. Treatment of pain in acutely burned children. *J Burn Care Rehabil*. 2002;23(2):135-156.

83. Luo H, Cao C, Zhong J, et al. Adjunctive virtual reality for procedural pain management of burn patients during dressing change or physical therapy: a systematic review and meta-analysis of randomized controlled trials. *Wound Repair Regen*. 2019;27(1):90-101.

84. Mott J, Bucolo S, Cuttle L, et al. The efficacy of an augmented virtual reality system to alleviate pain in children undergoing burns dressing changes: a randomised controlled trial. *Burns*. 2008;34(6):803-808.

85. Miller K, Rodger S, Kipping B, et al. A novel technology approach to pain management in children with burns: a prospective randomized controlled trial. *Burns*. 2011;37:395-495.

86. Taylor K. The management of minor burns and scalds in children. *Nurs Stand*. 2001;16(11):45-52.

87. Hurlin FK, Doyle B, Paradis P, et al. Use of an improved Watusi collar to manage pediatric neck burn contractures. *J Burn Care Rehabil*. 2002;23(3):221-226.

88. Ridgway CL, Daugherty MB, Warden GD. Serial casting as a technique to correct burn scar contractures: a case report. *J Burn Care Rehabil*. 1991;12:67-72.

89. Whitehead C, Serghiou M. A 12-year comparison of common therapeutic interventions in the burn unit. *J Burn Care Res*. 2009;30(2):281-288.

90. P. Ault P, Plaza A, Paratz J. Scar massage for hypertrophic burns scarring—A systematic review. *Burns*. 2018: 44; 24-38. https://doi.org/10.1016/j.burns.2017.05.006

91. Nedelec B, Couture MA, Calva V, et al. Randomized controlled trial of the immediate and long-term effect of massage on adult postburn scar. *Burns*. 2019;45(1):128-139. doi:10.1016/j.burns.2018.08.018

92. Nedelec B, Serghiou M, Niszczak J, et al. Practice guidelines for early ambulation of burn survivors after lower extremity grafts. *J Burn Care Res*. 2012;33:319-329.

93. Sakurai Y, Aarsland A, Herndon DN, et al. Stimulation of muscle protein synthesis by long-term insulin infusion in severely burned patients. *Ann Surg*. 1995;222:283-297.

94. Celis MM, Suman OE, Huang TT, et al. Effect of a supervised exercise and physiotherapy program on surgical interventions in children with thermal injury. *J Burn Care Rehabil*. 2003;24(1):57-61.

95. Cucuzzo NA, Ferrando A, Herndon DN. The effects of exercise programming vs. traditional outpatient therapy in the rehabilitation of severely burned children. *J Burn Care Rehabil*. 2001;22(3):214-220.

96. Yohannon S, Tufaro P, Hunter H, et al. The utilization of Nintendo® Wii™ during burn rehabilitation: a pilot study. *J Burn Care Res*. 2012;33(1):36-45.

97. Edwards J. Scar management. *Nurs Stand*. 2003;17(52):39-42.

98. Williams F, Knap D, Wallen M. Comparison of the characteristics and features of pressure garments used in the management of burn scars. *Burns*. 1998;24:329-335.

99. Van den Kerckhove E, Stappaerts K, Boeckx W, et al. Silicones in the rehabilitation of burns: a review and overview. *Burns*. 2001;27(3):205-214.

100. Harte D, Gordon J, Shaw M, et al. The use of pressure and silicone in hypertrophic scar management in burns patients: a pilot randomized controlled trial. *J Burn Care Res*. 2009;30(4):632-642.

101. Serghiou MA, Holmes CL, McCauley RL. A survey of current rehabilitation trends for burn injuries to the head and neck. *J Burn Care Rehabil*. 2004;25(6):514-518.

102. Rivers EA, Strate RG, Solem LD. The transparent facemask. *Am J Occup Ther*. 1979;33:109-113.

103. Anderson RR, Donelan MB, Hivnor C, et al. Laser treatment of traumatic scars with emphasis on ablative fractional laser resurfacing: consensus report. *JAMA Dermatol*. 2014;150:187-193.

104. Hultman CS, Friedstat JS, Edkins RE, et al. Laser resurfacing and remodeling of hypertrophic burn scars: the results of a large, prospective, before-after cohort study, with long-term follow-up. *Ann Surg*. 2014;260:519-529.

105. Donelan MB, Parrett BM, Sheridan RL. Pulsed dye laser therapy and z-plasty for facial burn scars: the alternative to excision. *Ann Plast Surg*. 2008;60:480-486.

106. Zuccaro J, Muser I, Singh M, et al. Laser therapy for pediatric burn scars: focusing on a combined treatment approach. *J Burn Care Res*. 2018;39:457-462.

107. Everett T, Parker K, Fish J, et al. The construction and implementation of a novel postburn pruritus scale for infants and children aged five years or less: introducing the Toronto Pediatric Itch Scale. *J Burn Care Res*. 2015;36:44-49.

108. Sheridan RL, Hinson MI, Liang MH, et al. Long-term outcome of children surviving massive burns. *JAMA*. 2000;283(1):69-73.

109. Landolt MA, Grubenmann S, Meuli M. Family impact greatest: predictors of quality of life and psychological adjustment in pediatric burn survivors. *J Trauma*. 2002;53(6):1146-1151.

110. Murphy ME, Holzer CE 3rd, Richardson LM, et al. Quality of life of young adult survivors of pediatric burns using World Health Organization Disability Assessment Scale II and Burn Specific Health Scale-Brief: a comparison. *J Burn Care Res*. 2015;36(5):521-533. doi:10.1097/BCR.0000000000000156

111. Mancuso MG, Bishop S, Blakeney P, et al. Impact on the family: psychosocial adjustment of siblings of children who survive serious burns. *J Burn Care Rehabil*. 2003;24(2):110-118.

112. Duke JM, Randall SM, Vetrichevvel TP, et al. Long-term mental health outcomes after unintentional burns sustained during childhood: a retrospective cohort study. *Burns Trauma*. 2018;6:32. 2018. doi:10.1186/s41038-018-0134-z

113. *Section 504 of the Rehabilitation Act of 1973, 29 USC §794*. Accessed July 22, 2020. https://www.dol.gov/agencies/oasam/centers-offices/civil-rights-center/statutes/section-504-rehabilitation-act-of-1973

23

Autism Spectrum Disorders

Anjana Bhat, Deborah Bubela, and Rebecca Landa

⟫ Introduction

The broad objectives of this chapter are to increase awareness among physical therapists (PTs) about the various multisystem impairments of autism spectrum disorder (ASD), including motor impairments; propose examinations that will increase our understanding of the child with ASD; and propose possible motor interventions for infants, children, and adolescents with ASD that are supported by available evidence.

⟫ Defining autism spectrum disorder

ASD is a neurodevelopmental disorder in which persons present with a range of impairments in social communication skills and restrictions in behaviors and interests.[1] Social communication impairments include poor social–emotional reciprocity or the ability to go back and forth during conversations with others; reduced sharing of experiences, interests, and emotions with others; and poor initiation of and response to social bids. Both nonverbal communication deficits in use of gestures or eye gaze during social interactions and verbal communication deficits such as atypical or reduced language skills are hallmarks of ASD. Individuals with ASD have difficulties developing and maintaining relationships with peers

and caregivers. For example, they may have difficulties making friends. In terms of restricted and repetitive behaviors, children may present with motor stereotypies (e.g., finger flicking, arm flapping, and body rocking) or they may insist on sameness, rituals, and fixed routines, or highly restricted interests (e.g., preoccupation with certain objects or certain topics). Children with ASD also have hyper- or hyporeactivity to sensory inputs or unusual interest in certain sensations (e.g., indifference to pain, adverse response to specific sounds or textures, excessive smelling or touching of objects, visual fascination with lights or movement). In addition, the majority of the children with ASD have significant motor impairments that deserve examination and intervention, which is the focus of this chapter. In fact, recent work shows that 75% to 87% of children with ASD have significant motor delays and risk for a motor impairment.[2,3]

⟫ Prevalence

According to the latest report from the Centers for Disease Control and Prevention, 1 in 59 children in the general population will be diagnosed with ASD, an incidence significantly greater than the 1 in 110 reported in 2000.[4] The prevalence of ASD is five times more common in boys (1 in 54) than in girls (1 in 252).[4] ASD has become the most commonly diagnosed pediatric condition in the United States, with 36,500 new cases per year, adding to a total of 730,000 cases.[4] Families of children with ASD incur an average of $3.2 million in lifetime costs, with an estimated $34.8 billion in societal costs for all families having individuals with ASD.[5] Specifically, average medical expenditures for individuals with an ASD were 4.1 to 6.2 times greater than for those without an ASD. In addition to medical costs, intensive behavioral interventions for children with ASD could cost up to $40,000 to $60,000 per child per year.[6] Taken together, the rising incidence and the growing costs of treating ASD are an urgent call for clinicians to diagnose and treat this disorder early to improve the future outcomes of individuals with ASD.

» Etiology and risk factors

The neuropathology of autism begins during the prenatal or perinatal period of development.[7] Although there is no clear etiology, twin studies point to genetics as one of the risk factors.[8] Twin studies have shown that among identical twins, the occurrence of ASD in one child increases the chance of the other having ASD by 36% to 95%.[8] Among siblings, if one child has ASD, then the other child has a 31% risk of developing ASD.[8] Furthermore, siblings of children with ASD are reported to have a 25% to 50% risk of developing other developmental delays that warrant intervention, for example, social, language, sensory, or motor delays or abnormalities.[9] For this reason, researchers often conduct a prospective follow-up of infant siblings of children with ASD to understand the early development of infants at risk for ASD.[9] Other populations at risk for developing ASD include infants who were born prematurely,[10] were born to older parents,[11] or who were exposed to prescription medications such as valproic acid and thalidomide during gestation.[12]

» Neuropathology of autism spectrum disorder

Brain development in individuals with ASD typically goes through three stages: (1) overgrowth in infancy and early childhood; (2) slowing and arrest of growth in late childhood; and (3) degeneration in preadolescence and adulthood.[13–15] Head circumference of 1- to 2-year-old children who later developed autism was significantly greater than that in typically developing children.[13–15] Head size is near normal at birth, thus indicating that brain overgrowth may occur in the first 2 years of life. Brain overgrowth continues into early childhood and is observed in children with autism with a mean age of 4 years.[16] The brain overgrowth period mainly affects the frontal lobes, temporal lobes, and the amygdala. In particular, there is an overconnectivity in the short-range neuronal fibers and an underconnectivity of the long-range neuronal fibers.[17] The lack of long-range connectivity within the brain leads to the poor integration of sensorimotor, social communication, and cognitive functions. These neuroanatomic findings align with the complex information processing theory of autism in that basic associative learning or simple motor tasks are intact in children with ASD, whereas complex cognitive functions such as executive functioning (EF) or complex motor planning is impaired.[18] In addition, a recent functional magnetic resonance imaging (fMRI) study revealed that children with autism showed persistent frontal lobe activation and reduced cerebellar activation during a finger-tapping task.[19] In contrast, typically developing peers had increased cerebellar activation compared with frontal lobe activation once the motor pattern was learned and became automated.[19] This lack of transition in neural activation from the prefrontal regions to the cerebellum could be attributed to the lack of long-range neuronal connections between the cortical and subcortical regions, and may be the neural basis for incoordination and related motor difficulties observed in children with autism.[18,19] Other researchers have reported deficits in basal ganglia functioning in individuals with Asperger syndrome, as seen by the shorter step length and higher cadence during walking.[20–22] Lastly, children with ASD may have impaired mirror neuron systems found in the frontoparietal cortices of the brain.[23,24] Mirror neuron systems are a group of neurons that activate during action production and action observation, and may play a role in observation-based motor learning.[23] These impairments may explain why children with ASD have poor imitation skills and difficulties learning motor and social skills through observation of others.[24]

» Diagnosis and prognosis

The recent diagnostic criteria for ASD[1] have merged the subcategories of ASD that were often used in the past (Figure 23.1). However, presently, children meeting criteria for ASD only receive a singular diagnosis of ASD. The developmental history of children with ASD will differ depending on the severity of their symptoms. Some children present with language delays any time between the second and third years of life.[25] However, parents often report other perceptuomotor or language delays earlier in life.[26–29] Children with milder forms of ASD, for example, children with Asperger syndrome (i.e., diagnosis offered on the basis of past criteria) usually present with typical to near-typical development until around 5 to 6 years of age. Parents later report their children having difficulties in social interaction in spite of typical language and average to above-average intellectual capacity.

Trained clinicians are able to diagnose ASD using the gold-standard tool called the Autism Diagnostic Observation Schedule (ADOS)[30] and the companion parent

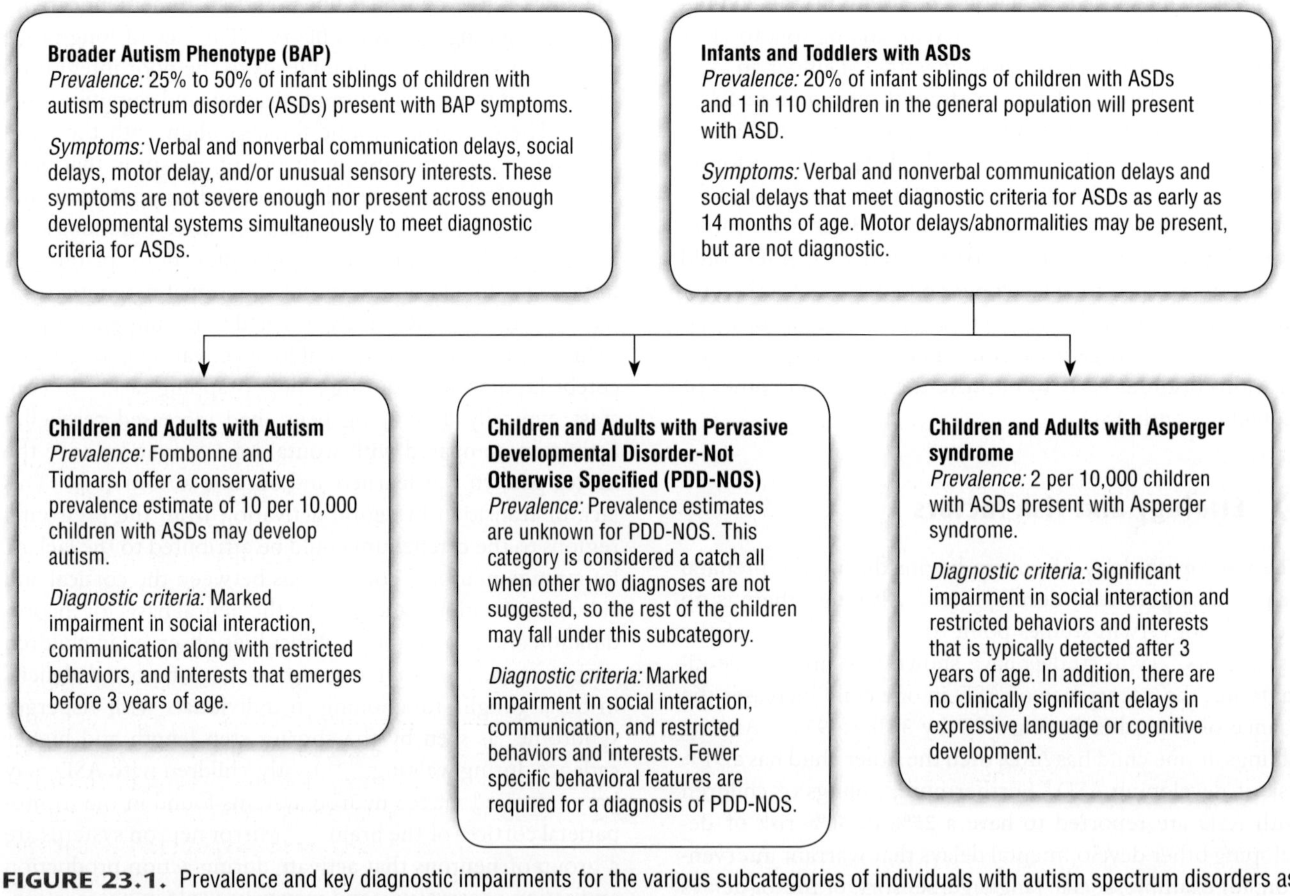

FIGURE 23.1. Prevalence and key diagnostic impairments for the various subcategories of individuals with autism spectrum disorders as well as early symptoms in infants at risk for autism spectrum disorders.

Adapted from Bhat A, Landa R, Galloway J. Perspectives on motor problems in infants, children, and adults with autism spectrum disorders. *Phys Ther.* 2011;91(7):1116-1129 with permission from American Physical Therapy Association. This material is copyrighted, and any further reproduction and distribution requires written permission from APTA.

interview called the Autism Diagnostic Interview–Revised (ADI-R).[31] The ADOS is a 45-minute to 1-hour standardized qualitative assessment that evaluates a child's social reciprocity, nonverbal and verbal communication, and stereotypical behaviors and interests using various play-based activities with an adult tester. The ADOS can be administered to individuals from 12 months of age to adulthood. For each coding item within the three domains of interest (social, communication, and repetitive behaviors), a child is given scores ranging from 0 to 3, with 0 signifying typical or near-typical performance. A diagnostic algorithm is developed on the basis of a subset of coding items. For example, in verbal children, the sum of ten social communication items and four repetitive behavior items provides a total score ranging from 0 to 28. A score of 9 and above is termed *autism* and a score from 7 to 9 is termed autism *spectrum*. Comparison scores ranging from 0 to 10 have been developed to describe the symptom severity of a child with ASD. Comparison scores have prognostic value because they can help evaluate long-term improvements following treatments.

Other differential diagnoses that should be considered in children who present with a range of social, communication, and sensorimotor difficulties include Rett disorder, childhood disintegrative disorder (CDD), and fragile X syndrome. Rett disorder is a neurologic disorder with defined genetic origin involving the gray matter of the brain and leading to decelerated brain growth between 5 months and 4 years of age.[32] It occurs only in females, and leads to loss of hand function and emergence of stereotypical arm movements within the first year of life.[1,32] Poor whole-body coordination and balance, impaired language skills, and poor psychomotor development are also observed. In contrast, CDD presents as ASD with typical development until developmental regression occurs with sudden loss of language skills before 10 years of age.[1] Lastly, fragile X syndrome is a clearly defined genetic disorder found in males with clinical presentation similar to that of ASD, with the exception that the etiology can be confirmed through genetic testing.[1,33] Important physical features associated with fragile X syndrome include large body size, forehead, face, and ears, as well as low muscle tone and increased joint laxity.

» Impairments

In this section, the cognitive, social communication, sensory-perceptual, and motor impairments found in infants and children with ASD are described.

Cognitive Impairments

Attention and Other Social Skills

Children and adults with ASD have attentional impairments such as difficulty disengaging attention and increased focus on objects.[34,35] These impairments may contribute to social functional deficits such as lack of or delayed response to name and/or delays in joint attention (the ability to shift attention to the attentional focus of a social partner).[36] Theories of social impairment suggest that children with autism may prefer nonsocial cues over social cues and may avoid eye contact and looking at faces owing to the complexity of social stimuli.[37,38] These basic attentional preferences may give rise to complex social deficits such as difficulties in understanding others' mental states (emotions, intentions, and desires) and lack of empathy.[39] During development, children with ASD show delays in responding to attentional bids of others. Spontaneous sharing of attention with others continues to be deficient until late childhood.[39]

Language

Language is clearly affected in children with autism, with some children never acquiring functional speech.[40–42] Language impairments include impaired pragmatic language such as poor use of nonverbal cues such as gaze, facial expressions, turn-taking, and body language during communication with others, poor prosody (i.e., rhythm, stress, and intonation during speech), poor phonology (i.e., word articulation), and atypical linguistic forms such as echolalia (i.e., immediate or delayed imitation of words).[41,42]

Executive Functioning

EF is defined as the ability to maintain a problem-solving set related to a goal that requires skills such as planning, impulse control, response inhibition, organized search, and flexibility in thought process.[43] In terms of perceptual inflexibility, children with ASD may show resistance to distraction and an inability to shift attention between activities or stimuli.[34] In terms of motor inflexibility, children with ASD may show repetitive behaviors or have difficulty inhibiting movements.[1] In terms of inflexibility in social communication, children with ASD will show a lack of reciprocity leading to one-sided conversations and lack of turn-taking during nonverbal and verbal communication.[1]

Sensory-Perceptual Impairments

Sensory-perceptual processing impairments can be categorized into sensory modulation disorders and enhanced/atypical sensory perception.

Sensory Modulation Disorders

Sensory modulation disorders are difficulties in regulating and organizing the nature and intensity of responses to specific sensory inputs, including tactile, olfactory, visual, auditory, proprioceptive, and vestibular inputs.[44] Children with ASD can be "underresponsive" such that they are slow to respond or may fail to respond to name or react to pain.[44] "Overresponsive" children may have exaggerated or prolonged responses to sensory inputs such as covering of ears to loud sounds or background noise.[44] Sensation-seeking children may crave for sensory input for extended periods by performing stereotypical movements of body rocking or arm flapping, and so on.[44] Various parent questionnaires have been used to report sensory modulation issues, for example, the Short Sensory Profile or the Infant and Toddler Sensory Profile.[45] The severity of sensory modulation impairments appears to directly correlate with overall symptom severity and level of functioning of children with autism.[46] Recently, mixed patterns of sensory processing have also been reported in children with ASD between 3 and 10 years of age: (1) "inattention/excessive attention"; (2) "atypical tactile/smell sensitivity"; and (3) "atypical movement sensitivity/low energy and weak motor responses."[47] These subgroups include underresponsive and overresponsive children with ASD within specific sensory domains. The third subgroup included children with ASD who had clear motor impairments. For example, children with "atypical movement sensitivity" are usually overresponsive to proprioceptive and vestibular input, whereas children with "low energy/weak motor responses" may present with fine and gross motor difficulties.[47] Therefore, children who perform poorly on the "movement sensitivity/low energy" sections of the Sensory Profile questionnaire may be at a greater risk for motor delays and long-term motor impairments.

Enhanced/Atypical Visual and Auditory Perception

Children with ASD show enhanced local processing compared with global processing of perceptual information.[48] They are unable to understand the interelement relationships between the parts of a complex presentation of stimuli, and are hence unable to understand the overall context and meaning of a complex picture or a piece of music. The enhanced local processing may contribute to their heightened perception of visual and auditory information. For example, during visual search tasks involving several similar-looking objects, typically developing children use a serial search strategy to find the odd object, whereas children with ASD will encounter a pop-out phenomenon where they perceive each individual object in parallel and immediately identify the outlier.[49] Similarly, children with ASD have heightened pitch perception, greater pitch discrimination, and better memory of musical pitch; however, they may lack emotion perception within the musical content.[50,51] Interestingly, evidence indicates that these perceptual skills can be developed with age and may be intact in adults with ASD. It is not surprising that music education and music therapy are often used as training tools to facilitate social communication skills in children with ASD owing to their advanced musical abilities.[52,53]

Motor Impairments

Although social communication impairments are considered hallmarks of ASD, there is substantial evidence to consider motor impairments as a core deficit of ASD owing to its widespread prevalence and its correlation with other social communication impairments.[3,54,55] For example, the large effect sizes calculated in a recent meta-analysis on motor impairments in individuals with ASD suggested that this group has significantly greater motor impairments compared with healthy controls.[55] Moreover, recent reviews indicate clear impairments in arm motor functions, bilateral coordination, gait and balance, as well as praxis/motor planning in young and older children with ASD.[3,54,55] A comprehensive listing of motor impairments is provided in Table 23.1.

Motor Stereotypies

Children and adolescents with autism may show several different motor stereotypies, including repetitive behaviors such as whole-body rocking, twirling, jumping, bouncing, and arm flapping. Object-related behaviors such as poking, rubbing, or spinning objects are also commonly demonstrated by children with ASD.[56] Children with ASD may show covering of eyes or ears because they are "overresponsive" to certain visual and auditory inputs from a very young age.[56,57] Individuals with ASD may also show resistance to change and compulsive behaviors such as inflexible routines during their daily activities.[31,56] Motor stereotypies often correlate with level of functioning and autism severity, with a greater presence of stereotypies in the more affected children.[31,58] Repetitive behaviors are often clearly present by 2 years of age because of the difficulty of distinguishing them from typical motor stereotypies of infants within the first year of life.[55,57] Specifically, toddlers who later developed autism showed more atypical hand and finger movements and more stereotypical object play, such as excessive banging or preoccupation with spinning objects or with part of an object, compared with toddlers with milder forms of ASD such as pervasive developmental disorder-not otherwise specified (PDD-NOS).[59] Interestingly, reduced spontaneous movement exploration or limited change in body postures is often present in infants at risk for ASD.[60] Repetitive behaviors may also be considered as a child's means of obtaining different forms of visual or kinesthetic stimulation and may be a function of the sensory modulation impairments found in children with ASD.[44]

Motor Coordination and Arm Function

School-age children and adolescents with ASD often show impairments in running speed and agility, bilateral coordination, manual dexterity, and ball skills, as based on various standardized motor measures.[61-64] A recent population database review conducted by the first author found that 87%

TABLE 23.1.	Motor Impairments in Children and Adults with Autism Spectrum Disorder	
Motor Impairments/Motor Delays	Impairments in School-Aged Children and Adults with Autism Spectrum Disorders (ASDs)	Delays in Infants at Risk for ASD, and Toddlers and Preschoolers with ASDs
Gross motor coordination	Poor upper and lower limb coordination, including bilateral coordination and visuomotor coordination	Gross motor delays in supine, prone, and sitting skills in the first year of life. Delayed onset of walking in the second year of life. Gross motor delays are present in preschoolers recently diagnosed with ASD.
Fine motor coordination	Poor fine motor coordination such as performance on manual dexterity tasks, for example, Purdue pegboard task	Reaching and grasping delayed in infants at risk for ASDs. Fine motor delays persist in the second and third years of life.
Motor stereotypies	Motor stereotypies are common in older children and adults with ASDs.	Motor stereotypies such as repetitive banging of objects or unusual sensory exploration may appear in the first year of life, but most often emerge in the second year of life.
Postural	Feed-forward and feedback control of posture is affected in children and adults with ASDs. Overall, deficient postural control persists in adults with ASDs.	Postural delays in rolling, sitting, and so on. Unusual postures may be held for brief to long periods in infants who later developed ASDs.
Imitation and praxis	Imitation impairments are present during postural, gestural, and oral imitation. Performance of complex movement sequences is poor during imitation, on verbal command, and during tool use, suggesting generalized dyspraxia not specific to imitation.	

of children with ASD between 5 and 15 years of age are at risk for a motor impairment; however, only 15% of the children received a dual diagnosis of developmental coordination disorder (DCD), highlighting that a substantial number of children with ASD are in need of motor evaluations and interventions.[61] Past studies have reported greater motor deficits in children with low intelligence quotient (IQ) compared with children with average and above-average IQ.[63] However, recent studies in our laboratory and others recognize that motor impairments are observed across the spectrum, including in children with ASD with low and high IQ.[2,64] Coordination impairments are also observed during functional activities such as walking, reaching, writing, and gestural communication.[20,22,65–67] Poor use of hand and body gestures such as pointing, showing, and reaching out to caregivers is, in fact, one of the core social impairments in autism.[1] Furthermore, lack of associated gestures during story telling leading to asynchrony between hand gestures and language production is coded for within the ADOS administration, the diagnostic tool for ASD.[30]

Motor Delay

Motor incoordination in children with ASD may emerge as early as infancy. Retrospective and prospective studies tracking the motor development of high-risk infants who later developed ASD or language delays have reported gross motor and fine motor delays as early as 6 months of age.[26,27,68–70] For example, infants who later develop ASD may show delays in gross motor milestones such as head holding, rolling, sitting, crawling, and walking.[26–28] Infants who later developed ASD were also reported to have early motor delays in reaching, banging, clapping, block stacking, scribbling, pointing, and turning door knobs.[70] In addition, these early manual–motor skills of children with autism correlated with their later speech fluency at school age.[70] Fine motor delays have been more thoroughly studied than were gross motor delays owing to their relationships with nonverbal communication. There is recent evidence that preschoolers diagnosed with ASD have comparable impairments in fine and gross motor performance.[70] Therefore, it is extremely important to examine early motor performance of infants and toddlers at risk for autism, including infant siblings of children with autism or preterm infants.

Gait and Balance

Walking patterns of children with ASD have been described as "ataxic" owing to the inconsistency between strides or "parkinsonian" shuffling nature of steps and lack of alternating arm swing.[20,22] Toe-walking is often reported by clinicians, although it is not well studied by researchers. On the basis of standardized testing, static and dynamic balance is found to be affected in children with ASD.[61,71] Moreover, deficits in feedback (responding to postural perturbations) and feed-forward (anticipatory postural adjustments) mechanisms have been reported in individuals with ASD, which

may account for the poor balance observed during clinical examination.[72] Furthermore, infants who later develop ASD show delays in acquiring advanced postures such as standing and sitting compared with typically developing infants.[28,60] Delayed onset of walking was one of the first gross motor delays observed in toddlers who developed language delays later in life.[25] It has been reported that some at-risk infants who showed delayed onset of autism symptoms did not present with motor delays within the first year.[73] The delayed onset of autism symptoms may present as a developmental regression in the second and third years of life.[73] Therefore, it would be important to monitor motor development and social communication development over the first 3 years of life in infants at risk for ASD.

Motor Planning, Praxis, and Imitation

Praxis refers to one's ability to plan, coordinate, and execute complex movement sequences.[74] Children with ASD often present with dyspraxia (difficulty with planning, coordinating, and executing movement sequences) during oromotor, fine motor, and gross motor activities.[75] These deficits typically represent more complex processing and are not simply related to basic motor abnormalities such as abnormal tone or muscle weakness. Individuals with ASD usually acquire the ability to perform simple motor tasks, for example, fundamental motor milestones, walking, and reaching skills, although delays may be experienced. However, complex motor tasks such as complex sports, handwriting, daily living skills such as dressing and tying shoe laces, or other movement sequences associated with broader goals persist for school-age children with ASD. Praxis is often measured during gesture production, in response to verbal command, on imitation, or during tool use.[76] Children with ASD showed similar errors within each of these conditions, indicating a generalized praxis impairment that is not limited to movement imitation.[76] Studies of imitation of oromotor, fine motor, and gross motor actions in this population have verified that children with ASD have difficulties with various forms of imitation from early on in life.[75,77–79] Poor imitation skills put children with ASD at a clear disadvantage when learning daily living skills from their peers and caregivers.

Strength and Tone

The only study evaluating muscle strength in children with ASD reported that hand muscle strength was poor in children with ASD compared with typically developing children.[80] The presence of abnormal reflexes has been reported in infants who later developed ASD.[81] Tonal abnormality resulting in toe-walking has also been observed in children with ASD.[81] Hypotonia is also often reported in retrospective studies of infants who later developed ASD and is often observed in school-age children with ASD.[81,82] In fact, clinicians often report postural muscle hypotonia in children with ASD.

Endurance and Physical Activity Levels

Children and adults with ASD are at a high risk of developing obesity in view of their low physical activity levels, poor dietary intake, and significant barriers to accessing opportunities for physical activity.[83,84] Two different retrospective analyses of survey databases conducted in the United States reported that 23.4% of older children and adolescents with ASD were obese (body mass index [BMI] greater than 95th percentile), 19% were overweight (BMI >85th percentile), and 35.7% were at risk for overweight.[85] It is reported that obesity is either equally likely or three times more likely in children with ASD than in the general population.[85] Although there is little known about factors leading to obesity in children with ASD, it is suggested that less time spent in physical activity programs and more time spent in sedentary activities such as working at a computer may be contributing factors.[84,86-88] This pattern could be directly related to the social impairments and motor impairments and to their preference to engage in solitary, technology-based activities such as watching television or playing video games. Unusual dietary patterns in children with ASD may occur owing to restricted food habits, which is also a function of the ASD diagnosis.[84,85] Long-term use of anti-seizure medications such as valproate has been implicated in cases of obesity in children with developmental disorders.[84] Taken together, there is a clear need to enhance motor participation, physical activity levels, and cardiorespiratory endurance in children and adults with ASD to improve their quality of life.

» Examination

The components of an examination for a child with autism will vary on the basis of the child's age, level of functioning, and range of impairments. In this section, we offer ideas for appropriate history taking as well as nonstandardized and standardized assessments.

History Taking

After obtaining basic identifying information, including date of birth, age, gender, height, weight, and handedness, one should collect birth history, including prenatal, perinatal, and postnatal history, family history, developmental history, medical history, treatment history, as well as the child's current level of functioning and expectation of the caregiver and/or child. Prenatal, perinatal, and postnatal history may provide some insight into the etiologies of the diagnosis (see section "Etiology and Risk Factors"). When obtaining family history, ask for presence of ASD diagnosis in other family members such as siblings or relatives. When obtaining developmental history, ask about the child's overall development, for example, whether motor and communication milestones were achieved at appropriate ages. Specifically, onset ages for motor milestones such as reaching, sitting, crawling, standing, and walking are important

in identifying the degree and length of motor delay. In addition, onset ages for communication milestones such as production of vowel sounds, consonant sounds, variegated babbling, first words, two- to three-word phrases, and complex language are important. As part of the medical history, ask when the diagnosis was obtained, any medications the child may be taking, presence of motor stereotypies, and any dietary modifications. Children with ASD may have food allergies for which gluten-free and casein-free diets may have been recommended. This is especially important to know if use of edible treats is considered for rewards. In terms of treatment history, it is important to know about the other services the child has received or is receiving (e.g., behavioral therapies, social skills training, speech or occupational or music therapy), including their intensity, frequency, and duration, because this will directly affect the family's ability to engage in physical therapy. It is important to identify the child's current level of functioning in performing activities of daily living, including the level of caregiver support throughout the day. It is important to ask about the child's present communication, cognitive, and sensorimotor abilities and difficulties. Last but not the least, ask the caregiver's expectations for their child and the child's expectations for himself or herself, when the child has adequate communication.

Observations of Naturalistic Play

Children often need time to warm up to strangers, and allowing a 10- to 15-minute period where the child explores the toys within the examination space would be a nice icebreaker for the child. During this period, the examiner could complete history taking and move onto observing the child's play for nonverbal and verbal communication, repetitive behaviors, and motor performance. In terms of nonverbal communication skills, observe the child's use of gestures, reciprocal interactions and turn-taking, the use of spontaneous versus responsive communication with the caregiver or tester, as well as rapport between the child and the caregiver. Gestures could be "instrumental" such as showing, pointing, and giving, or "descriptive" such as actions describing verbs or adjectives within a sentence. In terms of verbal communication skills, collect a language sample to understand the level of verbal communication: specifically, the number of words used within phrases and the appropriateness of the language based on the child's developmental level. Review of the speech evaluation can provide more specific insight into the child's level of language.

The complexity and variability of the child's play should be considered. Is the child using objects for their intended purpose and demonstrating any imitation within the play schemes? Alternately, does the child only focus on the mechanical characteristics of play objects? For example, a typically developing child playing with trains may build tracks and pretend to bring cargo to the station, whereas a child with ASD may become preoccupied with the spinning of the train wheels. The evaluator should also consider whether the child demonstrates curiosity and variability within play activities offered by the environment.

In terms of motor skills, observe the child's ability to perform those motor tasks expected of his or her age with attention to movement control and sophistication of movement patterns. Observe the child's fine motor skills such as reaching, transfers, use of two hands for symmetrical and asymmetrical activities, as well as gross motor skills such as basic walking patterns, balancing on one leg (static balance), and balancing while walking on narrow surfaces (dynamic balance). Complex motor skills such as clapping, marching, jumping, skipping, galloping, hopping, and so on (dual and multilimb coordination) provide insight into the child's bilateral coordination abilities. For children with ASD needing more support, it might be best to observe them during functional tasks such as climbing stairs and kicking a ball to infer balance and coordination skills. Simple instructions such as "can you do this" within an imitation game could offer appropriate visual cues to complete the task. Note: if some of the activities are part of a standardized assessment, then they do not have to be repeated here.

Cognitive Examination

Intellectual abilities of children with ASD are evaluated using various cognitive assessments, typically administered by clinical psychologists or educators. For example, the Stanford–Binet Intelligence Test (SBIT) can be administered to individuals between 2 and 85 years of age to examine nonverbal and verbal IQ. The Kaufman Brief Intelligence Test (KBIT) is often administered in individuals between 4 and 90 years of age and within school settings because various professionals can administer it. The Wechsler Intelligence Scale for Children (WISC) offers similar information for children between 6 and 16 years of age. Although the KBIT is used widely across professions and is a quick IQ measure, it is considered unreliable when measuring IQ in nonverbal children. To understand a child's verbal and nonverbal abilities, it would be valuable to obtain reports on IQ measures, when available. However, in the absence of these measures, instructing the child to follow simple one-step or two-step commands to bring something to you or the child's conversational abilities can offer you information on the child's current abilities. Secondly, observe for inattention and hyperactivity during the child's play because it will dictate the amount of time the child can actively engage with you during examination and treatment sessions.

Sensory-Perceptual Examination

First, rule out hearing and vision impairments by asking the caregiver during history taking and then by reviewing medical and speech and language evaluation reports. The child's records may include hearing tests such as the brain stem auditory-evoked response (BAER) audiometry or pure tone testing conducted by audiologists. Secondly, obtain caregiver reports on whether the child has sensory modulation

issues such as hypo- or hyperresponsiveness to various sensory stimuli. Some children may be using noise-canceling earphones to reduce the noise levels in their environment. Parent questionnaires such as the Infant and Toddler Sensory Profile or the Short Sensory Profile can be used.[45] A detailed Sensory Integration and Praxis Test (SIPT)[89] is typically administered by the occupational therapist (OT) on the team, and reviewing that report would offer ideas for supporting the child's sensory responses during therapy sessions.

Motor Examination

Motor performance can be examined by obtaining parent responses through motor questionnaires, by administering standardized and/or developmentally appropriate measures of motor performance, and through observation of the child's current levels of motor functioning during functional activities of daily living as well as standardized functional assessments. Table 23.2 provides a full listing of questionnaires and assessment for children with ASD.

Motor Questionnaires/Parent Interviews

Motor-related instruments include the Movement Assessment Battery for Children (MABC)–questionnaire version or the Developmental Coordination Disorders Questionnaire (DCDQ).[61,90] A typical administration lasts about 15 to 30 minutes. These questionnaires provide therapists with the parent's and/or teacher's impressions of what the child can do in terms of fine motor and gross motor skills, as well as static and dynamic activities occurring in home and school environments. Other factors that might affect a child's motor performance, such as attention, anxiety, and so on, are also considered within these instruments. The DCDQ allows one to compare a child's motor performance with that of children with DCDs to determine the severity of the motor impairment. The Children's Assessment of Participation and Enjoyment (CAPE)[91] is a useful measure to examine how children between 5 and 21 years of age participate in everyday activities outside of the mandated school activities. The measure targets whether the child has opportunities and interest to engage in any of the 55 different activities, including information on (1) whom they typically do the activity with (e.g., parent, friend), (2) where they do the activity (e.g., home, at a friend's house), and (3) how much they enjoy doing the activity. Each activity is presented to the child/youth on a card with a drawing of the activity and a phrase (in words) describing the activity. Overall, motor questionnaires are a caregiver's reflection about the child's motor abilities and interest and could be a useful measure to determine activity themes that would be relevant and motivating to the child.

Standardized Assessment

There are multiple measures of overall motor performance such as the Peabody Developmental Motor Scales, MABC, or the Bruininks–Oseretsky Test of Motor Performance (BOTMP), which include subtests to quantify the child's

TABLE 23.2.	Reliability and Validity Data on Motor Assessments for Autism Spectrum Disorders

Motor Assessments	
For Young and Older Children	**For Infants and Toddlers**
Movement Assessment Battery for Children (MABC) Concurrent validity with Bruininks Test: 0.76 Interrater reliability: 0.96 Test–retest reliability: 0.77	Gross and fine motor subtests of Mullen Scales of Early Learning (MSEL) Validity: 0.5 or higher Reliability: 0.65 or higher
Bruininks–Oseretsky Test of Motor Proficiency (BOTMP) Concurrent validity with MABC: 0.88 Reliability: 0.90	Alberta Infant Motor Scale (AIMS) Concurrent validity with PDMS-2: >0.9 Interrater reliability: 0.99 Test–retest reliability: 0.99
Peabody Motor Developmental Scales (PDMS)-2 Concurrent validity with Bayley Scales of Infant Development (BSID): high to very high Test–retest reliability: 0.73–0.89 across subtests	
	Autism Observation Schedule for Infants (AOSI) has a motor control component that predicts ASDs at 3 years of age Interrater reliability: 0.7–0.9 Test–retest reliability: 0.7
Praxis and Imitation Batteries Modified Florida Apraxia Battery Interrater reliability: 0.85–0.95 Sensory Integration and Praxis Testing Concurrent validity: 0.46–0.71 for some subtests Interrater reliability: moderate to high	

Adapted from Bhat A, Landa R, Galloway J. Perspectives on motor problems in infants, children, and adults with autism spectrum disorders. *Phys Ther.* 2011;91(7):1116–1129 with permission from American Physical Therapy Association. This material is copyrighted, and any further reproduction and distribution requires written permission from APTA.

performance within various motor domains, including fine and gross motor coordination, balance, strength, and so on.[55] The typical administration time is about 1 to 1.5 hours to complete the full assessment. For example, the BOTMP-2 has eight subtests: running speed and agility, balance, bilateral coordination, strength, upper limb coordination, response speed, visual-motor control, and upper limb speed and dexterity.[92] It provides raw, standard, and percentile scores for the subtests as well as the overall assessment. A short-form version of the full assessment is also provided to conduct an initial examination of motor performance in about a half hour.

Motor impairments are observed in children with ASD with various levels of cognitive functioning; hence, one clear limitation of all motor assessments is that we are unable to discern whether poor motor performance is reflective of primary motor impairment or an artifact of poor comprehension. This is especially true for children with ASD who not only have known verbal comprehension limitations but also present with difficulties in imitating actions. There is a clear need to further develop observational motor measures during functional tasks for children who are nonverbal and low functioning.

Developmental Screening

Children younger than 3 years of age who are screened for ASD receive screening for developmental delays and autism-specific signs. Screening tools take about 15 minutes to complete and may include general parent questionnaires such as the Ages and Stages Questionnaire (ASQ)[93] or the autism-specific parent questionnaires such as the Modified Checklist for Autism in Toddlers (MCHAT).[94] Recently, researchers have developed a multisystem observational tool called the Autism Observation Schedule for Infants (AOSI) in young infants at risk for ASD, and it is inclusive of a motor component.[95]

Developmental Assessments

Multidomain developmental assessments such as the Bayley Scales of Infant Development (BSID)[96] or Mullen Scales of Early Learning (MSEL)[97] could be used to obtain the child's overall cognitive and motor performance. A single domain may take about 15 to 20 minutes to complete, and a full assessment could be well over 1 hour. The BSID can be used for children from birth to 3 years of age, and the MSEL is normed from birth to 5 years of age. Both have subdomains for gross motor, fine motor, visual reception, receptive, and expressive language. Raw scores, scaled scores, composite scores, and percentile scores can be calculated for each subtest as well as overall development. Single-domain assessments such as the Alberta Infant Motor Scale may also be used to identify gross motor delays using raw subscale scores or overall percentile scores. The Vineland Adaptive Behavior Scale (VABS)[98] is a caregiver interview and observational measure or a parent/caregiver questionnaire to help evaluate individuals across the gamut of functional skills from preschool to 18 years of age. This scale measures adaptive behaviors, including the ability to cope with environmental changes, to learn new everyday skills, and to demonstrate independence. The test measures five domains: communication, daily living skills, socialization, motor skills, and maladaptive behavior. The communication domain evaluates the receptive, expressive, and written communication skills of the child. The daily living skills domain measures personal behavior and the domestic and community interaction skills. The socialization domain covers play and leisure time, interpersonal relationships, and various coping skills. The motor skills domain measures both gross and fine motor skills.

Praxis and Imitation Examination

Imitation and praxis can be measured using the Modified Florida Apraxia Battery[99] or subtests of the SIPT.[89] Both these tests typically measure praxis at three levels: during imitation, following verbal command, or during tool use. Gestures or actions range from fine motor to gross motor, simple to complex, and meaningful to meaningless. The child's motor responses are scored for spatial, temporal, and reversal errors. Furthermore, SIPT is a standardized and normed measure for examining various sensorimotor skills, including motor coordination, sensory integration (SI), and praxis in children between 4 and 9 years of age. Specifically, subtests of postural praxis, praxis on verbal command, sequencing praxis, bilateral motor coordination, and kinesthesia might be relevant. Note that among the standardized measures for imitation, SIPT is the only one that is normed.

Strength and Tone Examination

Abnormal tone is often reported in infants who later developed ASD and in children with ASD. For example, hypotonia has been reported in young infants who later developed autism and is often found in children with autism. It most often affects posture and balance of the child with autism and is measured during observation of the child's posture and movement. For example, observe for slouched or swayback postures, hyperextended knees or elbows, toe-walking, and so on. Strength is not often measured in children with autism. Only one study has reported muscle weakness in hand muscles of children with autism;[80] hence, it is important to consider measuring pinch and grip strength using hand and finger dynamometry, especially when the child has significant fine motor difficulties such as poor handwriting.

Physical Activity Level Measurement

These could be measured subjectively using activity diaries or self-report surveys, or objectively using pedometers, accelerometers, and so on. Parents will need to record the information for children or for those children who are not capable; and self-report may be reliable for adolescents. Although subjective measures are prone to errors owing to recall bias, the objective measures are expensive and could be bothersome to children with ASD who have associated sensory issues.

Functional Performance Examination

Functional performance can be measured using the Pediatric Evaluations of Disability Inventory (PEDI)[100] or the School Functional Assessment (SFA).[101] The PEDI is a standardized measure to identify functional capabilities and performance in the areas of self-care, mobility, and social function. It is designed for young children between 6 months and 7 years or older children who present with functional abilities lower than those of a typically developing 7-year-old. Scores are assigned on the basis of observation or parent/caregiver report. The PEDI allows calculation of both standard and scored performance scores. Results of the PEDI can be used to monitor a child's performance over time and develop intervention plans. The SFA[101] is a criterion-referenced instrument used to quantify and monitor a child's performance of nonacademic activities within the elementary school setting—kindergarten through sixth grade. The educational team members familiar with the child complete the scoring in three areas: participation, task supports, and activity performance. This instrument yields criterion cutoff scores that help establish eligibility for special education services and monitor a child's performance while promoting team collaboration.

Evaluation Synthesis

a. Convey evaluation instructions in a manner the child can comprehend. Use picture schedules, simplify verbal commands, hand-on-hand instruction, visual models, breaks, and rewards to ensure that the child complies, understands your instructions, and demonstrates what is asked of him or her (see Table 23.3 for specific strategies).

b. Identify cognitive impairments that govern the motor activities planned. For example, level of focus (i.e., overfocused attention or inattention), presence of hyperactivity, and intellectual level (i.e., nonverbal, verbal but delayed, verbal/hyperverbal, and age-appropriate).

c. Identify sensory modulation impairments that will affect the child's engagement in the intervention plan.

d. Identify the child's key motor impairments: coordination, balance, praxis, and so on, and plan for treatment activities that are addressing the needs of the whole child (i.e., social-motor or cognitive-motor needs). Prioritize goals depending on the child's and the family's highest need. Most likely, the family has been asked to participate in multiple therapies and has little time to focus on a range of motor activities.

TABLE 23.3.	Strategies for Structuring Physical Therapy Treatment Sessions for Children with Autism

Principles	Specific Strategies
1. Structuring the environment	1. Use just the right amount of space for the motor activities to be performed 2. Use the same space to ensure predictability 3. Limit the materials to the ones required for the session 4. Remove or cover the other distractors in the room 5. Put up rules sheet, listing of activities, or picture schedules to describe the expectations from the child and the structure of the sessions, whenever appropriate 6. Follow a predictable routine. You could vary the routine of the child if that is a treatment goal. Begin with small (versus large) changes to the routine. When these changes are made, be sensitive to its effects on the child. 7. Promote transitions with the use of picture schedules or predictable verbal or gestural commands, for example, "a good job and a hi-five at the end of each trial." Within a session, if the activities break up into warm-up, whole-body, and walking themes, then use pictures to define those activities, and have the child either move the picture schedule off the board or have him or her check off the activity from an available list. This helps the child keep track of the session
2. Instructions for the activity	Use the various means of communication available to the child. For example, for a verbal child, verbal instructions are appropriate. However, for a nonverbal child, sign language/gestural communication, visual picture schedules, and short verbal commands may be needed
3. Prompting/modeling/ feedback	1. Models could be the PT, peers, paraprofessionals, or caregivers who join the child. Your child may benefit from parallel and/or mirrored motions, so you will need to determine what works best for your child and for the actions being practiced 2. When possible, use group activities because they are valuable for learning social monitoring. This may also reduce the child's anxiety because he or she is not put on the spot. On the other hand, distracting peers may increase the anxiety in some children. It is important to judge what will meet the individual needs of the child. Both group and individual activities provide different important experiences for the child 3. Make sure that the child is attending to you before you begin your instructions. He or she may use foveal/peripheral vision to attend to you 4. First say, "Child's name, do this?" then show the action. If he or she did not move correctly, then hand-on-hand feedback could be provided. Determine whether this helps the child's performance by asking them to repeat the action on their own. Some children may not like "hand-on-hand" feedback or may not improve performance with such feedback 5. Use external props to clarify the goals of the activity
4. Repetition	1. Practice is important for motor learning and should be encouraged within a session but also across sessions 2. Caregivers should practice the same activities between the two physical therapy sessions 3. Generalization to a different space and a different caregiver will be facilitated through such practice
5. Active engagement	1. It is important to allow for free movement and improvisational activities 2. Waiting is critical for the child to explore spontaneously and actively problem-solve. After the initial instructions are provided, allow the child to move freely (without excessive prompting) 3. Prompting could be used in the second trial of the same activity. For low-functioning children, more prompting will be required 4. Allow the child to choose a theme or a set of activities for the session. Encourage them to move differently than you. Promote movement creativity and spontaneity
6. Progression	1. In terms of progression, it is important to create the just-right challenge for the child. It is important to allow for success. You could choose to increase the complexity of activities across sessions or within a session for a given activity. Note that trial-and-error learning is important, so the child does not have to achieve 100% success. If the child is not discouraged by his or her motor performance, then adding complexity to the activity is okay. However, if the child is easily frustrated by failure, then it is important to create a safe environment for the child that allows for success and avoids excessive feedback and prompting 2. Look out for negative behaviors such as tantrums, noncompliance, and self-injurious behaviors. If these are observed, then ask the child to communicate in appropriate ways—verbalizing or signing that the activity be stopped. This will imply that the task is difficult for the child and should be simplified
7. Reinforcement/rewards	1. Various rewards could be provided 2. Verbal and gestural reinforcement in the form of "good jobs" and "hi-fives" 3. Breaks from activity to do favorite sensory activities—spinning, containment, or deep pressure or free play 4. Stickers or small toys. Provide if the aforementioned ideas do not seem to work 5. Edibles. Provide if the aforementioned ideas do not seem to work. This may be more appropriate for children with ASD needing more support. It is important to use healthy snacks; otherwise, it will affect the overall health and wellness of the child

ASD, autism spectrum disorder; PT, physical therapist.

» Intervention

The multiple motor impairments listed in the earlier sections may significantly contribute to the functional limitations of children with ASD. The early motor delays, the continued motor deficits later on in life, and their long-term ramifications deserve the attention of motor specialists such as PTs who can contribute to the overall treatment programs of children with ASD. It is difficult to separate the dynamic interplay of movements, sensory processing, and social communication as a child continuously interacts with his or her environment and caregivers. Bhat et al. have suggested that motor impairments will lead to reduced movement exploration, difficulties in keeping up with peers during playtime, and missed opportunities during social interactions.[55] Together, these problems will limit the initiation and maintenance of social relationships and will ultimately contribute to delayed social skills and long-term social impairments.[55]

Despite the implicit and explicit relation of motor abilities and overall development, the majority of autism interventions are focused on enhancing the social communication and academic skills of children with ASD. Over the years, various interventions have evolved to address the sensory and motor needs of children with ASD. Although these interventions are frequently practiced, more empirical research is needed to support the use of these interventions to enhance sensorimotor performance, social engagement, and long-term quality of life.[55,102] The majority of the sensorimotor intervention studies involve small sample sizes or single cases or case series. Moreover, research in this population is also challenged by the variability among the children with ASD and the complexity of the multiple factors that affect treatment outcomes.

Team Approach to Autism Spectrum Disorder Treatment

Children with ASD present with multiple, complex developmental variations that are best addressed through a team approach. Given the variability of presentation within the autism spectrum, individualized programs with different types of therapies are imperative to meet the unique needs of each child with ASD. Family members provide essential information about the child's behavior, current level of functioning, and areas of interest that can be utilized in program development. The family, along with the trained professionals, identifies skills and behaviors to be developed. Special educators and psychologists help understand and address the cognitive and behavioral challenges demonstrated by children with ASD. Speech and language pathologists will help the child with ASD to communicate with family, educators, and caregivers through verbal or alternative means and to gain nonverbal and verbal communication skills. OTs and PTs can provide insight and programming to address sensory-perceptual processing and enhance motor performance. Other medical personnel can provide information about the child's health that is critical to program planning. Coordinated efforts of these trained professionals, along with the family and other caregivers, can provide structured and consistent interactions for the child with ASD that will promote positive and meaningful social engagement as well as learning of important skills.

Sensorimotor Treatment Approaches for Children with Autism Spectrum Disorder

The standard-of-care treatment approaches for children with autism include the Applied Behavioral Analysis (ABA),[102,103] the Treatment and Education of Autistic and related Communication-handicapped Children (TEACCH),[104,105] the Picture Exchange Communication System (PECS),[106] and the SI therapy,[107] as well as some others that lack substantial research evidence to support their use.

Applied Behavioral Analysis

ABA is the current intervention standard for children with ASD, and is accepted as an effective means for reducing negative behaviors while improving appropriate communication and prosocial behaviors, and teaching new skills to children with ASD.[102,103] The broader goals of ABA programs are to reinforce desirable behaviors and reduce those that are undesirable. This is accomplished by breaking down a complex task into a series of simple steps and providing positive reinforcement in a predictable manner in response to the child successfully meeting the criteria established for each step. Traditional ABA practices of discrete trial training are performed in a 1:1, controlled setting using a blocked practice format using adult-developed materials and tasks with several repetitions.[108,109] These traditional approaches have received significant criticism because they do not promote naturalistic interactions involving child-preferred and child-centered activities. More contemporary ABA models such as incidental teaching approaches promote spontaneity during motivating contexts that involve natural rewards within naturalistic environments.[110,111] These approaches promote child-preferred and child-selected activities to increase repetition and to sustain engagement. Principles of ABA are typically applied to academic, social, communication, and vocational skills. PTs could incorporate the principles of task analysis, repetition, and positive reinforcement using contemporary approaches to promote acquisition of specific motor skills, activities of daily living, or specific vocational skill sets. Communication among all team members is important to establish acceptable criteria, use of reinforcements, and reinforcement scheduling.

In this section, ABA strategies are compared to motor learning principles that are often used within physical therapy interventions. Specifically, principles of task analysis, repetition/practice, feedback, reinforcement, and generalization are similar across the two treatment approaches; however, the value for trial-and-error learning and self-produced behaviors may differ. First, task analysis is a critical component of both ABA and motor learning.[102,112] Both approaches promote breaking down complex activities into simpler parts and practicing each part as well as the whole. Children with ASD are capable of learning simple cause-and-effect relationships[38] and simple motor skills in an implicit manner using a "learning-by-doing" approach.[113,114] For example, if a child is practicing jumping jacks, you can break up the activity into multiple steps and practice it in parts. The repetition with active engagement inherent in the contemporary ABA programs is equivalent to the high levels of self-produced practice promoted by the current motor learning theories. Repetition is critical for mastering skilled behaviors. Both approaches also promote the use of positive reinforcement upon successful task completion. Although motor learning theories limit reinforcement to verbal and gestural reinforcers, traditional ABA programs also promote the use of materialistic reinforcers such as toys and edibles. However, contemporary ABA approaches promote the use of "access to desired activities" as the reinforcement and discourage the use of materialistic reinforcers. For example, improved proficiency while doing jumping jacks could be a naturally occurring reinforcement and an intrinsic motivation for the child. Activities designed must create the appropriate level of challenge so that the child experiences success. The intervention program can gradually include more complex activities based on the child's skill level and can be practiced in varying environments to maximize generalization. Activities should be not only developmentally appropriate but also intrinsically motivating, tailored to meet the functional needs of child and family, and able to serve a lifelong purpose.

Prompting or providing feedback is also common to both ABA and motor learning approaches. Motor learning theories propose that actions are reinforced when the end goal is emphasized through immediate visual, kinesthetic, or verbal feedback.[112] Although ABA programs promote the use of graded prompting, including visual, verbal, and hand-on-hand instruction, motor learning theories promote the use of both internal (self-produced) and external feedback (provided in the environment/by the caregiver). Children with ASD are able to use both proprioceptive and visual feedback, but it is unclear whether they have a preference for one or the other.[115] Glazebrook et al. indicated that children with ASD took longer to process information presented through visual rather than through proprioceptive channels.[115] These findings may indicate that physical guidance through an action, if tolerated by the child, may be more effective than is providing visual

feedback. There is some evidence that visual modeling using two-dimensional maps of each step or computerized video feedback may also promote skill development.[116] For example, you could either show the components of a jumping jack action sequence in parts, or offer key verbal cues for the missing components, or take the child through the action manually. Children with ASD also have difficulty understanding movement goals.[117] Therefore, it is important to couple the feedback provided with the appropriate end goal of the task to promote motor learning. For example, for the two key postures within a jumping jack sequence, you could use verbal cues such as "pencil" for the hands down and feet together posture and "rocketship" for the hands up and feet-apart posture. This would help improve the child's understanding of what is expected of him or her.

One tenet that clearly differs between ABA and motor learning approaches is the value placed on trial-and-error learning. Observations of school-based ABA programs suggest that they promote predominantly errorless, prompted teaching. In contrast, motor learning principles promote active, self-produced exploration wherein errors are allowed and spontaneity is encouraged. In fact, trial-and-error learning is considered vital for greater generalization of motor skills. Therefore, PTs must be careful to allow opportunities for spontaneous movement exploration such as free, unprompted movement because that is often lacking in children with ASD. The dynamical systems theory of motor control reminds clinicians that the child with ASD, with his or her unique qualities, is embedded within an environment that can be molded to reduce or increase the complexity of motor activities. Once you use the environment to create the just-right challenge for the child, remember to wait for the child to respond spontaneously before beginning prompting or providing feedback and reinforcement. Specific recommendations for implementing ABA strategies within a physical therapy treatment session are provided in Table 23.3.

Sensory Integration Therapy

Sensory-perceptual information, including tactile, visual, and auditory stimuli created in the child's environment, can have profound effects on the child with ASD. A child who is experiencing a fight-or-flight response will not be open to learning. Hence, it is important that the child feel safe and comfortable within the treatment environment. Children with ASD are known to process sensory stimulation differently than do typically developing children, with atypical patterns emerging as early as within the first year of life.[46,68] Sensory modulation disorders of hyper- or hyposensitivity are often present in children and adults with ASD.[46] A variety of SI therapy techniques have been proposed to address the sensory impairments in children with ASD.[46] First, the classic SI therapy purports to focus directly on the neurologic processing of sensory information by providing somatosensory and vestibular activities sought out and controlled by the child to allow the child to better modulate, organize, and integrate environmental stimuli.[118] Empirical studies investigating this treatment method have consisted of case or case series design with weak evidence for efficacy.[119] This form of treatment has come under criticism, with a call for greater evidence-based treatment.[107] Second, the "sensory diet" provides more adult-structured, passively applied, and cognitively focused sensory-based activities than does the traditional SI therapy to meet the individual needs of a child.[119,120] The "diet" may include activities such as brushing with a surgical brush, joint compression, and deep pressure. However, there is weak empirical evidence to support the use of sensory diets in children with ASD.[119,120] Third, specific sensory stimulation techniques have been used to promote positive behaviors, reduce stereotypies, and to modulate arousal. Deep pressure is commonly used to elicit a calming effect, with delivery through therapeutic touch or devices such as the Hug Machine (a deep pressure–generating device), pressure garments, or weighted vests.[121,122] However, there are a limited number of studies to support their use. Children receiving touch therapy at a frequency of 15 minutes per day, 2 days per week for 4 weeks showed improvements in responsiveness to sounds and social communication.[121] Investigation of the Hug Machine twice weekly for 20 minutes per session over a 6-week period showed a statistically significant decrease in scores on a tension scale and marginal reduction in anxiety.[122] When implementing such sensory techniques, especially those that are adult-guided ones, it is important to monitor the child's stress levels as a means of determining the effects of such programs.[46,119]

Treatment and Education of Autistic and Related Communication-Handicapped Children

TEACCH emphasizes a very structured organization of the environment along with an activity sequence that allows some flexibility within a predictable routine.[105] Specifically, the space of the teaching environment is uniquely organized, the activity schedules are used to increase organization and predictability, individual workstations are used to promote independent and goal-directed activities, and appropriate visual cues are offered for successful task completion. A controlled trial found that children who participated in a TEACCH-based program for 4 months along with their typical day program demonstrated significantly greater improvements than did their peers who participated in day programs only.[104] Specific ideas on structuring the environment within a physical therapy treatment session are provided in Table 23.3.

The Picture Exchange Communication System

PECS facilitates communication using elaborate picture exchange techniques. It is often used to provide visual cues for word learning and also helps structure a child's daily schedule.[106] Specifically, picture schedules can be used throughout the day or within an activity to inform the child of the activities and the transitions between activities. Evidence suggests that the use of PECS increases the duration of spontaneous, nonverbal and verbal communication and facilitates skill generalization in children between 18 months and 12 years.[71,123] More specifics on how to incorporate picture schedules within a physical therapy treatment session are provided in Table 23.3.

Other Approaches

There are other approaches that promote the development of sensorimotor skills; however, there is weak evidence to support their use.[71,124] Greenspan and Wieder's "floortime" play is intended to enhance social–emotional relationships and cognitive growth.[71] Gutstein and Sheeley's relationship development intervention (RDI)[125] and Mahoney et al.'s responsive teaching (RT) address auditory processing, language, motor planning, sequencing, and sensory modulation and visual processing impairments in children with ASD.[124,126] Currently, there is limited empirical research being done to support claims for these interventions.[127]

Physical Therapy in Early Intervention

The Infant Sibling Research Consortium confirms the limited evidence to guide optimal programming in infancy and toddlerhood. They recommend the use of caregiver-facilitated, reciprocal social play contexts, particularly infant-initiated social interactions that require the child to actively engage with the caregiver.[128] They too recommend promoting social communication and motor systems of the at-risk infant. Moreover, they advocate individualized interventions based on the delays observed in the infant. Given these recommendations, a multisystem approach through caregiver handling is recommended. Infants at risk for ASD can receive a variety of social, object-based, and postural experiences that facilitate general and specific movement patterns, positive affect, as well as social communication.[55] In the first half-year of life, parents can provide cues through verbal reinforcement and physical handling of the infant.[129] Similarly, object-based cues can be provided by cause-and-effect toys.[129,130] Parents should encourage hands and feet reaching by offering objects near the infant's arms or legs as well as age-appropriate locomotor and object exploration skills. During object-based interactions, caregivers must incorporate triadic contexts wherein relevant social behaviors such as joint attention, that is, sharing of object play with caregivers, are encouraged.[38] Postural experiences can be provided by passively placing or by actively moving the child within the postures that appear to be delayed in the infant.[131]

If the child is diagnosed with ASD or presents with concerns leading to that diagnosis before age 3, early intervention should be recommended. Early intervention is typically conducted in the home or other natural environment with family-directed goals outlined on the Individualized Family Service Plan. Such a model of intervention is centered on functional activities, many of which require a child to perform coordinated actions and maximizes the likelihood of generalizing to naturally occurring situations.

Physical Therapy in School Systems

The public school system is responsible for children carrying the diagnosis of ASD at 3 years of age and older who require special education services. In addition to the family, the educational team may consist of the regular education teacher, special education teacher, speech-language pathologist, psychologist, OT, PT, and school nurse, depending on the child's needs to engage in the educational program. The goals of the program will be developed by the team specifically for that student and outlined on the Individualized Education Plan (IEP). Direct and/or consultative physical therapy service is appropriate for many students with ASD.

The Individuals with Disabilities Education Act (IDEA) requires that students receive educational program in the least restrictive environment. Because of the range of abilities and behavior, appropriate settings for children with ASD range from specialized programs and self-contained classrooms to full inclusion in regular classrooms. As with other students receiving special education services, transition planning for students with ASD formally begins as early as 14 years of age, and by age 16, a formal plan must be included in the IEP. The student, parents, educators, and all community agencies should be involved in developing a comprehensive transition plan that may include preparation for secondary education or competitive, supported, or sheltered employment depending on the student's interests, abilities, and behavior.[127] All members of the educational team may play a role in preparing the student with ASD to enter the community as independently as possible.

Recreational Activities and the Use of Technologies

There is growing empirical evidence to support alternative therapeutic approaches such as music and movement,[53] hippotherapy,[132] aquatic therapy,[133] yoga,[134] as well as sport and small group-based physical play for children with ASD.[135] These activities may be incorporated within PT-provided intervention sessions or could serve as a means of community involvement and preparation for lifelong fitness activities for some children with ASD. Community-based yoga, music, dance, and martial arts are often available in the community and could be alternatives for physical activities

if necessary modifications and accommodations can be made to create a positive learning environment. Special consideration should be given to the child's safety, interest, ability level, and tolerance to environmental stimuli. Therapists could be involved in making recommendations to promote positive experiences in these alternative community experiences.

Children with ASD have a predilection for using advanced technologies; hence, these have been used in meaningful ways to promote social, communication, and motor skills in children with ASD.[136] Specifically, computer technologies such as Wii boards,[136] Dance Dance Revolution,[136] and robotic technologies[137,138] could be used to facilitate social and motor skills, as well as physical fitness in children with ASD. Evidence to support their use is currently limited. But, when appropriate, these technologies could be employed in home and school environments to provide the required motor practice and generalization to other environments, to standardize the activities, and to intrinsically motivate a child during the activity.

» Conclusions

In this chapter, evidence has been offered for qualitative and quantitative differences in motor development among children and adolescents with ASD as compared with those without ASD. Significant impairments in motor coordination, postural control, imitation, and praxis are present in individuals with ASD. These areas of need can be addressed using fundamental principles of current motor learning and dynamic systems theories, along with standard autism intervention approaches such as ABA, TE-ACCH, and PECS principles through direct intervention and/or consultation with family, caregivers, and educators. Strategies to implement various intervention approaches within a physical therapy session have also been provided. Given the heterogeneity of presentation in individuals with ASD, each child must be considered individually with respect to motor abilities, sensory responses, social communication, and cognition. The PT can make a valuable contribution to the team working with the child with ASD by providing information about the child's sensorimotor abilities, recommending activities to address the individual's unique social-motor (i.e., movements with others) and cognitive-motor needs (i.e., movements requiring planning), and suggesting modifications to promote the child's ability to learn in his or her typical environments, school, and home. Suggestions may take the form of changing expectations, addressing motor challenges, modifying classroom activities to minimize negative sensory responses, teaching compensatory strategies, and promoting more active engagement with peers and caregivers within various learning situations at home, in the school, and in the community.

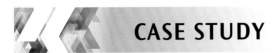

CASE STUDY

CHRIS—A 4-YEAR-OLD BOY WITH AUTISM

Chris is a 4-year-old boy who lives with his parents in a midsized home in a suburban area. He attends the preschool program of his local elementary school, where he receives special education support services. He was diagnosed with autism at 30 months of age.

History

Chris' mom reported having a full-term pregnancy and a delivery that was without any notable problems. However, there is a family history of ASD because his uncle had the same diagnosis. Chris sat independently by 9 months, walked without assistance at 16 months, and would often fall while walking for several months. When Chris was 20 months old, his mother prompted evaluation by their pediatrician, and eventually a specialist, because she was concerned that Chris appeared to have a language delay and behaved "differently" than did her friend's children. Although he did not always attend to people calling his name or talking with him, Chris seemed very sensitive to sounds such as kitchen timers, constructions sounds, and so on, as demonstrated by tantrums when such sounds occurred. He would sit watching moving objects for extended time periods, such as the fan, so much so that it was difficult for him to stop that activity. At 20 months, he had not produced words, but grunted, growled, or cried to convey distress. He would not convey his needs or his feelings through gestures such as pointing to something he wanted or showing the toys that he played with. When they went to play dates with other children, Chris did not interact and would often remove himself from where the other children were playing, sometimes hiding behind the couches. He would repeatedly activate toys with flashing lights. His mother was very concerned because Chris would eat only macaroni and cheese and applesauce, and would refuse to even try most other foods.

Birth-to-three programming began shortly after the diagnosis was made. Educational, speech, and occupational therapy services were provided on a regular basis until Chris' third birthday. Interestingly, his parents insisted on physical therapy services for the overt gross motor issues they observed; hence, those services were later added to his program. The early intervention staff provided the family with strategies to promote social communication and motor skills, modulate his sensory responses, engage Chris in the family's routine, and plan transition into the preschool program.

Current Status

Chris is currently enrolled in the morning preschool program at the local elementary school. On the basis of birth-to-three recommendations and initial examination by the educational team, Chris receives specialized educational instruction, including one-on-one paraprofessional support, along with direct speech and language, occupational, and physical therapy services infused in the typical preschool activities. His individualized educational program addresses receptive and expressive language, social interaction, sensorimotor development, and self-help skills. The parents and the educational team meet once monthly to discuss Chris' progress and to coordinate efforts to maximize consistency of expectations and interactions.

Language and Social Interaction

Chris demonstrates echolalic speech, that is, he repeats a few words uttered by adults or on television shows. All staff model appropriate verbal responses to situations clearly with emphasis and praise Chris when he imitates the correct response. He has very little spontaneous interaction with his peers, and tends to engage in activities that do not involve interaction with others. Teachers and therapists have paired him with the least threatening peers for play and academic activities, with favorable results. Chris does enjoy his time with the other children. He is able to stay in the desired location and concentrate on the task at hand with support. Chris demonstrates signs of anxiety (increased stereotypies and raised vocalizations) during transitions between activities and locations. A picture schedule is used to help Chris orient to his daily schedule. All classroom and related services are represented on the schedule. Pictures are also available to represent activities within each center and to allow choices. He consistently looks toward the picture schedule to determine the next step in his routine, and he seems to make transitions more easily in response to prior notification through pictures than if no or little warning is provided. A similar picture system is used for the different home routines. Chris has recently begun spontaneously pointing to pictures of objects he would like on occasion. When Chris successfully performs the desired behavior, those involved with programming provide rewards that have been agreed upon by parents and educators. Each team member is aware of the plan and provides the reinforcement for a job well done and additional wagon time (Chris' preferred activity) for successful completion of the activities asked of him.

Sensorimotor Development

Chris has developed stereotypic behavior of rocking and occasionally spinning. He flaps his hands and watches them at times. He continues to become distressed with loud sounds; he often covers his ears and increases rocking motion. Such responses also occur if adults or peers touch him. He prefers to play with the computer and toys that have lights.

He will sit in circle time for only a few minutes before he wants to get up and move quickly about the classroom. On the playground, he enjoys activities that provide movement such as the swings, slides, and rotary equipment. It is sometimes a challenge for Chris to end such activities. In physical education (PE), Chris typically runs around the space, behavior escalates, and he sometimes tries to hide under the mats that are stacked against the wall.

Chris is ambulatory without physical assistance around the interior and exterior of the school; he needs supervision and cuing for safety and direction. His gait pattern is usually characterized by toe-walking. He is able to run and change directions, but his motor planning is clearly affected. He is unable to perform actions involving multiple steps required for using the stepper, scooter, or the bicycle. He has not demonstrated multilimb actions such as galloping and skipping, and has difficulty maintaining one-leg stance. He usually does not respond to the request of copying the demonstrations of the PT/OT. He cannot ascend and descend stairs without the support of a railing and appears to lack balance in situations that require a narrow base of support. He presents with diminished muscle tone as demonstrated by joint laxity and difficulty maintaining antigravity positions for extended periods.

Chris' performance on the MABC indicated that he functions in the ninth percentile for manual dexterity, fifth percentile for aiming and catching, and first percentile for balance. Using the Sensory Profile, parents and educators provided information about Chris' responses to sensory stimuli. On the basis of their responses, definite differences with hypersensitivity were identified in the following areas: tactile sensitivity, taste/smell sensitivity, auditory filtering, and visual/auditory sensitivity.

On the basis of observations throughout the school day, input from all team members, and results of standardized testing, the PT and OT have collaboratively made recommendations for strategies to help regulate sensory responses and promote gross and fine motor development. The OT and paraprofessional have found that Chris tends to sit longer in the circle activities when deep pressure input is provided. Use of a weighted lap blanket also seems to lengthen periods of quiet sitting. Chris tends to be more engaged in the PE activities when the lesson is conducted in a room smaller than the gymnasium. The staff is currently in the process of collecting data about time-on-task and signs of anxiety when wearing a weighted vest with special attention to performance during PE.

A designated time is now built into Chris' routine to use the swing on the playscape. Since adding this opportunity for Chris to get vestibular input, the rocking and flapping stereotypies have diminished. A rocking chair is available in the listening/story center, and Chris is usually allowed to use it for short periods as a reward for completing his therapeutic/academic activities. A rocking horse is occasionally included as a gross motor option at recess. He has a cart that he loads with various objects and pushes at home and at school. The parents and school staff have developed a plan for after-school hours that allows Chris to play on his swing set and run in the yard with supervision shortly after he comes home.

The speech therapist and OT are currently working closely with the parents to systematically introduce textures and flavors into Chris' diet to expand his food choice repertoire. Chris' mother follows through by sending in snacks of various textures that can be trialed under the supervision of the trained related service providers.

The PT recommended a trial of wearing high-top work boots to help improve Chris' gait pattern with positive results; consistent foot-flat and occasional heel strike have been noted. Balance, coordination, and gross motor planning are being addressed within his physical therapy program. He is encouraged to walk on different ambulation surfaces that vary by texture, size, pitch, compliance, and stability. On more challenging surfaces, Chris' performance is enhanced if the PT provides some manual support for him to hold onto gently and guards him. As carryover, the paraprofessional

walks with Chris along the railroad ties surrounding the playscape each day during recess while providing guarding and some manual support. His classroom teacher, music teacher, and PE teachers have been advised to ensure he has opportunities to move while singing, move with his peers, and engage in movement games within small groups of one to three peers.

Motor planning is addressed by engaging in throwing and catching through the use of beanbags and balls that vary in size, texture, and compliance. Targets that will yield activation of lights or motion when successfully reached have been chosen. Similar activities are done at school and during play at home. He is also learning to use exercise equipment such as a stepper and a tricycle, but needs significant instruction and physical support to complete the activity. The paraprofessional is typically supporting the PT during these activities.

Self-Help Skills

Chris requires assistance to manage dressing and toileting at school and at home. He uses pull-ups because he does not indicate when he needs to use the toilet. He is able to use his hands or utensils to feed himself, and he is able to independently use a cup with a spout to drink. His diet is limited to a few preferred food choices.

The PEDI was done with observation and report by parent and educational staff, yielding normative standard scores for self-care of less than 10 (Caregiver Assistance <10), Mobility 20.4 (Caregiver Assistance 60.7), and Social Function less than 10 (Caregiver Assistance <10).

The family identified washing and bathing as being particularly challenging because Chris seems genuinely fearful. The school staff plans to perform the SFA when Chris enters kindergarten.

Family and educators identified hand washing and toileting as priorities. The special educator, the OT, and the PT broke each task into concrete steps and developed specific instructions for each step. The steps were described using a picture schedule placed at a location near the sink where he washes his hands. Everyone in school and at home who assists Chris with the hand washing and toileting go through the picture schedule in the specified manner using the same terminology, provide praise along the way, and reward him when he successfully completes the task. Proper participation in self-help skills is also reinforced through stories that are part of the preschool curriculum.

Collaborative input and efforts of the family, educators, caregivers, and medical personnel are imperative to optimize the programming for a child with ASD. The likelihood of the child acquiring important lifelong functional skills is enhanced when:

a. The activities are meaningful to the child and family and serve a long-term function.
b. The activities are individualized to the child's ability level.
c. The program accounts for and is respectful of the child's ability to take in information from the caregivers within the child's environment.
d. The people who interact with the child with ASD are consistent in their expectations and implementation of the program.

REFERENCES

1. American Psychiatric Association. *Diagnostic and Statistical Manual of Mental Disorders.* 5th ed. American Psychiatric Association; 2013.

2. Jansiewicz E, Goldberg M, Newschaffer C, et al. Motor signs distinguish children with high functioning autism and Asperger's syndrome from controls. *J Autism Dev Disord.* 2006;36(5):613-621.

3. Fournier K, Hass C, Naik S, et al. Motor coordination in autism spectrum disorders: a synthesis and meta-analysis. *J Autism Dev Disord.* 2010;40(10):1227-1240.

4. Centers for Disease Control. Prevalence of autism spectrum disorders—Autism and Developmental Disabilities Monitoring Network (ADDM), United States, 2008. *MMWR Surveill Summ.* 2012;61(3):1-24.

5. Ganz M. *Understanding Autism.* Taylor & Francis; 2006.

6. Centers for Disease Control and Prevention. *Autism Spectrum Disorders.* Accessed January 15, 2021. http://www.cdc.gov/NCBDDD/autism/facts.html

7. Bauman M, Kemper T. Neuroanatomic observations of the brain in autism: a review and future directions. *Int J Dev Neurosci.* 2005;23(2-3):183-187.

8. Sumi S, Taniai H, Miyachi T, et al. Sibling risk of pervasive developmental disorder estimated by means of an epidemiologic survey in Nagoya, Japan. *J Hum Genet.* 2006;51(6):518-522.

9. Zwaigenbaum L, Thurm A, Stone W, et al. Studying the emergence of autism spectrum disorders in high-risk infants: methodological and practical issues. *J Autism Dev Disord.* 2007;37(3):466-480.

10. Guinchat V, Thorsen P, Laurent C, et al. Pre–, peri–, and neonatal risk factors for autism. *Acta Obstet Gynecol Scand.* 2012;91(3):287-300.

11. Sandin S, Hultman C, Kolevzon A, et al. Advancing maternal age is associated with increasing risk for autism: a review and meta-analysis. *J Am Acad Child Adolesc Psychiatry.* 2012;51(5):477-486.

12. Narita M, Oyabu A, Imura Y, et al. Nonexploratory movement and behavioral alterations in a thalidomide or valproic acid-induced autism model rat. *Neurosci Res.* 2010;66(1):2-6.

13. Courchesne E, Redcay E, Kennedy D. The autistic brain: birth through adulthood. *Curr Opin Neurol.* 2004;17(4):489-496.

14. Dementieva Y, Vance D, Donnelly S, et al. Accelerated head growth in early development of individuals with autism. *Pediatr Neurol.* 2005;32(2):102-108.

15. Dawson G, Munson J, Webb SJ, et al. Rate of head growth decelerates and symptoms worsen in the second year of life in autism. *Biol Psychiatry.* 2007;61(4):458-464.

16. Sparks B, Friedman S, Shaw D, et al. Brain structural abnormalities in young children with autism spectrum disorder. *Neurology.* 2002;59(2):184-192.

17. Casanova M, Buxhoeveden D, Switala A, et al. Minicolumnar pathology in autism. *Neurology.* 2002;58(3):428-432.

18. Williams D, Goldstein G, Minshew N. Neuropsychologic functioning in children with autism: further evidence for disordered complex information-processing. *Child Neuropsychol.* 2006;12(4-5):279-298.

19. Mostofsky S, Powell S, Simmonds D, et al. Decreased connectivity and cerebellar activity in autism during motor task performance. *Brain.* 2009;132(pt 9):2413-2425.

20. Hallett M, Lebiedowska M, Thomas S, et al. Locomotion of autistic adults. *Arch Neurol.* 1993;50(12):1304-1308.

21. Rinehart N, Bradshaw J, Brereton A, et al. A clinical and neurobehavioural review of high-functioning autism and Asperger's disorder. *Aust N Z J Psychiatry.* 2002;36(6):762-770.

22. Vilensky J, Damasio A, Maurer R. Gait disturbances in patients with autistic behavior: a preliminary study. *Arch Neurol.* 1981;38(10):646-649.

23. Cattaneo L, Rizzolatti G. The mirror-neuron system. *Arch Neurol.* 2009;66(5):557-560.

24. Dapretto D, Pfeiffer P, Scott A, et al. Understanding emotions in others: mirror neuron dysfunction in children with autism spectrum disorders. *Nat Neurosci.* 2006;9(1):28-30.

25. Landa R, Garrett-Mayer E. Development in infants with autism spectrum disorders: a prospective study. *J Child Psychol Psychiatry.* 2006;47(6):629-638.

26. Bhat A, Galloway J, Landa R. Relation between early motor delay and later communication delay in infants at risk for autism. *Infant Behav Dev.* 2012;35(4):838-846.

27. Flanagan J, Landa R, Bhat A, et al. Head lag in infants at risk for autism: a preliminary study. *Am J Occup Ther.* 2012;66(5):577-585.

28. Ozonoff S, Young G, Goldring S, et al. Gross motor development, movement abnormalities, and early identification of autism. *J Autism Dev Disord.* 2008;38(4):644-656.

29. Paul R, Fuerst Y, Ramsay G, et al. Out of the mouths of babes: vocal production in infant siblings of children with ASD. *J Child Psychol Psychiatry.* 2011;52(5):588-598.

30. Lord C, Rutter M, DiLavore PC, et al. *Autism Diagnostic Observation Schedule (ADOS).* Western Psychological Services; 1999.

31. Lord C, Rutter M, Le Couteur A. Autism diagnostic interview-revised: a revised version of a diagnostic interview for caregivers of individuals with possible pervasive developmental disorders. *J Autism Dev Disord.* 1994;24(5):659-685.

32. MedlinePlus. Rett Syndrome, National Library of Medicine. Accessed March 6, 2021. https://medlineplus.gov/genetics/condition/rett-syndrome/

33. Genetics Home Reference. Fragile X syndrome. 2007; Accessed June 8, 2012. http://ghr.nlm.nih.gov/condition/fragile-x-syndrome

34. Townsend J, Harris N, Courchesne E. Visual attention abnormalities in autism: delayed orienting to location. *J Int Neuropsychol Soc.* 1996;2(6):541-550.

35. Wainwright J, Bryson S. Visual-spatial orienting in autism. *J Autism Dev Disord.* 1996;26(4):423-438.

36. Mundy P, Thorp D. *New Developments in Autism: The Future Is Today.* Jessica Kingsley Publishers; 2007.

37. Dawson G, Webb S, McPartland J. Understanding the nature of face processing impairment in autism: insights from behavioral and electrophysiological studies. *Dev Neuropsychol.* 2005;27(3):403-424.

38. Bhat AN, Galloway JC, Landa RJ. Social and non-social visual attention patterns and associative learning in infants at risk for autism. *J Child Psychol Psychiatry.* 2010;51(9):989-997. doi:10.1111/j.1469-7610.2010.02262.x

39. Mundy P, Sigman M. Joint attention, social competence, and developmental psychopathology. In D. Cicchetti & D. J. Cohen (Eds.), *Developmental psychopathology: Theory and method.* 2006:293–332. John Wiley & Sons, Inc.

40. Mundy P, Sigman M, Kasari C. A longitudinal study of joint attention and language development in autistic children. *J Autism Dev Disord.* 1990;20(1):115-128.

41. Eigsti I-M, de Marchena A, Schuh J, et al. Language acquisition in autism spectrum disorders: a developmental review. *Res in Autism Spectr Disord.* 2011;5(2):681-691.

42. Tager-Flusberg H, Paul R, Lord C. Language and communication in autism. In: Cohen D, Volkmar F, eds. *Handbook of Autism and Pervasive Developmental Disorders.* 3rd ed. John Wiley & Sons; 1997:195-225.

43. Ozonoff S, Pennington B, Rogers S. Executive function deficits in high-functioning autistic individuals: relationship to theory of mind. *J Child Psychol Psychiatry.* 1991;32(7):1081-1105.

44. Ben-Sasson A, Hen L, Fluss R, et al. A meta-analysis of sensory modulation symptoms in individuals with autism spectrum disorders. *J Autism Dev Disord.* 2009;39(1):1-11.

45. Tomchek S, Dunn W. Sensory processing in children with and without autism: a comparative study using the short sensory profile. *Am J Occup Ther.* 2007;61(2):190-200.

46. Baranek G, Parham L, Bodfish J. Sensory and motor features in autism: assessment and intervention. In: Volkmar FR, Paul R, Klin A, et al., eds. *Handbook of Autism and Pervasive Developmental Disorders.* Wiley; 2005:831-857.

47. Lane A, Young R, Baker A, et al. Sensory processing subtypes in autism: association with adaptive behavior. *J Autism Dev Disord.* 2010;40(1):112-122.

48. Bölte S, Holtmann M, Poustka F, et al. Gestalt perception and local-global processing in high-functioning autism. *J Autism Dev Disord.* 2007;37(8):1493-1504.

49. Gernsbacher M, Stevenson J, Khandakar S, et al. Why does joint attention look atypical in autism? *Child Dev Perspect.* 2008;2(1):38-45.

50. Heaton P. Pitch memory, labelling and disembedding in autism. *J Child Psychol Psychiatry.* 2003;44(4):543-551.

51. Bhatara A, Quintin E, Levy B, et al. Perception of emotion in musical performance in adolescents with autism spectrum disorders. *Autism Res.* 2010;3(5):214-225.

52. Whipple J. Music in intervention for children and adolescents with autism: a meta-analysis. *J Music Ther.* 2004;41(2):90-106.

53. Srinivasan S, Kaur M, Park I, et al. The effects of rhythm and robotic interventions on the imitation/praxis, interpersonal synchrony, and motor performance of children with Autism Spectrum Disorder (ASD): a pilot randomized controlled trial. *Autism Res Treat.* 2015: 1-18. Article ID 736516.

54. Dzuik M, Gidley Larson J, Apostu A, et al. Dyspraxia in autism: association with motor, social, and communicative deficits. *Dev Med Child Neurol.* 2007;49(10):734-739.

55. Bhat A, Landa R, Galloway JC. Perspectives on motor problems in infants, children, and adults with autism spectrum disorders. *Phys Ther.* 2011;91(7):1116-1129.

56. Bodfish J, Symons F, Parker D, et al. Varieties of repetitive behavior in autism: comparisons to mental retardation. *J Autism Dev Disord.* 2000;30(3):237-243.

57. Loh A, Soman T, Brian J, et al. Stereotyped motor behaviors associated with autism in high-risk infants: a pilot videotape analysis of a sibling sample. *J Autism Dev Disord.* 2007;37(1):25-36.

58. Walker D, Thompson A, Zwaigenbaum L, et al. Specifying PDD-NOS: a comparison of PDD-NOS, Asperger syndrome, and autism. *J Am Acad Child Adolesc Psychiatry.* 2004;43(2):172-180.

59. Chawarska K, Klin A, Paul R, et al. Autism spectrum disorder in the second year: stability and change in syndrome expression. *J Child Psychol Psychiatry.* 2006;48(2):128-138.

60. Nickel L, Thatcher A, Iverson J. Postural development in infants with and without risk for autism spectrum disorders. Paper presented at: 9th Annual International Meeting for Autism Research; May 20–22, 2010; Philadelphia, PA. 2010.

61. Bhat AN. Is motor impairment in Autism Spectrum Disorder distinct from Developmental Coordination Disorder? A report from the SPARK study. *Phys Ther.* 2020;100(4):633-644.

62. Green D, Baird G, Barnett A, et al. The severity and nature of motor impairment in Asperger's syndrome: a comparison with specific developmental disorder of motor function. *J Child Psychol Psychiatry.* 2002;43(5):655-668.

63. Miyahara M, Tsujii M, Hori M, et al. Brief report: motor incoordination in children with Asperger syndrome and learning disabilities. *J Autism Dev Disord.* 1997;27(5):595-603.

64. Kaur M, Srinivasan S, Bhat A. Comparing motor performance, praxis, coordination, and interpersonal synchrony between children with and without Autism Spectrum Disorder (ASD). *Res Dev Disabil.* 2018;72:79-95. doi: 10.1016/j.ridd.2017.10.025.

65. Mari M, Castiello U, Marks D, et al. The reach–to–grasp movement in children with autism spectrum disorder. *Philos Trans R Soc Lond B Biol Sci.* 2003;358(1430):393-403.

66. Glazebrook CM, Elliott D, Lyons J. A kinematic analysis of how young adults with and without autism plan and control goal-directed movements. *Motor Control.* 2006;10(3):244-264.

67. Fuentes CT, Mostofsky SH, Bastian A. Children with autism show specific handwriting impairments. *Neurology.* 2009;73(19):1532-1537.

68. Baranek G. Autism during infancy: a retrospective video analysis of sensory-motor and social behaviors at 9-12 months of age. *J Autism Dev Disord.* 1999;29(3):213-224.

69. Bryson S, Zwaigenbaum L, Brian J, et al. A prospective case series of high-risk infants who developed autism. *J Autism Dev Disord.* 2007;37(1):12-24.

70. Gernsbacher M. Infant and toddler oral-and manual-motor skills predict later speech fluency in autism. *J Child Psychol Psychiatry.* 2008;49(1):43-50.

71. Greenspan SI, Wieder S. Developmental patterns and outcomes in infants and children with disorders in relating and communicating: a chart review of 200 cases of children with autistic spectrum diagnoses. *J Dev Learn Disord.* 1997;1:87-141.

72. Minshew N, Sung K, Jones B, et al. Underdevelopment of the postural control system in autism. *Neurology.* 2004;63(11):2056-2061.

73. Landa R, Gross A, Stuart E, et al. Developmental trajectories in children with and without autism spectrum disorders: the first 3 years. *Child Dev.* 2013;84(2):429-442.

74. Dewey D. What is developmental dyspraxia? *Brain Cogn.* 1995;29(3):254-274.

75. Demyer M, Hingtgen I, Jackson R. Infantile autism reviewed: a decade of research. *Schizophr Bull.* 1981;7(3):388-451.

76. Mostofsky SH, Dubey P, Jerath VK, et al. Developmental dyspraxia is not limited to imitation in children with autism spectrum disorders. *J Int Neuropsychol Soc.* 2006;12(3):314-326.

77. Charman T, Baron-Cohen S. Brief report: prompted pretend play in autism. *J Autism Dev Disord.* 1997;27(3):325-332.

78. Rogers SJ, Bennetto L, McEvoy R, et al. Imitation and pantomime in high-functioning adolescents with autism spectrum disorders. *Child Dev.* 1996;67(5):2060-2073.

79. Stone W, Yoder P. Predicting spoken language level in children with autism spectrum disorders. *Autism.* 2001;5(4):341-361.

80. Kern J, Geier D, Adams J, et al. Autism severity and muscle strength: a correlation analysis. *Res Autism Spectr Disord.* 2011;5(3):1011-1015.

81. Teitelbaum P, Teitelbaum O, Nye J, et al. Movement analysis in infancy may be useful for early diagnosis of autism. *Proc Natl Acad Sci USA.* 1998;95(23):12987-13982.

82. Adrien J, Lenoir P, Martineau J, et al. Blind ratings of early symptoms of autism based upon family home movies. *J Am Acad Child Adolesc Psychiatry.* 1993;32(3):617-626.

83. Srinivasan S, Pescatello L, Bhat A. Current perspectives on physical activity and exercise recommendations for children and adolescents with Autism Spectrum Disorders. *Phys Ther.* 2014;94(6):875-889.

84. Curtin C, Anderson SE, Must A, et al. The prevalence of obesity in children with autism: a secondary data analysis using nationally representative data from the National Survey of Children's Health. *BMC Pediatr.* 2010;10(1):11.

85. Bandini L, Anderson S, Curtin C, et al. Food selectivity in children with autism spectrum disorders and typically developing children. *J Pediatr.* 2010;157(2):259-264.

86. Matson M, Matson J, Beighley J. Comorbidity of physical and motor problems in children with autism. *Res Dev Disabil.* 2011;32(6):2304-2308.

87. Chen A, Kim S, Houtrow A, et al. Prevalence of obesity among children with chronic conditions. *Obesity.* 2009;18(1):210-213.

88. Rimmer J, Yamaki K, Lowry B, et al. Obesity and obesity-related secondary conditions in adolescents with intellectual/developmental disabilities. *J Intellect Disabil Res.* 2010;54(9):787-794.

89. Ayres J. *Sensory Integration and Praxis Tests (SIPT).* Western Psychological Services; 1996.

90. Henderson SE, Sugden DA. *Movement Assessment Battery for Children.* Psychological Corporation; 1992.

91. King G, Law M, King S, et al. *Children's Assessment of Participation and Enjoyment (CAPE) Manual.* Hartcourt Assessment; 2004.

92. Bruininks R. *The Bruininks-Oseretsky Test of Motor Proficiency (BOTMP) Manual.* American Guidance Service; 1978.

93. Squires J, Bricker D. *Ages & Stages Questionnaires, Third Edition (ASQ-3).* Brookes Publishing; 2009.

94. Robins DL, Fein D, Barton ML, et al. The modified checklist for autism in toddlers: an initial study investigating the early detection of autism and pervasive developmental disorders. *J Autism Dev Disord.* 2001;31(2):131-144.

95. Bryson S, Zwaigenbaum L, McDermott C, et al. The autism observation scale for infants: scale development and reliability data. *J Autism Dev Disord.* 2008;38(4):731-738.

96. Bayley N. *Bayley Scales of Infant and Toddler Development.* 3rd ed. Pearson Assessment; 2005.

97. Mullen E. *Mullen Scales of Early Learning.* American Guidance Service; 1995.

98. Volkmar F, Sparrow S, Goudreau D, et al. Social deficits in autism: an operational approach using the Vineland adaptive behavior scales. *J Am Acad Child Adolesc Psychiatry.* 1987;26(2):156-161.

99. Rothi L, Gonzalez R, Heilman K. Limb praxis assessment. In: Hove E, ed. *Apraxia: The Neuropsychology of Action.* Psychology Press/Taylor & Francis; 1997:61-73.

100. Haley SM, Coster WJ, Ludlow LH, et al. *Pediatric Evaluation of Disability Inventory (PEDI).* Psychological Corporation; 1992.

101. Coster W, Deeney T, Haltiwanger J, et al. *School Function Assessment (SFA).* The Psychological Corporation; 1998.

102. Landa R. Early communication development and intervention for children with autism. *Ment Retard Dev Disabil Res Rev.* 2007;13(1):16-25.

103. Sallows G, Graupner T. Intensive behavioral treatment for children with autism: four-year outcome and predictors. *Am J Ment Retard.* 2005;110(6):417-438.

104. Ozonoff S, Cathcart K. Effectiveness of a home program intervention for young children with autism. *J Autism Dev Disord.* 1998;28:25-32.

105. Mesibov GB, Shea V, Schopler E. *The TEACCH Approach to Autism Spectrum Disorder.* Kluwer Academic/Plenum; 2005.

106. Bondy A, Frost A. Communication strategies for visual learners. In: Lovaas OI, ed. *Teaching Individuals with Developmental Delays: Basic Intervention Techniques.* Pro-Ed; 2003:291-304.

107. Bundy AC, Murray EA. Sensory integration: a Jean Ayre's theory revisited. In: Bundy AC, Murray EA, Lane S, eds. *Sensory Integration: Theory and Practice.* FA Davis; 2002.

108. Lovaas OI. Behavioral treatment and normal educational and intellectual functioning in young autistic children. *J Consult Clin Psychol.* 1987;55(1):3-9.

109. McEachin JJ, Smith T, Lovaas OI. Long-term outcome for children with autism who received early intensive behavioral treatment. *Am J Ment Retard.* 1993;97:359-372.

110. Stahmer A, Ingersoll B. Inclusive programming for Toddlers with autism spectrum disorders: outcomes from the children's Toddler school. *J Posit Behav Interv.* 2004;6(2):67-82.

111. Pierce K, Schreibman L. Increasing complex social behaviors in children with autism: effects of peer-implemented pivotal response training. *J Appl Behav Anal.* 1995;28(3):285-295.

112. Shumway-Cook A, Woollacott M. *Motor Control: Translating Research in Clinical Practice.* 3rd ed. Lippincott Williams & Wilkins; 2007.

113. Gidley Larson JC, Bastian AJ, Donchin O, et al. Acquisition of internal models of motor tasks in children with autism. *Brain.* 2008;131(11):2894-2903.

114. Mostofsky SH, Bunoski R, Morton SM, et al. Children with autism adapt normally during a catching task requiring the cerebellum. *Neurocase.* 2004;10(1):60-64.

115. Glazebrook C, Gonzalez D, Hansen S, et al. The role of vision for online control of manual aiming movements in persons with autism spectrum disorders. *Autism.* 2009;13:411-433.

116. Maione I, Mirenda P. Effects of video modeling and video feedback on peer-directed social language skills of a child with autism. *J Posit Behav Interv.* 2006;8:106-118.

117. Fabbri-Destro M, Cattaneo L, Boria S, et al. Planning actions in autism. *Exp Brain Res.* 2009;192(3):521-525.

118. Miller L, Anzalone M, Lane S, et al. Concept evolution in sensory integration: a proposed nosology for diagnosis. *Am J Occup Ther.* 2007;61(2):135-140.

119. Baranek G. Efficacy of sensory and motor interventions for children with autism. *J Autism Dev Disord.* 2002;32(5):397-422.

120. Stagnitti K, Raison P, Ryan P. Sensory defensiveness syndrome: a paediatric perspective and case study. *Aust Occup Ther J.* 1999;46:175-187.

121. Field T, Lasko PM, Henteleff T, et al. Brief report: autistic children's attentiveness and responsivity improve after touch therapy. *J Autism Dev Disord.* 1997;27:333-339.

122. Edelson SM, Goldberg M, Edelson MG, et al. Behavioral and physiological effects of deep pressure on children with autism: a pilot study evaluating the efficacy of Grandin's Hug Machine. *Am J Occup Ther.* 1999;53:143-152.

123. Yoder PJ, Stone WL. Randomized comparison of two communication interventions for preschoolers with autism spectrum disorders. *J Consult Clin Psychol.* 2006;74(3):426-435.

124. Mahoney G, Perales F. Relationship-focused early intervention with children with pervasive developmental disorders and other disabilities: a comparative study. *J Dev Behav Pediatr.* 2005;26:77-85.

125. Gutstein SE, Sheeley RK. *Relationship Development Intervention with Children, Adolescents, and Adults.* Jessica Kingsley; 2002.

126. Mahoney G, McDonald J. *Responsive Teaching: Parent-Mediated Developmental Intervention.* Paul H. Brookes; 2003.

127. Zwaigenbaum L, Bauman ML, Choueiri R, et al. Early intervention for children with Autism Spectrum Disorder under 3 years of age: recommendations for practice and research. *Pediatrics.* 2015;136:S60-S81.

128. Zwaigenbaum L, Bryson S, Lord C, et al. Clinical assessment and management of toddlers with suspected autism spectrum disorder: insights from studies of high-risk infants. *Pediatrics.* 2009;123(5):1383.

129. Heathcock J, Lobo M, Galloway J. Movement training advances the emergence of reaching in infants born at less than 33 weeks of gestational age: a randomized clinical trial. *Phys Ther.* 2008;88(3):1-13.

130. Lobo MA, Galloway JC, Savelsbergh GJP. General and task-related experiences affect early object interaction. *Child Dev.* 2004;75(4):1268-1281.

131. Lobo M, Galloway J. Postural and object-oriented experiences advance early reaching, object exploration, and means–end behavior. *Child Dev.* 2008;79(6):1869-1890.

132. Srinivasan S, Cavagnino D, Bhat A. Effects of equine therapy on individuals with autism spectrum disorder: a systematic review. *Rev J. Autism Dev Disord.* 2018;5(2)156-175.

133. Pan C. The efficacy of an aquatic program on physical fitness and aquatic skills in children with and without autism spectrum disorders. *Res Autism Spectr Disord.* 2011;5(1):657-665.

134. Kaur M, Bhat A. Creative yoga intervention improves motor and imitation skills of children with Autism Spectrum Disorder. *Phys Ther.* 2019;99:1520-1534.

135. Bremer E, Balogh R, Lloyd M. Effectiveness of a fundamental motor skill intervention for 4-year-old children with autism spectrum disorder: a pilot study. *Autism.* 2015;19(8):980-991. doi:10.1177/1362361314557548. Epub 2014 Nov 28. doi:10.1177/1362361314557548

136. Getchell N, Miccinello D, Blom M, et al. Comparing energy expenditure in adolescents with and without autism while playing nintendo—Wii Games. *Games Health J.* 2012;1(1):58-61.

137. Diehl JJ, Schmitt LM, Villano M, et al. The clinical use of robots for individuals with autism spectrum disorders: a critical review. *Res Autism Spectr Disord.* 2011;6(1):249-262.

138. Robins B, Dautenhahn K, te Boekhorst R, et al. *Effects of repeated exposure to a humanoid robot on children with autism.* Paper presented at: Universal Access and Assistive Technology; March 22-24, 2004; Cambridge, UK.

Down Syndrome and Intellectual Disorders

Christine G. Paris

>> Introduction

The physical therapist plays a challenging and important, multifaceted role in the management of children with intellectual disability (ID) because the clinical presentation of this group of children includes simultaneous and interactive impairments in the neuromotor, musculoskeletal, developmental, cognitive, and affective domains. The physical therapist must be able to accurately examine the child and must also innovatively develop, implement, modify, and share with parents and other providers of service an appropriate plan of care in order to maximize

the child's abilities and participation. In this chapter, an approach is offered to assist the entry-level physical therapist with examination, intervention, and management of the child with ID. The strategy presented is from a functional perspective, delineating the interactive effects of common impairments associated with such disabilities and the role of the physical therapist in managing these impairments to promote the maximum best function of the child within his or her environment. ID results from a variety of etiologies. This chapter presents the physical therapy management strategy for the child with Down syndrome (Fig. 24.1).

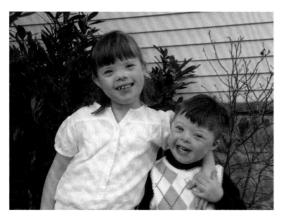

FIGURE 24.1. Introducing Angelo and Juliana, siblings with Down syndrome. Julianna was adopted by her family when Angelo was 3 years old.

» Historical review

The history of society and its treatment of people with intellectual disabilities has had an intriguing, interesting, and still unfolding, interactional relationship. As societal trends followed a path of increased education and understanding, the quality of these interactions wandered along a pathway from severe humiliation to tolerance and protection, to understanding and acceptance, and is now evolving along a pathway that promotes full inclusion and self-determination. In the earliest of recorded interactions between the two groups, people with ID were ignored, received little or no care, or were even left to die.[1] Spartan society believed in survival of only the fittest, and many people, including the physically and mentally impaired, were left to perish.

Conversely, during the Middle Ages and in ancient Rome, it was not uncommon for wealthy people to keep a "fool" or "court jester" in return for the amusement these people provided for the household and its guests.[1] Artistic work of the Middle Ages shows people serving as clowns and jesters who depict the physical characteristics of what we now identify as Down syndrome.[2] In the later Middle Ages, particularly in Europe, superstitious beliefs led to the execution of many people who were considered to be "witches and warlocks." People with intellectual and other disabilities were undoubtedly included in these groups.[1] This idea that people with disabilities were social menaces persisted throughout the 19th century, with the eventual trend away from execution but still toward punishment, imprisonment, and isolation.[3]

In the early 20th century, there was a publicly perceived need to shelter and protect people with ID from the misunderstanding, abuses, and wrath of society. Consequently, people perceived as having a mental deficiency were isolated in asylums, shelters, and farm communities. These communities, however, rapidly became overcrowded. The goal of this public effort was clearly housing, not the provision of services, let alone education.

Interest in providing services to assist people with ID had a difficult beginning. In the early 1800s, Jean Marc Itard, a French physician, became intrigued with an intellectually challenged youngster whom the physician had captured in the forests of Aveyron in France. Acting on his then revolutionary premise that intellectual performance could be affected by environmental stimulation, Itard succeeded in teaching this "Wild Boy of Aveyron." Although Itard's work helped the boy improve over a 5-year period, the gains were not sufficient for acceptance of the boy into Parisian society at that time. Society frowned on the child, and Itard believed he had failed.[4]

In 1840, Johann Jacob Guggenbuhl established a center in Switzerland for a then innovative approach involving group teaching for children with ID. His work received worldwide acclaim as a major reform. This reform influenced the work, in Europe and in the United States, of Edouard Sequin, who was a world leader in the development of educational and residential services for people with ID. In 1876, Seguin was made president of the newly formed Association of Medical Officers of the American Institutions for Idiotic and Feeble-Minded Persons. This association later (1876) became the American Association of Mental Deficiency (AAMD), which renamed itself in 2006 as the American Association on Intellectual and Developmental Disabilities (AAIDD).

In the United States, the social organization accompanying the Industrial Revolution reinforced this concept of group care of children, as well as stimulating a sense of social responsibility.[1] Throughout the 1800s, small gains fluctuated with a sense of frustration and futility, and there was a large-scale movement to house the "incurables" in large, overcrowded facilities in isolated areas.[2] As such, education first promoted for use with individuals with severe disabilities, including those with ID, was generally provided in large institutions designed as much to protect persons with disabilities from the public as to protect the public from them.

During the mid-19th century, an interesting development began that was referred to as "special education." Samuel Gridley Howe and Horace Mann aided this development through publicizing the educational experiences of Laura Bridgman, a child who was blind and came to be educated at school for the blind housed at the Perkins Institute in Massachusetts. Howe's description of the processes used at the Institute with Bridgman was further circulated in reports written by Charles Dickens. Dickens' articles were widely read, aided by his popularity at that time, and helped give fuel to the special education movement.[5,6]

This treatment model, delivered in large, segregated settings, persisted through the end of World War II, when the emphasis on care of people with ID evolved to include "programming." This shift to a plan of activity was mainly the result of efforts by the National Association for Retarded Citizens (NARC) and other parent or professional advocacy groups.[2] Increasing awareness of the negative effects of residential segregation and the limitations of existing programs led to a critical reappraisal of existing kinds of care available for people with ID. Influenced by the Civil Rights Movement, the 1960s represented a time of expansion in program legislation and funds allocation for all persons with disabilities. Discrimination against and segregation of people with ID were finally recognized as negative and undesirable.[2]

In the early 1970s, American visitors to Scandinavian countries encountered the concept of "normalization," which was defined as the principle of educating persons with handicaps to the maximum extent feasible within the "normal" environment of the nonhandicapped.[7] This process obviously required major development and use of community support systems. This era became known as the era of "deinstitutionalization." As an example, in 1972 the Association for Retarded Citizens won a landmark decision against the Commonwealth of Pennsylvania that provided access to public education for children with ID. This decision stated that "[i]t is the Commonwealth's obligation to place each mentally retarded child in a free, public program of education and training appropriate to the child's capacity...placement in a regular school class is preferable to placement in a special public school class and placement in a special public school is preferable to placement in any other type of program of education and training."[7] Similar landmark cases were happening in states across the country. This deinstitutionalization movement continued into the 1980s, and public interest was further stirred by a series of investigations and publications of the conditions of several institutions. Televised broadcasts "exposed abuse, neglect, and lack of programming at Willowbrook, a state institution for persons with ID on Staten Island."[8] This spurred the interest of Jacob Javits, a state senator from New York, to propose legislation to regulate practices in institutions.[7] Since then, many changes have occurred as a result of public interest and educators. Most of the nation's institutions serving the population with ID have closed, and other types of educational facilities and housing have been developed. Living arrangements in the community have now become the norm for the long-term care and support of people with ID. As a result of these changes, physical therapists now serve individuals with intellectual disabilities in a variety of settings. These include in the home, in a day-care or preschool setting, in elementary and secondary schools as a related service as well as in more traditional settings such as a hospital or outpatient clinic.

The most current approach to programming in the field of ID is a functional, integrated treatment model. Society as a whole, and therefore the countless legislatures and service providers of today's society, view ID along a changing paradigm, with a more functional definition and a focus on the interaction between the person, the environment, and the intensities and patterns of needed supports. The term readers will hear most frequently now is "support," including needed level of support for maximum function of the individual with ID in the environment.[8]

» Definition

ID is characterized by significant limitations in both intellectual functioning and adaptive behavior expressed in conceptual, social, and practical adaptive skills that originate before the age of 18.[9] According to the *Diagnostic and Statistical Manual, 5th edition (DSM-5)*, published by the American Psychiatric Association, there are three criteria that must be met in order for an individual to receive the diagnosis of ID. First, there should be documented limitations in intellectual functioning such as reasoning, comprehension, problem solving, or the use of working memory. These limitations would generally fall at least 2 standard deviations below the mean for a given population on a standardized test of intelligence. This would correspond to an IQ score of 65 to 75 or lower. The second criterion is that there is a limitation in adapted functioning. This would be caused by the intellectual impairments that require the individual to need ongoing support in order to function as would be expected for their age and sociocultural background. These need to be in one or more of their societal roles, for example, in school, at home, or in the workplace. This limitation in adapted functioning results from difficulty in the ability to reason and function in the academic, social, or practical realms. The third criterion is that these limitations have their origin before the individual's 18th birthday. The *DSM-5* criteria are clear that given the multifaceted nature of this diagnosis, the decision to classify this learning difficulty should be informed by clinical judgment and should not rely on standardized tests of intelligence alone.[10]

This definition reflects a continued emphasis on the adaptive behavior dimensions but differs from earlier definitions by adding that these limitations result in the need for ongoing support. For example, an individual with an ID may require intermittent, limited, extensive, or pervasive support to function competently in their daily routines of life. ID are generally regarded as a condition existing in an individual that is described by the specific performance of the individual not resulting from a specific trait, although it is influenced by certain characteristics or capabilities of the individual. Rather, ID describe a performance *state* in which functioning is impaired. This distinction is central to understanding how the present definition broadens the concept of ID and how it shifts the emphasis from measurement of traits to understanding the individual's actual functioning in everyday living within their own sociocultural context. For any individual with ID, the description of its current state of functional behavior requires knowledge of the individual's capabilities as well as an understanding of the behavior within the structure and expectations of the individual's personal, social, and cultural environment.

❱❱ Incidence

Using the identifier of two or more standard deviations below the mean as part of the definition, about 3% of the population of the United States is assumed to have ID, but only 1% to 1.5% are actually diagnosed with this condition.[10] Approximately 80% of the causes of ID are unknown. ID are four times more prevalent among males than females. Seventy-five percent of all people with ID have a mild form, 20% a moderate form, and 5% have a severe or profound form.[10] One of the most prevalent forms of ID is Down syndrome, which is discussed later in this chapter.

❱❱ Diagnosis and classification

A diagnosis of ID is based on the criteria embodied within the definition reflecting intellectual functioning level, adaptive skill level, and age of onset of the disability.

Assessment of Intellectual Functioning

A child's intellectual functioning is determined to be significantly below average on the basis of a standardized intelligence test, usually administered by a psychologist. Fulfillment of this criterion for the diagnosis of ID is made on the basis of two or more standard deviations below an IQ of 100, considered "normal," or an IQ of 70 or 75 or below.[10] The instruments most commonly used for the assessment of intellectual functioning in children are the Stanford-Binet Intelligence Scale[9,11]; one of the Wechsler Scales, such as Wechsler Intelligence Scale for Children-IV[9,12] or Wechsler Preschool and Primary Scale of Intelligence III,[13] and the Kaufman Assessment Battery for Children.[14] In nonverbal individuals, the Comprehensive Test of Nonverbal Intelligence, second edition (C-TONI-2), may be a useful diagnostic tool,

and at times the Bayley Scales of Infant Development have been used in place of intelligence testing on children with profound intellectual impairment.[9] These tests are usually administered by a trained school or clinical psychologist and should be used in coordination with clinical judgment to make a diagnosis.[9]

Assessment of Adaptive Skill Level

Impairments in adaptive functioning, rather than low IQ, are usually the presenting symptoms in individuals with ID.[10] Adaptive skills are those skills considered to be central to successful life functioning and are frequently related to the need for support for persons with ID. The adaptive areas in which limitations are specifically exhibited are in the following areas: communication, self-care, home living, social skills, community use, self-direction, health and safety, functional academics, leisure, and work. In order to fulfill the diagnostic criteria for ID, deficits in one or more areas of adaptive functioning must be present, thus showing a generalized limitation in adaptive skill level.[10] In order to address the level of adaptive behaviors, the practitioner must perform a standardized functional assessment of the child's behavior across all environmental settings. Several scales are available to measure adaptive functioning, such as the Vineland Adaptive Behavior Scales[15] and the American Association on Intellectual Disabilities Adaptive Behavior Scale.[16] Any decision made using a standardized measure should also be informed by clinical reasoning and should take into consideration the typical functioning of an individual, not the person's best or maximum performance.[9] Additional sources of information regarding adapted skill level may be taken from parent report or developmental, educational, and mental health evaluations.[10] Table 24.1 describes the general adaptive behavioral characteristics of children and adults with different levels of ID.[16]

TABLE 24.1.	Adaptive Behavior Characteristics of Persons with Intellectual Disability Chronological Age of the Person with Intellectual Disability		
IQ	Preschool	School-Aged	Adult
50–55 to 70	Often appears unimpaired; develops functional social and communication skill	Academic skills of 6th grade are possible; special education support is needed for secondary—school	Can learn social and vocational skills
35–40 to 50–55	Impaired social skills; can communicate; may need supervision	Can develop up to 4th grade academic skills with special training/modification	Unskilled or semiskilled vocation
20–25 to 35–40	Severely impaired communication; impaired motor skills	May learn to communicate; basic personal health habits; limited academic skills	Needs complete support and supervision for any self-support activity
<20–25	Requires full support; dependent for care; limited sensorimotor development	Some motor development; continues to be dependent for care; limited success with training	Limited motor ability and communication; continued dependency for care

Updated by authors from original source.[16]

» Classification

In keeping with contemporary disablement models,[17–19] the key elements in the definition of ID include *capabilities, environment, functional limitations, and participation restriction.* Current classification carries with it an application of the new diagnostic criteria directly correlated with need for support. Needed support will vary along many dimensions: First, support may be necessary in some areas of adaptive skills but not in others. Second, support requirements may be time limited or ongoing. Third, the intensities of the support required, the types of support resources, and the support functions will be specific to the individual and the life cycle. It is important to note that the need for support may vary across environments as well as the life span. There are basically four intensities of support: intermittent, limited, extensive, and pervasive. Similarly, support services may come to the child with ID from four sources: the individual child (e.g., ability to make choices), other people (e.g., parent, teacher), technology (e.g., an augmentative communication device or a tablet with alarms and schedules), or habilitation services (e.g., PT, OT, Speech Therapy).[9]

Educational Classification

Current special education practices are shaped by both the definition of ID and the need for support services. Contemporary educational placement terms follow a more functional approach, highlighting the need for support and thereby being descriptive of the child's needs for educational success. This descriptive terminology for educational programs through which many children with ID may be served, depending on the child's priority needs, include support described as follows:

- Autistic support
- Learning support
- Life skills support
- Emotional support
- Visual support
- Hearing support
- Speech and language support
- Physical support
- Multiple disabilities support[20]

Physical therapy in the educational setting is considered to be a related service to special education and is discussed in another chapter of this text.

Medical Classification

Medical classification, according to the *Diagnostic and Statistical Manual of Mental Disorders, 5th ed. (DSM-5),*[10] has evolved to be more comprehensive of the child's presentation and is not based on IQ levels as had been the case in previous editions.

The World Health Organization's ICD 10 code system also classifies the severity of ID using IQ score but with adapted functioning as a supplement to IQ in designating a classification.[9] However, the most current view of intellectual functioning uses a multidimensional approach rather than relying on IQ scores alone.[9,10] The *DSM-5* categorizes the severity of disability as mild, moderate, severe, or profound by considering the ability of the individual to function within their environment in three domains. These are the conceptual, social, and practical demands.[10]

» Etiology and pathophysiology

Over 350 etiologies for ID have been identified.[21,22] There are four categories of risk factors that can lead to an ID, including biomedical, social, behavioral, and educational factors.[9] These factors often interact with one another and may change over time. The etiologic causes of ID could be divided into two broad categories. These are ID resulting from psychosocial disadvantage such as poverty, abuse or neglect and ID resulting from biologic causes.[9] Etiologic causes with examples are depicted in Table 24.2. Movement disorders are associated more with some etiologies than with others. Many children also present with a variety of associated disorders such as visual, hearing, or additional medical problems. In approximately 30% to 40% of individuals with ID seen in educational or clinical settings, no clear etiology can be determined despite extensive evaluation efforts.[10] When working with the child with intellectual disability, it is important for the physical therapist to understand what the cause of the impairment is and to become familiar with what particular challenges and impairments are associated with the etiology. With modern genetic testing, many new chromosomal anomalies are being identified, and our understanding on how this affects individuals is continually evolving.

» Primary impairments

Neuromotor Impairments

Many types of ID have associated neuromuscular, musculoskeletal, and cardiopulmonary impairments. Table 24.3 details the most common ID conditions and their associated neuromotor impairments.[23–38] Most neuromuscular impairments result from primary pathology in the central nervous system (CNS). Secondary impairments include deficits typically of concern to the physical therapist such as deficits in motor control, coordination, postural control, force production, flexibility, and balance.[39] Physical therapy evaluation and treatment of these impairments

TABLE 24.2. Etiologic Classification of Intellectual Disabilities

Prenatal Onset	Examples
1. Chromosomal disorder	Down, Turner, or Klinefelter syndrome
2. Syndrome disorders	Neurofibromatosis, myotonic muscular dystrophy, Prader-Will, tuberous sclerosis
3. Inborn errors of metabolism	Phenylketonuria, carbohydrate disorders, mucopolysaccharide disorders (e.g., Hurler type), nucleic acid disorders (e.g., Lesch-Nyhan syndrome)
4. Developmental disorders of brain formation	Neural tube closure defects (e.g., anencephaly), hydrocephalus, porencephaly, microcephaly
5. Environmental influences	Intrauterine malnutrition, drugs, toxins, alcohol, narcotics, maternal diseases
Perinatal Causes	
6. Intrauterine disorders	Placental insufficiency, maternal sepsis, abnormal labor or delivery
7. Neonatal disorders	Intracranial hemorrhage, periventricular leukomalacia, seizures, infections, respiratory disorders, head trauma, metabolic disorder
Postnatal Causes	
8. Head injuries	Intracranial hemorrhage, contusion, concussion
9. Infections	Encephalitis, meningitis, viral infections
10. Demyelinating disorders	Postinfectious and postimmunization disorders
11. Degenerative disorders	Syndromic disorders (e.g., Rett syndrome), poliodystrophies (e.g., Friedreich ataxia), basal ganglia disorder, leukodystrophies
12. Seizure disorders	Infantile spasms, myoclonic epilepsy
13. Toxic-metabolic disorders	Reye syndrome, lead intoxication, metabolic disorders (e.g., hypoglycemia)
14. Malnutrition	Protein-calorie, prolonged IV alimentation
15. Environmental deprivation	Psychosocial disadvantage, child abuse/neglect

From American Association on Intellectual Disabilities (AAID). 1719 Kalorama Road, NW, Washington, DC, 20009-2683; and International Classification of Functioning, Disability and Health (ICF). Geneva, Switzerland World Health Organization; 2001.

TABLE 24.3. Neuromuscular, Musculoskeletal, and Cardiopulmonary Impairment Associated with Selected Conditions of Intellectual Disability

Condition	Neuromuscular	Musculoskeletal	Cardiopulmonary
Cri-du-chat syndrome[23]	Hypotonia in early childhood sometimes later hypertonia	Minor upper extremity anomalies, scoliosis	Congenital heart disease common
Cytomegalovirus[24] (prenatal infection)	Hypertonia, seizures, microcephaly	Secondary to neuromuscular problems	Mitral stenosis, pulmonary valvular stenosis, atrial septal defect
De Lange syndrome[25,26]	Spasticity, seizures, intention tremor, microcephaly	Decreased bone age, small stature, small hands and feet, short digits, proximal thumb placement, clinodactyly fifth digit, other hand and finger defects, limited elbow extension	Neonatal respiratory problems, cardiac malformations, recurrent upper respiratory tract infections
Down syndrome[27,28]	Hypotonia, low muscle force production, slow postural reactions, slow reaction time, motor delays increasing with age	Joint hyperflexibility, ligamentous laxity, foot deformities, scoliosis, atlanto-hypertension axial instability (20%)	Congenital heart disease (40%), lung hypoplasia with pulmonary
Fetal alcohol syndrome[26,29]	Fine motor dysfunction, visual-motor deficits, weak grasp, ptosis	Joint anomalies with abnormal position or function, maxillary hypoplasia	Heart murmur- often disappears after first year
Fragile X syndrome[30,31]	Hypotonia, poor coordination and motor planning, seizures	Hyperextensible finger joints, prominent jaw, scoliosis	Mitral valve prolapse
Hurler's syndrome[22,26]	Hydrocephalus	Joint contractures, claw-like deformities of hands, short fingers, thoracolumbar kyphosis, shallow acetabular and glenoid fossae, irregularly shaped bones	Cardiac deformities such as cardiac enlargement due to right ventricular hypertension, death frequently due to cardiac failure

(continued)

TABLE 24.3.	Neuromuscular, Musculoskeletal, and Cardiopulmonary Impairment Associated with Selected Conditions of Intellectual Disability (*continued*)		
Condition	**Neuromuscular**	**Musculoskeletal**	**Cardiopulmonary**
Lesch-Nyhan sydrome[32]	Hypotonia followed by spasticity, chorea, and athetosis/dystonia; compulsive self-injurious behavior	Secondary to neuromuscular problems	
Prader-Willi syndrome[33,34]	Severe hypotonia and feeding problems in infancy, excessive eating and obesity in childhood, poor fine and gross motor coordination	Short stature, small hands and feet	May be associated with cor pulmonale (most common cause of death)
Rett syndrome[35–38]	Hypotonia in infancy, than gradually increasing hypertonia and lack of acquired skill; ataxia, apraxia, choreoathetosis and/or dystonia, progression from hyperkinesia to bradykinesia with age, slow reaction time, stereotypic hand movements (clapping, wringing, clenching) drooling, involuntary rhythmic tongue movement/deviation, seizures	Scoliosis, kyphosis, joint contractures, hip subluxation or dislocation, equinovarus deformities	Immature respiratory patterns, breathing irregularities, such as hyperventilation, apnea
Williams syndrome[26,29] (elfin facies)	Mild neurologic dysfunction, poor motor coordination	Hallux valgus	Variable congenital heart disease

Adapted with permission from McEwen I. Intellectual Disabilities. In: Campbell SK, ed. *Physical Therapy for Children*, ed. 4. Philadelphia: WB Saunders, 2011.

for children with ID are similar to those procedures used in any pediatric setting. The use of Table 24.3 can guide the pediatric physical therapist in anticipating typical management concerns associated with common ID disorders. The ID itself, viewed as an additional or confounding impairment, requires some adaptation in evaluation and treatment application because of the specific cognitive limitations presented by the child.

Learning Impairment

Learning is impaired in children with ID. Children with ID demonstrate an impaired ability to utilize advanced cognitive processes, manage simultaneous or multiple demands, and successfully organize complex information, with subsequent effects on task performance as well as task mastery.[40] Poor memory, limited generalization (i.e., the inability to perform a learned task across different environments), and poor motivation may also impair the learning of a child with an ID.[41] Memory impairment is seen when these individuals have difficulty recalling multistep directions or steps to complete a task. When an individual cannot generalize, a change in settings may be extremely challenging. Finally, the slow learning rate and frequent failure to learn experienced by individuals with ID can produce a low level of motivation and self-determination in the acquisition of many necessary life skills.

Physical therapists must be able to adapt examination and intervention approaches to accommodate the impaired intellectual functioning. Clearly, the range of cognitive deficit and ability found in children with ID is indicative of variant levels of performance, functioning, and potential.[42] It is the task and the challenge of the therapist to assist the child to maximize his or her potential for optimum functioning and participation across environments.

» Physical therapy examination and intervention principles

Key Elements of Examination

Meaningful examination always maintains a focus on the child's functioning as the key issue. A successful and effective physical therapy examination of the child with ID depends largely on the therapist's approach to the child. Four important elements should facilitate the process of examination.

First, throughout the examination, the therapist must analyze not only what the child can do but also the *processes underlying the observed skills and behaviors.*[43] Thus, the therapist must determine not only what tasks the child can do but also why the child can do those specific tasks and not others. Movements must be broken down into components, and basic mental, physiologic, and physical processes must be analyzed in relation to those tasks.

Second, examination procedures used for children, particularly children with ID, often differ from the more rigid clinical procedures used for adults. In pediatrics, much information can be gathered by interacting with the child through observation and during play. In view of challenges with following directions, attention, or behavior, it can be challenging to perform standardized testing with a child with an ID; however, standard examination tests and outcome measures are important tools for identifying the need for physical therapy intervention, setting and monitoring progress toward goals, and evaluating the effectiveness of a particular intervention. At times it may be necessary to complete examination and testing over several sessions, as trust and rapport with the child is established. Consistent with the functional approach to curriculum and intervention planning, the physical therapist should perform an examination with as many *functional aspects,* using age-appropriate materials, as is reasonable.

The third important element necessary for appropriate examination is related to the basic orientation of the therapist. As with other areas of physical therapy, but more importantly with the child with multiple disabilities, the therapist must be able to identify not only the disability but also the child's abilities, however minimal. The skilled therapist will identify even the smallest of abilities and effectively communicate the importance of those abilities to the child, parents, and other professionals working with the child. A major focus of intervention involves attempts to increase those abilities. This *"positive" orientation and approach* will have a beneficial effect on the child's self-image and on those people working with the child.[44] If our actions suggest a true concern and expectation for progress, however limited that progress may be, the effect of this attitude should encourage the child, the teachers, and the family to strive toward goals that have been identified.[44]

The fourth important element in examination is that the therapist must always concurrently address *sensory processes and attention*. Children experience their world through their senses and the feedback they receive from sensory input as well as their interaction with the information. They assimilate the information; they take action; and they consequently modify any subsequent actions. Children with ID have been shown to have difficulty utilizing sensory information, resulting in an increased reaction time and increased time to complete a motor task.[45] The therapist must understand by what means—or even whether—the child perceives the world, including the examiner, before continuing with the examination.

Sensory Examination and Intervention

The therapist must determine the basic responsiveness of the child before deciding on an appropriate interaction strategy for the rest of the examination. An early educator, Kinnealy, distinguished two broad categories of behaviors typical of children with ID on the basis of their reactions to various sensory stimuli or environmental input.[46] She described one group as having difficulty monitoring the intensity of sensory input and, therefore, difficulty in modulating the response. The other group was described as having reduced perception of the incoming stimuli and required more intense input for arousal or elicitation of a response. This initial difference in perception of sensory stimulus is a critical point of departure that the therapist must ascertain during the first attempt at interaction with the child.

Visual

When examining the child's visual sense, the therapist should note the ability of the child to orient to, focus on, and track a visual stimulus. Notable responses include difficulty in tracking across the midline and noting the presence or absence of resting eye movements (nystagmus). During intervention and integration into classroom activities, visual stimulation activities can be used to provide practice in both focusing and tracking. Children who have poor head control may have an inadequate base of support for eye movements. Intervention aimed at improving postural mechanisms may improve visual skill.[43] Children with ID have limited ability to use visual information to prepare for and execute motor tasks, and, therefore, physical prompts or guiding an individual through a task as well as adaptive aids to ensure proper body positioning should be used as needed.[45] Vestibular input may also improve visual focusing and processing because vestibular reflexes, in combination with optic and tonic neck reflexes, maintain a stable image on the retina while the head and body are in motion.[43] The vestibulo-oculomotor pathways contribute to skilled movements of the eyes that can be used for educational skills, including reading and writing (Fig. 24.2).

Auditory

The child's response to auditory stimuli may range from an absence of response to simple orientation to and movement toward the stimulus to a startle response.[43] Although it is difficult to examine hearing loss in a child with ID or multiple handicaps, referral for a complete audiologic evaluation is indicated whenever there is a possibility of a hearing loss. Audiologic testing can be used to identify a hearing loss, to differentiate between conductive and sensorineural loss, and to quantify the degree of loss. Tympanometry (an objective measure of eardrum function) helps identify a conductive hearing loss when behavioral testing is unreliable. Testing for brain stem–evoked response traces the passage of an auditory stimulus from the ear to the brain stem. Central or cortical deafness describes a lack of interpretation of auditory information caused by brain damage.

Vestibular stimulation is a component of intervention aimed at enhancing auditory integration. Although the

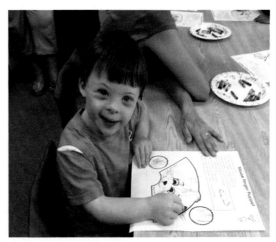

FIGURE 24.2. Angelo engaged in visual-motor and fine motor activity.

vestibulocochlear nerve (cranial nerve VIII) has been described as comprising two separate entities (vestibular and auditory), it developed phylogenetically as a unit, and its portions appear to be related functionally.[43] There is clear clinical evidence that difficulties in hearing interfere with equilibrium responses. Vestibular input, such as the use of ride-on toys, swings, or therapy balls, may not only improve equilibrium reactions but may also sometimes enhance auditory attention and integration.[47]

Tactile

The tactile system is the largest sensory system, and it plays a major role in both physical and emotional behavior.[48,49] The tactile system develops earliest in utero, and the ability to process tactile input is important for neural organization. The sensation of touch is, in fact, the "oldest and most primitive expressive channel" and is a primary system for making contact with the external environment.[49,50] When threatened, there is a predominant response of increased alertness and increased affect. When not challenged, however, the person is free to explore and manipulate the environment.[51,52] Many children with developmental disorders have a disordered tactile system. With neurologic impairment, many children demonstrate an aversive response to some types of tactile stimulation. This aversion to tactile stimuli, called *tactile defensiveness,* is often manifested by such behavior as hyperactivity or distractibility.[51] Children who demonstrate tactile defensiveness may display avoidance reactions around the hands, feet, and face. This behavior has obvious implications for the manner in which a child explores the environment, appreciates tactile sensation, and thus learns. Tactile defensiveness in the oral area may cause the child to reject textured or flavored food in preference to smoother, blander foods.

It has been suggested that tactile defensiveness is part of a generalized "set" of the nervous system by which the child interprets stimuli as "danger."[51] Tactile functions were among the first means by which the child received information about his or her environment in order to adapt appropriately. The result of a developmental disorder is often behavior that appears to be less sophisticated and less discriminatory than normal. Tactile defensiveness or overresponsiveness may be seen in this context as poorly developed mechanisms for the interpretation of information. Clinically, the child may appear anxious, emotionally labile, or threatened and unable to cope. Compensatory behavior may be characterized by withdrawal, irritability, or distractibility.[51] Ayres has suggested various intervention approaches designed to facilitate increased organization of the tactile system and increased integration of this subsystem into effective environmental interaction. The proprioceptive system plays a cooperative role in this functional scheme.[51] The physical therapist can easily incorporate appropriate activities for both the tactile and the proprioceptive systems into intervention. Heavy touch or weight bearing are excellent activities for decreasing tactile

hypersensitivity and promoting proximal joint stability. Light touch or stimuli that tickle or irritate the child should be avoided in favor of activities that offer deep pressure.

The response of the child with ID to tactile input must be observed and monitored during examination and intervention. The therapist must note whether the child responds to the stimulus (i.e., the touch of the therapist's hand), and if a response is noted, the therapist must identify the type of response. If the input is noxious, does the child respond with a grimace, or does the child move actively to avoid the stimulus? One might surmise that the child who actively removes or withdraws from the noxious stimulus is not only aware of the stimulus but also has some proprioceptive sense by which to locate and remove the stimulus. Conversely, the therapist must be aware of the child who is so totally unaware of sensory input that the therapist is unable to penetrate and reach the child by any means. Clearly, knowing the level of awareness of the child will direct the therapist through subsequent stages of the evaluation and intervention process.[52]

Vestibular

Along with the tactile system, the vestibular system is one of the earliest developing sensory systems in the human being. The tracts within the vestibular system are fully myelinated by 20 weeks of gestation.[51] Information from the vestibular system tells us our position exactly in relation to gravity, whether or not we are moving, and our speed and direction of movement.[48] The vestibular system is so sensitive that changes in position and movement have a powerful effect on the brain, and this effect changes with even the most subtle adjustments of movement or posture.[51]

The vestibular system has a strong effect on muscle tone and movement. This influence is mediated through the lateral and medial vestibular nuclei and affects efferent transmission to both intrafusal and extrafusal muscle fibers. Vestibular influence usually exerts a facilitatory effect on the gamma motoneuron to the muscle spindle and may influence the alpha motor neurons supplying skeletal muscle. By activating the gamma efferent to the muscle spindle, the afferent flow from the spindle is maintained and regulated for assistance with motor function. This basic role in muscle function and mobility gives the vestibular system an important role in the development and maintenance of body scheme that depends on interpretation of movement.[50,51] Impulses ascending to brain stem and cortical levels synapse with tactile, proprioceptive, visual, and auditory impulses to provide both perception of space and orientation of the body within that space.[48] Vestibular input seldom enters conscious thought or awareness except when the stimulus is so intense that we are rendered dizzy. It is important to know whether the child overreacts to or is threatened by movement or has difficulty in attending to and assimilating movement experiences.[53] With a knowledge of the child's response to vestibular stimulation, activities can be chosen to improve balance, simulate experience of movement, activate muscle contraction, promote awareness and eye contact, and increase spatial awareness and perception. Examples of equipment used in these movement activities include swings, barrels, and scooter boards.

Self-Stimulation

Self-stimulation in some children with ID is an area of concern. This type of behavior can take many forms, including self-abuse. Examples of self-stimulation include constant mouthing of objects or the hand, spinning, head banging, hand or arm flapping, teeth grinding, rocking, and self-biting. Evaluation of the sensory status of the child may identify the reason for self-stimulation. The behavior could have a function or goal, such as to attain attention or avoid a demand, or the child may be performing self-stimulation to fulfill a basic sensory need, or he or she may be overstimulated and may be reacting out of frustration or an inability to cope with sensory overload.[42,54]

In educational programs, the tendency is to discourage self-stimulation, especially when the stimulation is abusive or socially unacceptable. An appropriate sensory input must be substituted or the child may substitute another form of self-stimulation. A child who cannot cope with the sensory stimuli in the environment and is being overstimulated needs to have sensory input graded to tolerance.[42,54] As in all other areas of evaluation and intervention, the therapist must look beyond the behavior to the processes that are initiating it. Underlying sensory abnormalities or deficiencies must be recognized and intervened before a change in behavior can be expected.

The manner in which the child provides self-stimulation can suggest strategies that may be effective in improving or eliminating the behavior. Slow, rhythmic rocking may be the distractible child's method of calming himself or herself, whereas violent, irregular rocking may be the hypotonic child's method of providing sensory input that will increase muscle activation and alertness. The type of behavior must also be considered in light of the developmental age of the child. Constant mouthing of objects and hands is socially unacceptable for a school-aged child. If, however, that child is functioning at a lower developmental and functional level than age would dictate, oral exploration is a primary component of the learning process.[42,54] Rather than restricting such oral exploration and stimulation, the child must be provided means of oral stimulation, such as toothbrushing, the use of an appropriate substitution such as a chewable toy or tubing and foods of various textures, in order to help facilitate progression to the next developmental and functional level.[54,55]

To summarize, the physical therapist examining the child with ID must have various skills and must approach the evaluation with a flexible but organized strategy. Examination must include not only developmental, functional, musculoskeletal, postural and strength tests and measures but also an evaluation of the sensory systems. Because the main goal of intervention is to enhance developmental skill attainment and to improve function, there must be a thorough examination of all sensory and motor components of development. It is challenging and rewarding to examine such a complex group of skill areas and still have a concise picture of the whole child.

» Key elements of physical therapy intervention

General Principles

Intervention with and management of the child with ID must be directed toward the development of the child's full potential in all areas of learning: motor, cognitive, and affective. The child's ability to respond appropriately and effectively in terms of movement, intellectual function, and attitudes and feelings serves as the major long-range goal of intervention. This concept of intervention applies to the total function of the child. A deficit in one type of behavior may influence all other types. The child who needs motor stability may also benefit from psychological stability. Influences used to change the former may also have an effect on the latter and vice versa.[44,56]

Several important elements need to be remembered when designing effective intervention programs for children with ID. The therapist must recognize the importance of choosing activities that not only accommodate the cognitive capabilities of the child but that are also as age-appropriate as possible. Activities in the intervention program should be interesting, fun, and meaningful. Because children with ID often have a poor attention span, therapeutic activities should be chosen that most effectively and efficiently meet the identified goal. Rather than asking a child to do standard physical therapy exercises for strengthening, the necessary therapeutic activities can be translated into a functional task or social game, often including other family members. This approach not only sustains interest, cooperation, and enthusiasm, but also emphasizes carryover into activities of daily living. It may also promote achievement of goals in other areas, such as social, emotional, self-help, and cognitive skills. Children with ID have difficulty generalizing a skill from one activity to a different context, setting, or location. Ideally, skills should be practiced in the natural location where they typically take place, such as the school or home. If this is not possible, the therapist should strive to ensure that any skill practiced should resemble as closely as possible the context in which it will be functionally used. If a child is seen in a clinical setting, families and others providing support to an individual should be instructed to practice the skill in the home or other locations to encourage carryover to these settings. The therapist must be imaginative and should integrate many different approaches in order to develop an effective intervention approach for a particular child in a particular situation (Fig. 24.3).

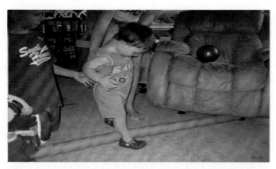

FIGURE 24.3. Two-year-old Angelo navigating his way around environmental obstacles and refining his postural control and balance.

Repetition and consistency are crucial aspects of any program in which learning is expected to occur. Because repetition is important for learning any task, the therapist must design several activities that teach the same component task but do so in different ways. For example, if the goal is to improve extension strength of the trunk, the therapist may use activities such as a basketball drop or scooter board games. These activities are varied but enjoyable methods of attaining the same goal. This approach to program planning not only ensures the necessary repetition of activities, but also offers the dimensions of interest and fun for a child with limited comprehension or attention.

One of the most important yet most difficult skills for the therapist to master is the ability to delineate priorities for intervention and to establish effective and appropriate long-term plans. When the therapist is faced with the challenge of a child with numerous deficits in many areas of development, it is easy for the therapist to become overwhelmed. When developing intervention plans, it is important to consider the child as a whole person. All pieces of the evaluation puzzle should merge to provide the therapist with a composite picture of how the child is or is not functioning within the child's world. The priorities for programming should become clear by looking at the child's overall development in this functional sense.

Learning Characteristics

Differences in the Child with ID

An overview of cognitive development is necessary in order to understand the cognitive limitation of the child with ID and to design effective treatment programs to overcome those cognitive limitations.

Piaget's Theory of Intellectual Development

Jean Piaget, in order to explain normal and abnormal intellectual development, divided the developmental process into four stages: the sensorimotor period (0 to 18 months); the preoperational stage (2 to 7 years); the stage of concrete operations (7 to 12 years); and the period of

formal operations (12 years and older).[57] The delineations offered by Piaget's stages provide a basis for understanding the sequence of normal development and the limitations that are typical at each stage of cognitive development. The Piagetian theory of development can be useful in understanding the various degrees of cognitive impairment seen in ID.

Children learn mainly through exploration of the senses and through movement during the sensorimotor stage, which Piaget explained as an equilibration process. The unknown is presented as a confrontation with the unexplained and less understood, and the child learns by his or her attempts to manipulate the environment with strategies with which to create new understandings, called accommodations. The inability to coordinate sensorimotor activity to reach certain goals is displayed by children with behaviors reflective of seriously impaired cognitive abilities, many of whom have coexisting physical and sensory impairments. Children thought to be functioning at this early stage explore their environment through much experimentation, which may even be repeated over and over. Accommodations to manage the environment when not routinely understood cannot be generalized to new situations. In fact, most learning involves discoveries made by trial and error. The preoperational stage is characterized by the development of language and the beginnings of abstract thought. Children at this stage can use symbols to represent objects that are not present and may be able to classify and group objects, although not proficiently. A child with an IQ between 35 and 55 may not develop beyond this stage.[57]

During the concrete operations stage, the ability to order, classify, and relate experience to an organized whole begins to develop.[57] The child can solve some mathematical problems and can read well. The child can generalize learning to new situations and can begin to recognize another person's point of view. There is still an inability to deal with hypothetical or abstract problems. Persons with mild cognitive impairments often remain at this level of development.[57]

Piaget's final stage—formal operations—normally begins at 12 years of age and continues throughout life. The abilities to reason and hypothesize are characteristic of this stage. The child with ID seldom reaches this level of development. Cognitively, these children have characteristically limited memory, general knowledge, and abstract thinking, all combined with a slower learning rate.[58]

Intervention to Limit Cognitive Impairment

Concrete Concepts Compared with Abstract Concepts

Children with ID are less able to grasp abstract concepts than concrete concepts. When working with children with ID, the therapist must present concepts using meaningful, concrete directions. Activities are best understood when demonstrated, done passively first or translated into familiar functional activities pertaining to daily life. Using step-by-step examples and pictures to represent activities would be useful to building understanding of the expectations. The child learns from telling, retelling, demonstrating, practicing, and ultimately actually performing in the "real" environment. Therapists need to understand the performance level in order to plan and direct the intervention plan.

Memory

The ability of a person with ID to remember is related to the type of retention task involved. Use of short-term memory is consistently difficult for the child with ID.[56,59] There is a high level of distractibility caused by external, irrelevant stimuli associated with these short-term memory deficits. However, overcoming this short-term memory problem can be dealt with by repetitions to enhance the use of long-term memory, an area that tends to be a relative strength for children with ID. In light of this knowledge, some of the following strategies can be used during physical therapy sessions.

- Remove irrelevant, distracting material from the activity area. Do not work with the child in distracting surroundings, even if room dividers or curtains must be used to separate a small space from a larger, busy area.
- Present each component of the task clearly and separately.
- Begin with simple tasks and then progress to more difficult tasks.
- Explain your expectations of the child at each stage of the intervention.
- Try to support the tasks with visual aids, or model the task repeatedly.
- Give immediate and consistent positive reinforcement.
- Repeat directions as often as necessary.
- Check the accuracy of performance frequently.
- Keep the child informed of progress, and give the child an opportunity to demonstrate or practice the new skill independently.

Most educators agree that practice, review, and overlearning help the child with ID with long-term retention of skills. The therapist can promote learning and retention with repetition of both the directions and the steps needed to complete the intended skill. It is important to provide ample opportunity to practice and use the newly learned material. Physical therapists inform parents and teachers of a child's progress and should encourage practice of the newly learned task at home or in the classroom. Learning cannot occur or be retained when the physical therapy sessions are an isolated segment of the child's day. Here again, the use of pictures and examples to extend the learning could be developed for the child to use in the home or community. Extended practice and communication with other team members are both vital.

Transfer of Learning

Transfer of learning is the ability to apply newly learned material to new situations having components that are similar to those of the material that was newly learned.[60] The Piagetian term for this process is assimilation. The learning challenge has been understood, and the child has invented new strategies that are found to be useful in performing within the environment. The literature on transfer of learning suggests that two factors, in particular, be considered when formulating a plan for intervention.

Meaningfulness is an important element in transfer of learning for the child with cognitive impairment. A meaningful task is both easier to learn at the outset and easier to transfer to a second setting than one that has no meaning for the learner. This concept strongly supports the use of functional activities during physical therapy as opposed to meaningless "splinter skills."

Moreover, learning can be transferred best when both the initial task and the transfer task are *similar*. If, for example, the therapist is working on the ability to push rather than to pull on an assistive device, all of the therapy tasks, such as pushing in a prone position, sitting push-ups, and other tasks, can be transferred more readily to the task of pushing on the assistive device. *Consistency* also helps the child see the connection between therapy tools and their function.

Knowledge of basic learning concepts and an understanding of cognitive development are crucial for the physical therapist working with a child who is intellectually impaired. Learning is enhanced through repetition and the use of visual aids, with demonstrations of the usefulness of the habilitation skill, all of which support the accommodation and the understanding, and thus fosters generalization of the skill. Physical therapy is a learning situation, and some modifications in approach will be necessary to accommodate the differences in performance seen in the child with ID.

Motor Learning Research and ID

Motor learning can be described as the process of producing "permanent changes in the capacity for producing action" through practice and experience.[61,62] This is an important line of research for pediatric physical therapists to be familiar with, in that it can help a therapist to design effective teaching methods for the practice of functional motor tasks. It has already been established that individuals with ID are thought to have limited ability to process complex information and learn new skills.[9] It is important for physical therapists to understand how those limitations affect the ability to learn functional motor tasks and how to best design intervention.

Implicit vs Explicit Feedback Individuals with ID have been found to benefit from practice that encourages the use of implicit information rather than the use of extrinsic feedback. For example, in learning a basic throwing task it is more effective for a child with an ID to focus on the success or failure of their movements than to receive feedback on the kinematics such as the position of their hands. This may be because practice with such internal factors such as hand position during a throw may rely on conscious control of the movement instead of a more automatic mode of control.[63] Therapists should use feedback regarding the success of individual trials during practice rather than providing specific instruction about body position or the quality of movement.

Frequency of Knowledge of Results—Receiving more frequent feedback will enhance the performance of a particular motor task over the short term but may interfere with the learning, retention, and transfer of a skill to a different setting or activity.[61]

Error Reduced Practice—Error Free or Error Reduced practice has also been shown to enhance motor learning in subjects both with and without ID. This suggests that it is more effective to design treatment and practice sessions so that the individual is successful in most of the initial trials and then gradually introduce the difficulty of the task. This error-free learning requires fewer cognitive resources, resulting in improved performance in children with ID, who possess reduced working memory skills.[64,65]

The therapist can use this information to enhance the motor learning of individuals with intellectual delays by:

- Structuring practice sessions with constraints that facilitate initial success and gradually increase difficulty over time
- Focus feedback on the overall goal and success of the task, rather than on providing coaching on the kinematics of the task
- Provide enough feedback on the outcome of the task in order to provide motivation but refrain from providing feedback on every or most trials, which can limit the retention of the task.

Intervention to Limit Physical Impairments and Functional Limitations

Pediatric physical therapists have traditionally focused their efforts on interventions designed to limit musculoskeletal, neuromuscular, and cardiopulmonary impairments; reduce functional limitations; and prevent secondary impairment.[39] Early identification of these musculoskeletal, neuromuscular, and cardiopulmonary problems and anticipation of their recognition as associated within specific diagnoses give the therapist an insight into appropriate life span management of the child with ID. A glance again at Table 24.3 gives the therapist familiarity with some of the specific musculoskeletal, neuromuscular, or cardiopulmonary risks associated with common types of ID. Within this chapter, a focus on physical therapy management for the child with Down syndrome will offer the entry-level therapist a strategy for applying this management model to any child with any type of intellectual disabilities diagnosis. The child's needs change throughout the life span and will determine the level of support intervention required by physical therapy. Although this text is a pediatric physical therapy resource, this author will discuss life span management issues relevant to the client with developmental disabilities as he or she moves into and through adulthood.

The Importance of Focused Intervention

Interventions designed by the therapist should be directed by the results of the multifaceted examination and guided by the findings of the functional examination. Together these findings will provide the therapist and the intervention team with direction in order to design focused interventions that address not only skills but also their application in the various environments interfaced by the child. Following the design of the intervention plan, multiple task analyses will guide the specific intervention strategies.

To ensure the desired learning, the therapist is encouraged to design discrete tasks that reflect the child's participation within the current environments and to set goals that increase the participation levels. Goals should be established by the physical therapist in coordination with the child and the child's family. This will address the child's need for meaningful, purposeful, and concrete activities to more naturally provide the motivation to learn. As mentioned earlier, children with cognitive impairment learn better through multimodal teaching. Therapists are encouraged to use these techniques while teaching new tasks and practicing those previously introduced. In order to do this, we encourage the use of the "Practitioner's P's" methodology: plan, present, picture, practice, perform. First, it is important to *plan* the procedures for learning in specific discrete steps. Next, the therapist needs to be *present* in ways that are understood by the child, being aware of any communication needs uncovered during the evaluation stages. Following the presentation of the tasks to be learned during the session, the *picture* of the task to be performed should be presented, as well. This can be done through the use of pictures taken of the specific skill performance, through the use of available commercially produced stick-figure diagrams, or by showing a video clip. Another form would be the therapist modeling the task in step-by-step fashion. The fourth step is to have the child *practice* the task. In this portion of the session, the therapist guides the child through the steps of the task using the hand-over-hand methodology. The fifth and final P is for the child to *perform* the task. Using these P's, the therapist will be encouraged to use the multimodal methods more routinely.

≫ The team concept and collaboration

When working with the child with ID, physical therapists must view themselves and their intervention goals as part of a total management plan. Use of a transdisciplinary team of professionals is the standard approach for children with special needs. The child's parents or caregivers are also a crucial part of this team because they are most familiar with the child's development and needs across their life span. The current inclusion model offers strong support for the team concept. Comprehensive delivery of services for the child with ID is beyond the scope of any single professional discipline. One of the main values of a transdisciplinary approach is the pooling of knowledge so that a composite and relevant course of action can be made. Because the child with ID will have delays in many areas of development, the skills of many professionals can be used. No single professional has the necessary scope of expertise or the resources to effectively provide care and education throughout the life of the child with ID.

In order to be effective, each professional on the team must understand the periodic shift of authority and emphasis at different times and different stages of development. Input from the physical therapist will sometimes be of paramount importance, whereas at other times, the priorities will lie in other areas of care. During these latter periods, the physical therapist may play a consultative or advisory role. Success of the team in its primary purpose of helping the child achieve his or her maximum potential will depend on each professional considering the whole child, while offering the needed expertise to alleviate specific problems. Communication among team members and respect for one another's unique knowledge and skills are keys to making the team process truly collaborative and therefore effective.

Effective use of all team members will ensure that consistency and reinforcement are present throughout the child's total program. For example, if certain sounds are being taught in speech therapy, the learning of these sounds can be reinforced by using them during physical therapy sessions. The physical therapist and special education teacher must work as partners in working with the child. The therapist is uniquely qualified to assist the teacher in understanding the impact of impaired sensorimotor function on the achievement of cognitive milestones. For example, consider the child with severely impaired movement control, average head control, and preferred movement patterns dominated by poor motor control patterns and strong tonic reflex patterns. In such a case, knowledge of the basics of normal movement control development could be invaluable to the teacher when working on a cognitive skill with the child, such as performing a simple cause-and-effect activity. A simple suggestion from the therapist that the child be side-lying rather than supine could enable the child to reach for and manipulate the toy or utensil. Such a cooperative approach both facilitates the child's accomplishment of the educational goal and reduces the frustration of the teacher. The physical therapist must communicate and work with all members of the team, including the nurse, occupational therapist, psychologist, physician, teacher, physical education teacher, speech therapist, and parent. The present day model of inclusion certainly facilitates this collaborative team concept.

When working with children, physical therapists must recognize the importance of the parents as part of the

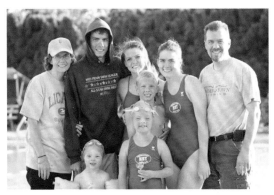

FIGURE 24.4. A family engaged in common fun physical activity, inclusive of Angelo and Julianna's interests and capabilities.

therapeutic team. Program carryover into the home and in daily life is important for maximum effectiveness. The parents must learn how to work effectively with the child and must be able to help achieve the goals of the program. This concept is true not only for physical therapy, but for all areas of intervention and education. When asking parents to participate in a home program of care, physical therapists must be able to evaluate the family's abilities, must respect the family's values and cultural beliefs and practices, and must recognize problems or conditions in the home that may limit the successful participation in the program. Suggestions and training to families should be realistic and meaningful and should be embedded in the daily routines of the family. Referral to appropriate agencies may help parents alleviate or resolve any problems or conditions that impede a family from supporting the child's development. The long-term nature of problems associated with ID and management of those problems requires a major commitment from the family (Fig. 24.4).

» A management model for physical therapists for the child with Down syndrome

Definition

Down syndrome is a chromosomal disorder resulting in 47 chromosomes instead of 46.[66] Commonly called trisomy 21, Down syndrome results from faulty cell division affecting the 21st pair of chromosomes, either owing to a nondisjunction (95%), translocation (3% to 4%), or, least commonly, as a mosaic presentation (1%).[66]

History and Incidence

Down syndrome is the most common cause of ID and is a diagnosis frequently encountered by pediatric physical therapists. Approximately 4,000 infants with Down syndrome are born annually in the United States at a rate increasing with maternal age, from 1 in 2,000 when the mother is aged 20, to 1 in 10 when the mother reaches the age of 49, with an overall incidence of 1 in 800 to 1 in 1,000 live births.[67]

Evidence of an awareness of Down syndrome dates back to early times, with the earliest anthropologic record stemming from excavations in the 7th century of a Saxon skull that had many of the structural changes associated with Down syndrome.[68] Artwork throughout the Middle Ages contains depictions of children with the now recognized facial characteristics of Down syndrome. Despite these early historical conjectures, there are no published documented reports of Down syndrome until the 19th century. This is understandable from a historical perspective because of the prevalence of infectious diseases and malnutrition that overshadowed research into genetic problems. Also, until beyond the mid-19th century, many children who were indeed born with Down syndrome probably died in early infancy.[68]

In 1846, Edouard Sequin described a patient with features suggestive of Down syndrome. In 1866, John Langdon Down published an article describing the characteristics of the then recognizable syndrome, which has since borne his name.[68] It was not until the mid-1950s that progress in methodologies to visualize chromosomes allowed more accurate studies of human chromosomes, leading to Lejeune's discovery that an alteration in the 21st chromosomal pair is the characteristic hallmark of Down syndrome.[69]

Pathophysiology and Associated Impairments of the Child with Down Syndrome

Down syndrome results in neuromotor, musculoskeletal, and cardiopulmonary pathologies, all of which require management by pediatric physical therapists. As with any etiology of ID, an awareness of the pathologies and impairments indigenous to that specific etiology will offer the practicing therapist a model for life span management for the child.

Neuropathology

The primary neuropathology underlying the CNS disorder in children with Down syndrome results from several well-documented brain abnormalities. Overall brain weight in individuals with Down syndrome is 76% of normal, with the combined weight of the cerebellum and brain stem being even smaller—66% of normal. There is also microcephaly, and the brain is abnormally rounded and short with a decreased A-P diameter, specifically called microbrachycephaly.[65] The number of secondary sulci is reduced, resulting in a simplicity of convoluted patterns in the brains of children with Down syndrome.[70] Several cytologic distinctions of the brain in Down syndrome include a paucity of small neurons, a migrational defect involving small neurons, and decreased synaptogenesis caused by altered synaptic morphology.[70] There are also structural abnormalities in the dendritic

spines in the pyramidal tracts of the motor cortex that possibly underlie the motor incoordination so often seen in children with Down syndrome.[66] Research also shows evidence of a lack of myelination as well as a delay in the completion of myelination between 2 months and 6 years of age, which may explain the overall developmental delay typically seen in children with Down syndrome.[71] Some studies claim that up to 8% of children with Down syndrome also have some form of seizure disorder.[72]

Sensory Deficits

Visual and hearing deficits, as well as speech impairments, are common in children with Down syndrome and have a direct impact on physical therapy examination and intervention. Visual deficits include congenital as well as adult onset cataracts, myopia (50%), farsightedness (20%), strabismus, and nystagmus.[72] Other ocular findings of less clinical significance include the presence of Brushfield spots in the iris and the classic presence of epicanthal folds.

Many children with Down syndrome (60% to 80%) are found to have a mild to moderate hearing loss.[72] Otitis media is a frequently occurring medical problem that may contribute to intermittent or persisting hearing loss in children with Down syndrome.[66]

Cardiopulmonary Pathologies

Forty percent of children with Down syndrome are born with congenital heart defects, most commonly atrioventricular canal defects and ventriculoseptal defects.[67] Although usually repaired in infancy, heart defects not corrected by age 3 are closely associated with greater delays in motor skill development.[73]

Musculoskeletal Differences

Children with Down syndrome demonstrate many musculoskeletal differences that are of concern to the physical therapist. Linear growth deficits are observed, including a decrease in normal velocity of growth in stature, the greatest deficiency being between 6 and 24 months of age,[74,75] leg length reduction,[76] and a 10% to 30% reduction in metacarpal and phalangeal length. Muscle variations may also be present including an absent palmaris longus and supernumerary forearm flexors. There is also a lack of differentiation of distinct muscles bellies for the zygomaticus major and minor and the levator labii superior, which may account for the typical facial appearance of the child with Down syndrome.[77]

The most significant musculoskeletal differences, however, are caused largely by the hypotonia and ligamentous laxity characteristic of this disorder. Ligamentous laxity is thought to be attributable to a collagen deficit and commonly results in pes planus, patellar instability, scoliosis (52%), and atlantoaxial instability.[78,79] Atlantoaxial subluxation with risk for atlantoaxial dislocation is caused by laxity of odontoid ligament, whereby there may be excessive motion of C1 on C2 (12% to 20% incidence).[80] Hip subluxation is also commonly seen in children with Down syndrome.

Generalized hypotonia, found in all muscle groups of extremities, neck, and trunk, is a hallmark feature in children with Down syndrome and is a major contributing factor to developmental motor delay.[27] Grip strength, isometric strength, and ankle strength have all been found to be deficient in studies on school-age children with Down syndrome.[81,82]

Additional Physical Characteristics

The back of the head is slightly flattened (brachycephaly), and the fontanels are frequently larger than normal and take longer to close. There may be areas of hair loss, and the skin is often dry and mottled in infancy, rough in the older child. The face of the child with Down syndrome has a somewhat flat contour, primarily because of the underdeveloped facial bones, facial muscles, and a small nose. Typically, the nasal bridge is depressed, and the nasal openings may be narrow. The eyes are characterized by narrow, slightly slanted eyelids, with the corners marked by epicanthal folds. The mouth of the child with Down syndrome is small, the palate narrow, and the tongue may take on a furrowed shape in later childhood. Dentition is often delayed and may be spotty. The abdomen may be slightly protuberant secondary to hypotonia, and the chest may take on an abnormal shape secondary to congenital heart defect. More than 90% of children with Down syndrome develop an umbilical hernia. Hands and feet tend to be small, and the fifth finger is curved inward. In about 50% of children with Down syndrome, a single crease is observed across the palm on one or both hands (simian crease). The toes are usually short, and in the majority of cases there is a wide space between the first and the second toes, with a crease running between them on the sole of the foot.

>> Physical therapy examination and intervention for the child with Down syndrome

Physical therapy examination of the child with Down syndrome should be holistic, viewing the child from multiple perspectives. The therapist must be aware of coexisting medical problems and especially alert to those typically associated with Down syndrome such as cardiac status, atlantoaxial stability, hearing and visual status, and the presence of seizure disorders. Speech difficulties may be present, and therapists may be additionally challenged to effectively communicate during examination and subsequent intervention. The therapist must also integrate the child's cognitive capabilities into the evaluation process, including discussion of

formal intelligence tests with appropriate team members and parent interviews, as well as conducting a brief cognitive assessment as part of a comprehensive developmental test battery. Examination includes any or all of the following measures as appropriate for the age and clinical or educational setting: comprehensive developmental testing, component testing of gross and fine motor skills, including qualitative observational examination of movement, musculoskeletal examination, examination of automatic reactions and postural responses, and, ultimately, a functional examination. These pediatric evaluation procedures are discussed elsewhere in this text. Evaluation of the child with any type of ID disorder, including Down syndrome, additionally encompasses examination of the musculoskeletal, neuromotor, and cardiopulmonary impairments associated with the specific diagnosis (Table 24.3) and knowledge of the coexistence of the cognitive deficit associated with ID and how that affects physical therapy evaluation and intervention.

Learning Differences

Generally, children with ID such as Down syndrome have been found to:

1. be capable of learning.
2. benefit from frequent repetitions in order to learn.
3. have difficulty generalizing skills.
4. need to have more frequent practice sessions in order to maintain learned skills.
5. need extended time in order to respond.
6. have a more limited repertoire of responses.[83]

The levels of cognitive impairment seen in children with Down syndrome vary from profoundly to mildly impaired, mild to moderate impairment being most common. As with any child with coexistent visual or hearing deficits, therapists must adapt interaction, examination, and teaching to accommodate these coimpairments. Children with Down syndrome typically demonstrate attention difficulties and difficulties with information processing. Research also shows a myriad of specific cognitive problems encountered in children with Down syndrome, including difficulties in sequential verbal processing, social-cognitive skills, auditory memory, and motor planning.[42,84–86] Children with Down syndrome appear to have significant impairments in verbal–motor interactions, learning being least proficient when the mode of response or reception calls for auditory or vocal skill.[87] It is important, therefore, for therapists to utilize frequent visual demonstration, practice and rehearsal, and perhaps multimodal sensory avenues in order to best interact with the child with Down syndrome. The child may benefit from hand-over-hand demonstrations to aid in movement pattern development. The child with Down syndrome is more likely to remember the rules and patterns of a new activity if he or she is presented with input over many modalities—visual and kinesthetic as well as verbal.

Associated Motor Deficits

The ligamentous laxity and generalized muscular hypotonia associated with Down syndrome contribute the most to the motor delays and secondary musculoskeletal impairments that are of utmost concern to pediatric physical therapists. The degree to which muscular hypotonia is present will vary, but most investigators agree that it is the most frequently observed characteristic in children with Down syndrome.[27] Hypotonia is distributed to all major muscle groups, including neck trunk, and all four extremities.

Developmental Delay

Clinically, muscular hypotonia has been well established to be highly correlated with developmental delay, including delay in attainment of gross motor and fine motor milestones,[73,88] as well as with delay in other areas of development such as speech acquisition and cognitive development.[89,90] A slower rate of development of postural reactions has been noted in children with Down syndrome.[91] Additional studies by Harris and Rast and Shumway-Cook also demonstrated difficulties in postural control, antigravity control, deficits in postural response synergies when balance perturbations were introduced, and, consequently, the development of compensatory movement strategies as children with Down syndrome attempted to learn to move and stabilize themselves.[84-86] These investigators attribute the movement deficiencies seen in children with Down syndrome primarily to disturbances in postural control and balance. Another difference in movement ability is that persons with Down syndrome are usually slower to initiate a movement and that the velocities of movement tend to be slower.[92] Persons with Down Syndrome are also more likely to use motor patterns that involve cocontractions or simultaneous firing of opposing muscle pairs in movements requiring stabilization of one limb segment while another is moving, possibly an adapted change resulting from differences in brain structure and function.[92]

Not only is developmental delay to be anticipated when evaluating children with Down syndrome, but there is also some evidence to suggest that the underlying muscular hypotonia, ligamentous laxity, and postural difficulties contribute to some of the movement differences frequently observed in children with Down syndrome. Examples include "W" sitting, where the child will characteristically spread his or her legs to a full 180-degree split while in prone and then advance to a sitting posture by pushing up with his or her hands into sitting.[93] Gait acquisition is delayed and is immature, characterized by a persistent wide base and out-toeing.[93,94] It has been suggested that these differences in movement qualities are caused by muscular hypotonia, ligamentous laxity, and a resultant lack of trunk rotation. Hypotonia is thought to contribute to slower reaction time and depressed kinesthetic feedback. Children who have motor impairments are at subsequent risk for secondary impairments because of their restricted ability to explore the environment, affecting, in turn, cognition, communication, and psychosocial development.[95,96]

Physical Therapy Examination and Intervention Implications

Examination should include administration of a comprehensive or component test to measure and track the developmental delay.[97] Qualitative observation of movement will alert the therapist to movement differences and possible emergent compensatory strategies. Intervention must include an understanding from a functional, dynamic systems perspective; the control parameters most likely to cause a responsiveness shift when attempting to influence developing motor strategies.[97] The goal is broadly to anticipate gross and fine motor delay and provide interventions to minimize it by:

- Teaching the caregivers appropriate positioning and handling activities to use throughout early infancy and childhood to promote antigravity control and weight bearing
- Designing activities to encourage the development of antigravity muscle strength in all positions
- Emphasizing trunk extension and extremity loading, which tend to increase axial muscle tone
- Encouraging the emergence of righting and postural reactions through use of rotation within and during movement
- Encouraging dynamic rather than static exploration of movement
- Facilitating the emergence of developmental milestones when chronologically appropriate, including supported sitting and standing, when trunk control and alignment are able to be established; for example, supported treadmill training has been shown to be effective in encouraging earlier onset of independent ambulation.[98-100]
- Anticipating the delay in postural control responses and providing functional opportunities to enhance development in areas of cognition, language, and socialization
- Teaching parents and other team members activities and position choices that will enhance the child's overall development (Fig. 24.5).[101]

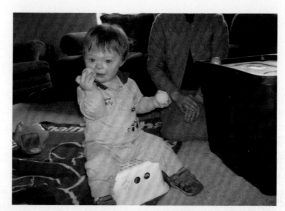

FIGURE 24.5. Incorporating play within the natural home environment as Angelo develops and practices balance and postural control.

Musculoskeletal Impairments

In addition to generalized muscular hypotonia, ligamentous laxity is a hallmark musculoskeletal characteristic of Down syndrome and commonly results in pes planus, patellar instability, scoliosis (52%), and atlantoaxial instability.[78,79] The previously noted atlantoaxial relationship is identified by sagittal plane radiographs of the cervical spine in three different positions: flexion, neutral, and extension.[102–104] A joint interval of 6 to 10 mm is considered symptomatic. A joint interval of more than 4.5 mm carries precautions with it. Early signs of atlantoaxial dislocation include gait changes, urinary retention, reluctance to move the neck, and increased deep tendon reflexes (DTRs).[80] In cases of dislocation with symptomatic atlantoaxial instability, posterior arthrodesis or fusion of C1 and C2 is recommended.[102] In addition to atlantoaxial instability, thoracolumbar scoliosis is also an associated vertebral column musculoskeletal impairment frequently seen in children and adolescents with Down syndrome, usually defined as a mild to moderate degree.[79]

In the lower extremities, hip instability, patellar instability, and foot deformity are the most common musculoskeletal concerns for the physical therapist managing the child with Down syndrome. Hip subluxation is secondary to developmental acetabular dysplasia and long, tapered ischia that result in decreased acetabular and iliac angles as well as laxity of ligamentous support.[78] Pes planus and metatarsus primus varus are the major foot deformities seen in children with Down syndrome.

Physical Therapy Examination and Intervention Implications for Musculoskeletal System

Ligamentous laxity makes any joint less resistant to any trauma, malalignment, or uneven forces. Alignment and support are crucial. At the atlantoaxial joint, this laxity makes the joint less resistant, especially to superimposed flexion, where the joint interval is already widened. Therapists should avoid exaggerated neck flexion, extension, rotation, and positions or movements that may cause twisting or undue forces. Therapists should use caution when placing a child in the inverted position or in other positions that increase risk of a fall onto the head.[80] In the infant and child under the age of 3 years, a radiograph will not reliably detect atlantoaxial instability.[105] Extreme caution must be taken, and any activity that may result in cervical spine injury may be contraindicated in most children with Down Syndrome. Physical therapists must closely monitor children with Down syndrome for changes in neurologic status such as neck pain, torticollis, a change in gait or bowel and bladder function, or any other symptom suggestive of spinal impingement, and refer any child immediately for medical evaluation.[105] Parent education should include issues of atlantoaxial instability; symptoms of neurologic compromise, periods, and activities that may carry increased risk; and activities to avoid if instability is identified.[74]

In children without symptoms of spinal atlantoaxial instability, such as neck pain or neurologic symptoms, the American Academy of Pediatrics does not recommend routine radiographs of the cervical spine. This is because prior to age 3 there is insufficient ossification and epiphyseal development to accurately view the cervical spine using radiography, and plain routine radiographs have been shown to be ineffective at predicting which children will develop instability at a later age.[105] Therefore, it is necessary to explain to parents that contact sports may put children with Down syndrome at risk for spinal cord injury.[105] The following activities are considered to be restricted for children with even asymptomatic atlantoaxial intervals of greater than 4.5 mm: gymnastics (somersaults), diving, high jump, soccer, butterfly stroke in swimming, exercises that place pressure on the head and neck, and high-risk activities that involve possible trauma to the head and neck.[102–107]

Screening for scoliosis should be a routine part of life span management of the child with Down syndrome, especially during periods of increased risk such as growth spurts, puberty, and throughout adolescence. Parents should be taught to perform routine screening for scoliosis. Activities and exercises should promote symmetry and alignment.

Musculoskeletal examination should also include biomechanical examination of the lower extremity and orthotic management, if indicated, for pes planus. In the infant, evaluation of hip stability is a routine part of a physical therapy examination, and referral to orthopedics if hip instability is suspect. Supported standing in a stander should not be instituted unless hip stability and proper alignment has been established.

Broadly, the goal is to maintain alignment and encourage normal movement forces in order to promote optimal biomechanical forces for best musculoskeletal development and prevention of anticipated malalignment and instabilities. Suggestions include:

1. Use of aligned compression or weight-bearing forces in order to stimulate longitudinal bone growth as well as thickness and density of the bone and shaft
2. Promotion of aligned, supported weight bearing in order to promote joint stability and formation; consider the use of orthotic devices such as supramalleolar orthosis to improve alignment after the child has learned to walk.[98–100]
3. Facilitation of muscular strength, force production, and increased muscle tone

In summary, the impact of all of these associated motor deficits in Down syndrome on physical therapy can be viewed in terms of how they affect the child's development and overall functioning. Most of these movement problems have their basis in CNS pathology or primary musculoskeletal differences, which then often lead to secondary impairments in flexibility, stability, force production, coordination, postural control, balance, endurance, and overall efficiency. The specific intervention used will depend on the problems identified and on the consequences that can be predicted and perhaps prevented.

Neuromuscular Impairments Functional Implication

• Hypotonia, low force production Movement paucity	Motor delay, poor contraction
• Slow automatic postural reactions Slow reaction time, decreased speed,	Balance limitations
• Joint hypermobility	Instability, movement anxiety
• Atlantoaxial instability, scoliosis, foot deformities	May preclude access to activities or limit participation level in activity

Cardiopulmonary Fitness

General physical fitness is often below the desired levels in children with ID, and, specifically, in children with Down syndrome.[108] Children with Down syndrome are at risk for restrictive pulmonary disease with concomitant decreased lung volumes and a weak cough, because of generalized trunk and extremity weakness.[109–111] Reduced cough effectiveness may contribute to a high incidence of respiratory infections. Decreased lung volumes including vital capacity and total lung capacity may contribute to a deficiency of the pulmonary system to oxygenate the mixed venous blood or remove the carbon dioxide from the same blood.[112] If there is a reduction in the maximum amount of oxygen available for transport, the energy available for activities is lowered, and consequently a poorer level of physical fitness is achieved.

Physical Therapy Life Span Examination and Intervention Implications

The implications for life span management of the child with Down syndrome are obvious.

Greater emphasis needs to be placed on physical fitness that may increase cardiopulmonary endurance and muscular strength. Programming should begin with children of primary school age in order to prevent a slowing of activity and the subsequent onset of obesity and long-term atherosclerotic risk profiles.[108] Knowledge of improvement reported from training programs for children with Down syndrome supports the ability of these children to respond to early intervention.[113,114] Physical therapists have an excellent opportunity to impact on the health of children with Down syndrome through direct intervention or in consultation with special educators or physical/recreational educators. The general goals are to encourage commitment to wellness by promoting cardiopulmonary endurance, overall physical fitness, and parent/caregiver/client education. Participation in sports and recreational activities such as swimming, dancing, and martial arts should be encouraged and supported from early childhood and onward (Fig. 24.6).

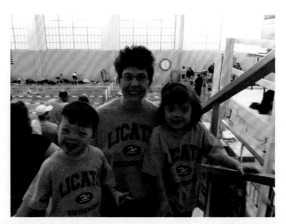

FIGURE 24.6. Mom encouraging participation in group recreational activities, such as swimming, for the multiple benefits of physical fitness and socialization.

» The person with ID moving into and through adulthood: key management issues

ID and Down syndrome both fall under the broad descriptive definition as types of developmental disabilities. The Developmental Disabilities Assistance and Bill of Rights Amendment of 1987 defines a "developmental disability" as a severe and chronic disability that manifests before age 22, is attributable to a mental and/or physical impairment, results in substantial functional limitations in three or more major life activities, and reflects a need for a combination and sequence of special, individualized services that are of extended duration or lifelong.[115,116] With increased sensitivity to life span issues and the recent availability of both retrospective reviews and good clinical case reports, the literature is now available documenting typical life span management concerns. Concurrently, the current practice of physical therapy focuses attention on wellness and preventative management. It is imperative that practitioners integrate a proactive, wellness focused preventative bias into a client's management plan. Because persons with ID, including Down syndrome, typically begin intervention in childhood, the pediatric physical therapist is most likely to be the clinician who will have contact with that client throughout childhood and should be prepared to assist with the transition to adult services by developing relationships with providers of adult services who are interested in and equipped to deal with adults with developmental disabilities.[117]

Persons with ID and other developmental disabilities, including Down syndrome, are enjoying a lengthened life expectancy and will experience the same age-related changes that occur in the general population.[118–120] The aging process does, however, start earlier in persons with ID, perhaps as early as age 35, and generally at around age 55.[105–108] The onset and the impact of the age-related changes are influenced by the severity of the person's existing disabilities and are likely to have a more significant effect if the person has multiple coimpairments.[121]

A review of the literature reveals several features of the aging process that are pertinent for integration into a life span physical therapy management approach. Therapists should be alert to the following anticipated issues: early menopause with the related secondary effects, such as increased risk for osteoporosis, thyroid dysfunction, obesity, diabetes mellitus, late onset of seizure disorder, increased visual or hearing impairment, cardiac disease, depression, dementia, and Alzheimer's disease.[117,122–129] Physical therapy examination and intervention should include proactive preventative management for the possible early onset of any number of these disorders. Examination methods may require that standardized tests be modified for use with the cognitively impaired individual.[115]

The physical therapy management of adults with ID should also focus on the prevention of secondary impairments, for example obesity, or osteoporosis. Exercise and fitness activities including strength and interval training have been shown to improve cardiovascular fitness, muscle strength, and functional mobility[130,131] as well as improving social opportunities. Physical therapists can play a pivotal role in the development and monitoring of physical fitness programs for adults with ID as well as in educating their clients and caregivers about the importance of activity in the maintenance of health and the prevention of secondary disability.

As emphasized throughout this chapter, a main focus of examination and intervention is always on the preservation of safe, independent function or caregiver assistance, as required. Therapists need to use a holistic and multidimensional approach to meet these wide-ranging needs of adults with developmental disabilities.[132]

Summary

In the management of the child with ID, the physical therapist is challenged to use various skills. The many complex and persistent difficulties encountered by children with ID often require innovative methods of physical therapy evaluation and intervention. It is easy to understand that physical therapists may feel overwhelmed by the complexity of this population.

This chapter has attempted to give therapists a "user-friendly" strategy for physical therapy management, including examination and intervention, for *any* child with a diagnosis of ID. Therapists are reminded to view the ID themselves as only a partial description of that child's learning impairment, whose impact on that child's functional learning capabilities may vary from mild to profound. This may be further compounded by other concomitant sensory deficits, including visual, hearing, or sensory organizational problems. Physical therapy examination and intervention must incorporate not only the basic principles of pediatric physical therapy but also an understanding of the principles of teaching and learning as they relate to the child with ID.

Additionally, although there are at least 350 known etiologies for ID, the therapist can easily investigate any of those specific etiologies and acquaint themselves with any commonly associated neuromuscular, musculoskeletal, or cardiopulmonary impairments. This investigative approach will sharpen the therapist's examination skills and alert the PT to the presence of likely coimpairments or associated medical problems as well as to form a prognosis to help with planning for future needs. An understanding of the primary pathology and associated motor deficits readily assists the therapist in establishing treatment goals and priorities. Effective life span physical therapy management of the child can then encompass the anticipation of secondary impairments and risks for that child, which can then be shared with parents and other team members. This chapter illustrated the application of this investigative strategy to the physical therapy management of a child with Down syndrome. This same investigative strategy can be utilized for any ID diagnosis encountered in pediatric physical therapy practice.

Communication of the changing needs of children with ID to parents and other professionals requires not only technical expertise on the part of the therapist but also the ability to be a sensitive listener and creative teacher. Through an effective transdisciplinary approach to the child and his or her family, we can strive to help the child with ID to function at his or her best in society.

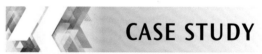

CASE STUDY

This case study will summarize the use of physical therapy with two children with Down syndrome in the same family. (Written by Ann Marie Licata, PhD, Assistant Professor of Education, Alvernia University, Parent of Children with Down syndrome)

"Heel, toe, let's go," I heard our son, Vincent, echo as he helped his younger brother Angelo take strides along the path to the mailbox, a scene typical of our family as we work together in an effort to help Angelo and Julianna, the two youngest members of our family. Angelo and Julianna were born with trisomy 21, more commonly known as Down syndrome. Although it is true that two of our six children have the same medical diagnosis, each is an individual, possessing a charm-like quality that wins the hearts of their family members and those whom they encounter. Like their personalities, Angelo and Julianna's unique stories of development are vastly different, presenting a rich contrast and heartwarming account that gives greater depth to our family experiences, and are a testament to the individuality of all persons, with or without Down syndrome (Fig. 24.7).

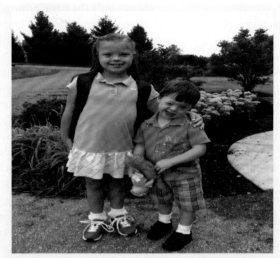

FIGURE 24.7. Julianna and Angelo, two unique individuals.

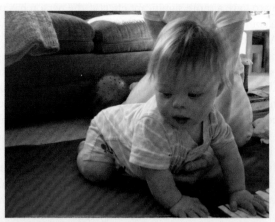

FIGURE 24.8. Angelo actively investigates and navigates his home environment as the therapist uses that natural environment to facilitate development.

Our story begins on a beautiful October day in the early afternoon when our fifth child, a little boy, whom we named Angelo, was born. As an older mother, I carefully counted his ten toes and fingers and pronounced him "perfect." His Apgar score was strong, and we were elated to now be parents of three boys and two girls. It was not until later that day that we were quite surprised to learn that our "perfect" little boy had Down syndrome. As a professional educator who had worked in different capacities throughout my career and had supported many children with disabilities and their families, I had never imagined that I would be a mother to a child with special needs.

Once we were over the initial surprise that news of this nature often delivers, we began to immediately discern the supports that Angelo would need. Children born with Down syndrome tend to have more related health concerns with their heart, eyes, and ears. Within the first 24 hours of his life, Angelo's heart was measured and found to be normal. Several days later, Angelo's hearing was also found to be within the normal range. While we knew Angelo's vision must be addressed, that task happened three months into his short life with again, a positive affirmation that he had normal vision. With these initial physical concerns addressed, we then quickly moved on to Angelo's considering the overall developmental supports that Angelo would need. At 2 weeks of age, a phone call was made to the office of Early Intervention seeking an evaluation to determine the need for supportive services. What we did not know at the time was that Angelo's medical diagnosis of Down syndrome automatically qualified him for the therapies that he would need.

By Angelo's fifth week of life, he had been evaluated by a team and found to be in need of two services, one of which was physical therapy. A selection process allowed us to choose the person whom we would grow to trust, Angelo's physical therapist, Nancy. With very limited knowledge of the adventure in which our family was about to embark, Nancy began Angelo's weekly one-hour therapy sessions in our home initiating the process with a formal plan for his development, an individual family services plan (IFSP). We did not realize the hours of

effort that it would take to help Angelo achieve the developmental tasks that we take for granted, such as rolling over, sitting independently, crawling, and walking. Because of Angelo's low muscle tone and motor delays, we were coached by his physical therapist on how to teach or train his muscles to become strengthened so that they could support and move him as he wanted to move (Fig. 24.8).

We had confidence that he would accomplish these tasks, knowing that his delays in motor development were impacting his cognitive growth. Nancy had explained that Angelo's delay in crawling and walking would also slow down his ability to explore the world around him. We knew he would reach these developmental milestones that would support his overall development but the question that plagued us was "when?"

Being a professional educator and mother of four other children who all displayed typical development, I thought I understood how children grew and matured. It was only when Angelo began to crawl and later walk for the first time, when more than 2 years of age, that Nancy's subtle reminders helped us to realize that typical development was truly a miracle. How could I have missed this fact all these years? This revelation was cause for celebration and celebrate we did. Angelo's attainments of the developmental milestones were viewed as huge victories— a realization of much greater joy than I had ever experienced or appreciated for my four older children. Even now, at age 5, we commemorate the small wins along the way, as Angelo has recently learned the skill of jumping and yes, even running and playing soccer (Fig. 24.9).

Helping us to recognize the joys and celebrations of achievement were a part of what Angelo's therapists did naturally, by building a relationship with not just Angelo, but all the members of our family, Nancy gave us the confidence that we needed as parents of a child born with Down syndrome. She encouraged our interactions, connected us with resources, and used us as resources for other families who needed support. She frequently looked for opportunities to include Angelo's brothers and sisters in his therapy sessions, recognizing the significance of the

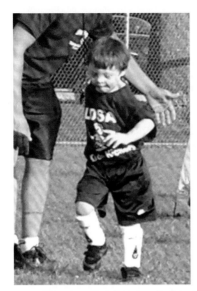

FIGURE 24.9. Team member Angelo enjoying playing soccer!

support that he needed and the enduring bond that Angelo had made with each one of us. These weekly interactions, while not designed for this purpose, helped the members of our family grow closer to one another, forming a single family unit, stronger than we could have imagined (Fig. 24.10).

Nancy's friendly demeanor and genuine interest in not just Angelo and his development, but our entire family extended beyond the scheduled one-hour therapy sessions. Frequently, she brought newspaper clippings of the older children's swimming achievements, building rapport and establishing a relationship that would last for a long time. Nancy, like Angelo's other therapists, gave us support and encouragement as parents. She

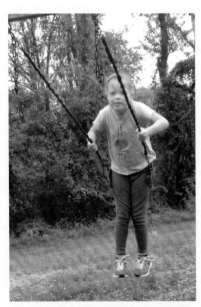

FIGURE 24.10. Julianna learns how to propel herself on a swing!

helped us to recognize the strengths that we had as a family and that my husband Kenny and I shared as parents.

During the first two years of Angelo's life, we were blessed with many competent caring individuals who supported us along the way. What Angelo also helped us to realize was that there were others like him in this world that needed a mom and dad, especially due to their disabilities. Angelo helped us to conquer our fears when considering the possibility of helping another child to find a family—our family. After much thought, prayer, and many sleepless nights, our family began the international journey shortly before Angelo's second birthday to adopt Julianna, our daughter who was born with Down syndrome. Nine months later, we brought our eight year old daughter home to her five siblings. Her homecoming was another opportunity for our family to celebrate.

Unlike Angelo, Julianna had no therapeutic intervention as a baby. She had lived initially in a baby house orphanage and later was sent to a mental institution in her home country. Despite her lack of educational experiences, Julianna was amazingly physically coordinated, drop-kicking a ball better than most of her typically developing peers. Julianna quickly taught herself many of the developmental skills that she may have missed, including how to alternate feet while descending stairs, snap her fingers, and swing. As parents we observed firsthand that no two individuals with Down syndrome are alike; their strengths and needs were very different (Fig. 24.10).

Angelo continues to receive physical therapy, as well as other supportive services that meet his needs at this stage of his life. Julianna, too, receives services, and continues to thrive in the physical domain, playing soccer on an age group club team and swimming competitively. Their abilities differ, as do their personalities. It is so true that no two individuals are the same regardless of the conditions or labels that they might share.

As the members of our family continue to grow older, we become closer to one another, supporting each other along the journey. An appreciation for each other's strengths and differences has become the norm in our home, noting what makes each of us uniquely special. Our life experiences with one another have given us a connection that cannot be broken. The therapeutic terms, jargon and skills that have been acquired through our experiences with initially, Angelo and now with Juliana, help us all to be grateful for the simple joys in life, acknowledging that not only are our lives a gift; we are a gift to one another.

Acknowledgments

This chapter is dedicated to the children and young adults with ID with whom I have had the privilege of working and to the parents and caregivers who have let me into their lives and often their homes to come together to maximize their child's potential and opportunities. A special thank you to Ann Marie Licata, as she shares her family's story in the case study in this chapter. Their family story offers inspiration for countless families and therapists.

REFERENCES

1. Nichtern S. *Helping the Retarded Child.* Grosset and Dunlap; 1974.
2. Historic England. Disability in the medieval period 1050-1485. Accessed March 10, 2021. https://historicengland.org.uk/research/inclusive-heritage/disability-history/1050-1485/
3. National Institute on Intellectual Disabilities. *Orientation Manual on Intellectual Disabilities.* York University; 1981.
4. Itard J. *The Wild Boy of Aveyron.* Prentice-Hall; 1962.
5. Sorrells AM, Rieth HJ, Sindelar PT. *Critical Issues in Special Education: Access, Diversity, and Accountability.* Pearson Education; 2004.
6. Winzer MA. A tale often told: the early progression of special education. *Remedial Spec Educ.* 1998;19(4):212-219.
7. Heward WL. PARC v. Commonwealth of Pennsylvania, 1972. *Exceptional Children.* Merrill Prentice Hall; 2003.
8. Dalton KF. The horrors of Willowbrook State School. 2017. Accessed March 10, 2021. https://www.silive.com/news/2017/01/the_horrors_of_willowbrook_sta.html
9. Schalock RL, Yeager MH, Wehmeyer ML, et al. *Intellectual Disability: Definition, Classification, and Systems of Supports.* 11th ed. American Association on Intellectual and Developmental Disabilities; 2010.
10. *Diagnostic and Statistical Manual of Mental Disorders.* 5th ed. American Psychiatric Association; 2013.
11. Roid GH. *Stanford-Binet Intelligence Scale.* 5th ed. Riverside; 2003.
12. Wechsler D. *Wechsler Intelligence Scale for Children-IV.* Psychological Corp; 2003.
13. Wechsler D. *Wechsler Preschool and Primary Scale of Intelligence III.* Psychological Corp; 2002.
14. Kaufman AS, Kaufman NL. *Kaufman Assessment Battery for Children.* American Guidance Service; 2003.
15. Adams GL. *Comprehensive Test of Adaptive Behavior.* Merrill; 1984.
16. Sloan W, Birch JW. A rationale for degrees of retardation. *Am J Ment Defic.* 1955;60:262.
17. Jette AM. Toward a common language for function, disability, and health. *Phys Ther.* 2006;86(5):726-734.
18. World Health Organization. *International Classification of Functioning, Disability, and Health.* Geneva, Switzerland: WHO; 2001.
19. National Institutes of Health. *Draft V: Report and Plan for Rehabilitation Research.* National Institutes of Health, National Center for Rehabilitation and Research; 1992.
20. Chinn PC, Drew CJ, Logan DR. *Intellectual Disabilities: A Life Cycle Approach.* CV Mosby; 1979.
21. World Health Organization. *International Classification of Diseases (ICD).* WHO; 1992.
22. Leonard H, Xingyan W. The epidemiology of mental retardation: challenges and opportunities in the new millennium. *Ment Retard Dev Disabil Res Rev.* 2002;8:117-134.
23. Nyhan WL, Sakati NO. *Genetic and Malformation Syndromes in Clinical Medicine.* Year Book Medical Publishers; 1976.
24. Kingston HM. ABC of clinical genetics. Dysmorphology and teratogenesis. *BMJ.* 1989;298(6682):1235-1239.
25. Liu J, Krantz I. Cornelia de Lange syndrome, cohesin, and beyond. *Clin Genet.* 2009;76(4):303-314.
26. Jones KL, Jones MC, Del Campo M. Recognizable patterns of malformation. In *Smith's Recognizable Patterns of Human Malformation.* 7th ed. WB Saunders; 2013: 118-123.
27. Harris SR, Shea AM. Down syndrome. In: Campbell SK, ed. *Pediatric Neurologic Physical Therapy.* 2nd ed. Churchill Livingstone; 1991:131-168.
28. Shumway-Cook A, Woollacott MH. Dynamics of postural control in the child with Down syndrome. *Phys Ther.* 1985;65: 1315-1322.
29. American Association for Pediatric Ophthalmology and Strabismus. Williams syndrome. https://aapos.org/glossary/williams-syndrome
30. Keenan J, Kastner T, Nathanson R, et al. A statewide public and professional education program on fragile X syndrome. *Ment Retard.* 1992;30(6):355-361.
31. Rinck C. *Fragile x Syndrome: Dialogue on Drugs, Behavior and Developmental Disabilities.* University of Missouri; 1992;4(3):1-4.
32. Anderson LT, Ernst M. Self-injury in Lesch-Nyhan disease. *J Autism Dev Disord.* 1994;24:67-81.
33. Aughton DJ, Cassidy SB. Physical features of Prader-Willi syndrome in neonates. *Am J Dis Child.* 1990;144:1251-1254.
34. Dykens EM, Cassidy SB. Prader-Willi syndrome: genetic, behavioral and treatment issues. *Child Adolesc Psychiatr Clin N Am.* 1996;5:913-927.
35. Guidera KJ, Borrelli J, Raney E, et al. Orthopaedic manifestations of Rett Syndrome. *J Pediatr Orthop.* 1991;11:204-208.
36. Holm VA, King HA. Scoliosis in the Rett syndrome. *Brain Dev.* 1990;12:151-153.
37. Nomura Y, Segawa Y. Characteristics of motor disturbance in Rett syndrome. *Brain Dev.* 1990;12:27-30.
38. Stewart KB, Brady DK, Crowe TK, et al. Rett syndrome: a literature review and survey of parents and therapists. *Phys Occup Ther Pediatr.* 1989;9(3):35-55.
39. McEwen I. Children with motor and intellectual disabilities. In: Campbell SK, ed. *Physical Therapy for Children.* 4th ed. WB Saunders; 2011: 539-576.
40. Detterman DK, Mayer JD, Canuso DR, et al. Assessment of basic cognitive abilities in relation to cognitive deficits. *Am J Ment Retard.* 1992;97:251-286.
41. Turnbull A, Turnbull R, Wehmeyer ML, et al. *Exceptional Lives.* Pearson; 2013.
42. Horvat M, Croce R. Physical rehabilitation of individuals with intellectual disabilities: physical fitness and information processing. *Crit Rev Phys Rehabil Med.* 1995;7(3):233-252.
43. Montgomery PC. Assessment and treatment of the child with intellectual disabilities. *Phys Ther.* 1981;61:1265-1272.
44. Shields N, Bruder A, Taylor N, et al. Influencing physiotherapy student attitudes toward exercise for adolescents with Down syndrome. *Disabil Rehabil.* 2011;33(4):360-366.
45. Horvat M, Croce R, Zagrodnik J. Utilization of sensory information in intellectual disabilities. *J Dev Phys Disabil.* 2010;22(5):463-473. doi:10.1007/s10882-009-9182-4
46. Kinnealy M. Aversive and nonaversive responses to sensory stimulation in mentally retarded children. *Am J Occup Ther.* 1973;27:464-472.
47. Moore J. Cranial nerves and their importance in current rehabilitation techniques. In: Henderson A, Coryell J, eds. *The Body Senses and Perceptual Deficit.* Boston University; 1973:102-120.
48. Ayres AJ. *Sensory Integration and the Child, 25th Anniversary Ed.* Western Psychological Services; 2005.
49. Collier G. *Emotional Expression.* Lawrence Erlbaum Associates; 1985.
50. Royeen CB, Lane SJ. Tactile processing and sensory defensiveness. In Fisher AG, Murray EA, Bundy AC, eds. *Sensory Integration: Theory and Practice.* FA Davis; 1991.
51. Ayres AJ. *Sensory Integration and Learning Disorders.* Western Psychological Services; 1973.
52. Clark RG, Gilman S, Wilhaus-Newman S. *Essentials of Clinical Neuroanatomy and Neurophysiology.* 10th ed. FA Davis; 2002.
53. Westcott SL, Lowes LP, Richardson PK. Evaluation of postural stability in children: current theories and assessment tools. *Phys Ther.* 1997;77:629-645.
54. Minshawi NF. Behavioral assessment and treatment of self-injurious behavior in Autism. *Child Adolesc Psychiatr Clin N Am.* 2008;17(4):875-886.
55. Scheerer CR. Perspectives on an oral motor activity: the use of rubber tubing as a "chewy." *Am J Occup Ther.* 1992;46(4):344-352. http://search.ebscohost.com/login.aspx?direct=true&db=ccm&AN=107484341&site=eds-live
56. Harvey B. Down's syndrome: a biopsychosocial perspective. *Nurs Stand.* 2004;18(30):43-45.
57. Piaget J. Part I: cognitive development in children-Piaget development and learning. *J Res Sci Teach.* 2003;40(S1):S8-S18.

58. Algozzine B, Ysseldyke J. *Teaching Students with Mental Retardation: A Practical Guide for Every Teacher.* Corwin Press; 2006.

59. Bird EKR, Chapman RS. Sequential recall in individuals with Down syndrome. *J Speech Hear Res.* 1994;37:1369-1381.

60. Hale CA, Borkowski JG. Attention, memory, and cognition. In: Matson JL, Mulick JA, eds. *Handbook of Intellectual Disabilities.* Pergamon Press; 1991:505-528.

61. Rice MS, Hernandez HG. Frequency of knowledge of results and motor learning in persons with developmental delay. *Occup Ther Int.* 2006;13(1):35-48. doi:10.1002/oti.206

62. Schmidt RA, Lee S. *Motor Control and Learning, a Behavioral Emphasis.* Human Kinetics; 1999.

63. Chiviacowsky S, Wulf G, Ávila LT. An external focus of attention enhances motor learning in children with intellectual disabilities. *J Intellect Disabil Res.* 2012;57(7):627-634. doi:10.1111/j.1365-2788 .2012.01569.x

64. Capio CM, Poolton JM, Sit CH, et al. Reduction of errors during practice facilitates fundamental movement skill learning in children with intellectual disabilities. *J Intellect Disabil Res.* 2012;57(4): 295-305. doi:10.1111/j.1365-2788.2012.01535.x

65. Capio CM, Poolton JM, Eguia KF, et al. Movement pattern components and mastery of an object control skill with error-reduced learning. *Dev Neurorehabil.* 2016;20(3):179-183. doi:10.3109/1751842 3.2016.1140844

66. Dykens EM, Hodapp RM, Finucane BM. *Genetics and Mental Retardation Syndromes.* Paul H Brookes Publishing; 2000.

67. National Down Syndrome Society. Website for incidence of Down syndrome given by the National Down syndrome Society. Retrieved May 5, 2019. https://www.ndss.org/about-down-syndrome/down-syndrome/

68. Pueschel SM. Cause of Down syndrome. In: Pueschel SM, ed. *A Parent's Guide to Down Syndrome: Toward a Brighter Future.* Paul H Brookes Publishing; 1990:9-16.

69. Lejeune J, Gauthier M, Turpin R. Les chromosomes humain en culture de tissus. *C R Acad Sci (D).* 1959;248:602.

70. Scott BS, Becker LE, Petit TL. Neurobiology of Down's syndrome. *Prog Neurobiol.* 1983;21:199.

71. Wisniewski KF, Schmidt-Sidor, B. Postnatal delay of myelin formation in brains from Down's syndrome. *Clin Neuropathol.* 1989;6(2):55.

72. Pueschel SM. Medical concerns. In: Pueschel SM, ed. *A Parent's Guide to Down Syndrome: Toward a Brighter Future.* Paul H Brookes Publishing; 1990:59-74.

73. Zausmer EF, Shea A. Motor development. In: Pueschel SM, ed. *The Young Child with Down Syndrome.* Human Sciences Press; 1984:143-226.

74. Castells S, Beaulieu I, Torrado C, et al. Hypothalamic versus pituitary dysfunction in Down's syndrome as a cause of growth retardation. *J Intellect Disabil Res.* 1996;40:509-517.

75. Cronk CE, Crocker AC, Pueschel SM, et al. Growth charts for children with Down syndrome; 1 month to 18 years of age. *Pediatrics.* 1988;81:102-110.

76. Rarick GG, Seefeldt V. Observations from longitudinal data on growth and stature and sitting height of children with Down syndrome. *J Ment Defic Res.* 1974;18:63-78.

77. Bersu ET. Anatomical analysis of the developmental effects of aneuploidy in man: the Down syndrome. *Am J Med Genet.* 1980;5:399.

78. Dummer GM. Strength and flexibility in Down's syndrome. In *American Association for Health, Physical Education and Recreation: Research Consortium Papers: Movement Studies.* Vol. 1, Book 3. American Association for Health, Physical Education and Recreation; 1978.

79. Diamond LS, Lynne D, Sigman B. Orthopedic disorders in patients with Down's syndrome. *Orthop Clin North Am.* 1981;12:57.

80. Gajdosik CG, Ostertag S. Cervical instability and Down syndrome: review of the literature and implications for physical therapists. *Pediatr Phys Ther.* 1996;8(1):31-36.

81. Morris AF, Vaughan SE, Vaccaro P. Measurements of neuromuscular tone and strength in Down syndrome children. *J Ment Defic Res.* 1982;26:41-47.

82. MacNeill-Shea SH, Mezzomo JM. Relationship of ankle strength and hypermobility to squatting skills of children with Down syndrome. *Phys Ther.* 1985;65:1658-1666.

83. Orelove FP, Sobsey D. Designing transdisciplinary services. In: Orelove FP, Sobsey D, Silberman RK. *Educating Children with Multiple Disabilities: A Transdisciplinary Approach.* Paul H Brooks; 1991:9-27.

84. Marcel MM, Armstrong V. Auditory and visual sequential memory of Down syndrome and non-retarded children. *Am J Ment Defic.* 1982;87:86.

85. Edwards JM, Elliott D, Lee TD. Contextual interference effects during skill acquisition and transfer in Down's syndrome adolescents. *Adapt Phys Act Quart.* 1986;3:250.

86. Elliott D, Weeks DJ. A functional systems approach to movement pathology. *Adapt Phys Act Quart.* 1993;10:312.

87. Griffiths MI. Development of children with Down's syndrome. *Physiotherapy.* 1976;62:11-15.

88. Harris SR. Relationship of mental and motor development in Down's syndrome infants. *Phys Occup Ther Pediatr.* 1981;1:13.

89. Canning CD, Pueschel SM. Developmental expectations: an overview. In: Pueschel SM, ed. *A Parent's Guide to Down Syndrome: Toward a Brighter Future.* 2nd ed. Paul H Brookes Publishing; 2001:83-96.

90. Cicchetti D, Sroufe LA. The relationship between affective and cognitive development in Down's syndrome infants. *Child Dev.* 1976;47:920.

91. Haley SM. Postural reactions in children with Down syndrome. *Phys Ther.* 1986;66(1):17-31.

92. Latash ML. Learning motor synergies by persons with Down syndrome. *J Intellect Disabil Res.* 2007;51(12):962-971. doi:10.1111/j.1365-2788.2007.01008.x

93. Lydic JS, Steele C. Assessment of the quality of sitting and gait patterns in children with Down's syndrome. *Phys Ther.* 1979;59(12):1489-1494.

94. Parker AW, Bronks R. Gait of children with Down syndrome. *Arch Phys Med Rehabil.* 1980;61:345-351.

95. Affoltier FD. *Perception, Interaction and Language: Interaction of Daily Living: The Root of Development.* Springer; 1991.

96. Kermonian R, Campos JJ. Locomotor experience: a facilitator of spatial cognitive development. *Child Dev.* 1988;59:908-917.

97. Ulrich BD, Ulrich DA, Collier DH, et al. Developmental shifts in the ability of infants with Down syndrome to produce treadmill steps. *Phys Ther.* 1995;75:20-29.

98. Looper J, Ulrich DA. Effect of treadmill training and supramalleolar orthosis use on motor skill development in infants with Down syndrome: a randomized clinical trial. *Phys Ther.* 2010;90(3):382-390. doi:10.2522/ptj.20090021

99. Looper J, Ulrich D. Does orthotic use affect upper extremity support during upright play in infants with Down syndrome? *Pediatr Phys Ther.* 2011;23(1):70-77. doi:10.1097/pep.0b013e318208cdea

100. Paleg G, Romness M, Livingstone R. Interventions to improve sensory and motor outcomes for young children with central hypotonia: a systematic review. *J Pediatr Rehabil Med.* 2018;11(1):57-70. doi:10.3233/prm-170507

101. Long TM, Cintas HL. *Handbook of Pediatric Physical Therapy.* 2nd ed. Williams & Wilkins; 2001.

102. American Academy of Pediatrics, Committee on Sports Medicine. Atlantoaxial instability in Down syndrome. *Pediatrics.* 1984;74: 152-154.

103. Pueschel SM, Scola FH. Atlantoaxial instability in individuals with Down syndrome: epidemiologic, radiographic, and clinical studies. *Pediatrics.* 1987;80:555-560.

104. Singer SJ, Rubin IL, Strauss KJ. Atlantoaxial distance in patients with Down syndrome: standardization of measurement. *Radiology.* 1987;164:871-872.

105. Bull MJ. American academy of pediatrics. Health supervision for children with Down syndrome. *Pediatrics.* 2011;128(2):393-406. doi:10.1542/peds.2011-3113

106. Giblin PE, Micheli, LJ. The management of atlanto-axial subluxation with neurological involvement in Down syndrome. *Clin Orthop.* 1979; 5(140):66-71.

107. Cooke RE. Atlantoaxial instability in individuals with Down syndrome. *Adapt Phys Activ Q.* 1984;1:194-196.

108. Dichter CG, Darbee JC, Effgen SK, et al. Assessment of pulmonary function and physical fitness in children with Down syndrome. *Pediatr Phys Ther.* 1993;5(1):3-8.

109. Polacek JJ, Wang PY, Eichstaedt CB. *A Study of Physical and Health Related Fitness Levels of Mild, Moderate, and Down Syndrome Students in Illinois.* Illinois State University Press; 1985.

110. DeCesare J. Physical therapy for the child with respiratory dysfunction. In: Irwin S, Tecklin JS, eds. *Cardiopulmonary Physical Therapy.* 3rd ed. Mosby–Yearbook; 1995:516-562.

111. Connolly BH, Michael BT. Performance of retarded children, with and without Down syndrome, on the Bruinicks Oseretsky test of motor proficiency. *Phys Ther.* 1986;66:344-348.

112. Ruppel G. *Manual of Pulmonary Function Testing.* 3rd ed. CV Mosby; 1982.

113. Skrobak-Kaczynski J, Vavik T. Physical fitness and trainability of young male patients with Down syndrome. In: Berg K, Eriksson BO, eds. *Children and Exercise IX.* University Park Press; 1980:300-316.

114. Weber R, French R. *The Influence of Strength Training on Down Syndrome Adolescents: A Comparative Investigation.* Texas Women's University.

115. Herge E, Campbell JE. The role of the occupational and physical therapist in the rehabilitation of the older adult with mental retardation. *Top Geriatr Rehabil.* 2004;13(4):12-22.

116. Amadio AN, Lakin KC, Menke JM. *Chartbook Services for People with Developmental Disabilities.* Center for Residential and Community Services; 1990.

117. Orlin MN, Cicirello NA, O'Donnell AE, et al. The continuum of care for individuals with lifelong disabilities: role of the physical therapist. *Phys Ther.* 2014;94(7):1043-1053. doi:10.2522/ptj.20130168

118. Lubin RA, Kiley M. Epidemiology of aging in developmental disabilities. In: Janicki MP, Wisniewski HM, eds. *Aging and Developmental Disabilities: Issues and Approaches.* Paul H. Brookes Publishing; 1985:95-113.

119. Connolly BH. General effects of aging on persons with developmental disabilities. *Top Geriatr Rehabil.* 1998;13(3):1-18.

120. Campbell JE, Herge E. Challenges to aging in place: the elder adult with MR/DD. *Phys Occupat Ther Geriatr.* 2000;18:75-90.

121. Nochajski SM. The impact age-related changes on the functioning of older adults with developmental disabilities. *Phys Occupat Ther Geriatr.* 2000;18:5-21.

122. Seltzer MM, Seltzer GB. The elderly mentally retarded: a group in need of service. *J Gerontol.* 1985;8:99-119.

123. Gill CJ, Brown AA. Overview of health issues of older women with intellectual disabilities. *Phys Occupat Ther Geriatr.* 2000;18:23-36.

124. Rapp C. Improved lifespan for persons with Down syndrome: implications for the medical profession. *Except Parent.* 2004;34:70-71.

125. Finesilver C. Down syndrome. *RN.* 2002;65:43-49.

126. Platt LS. Medical and orthopaedic conditions in special Olympics athletes. *J Athl Train.* 2001;36:74-80.

127. Post SG. Down syndrome and Alzheimer disease: defining a new ethical horizon in dual diagnosis. *Alzheimer Care Quart.* 2002;3:215-224.

128. Barnhart RC, Connolly B. Aging and Down syndrome: implications for physical therapy. *Phys Ther.* 2007;87(10):1399-1406. doi:10.2522/ptj.20060334

129. Foley JT, Lloyd M, Temple VA. Body mass index trends among adult U.S. Special Olympians, 2005-2010. *Adapt Phys Activ Q.* 2013;30(4):373-386. doi:10.1123/apaq.30.4.373

130. Sugimoto D, Bown S, Meehan WP. Stracciolinie, a effects of neuromuscular training on children and young adults with Down syndrome: systemic review and meta-analysis. *Res Dev Disabil.* 2016;55:197-206.

131. Boer PH, Moss SJ. Effect of continuous aerobic vs. interval training on selected anthropometrical, physiological and functional parameters of adults with Down syndrome. *J Intellect Disabil Res.* 2016;60(4):322-334. doi:10.1111/jir.12251

132. Hotaling G. Rehabilitation of adults with developmental disabilities: an occupational therapy perspective. *Top Geriatr Rehabil.* 1998;13:73-83.

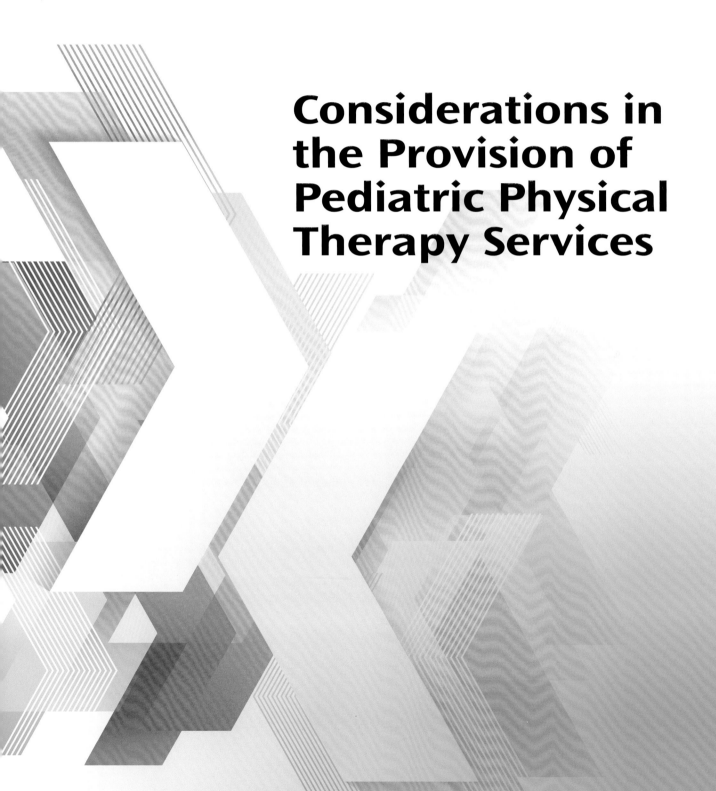

Considerations in the Provision of Pediatric Physical Therapy Services

VII

Transitioning to Adulthood

Mark Drnach

» Introduction

Congress periodically reauthorizes legislation, such as *the Individuals with Disabilities Education Act* (IDEA) and *the Americans with Disabilities Act of 1990* (ADA), that reflects the nation's commitment to children and adults with disabilities. In a reauthorization of IDEA, Congress stated, "disability is a natural part of the human experience and in no way diminishes the right of individuals to participate in or contribute to society. Improving educational results for children with disabilities is an essential element of our national policy of ensuring equality of opportunity, full participation, independent living, and economic self-sufficiency for individuals with disabilities."[1]

Physical therapy is a service frequently utilized by families for their children as they grow into adulthood. For children with a disability, services are available from birth until the age of majority, at which time the now young adult is expected to participate, as independently as possible, in society. With the passage of the ADA, there has been a greater public awareness of the barriers to employment opportunities and public services for millions of people with a disability. Although public awareness has increased in these areas, there still remains a significant gap between employment, independent living, and economic self-sufficiency (annual household income) for individuals with disabilities when compared to those without a disability.[2]

This chapter explores the general framework in which physical therapy services are provided to people with disabilities to promote full participation in society as adults, who just happen to have a disability.

» Defining adulthood

The definition of adulthood is complex, as is the transition from childhood to adulthood. Traditionally, *adulthood* has been considered the age at which a person is a full member of society with responsibilities, not only for themselves but for the community as well.[3] These responsibilities include roles and rituals such as moving out of the family house, getting married, being employed, and voting. In addition to age, physical maturity, cultural and/or societal considerations, and mental capacity are common factors used to define the characteristics of an adult.[4] How a society defines adulthood has implications for the laws and rules that it adopts and follows.

Chronological age is used to describe an adult from a physical perspective. The period after puberty is considered in many cultures to be the beginning of adulthood. Girls will reach their adult size around age 17 to 18 years. Boys will reach their adult size between ages 18 and 21 years.[5] Changes in muscle distribution, fat, and circulatory and respiratory systems lead to increases in stamina and endurance during adolescence and a peak in cognitive, visual, auditory, and strength levels.[6] With these abilities, the young adult would be able to engage in social activities such as driving a motorized vehicle, entering into marriage, voting, caring for children, choosing to live independently, and working for financial gain, which are common characteristics of being an adult.

Cultural and/or societal definitions of adulthood include being *independent from parents* financially, structurally, and cognitively.[4] The ability of a person to live independently, pay bills, live in a place other than a parent's home, and be able to make autonomous decisions is a characteristic adulthood and a common goal that parents have for their child. Cognitive abilities are a major factor in the ability of a young adult to be able to make the decisions that could lead to independent living, gainful employment, and to make reasonably safe and rational choices. It is having the potential to live independently that is important. Many adult children may choose to live with their parents and share financial responsibilities, but the potential to live without that structure and support is the key characteristic reflective of adulthood.

Historically, *marriage* was a sign of being an adult and an expected part of adulthood. Cultural and societal influences can vary, making marriage either a necessity or nicety for being valued as an adult. Marriage is a reflection of the mental competence of the person who makes a decision to enter into a legally binding agreement. Although two people may love one another, their status as competent adults dictates the legal requirements to form this type of union. Although parents may disapprove of their adult child's choice of a spouse, a key difference for a person with a disability is that the parents may be able to legally stop the marriage by bringing into question the ability of the person with the disability to make such a decision.[4]

Consent is defined as the knowing, intelligent, and voluntary agreement to engage in a given activity.[7] Legal requirements that dictate the age of *sexual consent* are set up to protect children. In most states, the age of sexual consent is 16 years for a competent person. A person may be cognitively impaired, but it doesn't mean that the person is sexually impaired. It is the social rituals that lead up to consensual sexual encounters that are impaired. Developing social groups of same-age peers, which can lead to dating in groups, then to dating individuals, and, finally, to dating exclusively, which is seen in the adolescent period, is often absent for individuals with developmental disabilities.

Being able to *vote* is a right and another indication of being an adult. This behavior reflects the society's opinion that the person voting is capable of making a decision about a potential law or another person who will represent his or her beliefs and opinions in the government. This is a right granted to any non-felonious citizen of the United States who is 18 years old or older regardless of race, religion, gender, or intelligence quotient (IQ).[4] It is the *potential* to vote that is a characteristic of adulthood. Some adults may choose not to vote, but that choice doesn't make them any less of an adult.

Being an adult includes the characteristic of *self-determination*. Wehmeyer and Schalock[8] define *self-determination* as acting as the primary causal agent in one's life and making choices and decisions regarding one's quality of life free from undue external influence or interference. They describe four main characteristics of self-determination behavior: actions are autonomous; actions are self-regulated; the person initiates and responds to events in a psychologically empowered manner; and the person acts in a self-realizing manner. If a person is declared incompetent, such as a person

---

DISPLAY

25.1   Basic Characteristics and Abilities of Young Adults

Evaluate the following characteristics and abilities of a young adult:

1. Articulates his or her dreams and aspirations of the future
2. Has realistic goals for the future
3. Understands his or her abilities and capabilities in the framework of identified limitations
4. Demonstrates the optimal level of communication and personal mobility, by self, vehicle, or public transportation
5. Has the capacity to develop the strength, endurance, and skills needed to achieve the identified goals for the future
6. Demonstrates an optimal level of autonomy in decision making with regard to health care, finances, and decisions about the activities in a typical day
7. Demonstrates the optimal level of ADLs and IADLs
8. Has the ability to manage his or her medications, either over the counter (OTC) or those prescribed
9. Demonstrates the optimal level of autonomy in daily dietary intake
10. Demonstrates the optimal level of community involvement and access to public services
11. Consistently demonstrates adherence to basic safety behaviors both in the home, at work or school, and in the community

Developed by Drnach M. Basic Characteristics and Abilities of Young Adults. Unpublished. 2020.

---

with a severe cognitive impairment, then that person is considered unable to make reasonable choices regarding his or her life.[8]

Self-determination does not happen overnight. The characteristics of self-determination begin early in childhood and develop throughout a person's life. People who have a disability may be impaired in their ability to fulfill the rituals and roles that a society expects of an adult owing to innate factors of the disability itself or to factors imposed upon them by societal attitudes or beliefs. Understanding and identifying the differences between an innate inability and an imposed external constraint is the first step in creating equal opportunity for all people. Display 25.1 lists some of the basic characteristics and abilities of all young adults.

» Equality for the differently abled

According to the World Report on Disability, it is estimated, on the basis of the best available data, that 15% of people in the world have a disability.[9] The U.S. Census Bureau, Americans with Disabilities Report, estimates that 27% of people in the United States have a disability, with 17% of the population having a severe disability.[10] People with a disability are less likely to be employed when compared to their nondisabled peers. Among the adults with a disability, less than half

(47%) were employed. People reporting a severe disability had the lowest employment rate compared to those with a less severe disability and those with no reported disability (77% were employed). And, interestingly, adults with a disability reported that they were more likely to be limited in the type or amount of work they could perform than they were in finding a job or remaining in a job because of their disability.[10] The most common functional limitations were reported to be walking a quarter mile, getting out of a bed or a chair, leaving the home to perform errands, and lifting a 10-pound object. All are common activities and skills that can be addressed in physical or occupational therapy. In 2019, the employment participation rate for people (age 16 years and older) with a disability was 20.7% versus 68.3% for people without a disability.[11]

Both federal and state governments have been instrumental in facilitating the inclusion of people with disabilities in the workplace by the passage and implementation of various laws and programs that address the needs of people with disabilities. Having a general awareness and understanding of these external factors can assist the physical therapist (PT) in understanding the options and entitlements available to people with disabilities.

Key United States Legislation Impacting People with Disabilities

The federal government has responded to the need for social reform through the enactment of a number of laws that address the needs of people with disabilities (Table 25.1). As a

TABLE 25.1.	Key United States Laws Impacting People with Disabilities
Year Enacted	1911–1948
Title of Legislation	State Workers' Compensation laws
Impact	Social insurance system for industrial and work-related injuries. Provides financial benefits for medical care related to the injury and lost wages, and pays for vocational rehabilitation if the worker cannot return to the job occupied before the injury.
Year Enacted	1935
Title of Legislation	Social Security Act
Impact	Established federal aid for public health and welfare assistance, maternal and child health, children with disabilities services, federal vocational rehabilitation programs, Medicare, Medicaid, Supplemental Security Income (SSI), and Social Security Disability Insurance (SSDI).
Year Enacted	1965
Title of Legislation	Medicaid. An amendment to the SSA (Title XIX)
Impact	Medicaid is a federal and state government jointly funded, state-administered program that provides health services to eligible individuals. People with a disability can qualify for Medicaid assistance if they meet two criteria: one functional, the other financial.
Year Enacted	1968
Title of Legislation	Architectural Barriers Act
Impact	Required that buildings that receive federal funds for construction comply with the federal standards for physical accessibility. One of the first federal efforts to ensure access to the physical environment by people with disabilities.
Year Enacted	1973 (amended in 2015)
Title of Legislation	Vocational Rehabilitation Services. An amendment to the Rehabilitation Act (Title I)
Impact	Vocational rehabilitation programs provide or arrange for a wide array of training, educational, medical, and other services individualized to the needs of people with disabilities.
Year Enacted	1980
Title of Legislation	Civil Rights of Institutionalized Persons Act
Impact	Authorized the U.S. Attorney General to investigate conditions of confinement at state and local government institutions, including publicly operated nursing homes and institutions for people with disabilities.
Year Enacted	1984
Title of Legislation	Voting Accessibility for the Elderly and Handicapped Act
Impact	Requires polling places across the United States to be physically accessible to people with disabilities for federal elections.
Year Enacted	1988 amended. Originally passed in 1968.
Title of Legislation	Fair Housing Act
Impact	Prohibits housing discrimination on the basis of race, color, religion, sex, disability, familial status, and national origin. Also requires owners of housing facilities to make reasonable exceptions in their policies and operations to afford people with disabilities equal housing opportunities.
Year Enacted	2000
Title of Legislation	Developmental Disabilities Assistance and Bill of Rights Act

(continued)

TABLE 25.1.	Key United States Laws Impacting People with Disabilities (*continued*)
Impact	Provides funds to states to assist in providing comprehensive services and advocacy assistance to persons up to age 21 with developmental disabilities that promote self-determination, independence, productivity, and integration and inclusion in all facets of community life. Established the state's Developmental Disability Council and Protection and Advocacy organizations.
Year Enacted	2004
Title of Legislation	Assistive Technology Act of 2004. An amendment to Section 508 of the Rehabilitation Act of 1973.
Impact	Requires federal agencies to make their buildings, web sites, and services accessible to people with disabilities. The 2004 amendment provide states with financial assistance that supports programs designed to maximize the ability of individuals with disabilities and their family members to obtain assistive technology devices and services.
Year Enacted	2009 amended. Originally passed in 1990.
Title of Legislation	Americans with Disabilities Act
Impact	Prohibits discrimination on the basis of disability in employment, state and local government, public accommodations, commercial facilities, transportation, and telecommunications.
Year Enacted	2014
Title of Legislation	Achieving a Better Life Experience Act or ABLE Act
Impact	Permits states to establish a savings program for qualified individuals to support qualified disability expenses that can include funds for education, housing, transportation, employment training and support, assistive technology, health, financial, and other expenses related to the individual's disability.

Drnach M. Summary of legislation taken from chapter references 12 to 31. Compiled 2020.

federal law, citizens are entitled to the services or support that has been legislated. As a health care provider, PTs should have a basic awareness of these laws that influence the adult lives of people who live with a disability. In addition to the Rehabilitation Act of 1973 (PL 93–112) and the Education for All Handicapped Children Act of 1975 (PL 94–142; now IDEA), the following laws have also been passed to help people with a disability participate more fully in society as adults.

The *Social Security Act of 1935* (SSA; PL 74–271) was the most significant piece of social legislation passed by the U.S. government. This legislation established federal aid for public health and welfare assistance, maternal and child health, and children with disabilities services.[12] It also provided the first permanent authorization for the federal vocational rehabilitation program. The SSA would give rise in subsequent years to the programs of Medicare, Medicaid, and Supplemental Security Income (SSI).

The Social Security Amendments in 1956 (PL 84–880) established the Disability Insurance Trust Fund under Title II of the SSA and provided for payment of benefits to workers with disabilities under the *Social Security Disability Insurance* (SSDI) program.[13,14] Subsequent reauthorization extended the benefits to the dependents of the disabled worker.

Title XIX of the SSA (PL 89–97) is known as the *Medicaid* program, and was adopted in 1965. This medical assistance program is administered by the states with federal matching funds. The Medicaid program is available to all people receiving assistance under the public assistance titles (Title I, Title IV, Title X, and Title XIV) and to people whose income and resources are insufficient to meet their medical costs.[14]

Title XVI of the SSA (PL 92–603), SSI, provides cash benefits to those persons older than 65 years, are blind, disabled,

or poor, or to a child younger than 18 years of age with a disability or blindness. There are also benefits for persons who work despite a disabling impairment. It provides cash to meet basic needs for food, clothing, and shelter.[15] SSI is funded by general tax revenue, not social security taxes.

The *Architectural Barriers Act of 1968* (ABA) requires that buildings and facilities that are designed, constructed, or altered with federal funds, or leased by a federal agency, comply with federal standards for physical accessibility.[16] ABA requirements are limited to architectural standards in new and altered buildings and in newly leased facilities. This law marks one of the first efforts by the federal government to ensure access to the physical environment by people with disabilities.

The *Civil Rights of Institutionalized Persons Act of 1980* (CRIPA) authorizes the U.S. Attorney General to investigate conditions of confinement at state and local government institutions, publicly operated nursing homes, and institutions for people with psychiatric or developmental disabilities. Its purpose is to allow the Attorney General to uncover and correct widespread deficiencies that seriously jeopardize the health and safety of residents of institutions.[16] The Special Litigation Section investigates covered facilities to determine whether there is a pattern or practice of violations of the residents' federal rights. The Special Litigation Section is not authorized to represent individuals or to address specific individual cases.

The *Developmental Disabilities Assistance and Bill of Rights Act of 2000* (PL 106–402) allows for federal monies to be made available to the states to assist in providing comprehensive services and advocacy assistance, to persons up to age 21 with developmental disabilities, that promote self-determination, independence, productivity, and integration and inclusion in all facets of community life.[17] Each state's Developmental Disability Council plans and implements projects to assist people with developmental disabilities to live in the least restrictive environment and to actively participate in their communities. State Councils pursue systems change (e.g., the way human service agencies do business so that individuals with developmental disabilities and their families have better or expanded services), advocacy (e.g., educating policy makers about unmet needs of individuals with developmental disabilities), and capacity building (e.g., working with state service agencies to provide training and benefits to direct care workers) to promote independence, self-determination, productivity, integration, and inclusion of people with developmental disabilities in all facets of community life.[18] State Council members are appointed by the governor and are individuals with developmental disabilities, parents and family members of people with developmental disabilities, representatives of state agencies that administer funds under federal laws related to individuals with disabilities, and representatives of local and nongovernmental agencies. In addition, the Developmental Disabilities Act established Protection and Advocacy Organizations in each state charged with promoting and protecting the rights of individuals with developmental disabilities. These organizations provide legal assistance to individuals with developmental disabilities or to their families.[17]

The Voting Accessibility for the Elderly and Handicapped Act of 1984 generally requires polling places across the United States to be physically accessible to people with disabilities for federal elections. Where no accessible location is available to serve as a polling place, a political subdivision must provide an alternative means of casting a ballot on the day of the election. This law also requires states to make available registration and voting aids for voters who are elderly or disabled, including information by telecommunications devices for the deaf (TDDs), which are also known as teletypewriters (TTYs).[16]

The Fair Housing Act, as amended in 1988, prohibits housing discrimination on the basis of race, color, religion, sex, disability, familial status, and national origin. Its coverage includes private housing, housing that receives federal financial assistance, and state and local government housing. It makes it unlawful to discriminate in any aspect of selling or renting housing or to deny a dwelling to a buyer or renter because of the disability of that individual, an individual associated with the buyer or renter, or an individual who intends to live in the residence.[16]

The Fair Housing Act requires owners of housing facilities to make reasonable exceptions in their policies and operations to afford people with disabilities equal housing opportunities. For example, a landlord with a "no pets" policy may be required to grant an exception to this rule and allow an individual who is blind to keep a guide dog in the residence. The Fair Housing Act also requires landlords to allow tenants with disabilities to make reasonable access-related modifications to their private living space, as well as to common use spaces, although the landlord is not required to pay for the changes. The Act further requires that new multifamily housing with four or more units be designed and built to allow access for persons with disabilities. This includes accessible common use areas, doors that are wide enough for wheelchairs, kitchens and bathrooms that allow a person using a wheelchair to maneuver, and other adaptable features within the units.[16]

The ADA prohibits discrimination on the basis of disability in employment, state and local government, public accommodations, commercial facilities, transportation, and telecommunications.[16] To be protected by the ADA, a person must have a disability or have a relationship or association with an individual with a disability. An *individual with a disability* is defined by the ADA as a person who has a physical or mental impairment that substantially limits one or more major life activities, a person who has a history or record of such impairment, or a person who is perceived by others as having such impairment. The ADA does not specifically name all of the impairments that are covered.[16] In 2008, Congress passed the Americans with Disabilities Amendment Act (ADAA) that clarified, in part, the interpretation and application of the terms "disability" and "substantially limits" and also the intent and broad application of the original wording.

Title I of the ADA (Equal Opportunity Employment) requires employers with 15 or more employees to provide qualified individuals with disabilities an equal opportunity to benefit from the full range of employment-related opportunities available to others. It prohibits discrimination in recruitment, hiring, promotions, training, pay, social activities, and other privileges of employment. This Title restricts questions that can be asked about an applicant's disability before a job offer is made, and it requires that employers make reasonable accommodation to the known physical or mental limitations of otherwise qualified individuals with disabilities, unless it results in undue hardship.[16]

Title II covers all activities of state and local government regardless of the government entity's size or receipt of federal funding. Title II requires that state and local governments give people with disabilities an equal opportunity to benefit from all of the state's programs, services, and activities (e.g., public education, employment, transportation, recreation, health care, social services, courts, and town meetings).[16]

State and local governments are required to follow specific architectural standards in the new construction and alteration of their buildings. They also must relocate programs or otherwise provide access in inaccessible older buildings, and communicate effectively with people who have hearing, vision, or speech impairments. Public entities are required to make reasonable modifications to policies, practices, and procedures where necessary to avoid discrimination, unless they can demonstrate that doing so would fundamentally alter the nature of the service, program, or activity being provided.[16]

The transportation provisions of Title II cover public transportation services, such as city buses and public rail transit (e.g., subways, commuter rails, Amtrak). Public transportation authorities may not discriminate against people with disabilities in the provision of their services. They must comply with requirements for accessibility in newly purchased vehicles, make a good faith effort to purchase or lease accessible buses, remanufacture buses in an accessible manner, and, unless it would result in an undue burden, provide paratransit where they operate fixed-route bus or rail systems. *Paratransit* is a service in which individuals who are unable to use the regular transit system independently (because of a physical or mental impairment) are picked up and dropped off at their destinations.[16]

Title III covers businesses and nonprofit service providers that are public accommodations, privately operated entities offering certain types of courses and examinations, privately operated transportation, and commercial facilities. *Public accommodations* are private entities that own, lease, or operate facilities such as restaurants, retail stores, hotels, movie theaters, private schools, convention centers, physicians' offices, homeless shelters, transportation depots, zoos, funeral homes, day care centers, and recreation facilities including sports stadiums and fitness clubs. Title III also covers transportation services provided by private entities.[16]

Public accommodations must comply with basic nondiscrimination requirements that prohibit exclusion, segregation, and unequal treatment. They also must comply with specific requirements related to architectural standards for new and altered buildings; reasonable modifications to policies, practices, and procedures; effective communication with people with hearing, vision, or speech impairments; and other access issues. In addition, public accommodations must remove barriers in existing buildings where it is easy to do so without much difficulty or expense, given the public accommodation's resources.[16]

Title IV addresses telephone and television access for people with hearing and speech impairments. It requires common carriers (telephone companies) to establish interstate and intrastate telecommunications relay services (TRSs) 24 hours a day, 7 days a week. TRS enables callers with hearing and speech impairments who use TDDs, and callers who use voice telephones, to communicate with each other through a third-party communications assistant. The Federal Communications Commission (FCC) has set minimum standards for TRS services. Title IV also requires closed captioning of federally funded public service announcements.[16]

The Assistive Technology Act of 1998 was an amendment to Section 508 of the Rehabilitation Act of 1973. The Act covers access to federally funded programs and services. Its main purpose is to strengthen the already existing Section 508 of the Rehabilitation Act and access to technology provided by the federal government. Electronic and information technology are the focus. Federal agencies are required to make their buildings, web sites, and services accessible to people with disabilities.[19]

The Assistive Technology Act of 2004 is an amendment to the Assistive Technology Act of 1998. This amendment affects the states and their ability to provide assistance to people with disabilities who depend on assistive technologies in their daily lives. This includes, but is not limited to early intervention, K–12, postsecondary, vocational rehabilitation, community living, and aging services programs. The purpose of this Act is to "provide states with financial assistance that supports programs designed to maximize the ability of individuals with disabilities and their family members, guardians, advocates, and authorized representatives to obtain assistive technology devices and assistive technology services."[20]

An advisory council carries out "consumer-responsive, consumer-driven advice" for planning, implementing, and evaluating programs. At least 60% of the funds available are used for state finance systems, device utilization, loans, and demonstration programs. A 40% maximum of funds is used on state leadership activities. These activities can include training and technical assistance, public awareness, and coordination and collaboration.[20]

The device loan program involves loans to individuals or entities for devices. The device exchange program is for devices that are exchanged, repaired, recycled, or reutilized. Demonstration of devices is a program that benefits individuals, communities, and entities.[20] Funds are not used for direct payment for an individual person's assistive device.

According to information from the U.S. Centers for Disease Control and Prevention (CDC) on the trends and usage of assistive technology devices, mobility impairment was the number one reason for the use of an assistive device, with a cane being most commonly used.[21] The age group with the most assistive devices used (hearing, mobility, and vision) was the older than 65 years age group. The majority of people who use any anatomic assistive device (a brace for any part of the body, such as a back, hand, or knee brace) were in the age group 44 years or younger.[21]

State governments have also passed laws and implemented federally required programs that address the issue of employment and financial assistance for individuals with disabilities. The three most common of these state-run programs are workers' compensation, vocational rehabilitation, and Medicaid.

Workers' compensation was one of the first laws enacted that addressed work and disability. It is defined as the U.S. social insurance system for industrial and work-related injuries.[22] Workers' compensation is regulated at the state level. This statute requires the employer to pay benefits and to furnish care for job-related injuries sustained by employees, regardless of fault. It also requires payment of benefits to dependents of employees killed in the course of, and because of, their employment.

Each state has its own history on how its compensation laws were started. Workers' compensation laws were enacted to make litigation less costly and to eliminate the need for injured workers to prove their injuries were the employer's "fault." The first state workers' compensation law was passed in Maryland in 1902. By 1949, all states had enacted some kind of workers' compensation law.[23]

It is illegal in some states for an employer to terminate an employee for reporting a workplace injury or for filing a workers' compensation claim. Most states also prohibit refusing employment to a person who previously filed a workers' compensation claim. Those individuals who are disabled on the job and try to get another job somewhere else are protected from discrimination under the ADA.

Persons who are disabled on the job receive benefits depending on the resulting level of disability. The levels or categories of disability include permanent total disability, permanent partial disability, and temporary total disability. Each category has its own amount of compensation awarded and a specified length of benefit.

Workers' compensation provides financial benefits for medical care related to the injury and lost wages, and pays for vocational rehabilitation if the worker cannot return to the job that he had before the injury. Putting people with disabilities to work, or enabling them to remain in their jobs with the onset of a disability, is one of the key elements of the U.S. disability policy.[24]

Vocational rehabilitation refers to programs conducted by state vocational rehabilitation agencies operating under the Rehabilitation Act of 1973. Vocational rehabilitation programs provide or arrange for a wide array of training, educational, medical, and other services individualized to the needs of people with disabilities. The services are intended to help people with disabilities acquire and maintain gainful employment.[25] Services may include restoration of physical or mental functioning; academic, business, or vocational training; personal or vocational adjustment training; employment counseling; and job placement and referral.

Vocational rehabilitation programs are eligibility programs, not entitlements. The person must have a physical or mental disability, the disability must substantially impair the person's ability to work, and a reasonable expectation that the provision of services will make the person employable must exist.[26]

Probably the most well-known of the federally mandated, state-run programs is the *Medicaid* program. Medicaid is a state-administered program, with each state having its own guidelines regarding eligibility and services. People with a disability can qualify for Medicaid assistance (under the Optional Eligibility Groups) if they meet two criteria: one functional, the other financial. First, they have to be considered disabled, as defined by the Social Security Administration's definition of disability (Display 25.2). To be financially eligible for disability benefits, a person must be unable to engage in substantial gainful activity (SGA). A person who is earning more than a certain monthly amount (net of impairment-related work expenses) is ordinarily considered to be engaging in SGA. The amount of monthly earnings considered as SGA depends on the nature of a person's disability.[27] In most states, an individual is automatically eligible

---

DISPLAY 25.2 Social Security Administration's Definition of Disability

The SSA defines disability (for adults) as "inability to engage in any substantial gainful activity by reason of any medically determinable physical or mental impairment which can be expected to result in death or which has lasted or expected to last for a continuous period of not less than 12 months" (Section 223[d][1]). Amendments to the Act in 1967 further specified that an individual's physical and mental impairment(s) must be "… of such severity that he is not only unable to do his previous work but cannot, considering his age, education, and work experience, engage in any other kind of substantial gainful work which exists in the national economy, regardless of whether such work exists in the immediate area in which he lives, or whether a specific job vacancy exists for him, or whether he would be hired if he applied for work" (Sections 223 and 1614 of the Act).

Social Security. Compilation of the Social Security Laws. Disability Benefits. SSA. Section 223 (d) (1). Accessed June 10, 2020. https://www.ssa.gov/OP_Home/ssact/title02/0223.htm#ft282 and https://www.ssa.gov/OP_Home/ssact/title16b/1614.htm

---

for Medicaid if he or she is eligible for SSI.[28] Services offered by Medicaid are extensive and usually free. States are allowed to provide a variety of services, but the federal government requires each state to make available certain basic services. Display 25.3 lists those services required by federal law.

Optional services that are important to people with disabilities may include prescription drug coverage; physical,

---

DISPLAY 25.3 Medicaid Mandatory State Plan Services

Medicaid eligibility groups classified as categorically needy are entitled to the following services under federal law:
  Inpatient hospital services
  Outpatient hospital services
  EPSDT: Early and Periodic Screening, Diagnostic, and
    Treatment Services
  Nursing Facility Services
  Home health services
  Physician services
  Rural health clinic services
  Federally qualified health center services
  Laboratory and X-ray services
  Family planning services
  Nurse-Midwife services
  Certified Pediatric and Family Nurse Practitioner services
  Freestanding Birth Center services (when licensed or otherwise recognized by the state)
  Transportation to medical care
  Tobacco cessation counseling for pregnant women

Centers for Medicare & Medicaid Services. Mandatory and optional Medicaid benefits. Accessed May 17, 2020. https://www.medicaid.gov/medicaid/benefits/mandatory-optional-medicaid-benefits/index.html

occupational, and speech therapy services; prosthetic devices; eyeglasses; rehabilitation; Intermediate Care Facilities for Individuals with Intellectual Disabilities (ICF/ID); and personal care.[28] In 1971, Medicaid benefits were extended to cover services provided by ICFs, commonly known as group homes. The purpose of this amendment was to provide a less costly alternative for medically indigent persons, who do not need the institutional or intensive care provided in hospitals and skilled nursing facilities.[29]

The Omnibus Reconciliation Act of 1981 (PL 97–35) further expanded the services provided by Medicaid, allowing states to apply for a waiver from the federal regulations to provide home- or community-based service packages to specific Medicaid populations.[28] These *waiver programs* (Section 1915[c] of the SSA) would allow an individual who meets the state requirements for the Medicaid nursing home benefit to receive services at home or in the community. The number of individuals served under a waiver program is limited by the state's ability to prove to the federal officials that the savings on nursing home care offsets waiver expenditures.[28] Most states share the cost of Medicaid services with the federal government at approximately a 50:50 ratio.[30]

The Achieving a Better Life Experience Act or ABLE Act of 2014 permits states to establish a savings program for qualified individuals.[31] The law encourages individuals with disabilities to save money to support qualified disability expenses that can include funds for education, housing, transportation, employment training and support, assistive technology, and health, financial, and other expenses related to the individual's disability. To be eligible the individual must have a significant disability, as defined by the Social Security Administration, that began before the individual turned 26 years of age. ABLE accounts are modeled after college saving plans (529 Plans, named in reference to Section 529 of the Internal Revenue Code).

» Transitioning out of high school

Transitioning is not an event but a process that requires knowledge, opportunity, skills, and courage. As for all children, and their parents, the process of moving from one program to another, and from one stage of life to the next, is made easier when both the parent and child are comfortable with their own knowledge and skills, and understand how they can successfully navigate the next environment given the basic set of possibilities that they may encounter. Bringing an infant home from the hospital after birth, placing a child in a daycare program, sending a child to school, or entering society as an adult, are all transitions in a child's and parent's life. The process of transitioning is always developing in both the child and parent. As a member of the health service in the hospital, an early intervention service under Part C of IDEA, and a related service under Part B of IDEA, the PT can play an integral part in the preparation of any transition. PTs should keep in mind that they are not only providing a service in a specific environment for a specific period of time but also are providing the parents and child with knowledge and skill training to become self-sufficient and are promoting self-determination in both the child and parent. It is important that the PTs keep this in mind and help the family become informed decision makers in their child's life. It is not only information acquisition but thoughtful, timely, and informed planning, with available opportunities identified and understood, that make the transition process less stressful. One way to facilitate the process is to use a list or worksheet that will allow the young adult and family to discuss and explore the options available to them. Display 25.4 contains an example of a Transition Worksheet.

Transitioning out of high school is a critical time for all individuals and their families. For young people with disabilities, the transition is an ending of entitlement programs

---

DISPLAY 25.4   Basic Transition Worksheet

Name:
Date of Birth:
Today's Date:
This worksheet is intended to assist you in planning for your transition to adult life and services. Please take time to discuss the questions with your parent or guardian. Check the boxes below that apply to you today.

Health

( ) I understand my medical condition.
( ) I am able to manage my medications.
( ) I am able to perform daily medical treatments, if necessary.
( ) I understand my health insurance and coverage.
( ) I am able to use and care for the medical/health equipment that I own.
( ) I can advocate for myself with my health care providers.

Living

( ) As an adult I plan to live with (circle those that apply): Self   Parent   Assisted Living   Residential Care/ICF
( ) I will need assistance for (circle those that apply): Self care   Shopping   Home management   Food acquisition and/or preparation   Nutrition advice
( ) To access public services, I will (circle those that apply): Drive myself   Require someone to transport me   Access public transportation
( ) I can access communication devices to contact my family, friends, or emergency assistance if needed.
( ) I am aware of the public services that are available to help me live as independently as possible.

Working

( ) I plan to work in the following employment setting (circle the one that applies):   competitive   competitive/integrative   sheltered
( ) I plan on working (circle that which applies): full time   part time   hourly, as needed   volunteer
( ) I have a written resume.
( ) I can fill out a work application.
( ) I know the accommodations that I will need to help me do my intended job.
( ) I am aware of my civil rights under the ADA.

College

( ) I know how to enroll in an educational program and courses.
( ) I am aware of my civil rights for reasonable accommodations under Section 504 of the Rehabilitation Act.
( ) I can access transportation to campus and safely negotiate the campus environment.
( ) I am able to manage the tools that are necessary for my education (e.g., computers, Internet, bookbags).
( ) I can manage my time for homework and other classroom assignments.
( ) I can advocate for myself with teachers, school administrators, and classmates.

Finances

( ) I can manage money to make purchases.
( ) I can manage my bank accounts.
( ) I can manage paying my bills.
( ) I understand how to budget.
( ) I understand what taxes are and my responsibility in filing the necessary forms.
( ) I am aware of the government programs for income support (e.g., SSI, SSDI, TANF).

Social/Recreational Activities

( ) I am interested in the following hobbies, topics, or activities (please list):

_____
( ) I am aware of the programs/groups in my community that are centered around my interests.
( ) I feel that I am understood when I express myself to others.
( ) I know how to stay safe when I am away from home (e.g., making appropriate choices, understanding unsafe situations, accessing assistance when needed).
( ) I can advocate for myself with others in social situations.

I would like more information on the following topics:

_____

I would like to work on my skills in the following areas:

_____

Developed by Drnach M. Basic Transition Worksheet. Unpublished. 2020. Adapted in part from The University of Illinois at Chicago's Division of Specialized Care for Children. Transition Tools. Transition Toolkit. Revised ed. 2017. Accessed June 10, 2020. https://dscc.uic.edu/browse-resources/transition-resources/

and the related services they provided into the adult world of working, or postsecondary education, and possibly establishing living arrangements as a young adult. The student and family are leaving the relatively organized service delivery system of education, and entering one in which they are solely responsible for identifying, obtaining, and coordinating the services needed for employment and independent living.[26] All those years of educational instruction and planning have reached their zenith.

Section 504 of the Rehabilitation Act states that "No otherwise qualified individual with a disability in the United States, as defined in section 706(8) of this title, shall, solely by reason of her or his disability, be excluded from the participation in, be denied the benefits of, or be subjected to discrimination under any program or activity receiving Federal financial assistance" (29 USC §794[a], 34CFR104.4[a]).[32] Nearly all postsecondary institutions receive federal financial assistance and would fall under this civil rights law. Many college campuses have an office for Disabled Student Services or Special Services.[26] But unlike education law (IDEA), colleges and universities are not mandated to provide services in accordance with an Individualized Education Program (IEP). Accommodations, as identified under civil rights law, such as the Rehabilitation Act and the ADA, do come into play. Table 25.2 lists some of the general differences between secondary and postsecondary requirements for individuals with disabilities under Section 504 of the Rehabilitation Act.

PTs can play an important role in preparing students for life after high school. Display 25.5 identifies some of the key aspects of transitioning that the PT could adopt. Promoting functional skills that will carry over into the workplace or daily life of a student is an important aspect of a student's education. Such activities may include developing the strength and coordination necessary to dress and perform daily hygiene tasks; the ability to manipulate the tools of education, work, and home; the ability to access communities, buildings, and classrooms; the ability to drive or access public transportation; developing endurance to attend to a job or academic program for several hours a day; and the ability to participate meaningfully in a life activity that goes beyond ADLs or IADLs (see Display 25.6). Meaningful participation can be defined as the involvement in a complex activity, with at least one other person, that contributes to the person's sense of well-being and fulfillment of his or her societal role. Unfortunately, these skills and activities are not easily acquired in a year or two before graduation from high school; it may take years to identify the student's capacity and then subsequent mastery of the life skills that are necessary to participate in life after high school. Many of them begin in early childhood, but, at a minimum, the PT should be addressing these identified skills when the student is 14 years of age.

Living Options

After high school, many young adults continue to live at home with their parents as they continue to mature socially, and then other living arrangements become desired or required. For a person with a severe disability, the options for living arrangements are dependent on caregiver availability and community resources. For many, the parent is the primary caregiver and the family home is the first choice for housing.

It is reported that approximately 43.5 million adults in the United States provide some level of unpaid care to a child or adult, with 4% of the recipients identified as individuals with developmental or intellectual disorders.[33] The caregiver

TABLE 25.2.	A Comparison of Various Aspects of the Section 504 Regulations for School-Aged Children versus Postsecondary Education	
	Preschool, Elementary, and Secondary	Postsecondary
Identification	Schools have an obligation to identify and locate students entitled to Section 504 protections.	No comparable obligation.
Evaluation	Schools must undertake evaluation of students that they believe may be covered under Section 504.	Student is responsible for documentation concerning disability.
Entitlement to Education	Every student must be provided a free and appropriate public education. The educational program must be designed to meet an individual's needs.	Student has the right not to be excluded from educational programs or activities by reason of disability.
Planning Process	Schools must have in place policies and procedures that ensure the documentation and consideration of evaluative information.	No comparable provision for comprehensive planning for individuals.
Grievances	Schools must have in place grievance procedures and designate individuals responsible for 504 compliance.	Same
Due Process Rights	Schools need to provide notice to parents, an opportunity to examine records, an impartial hearing with opportunity for parental participation and representation by counsel, and a review procedure.	No comparable provision.

Adapted from 504 Training. The Iowa Program for Assistive Technology. Training provided by John Allen (Clinical Professor of Law, University of Iowa), Mary Quigley (Co-Director, Iowa Program for Assistive Technology), and Lisa Heddens (Parent Training and Information Center of Iowa). Iowa City, Iowa. September 20, 2000.

DISPLAY 25.5 Fostering Transitioning by the Physical Therapist

1. Begin transitioning interventions and goals as early as possible. This should be part of a student's Individualized Education Plan or a factor in an outpatient program by the age of 14 years.
2. Focus on the attributes of an adult to the extent possible: Talk directly to the person instead of the parent; ask the person questions directly; ask parent/guardian if you can speak to the person privately; frequently discuss options that are available after the person exits the school system; treat the person as a responsible individual to the level appropriate; foster self-determination to the extent possible.
3. Look at predictors and skills for living and working independently and include those goals into the student's educational plan or outpatient program.
4. Make assisted walking or mobility functional. Once the student can move in a device for 20 feet, encourage the student to participate in routine activities in the classroom or at home such as emptying trash, setting up or clearing up spaces for learning or family routines, caring for the space. After the student moves 50 feet, have the student deliver items to locations outside the classroom or from one room of the house to another; attach a broom to the walker and have the student sweep the floor; attend to a family pet or house plant. After 100 feet, have the student move about the immediate environment with reasonable accommodations for time. After 200 feet, have the student begin chores for the school or home such as mail pick up, trash removal, dusting the furniture, delivering or retrieving items for education or family routines and daily rituals.
5. Improving performance does not equate to meaningful participation. Start early to involve children in activities that they identify, enjoy, and find meaningful. Help identify their options given their unique capabilities. Encourage children to explore the variety of activities that are possible and available.

Developed by Drnach M. Fostering Transitioning by the Physical Therapist. Unpublished. 2020.

DISPLAY 25.6 Desired Skills When Transitioning Out of High School

Living
Safely access and utilize the physical environment.
Communicate effectively.
Participate in family activities (dinner, care of the house, family events).
Demonstrate some level of participation with IADLs (creating shopping lists, preparing meals, scheduling events for the weekend).
Assist with personal care, including transfers.

Employment
Access transportation to and from the work site.
Safely access and utilize the physical environment.
Use the tools necessary to complete the job.
Communicate effectively and as efficiently as possible.
Attend to a task sufficiently to complete the work assignment.
Endurance to participate for at least 4–8 hours a day in work activities.
Ability to attend to personal needs (dressing skills, eating, medication management, personal hygiene).

College
Access transportation to a campus.
Safely access and utilize the physical environment.
Use the technology for distance learning and academic work.
Communicate effectively and as efficiently as possible.
Attend to a task sufficiently to complete the academic requirements.
Endurance to participate for at least 3–5 hours a day in educational activities.
Ability to attend to personal needs (dressing skills, eating, medication management, personal hygiene).

Developed by Drnach M. Desired Skills When Transitioning Out of High School. Unpublished. 2020.

is, on average, 49 years of age, a woman (60%), and is caring for a relative (85%). The idea of a person with a disability living at home with his or her parents as the primary caregivers is socially acceptable and understandable, but several aspects of this arrangement should be clarified. First, does the person with a disability desire to live at home with his or her parents? Young adults, as they develop and mature, may desire their own living space and environment in which they have more autonomy and privacy. The responsibility of maintaining one's own space also reflects independence and self-determination. Many children with disabilities may not see this as an option as they are growing up, because they are seldom exposed to the possibility. Also, do the parents of the adult child desire to have the child live with them? This is not the same as "will they," for the majority of parents will welcome their children to live in the same house

as they do. But do the parents of a young adult with a disability have the awareness and comfort of transitioning their child, who is more dependent on them than is a young adult without a disability, into a new living arrangement? Are they knowledgeable of the services and support systems available that would allow their child to live in a type of arrangement other than the family home? Do the parents feel that this is important? Another obvious, but often not discussed, issue is the fact that as the parents age, they may find it more difficult to care for their adult child at home. In the event that one or both parents die, the care for the adult child becomes an urgent issue, necessitating the need for community services or placement. Individuals and parents should be aware of their state programs and the various opportunities that may be available in their community. These can include such arrangements as independent living, the use of in-home services, and assisted or residential living.

Independent living is a philosophy for self-determination and equal opportunity. It does not mean that a person lives independently of everyone else. No one in society truly lives independently. Everyone has family, friends, and neighbors and lives in a community with grocery stores, parks, and shopping malls. Independent living for people with disabilities is the ability to live with the same opportunities and choices as people who do not have a disability. Many adults with disabilities choose to live in their own homes and use a variety of community resources and supports. Adults who meet the criteria for Developmental Disabilities Waiver services are eligible for additional supports, such as chore services, environmental modifications, and home-delivered meals. The National Council on Independent Living (NCIL) was founded in 1982 and represents many organizations and individuals including the Centers for Independent Living (CILs), Statewide Independent Living Councils (SILCs), individuals with disabilities, and other organizations that advocate for the human and civil rights of people with disabilities throughout the United States.[34]

Attendant services provide *in-home assistance* with activities of daily living (ADLs) and basic health maintenance activities. The goal is to provide support that enables a person with a disability to live in his or her own home. Some states offer Medicaid Waiver Assisted Living Services, which are provided in the home to Medicaid-eligible residents and can include such services as housekeeping, meal preparation, escort services, essential shopping, and medication assistance.

Assisted living usually refers to a facility that is used by people who are not able to live on their own, but do not need the level of care that a skilled nursing facility offers. The term *assisted living* can have several different meanings, depending on the targeted population and services available. The U.S. Senate's Assisted Living Workgroup developed recommendations to assure consistent quality in assisted living services nationwide. One recommendation is the following definition of assisted living:

> Assisted living is a state-regulated and monitored residential long-term care option. It provides or coordinates oversight and services to meet the residents' individualized scheduled needs, based on the residents' examinations, service plans, and unscheduled needs as they arise. Services that are required by state law and regulation to be provided or coordinated must include (but are not limited to):
>
> - 24-hour awake staff to provide oversight and meet scheduled and unscheduled needs
> - Provision and oversight of personal care and supportive services
> - Health-related services (e.g., medication management services)
> - Meals, housekeeping, and laundry
> - Recreational activities
> - Transportation and social services
>
> These services are disclosed and agreed to in the contract between the provider and resident. Assisted living does not generally provide ongoing, 24-hour

skilled nursing. It is distinguished from other residential long-term care options by the types of services that it is licensed to perform in accordance with a philosophy of service delivery that is designed to maximize individual choice, dignity, autonomy, independence, and quality of life.[35]

Residential care is an option for individuals who cannot live alone and require more supervision than is available through in-home community services. An ICF, commonly known as a group home, as defined by the Centers for Medicare & Medicaid Services, is a facility that primarily provides health-related care and services above the level of custodial care to individuals with disabilities, but does not provide the level of care available in a hospital or skilled nursing facility.[36] It is an optional Medicaid benefit. These residential facilities are licensed in accordance with state law and certified by the federal government as a provider of Medicaid services to ICF/ID in accordance with federal standards of operations. Hired staff provide, in a protected residential setting, ongoing evaluation, planning, 24-hour supervision, coordination, and integration of health or rehabilitative services to help each individual function at his or her greatest ability. Admission criteria will vary depending on the state program, but general criteria include the need for basic nursing care, assistance with ADLs, and care with physical and cognitive functioning or behavior problems. Most states do not allow admission of a person who needs 24-hour-a-day skilled nursing oversight. They are more appropriately referred to a skilled nursing facility.

Employment Options

Employment can be classified into three levels: competitive, supported, or sheltered. *Competitive employment* is defined as a full- or part-time job in the labor market with competitive wages and responsibilities in which the individual maintains the job with no more additional outside support than a coworker without a disability.[26] Many adolescents with disabilities leave high school with sufficient academic or vocational preparation to maintain competitive employment. These individuals only need assistance from an outside agency to locate an appropriate job.[26]

According to the Rehabilitation Act Amendments of 1986, *supported employment* is defined as competitive work in integrated work settings (with nondisabled peers) for individuals with the most significant disabilities. The provision of ongoing support distinguishes supported employment from competitive employment. Support is provided as long as the individual holds the job, allowing the person with a disability the opportunity to earn wages in job sites with nondisabled peers. The Workforce Innovation and Opportunity Act of 2014 amended Title I of the Rehabilitation Act with significant changes for people with disabilities with increasing access to workforce services and making available preemployment transition services to students with a disability.[37] It also provides a new definition for supported employment as *competitive integrated employment.*

Sheltered employment is the employment of individuals with disabilities in a self-contained work site, without integration with nondisabled coworkers. These employment sites can range from an adult day program, where the individual receives training in ADLs, social skills, and prevocational skills, to a sheltered workshop where the individual performs subcontracted tasks such as packaging, collating, or machine assembly.[26]

Physical therapy can be instrumental in fostering the success of the individual in any of the employment classifications. Early identification of the desires of the individual and early training to better prepare the individual for employment once out of high school are vital. Encouraging some level of employment while the individual is still in high school has also been shown to be a possible predictor of employment after graduation.[38] Volunteering, or being responsible for certain household chores, should also be encouraged in the adolescent.

The PT can evaluate the ability of the individual to perform the manual tasks required of the job such as bilateral manual dexterity, lifting overhead, or standing for periods of time. Job-specific training that analyzes the tasks of the job into its' component parts and then addresses those components individually, and then collectively, to make the job performance more efficient can also be done. This could include environmental modifications to optimize workplace ergonomics, appropriate job organization to optimize productivity, or the utilization of assistive technology.

The ability to work, whether that is paid or unpaid, provides a sense of well-being to the individual and can improve the individual's sense of well-being. Future work after high school should be a consideration in every student's educational plan.

Financial Assistance

In addition to the income generated through employment, common financial assistance programs available to adults include the federal government's welfare program, SSDI, and SSI.

The *Merriam-Webster* dictionary defines *welfare* as aid in the form of money or necessities for those in need and an agency or program through which aid is distributed.[39] Welfare has different meanings. What is generally considered welfare by politicians and the general public is the Aid for Families with Dependent Children (AFDC), which is today called *Temporary Assistance to Needy Families* (TANF).[40] The other meaning for welfare is the broad general term of all government programs providing benefits to needy Americans. These programs can include Medicaid, food stamps, SSI, and Housing and Urban Development (HUD) programs.[40]

TANF provides financial assistance and work opportunities to eligible families by granting states the federal funds to develop and implement welfare programs in the state. Citizens are able to apply at their local TANF agency. TANF is run through the U.S. Department of Health and Human Services, Office of Family Assistance.[41] It has four purposes: to assist families so that children can be cared for in their own homes; to reduce the dependence of parents by promoting job preparation, work, and marriage; to prevent and reduce the incidence of out-of-wedlock pregnancies; and to encourage the formation and maintenance of two-parent families.[41]

The Supplemental Nutrition Assistance Program, or SNAP, is another form of public assistance that is based on household size and household income after deductions are applied. Those households that have an elderly or disabled person are given special consideration. Financial assistance is provided for the purchase of food for human consumption and seeds and/or plants to grow food at home. There are limitations on the types of items that can be purchased, which may include certain household items, grooming products, tobacco, alcohol products, or pet food, to name a few.[42] Most nutritional assistance programs are administered at the state or local level, and therefore eligibility requirements may vary slightly, by state.

The Social Security Administration has two disability programs, SSDI and SSI. SSDI is funded through employees', employers', and self-employed persons' contributions, and it covers injured workers, their widows or widowers and dependents, and people with disabilities. To be eligible, a person must meet certain criteria. Income is one criterion and is based on the amount of benefit tied to a person's work history and earnings. Being disabled is another criterion.[43] A person has to meet the definition of disability according to the Social Security Administration's standards that uses a series of questions related to earned income and "a condition that significantly limits the person's ability to do basic work."[43] The disability must also last, or be expected to last, for at least 1 year, and the person has to have a work history long enough and recent enough under Social Security to qualify.[43] Other members of a family that may also qualify for SSDI may include a spouse, children, and children with a disability.[43]

SSI is a program administered by the Social Security Administration for eligible individuals (adults or children) who are disabled or blind, or who are 65 years old or older with limited income and resources (things they own). This program is funded by general tax revenue, not social security taxes. With SSI, a fixed monthly payment is provided, with some states supplementing this amount. The money from SSI is used to meet the basic needs of the individual for food, clothing, and shelter.[44]

Driving

Access to public services and the community is a key aspect of independence and can be accomplished by accessing public transportation or private taxi services or by driving oneself. Obtaining a license to drive a car on public roads is a major activity in adolescence that adds to the teenager's independence and socialization. People who are disabled may require adaptive training or equipment to acquire this much sought-after skill. Learning to drive or relearning to drive after becoming disabled can aid in independence, return to work, and accessing public markets as well as providing an overall sense of autonomy and self-determination.

Learning to drive is not solely a physical skill. Driving is a multitask type of activity with a lot of visual processing and safety factors associated with it. No one test can determine the ability of a person to safely operate an automobile on public highways. This determination can only be made by taking a multidisciplinary examination and a "hands on" driving test. The ability to operate the car is only one aspect of driving. Appropriate mental actions and reactions and appropriate interactions with the highway environment while operating a car are crucial aspects of this highly skilled activity.[45] Awareness and observation of the activity in a person's immediate environment, visual scanning while moving, knowledge of the rules of driving, and eye–foot coordination are some of the key factors to consider when discussing the possible goal of driving.[46]

» Service provision for adults with disabilities

Unlike referral and eligibility under IDEA or Section 504 of the Rehabilitation Act, adults with disabilities are referred to a PT as any other adult would be in the given state, under the state's practice act. The obvious difference is the underlying developmental disability that must be taken into consideration when examining and evaluating the primary reason for the referral. Consultation and collaboration with other health care providers, the person's guardian, if applicable, and personal care providers are always important, as with any patient/client. But unlike an individual who possess full autonomy over his or her decisions and actions, some individuals may not have full autonomy, making the inclusion of others necessary. The identification of goals, education of care givers or work supervisors, identification of agreed upon appropriate interventions and home exercise programs, becomes a group process. People with a disability must be treated the same as a person without a disability.

The assistance of a physical therapist assistant (PTA) can be valuable, provided that a good working relationship between the PT and PTA has been established and the skill set is appropriate. The delegation of care would be no different as with any other patient, under state law, with the exception of the underlying developmental disability for which any provider of care should have a basic understanding. The challenge is to be adaptable and observant in the delivery of interventions to obtain a desired outcome. It is the patient's right, and the professional's responsibility.

Examination/Evaluation of an Adult with a Developmental Disability

Comprehensive evaluations are performed to identify the capabilities and impairments that may influence a person's ability to live as independently as possible as an adult member of society. The physical therapy evaluation can add to a comprehensive plan that should address not only the personal factors that affect the disability but also the environmental and social factors as well. As with other formal plans, such as the Individualized Family Service Plan (IFSP) and IEP, the outcome of the physical therapy evaluation is not to establish discipline- or impairment-specific goals, but rather to develop meaningful individualized goals and outcomes that will facilitate independence and autonomy for the person with a disability. These goals can include the identification and modification of environmental barriers, to independence with self-care and basic ADLs, to the identification of appropriate employment environments and activities.

The examination can include those common elements of any physical therapy evaluation, which are the demographic information, the medical diagnosis, current medications, current complaint or issue, and a systems review (see the Case Study). Examination of the person's ability to perform ADLs, instrumental activities of daily living (IADLs), and functional activities is vital to the evaluation of a person's capabilities and the development of strategies to promote independence (Display 25.7). The ability to perform these activities can lead to the ability to hold a job and use public services, which in turn can lead to meeting people and developing relationships with others.

Part of the evaluation of a person's capability can include the use of *standardized tests*. By collecting objective information regarding functional skills, the PT will have documentation that can be used to help evaluate a person's functional capabilities over time. Two commonly used standardized tests that can aid in this process are the Functional Independence Measure (FIM) and the Barthel Index (Display 25.8).

In addition to a person's functional capabilities, the type of *work* that the person is expected to perform can be evaluated with regard to the physical space and/or access as well as the specific tasks and body mechanics needed to perform the job. The physical space could be examined using the guidelines from the ADA regarding physical accessibility (a walk-through screen can be found in Display 25.9). An examination of the physical space begins with the approach to the work site and the ability to park a car or exit a transport vehicle and approach the building. Entrance into the building includes the ability to access the entrance doors and successfully open and pass through them into the building. Once inside, physical access to the primary work site and the ancillary sites, such as the lunchroom, rest rooms, emergency evacuation routes, and employee lounge, should be examined for accessibility. The actual task of work should also be examined for the biomechanics needed to perform the task and the use of equipment or tools

DISPLAY 25.7 Definitions of ADLs, IADLs, and Function

ADLs: Everyday routines generally involving functional mobility and personal care and preparation[1]

Examples:

Personal Hygiene—Bathing, bowel and bladder management, brushing hair, brushing teeth, shaving

Dress—Getting dressed and undressed; donning shoes, socks, coat, gloves; manipulating fasteners (Velcro, hooks, buttons, zippers)

Feeding and Hydration—Eating, drinking, being able to cut meat, using utensils such as a spoon, fork, and knife

IADLs: Activities oriented to interactions with the environment, more complex than ADLs; optional (at times) or can be delegated[1]

Examples:

Financial Management—Going to the bank, keeping a checkbook, paying bills, managing spending

Meal Preparation—Preparing and cooking food, cutting, opening cans and jars, washing food, measuring items, keeping track of time

Shopping—For food, clothes, toiletries, household items

Medications—Preparing, organizing, buying, ordering, and managing medications, including safe and proper care, ability to dispense from container, and to take the proper dosage as prescribed

Telephone Use—Ability to operate a phone, call a person to talk, have appropriate conversations on the phone, call and talk in an emergency

Transportation—Ability to access public transportation, call taxi, or drive self

Housekeeping—Clean and maintain apartment, home, or living area

Function: Those activities identified by an individual as essential to support physical, social, and psychological well-being and to create a personal sense of meaningful living[1]

Functional activities can include ADLs and IADLs, in addition to activities such as standing, walking, carrying, squatting, and lifting or manipulating objects.

Reference

1. American Physical Therapy Association. *Guide to Physical Therapist Practice.* 2nd ed. APTA; 2003.

DISPLAY 25.8 Standardized Tests

The *FIM* is a criterion-referenced test that measures physical and cognitive disability in terms of burden of care.[1] Items are scored on a scale of 1–7, based on the amount of assistance a person needs to complete the item (1 = total assist to 7 = complete independence). The FIM includes 18 items categorized into areas of self-care, sphincter control, mobility, locomotion, communication, and social cognition. Ratings are based on observation or report. Total scores range from 18 to 126, with higher scores indicating more independent function in these areas. The psychometric properties of the FIM have been studied with several different populations, and the test has been shown to have good inter-rater reliability (0.86–0.96), content validity, and a strong correlation with the Barthel Index (0.84).[2-4]

The Barthel Index measures functional independence in personal care and mobility.[2] It can be done by a review of the person's medical record or from direct observation. Weighting of the items in the test reflects the aspect of disablement in impairment and disability as well as identifies the relative importance of that item in terms of care needed and social acceptability.[5] Total scores range from 0 to 100, with higher scores indicative of greater independence.

In the modified Barthel Index, eating and drinking are included as separate functions.[6] The modified version also has a range of total scores from 0 to 100. A total score of 60 is typically used as the threshold between marked dependence and independence. Shah et al.[7] suggest that scores of 0–20 (on either version) indicate total dependence, 21–60 severe dependence, 61–90 moderate dependence, and 91–99 slight dependence.

Reliability and validity have been established for both the 10- and 15-item tests with specific patient populations, namely, inpatient rehabilitation for patients with traumatic brain injury or cerebral vascular accident and for adults with severe disabilities (inter-rater reliability = 0.89).[6,8] Two noted limitations of the Barthel Index are in the structure of the test, which may not detect low levels of disability, and that, unlike the FIM, the Barthel test has no specific cognitive test items.[9]

References

1. *Guide for the Uniform Data Set for Medical Rehabilitation (Adult FIM).* Version 4.0. State University of New York at Buffalo; 1993.
2. Hamilton B, Laughlin J, Granger C, et al. Interrater agreement of the seven level Functional Independence Measure (FIM). *Arch Phys Med Rehabil.* 1991;72:790.
3. Keith R, Granger C, Hamilton B, et al. The Functional Independence Measure: a new tool for rehabilitation. In: Eisenberg M, Grzesiak R, eds. *Advances in Clinical Rehabilitation.* Vol 1. Springer; 1987:6-18.
4. Rockwook K, Stolee P, Fox RA. Use of goal attainment scaling in measuring clinically important change in the frail elderly. *J Clin Epidemiol.* 1993;46:1113-1118.
5. Granger C. Outcome of comprehensive medical rehabilitation: an analysis based upon impairment, disability, and handicap model. *Int Rehabil Med.* 1985;7:45-50.
6. Granger C, Albrecht G, Hamilton B. Outcome of comprehensive medical rehabilitation: measurement of PULSES Profile and the Barthel index. *Arch Phys Med Rehabil.* 1979;60:145-154.
7. Shah S, Vanclay F, Cooper B. Improving the sensitivity of the Barthel Index for stroke rehabilitation. *J Clin Epidemiol.* 1989;42:703-709.
8. Houlden H, Edwards M, McNeil J, et al. Use of the Barthel Index and Functional Independence Measure during early inpatient rehabilitation after single incident brain injury. *Clin Rehabil.* 2006;20:153-159.
9. Mahoney F, Wood O, Barthel D. Rehabilitation of chronically ill patients: the influence of complications on the final goal. *South Med J.* 1958;51:605-609.

25.9   Quick Screen of Accessibility

Building Access

1. People with disabilities should be able to arrive at and approach the building and enter as freely as anyone else.
2. Are there enough identified accessible parking spaces? (For every 25 under 100 spaces, there should be one identified accessible space.)
3. Are the accessible parking spaces close to the accessible entrance?
4. Is there a route of entrance that does not require a step or stairs?
5. If there is a ramp for access, is the slope at least 1:12?
6. Is the entrance door at least 32 inches wide?
7. Is the door handle no higher than 48 inches? (Can you open the door with one hand?)
8. Is the threshold no more than 1/4-inch high?

Building Corridors

1. Ideally, the layout of the building should allow people with disabilities to access services without any more assistance than would be required by a person without a disability.
2. Is the path of travel at least 36 inches wide?
3. Are controls for public use accessible?
   a. Maximum height for side reach is 54 inches.
   b. Maximum height for forward reach is 48 inches.
4. Is the height of the elevator call button no more than 42 inches from the ground?
5. Do elevators provide an audible and visual signal?
6. At the cashier counter, is there a portion that is no more than 36 inches high?
7. Is there a water drinking fountain with a spout no higher than 36 inches from the ground?
8. If there are four or more public phones in the building, is one phone equipped with a text telephone (TT or TDD)?

Public Rest Rooms

Public rest rooms should be available to all members of the public, including people with disabilities.

1. If public rest rooms are available, is there at least one accessible rest room?
2. Can the door to the rest room be easily opened (5 lbf maximum force)?
3. Is there a 5-foot-diameter space/stall available in the rest room for a wheelchair to turn?
4. Is the toilet seat between 17 and 19 inches from the floor?
5. Is the sink 34 inches or lower above the floor?
6. Are the mirrors mounted with the bottom edge of the reflecting surface no higher than 40 inches from the floor?
7. Are soap and towel dispensers mounted no more than 48 inches from the floor?

Adapted from ADA homepage. http://www.usdoj.gov/crt/ada/

required for the job. The PT can be instrumental in modifying the work space and tools to make the specific tasks of the job more ergonomically efficient and to decrease the risk of injury. Another aspect of work that should be examined is the work schedule. General questions that should be addressed include the following: Does the person have the endurance to sit or stand, or perform the movements, for the period of time needed to perform the job? Does the person have the ability to concentrate for an appropriate amount of time to perform tasks associated with the job? Does the person demonstrate appropriate behavior to perform the job safely? These questions will address the issue of endurance and concentration needed to perform the job well. Timing of medications, meals, rest periods, and the tasks associated with the job should be examined to make sure that the schedule fits the individual person and meets the needs of both the worker and the employer.

Individual Habilitation Plan

When the examination of the person, the physical environment of home or work, and the activities needed to participate in these environments is complete, the PT can participate in the construction of an *Individual Habilitation Plan* (IHP), Individual Service Plan (ISP), or an Individual Program Plan (IPP). Much like the IFSP and IEP, the IHP is an individualized plan to address the needs and desires of a person who resides in an ICF. An interdisciplinary team, including the person with a disability (either in person or through his legal guardian), provides input into the development of the IHP, which "must be directed toward the acquisition of the behaviors necessary for the individual to function with as much self-determination and independence as possible and the prevention or deceleration of regression or loss of current optimal functional status" (42CFR483.440[a]).[47] The PT can provide key information on a variety of health-related issues, but most importantly on promoting functional skills in the areas of daily living and work ability. Display 25.10 provides some examples of the content found in a typical IHP.

When the team meets to construct an IHP, *goals* are identified and agreed upon. Goals on an IHP should be objective, measurable, and, most importantly, related to a functional activity in the person's life. According to Kettenbach,[48] appropriate goals in physical therapy should contain references to the audience, person, or caregiver (A), the identified behavior or what the person will do (B), the conditions under which the behavior will be observed (C), and the degree to which the behavior will be implemented (D). In addition, the PT should keep in mind the education required of the caregiver or person to perform the behavior (E) and the functional relevance of the behavior in the person's everyday life (F) (Display 25.11).

When the IHP has been established, appropriate services are provided. The *interventions* used by the PT when working with adults with disabilities is no different from any of the interventions used with adults without disabilities. The purpose is to

DISPLAY
25.10

Example of Basic Content Included in a Habilitation Plan

Demographic information
Diagnosis
Medications
Nursing needs
Behavior patterns or concerns
Effective communication style
Physical, mental, and emotional health
Level of safety awareness
Level of supervision required
Assistive technology used
Interests and activities
Life goals
Current services provided
Mobility status, including transfers
Capacity for self-care
Capacity for self-direction
Level of independence with ADLs and IADLs
Level of social participation
Employment status
Accommodations needed

Developed by Drnach M. Example of Basic Content Included in a Habilitation Plan. Unpublished. 2020.

maximize the person's ability to function in daily life. In many instances, when working with a person who has a chronic condition, the goal is not to change the underlying condition but to make the person more able to function. This can be done by addressing those impairments to a specific ability that are inherent in the person, in the home or work environment, or in society (what other people believe he can do). As in other settings, coordination, communication, and documentation are vital components of intervention. Patient/client-related instruction, as well as caregiver instruction if appropriate, is necessary to ensure implementation of the recommended interventions into the daily life of the individual. Specific procedural interventions may include functional training in self-care, home management, work, and leisure activities. As with all adults, physical activity and exercise can help promote a healthy lifestyle and maintenance of function for many years.

DISPLAY
25.11

Constructing Goals

Remember:
  A: Audience
  B: Behavior
  C: Condition
  D: Degree
  E: Education needed
  F: Functional relevance

Adapted from Kettenbach G. *Writing SOAP Notes with Patient/Client Management Formats.* 3rd ed. FA Davis Company; 2004.

Summary

Transitioning is often presented as the movement from one program into another with their unique rules and regulations and expected role of the PT. In this chapter, transitioning is discussed in its broader application, from one phase of life into the next. Children with disabilities grow into adults with disabilities, who in turn age into seniors with disabilities. In the natural course of human events, as one ages there is a decline in physical activity and capability, accompanied by the loss of friends and family either through distance or death. The loss of a parent is an especially difficult transition, made even harder when that parent has been the primary caregiver for a person with a disability. A key question arises at this time: Who will assume the role of caregiver? Death is not the only event that forces this question. Natural aging of both the parent and the dependent child will eventually lead to a decline in the physical capabilities of both. What happens when a 62-year-old mother can no longer lift her 37-year-old son? Who will assume this role?

A PT has a unique role in facilitating discussions on what can be a very emotional and oftentimes difficult topic about the future. Factors that affect an individual's ability to live as independently as possible, to participate in some form of employment, or to acquire other characteristics commonly attributed to adulthood, accumulate over years of growth and development on both the part of the individual and the parents. The PT can begin by educating the parents on the importance of fostering skills in their child that will develop into characteristics of self-determination and independence as a young adult. Speaking to a child at an appropriate cognitive level, respecting a child's reasonable decisions, letting the child experience the effect of the choices made, listening to the wants and needs of the child, can aid in the development of adult behaviors and characteristics.

Educating the young adult and family on the options and resources that are available in the community is an important aspect of the transitioning process. Each family is unique in their beliefs and in how they function as a family unit. Honest discussion on the role of the parents, siblings, and the child with a disability could facilitate a mutual understanding of each family member's needs. Periodic discussions on future plans and aspirations, caregiver support, and service options should be viewed as a natural part of life planning, just as many families discuss issues of the future for any child. What do you want to be when you grow up? Where would you like to live? Where would you like to work? Who, or what supports, will be needed to achieve these goals? All children, regardless of their ability, should be presented with his or her reasonable options, including those that involve sheltered workshops and residential living arrangements.

By planning for these major life transitions, the PT and other people involved in the life of a person with a disability can make one step toward "ensuring equality of opportunity, full participation, independent living, and economic self-sufficiency for individuals with disabilities."[1]

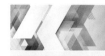

CASE STUDY

PHYSICAL THERAPY EXAMINATION: RESIDENT IN AN ICF/ID

Name:	Client A
Address:	1104 Some Road
	City, WV 12345
Date of Birth:	05-20-57
Date of Evaluation:	10-05-20
Age:	63 years
Insurance:	Medicaid
Guardian:	Joe. Phone: 123-56-7890
Physician: Luke Georgia	Luke. Phone: 234-156-0987
Place of Employment:	County Workshop
Supervisor:	Grace. Phone: 345-678-0098

Medical diagnosis: Mild intellectual impairment, arteriosclerosis, hyperlipidemia, intermittent explosive disorder, obesity, gastroesophageal reflux disease, history of seizure disorder, osteoarthritis

Medications: Lipitor 40 mg, Tegretol 200 mg, Oyster Shell 500 mg, Naproxen 500 mg, Zoloft 100 mg

Reason for referral: Annual review. Client A, guardian, and house staff report no concerns or needs at present.

Systems review

Height	5 feet 5 inches
Weight	197 lb
Vision	Wears glasses; nearsighted
Hearing	Intact
Behavior during examination	Cooperative; followed one-step request
Communication	Verbal; will communicate in complete sentences
Oral motor skills	Not impaired
Heart rate	71 bpm, regular
Shoe size	8½ wide
Edema	+1 in her lower extremities; capillary refill in distal extremity <3 seconds
Sensation	Appears intact to light touch in lower extremities
Integumentary	No obvious surgical scars noted upon visual examination of her extremities and trunk
Assistive devices	Bilateral flexible orthotics with arch supports; adaptive equipment for eating, which includes a nonskid placemat, plate guard, and built-up handled spoon and fork

Examination findings
Musculoskeletal Status
The range of motion in the upper extremities is within functional limits. Her spine presents with a kyphoscoliosis, with a rib hump in the right thoracic region. Curve does not change with forward

flexion. Passive range of motion in the lower extremities presents with symmetrical hip joint abduction with 45 degrees of external rotation bilaterally, 45 degrees of hip joint internal rotation on the left, and 30 degrees on the right. There is hip joint extension to neutral bilaterally, with a soft end feel noted. Hip joint flexion is 120 degrees bilaterally. Popliteal angles were 55 degrees measured bilaterally. Active ankle joint motions are within functional limits. She presents with pronated feet, for which she wears orthotics. The orthotics appear to fit well and were last replaced 4 months ago.

Calf girth measurements taken 10 cm distal to the tibial tubercle resulted in 39 cm on the right and 36 cm on the left. These measurements are unchanged from those taken 6 months ago. She has a long-standing history of edema in the lower extremities.

Neuromuscular Status
She tested negative for clonus in the ankles. There is no report of falling in the past 6 months. Balance responses in ankle and stepping strategies were noted in stance. Client does not report pain in her hips. Her caregivers report that she appears to have hip pain occasionally as noted by an increase in limping, especially after she returns from work.

Cardiopulmonary Status
No adventitious sounds were heard with auscultation of the lungs. The client reports no episodes of shortness of breath. Her caregivers do not report observing her having any episodes of shortness of breath. Her present level of endurance is sufficient for her level of activity; it does not impair her ability to participate in daily activities, work, or social outings. She does not have a history of respiratory infection over the past year.

Functional Status
Bed Mobility
Transfers: Independent in transfers from sit to stand. She is able to transfer into and out of the bathtub. She is able to transfer onto and off of a standard toilet. The client will step onto and out of the van with handrail assistance.

Gait/Mobility: The client can ambulate 200 feet in 75 seconds. Gait pattern demonstrates a decreased stance phase on the right, and hip and knee joint flexion when walking. Trunk flexed at hips. She is able to ascend (step over step) and descend (step to step) five steps with the assist of a handrail. (There are five steps at her place of employment.) She wears foot orthotics with a medial arch support.

Activities of Daily Living (by staff report): The client can dress herself, requiring minimal assistance for orientation and closure of fasteners. She requires assistance with bathing (preparing the washcloth and providing verbal cues) to complete the task sufficiently. She is able to eat her meals independently, using a plate guard and nonskid mat. She drinks from a regular cup. She will use the toilet when cued to do so. She requires only minimal assistance for hygiene. She does have episodes of bladder incontinence, approximately once a month by report. She is continent of bowel.

FIM Score: 63/126. Areas requiring the most assistance include sphincter control, self-care, and social cognition. Areas of most independence include locomotion, mobility, and communication.

Work

The client is employed by County Workshop where she works as a laborer. Her main job is putting labels on boxes. Her job requires long periods of sitting, the ability to transition from sit to stand, and the use of bilateral upper extremities to manipulate labels and empty cardboard boxes, with dimensions typically 2 feet by 1 foot by 6 inches. The job also requires the ability to rotate her trunk, to grasp and place boxes in front of her, and to stack boxes one on top of the other, three boxes high.

Leisure Activities

She enjoys rides in an automobile, watching movies at the local cinema, attending the County Fair, going on brief walks of approximately 15 to 30 minutes, and picking wildflowers.

Recommendations

Consult with physician regarding gait deviation. Possible radiograph of right hip joint may be appropriate. Arch supports in shoes fit well, but may need to be replaced in 6 months due to general wear.

Reflection Questions

1. Identify the specific movements needed for the client to perform her job. What are the key muscles associated with the identified movements? Prescribe three exercises that she could perform at home that would maintain her strength, flexibility, or endurance to perform her job.
2. Because she requires assistance with bathing, identify the features that would optimize safety for both the client and her caregiver during this task.
3. Identify appropriate assistive technology that would promote her independence in dressing.

REFERENCES

1. Individuals with Disabilities Education Improvement Act of 2004. 20 USC 1400. Title I. Sec. 601(c)(1).
2. Erickson W, Lee C, von Schrader S. *2017 Disability Status Report: United States.* Cornell University Yang Tan Institute on Employment and Disability (YTI); 2020.
3. Arnett J. Emerging adulthood—a theory of development from the late teens through the twenties. *Am Psychol.* 2000;55:469-480.
4. Jordan B, Dunlap G. Construction of adulthood and disability. *Ment Retard.* 2001;39:286-296.
5. Porter RE. Normal development of movement and function: child and adolescent. In: Scully RM, Barnes MR, eds. *Physical Therapy.* JB Lippincott; 1989.
6. Culbertson JL, Newman JE, Willis DJ. Childhood and adolescent psychologic development. *Pediatr Clin North Am.* 2003;50:741-764.
7. Kaeser F. Can people with severe mental retardation consent to mutual sex? *Sex Disabil.* 1992;10:33-42.
8. Wehmeyer M, Schalock R. Self-determination and quality of life: implications for special education services and supports. *Focus Except Child.* 2001;33:1-16.
9. World Health Organization, World Bank. *World Report on Disability.* World Health Organization; 2011.
10. Taylor DM. *Americans with Disabilities: 2014. Current Population Reports.* U.S. Census Bureau; 2018:70-152.
11. U.S. Department of Labor Statistics. The Employment Situation. Table A-6. Employment Status of the Civilian Population by Sex, Age, and Disability Status, not seasonally adjusted. 2019. Accessed January 18, 2021. https://www.bls.gov/news.release/archives/empsit_05032019.htm
12. Young K, Kroth P. *Health Care USA. Understanding Its Organization and Delivery.* 9th ed. Jones and Bartlett; 2018.
13. University of Iowa. Appendix 2: Major Disability-Related Legislation 1956–1999. Accessed May 22, 2020. http://disability.law.uiowa.edu/csadp_docs/APPENDIX_2_APR.txt
14. Kollmann G, Solomon-Fears C. Major decisions in the House and Senate on Social Security: 1935-2000. CRS Legislative Histories. Social Security Administration. Accessed May 22, 2020. http://www.ssa.gov/history/reports/crsleghist3.html
15. Supplemental Security Income Home Page—2020 Edition. U.S. Social Security Administration. Accessed May 22, 2020. https://www.ssa.gov/ssi/
16. U.S. Department of Justice, Civil Rights Division, Disability Rights Section. *A Guide to Disability Rights Laws.* 2020. Accessed May 22, 2020. http://www.usdoj.gov/crt/ada/cguide.htm
17. The Developmental Disabilities Assistance and Bill of Rights Act 2000 (PL 106–402). Accessed May 22, 2020. https://acl.gov/about-acl/authorizing-statutes/developmental-disabilities-assistance-and-bill-rights-act-2000
18. Administration for Community Living. State Councils on Developmental Disabilities. U.S. Department of Health and Human Services. Accessed: May 22, 2020. https://acl.gov/programs/aging-and-disability-networks/state-councils-developmental-disabilities
19. U.S. Department of Health and Human Resources. HHS Policy for Section 508 Compliance and Accessibility of Information and Communication Technology (ICT). Accessed January 18, 2021. https://www.hhs.gov/web/governance/digital-strategy/it-policy-archive/hhs-policy-section-508-compliance-accessibility-information-communications-technology.html#2
20. Association of Assistive Technology Act Programs. Accessed May 22, 2020. https://www.ataporg.org/
21. Russell JN, Hendershot GE, LeClere F, et al. Trends and differential use of assistive technology devices: United States, 1994. *Adv Data.* 1997:13(292):1-9. PMID: 10182811.
22. *Stedman's Medical Dictionary for the Health Professions and Nursing.* 7th ed. Lippincott Williams & Wilkins; 2012.
23. Boggs C. Workers' compensation history: the great tradeoff! *Insur J.* 2015. Accessed June 6, 2020. https://www.insurancejournal.com/blogs/academy-journal/2015/03/19/360273.htm
24. Kaye HS. *Vocational Rehabilitation in the United States. Disabilities Statistics Abstract Number 20.* U.S. Department of Education, National Institute on Disability and Rehabilitation Research; 1998.
25. Rehabilitation Act of 1973. As Amended through P.L. 114-95, Enacted December 10, 2015. 29 USC 701. Section 2 (a)(4). Accessed May 26, 2020. https://www2.ed.gov/policy/speced/leg/rehab/rehabilitation-act-of-1973-amended-by-wioa.pdf
26. Rehabilitation Act of 1973. As Amended through P.L. 114-95, Enacted December 10, 2015. 29 USC 701. Section 102 (a)(1). Accessed May 26, 2020. https://www2.ed.gov/policy/speced/leg/rehab/rehabilitation-act-of-1973-amended-by-wioa.pdf
27. U.S. Social Security Administration. Substantial Gainful Activity. Accessed May 26, 2020. https://www.ssa.gov/OACT/COLA/sga.html
28. Tanenbaum S. Medicaid and disability: the unlikely entitlement. *Milbank Q.* 1989;67(Suppl 2 Pt 2):288-310.
29. Social Security Administration. Social Security History. Accessed May 26, 2020. http://www.ssa.gov/history/nixstmts.html#amend
30. Clifton D. Disability management in long term care. In: Clifton D, ed. *Physical Rehabilitation's Role in Disability Management. Unique Perspectives for Success.* Elsevier Saunders; 2005:57.
31. Public Law 113-295, Stephen Beck, Jr, Achieving a Better Life Experience Act (ABLE Act) of 2014, Approved December 19, 2014. Accessed May 26, 2020. https://www.ssa.gov/OP_Home/comp2/F113-295.html
32. U.S. Department of Health and Human Services. Section 504 of the Rehabilitation Act of 1973, as amended. Accessed January 18, 2021.

https://www.govinfo.gov/content/pkg/USCODE-2010-title29/pdf/USCODE-2010-title29-chap16-subchapV-sec794.pdf

33. National Alliance for Caregiving and AARP Public Policy Institute. Caregiving in the U.S. Executive Summary. Published June 2015. Accessed May 26, 2020. https://www.caregiving.org/wp-content/uploads/2020/05/2015_CaregivingintheUS_Executive-Summary-June-4_WEB.pdf

34. National Council on Independent Living. *About NCIL.* Accessed January 18, 2021. https://ncil.org/about/

35. The Assisted Living Workgroup. Assuring quality in assisted living: guidelines for Federal and State Policy, State Regulation, and Operations. A report to the U.S. Senate Special Committee on Aging. 2003. Accessed May 26, 2020. http://www.aahsa.org/alw/intro.pdf

36. The U.S. Department of Health & Human Services, Centers for Medicare & Medicaid Services. Intermediate care facilities for individuals with intellectual disability. Accessed May 26, 2020. https://www.medicaid.gov/medicaid/long-term-services-supports/institutional-long-term-care/intermediate-care-facilities-individuals-intellectual-disability/index.html

37. United States Department of Labor. Workforce Innovation and Opportunity Act of 2014. Accessed May 19, 2020. https://www.dol.gov/agencies/eta/wioa/about

38. Carter EW, Austin D, Trainor AA. Predictors of postschool employment outcomes for young adults with severe disabilities. *J Disabil Policy Stud.* 2012;23(1):50-63.

39. *Merriam-Webster Online Dictionary.* Welfare. Accessed May 28, 2020. http://www.m-w.com/dictionary/welfare

40. News Batch. Welfare policy issues. Updated May 2011. Accessed May 28, 2020. http://www.newsbatch.com/welfare.htm

41. Administration for Children and Families. Office of Family Assistance (OFA). Accessed May 28, 2020. https://www.acf.hhs.gov/ofa/about/what-we-do

42. U.S. Department of Agriculture Food and Nutrition Service. https://www.fns.usda.gov/

43. Social Security Administration. Disability benefit. Accessed May 28, 2020. https://www.ssa.gov/planners/disability/

44. Social Security Administration. *Understanding Supplemental Security Income (SSI) Overview—2020 Edition.* Accessed May 28, 2020. https://www.ssa.gov/ssi/text-over-ussi.htm

45. Heikkila VM, Kallanranta R. Evaluation of the driving ability in disabled persons: a practitioners' view. *Disabil Rehabil.* 2005;17:1029-1036.

46. Marshall S, Man-Son-Hing M, Molnar R, et al. An exploratory study on the predictive elements of passing on-the-road tests for disabled persons. *Traffic Inj Prev.* 2005;3:235-239.

47. Govregs.com. U.S. Code of Federal Regulations. *Conditions of Participation: Active Treatment Services.* Updated January 2021. Accessed January 18, 2021. https://www.govregs.com/regulations/42/483.440

48. Kettenbach G. *Writing SOAP Notes with Patient/Client Management Formats.* 3rd ed. FA Davis Company; 2004.

ADDITIONAL ONLINE RESOURCES

A comprehensive overview of information on a state's Medicaid programs for the aged, blind, and disabled is available at https://www.medicaid.gov/. Accessed May 13, 2020.

Centers for Disease Control and Prevention, National Center for Health Statistics. Classification of diseases, functioning, and disability. Available at https://www.cdc.gov/nchs/icd/index.htm?CDC_AA_refVal=https%3A%2F%2Fwww.cdc.gov%2Fnchs%2Ficd.htm. Accessed May 13, 2020.

For more information on SSI, visit http://www.socialsecurity.gov/ssi/index.htm. Accessed May 13, 2020.

Information on vocational rehabilitation and other services for individuals with disabilities, in order to maximize their employment can be accessed through the U.S. Department of Education, Office of Special Education and Rehabilitation Services at http://www.ed.gov/about/offices/list/osers/rsa/index.html. Accessed May 13, 2020.

More information on the ADA is available at http://www.usdoj.gov/crt/ada/adahom1.htm. Accessed May 13, 2020.

The Centers for Medicare & Medicaid Services has information on the Medicaid programs in specific states available at http://www.cms.hhs.gov/home/medicaid.asp. Accessed May 13, 2020.

The National Center on Secondary Education and Transition (NCSET). Provides technical assistance in four areas: access in the secondary education curriculum; achieving positive results in accessing postsecondary education, meaningful employment, independent living, and participation in all aspects of community life; supporting student and family participation in educational and postschool decision making and planning; and improving collaboration and system linkages. Accessed May 13, 2020. http://www.ncset.org/

The National Council on Independent Living has information on local centers for independent living available at https://ncil.org/. Accessed May 13, 2020.

The Social Security Administration has information on employment support available at https://www.ssa.gov/redbook/eng/main.htm. Accessed May 13, 2020.

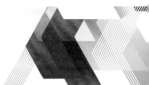
Note: Page numbers in italics denote figures; those followed by a t denote tables; those followed by a b denote display boxes.